Video Capsule Endoscopy

Martin Keuchel • Friedrich Hagenmüller
Hisao Tajiri

Editors

Video Capsule Endoscopy

A Reference Guide and Atlas

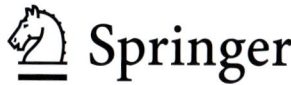
Springer

Editors
Martin Keuchel, MD, Dr. habil
Department of Internal Medicine
Bethesda Krankenhaus Bergedorf
Academic Teaching Hospital of the
University of Hamburg
Hamburg
Germany

Friedrich Hagenmüller, MD
Professor of Medicine
1st Medical Department
Asklepios Klinik Altona
Academic Teaching Hospital of the
University of Hamburg
Hamburg
Germany

Hisao Tajiri, MD, PhD
Professor of Medicine
Division of Gastroenterology and Hepatology
Department of Internal Medicine
The Jikei University School of Medicine
Tokyo
Japan

ISBN 978-3-662-44061-2   ISBN 978-3-662-44062-9   (eBook)
DOI 10.1007/978-3-662-44062-9
Springer Heidelberg New York Dordrecht London

Library of Congress Control Number: 2014957873

Printed on acid-free paper

Springer is part of Springer Science+Business Media (www.springer.com)

Foreword

Capsule endoscopy has been the most important innovation in endoscopy since video endoscopy replaced fiber optics. It has opened the whole of the small intestine to easy, direct, and safe endoscopic vision and in so doing has stimulated the development and increased the value of device-assisted enteroscopy. This has enabled minimally invasive intraluminal therapy to be performed throughout the whole of the gastrointestinal tract. The ability to visualize the small-bowel mucosa easily has also led to a better understanding of the pathological conditions that afflict the organ, has revolutionized the management of occult gastrointestinal hemorrhage, and has greatly improved the physician's ability to identify conditions such as Crohn's disease at an earlier stage and enables us to monitor its activity in response to treatment.

The development of enteroscopy however has highlighted some of the deficiencies inherent in endoscopic techniques and in particular the inability of optical visualization to provide information about disease within or outside of the bowel wall or, in the case of the small intestine, to determine exactly where in the intestine the pathology lies. The improvement of other imaging modalities, such as computed tomography and magnetic resonance, however has filled this gap, and our ability to link mucosal information to wider anatomical boundaries has further enhanced the contribution of enteroscopy to the study of the small intestine.

This remarkable book is more than an atlas of video capsule endoscopy. Its 52 chapters prepared by recognized experts comprehensively address all issues relating to capsule endoscopy, starting with the fascinating story of its development through the indications for its use, current equipment available, techniques, and training. A valuable chapter on the evaluation of capsule images brings the reader down to earth. Reading a huge number of images taken over the long period of the procedure requires software assistance, but even this cannot disguise the fact that the examination of images is time consuming for the reporting professional. Unlike real-time "hands-on" video endoscopy, it is not possible to view a lesion at leisure from different angles and distances or to touch it with biopsy forceps. Furthermore, the variety of different pathologies in the small bowel appears to be more extensive than those seen in the stomach or colon. Lesions are more difficult to identify than with video endoscopy as some of them are masked by the overlying villous mucosa. The images obtained are both fascinating and beautiful but not as crisp as those we have become used to with video endoscopy. Diagnosis is not a simple matter.

The second main section of the book addresses other modalities used to assess the small bowel. It includes excellent chapters on device-assisted enteroscopy as well as duodenoscopy and ileoscopy that detail the methodology and potential therapeutic applications again beautifully illustrated. Two chapters focus upon the use of computed tomography magnetic resonance and ultrasound, placing their use into the context of the management of small-bowel disease. The radiographs and scans, well annotated and labeled, enable the non-radiologist endoscopist reader to appreciate the abnormal findings with ease.

The central section of the book is devoted to the appearances of small-bowel lesions in a variety of conditions that include infections, systemic illness, and specific small-bowel conditions such as Crohn's, familial polyposis, rare lesions, and malignant tumors. The chapters comprise a cornucopia of high-quality common and uncommon small-bowel lesions accompanied by well-written explanation and background.

The next section of the book considers a variety of important areas, such as the prevention and management of complications and the use of capsule endoscopy in children. There is a particularly relevant and thoughtfully written chapter on the impact of capsule endoscopy on clinical outcome that puts the technique in context with other approaches to management and assesses its value in a variety of clinical conditions.

The last section first addresses the developing areas of esophageal capsule endoscopy and capsule endoscopy in the colon. It then moves on with two chapters that give a critical analysis of the deficiencies of the technology, among them considering the way that images might be improved and how the capsule could be independently controlled in real time. One chapter is on hardware, the other software.

This is altogether a most impressive book and one that should be available in all units that provide a capsule endoscopy service. It is of value both for reference purposes and as a learning experience for those starting in this area. It is particularly relevant for those in charge of endoscopy services if they are considering setting up a capsule endoscopy service. When capsule endoscopy was introduced, most endoscopists thought of it as a simple adjunct to conventional endoscopy and it would just be a matter of reviewing a number of images and making a diagnosis. This book pulls no punches. Capsule endoscopy is of great value, but those who are responsible for it require extensive training and experience. It is not for the dilettante.

The editors and authors are to be congratulated for this particularly important contribution to endoscopic literature.

Leeds, UK   Anthony Axon, MD, FRCP

Preface

Since the publication of the *Atlas of Video Capsule Endoscopy* (M. Keuchel, F. Hagenmüller, and D. Fleischer) in 2006, video capsule endoscopy has steadily and rapidly developed. Technical improvements, extended scientific evidence, and availability of new capsule systems including colon capsules have required this update. The present book follows its predecessor by combining state-of-the-art presentation of the different aspects of capsule endoscopy with a comprehensive collection of typical and rare capsule images. Once again, a board of world-renowned experts have agreed to contribute their experience, images, and enthusiasm, which is very much appreciated.

A major goal of this atlas is, again, to help readers interpret a capsule endoscopy examination by relating the images to corresponding histologic, endoscopic, radiologic, surgical, and clinical reference findings. We thank all colleagues who generously provided many rare images and videos.

The support by our teams at Bethesda Hospital Bergedorf, Asklepios Klinik Altona, and Jikei University School of Medicine is gratefully appreciated.

We also thank Lee Klein of Springer in Philadelphia for his excellent coordination throughout the creation of this atlas, Bernice Wissler for outstanding copyediting, Dr. R. Nithyatharani of spi-global in Chennai for perfect layout and production, Patrick Waltemate of le-tex in Leipzig for realizing all ideas related to the DVD and Dr. Ute Heilmann and Martina Himberger of Springer in Heidelberg for their guidance through the production of the work. Last but not least, we thank our families for their support and tolerance as we prepared this book.

Hamburg, Germany　　　　　　　　　　　　　　　　　Martin Keuchel
Hamburg, Germany　　　　　　　　　　　　　Friedrich Hagenmüller
Tokyo, Japan　　　　　　　　　　　　　　　　　　　　　Hisao Tajiri

Contents

Contributors

Samuel N. Adler Department of Gastroenterology, Shaare Zedek Medical Center, Jerusalem, Israel

Hiroyuki Aihara Department of Endoscopy, Jikei University School of Medicine, Tokyo, Japan

Jörg G. Albert Medical Clinic I, University Hospital Frankfurt, Frankfurt, Germany

Mark N. Appleyard Department of Gastroenterology and Hepatology, Royal Brisbane and Women's Hospital, Brisbane, QLD, Australia

Federico Argüelles-Arias Department of Gastroenterology, Hospital Universitario Virgen Macarena, Seville, Spain

Peter Baltes Department of Internal Medicine, Bethesda Krankenhaus Bergedorf, Hamburg, Germany

Dirk Bandorski Medical Clinic II, University Hospital of Giessen and Marburg, Giessen, Germany

Jamie Barkin Division of Gastroenterology, Mount Sinai Medical Center, University of Miami, Miami Beach, FL, USA

Eberhard Barth Gastroenterology and Rheumatology Practice, Hamburg, Germany

Robert Benamouzig Department of Gastroenterology, Avicenne Hospital, Bobigny, France

Ingvar Bjarnason Department of Gastroenterology, King's College Hospital, London, UK

Jan Bureš 2nd Department of Internal Medicine—Gastroenterology, University Hospital and Charles University Faculty of Medicine, Hradec Králové, Czech Republic

Carol Burke Department of Medicine, Cleveland Clinic Foundation, Cleveland, OH, USA

Jörg Caselitz Department for Pathology, Asklepios Klinik Altona, Hamburg, Germany

Carmela Cavallotti The BioRobotics Institute, Scuola Superiore Sant'Anna, Pontedera, Pisa, Italy

David R. Cave Department of Gastroenterology, University of Massachusetts Medical School, Worcester, MA, USA

Jean-Pierre Charton Medical Clinic, Evangelisches Krankenhaus, Düsseldorf, Germany

Michael W. Cheng Southern Gastroenterology Specialists, Locust Grove, GA, USA

Gastone Ciuti The BioRobotics Institute, Scuola Superiore Sant'Anna, Pontedera, Pisa, Italy

Pekka Collin Gastroenterology Outpatient Clinic, Tampere University Hospital, Tampere, Finland

Guido Costamagna Department of Surgical Endoscopy, Università Cattolica del Sacro Cuore, Rome, Italy

Dani Dajani Department of Internal Medicine, Bethesda Krankenhaus Bergedorf, Hamburg, Germany

Carolyn Davison Department of GI Services, South Tyneside NHS Foundation Trust, Tyne and Wear, UK

Roberto de Franchis Gastroenterology Unit, Luigi Sacco University Hospital, University of Milan, Milan, Italy

Gian Luigi de' Angelis Gastroenterology and Endoscopy Unit, University of Parma, Parma, Italy

Michel Delvaux Department of Gastroenterology and Hepatology, Nouvel Hôpital Civil, University Hospital of Strasbourg, Strasbourg, France

Edward J. Despott Centre for Gastroenterology, The Royal Free Hospital and UCL School of Medicine, London, UK

Martha H. Dirks Division of Gastroenterology, Hepatology and Nutrition, Hôpital Sainte-Justine, University of Montreal, Montreal, QC, Canada

Peter Draganov Division of Gastroenterology, Hepatology, and Nutrition, University of Florida College of Medicine, Gainesville, FL, USA

Gareth S. Dulai UCLA Digestive Disease Center, Los Angeles, CA, USA

Rami Eliakim Department of Gastroenterology, Sheba Medical Center, Sackler School of Medicine, Tel-Aviv University, Tel-Hashomer, Israel

Christian Ell Medical Clinic II, Sana Klinikum Offenbach, Offenbach, Germany

Evgeny D. Fedorov Digestive Endoscopy, Russia State Medical University, Moscow University Hospital No. 31, Moscow, Russia

Pedro Narra Figueiredo Department of Gastroenterology, University of Coimbra, Coimbra, Portugal

David E. Fleischer Division of Gastroenterology, Mayo Clinic Arizona, Scottsdale, AZ, USA

Christopher Fraser Wolfson Unit for Endoscopy, St. Mark's Hospital and Academic Institute, Imperial College London, London, UK

Lucia C. Fry Department of Internal Medicine, Gastroenterology, and Infectious Diseases, Marien Hospital, Bottrop, Germany

Gérard Gay Department of Gastroenterology and Hepatology, Nouvel Hôpital Civil, University Hospital of Strasbourg, Strasbourg, France

Ian M. Gralnek Department of Gastroenterology, Rambam Health Care Campus, Haifa, Israel

Juan Manuel Herrerías Gutiérrez Department of Gastroenterology, Hospital Universitario Virgen Macarena, Seville, Spain

Friedrich Hagenmüller 1st Medical Department, Asklepios Klinik Altona, Hamburg, Germany

James N. S. Hampton Radiology Department, Northern General Hospital, Sheffield Teaching Hospitals NHS Foundation Trust, Sheffield, UK

Dirk Hartmann Department of Internal Medicine, Sana-Klinikum Lichtenberg, Berlin, Germany

Francesca Iannuzzi Gastroenterology Unit, Luigi Sacco University Hospital, University of Milan, Milan, Italy

Gavriel J. Iddan Given Imaging Ltd., Yoqneam, Israel

Dennis M. Jensen UCLA Digestive Disease Center, Los Angeles, CA, USA

Victoria Alejandra Jiménez-Garcia Department of Gastroenterology, Hospital Universitario Virgen Macarena, Seville, Spain

Yasuo Kakugawa Endoscopy Division, National Cancer Center Hospital, Tokyo, Japan

Martin Keuchel Department of Internal Medicine, Bethesda Krankenhaus Bergedorf, Hamburg, Germany

Hirito Kita Department of Medicine, Teikyo University School of Medicine, Tokyo, Japan

Kiyonori Kobayashi Department of Gastroenterology, Kitasato University East Hospital, Sagamihara-city, Kanagawa Prefecture, Japan

Louis Y. Korman Chevy Chase Clinical Research, Chevy Chase, MD, USA

Asher Kornbluth Mount Sinai Hospital, New York, NY, USA

Torsten Kucharzik Department of Gastroenterology, Klinikum Lüneburg, Lüneburg, Germany

Niehls Kurniawan Department of Internal Medicine, Bethesda Krankenhaus Bergedorf, Hamburg, Germany

Peter E. Legnani Mount Sinai Hospital, New York, NY, USA

Jonathan A. Leighton Division of Gastroenterology, Mayo Clinic, Scottsdale, AZ, USA

Blair S. Lewis Mount Sinai Hospital, New York, NY, USA

Guntram Lock Clinic for Internal Medicine, Albertinenkrankenhaus, Hamburg, Germany

Ernst J. Malzfeldt Department of Radiology/Neuroradiology, Asklepios Klinik Nord, Hamburg, Germany

Christopher Marshall Department of Gastroenterology, University of Massachusetts Medical Center, Worcester, MA, USA

Fernando J. Martinez Division of Gastroenterology, Mount Sinai Medical Center, University of Miami, Miami, FL, USA

Uwe Matsui Department of Internal Medicine, Bethesda Krankenhaus Bergedorf, Hamburg, Germany

Vincent Maunoury Department of Gastroenterology, Hôpital Huriez, Lille Cedex, France

Andrea May Medical Clinic II, Sana Klinikum Offenbach, Offenbach, Germany

Mark E. McAlindon Gastroenterology and Liver Unit, Royal Hallamshire Hospital, Sheffield, UK

Arianna Menciassi The BioRobotics Institute, Scuola Superiore Sant'Anna, Pontedera, Pisa, Italy

Chris J. Mulder Department of Gastroenterology, VU University Medical Center, Amsterdam, The Netherlands

Joseph A. Murray Division of Gastroenterology and Hepatology, Mayo Clinic, Rochester, MN, USA

Tetsuya Nakamura Department of Medical Informatics, Dokkyo Medical University School of Medicine, Tochigi, Japan

Horst Neuhaus Medical Clinic, Evangelisches Krankenhaus, Düsseldorf, Germany

Marco Pennazio Division of Gastroenterology, San Giovanni Battista University Teaching Hospital, Turin, Italy

Christian P. Pox Department of Medicine, Ruhr-University Bochum, Knappschaftskrankenhaus, Bochum, Germany

D. Nageshwar Reddy Department of Medical Gastroenterology, Asian Institute of Gastroenterology, Hyderabad, India

Maria Elena Riccioni Department of Surgical Endoscopy, Università Cattolica del Sacro Cuore, Rome, Italy

Jürgen F. Riemann LebensBlicke Foundation for Prevention of Colorectal Cancer, Ludwigshafen, Germany

Emanuele Rondonotti Gastrointestinal Endoscopy Unit, Valduce Hospital, Como, Italy

Lisa Rundt Department of Internal Medicine, Bethesda Krankenhaus Bergedorf, Hamburg, Germany

Adriana Safatle-Ribeiro Department of Gastroenterology, University of Sao Paulo, Sao Paulo, Brazil

Yukata Saito Endoscopy Division, National Cancer Center Hospital, Tokyo, Japan

Choitsu Sakamoto Department of Gastroenterology, Nippon Medical School Graduate School of Medicine, Tokyo, Japan

Anna Sant'Anna McMaster University, Hamilton, ON, Canada

Jean-Christophe Saurin Department of Gastroenterology, Hôpital Edouard Herriot, Lyon, France

Wolff Schmiegel Department of Medicine, Ruhr-University Bochum, Knappschaftskrankenhaus, Bochum, Germany

Markus Schneider Medical Clinic, Evangelisches Krankenhaus, Düsseldorf, Germany

Hans-Joachim Schulz Department of Internal Medicine, Sana-Klinikum-Lichtenberg, Berlin, Germany

Detlef Schuppan 1st Medical Clinic, University Medical Center Mainz, Mainz, Germany

Ernest G. Seidman McGill IBD Research Group, Digestive Lab, Research Institute of McGill University Health Center, Montreal, QC, Canada

Uwe Seitz Internal Medicine/Gastroenterology, Kreiskrankenhaus Bergstrasse, Heppenheim, Germany

Warwick S. Selby AW Morrow Gastroenterology and Liver Centre, Royal Prince Alfred Hospital, Camperdown University of Sydney, Sydney, Australia

Virender K. Sharma Arizona Digestive Health, Gilbert, AZ, USA

Reena Sidhu Gastroenterology and Liver Unit, Royal Hallamshire Hospital, Sheffield, UK

Anupam Singh Department of Gastroenterology, University of Massachusetts Medical School, Worcester, MA, USA

Cristiano Spada Department of Surgical Endoscopy, Università Cattolica del Sacro Cuore, Rome, Italy

Ingo Steinbrück 1st Medical Department, Asklepios Klinik Altona, Hamburg, Germany

Joseph J. Y. Sung The Chinese University of Hong Kong, Hong Kong, The People's Republic of China

Ilja Tachecí 2nd Department of Internal Medicine–Gastroenterology, University Hospital and Charles University Faculty of Medicine, Hradec Králové, Czech Republic

Hisao Tajiri Division of Gastroenterology and Hepatology, Department of Internal Medicine, The Jikei University School of Medicine, Tokyo, Japan

Shinji Tanaka Department of Endoscopy, Hiroshima University Hospital, Hiroshima, Japan

Wolfgang Teichmann Hamburg, Germany

Michael Thomson Centre for Pediatric Gastroenterology, The Children's Hospital, Sheffield, UK

Ervin Tóth Department of Gastroenterology, Skåne University Hospital, Malmö, Sweden

Konstantinos Triantafyllou Hepatogastroenterology Unit, 2nd Department of Internal Medicine and Research Institute, Attikon University General Hospital, Medical School, Athens University, Haidari, Greece

Riccardo Urgesi Department of Surgical Endoscopy, Università Cattolica del Sacro Cuore, Rome, Italy

André Van Gossum Department of Hepato-Gastroenterology, Erasme Hospital—Free University of Brussels, Brussels, Belgium

Winfried A. Voderholzer Gastroenterology Practice, Berlin, Germany

Axel von Herbay Hansepathologie, Hamburg, Germany

Kenji Watanabe Department of Gastroenterology, Osaka City General Hospital, Osaka, Japan

Felix Wiedbrauck Department of Gastroenterology, Allgemeines Krankenhaus Celle, Celle, Germany

Hironori Yamamoto Division of Gastroenterology, Department of Medicine, Jichi Medical University, Tochigi, Japan

From Finding to Diagnosis

Synopsis of relevant findings in the small intestine: direct track to the image and video
See also:

Findings in the	
Normal small bowel	Chap. 19
Esophagus	Chaps. 42 and 43
Upper GI tract	Chap. 44
Colon	Chaps. 45 and 49
Postoperative GI tract	Chap. 39
Systematic description of findings	Chap. 10

Finding			Diagnosis	Image	Video
Stenosis	Extrinsic		Impression, bulge	10.2a	V19-20
	Duodenum		Peptic stenosis		V20-03
	Ulcerated		Crohn's	09.6	
			NSAIDs	30.9	
		Circular	NSAIDs	30.7	V16-02
		Edematous	Crohn's	25.10	V24.02
		Mucosal hemorrhage	Crohn's	25.9b	V25-01
		Petechiae	Crohn's	2.2	V24.03
			Ischemic enteropathy		V21-10
			Anastomotic stricture	39.13	
	Fibrotic		NSAIDs	30.8	V40-08
		White villi	Radiation enteritis	30.10	V30.06
	Erythematous, edema		Eosinophilic enteritis	27.8	
	Web like		NSAIDs	10.2b	V30-04
			Acute GI-GvHD	31.6	V31-01
			Follicular lymphoma	34.16	V34-11
			Anastomotic ulcer	39.14	V39-09
			EATL	34.19	
	Ulcerated infiltration		EATL	26.7	V34-12
			Centroblastic B-cell lymphoma	34.17	V40-07
	Mass		Adenocarcinoma	10.2c	V34-01
			Neuroendocrine carcinoma	34.6	V34-05
			Lymphoma	34.20	
			Metastasis	34.25-26	V34-16/17
Second lumen	Anastomosis		Roux-en-Y	10.3a	V39-03
	Circular ulcer		Side to side	39.14	V39-09
	Diverticulum		Duodenal	20.2	V20-01
			Jejunal	20.3	V20-02
			Meckel's	20.9	V20-05
			Anastomotic diverticulum	39.11	V39-06
			Side anastomosis	39.14	V39-09
			Duplication cyst	20.14	

	Fistula	Crohn's	49.8	V49-03 V25-02
	Artifact	Air bubble	05.19d	V05-17
Dilated lumen		Adhesion	39.22	V40-08
		Duodenojejunostomy	–	V39-02
		Roux-en-Y anastomosis	39.9	V39-03
Foreign body	Worm	Strongyloides	28.19	V28-06
	Tiny			
	Multiple, small, in colon	Pinworm	28.20	V28-07
	Multiple	Hookworm	28.23	
	Multiple, one thin end	Whipworm	28.21	V28-08
	Long	Roundworm	28.17	
	Long, multiple segments	Tapeworm	28.24-25	V28-09/10
	Capsules/remnants	Patency capsule	09.9	V09-01
		Patency capsule coating	09.10	V09-02
		PillCam	10.5b	V05-05
	Postinterventional	Intestinal suture	39.20c, d	
		Gastric suture	44.20	
		Staple	10.3b	V39-07
		Endoscopic clip	10.5a	V39-12
Intussusception	Idiopathic	Adolescent	38.15	V38-07
	Secondary	Ectopic pancreas	33.14-15	
		Lipoma	33.29	
		Hamartomatous polyp		V33-02
Edema	Diffuse	Portal hypertension	10.6b	V23-02
		Small-bowel transplantation	39.27	
	Glassy	Mycobacterium avium	28.2	V28-02
		Tuberculosis	28.3	
		Radiation enteritis	22.11	
	Erythema	Eosinophilic enteritis	27.8	
		IgA vasculitis	29.6c	V29-02
	Diffuse white villi	Whipple's disease	28.1	V28-01
		Yellow nail syndrome	22.15	
		Hypobetalipoproteinemia	29.18	
		Waldman's disease	38.14	
	Red spots	Systemic lupus erythematosus	29.13	
	Ulceration	Acute GI-GvHD	31.7	
	Bleeding	Acute ischemia	21.14	
	Segmental	Ileostoma	39.25a	
Abnormal mucosa	White, edematous	Primary lymphangiectasia	22.14	V22-02
		Hypobetalipoproteinemia	29.18	
		Yellow nail syndrome	22.15	
	Atrophic	Diverticulum	10.6d	
	Erosive	Acute GI-GvHD	31.3	
	Focally denuded	Crohn's	25.11	
		NSAIDs		V30-01/02
	Scalloped	Celiac	26.4	V26-03
	Reticulate	Portal hypertension	23.3-4	
	Nodular, ulcerated	Crohn's (cobblestone)	25.8b	V25-01
		Acute GI-GvHD	31.3-4	V31-01
		EATL	2.7	
	Granular	Autoimmune enteropathy	26.9	V26-10
	Hemorrhagic	Crohn's	25.9	
		Eosinophilic enteritis	27.9d	V27.01
		IgA vasculitis	29.5d	V29-02
	Ulcerated	IgA vasculitis	29.5f	V29-02
		Acute GI-GvHD	31.8	V31-01

	Friable	Eosinophilic enteritis	27.5	
		Noonan syndrome	29.22	
	Erythematous	Eosinophilic enteritis	27.5	
		NSAIDs	10.6c	V30-03
	Fibrotic	Panniculitis	28.10	V28-05
		Radiation enteritis	30.10	V30-05
	Atypical vessels	Systemic sclerosis	29.14d	
Atrophic villi	Patchy villous atrophy	NSAIDs	10.8	V30-01
	Patchy erythema	Crohn's	25.11	
	Patchy white villi	Crohn's	24.10	
		NSAIDs	30.1	
	Patchy erythema	Eosinophilic enteritis	27.3	
		NSAIDs		V30-03
	Erythema, edema, ulcer	Idiopathic chronic non-granulomatous jejunitis	50.11a	V26-11
		IgA vasculitis	29.5	V29-02
	Erosion	NSAIDs	30.2	
	Stenosis	NSAIDs	2.3b	
	Diffuse partial villous atrophy	Celiac	26.3b	
		Chemotherapy induced	30.12	
		Collagenous sprue	26.11	
	Nodules	CVID	29.16	
	Ulcerations	Ulcerative jejunoileitis	26.6	V26-08
	Diffuse total villous atrophy	Celiac sprue	26.3a	V26-01
	Fissures	Celiac sprue	02.6	V26-03
	White villi	Refractory sprue type II	26.5	
	Ulcerations	Refractory sprue type II		V26-06
		Autoimmune enteropathy		V26-09
	Ulceration, nodularity	EATL	02.7	
	Ulceration, stricture	EATL	34.19	
	Mass	EATL	34.20	
	Bleeding	Autoimmune enteropathy		V26-10
White villi	Diffuse white villi	Waldman's disease	22.14	V22-02
		Whipple's disease	28.1	V28-01
		Yellow nail syndrome	22.15	
		HIV	28.9	
	Nodular	Hennekam syndrome	22.16	V38-05
		Cronkhite-Canada syndrome	37.6	V37-04
	Granular	Sea blue histiocytosis	29.20	
	Patchy white villi	Atypical mycobacteriosis	22.6	V28-02
		Salmonellosis	22.7	
	Bleeding	Goldenhar syndrome	29.23	
	Nodules	Blastomycosis	28.14	
	Edema	Functional lymphangiectasia	22.1	
		Mycobacterium avium	28.2	V28-02
		Tuberculosis	28.3	
	Patchy villous atrophy	NSAIDs	30.1	V30-01
	Ulcer	NSAIDs	30.2	
	Ulcers, nodules	Idiopathic chronic non-granulomatous jejunitis	50.11a	V26-11
	Diffuse villous atrophy	Autoimmune enteropathy	26.9	V26-10
	Ulcers	Ulcerative jejunoileitis	26.6	V26-07
		Ischemic enteritis	21.15	V21-08
	Mucosal hemorrhage	Refractory sprue type II	26.5	
	Fibrosis	Radiation enteritis	30.10	V30-06
			22.12	

	Bleeding	Radiation enteritis	22.11	V30-05
	Aphthae, erosion	Crohn's disease	22.4	V24-01
		Collagenosis	22.5	
	Peritumorous	Adenocarcinoma	22.9	V34-01
		Lymphoma	22.8	V34-11
		Metastasis	22.10	V34-17
		Neuroendocrine carcinoma	34.6	V34-05
		GIST		V34-08
		MALT lymphoma	34.18	
White spots	Circumscript	Flat adenoma, sporadic	33.18	V33-03
Plaques		Flat adenoma (FAP)	35.6	V35-01
	Cystic	Lymph cysts	19.16	V19-16
	Solid, small	Lymph follicle	19.18a	V19-17
	Focal white villi	Focal lymphangiectasia	22.2	
	Plaque, irregular	Early duodenal carcinoma	34.1	
	Aphthae	Crohn's	25.6	V24-01
		Collagenosis	29.12	
	Patchy			
	Patchy white villi	Patchy lymphangiectasia	22.3	V22-01
	Patchy plaques	Acute GI-GvHD	31.9	V31-01
	Aphthae and nodules	Intestinal spirochetosis	28.6	V28-03
	Granula	Eosinophilic enteritis	27.9e	V27-01
	Segmental plaque, circular	Circular duodenal adenoma	33.19	V33-05
Black spot	Flat, large	Ink mark	39.31	V39-11
	Elevated	Melanoma	34.22	V34-13
	Multiple, diffuse	Hemosiderosis	29.17	V29-03
Red spots	Sharply demarcated	Angiectasia	10.9	V21-01 – 03
		In portal hypertension	23.5	
	Fern-like arborization	Angiectasia in HHT	21.2	V21-05
	With bleeding	Angiectasia, bleeding	21.3	
	Multiple, localized	Neuroendocrine carcinoma	5.23c	V34-06
	Unsharp	Atypical angiectasia	5.8cd	V05-06
		Crohn's	25.9a	
		Goldenhar syndrome	29.23	
		Refractory sprue type II	26.5	
	Erosion	NSAIDs	30.3	V30-02
	Ulcers	Amyloidosis	29.1	V29-01
		Cytomegalovirus	28.8	V28-04
		Crohn's	2.2	V24-03
	Erythema	Portal hypertension	23.4	
		Eosinophilic enteritis	27.3-4	
		Chemotherapy induced	30.12	
		Acute GI-GvHD	31.7	
		SLE	29.13	
	Edema	Portal hypertension	21.13	V23-02
	Mucosal hemorrhage	Radiation enteritis	22.11	
		Crohn's disease	25.9	
	Multiple red and white spots	Systemic mastocytosis	50.13	
Erythema	Patchy	NSAIDs	10.6c	V30-03
		Portal hypertension	21.13	
		Acute GI-GVHD	31.2	
	Distant tumor	Carcinoma involving mesentery	34.3	V34-01
	Fibrosis	Radiation enteritis	5.23b	
	Patchy villous atrophy	Eosinophilic enteritis	27.03	
	White villi	Eosinophilic enteritis	27.5	

	White villi, infiltration	Lymphoma EATL	26.7	
	Edema	Food allergy	38.1b	
	White villi	Healing IgA vasculitis	29.6c	
Aphthae		Crohn's	24.4	V24-01
		Systemic lupus erythematosus	29.12	
	Nodules	Intestinal spirochetosis	28.6	V28-03
Erosion		Crohn's	10.15b	V24-03
		NSAIDs	30.2-3	
		Intussusception	38.15	
	Villous atrophy	Celiac disease		V26-04
		Autoimmune enteropathy	26.9	
	Exudation	Acute GI-GVHD	31.4	
	Bleeding	Acute GI-GVHD	31.5	
	Mucosal hemorrhage	Collagenosis	22.5	
Ulcer	Aphthous	Crohn's	24.8	V24-03
		NSAIDs	38.3c	
			30.4	
	Fissural	Crohn's	24.7	
	Linear	Crohn's	25.7	
			41.7	
		Eosinophilic enteritis	27.9 g	
		Tuberculosis	28.5	
		IgA vasculitis	29.7	
		Behçet's	29.8	
		NSAIDs	30.5	
	Crater like	Crohn's	24.10	
		Eosinophilic enteritis	27.5c	
		Peptic duodenal ulcer	44.23	V44-07
		APC ulcer	39-29	
		Mucosectomy ulcer	39.30	
		Metastatic gastric cancer	34.28	
	(Semi)circular	Anastomotic ulcer	39.14	V39-09
		NSAIDs	30.5-7	
		NSAIDs stricture	30.7-8	V16-02
		Chronic nonspecific multiple ulcer of the small intestine	32.7-8	V32-01
		Meckel's diverticulum	20.11	V38-06
		EATL	41.15	
	Petechiae	Crohn's	2.2	V25-01
	Edematous stenosis	Crohn's disease	25.8	V24-02
	Second lumen	Diverticulitis	20.7	
		Meckel's diverticulitis	20.12	
		Anastomotic ulcer	39.12	V39-08
	Bleeding	Dieulafoy's ulcer	21.6	
		Peptic ulcer		V44-08
		Ischemic enteritis	21.15-16	V14-02
	Punched out	Cytomegalovirus	28.8	V28-04
		Cocaine abuse	30.14	
		Sarcoidosis	29.4b	
		PPI therapy	30.15	
		Biopsy ulcer	39.28	V39-10
	Necrotic	CMV/acute GI GvHD	31.11	
		Vasculitis	29.10	
	Multiple, diffuse	Amyloidosis	29.1	V29-01
		Vasculitis	29.10	

		Crohn's	25.8b	V24-02
		Acute GI-GvHD	31.8	
	With villous atrophy	Refractory sprue type II	26.5	V26-06
		Ulcerative jejunoileitis	41.14	V26-07-08
		EATL	34.19	V34-12
		Idiopathic chronic non-granulomatous jejunitis	50.11a	V26-11
		Ischemic enteritis	21.15	V21-08
	On submucosal tumor	Neurofibroma	33.32	
		GIST		V34-08
		Lipoma	33.29	V33-09
		Fibrolipoma	33.31	V33-10
		Amyloid tumor	29.3	
Diverticula	Proximal	Juxtapapillary diverticulum	20.1	
		Duodenal diverticula	20.2	V20-01
		Jejunal diverticulum	20.3	
	Multiple	Jejunal diverticulosis	20.4	V20-02
	Bleeding	Jejunal diverticulum	20.6	V20-03
	Distal	Meckel's diverticulum	20.8-9	V20-05
	Ulcerated, multiple	Diverticulitis	20.7	
	Ulcerated, single	Meckel's diverticulum, adult	20.11-12	
		Meckel's diverticulum, child	38.11	V38.06
	Gastric heterotopia	Meckel's diverticulum	20.10	V20-04
	Inverted	Meckel's diverticulum	20.13	V20-06
Scar		Ileocolostomy	39.17-19	V39-04
Nodules		Sarcoidosis	29.4a	
	Lymph follicular	Normal terminal ileum	19.18a	V19-17
	Ileum	Lymphoid hyperplasia	33.10a	V19-19
		Crohn's	24.11	
		HIV, CMV	28.12	
		Mycobacteriosis	33.10b	
	Entire small bowel	CVID	29.15	
		IgA deficiency	38.18	
		Giardiasis	28.15	
		Intestinal spirochetosis	28.6	V28-03
		IPSID	28.7	
Polyps	Sessile	Tubular adenoma	15.8	V15-02
	Flat, white	FAP	35.6	V35-03
		Sporadic duodenal adenoma	33.18b	V33-03
	Sessile, bleeding	Capillary hemangioma	33.21	V16-01
	Villous	Adenoma	10.14d	V33-05
	Ulcerated	Suture granuloma	33.2	
	Pedunculated	Peutz-Jeghers polyposis	10–12c	
	Large	Peutz-Jeghers polyposis	38.5	V38-03
	Medium	Peutz-Jeghers polyposis	10.13b	
		Juvenile polyp	33.13	
	Small	Hyperplastic polyp	33.6	V33-01
		Peutz-Jeghers polyposis	10.13a	
		Lynch syndrome	37.1b	
	White villi	Peutz-Jeghers polyposis		V36-01
	With ulcer	Juvenile polyposis	37.3	V37-02
		Inverted Meckel's diverticulum	20.13	V20-06
	Bleeding	Tubular adenoma	33.20	
	Probably pedunculated	Peutz-Jeghers polyposis	10.12d	V36-02
		Inflammatory pseudopolyp	33.3	
		Hamartomatous polyp	33.11-12	V33-02

	Multiple	Peutz-Jeghers polyposis	36.4	
	Various sizes	Peutz-Jeghers polyposis	10.13d	
	Large	Peutz-Jeghers polyposis	36.4	V36-01
	Small	Adenomas in FAP	35.10	V35-02
		Cowden syndrome	37.4-5	V37-03
		Cronkhite-Canada syndrome	37.6	V37-05
		Ganglioneuromatosis	37.8	V37-06
		Hennekam syndrome	22.16	V38-05
		IPSID	28.7	
	Terminal ileum	Lymph follicular hyperplasia	33-10a	V19-19
	Sessile and pedunculated	Sea blue histiocytosis	29.19	
Tumor/mass	Soft, bulging	Impression from outside	05.14	V19-20
	Polypoid	Kaposi's sarcoma	34.8	
		MALT lymphoma	34.18	
		Pleiomorphic cell sarcoma	34.12	
	Duodenal bulb	Brunner's gland hyperplasia	33.8	
		Ectopic gastric mucosa	44.21-22	V44-06
	Cystic	Lymphangioma	33.16	
	Crater like	Metastatic gastric cancer	34.28	
		Endemic Kaposi's sarcoma	34.9	
	In Meckel's diverticulum	Ectopic gastric mucosa	20.10	V20-04
	Anastomotic	Suture granuloma	33.2	
Submucosal	*Soft*, yellow	Lipoma	33.28	V33-06
	Yellow, multiple	Intestinal lipomatosis	33.30	
	Ulcerated	Ulcerated lipoma	33-29	V33-09
	Yellow, cystic	Lymphatic cyst	33.23-25	V19-16
	Dark, vascular	Hemangioma	2.4 33.21–22	V33-07
		Blue rubber bleb nevus	21.7	V38-04
		Varices	21.10-12 23.6	V21-06/07
		Venectasia	21.9	V19-16
	Firm			
	Whitish	GIST	41.3	V34-07
		Leiomyoma	33.27	V33-08
	Reddish	GIST	34.7	V34-08
	Dark, ulcerated	Amyloid tumor	29.3	
	Ulcerated	Neurofibroma	33.32	
	Bleeding ulcer	Fibrolipoma	33.31	V33-10
	Pathological vessels	Neuroendocrine tumor	05.8	V34-03
	Umbilicated, multiple	Neuroendocrine tumor	34.5	V34-04
Exophytic	Stenosing	Adenocarcinoma	34.3-4	V34-01
	Ulcerated	Adenocarcinoma	34.2	V40-05
		Amelanotic melanoma	34.24	V34-15
		Metastatic endometrian cancer	34.25	V34-16
	Livid	Metastatic ovarian cancer	34.26	V34-17
	White villi	Neuroendocrine carcinoma	34.6	
	Central depression	Mantle cell lymphoma	34.13	V34-09
	Eccentric nodules	Follicular lymphoma	34.14	V34-10
	Dark	Melanoma	34.21-23	V34-13/14
	Ulcerated	Angiosarcoma	34.10	
	Ulcerated, multiple	Epithelioid angiosarcoma	34.11	
	Multiple	Metastatic melanoma	34.22–23	
		Kaposi's sarcoma	34.8	

Infiltrating	Ulcerated	Lymphoma	38.13	
		Centroblastic lymphoma	34.17	V40-07
		EATL	2.7	V34-12
			34.19	
	Ulcer, focal erythema	Pancreatic head carcinoma	34.30	
	White villi	MALT lymphoma	34.18	
	Erythema, white villi	Metastatic lung cancer	34.27	
	Vesicular	Follicular lymphoma	34.15	V34-10

Image and Video Contributors

The following also contributed images and videos to this project:

Konstantin Ackers Given Imaging, Hamburg, Germany

Michael Amthor Department of Pathology, Diakonie Krankenhaus Rotenburg/Wümme, Rotenburg/Wümme, Germany

Jürgen Bauditz Department of Hepatology and Gastroenterology, Charité Universitätsmedizin Berlin, Berlin, Germany

Bakthiar Bejou Department of Gastroenterology, Avicenne Hospital, Bobigny, France

Christian Bojarski Medical Clinic for Gastroenterology, Infectiology, and Rheumatology, Charité Universitätsmedizin Berlin, Berlin, Germany

Stefanie Bosselmann Department of Internal Medicine, Bethesda Krankenhaus Bergedorf, Hamburg, Germany

Dorthe Bössow Clinic for General, Visceral, and Tumor Surgery, Albertinenkrankenhaus, Hamburg, Germany

Ruprecht Botzler Gastroenterology Practice, Lübeck, Germany

Marc Bota Department of Internal Medicine, Bethesda Krankenhaus Bergedorf, Hamburg, Germany

Philip Bufler Gastroenterology and Hepatology, Dr. von Haunersches Kinderspital, München, Germany

Jens-Peter Bruhn 1st Medical Department, Asklepios Klinik Altona, Hamburg, Germany

Federico Carpi Interdepartmental Research Centre "E. Piaggio" School of Engineering, University of Pisa, Pisa, Italy

Riccardo Carta Microelectronics and sensors, KU Leuven, Leuven, Belgium

Wolfgang Cordruwisch Medical Department III, Asklepios Klinik Barmbek, Hamburg, Germany

David Cummings University of Glasgow, Glasgow, Scotland

Henryk Dancygier Medical Clinic II, Klinikum Offenbach, Offenbach, Germany

Åke Danielsson Department of Medicine, University Hospital Umeå, Sweden

Gerd Diederichs Institut for Radiology, Charité Universitätsmedizin Berlin, Berlin, Germany

Lan-Rong Dung Department of Electrical Engineering, National Chiao Tung University, Hsinchu, Taiwan

Axel Eickhoff Medical Clinic II, Klinikum Hanau, Germany

Siegbert Faiss Medical Department III, Asklepios Klinik Barmbek, Hamburg, Germany

Britta Fiebig Pränatalzentrum Hamburg und Humangenetik im Gynaekologicum, Hamburg, Germany

Roman Fischbach Radiology, Asklepios Klinik Altona, Hamburg, Germany

Peer Flemming Institute for Pathology Celle, Celle, Germany

Christian Florent Fédération des Services d'Hépato-Gastro-Entérologie, Hôpital Saint-Antoine, Paris, France

Wolfgang Fortelny Gastroenterology Practice, Waldsassen, Germany

Ingo Franke Medical Clinic I, Klinikum Niederlausitz, Senftenberg, Germany

Folke Freudenberg Gastroenterology and Hepatology, Dr. von Haunersches Kinderspital, München, Germany

Helmut Erich Gabbert Institute of Pathology, University Hospital Düsseldorf, Düsseldorf, Germany

Soumitra Ghoshroy Electron Microscopy Center, University of South Carolina, Columbia, SC, USA

Andreas Gocht Pathology Center, Lübeck, Germany

Begoña González-Suárez Department of Gastroenterology, Hospital Sant Pau, Barcelona, Spain

Florian Graepler Department Internal Medicine I, University Hospital, Tübingen, Germany

Harald Grosse Department of Internal Medicine, Bethesda Krankenhaus Bergedorf, Hamburg, Germany

Arun Gupta Wolfson Unit for Endoscopy, St. Marks Hospital, Middlesex, UK

Udo Helmchen Institut for Pathology, Universitätsklinikum Hamburg-Eppendorf, Hamburg, Germany

Renate Höhne Department of Pathology, Asklepios Klinik Altona, Hamburg, Germany

Konstanze Holl-Ulrich Institut for Pathology, Universitätsklinikum Schleswig-Holstein, Lübeck, Germany

Tariq Iqbal University Hospitals Birmingham, Queen Elizabeth Hospital, Birmingham, UK

Matthias Joanowitsch Radiology, Asklepios Klinik Altona, Hamburg, Germany

Christian Jürgensen Department of Hepatology and Gastroenterology, Charité Universitätsmedizin Berlin, Berlin, Germany

Denise Kalmaz Division of Gastroenterology, University of California San Diego, La Jolla, CA, USA

Byungkyu Kim Microsystem Research Center, Korea Institute of Science and Technology, Seoul, Korea

Stefan Krüger Department of Pathology, Universitätsklinikum Schleswig-Holstein, Germany

Bernward Kurtz Clinic for Radiology, Evangelisches Krankenhaus Düsseldorf, Düsseldorf, Germany

Wilson Kwong Division of Gastroenterology, University of California San Diego, La Jolla, CA, USA

Otto Ljungberg Department of Pathology, Skåne University Hospital, Malmö, Sweden

Christoph Manegold Bernhard-Nocht Institute of Tropical Medicine, Hamburg, Germany

Virgilio Mattoli Center for Micro-Biorobotics at Scuola Superiore Sant'Anna, Istituto Italiano di Tecnologia, Pontedera, Italy

Emese Mihaly 2nd Department of Internal Medicine, Semmelweis University Medical School, Budapest, Hungary

Carsten Möllmann Clinic for Surgery, Bethesda Krankenhaus Bergedorf, Hamburg, Germany

Selva Mony University Hospitals Birmingham, Queen Elizabeth Hospital, Birmingham, UK

Morgan Moorghen St. Marks Hospital, Middlesex, UK

Daniela Müller-Gerbes Medical Clinic, Krankenhaus Holweide, Köln, Germany

Artur Nemeth Department of Gastroenterology, Skåne University Hospital, Malmö, Sweden

Bruno Neu 2nd Medical Clinic, Technical University of Munich, Klinikum Rechts der Isar, Munich, Germany

Jörgen Nielsen Department of Medicine, Skåne University Hospital, Malmö, Sweden

Ellen Nötzel Medical Clinic, Sana Klinik Lichtenberg, Berlin, Germany

Markus Oeyen Städtisches Krankenhaus St. Barbara, Attendorn, Bonn, Germany

Carolina Olano Department of Gastroenterology, Universidad de la República, Montevideo, Uruguay

Aine O'Rourke Wolfson Unit for Endoscopy, St. Marks Hospital, Middlesex, UK

Ilske Oschlies Department of Pathology, Universitätsklinikum Schleswig-Holstein, Lübeck, Germany

Simon Panter South Tyneside District Hospital, Tyne and Wear, UK

Carola Pflüger Department of Internal Medicine, Bethesda Krankenhaus Bergedorf Hamburg, Germany

Michael Philipper Gastroenterology Practice, Düsseldorf, Germany

Christopher Pohland 1st Surgical department, Asklepios Klinik Altona, Hamburg, Germany

Niall Power The Royal Free Hospital, London, UK

Brigitta Reinke Department for Internal Medicine and Gastroenterology, Klinikum Pinneberg, Pinneberg, Germany

Constantin Reinus Pathology Department, Sharee Zedek Medical Center, Jerusalem, Israel

Riccardo Ricci Institute for Histopathology, Università Cattolica del Sacro Cuore, Rome, Italy

Christoph Ruether 1st Medical Department, Asklepios Klinik Altona, Hamburg, Germany

Wolfgang Saeger Department of Pathology, Marienkrankenhaus, Hamburg, Germany

Marco Sailer Clinic for Surgery, Bethesda Krankenhaus Bergedorf, Hamburg, Germany

Jörg Sievers Radiology, Bethesda Krankenhaus Bergedorf, Hamburg, Germany

Masimiliano Simi The Biorobotics Institute of Scuola Superiore Sant'Anna Valdera, Pontedera, Italy

Annette Stelzer Clinic for Gastroenterology, Hepatology and Infektiology, Universitätsklinikum, Düsseldorf

Frank Stenschke Medical Clinic II, Klinikum Offenbach, Offenbach, Germany

Curosh Taylessani 1st Surgical Department, Asklepios Klinik Altona, Hamburg, Germany

Thomas Teuber Gastroenterology Practice, Freising, Germany

Henrik Thorlacius Department of Medicine, Skåne University Hospital, Malmö, Sweden

Nikolaos Viazis 2nd Department of Gastroenterology, Evangelismos Hospital, Athens, Greece

Marc Voss 1st Medical Department, Asklepios Klinik Altona, Hamburg, Germany

Wilko Weichert Pathology Institute, Charité Universitätsmedizin Berlin, Berlin, Germany

Doris Welger Radiology, Asklepios Klinik Altona, Hamburg, Germany

Axel Wellmann Pathology Institute Celle, Celle, Germany

Robert Wentrup Department of Hepatology and Gastroenterology, Charité Universitätsmedizin Berlin, Berlin, Germany

Hanns-Olof Wintzer Department of Pathology, Asklepios Klinik Harburg, Hamburg, Germany

Gabrielle Wurm-Johansson Department of Medicine, Skåne University Hospital, Malmö, Sweden

Cyrla Zaltman Gastroenterology Unit, HUCFF, Federal University, Rio de Janeiro, Brazil

Video Capsule Endoscopy: A Reference Guide and Atlas

A Short History of the Gastrointestinal Capsule

Gavriel J. Iddan

Contents

The origin of work on the gastrointestinal (GI) capsule can be traced back to 1981. At that time, I was on a sabbatical leave from my work as an electro-optical engineer at Rafael, a government defense lab in Israel, and was working in the United States for a medical instrument company in Boston, Massachusetts. A gastroenterologist friend, Prof. Eitan Scapa, explained to me some of the shortcomings of the fiber bundle endoscope, especially its rigidity and its inability to view the small intestine. At that time, I had no idea as to how to solve these intriguing and interesting problems.

Subsequently, small charge-coupled device (CCD) imagers had been developed and made available (mainly in Japan) for use in handheld video cameras. The endoscope manufacturers were quick to incorporate them into the endoscope, replacing the fiber bundle that was used for image transmission and making the device much more flexible. Nevertheless, there was still no satisfactory solution to the problem of how to view the small intestine.

My gastroenterologist friend kept querying me about ways to solve the problem, and while I was on another sabbatical in 1991, I started to think about the possibility of separating the CCD head from the endoscope, leaving it connected via an umbilical cable. It was explained to me that this method would be impossible because the cable would need to be about 5 m long, too long to be safely pulled out. Also, the process might last a few hours, and the endoscope would have to stay inside the patient all this time.

At that point, I intuitively asked, "Why not cut the CCD head from the endoscope and attach a minitransmitter to it, letting the head move free of any physical connection?" The chance of solving the problem then seemed more realistic, and in 1992 I started spending more time on the new idea. I realized, however, that the task I was facing was very far from having a solution.

Consultation with a CCD expert was very discouraging, as simple calculations indicated that a CCD camera head would be able to operate for only about 10 min on miniature batteries. It was also explained to me that because not too

The work was first published in 2006 by Springer Medizin Verlag Heidelberg with the following title: *Atlas of Video Capsule Endoscopy.*

G.J. Iddan
Given Imaging Ltd., Yoqneam, Israel
e-mail: iddan.gabi@gmail.com

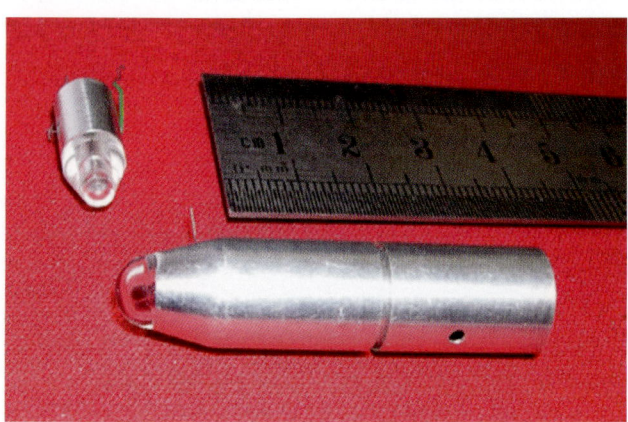

Fig. 1.1 Early, noningestible wired devices with a ¼-in. CCD used for testing the optics and the illumination

many pathologies are found in the small intestine, such a device would have only limited demand.

Because I was sure that the miniaturization problem would be solved in due time, I decided to continue my work on this very interesting and challenging problem and decided to focus on three major problems.

First, I figured that to avoid window contamination and obscuration, the optics would have to be designed in a way that would guarantee constant rubbing of the tissue on an ogive-shaped window to facilitate contact imaging and ensure self-wiping of the transparent window. A talented optical designer came up with a fine solution, and the prototype was built in 1993 (Fig. 1.1); a ¼-in. conventional CCD was used to test the optics and the results were good.

The next problem, long viewing hours, was solved by separating the system into three components: the *capsule*, containing the imager and transmitter; the *recorder*, containing an antenna array receiver and recording medium; and the *workstation*, incorporating the reader, processing software, and monitor. Simultaneously, we performed experiments to find the wavelength and power level required for wireless transmission of video through biologic tissue. (The experiments were done on a defrosted chicken bought in a nearby supermarket.) It seemed that we were on the right track but for one major obstacle—the power required by the CCD.

While casually reading a photonics magazine, I came upon an article written by Eric Fossum, a scientist at the Jet Propulsion Laboratory (Pasadena, California, USA), describing a new type of imager, the active pixel sensor (APS), which can be integrated on a single chip. Even more interesting, it was claimed to consume only 1 % of the power required by an equivalent CCD imager.

The APS was exactly what I was hoping for, and light appeared at the end of the tunnel. We submitted a patent application on 17 January 1994 and began to search for investment funds and start full-time work on the project. It

was difficult to find support because investors considered the project "science fiction, an Asimov-type adventure." During my search for investment, in 1995 I came upon a small company making miniature CCD cameras for medical applications and tried to interest its manager in the new video pill; the manager, Mr. Gavriel Meron, became excited and tried to raise money from his board but was refused.

At the same time, I succeeded in establishing a new start-up, 3DV Systems, in the area of three-dimensional (3-D) imaging, using funds from a new investment body, Rafael Development Corporation (RDC) Ltd.—an indication that the high-tech market was on the rise. While working at the imaging start-up, in 1997 we were awarded the first US patent on a video capsule: US 5604531, "In vivo video camera system." The patent approval triggered action by RDC, and Mr. Meron joined RDC and incorporated a new start-up, Given Imaging Ltd. I served simultaneously as a vice president at the 3-D imaging start-up and as a consultant at Given Imaging. With initial funds available, expert workers were hired and capsule development went on at full steam; Mr. Meron was able to attract more investors in Israel and abroad.

At a 1997 gastroenterology conference, Mr. Meron met Prof. C. Paul Swain from London, and they were both surprised to find that they were working independently on related subjects, as Professor Swain and his team were aiming at a wireless gastric camera. An agreement of cooperation resulted, and Prof. Swain joined the Given team and contributed extensively to the development and to the animal and clinical experiments. Professor Swain described his group's efforts in the historical review published in our article in *Gastrointestinal Endoscopy Clinics of North America* [1].

Work progressed rapidly under the supervision of Dr. Arkady Glukhovsky, who was at that time the research and development manager. A CMOS (complementary metal oxide semiconductor) camera chip was designed by Eric Fossum to specifications written by Mr. Dov Avni, our video expert, and it was manufactured at Tower Semiconductor (Figs. 1.2 and 1.3). In October 1999, at the private clinic of Prof. E. Scapa near Tel Aviv, the first real capsule was swallowed by Professor Swain, who insisted on being the first person to swallow the capsule. After some initial difficulties, clear images were received. A bottle of wine was opened, and the video capsule turned into reality.

As a result of our initial success, more funds became available and work accelerated. An article published in *Nature* in May 2000 described the new capsule [2]. Experiments on consenting patients started in Israel, Europe, and the United States, with encouraging results. By August 2001, Given Imaging was ready for an initial public offering (IPO) on the NASDAQ Stock Market, but this was delayed by the September 11 World Trade Center attacks. A couple of weeks later, Given's IPO was the first

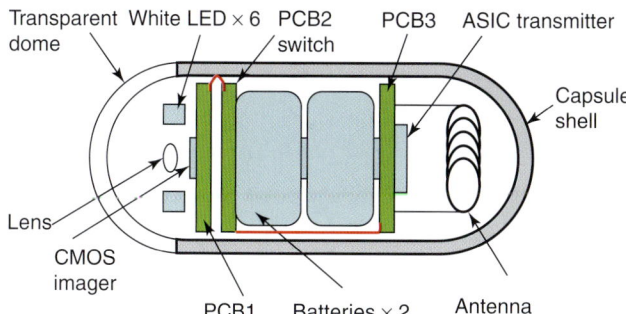

Transparent dome · White LED × 6 · PCB2 switch · PCB3 · ASIC transmitter · Capsule shell · Lens · CMOS imager · PCB1 · Batteries × 2 · Antenna

Fig. 1.2 A schematic view of the capsule and its components

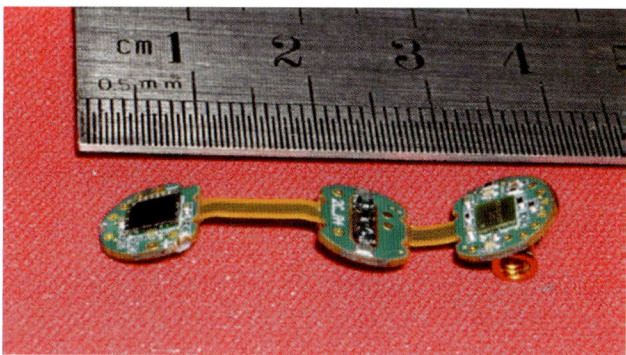

Fig. 1.3 Photo showing the three printed circuit boards: the left one holds the complementary metal oxide semiconductor (CMOS) imager, the central one holds the reed switch, and the right one holds the application-specific integrated circuit (ASIC) transmitter on the top and the antenna on the bottom

issue after the tower disaster. During the past decade, the video capsule has become a standard diagnostic tool used by gastroenterologists throughout the world; it is sold in more than 80 countries, and more than 1.8 million capsules have been ingested.

Since its introduction, researchers and practicing physicians have published more than 1,700 articles in professional journals describing all aspects of capsule usage. The fast-growing number of articles indicates that interest in the capsule is steadily growing.

The new capsule generation has an extended range of indications, and it is now considered as a leading diagnostic tool for intestinal bleeding, Crohn's disease, and other gastrointestinal disorders, as described elsewhere in this text. The new capsules incorporate a larger field of view, higher image quality, and a higher frame rate, all leading to superior performance and enabling a shorter viewing time. The new Data Recorder has new features such as a small monitor screen for real-time viewing and a two-way communication channel.

Most important, the colon capsule was introduced for cases in which conventional colonoscopy should be avoided. It is now being used mainly in Europe and has been submitted for approval by the US Food and Drug Administration (FDA).

At Given, we continue to develop better capsules with higher performance and new sensing capabilities that will enable the physician in the future to maneuver the capsule and control it from the outside of the body, thus improving the quality and increasing the speed of GI diagnostics.

Acknowledgment The pioneering contribution of Dov Avni, Eric Fossum, Arkady Glukhovsky, Gavriel Meron, Eitan Scapa, and Paul C. Swain to the capsule development work is greatly acknowledged.

References

1. Iddan GJ, Swain CP. History and development of capsule endoscopy. Gastrointest Endosc Clin N Am. 2004;14:1–9.
2. Iddan G, Meron G, Glukhovsky A, Swain P. Wireless capsule endoscopy. Nature. 2000;405:417.

Fields of Application

2

Mark E. McAlindon, Friedrich Hagenmüller,
and David E. Fleischer

Contents

The work was first published in 2006 by Springer Medizin Verlag Heidelberg with the following title: *Atlas of Video Capsule Endoscopy.*

M.E. McAlindon (✉)
Gastroenterology and Liver Unit, Royal Hallamshire Hospital, Sheffield, UK
e-mail: mark.mcalindon@sth.nhs.uk

F. Hagenmüller
1st Medical Department, Asklepios Klinik Altona, Hamburg, Germany
e-mail: f.hagenmueller@asklepios.com

D.E. Fleischer
Division of Gastroenterology, Mayo Clinic Arizona, Scottsdale, AZ, USA
e-mail: fleischer.david@mayo.edu

Video capsule endoscopy (VCE) is an established endoscopic modality that allows remote examination (without intubation) of almost the whole of the gastrointestinal (GI) tract. The first device was developed to examine the small bowel, previously inaccessible to endoscopic examination, for which it is now a first-line investigative modality. Most commonly, small bowel VCE is used in patients with suspected bleeding or to identify evidence of active Crohn's disease (in patients with or without a prior history of the disease). Conventionally, VCE is undertaken after upper and lower gastrointestinal flexible endoscopy has failed to make a diagnosis. (Small bowel radiology or a patency capsule test should be considered prior to VCE to minimize the risk of capsule retention in patients at high risk of strictures, such as those with Crohn's disease, a long history of ingestion of nonsteroidal anti-inflammatory drugs [NSAIDs], or obstructive symptoms.) VCE may also be used in patients with celiac disease, polyposis syndromes, and other small bowel disorders. Since the advent of small bowel capsule endoscopy (SBCE), dedicated esophageal and colon capsule endoscopes have expanded the fields of application to include the investigation of the upper and lower GI tract as well as midgut disorders. Esophageal capsule endoscopy (ECE) may be used to diagnose esophagitis, Barrett's esophagus, and varices, but it cannot be relied on to identify gastroduodenal disease. Colon capsule endoscopy (CCE) offers an alternative to conventional colonoscopy for symptomatic patients, and a possible role in colon cancer screening is intriguing. Current research is already addressing the possibility of controlling capsule movement and developing capsules that allow tissue sampling and the administration of therapy.

2.1 Small Bowel Capsule Endoscopy

2.1.1 Obscure Gastrointestinal Bleeding

Obscure GI bleeding is the commonest indication for small bowel capsule endoscopy (SBCE) [1–5]. The term is conventionally used when esophagogastroduodenoscopy

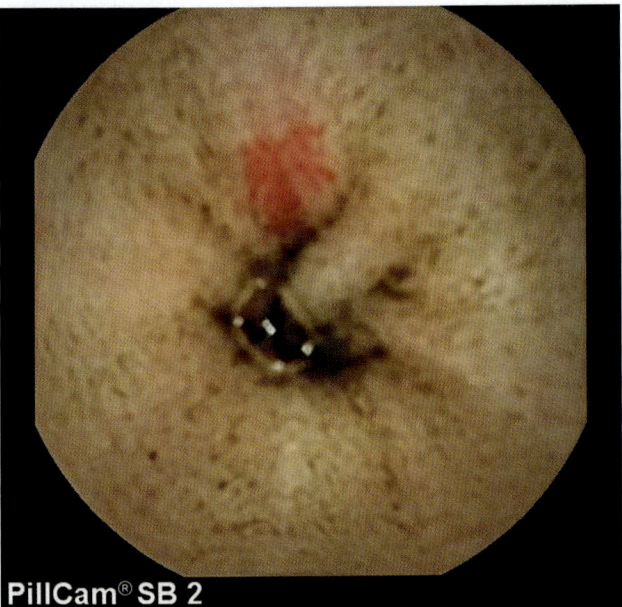

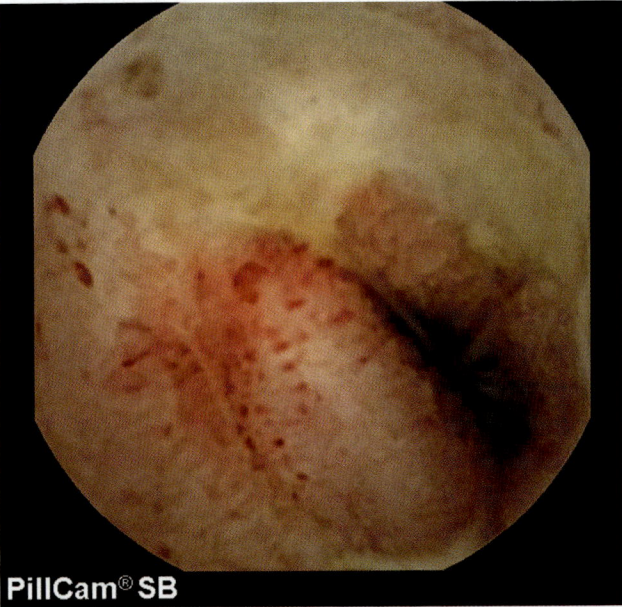

Fig. 2.1 Angioectasia

Fig. 2.2 Extensive ulceration and multiple petechiae caused by Crohn's disease

and colonoscopy have failed to identify a clear cause. Small bowel bleeding may be overt, manifesting with melena or hematochezia, or it may be occult, causing anemia. SBCE has a higher sensitivity than small bowel barium contrast radiology, small bowel CT, MRI, push enteroscopy, or angiography [6–11]. SBCE is recognized as a first-line investigative modality for obscure GI bleeding, with a diagnostic yield of 42–60 % [12, 13]. This yield is similar to that of double balloon enteroscopy [1, 4, 14, 15], which has the advantage of allowing biopsy or therapy, but the noninterventional nature and simplicity of SBCE mean that most clinicians use it to select patients (and target the lesion identified) for interventional endoscopy (see Chap. 41). Yield is improved if the procedure is performed during the episode of bleeding or as close to it as possible [16, 17]. Repeat VCE has a further yield of 35–75 % [18, 19], suggesting that, as with other modalities, lesions can be missed.

The reason that SBCE has greater sensitivity than other diagnostic modalities is that most lesions identified are flat vascular or mucosal lesions. Angioectasia—small, usually well-demarcated venous abnormalities that are often multiple—is the most commonly detected abnormality (Fig. 2.1) (see Chap. 21). Inflammatory lesions (ulcers and erosions) are also common findings [12, 13]. These may be due to Crohn's disease (Fig. 2.2), which occasionally presents with anemia or bleeding. However, an NSAID enteropathy may be indistinguishable from Crohn's disease and is probably under-recognized (Fig. 2.3) [20]. Vasculitis (Chap. 29), ischemia (Chap. 21) may cause small bowel ulcers, and infections like tuberculosis and cytomegalovirus (Chap. 28) should be considered in the appropriate clinical context. Finally,

minor mucosal breaks are recognized in 7–40 % of healthy volunteers [21, 22].

Small bowel tumors are the cause in about 4–10 % of patients with obscure gastrointestinal bleeding [12, 23, 24]. In addition to benign tumors such as hemangiomas (Fig. 2.4), these may include adenocarcinomas and gastrointestinal stromal tumors, neuroendocrine tumors, lymphoma, and metastases (particularly from melanoma (Fig. 2.5) and from breast, lung, and renal primary malignancies).

Less common causes include Meckel's or other diverticula, small bowel varices, and aortoenteric fistulae.

2.1.2 Suspected Active Crohn's Disease

VCE may be used to diagnose Crohn's disease de novo or to assess disease activity in patients known to have Crohn's disease. Meta-analyses suggest that VCE has a greater sensitivity in detecting inflammatory activity in both groups of patients than small bowel barium contrast studies, small bowel CT, push enteroscopy, and ileocolonoscopy [25, 26]. Fewer studies compare VCE with small bowel MRI, but available data suggest that they are equivalent. In clinical practice, the two studies are complementary: VCE detects early mucosal changes, whereas MRI is useful in assessing more established transmural disease and its complications without the need for irradiation or the risk of capsule retention. VCE may be at least as effective as ileocolonoscopy in detecting early postoperative relapse, is better tolerated [27–29], and can be used to reclassify a proportion of patients with unclassified inflammatory bowel disease as having

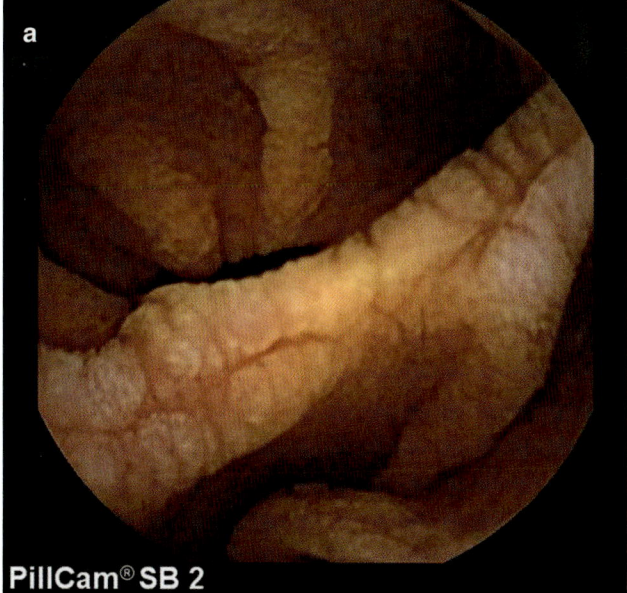

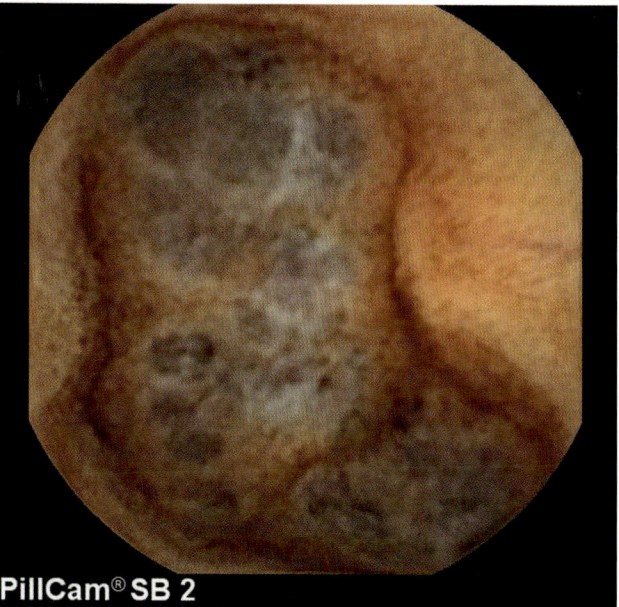

Fig. 2.4 Large hemangioma

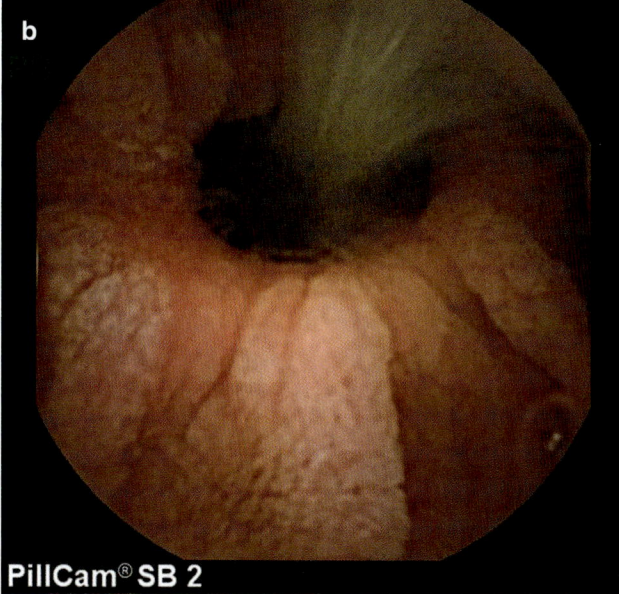

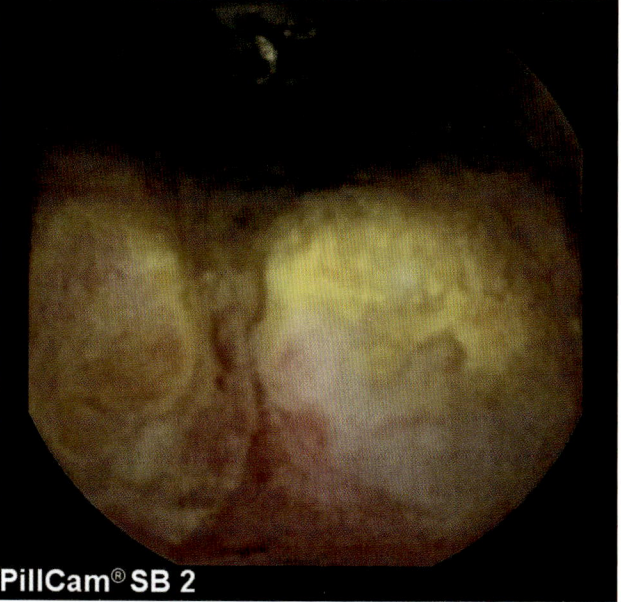

Fig. 2.3 (**a**) Villous atrophy with notching of folds and a linear mucosal break along the tip of a fold. (**b**) Stenosis with denuded mucosa and atrophic villi caused by ingestion of nonsteroidal anti-inflammatory drugs (NSAIDs)

Fig. 2.5 Ulcerated tumor mass with slight blue pigmentation owing to metastatic malignant melanoma

Crohn's disease by demonstrating small bowel inflammation [30–33]. A possible role in assessing mucosal healing after treatment requires further investigation [34].

The main concern about VCE is the risk of capsule retention, which is between 5 and 13 % in patients known to have Crohn's disease, although retention in those being investigated for suspected Crohn's disease and obscure GI bleeding is similar at about 1 % [4, 35, 36]. Existing radiologic methods do not always exclude the possibility of short strictures [1, 35]. Use of the swallowable PillCam® patency device

(Given Imaging, Yoqneam, Israel), which contains a radiofrequency tag, is effective in predicting safe passage of the capsule in the absence of a radiofrequency signal detected 30 h after ingestion (Chap. 9) [35]. Published guidelines recommend that prior investigation of the small bowel using the PillCam® patency device or alternative radiologic methods should be considered for patients with known or suspected Crohn's disease, particularly those with significant abdominal pain [1, 4, 37].

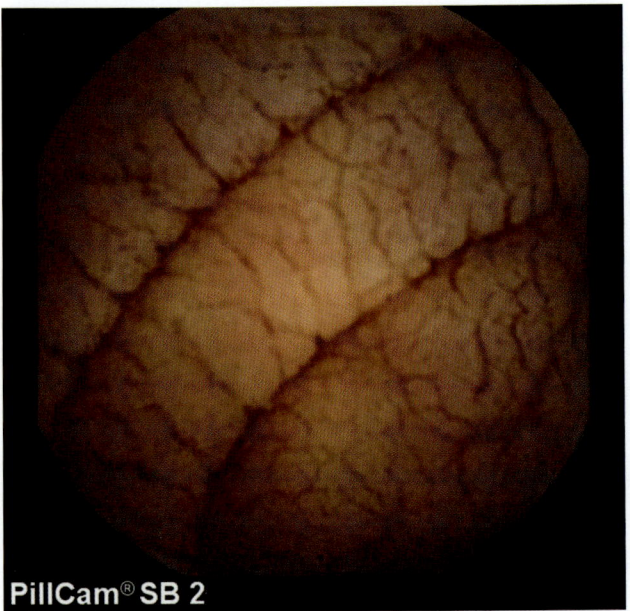

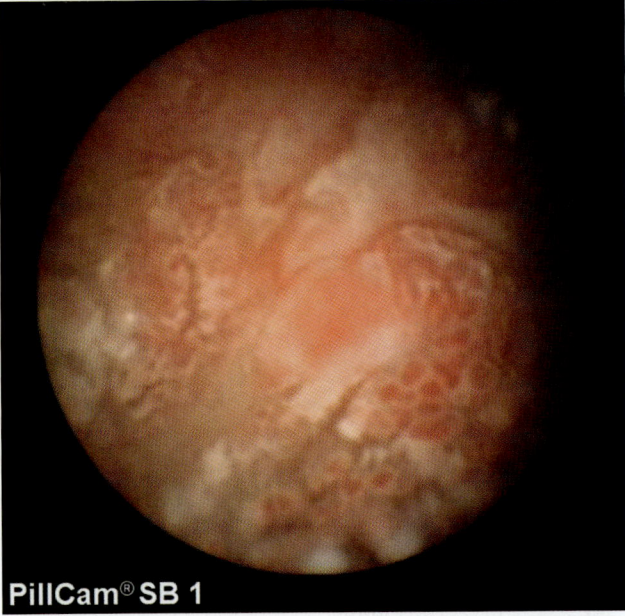

Fig. 2.6 Villous atrophy, with scalloping and notching of folds and a mosaic pattern due to celiac disease

Fig. 2.7 Enteropathy-associated T-cell lymphoma complicating celiac disease. Note the absence of normal villous surface, nodularity, and ulceration

2.1.3 Celiac Disease

Meta-analysis suggests that VCE has a sensitivity of 89 % in making a new diagnosis of celiac disease, recognized by reduced and scalloped folds, a mosaic pattern, and micronodularity of the mucosa (Fig. 2.6) [38, 39]. Clearly, it does not recognize those without villous atrophy (Marsh grades 1 and 2), and therefore, duodenal biopsy remains the gold standard for diagnosis. Because specificity is as high as 95 %, it would be reasonable to consider VCE as a diagnostic test in patients with raised tissue transglutaminase levels or endomysial antibody titers if they refuse to undergo esophagogastroduodenoscopy.

VCE may have a role in patients with antibody-negative villous atrophy, either providing supportive evidence of a diagnosis of celiac disease or identifying features more typical of Crohn's disease [40]. The main clinical use for VCE, however, is in patients who do not respond to a gluten-free diet or who relapse while on such a diet. The presence of villous atrophy alone may prompt a reassessment of dietary compliance or a consideration of immunosuppressive therapy. Severe inflammatory change, mucosal irregularity, or a tumor mass may suggest complications of ulcerative jejunitis, enteropathy-associated T-cell lymphoma (Fig. 2.7), or adenocarcinoma [40–42].

2.1.4 Polyposis Syndromes

VCE has a greater sensitivity in detecting the polyps of Peutz-Jeghers syndrome than barium studies; it also avoids irradiation and is preferred by patients [43, 44]. However, though VCE may identify more small polyps, it occasionally

misses very large polyps identified by MRI, which is of equivalent sensitivity in diagnosing clinically significant lesions (>10 mm) and appears to be as well tolerated [45].

For duodenal surveillance in familial adenomatous polyposis (FAP), current models of forward-viewing VCE detect the ampulla of Vater in 8.6–43.6 % of patients, so this method should not replace side-viewing duodenoscopy [46–48]. Polyps distal to the ligament of Treitz are much more likely in the presence of duodenal polyposis, and VCE is more sensitive than radiologic methods in detecting these lesions [49–52], but existing data suggest that the development of small bowel malignancy distal to the duodenum is extremely rare, so there seems to be little justification for monitoring FAP polyps using VCE in the absence of symptoms [53].

2.1.5 Miscellaneous

2.1.5.1 Abdominal Pain

In patients with abdominal pain alone, the diagnostic yield of VCE is between 6 and 21.4 %; it is higher in patients with weight loss or raised acute-phase proteins [54–58]. VCE may be useful in patients whose pain is thought to be obstructive in origin but whose diagnosis remains elusive despite multiple investigations. Diagnoses were made in 26 % of a small series of 19 patients thought to have small bowel obstruction based on symptoms alone or with supportive radiologic abnormalities [59]. VCE in this setting would, of course, require that the patient understand that the diagnosis may lead to either endoscopic or surgical retrieval of a retained capsule.

2.1.5.2 Graft-Versus-Host Disease

Graft-versus-host disease (GVHD) causes anorexia, nausea, vomiting, abdominal pain, and diarrhea in stem cell transplant patients. It is important to distinguish GVHD from drug toxicity and infection, which may require a reduction in immunosuppression. The small bowel is the commonest site for GVHD. Small studies suggest that VCE may be at least as effective in diagnosing GVHD as upper or lower GI endoscopy and biopsy [60–62] and it may be better tolerated. Microbiologic investigation remains important, however, as it is not known whether VCE can distinguish between GVHD and viral infection.

2.1.5.3 Nonsteroidal Anti-inflammatory Drug (NSAID) Enteropathy

As many as a third of the population may be using an NSAID at any given time [63]. Yet ingestion of diclofenac for 2 weeks causes small bowel inflammation in 68 % of those who use it [64], all NSAIDs (including low-dose aspirin) may cause mucosal injury [20, 64], and NSAID enteropathy is evident in 50–60 % of patients on long-term treatment [65]. Mild changes include reddened folds, petechiae, denuded mucosa, and mucosal breaks, but bleeding and deep ulceration may occur, along with stenoses in the longer term [64, 65]. As with many over-the-counter medications, patients may fail to declare their use, and NSAID enteropathy is likely to be underreported [20]. The relevance to the clinician is that NSAID enteropathy may be clinically and endoscopically indistinguishable from Crohn's disease and other causes of small bowel inflammation, so it should be considered in the differential diagnosis regardless of the indication for VCE.

2.2 Esophageal Capsule Endoscopy

2.2.1 Gastroesophageal Reflux Disease

When compared with conventional upper GI endoscopy, esophageal capsule endoscopy (ECE) has shown a sensitivity of 50–89 % in identifying erosive esophagitis [66–69]. ECE is significantly better tolerated [69, 70]. Perhaps because reflux symptoms are not associated with visible injury in as many as 60 % of patients [71] and other gastroduodenal disease is not excluded, ECE has not been widely adopted for this indication.

2.2.2 Barrett's Esophagus

Barrett's esophagus is a premalignant condition affecting 5–15 % of patients with reflux symptoms [72]; of those affected, 0.12–0.5 % of patients per year develop esophageal adenocarcinoma [73]. Meta-analysis suggests that ECE has a sensitivity of 78 % in identifying Barrett's esophagus, compared with conventional upper GI endoscopy [74]. The

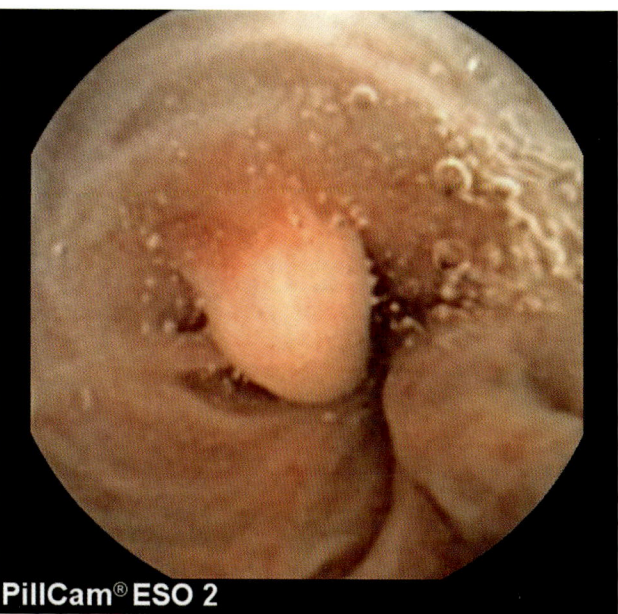

Fig. 2.8 Small varix, regenerative polyp, and scarring resulting from previous variceal banding in the esophagus

excellent tolerability profile of ECE may make it suitable for screening for Barrett's esophagus, but it is not routinely recommended for average-risk individuals [75]. Endoscopic surveillance is performed using imaging techniques and histologic analysis not currently possible with ECE [76], so at present ECE is not a suitable alternative for those known to have Barrett's esophagus.

2.2.3 Esophageal Varices

Of patients with compensated cirrhosis, 40 % have esophagogastric varices, and there is a further 5–10 % incidence per year. Variceal bleeding is associated with a 40 % 1-year mortality rate. Because bleeding risk can be reduced with pharmacologic or endoscopic intervention, these patients undergo regular endoscopic screening to detect varices [77]. Meta-analysis shows that ECE has 83 % sensitivity in screening for varices (Fig. 2.8) when compared with conventional upper GI endoscopy [78], so it may prove to be a viable alternative in this setting.

2.3 Colon Capsule Endoscopy

2.3.1 Colorectal Neoplasia

The second generation of the colon capsule includes an improved angle of view of 172° and an adaptive frame rate that allows acquisition of images at a rate between 4 and 35 frames per second, dependent on the speed of travel of the capsule. Two large multicenter studies comparing second-generation colon capsule endoscopy (CCE) with conventional colonos-

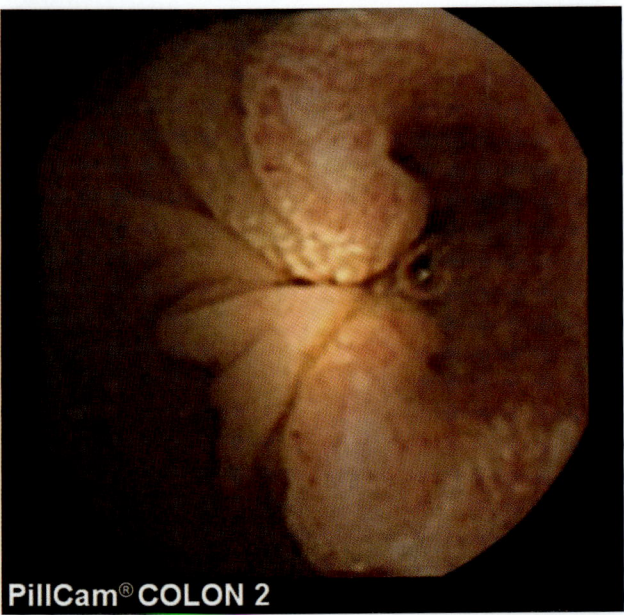

PillCam® COLON 2

Fig. 2.9 Adenocarcinoma of the colon

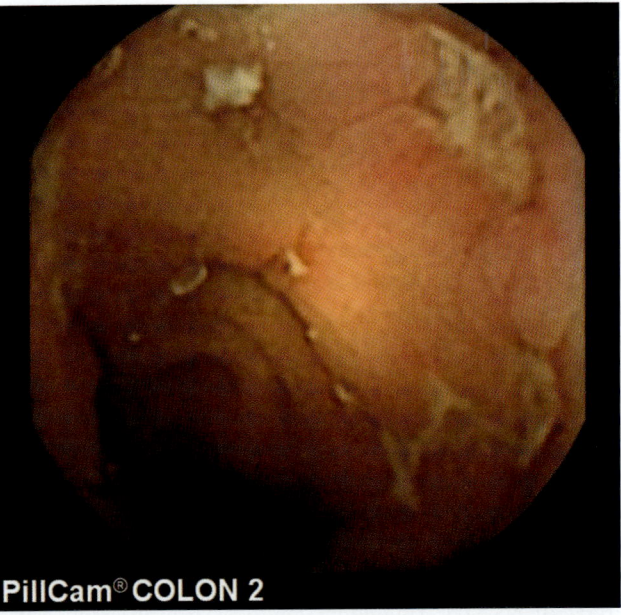

PillCam® COLON 2

Fig. 2.10 Deep and serpiginous ulcers caused by Crohn's colitis

copy showed 89 and 84 % sensitivity in detecting polyps measuring at least 6 mm [79, 80]. Such outcomes are not dissimilar from results of CT colonography when compared with colonoscopy [81] or indeed from colonoscopy when compared to itself (in "back-to-back" or "tandem" studies) [82]. Current European guidelines consider that although colonoscopy remains preferable for individuals at high risk of colorectal cancer (because of alarm symptoms, a family or personal history of colorectal cancer, or both), CCE may be a viable alternative for average-risk individuals in whom colonoscopy is not possible (Fig. 2.9) [83]. An interesting study using mathematical modeling suggested that CCE would be more cost-effective than colonoscopy in population screening if it were associated with a 30 % better compliance rate [84]. However, this study is based on outcomes from trials that used the first-generation colon capsule, and the second-generation device represents a measurable improvement. Therefore, further studies are needed to clarify the role of CCE versus colonoscopy and CT colonography in symptomatic patients and in population screening.

2.3.2 Inflammatory Bowel Disease

A multicenter study comparing the first-generation colon capsule with colonoscopy in assessing the activity of ulcerative colitis found 89 % sensitivity, 75 % specificity, 93 % positive predictive values, and 65 % negative predictive values [85]. A second small study identified a significant correlation with colonoscopy in monitoring the severity and extent of inflammation [86]. It has been suggested that CCE thus may be useful in assessing treatment-induced mucosal healing, a predictor of

better outcome (Fig. 2.10) [85]. However, even in a very small minority of patients with rectal sparing or patchy disease due to topical or other therapy [87], it seems likely that flexible sigmoidoscopy and biopsy usually will provide a relatively well-tolerated means of obtaining the required information.

2.4 Future Fields of Application of Capsule Endoscopy

The small bowel capsule was the first to be developed because of the clinical imperative: the inaccessibility of the small bowel meant that visualization of its mucosa was not possible without recourse to surgery. In addition, the size of the small bowel lumen lent itself to the possibility that a device small enough to be swallowed could visualize almost all of the surface area.

Visualization of the larger colonic lumen, part of which is obscured by the presence of haustral folds, was addressed by developing a double-headed capsule, which provides simultaneous antegrade and retrograde images that approach a 360° view.

The stomach provides a further challenge: optimal visualization requires distention such that the lumen develops substantial capacity. However, early studies have already demonstrated control of movement of a capsule in the stomach using magnets [88–90], and trials are under way to compare magnetically controllable VCE with conventional diagnostic upper gastrointestinal endoscopy.

It is now possible to examine the whole of the GI tract using VCE, and future technological developments may allow these devices to replace conventional upper GI diagnostic endoscopy. Devices that allow sampling of fluid or tissue or that even can administer therapy are already on the horizon [91].

References

1. Sidhu R, Sanders DS, Morris AJ, McAlindon ME. Guidelines on small bowel enteroscopy and capsule endoscopy in adults. Gut. 2008;57:125–36.

2. National Institute for Health and Clinical Excellence. Wireless capsule endoscopy for investigation of the small bowel. http://www.nice.org.uk/guidance/IPG101. Accessed 01 Oct 2014.

3. Rey JF, Ladas S, Alhassani A, Kuznetsov K. European Society of Gastrointestinal Endoscopy (ESGE). Video capsule endoscopy: update to guidelines (May 2006). Endoscopy. 2006;38:1047–53.

4. Ladas SD, Triantafyllou K, Spada C, Riccioni ME, Rey JF, Niv Y, et al. European Society of Gastrointestinal Endoscopy (ESGE): recommendations (2009) on clinical use of video capsule endoscopy to investigate small-bowel, esophageal and colonic diseases. Endoscopy. 2010;42:220–7.

5. Mishkin DS, Chuttani R, Croffie J, Disario J, Liu J, Shah R, et al. ASGE Technology Status Evaluation Report: wireless capsule endoscopy. Gastrointest Endosc. 2006;63:539–45.

6. Marmo R, Rotondano G, Piscopo R, Bianco MA, Cipolletta L. Meta-analysis: capsule enteroscopy vs. conventional modalities in diagnosis of small bowel diseases. Aliment Pharmacol Ther. 2005;22:595–604.

7. Triester SL, Leighton JA, Leontiadis GI, Fleischer DE, Hara AK, Heigh RI, et al. A meta-analysis of the yield of capsule endoscopy compared to other diagnostic modalities in patients with obscure gastrointestinal bleeding. Am J Gastroenterol. 2005;100:2407–18.

8. de Leusse A, Vahedi K, Edery J, Tiah D, Fery-Lemonnier E, Cellier C, et al. Capsule endoscopy or push enteroscopy for first line exploration of obscure gastrointestinal bleeding? Gastroenterology. 2007;132:855–62.

9. Neu B, Ell C, May A, Schmid E, Riemann JF, Hagenmüller F, et al. Capsule endoscopy versus standard tests in influencing management of obscure digestive bleeding: results from a German multicenter trial. Am J Gastroenterol. 2005;100:1736–42.

10. Saperas E, Dot J, Videla S, Alvarez-Castells A, Perez-Lafuente M, Armengol JR, Malagelada JR. Capsule endoscopy versus computed tomographic or standard angiography for the diagnosis of obscure gastrointestinal bleeding. Am J Gastroenterol. 2007;102:731–7.

11. Leung WK, Ho SS, Suen BY, Lai LH, Yu S, Ng EK, et al. Capsule endoscopy or angiography in patients with acute overt obscure gastrointestinal bleeding: a prospective randomized study with long-term follow-up. Am J Gastroenterol. 2012;10:1370–6.

12. Sidhu R, McAlindon ME, Drew K, Hardcastle S, Cameron IC, Sanders DS. Evaluating the role of small-bowel endoscopy in clinical practice: the largest single-centre experience. Eur J Gastroenterol Hepatol. 2012;24:513–9.

13. Liao Z, Gao R, Xu C, Li ZS. Indications and detection, completion, and retention rates of small-bowel capsule endoscopy: a systematic review. Gastrointest Endosc. 2010;71:280–6.

14. Chen X, Ran Z-H, Tong J-L. A meta-analysis of the yield of capsule endoscopy compared to double-balloon enteroscopy in patients with small bowel diseases. World J Gastroenterol. 2007;13:4372–8.

15. Pasha SF, Leighton JA, Das A, Harrison ME, Decker GA, Fleischer DE, Sharma VK. Double-balloon enteroscopy and capsule endoscopy have comparable diagnostic yield in small-bowel disease: a meta-analysis. Clin Gastroenterol Hepatol. 2008;6:671–6.

16. Pennazio M, Santucci R, Rondonotti E, Abbiati C, Beccari G, Rossini FP, de Franchis R. Outcome of patients with obscure gastrointestinal bleeding after capsule endoscopy: report of 100 consecutive cases. Gastroenterology. 2004;126:643–53.

17. Apostolopoulos P, Liatsos C, Gralnek IM, Kalantzis C, Giannakoulopoulou E, Alexandrakis G, et al. Evaluation of capsule endoscopy in active, mild-to-moderate, overt GI bleeding. Gastrointest Endosc. 2007;66:1174–81.

18. Bar-Meir S, Eliakim R, Nadler M, Barkay O, Fireman Z, Scapa E. Second capsule endoscopy for patients with severe iron deficiency anaemia. Gastrointest Endosc. 2004;60;711–3.

19. Jones BH, Fleischer DE, Sharma VK, Heigh RI, Shiff AD, Hernandez JL, Leighton JA. Yield of repeat wireless video capsule endoscopy in patients with obscure gastrointestinal bleeding. Am J Gastroenterol. 2005;100:1058–64.

20. Sidhu R, Brunt LK, Morley SR, Sanders DS, McAlindon ME. Undisclosed use of nonsteroidal anti-inflammatory drugs may underlie small-bowel injury observed by capsule endoscopy. Clin Gastroenterol Hepatol. 2010;8:992–5.

21. Goldstein JL, Eisen GM, Lewis B, Gralnek IM, Aisenberg J, Bhadra P, Berger MF. Small bowel mucosal injury is reduced in healthy subjects treated with celecoxib compared with ibuprofen plus omeprazole, as assessed by video capsule endoscopy. Aliment Pharmacol Ther. 2007;25:1211–22.

22. Hawkey CJ, Ell C, Simon B, Albert J, Keuchel M, McAlindon M, et al. Less small-bowel injury with lumiracoxib compared with naproxen plus omeprazole. Clin Gastroenterol Hepatol. 2008;6:536–44.

23. Cobrin GM, Pittman RH, Lewis BS. Increased diagnostic yield of small bowel tumors with capsule endoscopy. Cancer. 2006;107:22–7.

24. Rondonotti E, Pennazio M, Toth E, Menchen P, Riccioni ME, De Palma GD, European Capsule Endoscopy Group; Italian Club for Capsule Endoscopy (CICE); Iberian Group for Capsule Endoscopy, et al. Small-bowel neoplasms in patients undergoing video capsule endoscopy: a multicenter European study. Endoscopy. 2008;40:488–95.

25. Triester SL, Leighton JA, Leontiadis GI, Gurudu SR, Fleischer DE, Hara AK, et al. A meta-analysis of the yield of capsule endoscopy compared to other diagnostic modalities in patients with non-stricturing small bowel Crohn's disease. Am J Gastroenterol. 2006;101:954–64.

26. Dionisio PM, Gurudu SR, Leighton JA, Leontiadis GI, Fleischer DE, Hara AK, et al. Capsule endoscopy has a significantly higher diagnostic yield in patients with suspected and established small-bowel Crohn's disease: a meta-analysis. Am J Gastroenterol. 2010;105:1240–8.

27. Bourreille A, Jarry M, D'Halluin PN, Ben-Soussan E, Maunoury V, Bulois P, et al. Wireless capsule endoscopy versus ileocolonoscopy for the diagnosis of postoperative recurrence of Crohn's disease: a prospective study. Gut. 2006;55:978–83.

28. Pons Beltrán V, Nos P, Bastida G, Beltrán B, Argüello L, Aguas M, et al. Evaluation of postsurgical recurrence in Crohn's disease: a new indication for capsule endoscopy? Gastrointest Endosc. 2007;66:533–40.

29. Biancone L, Calabrese E, Petruzziello C, Onali S, Caruso A, Palmieri G, et al. Wireless capsule endoscopy and small intestinal contrast ultrasonography in recurrence of Crohn's disease. Inflamm Bowel Dis. 2007;13:1256–65.

30. Maunoury V, Savoye G, Bourreille A, Bouhnik Y, Jarry M. Value of wireless capsule endoscopy in patients with indeterminate colitis (inflammatory bowel disease type unclassified). Inflamm Bowel Dis. 2007;13:152–5.

31. Mehdizadeh S, Chen G, Enayati PJ, Cheng DW, Han NJ, Shaye OA, et al. Diagnostic yield of capsule endoscopy in ulcerative colitis and inflammatory bowel disease of unclassified type (IBDU). Endoscopy. 2008;40:30–5.

32. Lopes S, Figueiredo P, Portela F, Freire P, Almeida N, Lérias C, et al. Capsule endoscopy in inflammatory bowel disease type unclassified and indeterminate colitis serologically negative. Inflamm Bowel Dis. 2010;16:1663–8.

33. Di Nardo G, Oliva S, Ferrari F, Riccioni ME, Staiano A, Lombardi G, et al. Usefulness of wireless capsule endoscopy in paediatric inflammatory bowel disease. Dig Liver Dis. 2011;43:220–4.

34. Efthymiou A, Viazis N, Mantzaris G, Papadimitriou N, Tzourmakliotis D, Raptis S, Karamanolis DG. Does clinical response correlate with mucosal healing in patients with Crohn's disease of the small bowel? A prospective, case-series study using wireless capsule endoscopy. Inflamm Bowel Dis. 2008;14:1542–7.

35. Caunedo-Álvarez A, Romero-Vazquez J, Herrerias-Gutierrez JM. Patency and agile capsules. World J Gastroenterol. 2008; 14:5269–73.

36. Herrerias JM, Leighton JA, Costamagna G, Infantolino A, Eliakim R, Fischer D, et al. Agile patency system eliminates risk of capsule retention in patients with known intestinal strictures who undergo capsule endoscopy. Gastrointest Endosc. 2008;67:902–9.

37. Bourreille A, Ignjatovic A, Aabakken L, Loftus Jr EV, Eliakim R, Pennazio M, et al. Role of small-bowel endoscopy in the management of patients with inflammatory bowel disease: an international OMED–ECCO consensus. Endoscopy. 2009;41:618–37.

38. Spada C, Riccioni ME, Urgesi R, Costamagna G. Capsule endoscopy in coeliac disease. World J Gastroenterol. 2008;14:4146–51.

39. Rokkas T, Niv Y. The role of video capsule endoscopy in the diagnosis of celiac disease: a meta-analysis. Eur J Gastroenterol Hepatol. 2012;24:303–8.

40. Kurien M, Evans KE, Aziz I, Sidhu R, Drew K, Rogers TL, et al. Capsule endoscopy in adult celiac disease: a potential role in equivocal cases of celiac disease? Gastrointest Endosc. 2013;77:227–32.

41. Daum S, Wahnschaffe U, Glasenapp R, Borchert M, Ullrich R, Zeitz M, Faiss S. Capsule endoscopy in refractory celiac disease. Endoscopy. 2007;39:455–8.

42. Barret M, Malamut G, Rahmi G, Samaha E, Edery J, Verkarre V, et al. Diagnostic yield of capsule endoscopy in refractory celiac disease. Am J Gastroenterol. 2012;107:1546–53.

43. Brown G, Fraser C, Schofield G, Taylor S, Bartram C, Phillips R, Saunders B. Video capsule endoscopy in Peutz-Jegher's syndrome: a blinded comparison with barium follow-through for detection of small bowel polyps. Endoscopy. 2006;38:385–90.

44. Postgate A, Hyer W, Phillips R, Gupta A, Burling D, Bartram C, et al. Feasibility of video capsule endoscopy in the management of children with Peutz-Jegher's syndrome: a blinded comparison with barium enterography for the detection of small bowel polyps. J Pediatr Gastroenterol Nutr. 2009;49:417–23.

45. Gupta A, Postgate AJ, Burling D, Ilangovan R, Marshall M, Phillips RKS, et al. A prospective study of MR enterography versus capsule endoscopy for the surveillance of adult patients with Peutz-Jegher's syndrome. AJR Am J Roentgenol. 2010;195:108–16.

46. Kong H, Kim YS, Hyun JJ, Cho YJ, Keum B, Jeen YT, et al. Limited ability of capsule endoscopy to detect normally positioned duodenal papilla. Gastrointest Endosc. 2006;64:538–41.

47. Clarke JO, Giday SA, Magno P, Shin EJ, Buscaglia JM, Jagannath SB, Mullin GE. How good is capsule endoscopy for detection of periampullary lesions? Results of a tertiary-referral center. Gastrointest Endosc. 2008;68:267–72.

48. Koulaouzidis A, Plevris JN. Detection of the ampulla of vater in small bowel capsule endoscopy: experience with two different systems. J Dig Dis. 2012;13:621–7.

49. Caspari R, von Falkenhausen M, Krautmacher C, Schild H, Heller J, Sauerbruch T. Comparison of capsule endoscopy and magnetic resonance imaging for the detection of polyps of the small intestine in patients with familial adenomatous polyposis or with Peutz-Jeghers' syndrome. Endoscopy. 2004;36:1054–9.

50. Schulmann K, Hollerbach S, Kraus K, Willert J, Vogel T, Möslein G, et al. Feasibility and diagnostic utility of video capsule endoscopy for the detection of small bowel polyps in patients with hereditary polyposis syndromes. Am J Gastroenterol. 2005;100:27–37.

51. Mata A, Llach J, Castells A, Rovira JM, Pellise M, Gines A, et al. A prospective trial comparing wireless capsule endoscopy and barium contrast series for small bowel surveillance in hereditary GI polyposis syndromes. Gastrointest Endosc. 2005;61:721–5.

52. Iaquinto G, Fornasarig M, Quaia M, Giardullo N, D'Onofrio V, Iaquinto S, et al. Capsule endoscopy is useful and safe for small bowel surveillance in familial adenomatous polyposis. Gastrointest Endosc. 2008;67:61–7.

53. Dray X, Vahedi K, Valleur P, Marteau P. Is there any need for video capsule endoscopy evaluation in postduodenal small-bowel polyps detection in familial adenomatous polyposis? Gastrointest Endosc. 2007;66:634.

54. Spada C, Pirozzi GA, Riccioni ME, Iacopini F, Marchese M, Costamagna G. Capsule endoscopy in patients with chronic abdominal pain. Dig Liver Dis. 2006;38:696–8.

55. Fry LC, Carey EJ, Shiff AD, Heigh RI, Sharma VK, Post JK, et al. The yield of capsule endoscopy in patients with abdominal pain or diarrhea. Endoscopy. 2006;38:498–502.

56. Shim KN, Kim YS, Kim KJ, Kim YH, Kim TI, Do JH, et al. Abdominal pain accompanied by weight loss may increase the diagnostic yield of capsule endoscopy: a Korean multicenter study. Scand J Gastroenterol. 2006;41:983–8.

57. May A, Manner H, Schneider M, Ipsen A, Ell C. Prospective multicenter trial of capsule endoscopy in patients with chronic abdominal pain, diarrhea and other signs and symptoms (CEDAP-Plus Study). Endoscopy. 2007;39:606–12.

58. Katsinelos P, Fasoulas K, Beltsis A, Chatzimavroudis G, Paroutoglou G, Maris T, et al. Diagnostic yield and clinical impact of wireless capsule endoscopy in patients with chronic abdominal pain with or without diarrhea: a Greek multicenter study. Eur J Intern Med. 2011;22:e63–6.

59. Cheifetz AS, Lewis BS. Capsule endoscopy retention: is it a complication? J Clin Gastroenterol. 2006;40:688–91.

60. Shapira M, Adler SN, Jacob H, Resnick IB, Slavin S, Or R. New insights into the pathophysiology of gastrointestinal graft-versus-host disease using capsule endoscopy. Haematologica. 2005;90:1003–4.

61. Neumann S, Schoppmeyer K, Lange T, Wiedmann M, Golsong J, Tannapfel A, et al. Wireless capsule endoscopy for diagnosis of acute intestinal graft-versus-host disease. Gastrointest Endosc. 2007;65:403–9.

62. Varadarajan P, Dunford LM, Thomas JA, Brown K, Paplham P, Syta M, et al. Seeing what's out of sight: wireless capsule endoscopy's unique ability to visualize and accurately assess the severity of gastrointestinal graft-versus-host-disease. Biol Blood Marrow Transplant. 2009;15:643–8.

63. Motola D, Vaccheri A, Silvani MC, Poluzzi E, Bottoni A, De Ponti F, Montanaro N. Pattern of NSAID use in the Italian general population: a questionnaire-based survey. Eur J Clin Pharmacol. 2004;60:731–8.

64. Maiden L, Thjodleifsson B, Theodors A, Gonzalez J, Bjarnason I. A quantitative analysis of NSAID-induced small bowel pathology by capsule enteroscopy. Gastroenterology. 2005;128:1172–8.

65. Bjarnason I, Hayllar J, MacPherson AJ, Russell AS. Side effects of nonsteroidal anti-inflammatory drugs on the small and large intestine. Gastroenterology. 1993;104:1832–47.

66. Eliakim R, Sharma VK, Yassin K, Adler SN, Jacob H, Cave DR, et al. A prospective study of the diagnostic accuracy of PillCam ESO esophageal capsule endoscopy versus conventional upper endoscopy in patients with chronic gastroesophageal reflux diseases. J Clin Gastroenterol. 2005;39:572–8.

67. Gralnek IM, Adler SN, Yassin K, Koslowsky B, Metzger Y, Eliakim R. Detecting esophageal disease with second-generation capsule endoscopy: initial evaluation of the PillCam ESO 2. Endoscopy. 2008;40:275–9.

68. Galmiche JP, Sacher-Huvelin S, Coron E, Cholet F, Soussan EB, Sébille V, et al. Screening for esophagitis and Barrett's esophagus with wireless esophageal capsule endoscopy: a multicenter prospective trial in patients with reflux symptoms. Am J Gastroenterol. 2008;103:538–45.

69. Sharma P, Wani S, Rastogi A, Bansal A, Higbee A, Mathur S, et al. The diagnostic accuracy of esophageal capsule endoscopy in patients with gastroesophageal reflux disease and Barrett's esophagus: a blinded, prospective study. Am J Gastroenterol. 2008;103:525–32.

70. Lapalus MG, Dumortier J, Fumex F, Roman S, Lot M, Prost B, et al. Esophageal capsule endoscopy versus esophagogastroduodenoscopy for evaluating portal hypertension: a prospective comparative study of performance and tolerance. Endoscopy. 2006;38:36–41.

71. Modlin IM, Hunt RH, Malfertheiner P, Moayyedi P, Quigley EM, Tytgat GN, Vevey NERD Consensus Group, et al. Diagnosis and management of non-erosive reflux disease—the Vevey NERD Consensus Group. Digestion. 2009;80:74–88.

72. Watson A, Heading RC, Shepherd NA. Guidelines for the diagnosis and management of Barrett's columnar-lined oesophagus. 2005. Available at http://www.bsg.org.uk.

73. Hvid-Jensen F, Pedersen L, Drewes AM, Sørensen HT, Funch-Jensen P. Incidence of adenocarcinoma among patients with Barrett's esophagus. N Engl J Med. 2011;365:1375–83.

74. Bhardwaj A, Hollenbeak CS, Pooran N, Mathew A. A meta-analysis of the diagnostic accuracy of esophageal capsule endoscopy for Barrett's esophagus in patients with gastroesophageal reflux disease. Am J Gastroenterol. 2009;104:1533–9.

75. Gerson LB. Are we ready for gender-based guidelines for Barrett's esophagus screening? Gastroenterology. 2011;141:2271–3.

76. American Gastroenterological Association. Management of Barrett's esophagus. 2011. http://www.gastro.org/mobiletools/mobile-guidelines/aga-medical-position-statement-on-the-management-of-barrett-s-esophagus. Accessed 01 Oct 2014

77. Mehta G, Abraldes JG, Bosch J. Developments and controversies in the management of oesophageal and gastric varices. Gut. 2010;59:701–5.

78. Lu Y, Gao R, Liao Z, Hu LH, Li ZS. Meta-analysis of capsule endoscopy in patients diagnosed or suspected with esophageal varices. World J Gastroenterol. 2009;15:1254–8.

79. Eliakim R, Yassin K, Niv Y, Metzger Y, Lachter J, Gal E, et al. Evaluation of the second-generation colon capsule compared with colonoscopy. Endoscopy. 2009;41:1026–31.

80. Spada C, Hassan C, Muñoz-Navas M, Neuhaus H, Devière J, Fockens P, et al. Second-generation colon capsule endoscopy compared with colonoscopy. Gastrointest Endosc. 2011;74:581–9.

81. Johnson CD, Chen MH, Toledano AY, Heiken JP, Dachman A, Kuo MD, et al. Accuracy of CT colonography for detection of large adenomas and cancers. N Engl J Med. 2008;359:1207–17.

82. Heresbach D, Barrioz T, Lapalus MG, Coumaros D, Bauret P, Potier P, et al. Miss rate for colorectal neoplastic polyps: a prospective multicenter study of back-to-back video colonoscopies. Endoscopy. 2008;40:284–90.

83. Spada C, Hassan C, Galmiche JP, Neuhaus H, Dumonceau JM, Adler S, European Society of Gastrointestinal Endoscopy, et al. Colon capsule endoscopy: European Society of Gastrointestinal Endoscopy (ESGE) Guideline. Endoscopy. 2012;44:527–36.

84. Hassan C, Zullo A, Winn S, Morini S. Cost-effectiveness of capsule endoscopy in screening for colorectal cancer. Endoscopy. 2008;40:414–21.

85. Sung J, Ho KY, Chiu HM, Ching J, Travis S, Peled R. The use of Pillcam Colon in assessing mucosal inflammation in ulcerative colitis: a multicenter study. Endoscopy. 2012;44:754–8.

86. Ye CA, Gao YJ, Ge ZZ, Dai J, Li XB, Xue HB, et al. PillCam COLON capsule endoscopy versus conventional colonoscopy for the detection of the severity and extent of ulcerative colitis. J Dig Dis. 2013;14:117–24.

87. Glickman JN, Odze RD. Does rectal sparing ever occur in ulcerative colitis? Inflamm Bowel Dis. 2008;14(S2):S166–7.

88. Swain P, Toor A, Volke F, Keller J, Gerber J, Rabinovitz E, Rothstein RI. Remote magnetic manipulation of a wireless capsule endoscope in the esophagus and stomach of humans (with videos). Gastrointest Endosc. 2010;71:1290–3.

89. Rey JF, Ogata H, Hosoe N, Ohtsuka K, Ogata N, Ikeda K, et al. Feasibility of stomach exploration with a guided capsule endoscope. Endoscopy. 2010;42:541–5.

90. Keller J, Fibbe C, Volke F, Gerber J, Mosse AC, Reimann-Zawadzki M, et al. Inspection of the human stomach using remote-controlled capsule endoscopy: a feasibility study in healthy volunteers (with videos). Gastrointest Endosc. 2011;73:22–8.

91. VECTOR Project (Versatile Endoscopic Capsule for gastrointestinal TumOr Recognition and therapy). European Commission, Sixth Framework Programme, Information Society Technologies Priority. http://www.vector-project.com. Accessed 01 Oct 2014.

Technology

3

Niehls Kurniawan and Martin Keuchel

Contents

A number of video capsules are now commercially available. Many of these capsules are already in the second or third generation, with ongoing development. They differ, for example, in the number of cameras, rate of imaging, methods of data storage or transmission, battery power, and intended field of use [1, 2]. The basic technical specifications of the available video capsules are compiled on Table 3.1. Figure 3.1 shows the capsules and the corresponding radiograph images, with addition of the PillCam patency test capsule (see Chap. 9). The floating properties of the different capsules in water are demonstrated in Fig. 3.2.

The work was first published in 2006 by Springer Medizin Verlag Heidelberg with the following title: *Atlas of Video Capsule Endoscopy*.

N. Kurniawan (✉) • M. Keuchel
Department of Internal Medicine,
Bethesda Krankenhaus Bergedorf, Hamburg, Germany
e-mail: kurniawan@bkb.info; keuchel@bkb.info

M. Keuchel et al. (eds.), *Video Capsule Endoscopy: A Reference Guide and Atlas*,
DOI 10.1007/978-3-662-44062-9_3, © Springer-Verlag Berlin Heidelberg 2014

15

Table 3.1 Technical specifications of various video capsules

	PillCam			EndoCapsule		CapsoCam	OMOM	PillCam	PillCam
	SB2	SB3	MiroCam	EC1	EC-S10	SV1	capsule	ESO 2	COLON2
Length, *mm*	26	26	24	26	26	31	28	26	31.5
Diameter, *mm*	11	11	11	11	11	11	13	11	11
Weight, *g*	2.9	1.9	3.4	3.8	3.3	4	<6	2.9	2.9
Cameras, *n*	1	1	1	1	1	4	1	2	2
Frame rate (combined), *frames/s*	2	2/6	3	2	2	12/20	0.5/1/2	18	0.1/ 4/ 35
Image sensor	CMOS	CMOS	CMOS	CCD	CMOS	CMOS	CMOS	CMOS	CMOS
Viewing angle	156°	156°	150°	145°	160°	4×90°	140°	2×169°	2×172°
Minimal recording time, *h*	11	11	11	8	12	15	8±1	0.33	10 h

CCD charge-coupled device, *CMOS* complementary metal oxide semiconductor

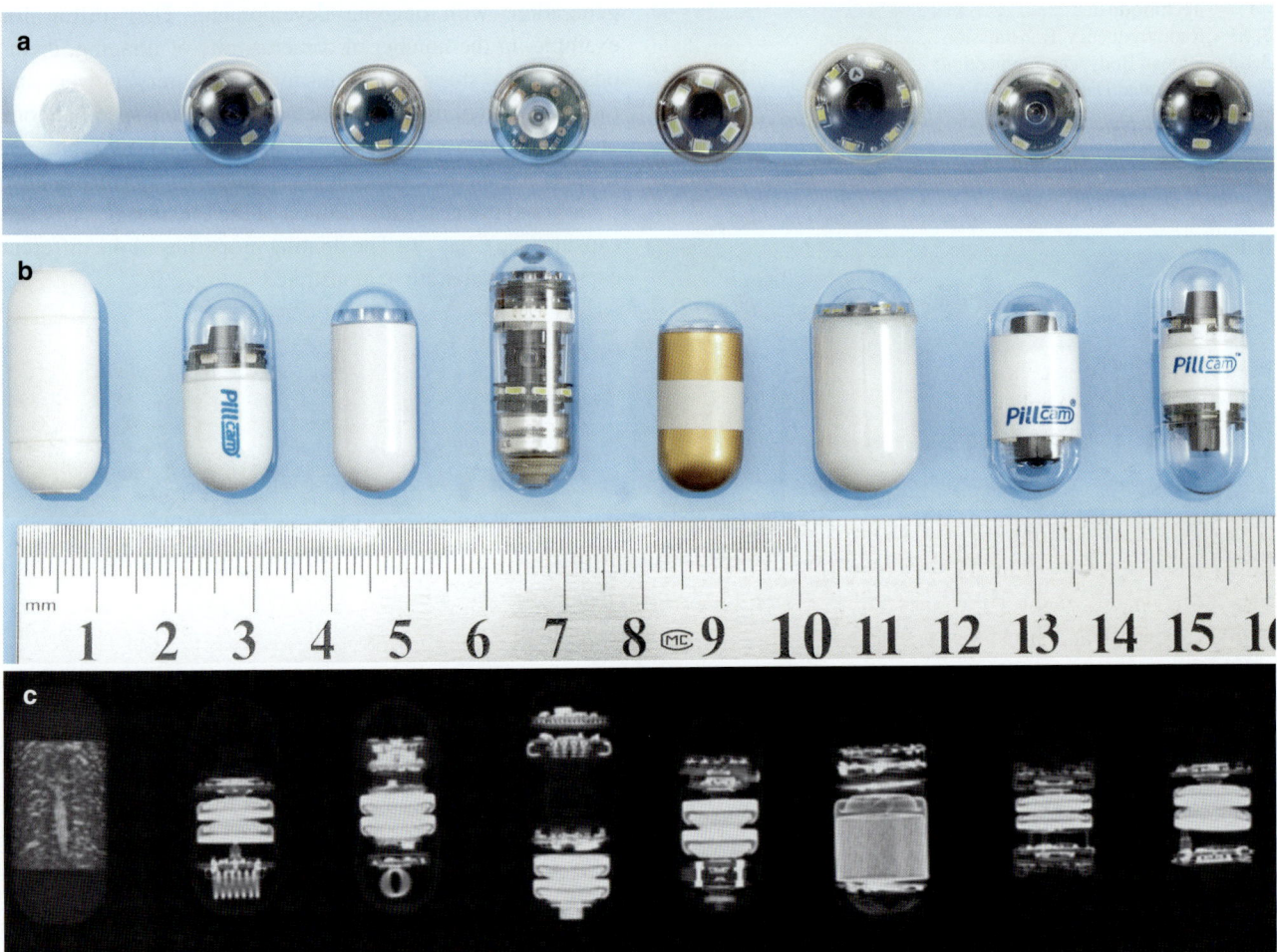

Fig. 3.1 Front view (**a**) and top view (**b**) of the capsules, with corresponding X-ray image (**c**). *Left to right*: Agile patency capsule, PillCam SB2, EndoCapsule, CapsoCam, MiroCam, OMOM capsule, PillCam ESO2, PillCam COLON2

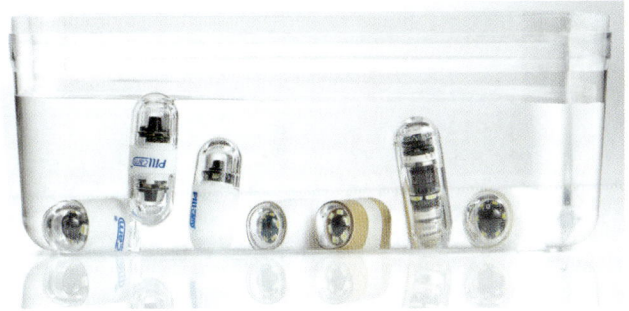

Fig. 3.2 Floating properties of different capsules in a water container

3.1 Capsule Configuration and Transmission Technique

Every video capsule has at least one camera with either a charge-coupled device (CCD) or a complementary metal oxide semiconductor (CMOS) chip as an imager. CCD chips convert light and charge in every single pixel to voltage, whereas CMOS imagers use an array of pixels requiring amplification for each pixel. As in digital photography, the discussion on the advantages of CCD versus CMOS is continuing. The CCD chip has a higher electric output with lower optical noise and consecutive stability to changes in illumination. CMOS chips have a lower space and power consumption that allows for longer work capacity and additional cameras. Both chips provide excellent gastrointestinal (GI) images for clinical use [3]. Application-specific integrated circuits (ASICs) further process the signal to a radiotransmitter, to a conductive casing, or to an internal storage device (Fig. 3.3).

The cameras generally are located on one or both ends of the capsule. An exception is the CapsoCam, which has four cameras located around the center axis in the midsection. This arrangement enables the cameras to take 360° panoramic images from the surrounding mucosa without forward- or backward-viewing optics (Fig. 19.2e).

Four to six light-emitting diodes (LEDs) serve as an illumination source for each camera. Every time an image is captured, these LEDs emit a flashing white light [4]. Most of the capsules include an adapted illumination control.

The energy source consists of two or three silver oxide button batteries, enabling images to be captured for up to 15 h or more.

All images are subsequently processed in one of three ways: radiofrequency transmission, human body communication, or integrated data storage.

3.1.1 Radiofrequency Transmission

All PillCam models (Given Imaging Ltd., Yoqneam, Israel), the EndoCapsule (Olympus Medical Systems Corp., Tokyo, Japan), and the OMOM capsule (Jinshan Science and

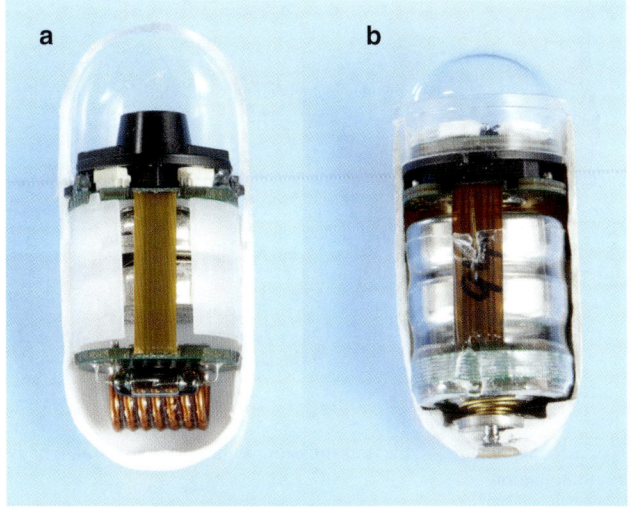

Fig. 3.3 (**a**) Interior of opened capsules. PillCam SB2 with antenna (*left*). (**b**) MiroCam with electrode connecting to conductive casing (*right*)

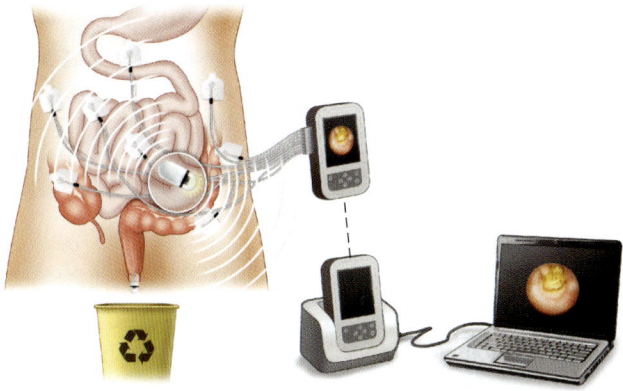

Fig. 3.4 Schematic of the radiofrequency transmission technique

Technology Co. Ltd., Chongqing, China) use the same transmission technique. The compressed images are sent via radiofrequency through an integrated antenna (Fig. 3.3a) to a sensor array. The patient wears this sensor array directly attached to the skin or integrated into a sensor belt or sensor vest. The array is connected to a portable storage device (Fig. 3.4). With the newest generations of video capsule endoscopy, every manufacturer using this method provides the possibility of real-time viewing through an integrated or connected display. Upon completion of the study, the storage device is connected via a docking station to the analysis computer for data transfer and processing for analysis. As these capsule types do not store any data by themselves, they can be discarded after excretion.

3.1.2 Human Body Communication

The MiroCam capsule (IntroMedic Co. Ltd., Seoul, Korea) transmits its data via a special exterior bipolar casing

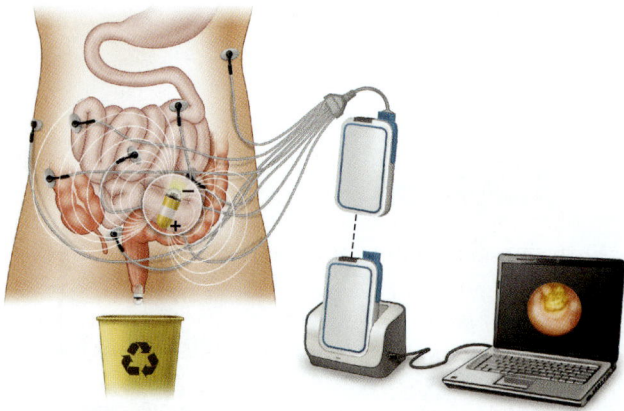

Fig. 3.5 Schematic of the transmission technique via human body communication

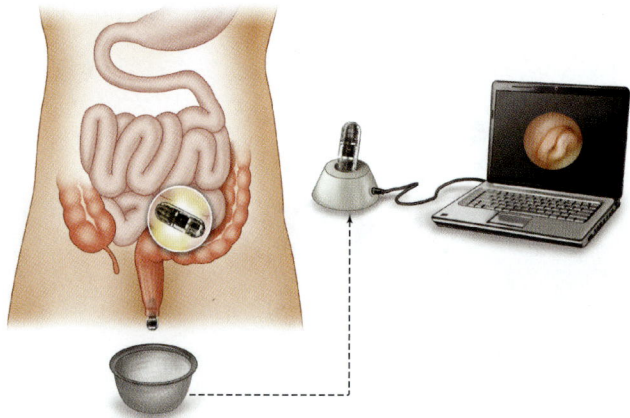

Fig. 3.6 Schematic of the transmission technique via integrated data storage

(Fig. 3.3b) to sensor electrodes on the skin, using the human body as a conductor (human body communication). This method uses less power than radiofrequency transmission [5]. Similar to radiofrequency transmission, the patient wears a portable storage device, which is subsequently connected to the analysis computer (Fig. 3.5). Upon completion of the study, the capsule does not need to be collected by the physician and can be discarded.

3.1.3 Integrated Data Storage

The CapsoCam (CapsoVision Inc., Saratoga, CA, USA) stores the captured images in an integrated Flash EPROM storage chip, avoiding the need for an integrated transmitter and an external receiver. After completion of the study, the patient returns the capsule to the medical staff for download of the data via a USB port in a docking station (Fig. 3.6). With this system, there is no possibility of real-time viewing.

3.2 Frame Rate

The esophagus capsule PillCam ESO2 [6] and the small bowel capsules PillCam SB2, EndoCapsule, and MiroCam use a static rate to acquire the images for the whole study. The CapsoCam has an overall frame rate of 20/s (5 per camera) for the first 2 h and then switches automatically to 12/s for the rest of the study.

With the capsules' limited power supply, it is possible that power may be depleted before examination of important areas (e.g., the small bowel or colon) is complete. Methods have been developed to conserve power while the capsule passes areas of less importance. For example, propulsion through the stomach usually takes less than an hour, but gastroparesis may delay it for several hours. Additionally, vari-

able bowel peristalsis may cause the capsule to be almost stationary for a longer time and then advance at a rapid pace, especially in the colon. As a result, dynamic methods to adjust the frame rate have been developed.

The PillCam COLON2 capsule reduces the frame rate after the first 3 min, when typically the Z-line has been passed, to 6/min. By this method, battery power is conserved as long as the colon capsule stays in the stomach. The recorded images are automatically analyzed in real time by the portable recorder. If the capsule stays in the stomach for more than 1 h, a signal (visual and vibration) is given and a prokinetic agent can be administered. Furthermore, the software recognizes small bowel mucosa and orders the capsule automatically and in real time to raise the frame rate to 4/s. If a rapid movement is detected, the frame rate is temporarily further raised to 35/s [7–9]. To make this two-way communication possible, the patient must wear an additional antenna (see Fig. 3.6).

Although the colon capsule has not been cleared for use in the small bowel, it has been applied successfully for this purpose [10]. With the present system, the frame rate must be switched manually via the recorder for small bowel detection while the capsule is still in the stomach, to avoid loss of images in the proximal small bowel, as automated small bowel detection may take some minutes [11]. PillCam SB3, with one camera, includes technology from PillCam COLON2 for the small bowel by adapting the frame rate in real time, acquiring 2 or 6 frames per second, depending on the capsule movement as analyzed by the DR3 recorder (Fig. 3.7).

The OMOM capsule uses a different method of interaction. The physician can view the captured images in real time via the display of the portable storage device and then can send a manual command to the capsule to change the frame rate to 0.5, 1, or 2 frames per second [12]. The necessary emitting antenna is integrated in the storage device (Fig. 3.8).

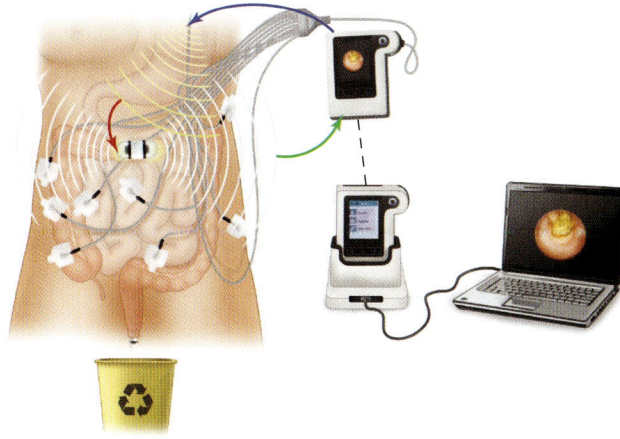

Fig. 3.7 Schematic of the automated interaction between the PillCam COLON2 or PillCam SB3 and the recorder

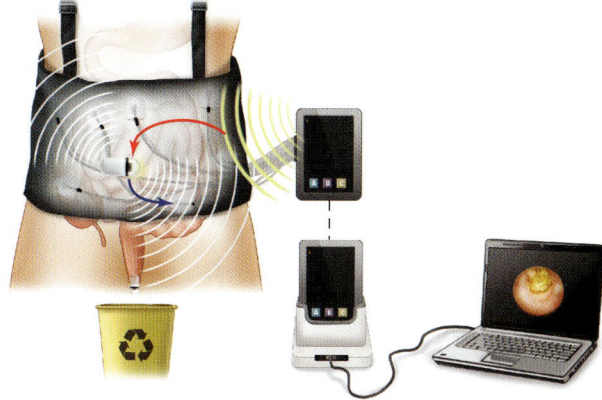

Fig. 3.8 Schematic of the manual interaction between the OMOM capsule and the recorder

3.3 Patency Capsule

To face the most important complication of video capsule endoscopy, the retention of the capsule due to a stenosis or stricture, Given Imaging Ltd. (Yoqneam, Israel) developed the Agile patency capsule (see Chap. 9, "Patency Capsule"). The application of the capsule is intended to precede the actual study in patients with an increased risk of stenosis. For optimal comparability, the capsule has the same diameter (11 mm) as almost all of the available video capsules. Only the OMOM capsule has a slightly larger diameter of 13 mm. The patency capsule consists of a lactose body with 10 % barium to enable radiologic detection. The body surrounds a small radiofrequency identification (RFID) tag, making the capsule also detectable by a handheld RFID tag scanner (sensing at 128 kHz, emitting at 64 kHz). After ingestion, the capsule sustains its full size for at least 30 h. If the capsule is not excreted by then, it dissolves, leaving just the flexible coating and the small RFID tag [13].

3.4 Comparative Studies

Numerous systematic, prospective, and randomized studies have documented the efficacy of individual small bowel video capsules. Most of these studies analyzed the PillCam series and its predecessor, the M2A by Given Imaging Ltd.

So far, only small comparative studies have been reported. No significant advantage of a specific video capsule system has been shown in regard to the diagnostic yield in patients with small bowel bleeding. These studies have compared PillCam SB1 versus EndoCapsule 1 [14, 15], PillCam SB1 versus MiroCam [16], PillCam SB2 versus MiroCam [17, 18], MiroCam versus EndoCapsule 1 [19], and CapsoCam versus PillCam SB2 [20]. Longer capsule working times might result in higher rates of completion of small bowel visualization. The applicability of studies is limited by the fast technical developments, often with new capsule properties, after the publication of comparative results.

References

1. Ciuti G, Menciassi A, Dario P. Capsule endoscopy: from current achievements to open challenges. IEEE Rev Biomed Eng. 2011;4: 59–72.
2. Eliakim R. Video capsule endoscopy of the small bowel. Curr Opin Gastroenterol. 2013;29:133–9.
3. Gerber J, Bergwerk A, Fleischer D. A capsule endoscopy guide for the practicing clinician: technology and troubleshooting. Gastrointest Endosc. 2007;66:1188–95.
4. Moglia A, Menciassi A, Dario P, Cuschieri A. Capsule endoscopy: progress update and challenges ahead. Nat Rev Gastroenterol Hepatol. 2009;6:353–62.
5. Bang S, Park JY, Jeong S, Kim YH, Shim HB, Kim TS, et al. First clinical trial of the "MiRo" capsule endoscope by using a novel transmission technology: electric-field propagation. Gastrointest Endosc. 2009;69:253–9.
6. Gralnek IM, Adler SN, Yassin K, Koslowsky B, Metzger Y, Eliakim R. Detecting esophageal disease with second-generation capsule endoscopy: initial evaluation of the PillCam ESO 2. Endoscopy. 2008;40:275–9.
7. Spada C, De Vincentis F, Cesaro P, Hassan C, Riccioni ME, Minelli Grazioli L, et al. Accuracy and safety of second-generation PillCam COLON capsule for colorectal polyp detection. Therap Adv Gastroenterol. 2012;5:173–8.
8. Bar-Meir S, Wallace MB. Diagnostic colonoscopy: the end is coming. Gastroenterology. 2006;131:992–4.
9. Adler SN, Metzger YC. PillCam COLON capsule endoscopy: recent advances and new insights. Therap Adv Gastroenterol. 2011;4:265–8.
10. Triantafyllou K, Papanikolaou IS, Papaxoinis K, Ladas SD. Can two cameras detect more lesions in the small-bowel than one? A small-bowel capsule endoscopy feasibility trial with PillCam Colon® [abstract W1081]. Gastroenterology. 2009;136 Suppl 1:A649.
11. Adler S, Hassan C, Metzger Y, Sompolinsky Y, Spada C. Accuracy of automatic detection of small-bowel mucosa by second generation colon capsule endoscopy. Gastrointest Endosc. 2012;76:1170–4.
12. Liao Z, Gao R, Li F, Xu C, Zhou Y, Wang JS. Fields of applications, diagnostic yields and findings of OMOM capsule

endoscopy in 2400 Chinese patients. World J Gastroenterol. 2010;16:2669–76.

13. Spada C, Spera G, Riccioni M, Biancone L, Petruzziello L, Tringali A, et al. A novel diagnostic tool for detecting functional patency of the small bowel: the Given patency capsule. Endoscopy. 2005;37:793–800.

14. Cave DR, Fleischer DE, Leighton JA, Faigel DO, Heigh RI, Sharma VK, et al. A multicenter randomized comparison of the Endocapsule and the Pillcam SB. Gastrointest Endosc. 2008;68:487–94.

15. Hartmann D, Eickhoff A, Damian U, Riemann JF. Diagnosis of small-bowel pathology using paired capsule endoscopy with two different devices: a randomized study. Endoscopy. 2007;39: 1041–5.

16. Kim HM, Kim YJ, Kim HJ, Park S, Park JY, Shin SK, et al. A pilot study of sequential capsule endoscopy using MiroCam and PillCam SB devices with different transmission technologies. Gut Liver. 2010;4:192–200.

17. Pioche M, Gaudin J-L, Filoche B, Jacob P, Lamouliatte H, Lapalus M-G, et al. Prospective, randomized comparison of two small-bowel capsule endoscopy systems in patients with obscure GI bleeding. Gastrointest Endosc. 2011;73:1181–8.

18. Choi EH, Mergener K, Semrad C, Fisher L, Cave DR, Dodig M, et al. A multicenter, prospective, randomized comparison of a novel signal transmission capsule endoscope to an existing capsule endoscope. Gastrointest Endosc. 2013;78:325–32.

19. Dolak W, Kulnigg-Dabsch S, Evstatiev R, Gasche C, Trauner M, Püspök A. A randomized head-to-head study of small-bowel imaging comparing MiroCam and EndoCapsule. Endoscopy. 2012;44: 1012–20.

20. Pioche M, Vanbiervliet G, Jacob P, Duburque C, Gincul R, Filoche B, et al. Prospective first comparison of an axial and a lateral viewing capsule endoscopic system in patients with obscure digestive bleeding [abstract]. Gastrointest Endosc. 2013;77(Suppl): AB173–4.

Internet: Capsule Manufacturers

www.capsovision.com
www.givenimaging.com
www.intromedic.com
www.jinshangroup.com
www.olympus-global.com

Procedure for Small Bowel Video Capsule Endoscopy

4

Carolyn Davison, Roberto de Franchis, and Francesca Iannuzzi

Contents

4.1   Equipment Requirements

The standard equipment necessary to perform a small bowel video capsule endoscopy (SBCE) procedure is summarized in Table 4.1. A video capsule designed for small bowel evaluation is required. Measuring 26 mm × 11 mm, current models operate at either a fixed frame rate of 4 frames per second (Fig. 4.1) or an adaptive frame rate of 2–6 frames per second. Each capsule is sealed in a small box and marked with an identifiable number and expiration date. The capsule is activated upon opening the box and has a minimum battery life of 12 h. Specific technological detail was discussed further in Chap. 3.

To receive and store data, a battery-operated data recorder (Fig. 4.2) is worn by the patient throughout the examination. The recorder is worn in a pouch held in place by either a waist or shoulder strap. A series of sensors connected to the patient transmit data to the recorder. Two sensor application methods are available: an eight-lead sensor array (Fig. 4.3), which is applied to the patient's abdomen using disposable adhesive sleeves, or a sensor belt (Fig. 4.4), within which fixed sensors are held in place on a removable insert. The belt is worn around the waist over a thin layer of natural fabric clothing, thus eliminating the need for shaving or other skin preparation. The belt is comfortable to wear and its preparation and application are time efficient. A disadvantage of this method, however, is the absence of a gastrointestinal (GI) tract localization function, which enables estimated tracking

The work was first published in 2006 by Springer Medizin Verlag Heidelberg with the following title: *Atlas of Video Capsule Endoscopy*.

C. Davison (✉)
Department of GI Services, South Tyneside NHS Foundation Trust, Tyne and Wear, UK
e-mail: carolyn.davison@stft.nhs.uk

R. de Franchis • F. Iannuzzi
Gastroenterology Unit, Luigi Sacco University Hospital, University of Milan, Milan, Italy
e-mail: roberto.defranchis@unimi.it; iannuzzifra@gmail.com

Table 4.1 Equipment required for small bowel video capsule endoscopy procedure

Small bowel video capsule
Fully charged data recorder with real-time viewer
Sensor belt or sensor array with adhesive sleeves and sensor location guide
Recorder pouch with shoulder or waist strap
Access to installed software system
Glass of water
Simethicone

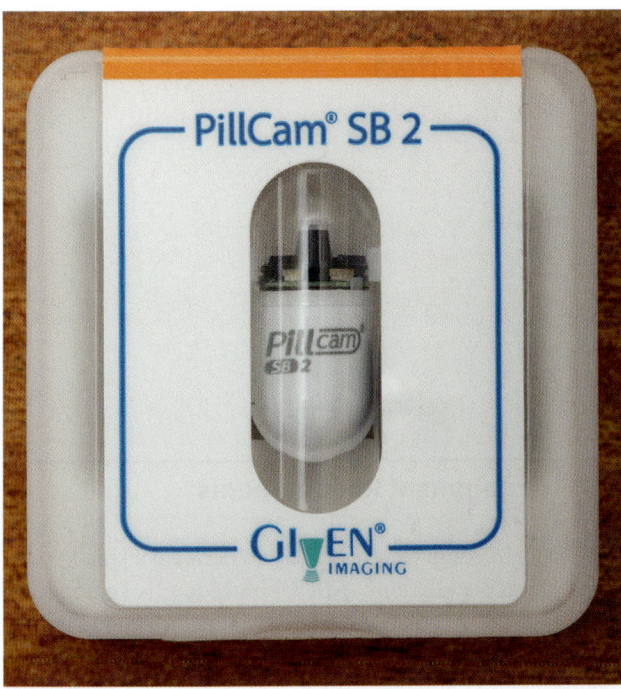

Fig. 4.1 PillCam SB2 small bowel video capsule

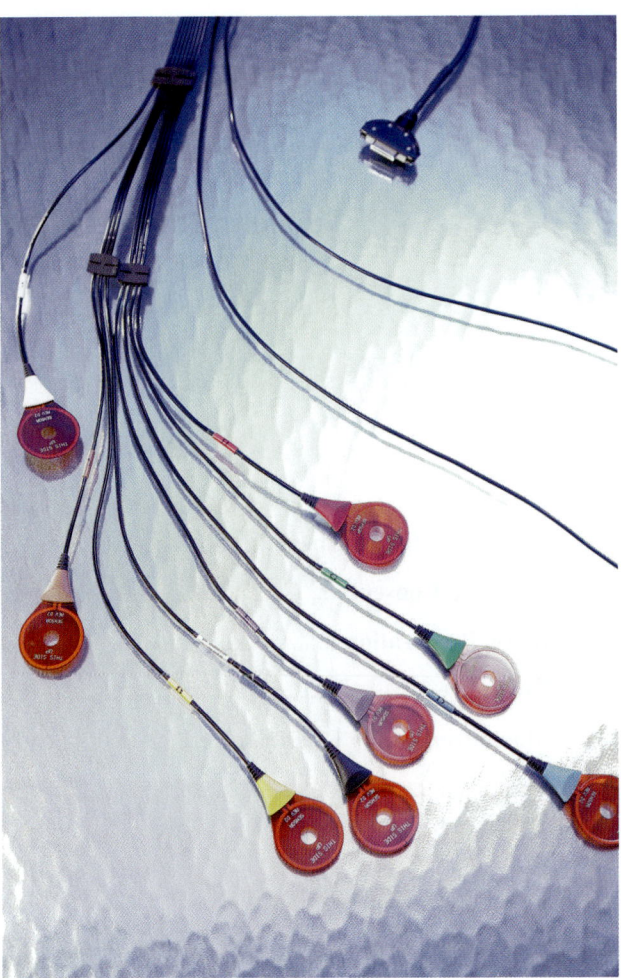

Fig. 4.3 Eight-lead sensor array for PillCam recorder DR3 (Courtesy of Given Imaging Ltd)

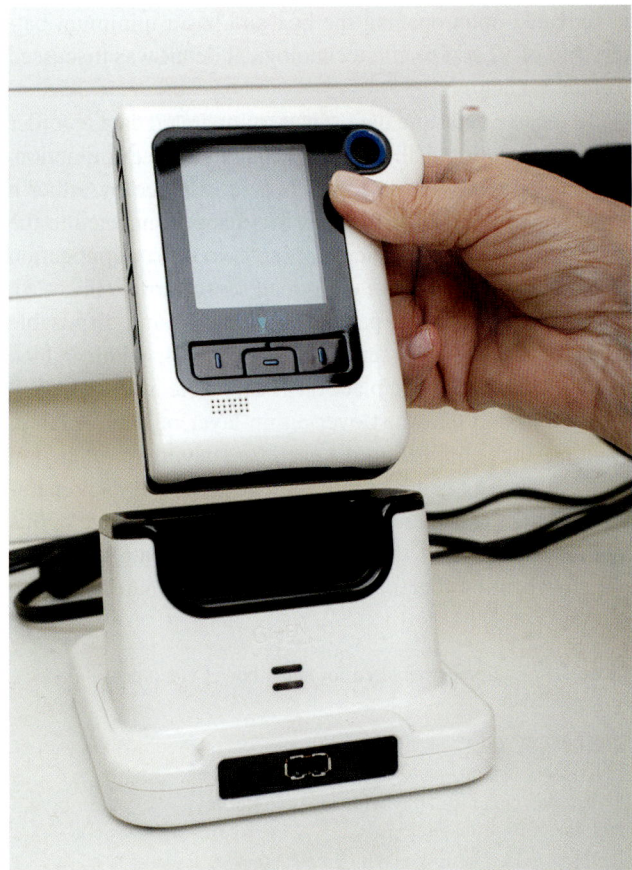

Fig. 4.2 PillCam data recorder (DR3)

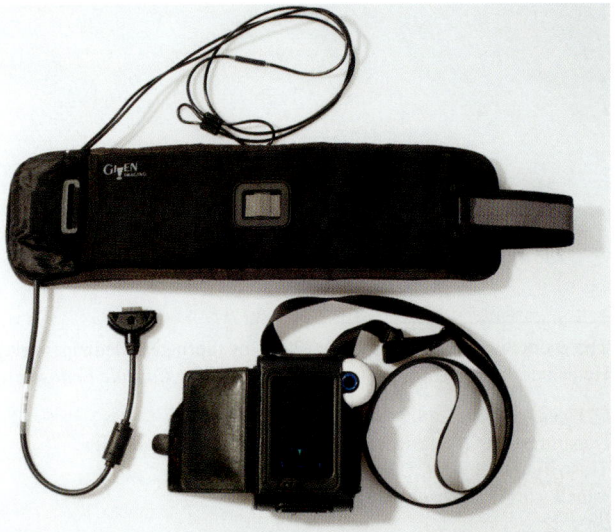

Fig. 4.4 PillCam sensor belt for use with PillCam recorder DR3

Fig. 4.5 Small bowel sensor location guide (DR3)

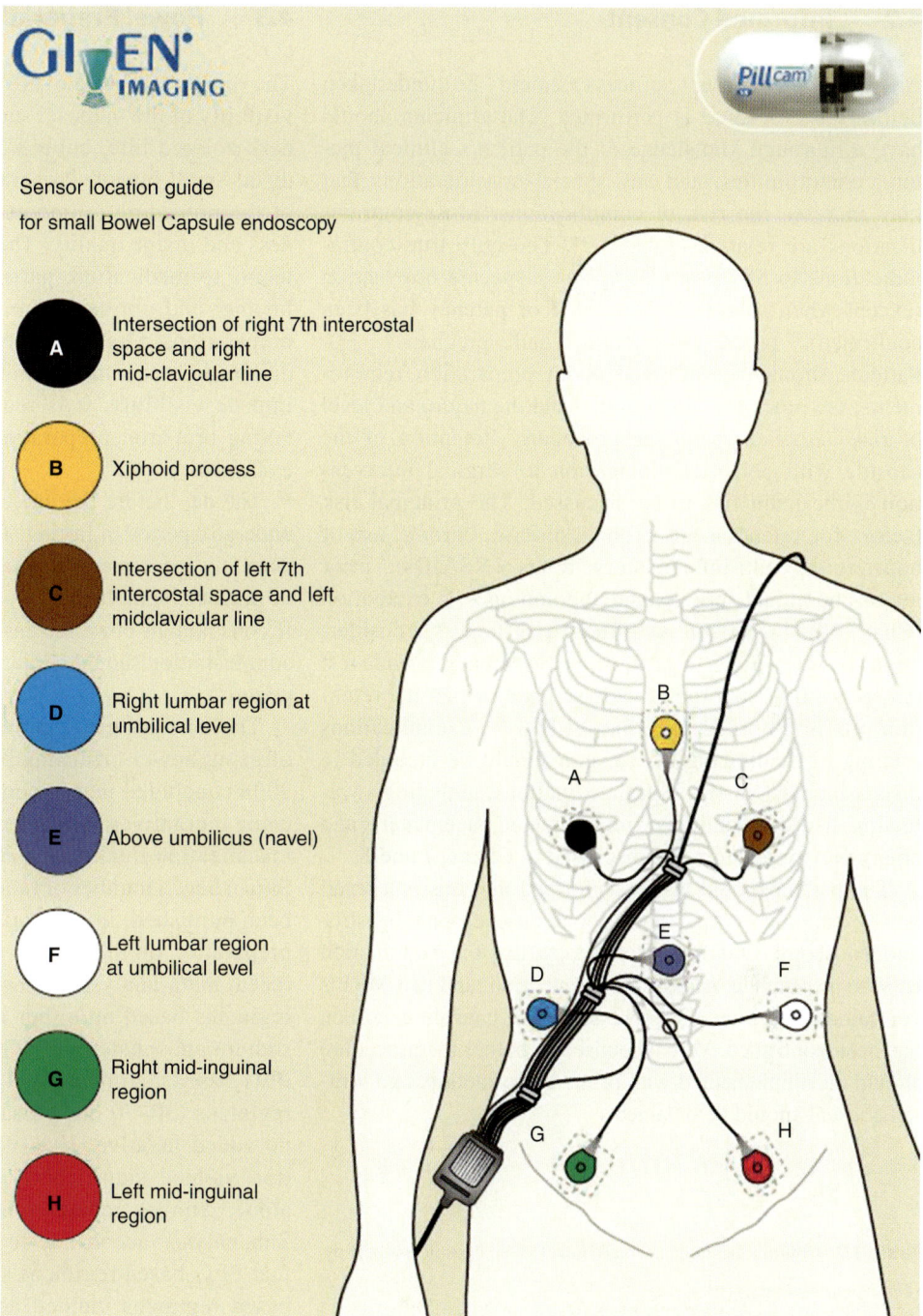

Sensor location guide
for small Bowel Capsule endoscopy

A Intersection of right 7th intercostal space and right mid-clavicular line

B Xiphoid process

C Intersection of left 7th intercostal space and left midclavicular line

D Right lumbar region at umbilical level

E Above umbilicus (navel)

F Left lumbar region at umbilical level

G Right mid-inguinal region

H Left mid-inguinal region

of the capsule in the GI tract during video review. This function is available only with the use of an eight-lead sensor array (Fig. 4.5). The sensor array is more practical to use for very obese patients. It is at the discretion of the individual or service to select the most appropriate sensor accessory.

The battery of the data recorder is charged in a cradle connected to a PC with a commercial software system installed. The software system (see Chap. 3) supports all aspects of the SBCE procedure, including patient check-in, download of data, video creation, image review, and generation of a SBCE report. Access to real-time viewing should also be available during the examination to monitor the progress of capsule transit, particularly entry into the small bowel and also the colon. Identifying transit delays and instituting early intervention can reduce the risk of an incomplete study. The latest generation of data recorders now has real-time viewing as an integral feature of the data recorder.

A glass of water and simethicone are also required for the procedure. Simethicone is reported to improve visibility by reducing intraluminal bubbles [1, 2].

4.2 Informed Consent

An informed consent process should be undertaken before the procedure is performed. The clinician should have a thorough knowledge of the patient's clinical picture, comorbidities, and any special considerations that may increase the risk of complications. Most contraindications are relative (Table 4.2). The only true contraindications to SBCE are known or suspected obstruction (except when surgery is warranted or patency has been confirmed), pseudo-obstruction, and pregnancy [3]. Patients should be informed about preparation requirements, the procedure, its benefits, and the nature and level of risk associated with the procedure. Retention of the capsule with potential progression to surgical intervention is the main risk to be discussed. The principal risk factors for retention are Crohn's disease, chronic use of nonsteroidal anti-inflammatory drugs (NSAIDs), prior major abdominal surgery, and abdominopelvic irradiation (Chap. 40). In patients with these risk factors, consideration should be given to performing the patency capsule test (Chap. 9). It is important to advise patients that the retention risk in a normal small bowel is 0 %. Complications relating to swallowing the capsule should be included in discussions (Chap. 40). Special situations, including swallowing disorders, patients with implanted pacemakers, and emergency procedures are discussed in Chaps. 7 and 8.

The patient should also be informed that this is a small bowel examination and does not replace esophagogastroduodenoscopy (EGD) or colonoscopy; that the examination may be incomplete, necessitating repetition; and that MRI is contraindicated after the procedure until capsule excretion has been confirmed. Verbal counseling before the procedure should be supplemented with printed information, and written consent should be obtained.

Table 4.2 Contraindications to small bowel video capsule endoscopy

Contraindications
Gastrointestinal obstruction, strictures, or fistulae, unless surgery is warranted or patency, is confirmed by patency test
Pseudo-obstruction
Pregnancy
Relative contraindications
Swallowing disorders
Cardiac pacemaker or defibrillator

4.3 Bowel Preparation

The diagnostic yield of SBCE can be limited by reduced visibility of the mucosal surface, which may be caused by dark-colored bile, bubbles, and debris, especially in the distal small bowel. Preparation of the bowel in advance of the procedure is important to ensure optimal cleanliness and image quality. This preparation involves adjustments to medication, particularly oral iron; a period of fasting; and optional administration of bowel-cleansing preparations. Oral iron formulations coat the mucosa in dark residue that may mimic melena and can significantly impede visibility. It is recommended that patients stop taking oral iron preparations at least 3 days before the examination [4].

The day before the procedure, the patient is required to undergo a period of fasting. The manufacturer of the PillCam currently recommends a simple 10-h overnight fast [5], but in practice, some units recommend fasting for 12 h [6–8]. If concomitant bowel-cleansing preparations are used, their administration should be started *after* the onset of the fasting period.

There is now good, cumulative evidence of the benefit of using bowel-cleansing purgatives. A meta-analysis in 2008 concluded that in comparison to a clear liquid diet, using purgatives before small bowel SBCE improves visualization quality and increases diagnostic yield [9]. Since then, a number of randomized controlled trials have been published, investigating further the effect of bowel preparation on the quality of mucosal visualization. In a recent meta-analysis, eight studies were identified, using regimens based on either polyethylene glycol (PEG) or sodium phosphate (NaP) [10]. Patients were treated with PEG-based regimens (1–4 L ± simethicone), NaP-based regimens (30–90 mL ± bisacodyl), or fasting alone, with no added laxative. Use of any form of bowel preparation yielded significantly better visibility than fasting alone. Similar results were seen for diagnostic yield. Subanalysis according to the treatment used showed that PEG-based regimens showed benefit, whereas NaP-based regimens yielded no significant difference compared with fasting alone. This analysis confirms the benefit of bowel purgatives together with fasting before SBCE. PEG-based regimens offer an advantage, but the currently available evidence does not support the use of NaP. For SBCE, lower-volume PEG (2 L) appears to be as effective as the higher volumes traditionally used for

Table 4.3 Small bowel video capsule endoscopy (SBCE) procedure

Stage	Steps
Day before the examination	Review indication, ensure that informed consent is documented
	Ensure that previous data have been downloaded
	Charge data recorder battery
	Patient should have no food for a minimum of 12 h before examination (may drink clear fluids until midnight)
	Evening: patient drinks 2 L of PEG solution (optional)
	Nil by mouth from midnight
Day of the examination	Check in patient by entering patient and capsule data into the computer and initializing the data recorder
	Attach sensors using either eight-lead sensor array or sensor belt:
	For eight-lead sensor array, place array according to location guide (Fig. 4.5)
	For sensor belt, place sensor belt around the patient's waist over clothing (a thin layer of natural fabric, *not* synthetic fabric)
	Fit the recorder pouch across the patient's shoulder, adjusting straps so that pouch hangs comfortably at waist height
	Confirm that the recorder is fully charged
	Confirm that correct patient and procedure data are displayed on LCD screen
	Insert data recorder into pouch; connect sensor cable to recorder
	Open capsule box and hold it with the blinking capsule close to the sensor leads or belt to enable the capsule to pair with the recorder (when the recorder receives transmission from designated capsule *before* ingestion). Pairing is confirmed by a green pairing icon on the LCD screen and blue flashing LED light on the top of the data recorder. Patients must never swallow an unpaired capsule, as data may be lost
	The patient swallows the VCE capsule with a glass of water and simethicone (80 mg)
	After 30 min, check the capsule position with real-time viewer to verify small bowel entry. If the capsule remains in the stomach, initiate interventions to assist passage into the small bowel (as described in 4.5)
	Patient is then free to leave the office or hospital
	Provide the patient with written instructions and contact details
	Patient is allowed to drink fluids (except carbonated beverages) 2 h after capsule ingestion
	Patient may eat and swallow tablets 4 h after capsule ingestion
	Examination is completed 8–9 h after capsule ingestion. If small bowel entry was delayed, recording may be extended until the end of battery life (12 h) or confirmation of colon entry
	Patient returns recorder and equipment
	Download the data from recorder to computer
	Clean all equipment in accordance with manufacturer instructions
Next day	Review and interpret examination
	Save SBCE data to intranet, compact disk, or external hard drive

colonoscopy preparation. The optimal timing of bowel preparation has not yet been determined. Most SBCE studies have examined the effects of bowel purgatives administered the day before the procedure, usually in the evening. One study has reported similar benefits for mucosal visualization and diagnostic yield when using a split-dose regimen. Using mannitol, the first dose was administered the evening before the examination, with the second dose given the following morning, prior to

capsule ingestion [11]. This approach may be particularly helpful for patients with poor tolerance of bowel purgatives.

4.4 Procedure

The SBCE procedure is outlined on Table 4.3 (Figs. 4.6– 4.17).

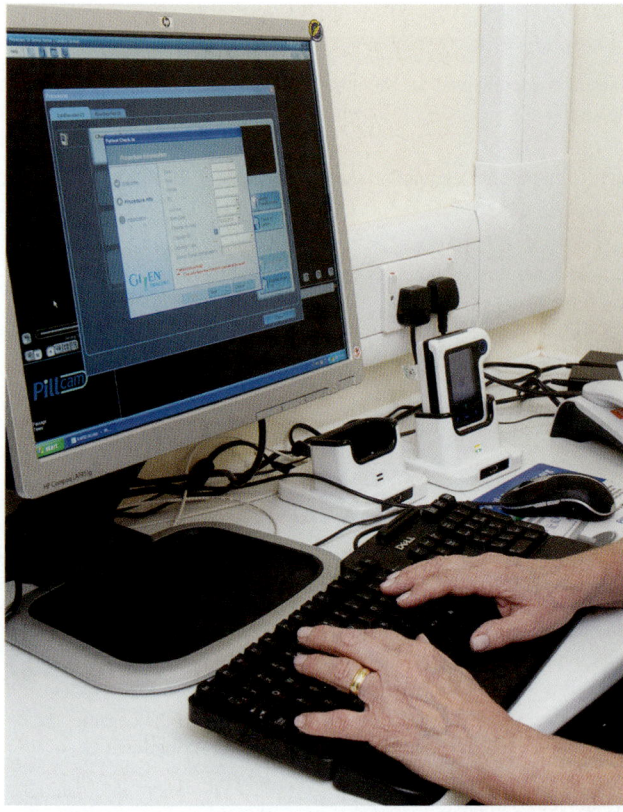

Fig. 4.6 In the check-in process, patient and capsule data are entered into the software template

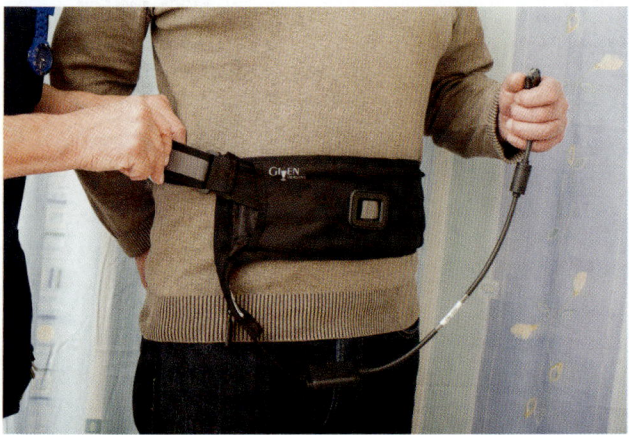

Fig. 4.7 The sensor belt is placed over natural fabric clothing around the patient's waist

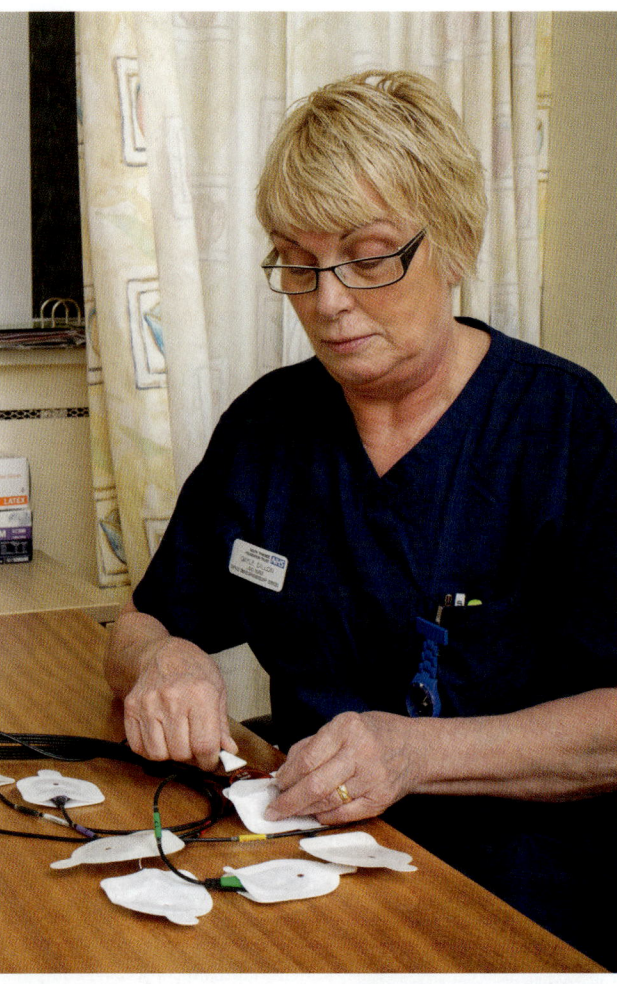

Fig. 4.8 An alternative to the sensor belt is an eight-lead sensor array; the leads are slipped into adhesive pouches

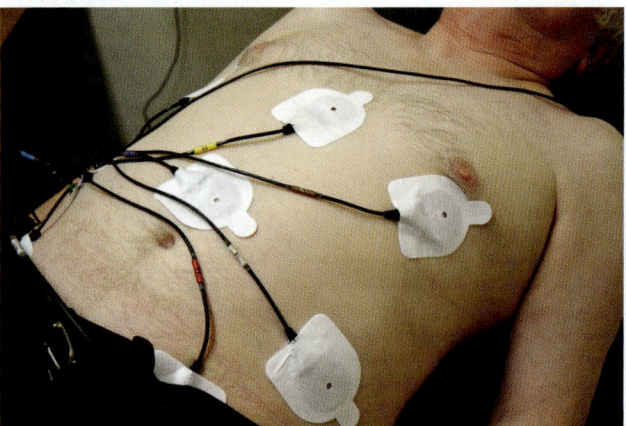

Fig. 4.9 The leads of the sensor array are affixed to the patient's abdomen

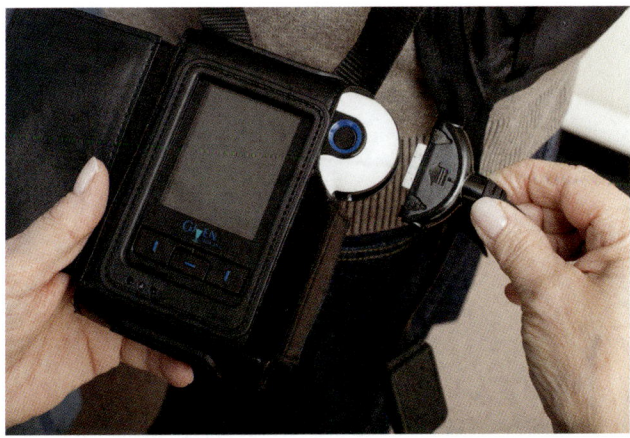

Fig. 4.10   The shoulder harness is placed on the patient, the recorder is placed into the pouch, and the sensor cable is connected to the recorder

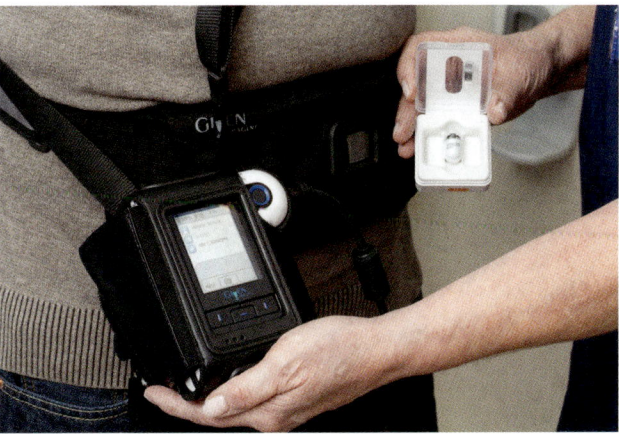

Fig. 4.12   The capsule is held close to the abdominal sensors to initiate the pairing of the capsule and recorder

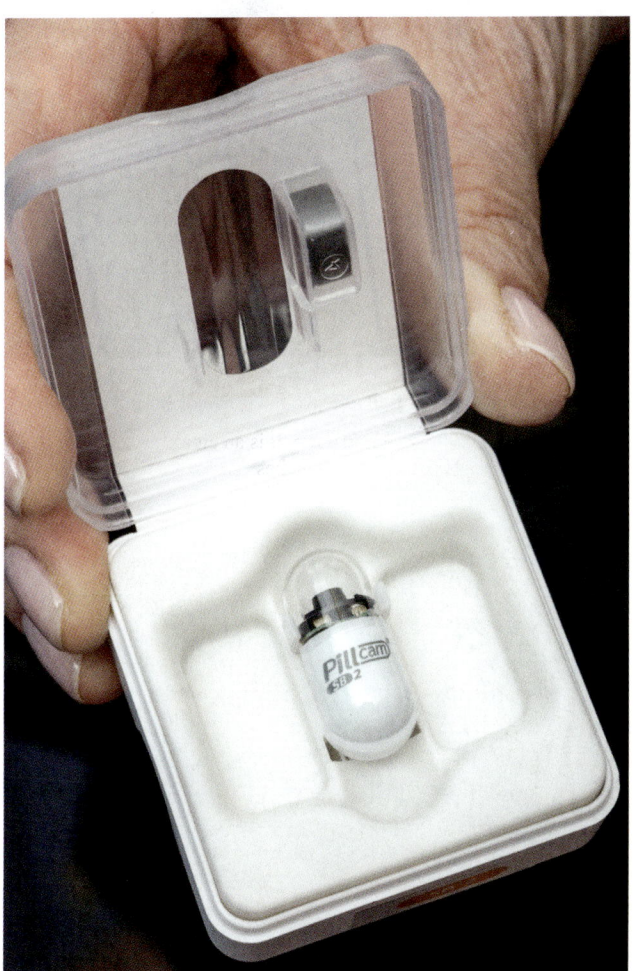

Fig. 4.11   The capsule is activated by opening the box

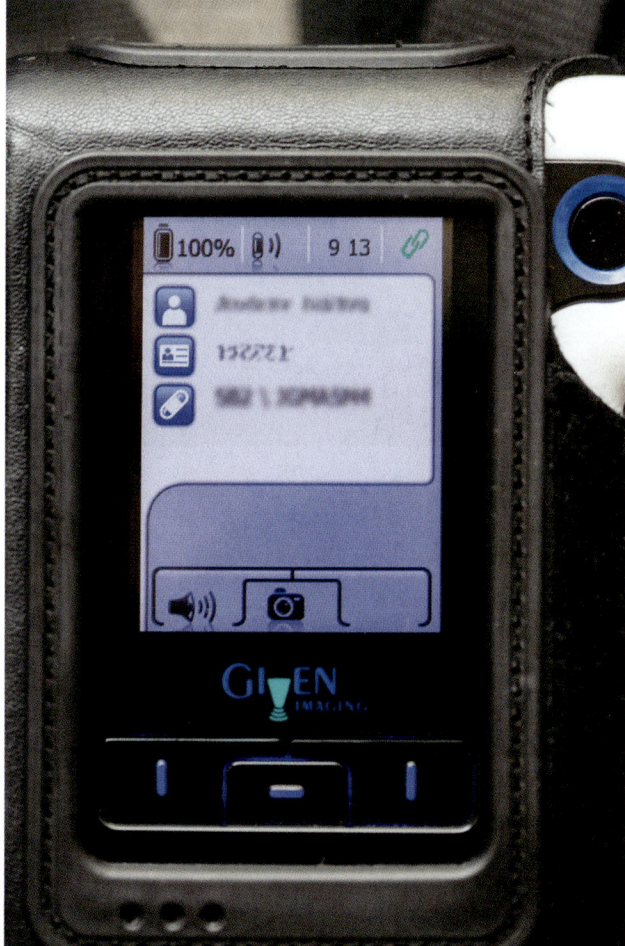

Fig. 4.13   Pairing is confirmed by a green icon in the upper right corner of the recorder screen, and the capsule LED on the top of the recorder should be blinking in blue

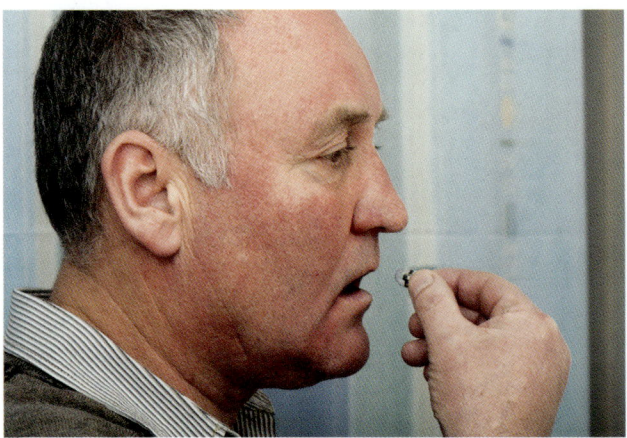

Fig. 4.14 The patient swallows the capsule with a glass of water containing simethicone

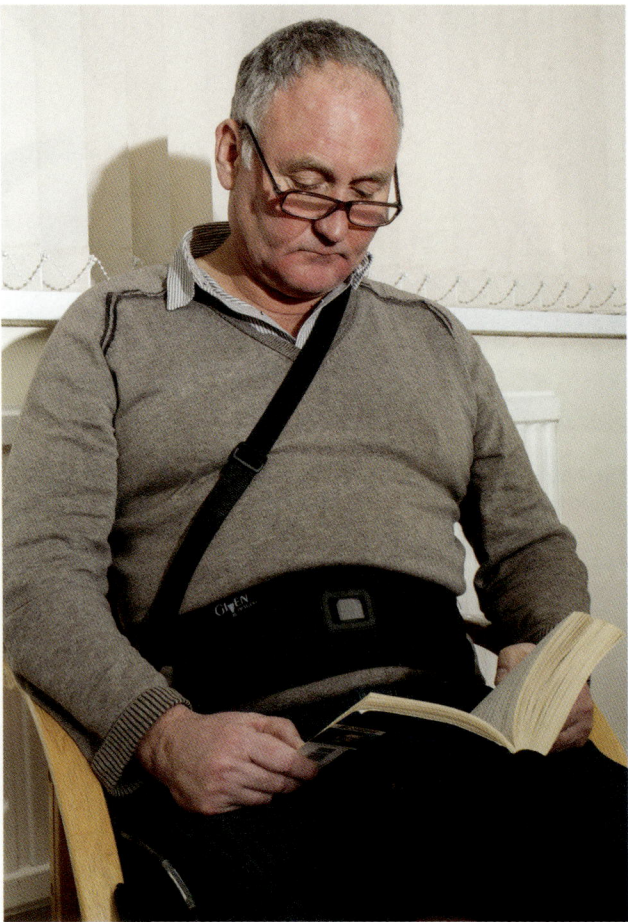

Fig. 4.16 The patient is free to leave the office or hospital during the examination and may resume light activity

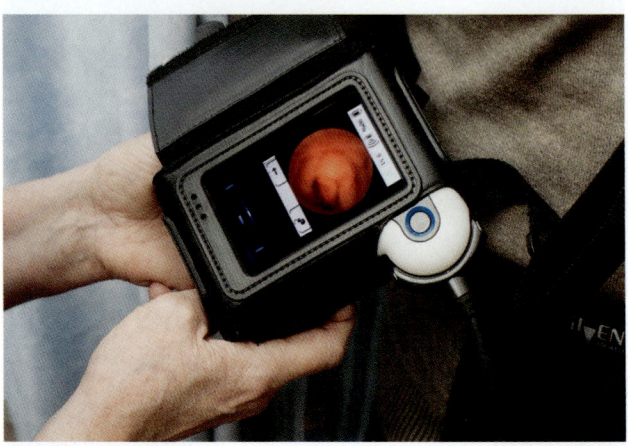

Fig. 4.15 After 30 min, the real-time viewer is used to check the position of the capsule and verify whether it has entered the small bowel

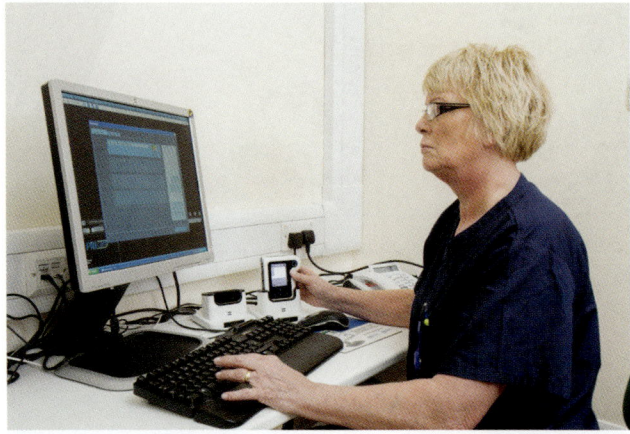

Fig. 4.17 On completion of the examination, the recorder is placed into the cradle to recharge the battery and download data to PC

4.5   Maximizing Study Quality

A quality SBCE study is the one that images the entire small bowel in a timely manner with clear mucosal visualization, thus providing the best conditions for optimal diagnostic value. In 20–30 % of capsule endoscopy procedures, the capsule does not reach the cecum within the recording time, so imaging of the small bowel is incomplete, and the value of the procedure is limited [12]. Several risk factors have been reported, including previous small bowel surgery, hospitalization, moderate or poor bowel cleansing, opiate use, older age, and hypothyroidism [12–15].

A key predictive factor for incomplete examinations is prolonged transit of the capsule through the stomach, which may result in insufficient time to visualize the whole small intestine before the capsule battery is exhausted. Gastric transit time (GTT) longer than 45 min has been postulated as an independent risk factor for incomplete SBCE studies [12]. Conditions that predispose to gastric emptying problems, such as known or suspected gastroparesis, particularly in patients with diabetes, vagotomy, or suspected scleroderma, should be identified during the assessment process. For these patients, use of a prokinetic agent before capsule ingestion should be considered [16]. Since the introduction of real-time viewing technology, it is now possible to identify prolonged GTT during the examination and initiate strategies to assist passage of the capsule into the duodenum [17–19]. Interventions include lateral positioning, asking the patient to take a short walk, use of oral purgatives or prokinetic agents, and endoscopic intervention to retrieve the capsule and move it through the pylorus.

Until recently, real-time viewers were optionally purchased as a handheld tablet that connected to the data recorder, but real-time viewing is now an integral data recorder function that is available to all users. It is recommended that every study include real-time viewing 30 min after capsule ingestion, to confirm gastric transit. Colon entry may also be verified prior to disconnection of the data recorder. Although rare, asymptomatic tracheal aspiration of the capsule can also be quickly detected with routine use of real-time viewing [20]. For patients with esophageal motility disorders or previous gastric surgery, the capsule may be electively placed endoscopically using a specifically designed device [21, 22]. Endoscopic placement techniques are discussed further in Chap. 7.

In practice, prokinetics are used to prevent or resolve prolonged GTT, but there is no consensus on indications for their use in SBCE [23]. Although the observed effects of prokinetic agents on small bowel transit time, completion rates, and diagnostic yield are inconsistent, there is sufficient evidence that metoclopramide [24–26], erythromycin [16, 27, 28], and domperidone [29] all significantly reduce GTT.

Other interventions reported to improve the quality of SBCE images include the use of a small amount (500 mL) of polyethylene glycol (PEG) 30–120 min *after* the ingestion of the capsule [30]. GTT was unaffected, but the small bowel transit time was significantly longer in the control group. This method did not enhance completion rate to the cecum, but image quality was maintained at the distal small bowel.

Clear mucosal visualization is the primary aim of preparing the small bowel for the examination. The use of 80 mg of simethicone to reduce intraluminal bubbles is recommended as standard practice, and purgative bowel-cleansing preparations should be considered, as discussed in Sect. 4.3 of this chapter.

References

1. Wu L, Cao Y, Liao C, et al. Systematic review and meta-analysis of randomized controlled trials of simethicone for gastrointestinal endoscopic visibility. Scand J Gastroenterol. 2011;46:227–35.
2. Albert J, Gobel CM, Lebke J, et al. Simethicone for small bowel preparation for capsule endoscopy: a systematic, single-blinded, controlled trial. Gastrointest Endosc. 2004;60:534–8.
3. Storch I, Barkin S. Contraindications to capsule endoscopy: do any still exist? Gastrointest Endosc Clin N Am. 2006;16:329–36.
4. Mishkin DS. Day of the procedure. In: de Franchis R, Lewis BS, Mishkin DS, editors. Capsule endoscopy simplified. Thorofare: SLACK Inc.; 2010. p. 15–24.
5. Given Imaging Ltd. PillCam SB: Information for health professionals. http://www.givenimaging.com/en-us/Innovative-Solutions/Capsule-Endoscopy/Pillcam-SB/HCP-Resources/Pages/What-Your-Patient-Can-Expect.aspx. Accessed 6 Nov 2013.
6. Spada C, Riccioni ME, Familiari P, et al. Polyethylene glycol plus simethicone in small-bowel preparation for capsule endoscopy. Dig Liver Dis. 2010;42:365–70.
7. Wi JH, Moon JS, Choi MG, et al. Bowel preparation for capsule endoscopy: a prospective randomized multicenter study. Gut Liver. 2009;3:180–5.
8. Wei W, Ge ZZ, Lu H, et al. Purgative bowel cleansing combined with simethicone improves capsule endoscopy imaging. Am J Gastroenterol. 2008;103:77–82.
9. Rokkas T, Papaxoinis K, Triantafyllou K, et al. Does purgative preparation influence the diagnostic yield of small bowel video capsule endoscopy? A meta-analysis. Am J Gastroenterol. 2009;104:219–27.
10. Belsey J, Crosta C, Epstein O, et al. Meta-analysis: efficacy of small bowel preparation for small bowel video capsule endoscopy. Curr Med Res Opin. 2012;28:1883–90.
11. Chen HB, Huang Y, Chen SY, et al. Small bowel preparations for capsule endoscopy with mannitol and simethicone: a prospective, randomized clinical trial. J Clin Gastroenterol. 2011; 45:337–41.
12. Westerhof J, Weersma RK, Koornstra JJ. Risk factors for incomplete small-bowel capsule endoscopy. Gastrointest Endosc. 2009;69:74–80.
13. Lee MM, Jacques A, Lam E, et al. Factors associated with incomplete small bowel capsule endoscopy studies. World J Gastroenterol. 2010;16:5329–33.
14. Fireman Z, Kopelman Y, Friedman S, et al. Age and indication for referral to capsule endoscopy significantly affect small bowel transit times: the Given database. Dig Dis Sci. 2007;52:2884–7.

15. Alim S, Matin S, Mann M, et al. Factors affecting capsule endoscopy transit time (abstract). Gastroenterology. 2007;132 Suppl 2:310.
16. Ben-Soussan E, Savoye G, Antonietti M, et al. Factors that affect gastric passage of video capsule. Gastrointest Endosc. 2005;62:785–90.
17. Lai LH, Wong GL, Lau JY, et al. Initial experience of real-time capsule endoscopy in monitoring progress of the videocapsule through the upper GI tract. Gastrointest Endosc. 2007;66:1211–4.
18. Spada C, Riccioni ME, Costamagna G. Rapid Access Real-Time device and Rapid Access software: new tools in the armamentarium of capsule endoscopy. Expert Rev Med Devices. 2007;4:431–5.
19. Delvaux M, Gay G. Real-time viewing of capsule endoscopy recordings: principle and clinical potential. Tech Gastrointest Endosc. 2006;8:160–3.
20. Despott E, O'Rourke A, Anikin V, et al. Tracheal aspiration of capsule endoscopes: detection, management and susceptibility. Dig Dis Sci. 2012;57:1973–4.
21. Holden JP, Dureja P, Pfau PR, et al. Endoscopic placement of the small-bowel video capsule by using a capsule endoscope delivery device. Gastrointest Endosc. 2007;65:842–7.
22. Skogestad E, Tholfsen JK. Capsule endoscopy: in difficult cases the capsule can be ingested through an overtube. Endoscopy. 2004;36:1038.
23. Postgate A, Tekkis P, Patterson N, et al. Are bowel purgatives and prokinetics useful for small-bowel capsule endoscopy? A prospective randomized controlled study. Gastrointest Endosc. 2009;69:1120–8.
24. Zhang JS, Ye LP, Zhang JL, et al. Intramuscular injection of metoclopramide decreases the gastric transit time and does not increase the complete examination rate of capsule endoscopy: a prospective randomized controlled trial. Hepatogastroenterology. 2011;58:1618–21.
25. Iwamoto J, Mizokami Y, Shimokobe K, et al. The effect of metoclopramide in capsule endoscopy. Hepatogastroenterology. 2010;57:1356–9.
26. Selby W. Complete small bowel transit in patients undergoing capsule endoscopy: determining factors and improvement with metoclopramide. Gastrointest Endosc. 2005;61:80–5.
27. Fireman Z, Paz D, Kopelman Y, et al. Capsule endoscopy: improving transit time and image view. World J Gastroenterol. 2005; 11:5863–6.
28. Leung WK, Chan FK, Fung SS, et al. Effect of oral erythromycin on gastric and small bowel transit time of capsule endoscopy. World J Gastroenterol. 2005;11:4865–8.
29. Keuchel M, Voderholzer WA, Schenk G, et al. Domperidone shortens gastric transit time of videocapsule endoscopy (VCE). Gastrointest Endosc. 2003;57:AB163.
30. Ito T, Ohata K, Ono A, et al. Prospective controlled study on the effects of polyethylene glycol in capsule endoscopy. World J Gastroenterol. 2012;18:1789–92.

Internet

www.capsuleendoscopy.org
www.givenimaging.com

Evaluation of Capsule Endoscopic Images

5

Blair S. Lewis and Martin Keuchel

Contents

The work was first published in 2006 by Springer Medizin Verlag Heidelberg with the following title: *Atlas of Video Capsule Endoscopy*.

B.S. Lewis (✉)
Mount Sinai Hospital, New York, NY, USA
e-mail: blairslewismdpc@me.com

M. Keuchel
Department of Internal Medicine,
Bethesda Krankenhaus Bergedorf,
Hamburg, Germany
e-mail: keuchel@bkb.info

5.1 The Task of Reading

Though capsule endoscopy has grabbed the attention of physician and layperson alike, most overlook the importance and intensity of examining the wirelessly obtained images. Typical examinations obtain images over at least 8 h and sometimes more than 13 h, and as images are obtained at a rate of at least two images per second, a total of 57,600 images are produced. The computer workstation allows images to be viewed singly or as a video stream (Fig. 5.1). Though the images are obtained at a rate of perhaps 2/s, they may be reviewed at a rate of up to 40/s. Given that an abnormality may be present on only one image, most physicians familiar with the system feel that lesions could easily be missed at the faster rates [1]. When viewing at 40 images per second, a single image is on the monitor for less than 0.02 s. A consensus conference of users in 2002 agreed that 15 frames per second is the fastest acceptable rate of review. At this rate, 57,600 images can be seen in 64 min—but only if they are run as a video without stopping to examine individual images.

In the beginning of capsule endoscopy, reviewing was reported to average between 50 and 120 min [2–4]. Average small bowel passage takes 4 h, and thus a physician had to review a minimum of 28,800 images without viewing the gastric and colonic portions of the examination. The time it takes to review the capsule study is extremely important, as it is a limiting factor to the acceptance of capsule endoscopy by gastroenterologists. In a 2002 editorial, Fleischer [5] stated, "the time required to read the studies (60–90 min) does not make economic or practice sense."

With further technical development of the hardware, such as movement-adapted frame rate, even more images are acquired. In an effort to shorten the review time, software has been developed to allow the reader to handle the increasing number of images (Fig. 5.2). A quad view mode places four images (2 full seconds of image collection) on one screen. This shortens the reading time by as much as 50 %. In addition to the length of time the review takes, physicians are also

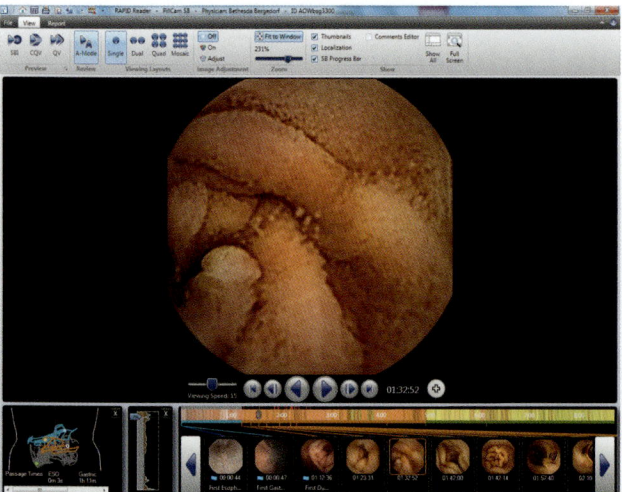

Fig. 5.1 Rapid 8 monitor (Given Imaging Ltd., Yoqneam, Israel) for small bowel capsule PillCam SB2 and SB3, showing endoscopic image (*top*); buttons for playback control under the image; tool bar (*top*); time bar in different colors, representing mean colors of the images in the corresponding segment and thumbnails of landmarks (*bottom*); localization (*left lower corner*); and small bowel progress indicator (between localization and thumbnails)

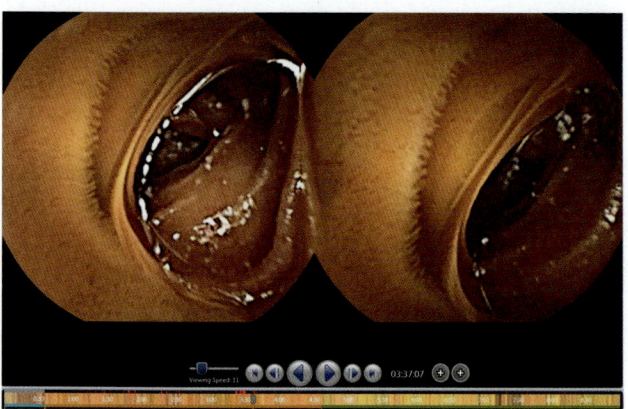

Fig. 5.2 Double image view. Rapid 8 monitor (Given Imaging)

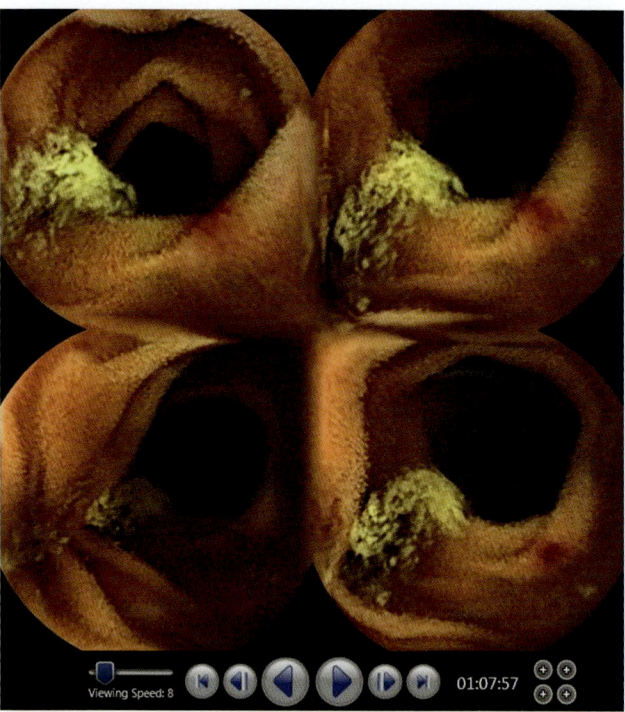

Fig. 5.3 Quadruple image mode, combining four different consecutive images

concerned about reading the studies properly and not missing lesions. By placing four images on one screen, each image changes at a slower pace to decrease the likelihood of missing abnormalities (Fig. 5.3). Other viewing modes include mosaic view (Fig. 5.4) and collage mode (Fig. 5.5).

Automatic variation of the playback speed according to the alteration of acquired images was implemented early. The next step was to omit redundant images. This mode had a miss rate of only 1 % [6]. Other software modules such as QuickView initially displayed a certain percentage of all images. Further developments included undisclosed intelligent algorithms to show all images with suspected pathology. Using QuickView, the mean reading time for 106 films was shortened to 11.6 min [7]; the QuickView mode missed seven lesions, the same number as were missed by the standard mode. Of the seven missed lesions, four were not displayed by the software, resulting in a "theoretical sensitivity" of 93.5 % for the QuickView mode.

With the Olympus EndoCapsule System (Olympus Medical Systems Corp., Tokyo, Japan), a miss rate of 8 % was found with an automated selection mode (overview function) in a retrospective analysis, while suppression of redundant images (express-selected mode) missed only 1 finding out of 40 images. This "single frame finding" was also missed with automated replay speed [8].

Presently, helpful algorithms are available to aid in quickly achieving a diagnosis, but the physician cannot yet rely on these algorithms. To cope with this limitation, software provides the possibility of looking at all rejected images (Complementary QuickView by Given, or express-skipped mode by Olympus).

Fleischer [5] also expressed concern that "without concentration on the part of the physician, a lesion could be missed." So, in the end, despite great technologic advances, it comes down to the physician and the act of observation.

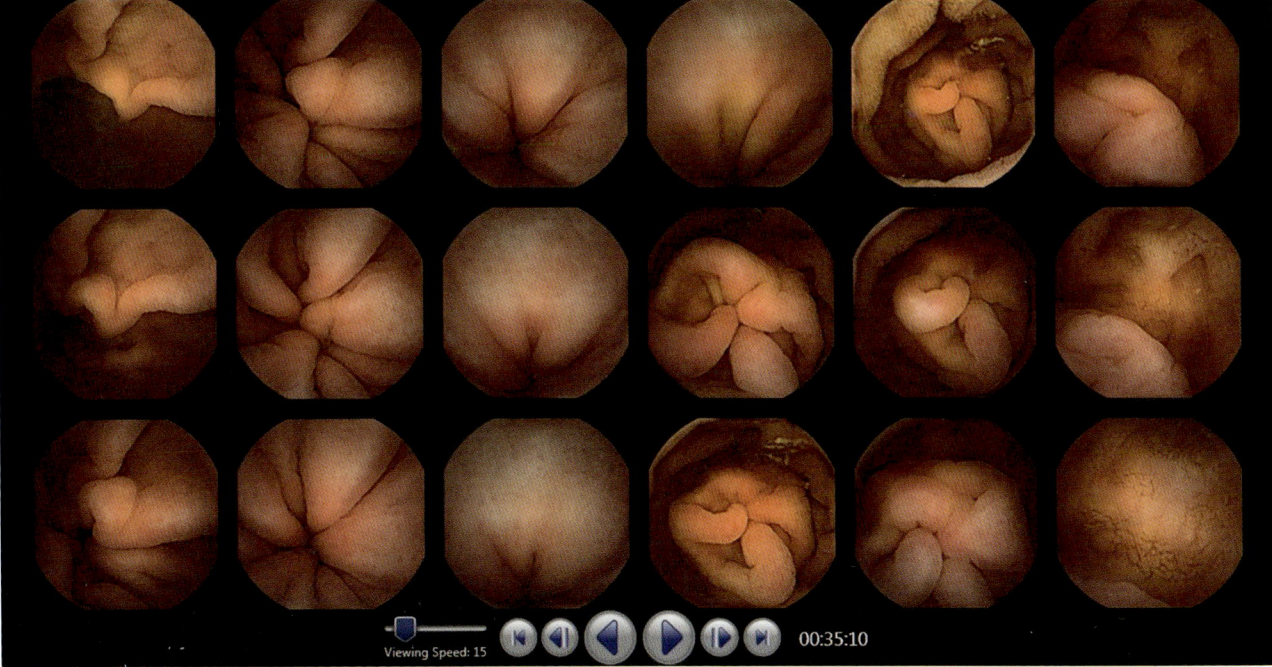

Fig. 5.4 Mosaic view provides a good overview of anatomic landmarks (here passage from antrum to the duodenal bulb) or distribution of lesions, but it is not applicable for reading a video capsule endoscopy (VCE) video

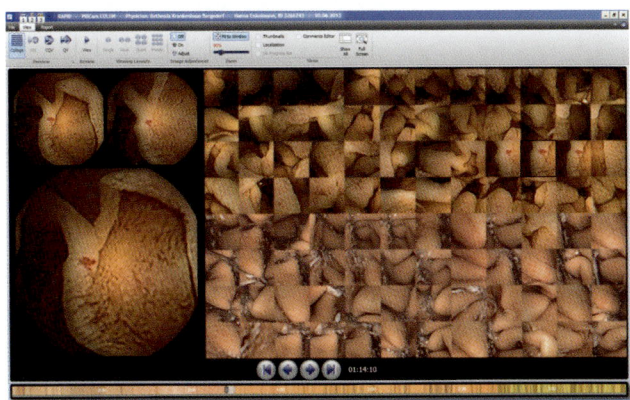

Fig. 5.5 Collage mode displays only regions of interest from each of multiple images in a compressed form. Pointing on a small image with the cursor displays this frame enlarged on the left, with the two images before and after. Presently this feature is active only in PillCam Colon 2 studies

5.1.1 Vigilance

Lessons learned from anesthesiology [9] and airline pilots during long flights [10] show that vigilance is especially necessary when the task is long and monotonous. The stress encountered by an individual being vigilant leads to fatigue and restlessness. This stress is determined by several factors, which include the type of event or cue that is being scanned for. Auditory cues are less stressful than visual events. The length of the period of observation is also important. Periods greater than 50 min increase the stress to the observer, no matter the cue or the event rate [11]. Indeed, the event rate is generally not related to creating stress: the same vigilance is required whether the thing being watched or listened for occurs frequently or rarely. Other important factors in an individual's vigilance include environmental factors such as background noise [12] and air temperature [13], nutrition [14], caffeine consumption [15], and physical activity during the time of observation. Based on these factors, several suggestions have been made to improve vigilance during reading of a video capsule endoscopy (VCE) examination [16]:

- Darkened but not black room
- Comfortable seating and clothing
- Carbohydrates (and caffeine?) prior to evaluation
- Auditory distraction (e.g., music)
- Sessions limited to 1 h
- Interruption of session in case of fidgetiness or restlessness

5.1.2 The Stress of Reading

It should also be remembered that the stress of reading a study depends on the indication for the study. Capsule exams performed for abdominal pain, malabsorption, or suspected Crohn's disease are generally less stressful to read than studies performed for obscure gastrointestinal bleeding. The lesions or visual cues being looked for in the former group are generally larger and less easily missed than a small vascular lesion that may be present on only a single image from a patient with bleeding. Most experienced physicians believe that the hardest study to read is the normal study, which requires the confidence of the reader that no lesion has been missed. With these issues in mind, physicians are reminded that before reading a capsule study, they should be familiar with the patient's medical history, including not only the indication for the study but also any surgical history. Prior knowledge of a surgical small bowel anastomosis (Chap. 39) can simplify the study's analysis.

5.1.3 Interpretation of Images

In addition to vigilance, physicians must have experience in interpreting endoscopic images. Only one part of capsule endoscopy is the vigilant reader, who is able to recognize an area that is abnormal or different from other areas examined. An equally important part of the examination is the proper identification of these abnormalities. The reader must be able to diagnose based on the images, dismissing normal variants and nonpathologic lesions and identifying specific pathologies requiring specific therapies. The images obtained at capsule endoscopy are slightly different from those of traditional endoscopy, as there is no air distention of the bowel wall, and the capsule is at times located within millimeters of the mucosa. This is so-called physiologic endoscopy, as the bowel is not altered by the process of the examination. In addition, no sedation is used, so there are no hemodynamic effects. There is no trauma caused by the capsule. There is no air insufflation to affect the microvasculature. Thus all findings are real, and their location has not been altered by the exam. Expertise must be obtained to allow review of the images in a manner that is not only efficient but also is able to provide a precise diagnosis.

5.1.4 The Steps to Efficient Reading

Very specific steps can be taken to ease the process of reading a capsule exam. The physician must develop a pattern of practice. Here we are describing the pattern we use when viewing an exam (Table 5.1). Initially, the very last image is examined to ensure that the colon has been entered. The presence of stool will confirm this finding. After returning to the very first image, the next task is to activate blood detection software if the exam was performed in the setting of obscure gastrointestinal bleeding. To scan the entire study including the stomach, the first image is falsely identified as the first duodenal image on a thumbnail edit. This turns on

Table 5.1 Steps in reading a video capsule endoscopy examination

Look at the last images first: has the colon been reached?
Activate SBI software by marking first duodenal image and view marked images
Falsely marking the esophagus as the first duodenal image enables SBI also for the stomach
Identify first gastric image; screen stomach with high speed
Correctly mark the first duodenal image
Mark the first cecal image
Thoroughly screen small intestine
Create thumbnails for abnormalities
Place a thumbnail every 30 min and save findings regularly to prevent data loss

SBI suspected blood indicator

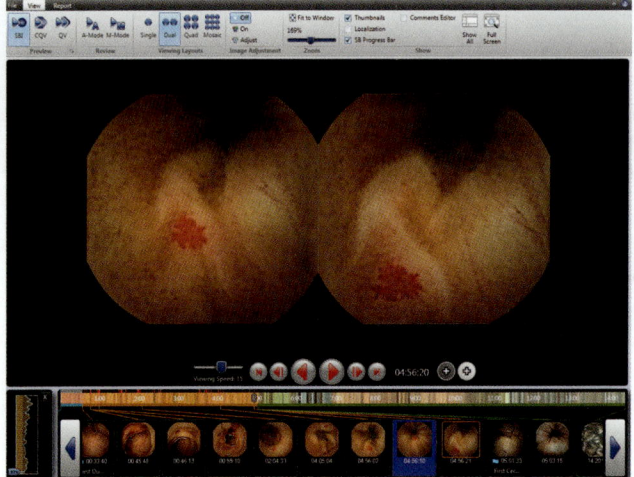

Fig. 5.6 Suspected Blood Indicator (SBI). After activation of this mode, only images with blood or red lesions suspected by the software are displayed. In this patient, fresh blood in the proximal small bowel and several angiectasias are detected (*thin red lines above the time/color bar*). Note that some angiectasias are missed by SBI, and some red bars are false positives

the Suspected Blood Indicator (SBI) software (Fig. 5.6). Any positive findings can be quickly examined and thumbnails created. Because of low sensitivity, however, the SBI software cannot replace careful personal examination of all images of the small intestine [17, 18]. In recent software versions, SBI accuracy has depended on capsule speed and background color [19]. Once the SBI function is completed, the first image thumbnail is deleted. The third task is to identify the three specific locations needed to determine both the gastric and small bowel emptying times. Using a single-view image but increasing the image rate to 25 frames per second, the images are played forward in an automatic mode. The esophagogastric junction is quickly seen, and the first gastric image is duly noted on a thumbnail edit. Using the time bar, the images are quickly advanced forward and backward until the first image of the duodenum is identified. This too is noted on a thumbnail edit. It should be remembered that the capsule can move backward and forward through the pylorus several times prior to its final passage and further advancement into the small bowel.

Again, the time bar is used to identify the ileocecal valve. This landmark proves to be quite difficult for many physicians. The presence of formed stool is a definite indicator of the colon. As bowel prep prior to VCE is increasingly used, this indicator may be less reliable. Hence, marking an image with clearly visible colonic mucosa reaffirms complete small bowel passage. It can take some time for the beginning reader to reliably identify this landmark and then note it on a thumbnail edit.

Once the landmarks have been thumbnailed, the images are viewed. The gastric portion of the exam should be examined but can be viewed at a rapid rate. In the small bowel, starting at the first image of the duodenum, one of the authors uses the multiviewer function to scan two images at a total rate of 20 frames per second or 10 frames per second of the individual images (Fig. 5.2). The other author scans with a single-image view at 10–15 frames per second. This difference demonstrates the need to find out and customize individual settings.

A mouse with a jogwheel is always at the ready. If reading is performed on a laptop computer, a mouse is attached, as this greatly eases the reading process. When an area moves by too quickly, or if a possible abnormality is seen, movement of the jogwheel will stop the progress of the images and allow review of the images that have passed. The capsule moves much more quickly in the proximal small bowel than in the distal sections. In the duodenum, the frame-to-finding ratio is quite high, so use of the jogwheel to examine each individual image is often required in the duodenum. The frame-to-finding ratio in the ileum is quite low, and the use of the jogwheel diminishes distally.

When an abnormality is identified, a thumbnail is created. This author routinely creates thumbnails for every 30 min of images viewed. Doing so allows the reader to stop and know where the reading stopped, and it prevents having to start over should the reader lose his or her place.

5.2   Use of Localization Software

In addition to interpreting individual images, localization data must also be learned. The advantage to localization data is that it allows a physician to know if an identified abnormality is within reach of a push enteroscope (Fig. 5.7). The information can also guide subsequent surgery. Generally, the localization drawing identifies the duodenum and ligament of Treitz well. The physician derives the location of an abnormality within the jejunum or ileum from a compilation of data, which includes the quadrant location provided by the

localization drawing with an accuracy of about 6 cm [20], the time of passage from the pylorus to the lesion, the amount of bowel visually passed by the capsule en route to the lesion, and the amount of bowel traversed from the lesion to the ileocecal valve. This information is difficult to quantify, but qualitative judgments by an experienced physician can be quite accurate in providing a location and thus in differentiating between patients who can be treated with push enteroscopy and those requiring device-assisted enteroscopy or surgical intervention.

Generally, lesions found within 30 min of passage from the pylorus and those located in the left abdomen (Fig. 5.7a, b) are generally within reach of a 2.5-m push enteroscope (Chap. 12). This statement is based on a typical small bowel passage time of 4 h and a normal progression of the capsule within the proximal small bowel. A small bowel progress bar aims to provide additional information on the percentage of small bowel traversed as calculated from the actual velocity of the capsule (Fig. 5.7e). This is especially helpful when the localization trace is not available because a sensor belt had been used instead of the sensor arrays (Chap. 4). Occasionally, a capsule can stay a prolonged time in the duodenal bulb, altering these generalizations. Device-assisted enteroscopy (Chaps. 13, 14, and 15) can be used to reach lesions further inside the small bowel. An oral insertion route has been suggested for lesions in the proximal 60 % of the small bowel, whereas a rectal approach is recommended for the distal 40 % [21].

5.3   Spectral Color Selection

The Rapid software has an integrated optional spectral color module for image post-processing (Fig. 5.8). The Flexible Spectral Imaging Color Enhancement (FICE) module (derived from Fujinon FICE for flexible endoscopy) enables an improved visualization of vascular pattern and surface structures [22]. Three settings (FICE 1, FICE 2, and FICE 3) are available with different spectral light compositions. In one study with 20 videos, the observer using FICE found more angiectasias (35 vs 32) and erosions (41 vs 24) than the observer using standard mode [23]. Better characterization of angiectasias with FICE was jeopardized by more irrelevant findings, resulting in a lower specificity [24]. With FICE, one group [25] obtained a higher number of findings but not an increase in diagnoses per patient. Using QuickView and FICE modes, sensitivity for angiectasias could be increased from 80 to 91 %, but with a reduction in specificity to 86 [26]. Kobayashi et al. [27] found no superiority of FICE in a per patient analysis. Two observers of 167 VCE images judged that another color modification mode, the "blue mode" (Fig. 5.8b), improved 83 % of images, whereas the three different FICE modes worsened a majority of images [28]. Thus FICE and blue mode may be helpful

Fig. 5.7 Localization software.
Progression of the capsule from the
duodenum (**a**), jejunum (**b**), and ileum
(**c**) to the colon (**d**). The *blue line* indicates
stomach, orange indicates small intestine,
and *green* indicates colon. Colors are
selected according to the first images of
the duodenum and cecum, as marked
manually by the examiner. The progress
indicator (**e**) shows the velocity of the
capsule and calculated percentage of
small bowel footage

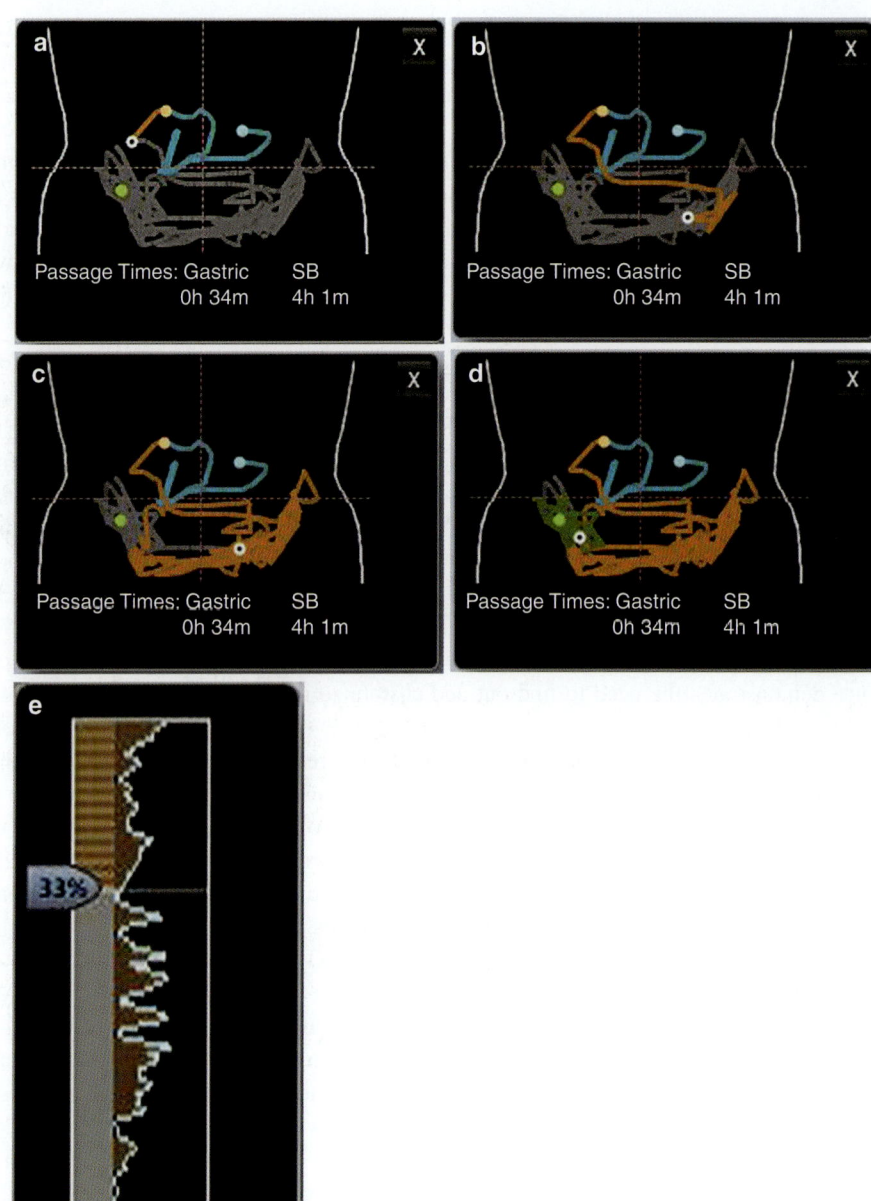

Fig. 5.8 Virtual chromoendoscopy. On the left are the original images, and on the right are images of spectral light selection in post-processing. (**a**, **b**) Carcinoid (**b** in blue mode). (**c**, **d**) Angiectasia (**d** in Flexible Intelligent Color Enhancement [FICE] 1 mode). (**e**, **f**) Adenocarcinoma (**f** in FICE 3 mode)

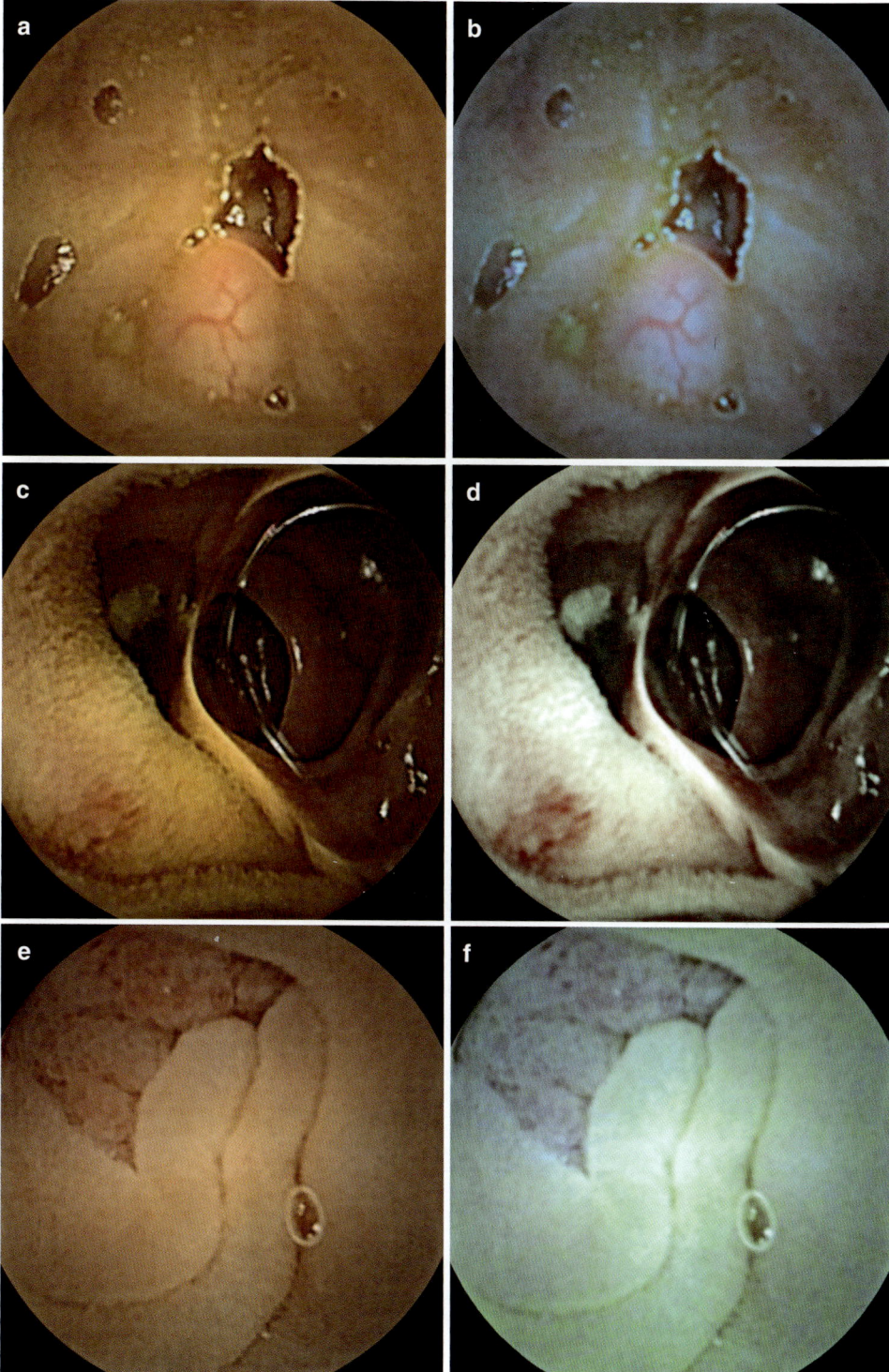

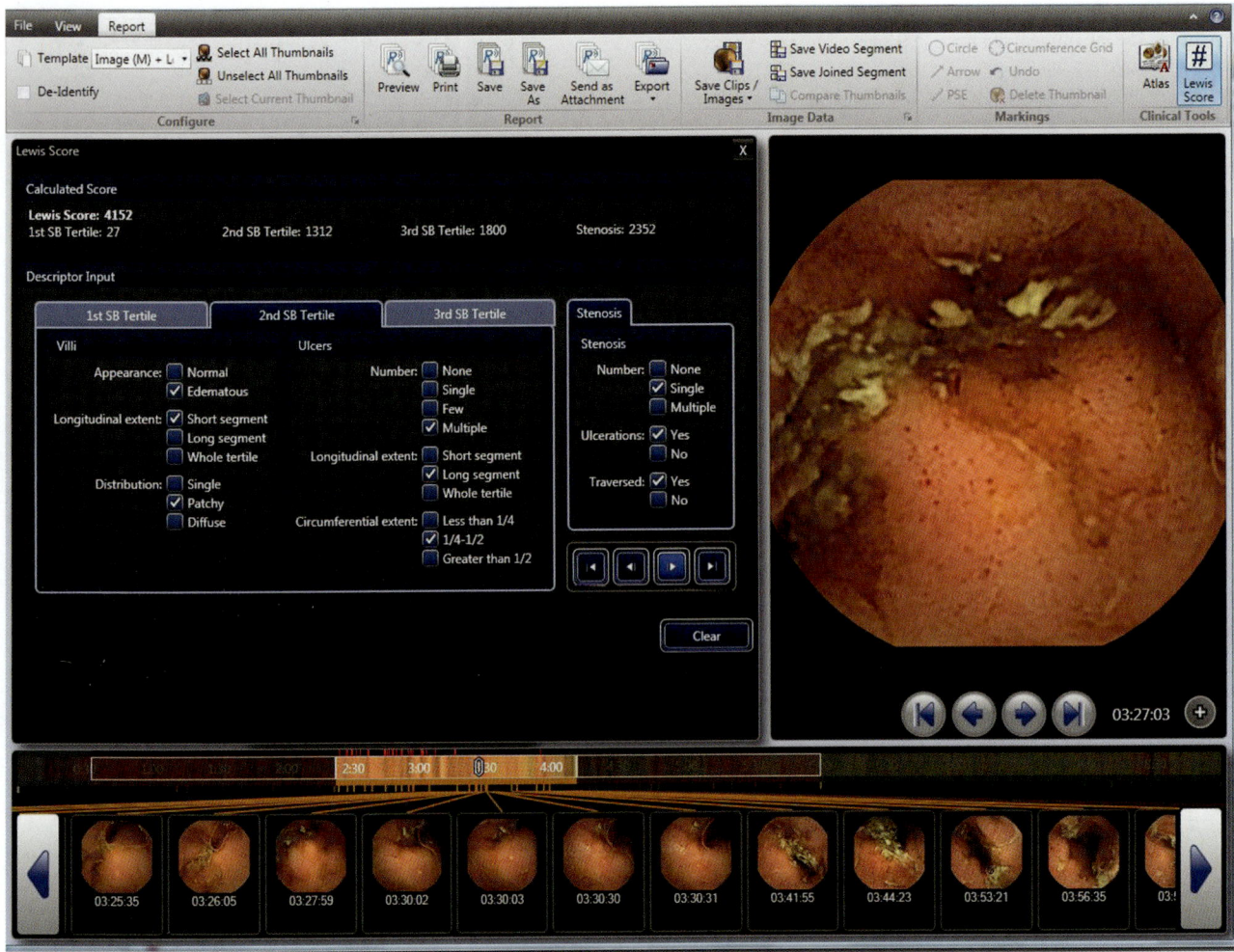

Fig. 5.9 Lewis score. This feature can be activated in the top right corner of the Rapid 8 report bar. The actual image on the right is assigned to the corresponding tertile. By clicking a few buttons for each tertile, the score is calculated automatically

in characterizing unclear lesions once they are detected in standard mode.

5.4 Lewis Score

After marking the first duodenal and first cecal image, the Lewis score button can be activated. The actual small bowel tertile (proximal, mid, and distal) is active (Fig. 5.9). This feature can be used to characterize the localization of any lesion. Additionally, for patients with Crohn's disease, an endoscopic score can be calculated from the terms villous edema, ulcers, and stenosis, with the attribute values distribution, longitudinal extent, and circumferential extent. This score has been validated in terms of correlation with overall capsule endoscopic impression of disease activity [29] and showed a correlation with fecal calprotectin [30]. A score of 135 is suggested as the cutoff between normal and active disease; this score does not provide a diagnosis, but only an estimation of activity.

5.5 Evaluation of Colon Studies

Evaluation of colon capsule endoscopy (CCE) studies using PillCam Colon is done with the same Rapid software as is used to evaluate small bowel capsule videos. The software automatically recognizes the type of capsule used, and the appropriate screen opens up (Fig. 5.10). For CCE studies, two different images are acquired simultaneously, one with the "yellow" and the other with the "green." The colors have been chosen, as it is generally not possible to determine which of the cameras looks forward and which looks backward.

Evaluation of CCE studies starts with thumbnailing the landmarks while looking at both images in a fast speed (Chap. 45). Suggested landmarks are the hepatic flexure, splenic flexure, and last rectal image. An adapted localization trace pictogram is again provided in the left bottom corner. With the yellow and green buttons, each camera can be selected separately, and both streams are reviewed carefully at slow speed, one after the other, looking for

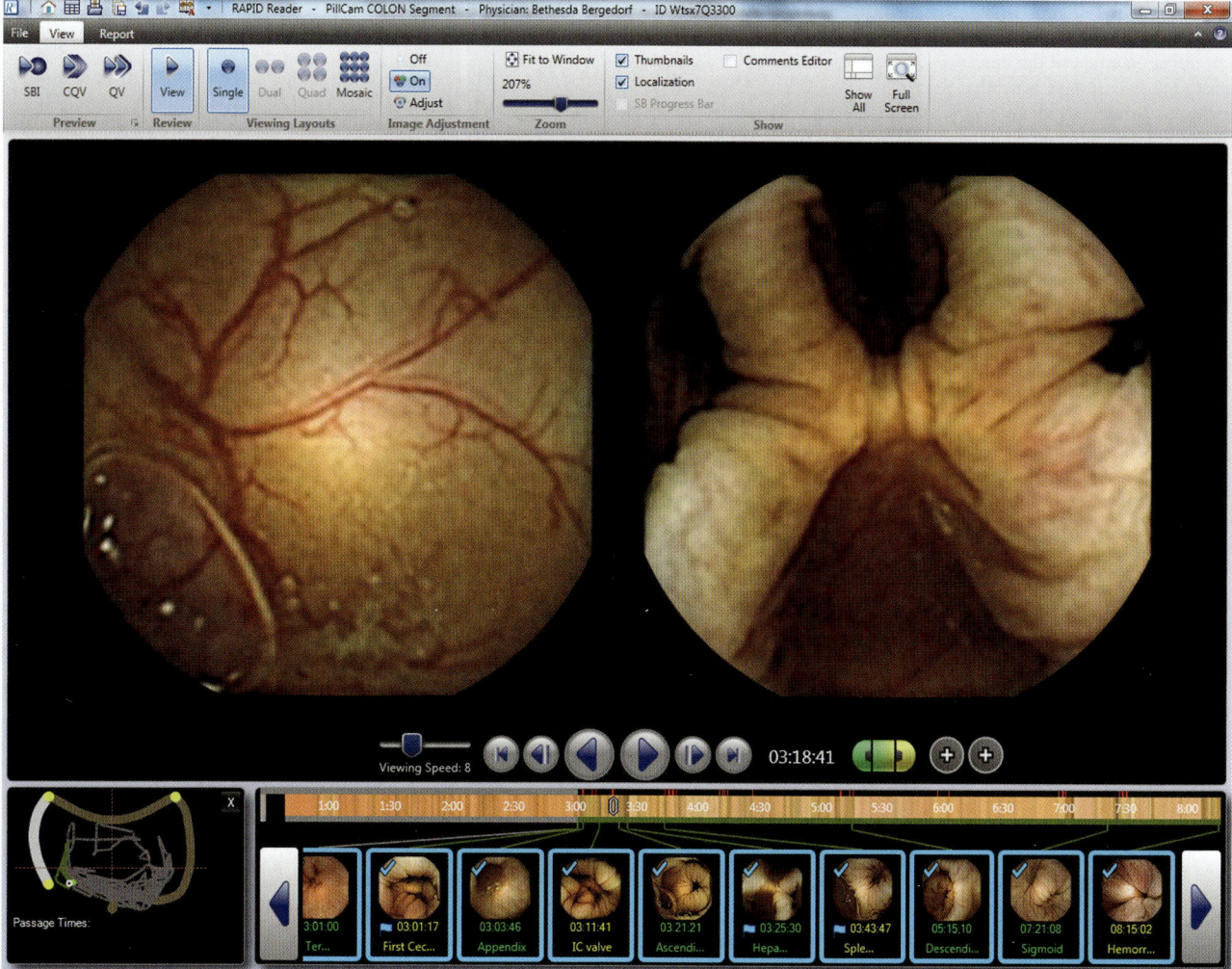

Fig. 5.10 Rapid 8 screen with PillCam Colon 2 study. Images of two cameras (yellow and green) can be displayed in parallel or separately, one after the other. Localization additionally provides landmarks for the hepatic and splenic flexure and last rectal image. The software can even suggest marks for the flexures

polyps. Small flat polyps displayed only in one image or a few images can easily be missed. Additionally, the anatomy of the colon, with larger folds, larger lumen, and often only minimal differences in color between polyps and normal mucosa (Fig. 5.11), requires more attention and a slower speed than small bowel videos. In the thumbnail editing pop-up, a polyp size estimation tool provides a measurement of polyp size corrected for the distance of the polyp from the capsule (Fig. 5.12). This estimate is important to classify whether the colonic polyps are significant (i.e., ≥6 mm). Electronic size correction for lesions more distant from the capsule is based on loss of illumination. However, when this tool was used in a trial comparing it with colonoscopy, some cases of size mismatch were observed [31].

As evaluation of capsule videos may be jeopardized by inadequate visualization limiting the diagnostic accuracy, cleanliness levels should be stated in every report. Judgment should be based on the overall cleanliness of a segment rather than on single images. Instead of a four-grade scale (excellent, good, fair, or poor) (Fig. 5.13), a two-point scale (adequate or inadequate) has been shown to be sufficient [32]. A computer-based scoring system has been suggested to analyze cleanliness from VCE images [33].

5.6   Interpreting Difficult Images

Specific problems occur when interpreting some capsule images. These problems include single-image abnormalities, proper identification of submucosal processes, and differentiating dark blood from dark bile. Unlike traditional endoscopy, a single-image abnormality cannot be viewed from different angles but rather must be identified by a single, half-second image. The identification depends on the experience and confidence of the reader. Equally troubling for the

Fig. 5.11 Polyp (8 mm) in the right colon. This flat polyp in the left upper quadrant of the image is easily missed, as there are only marginal differences in color and tissue texture compared with the normal mucosa. (**a**) Native image. (**b**) Structure enhancement. (**c**) FICE 1. (**d**) Blue mode

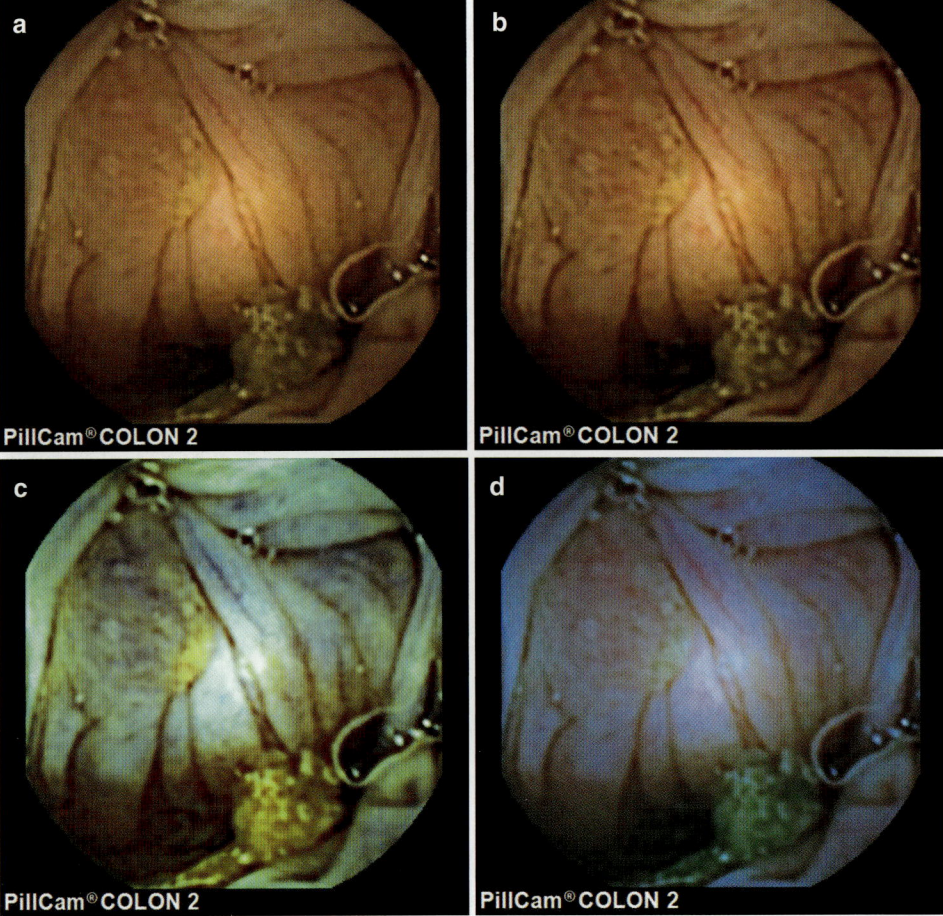

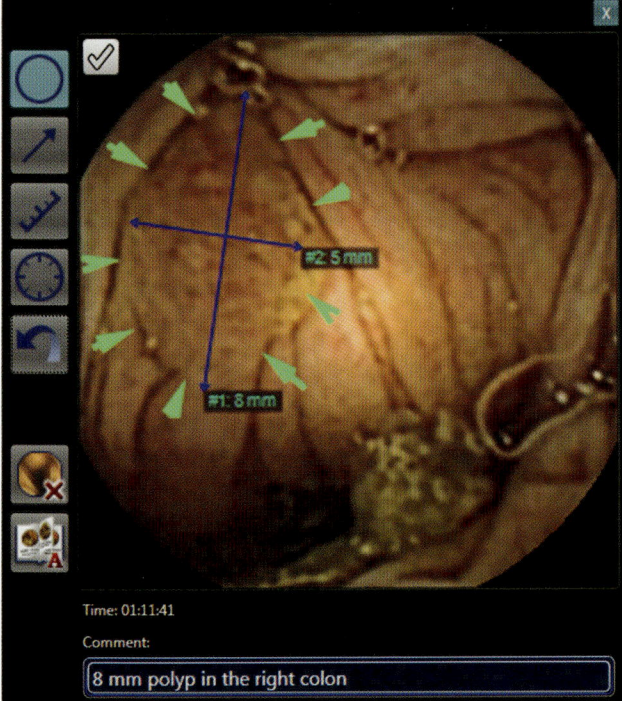

Fig. 5.12 Editing of thumbnail with the software tool for polyp size stimation (PSE; *blue arrows*) and manual delineation of the borders of the polyp (*green arrowheads*)

beginner, a bulge created by another loop of bowel overlying the loop being inspected can be mistaken for a submucosal lesion. Overlying loops or adjacent organs (Fig. 5.14) can be suspected when the indentation moves with peristalsis, indicating its softness. On the other hand, several visual cues attest to the presence of a submucosal lesion:

- Stretched or lobulated mucosa (Fig. 5.15d)
- Bridging folds (Fig. 5.15f)
- Central umbilication (Fig. 5.15b)
- Surface ulcerations (Fig. 5.15c)
- Villous alterations on surface (Fig. 5.15a)

Capsule images can clearly show the stretching of the mucosa as well as mucosal edema. A smooth, protruding lesion index on capsule endoscopy (SPICE) has been evaluated [34], based on ill-defined boundary, a diameter larger than its height, lumen filling, and visibility for less than 10 min. On the other hand, a scoring system for a mass lesion has been suggested, using the terms *bleeding, mucosal disruption, irregular surface, color,* and *white villi* [35].

Lymphangiectatic cysts typically appear softer, with yellow color shining through the mucosa above the entire mass, visible vessels on the surface, and sometimes whitish villi on their surface differentiating them from other solid submucosal tumors (Fig. 5.16b).

Fig. 5.13 Cleanliness levels.
(**a**) Excellent. (**b**) Good. (**c**) Fair.
(**d**) Poor

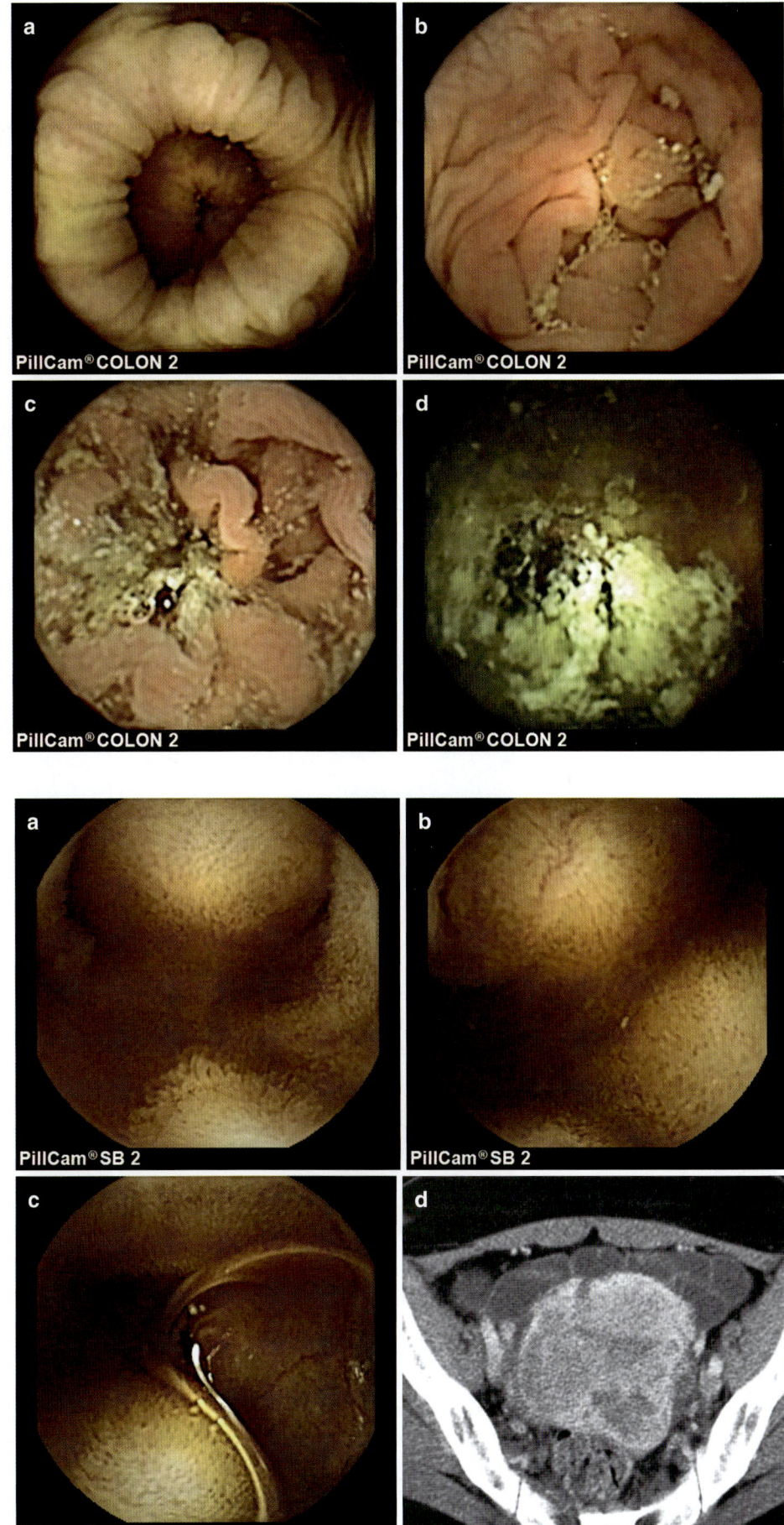

Fig. 5.14 (**a–c**) Bulges from
adjacent enlarged myomatous uterus
with normal mucosa and normal villi.
(**d**) Corresponding CT scan
(Courtesy of Roman Fischbach, MD)

Fig. 5.15 (**a**) Altered villi on surface. (**b**) Central umbilication. (**c**) Surface ulceration. (**d**) Lobulated and stretched mucosa. (**e**) Thickened fold. (**f**) Bridging folds come up to but not across the bulge

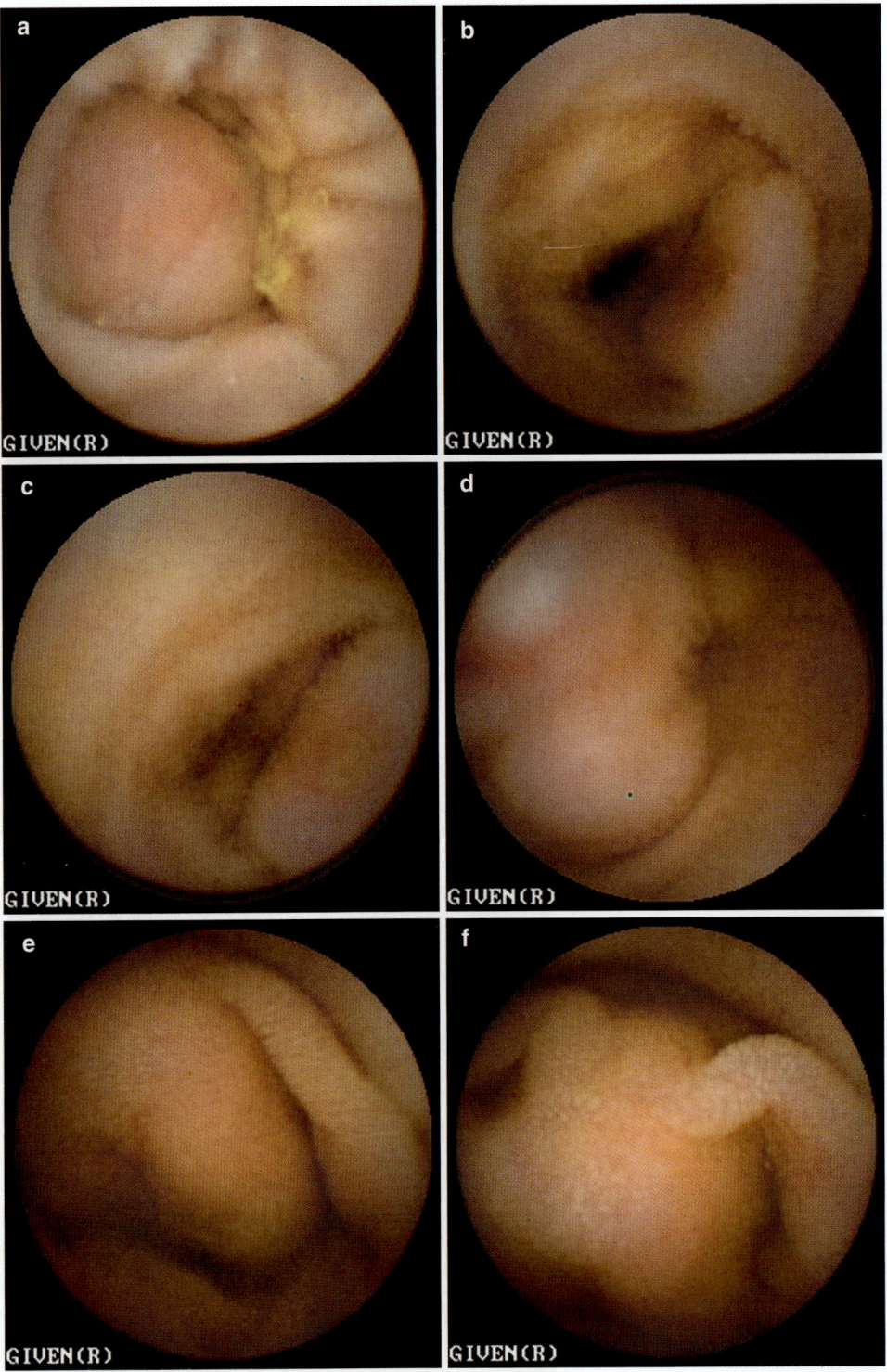

Overillumination may jeopardize visualization of the mucosa (Fig. 5.17a). If information on the patient's history and the capsule procedure is incomplete, interpretation of images with light from a flexible endoscope (Fig. 5.17b) may be challenging. Dark bile (Fig. 5.18a) is another situation that can be difficult for the beginning reader, who can mistake bile for dark blood. This error is avoided by examining the mucosa beyond the stained area to look for "coffee grounds" (Fig. 5.18b) or bloody material (Fig. 5.18c, d). Their absence indicates likely bile proximally. Air bubbles create light reflection and can give the false impression of absent villi (Fig. 5.19), and floating debris may resemble ulceration (Fig. 5.20). White lines on the edges of folds are a normal finding (Fig. 5.21).

Fig. 5.16 (**a**) Carcinoid (courtesy of Andre Van Gossum, MD). (**b**) Cystic lymphangiectasia

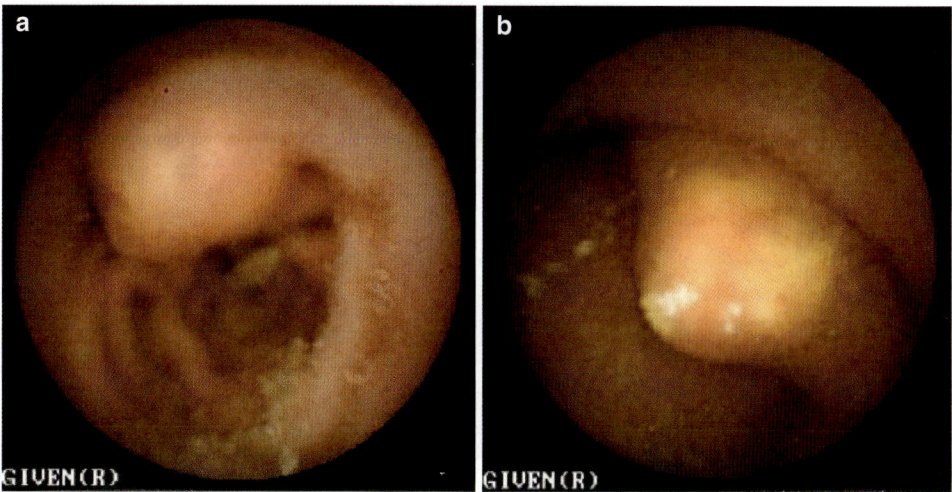

Fig. 5.17 (**a**) Overillumination. (**b**) Endoscope light as seen during endoscopic deployment of the capsule to the duodenum

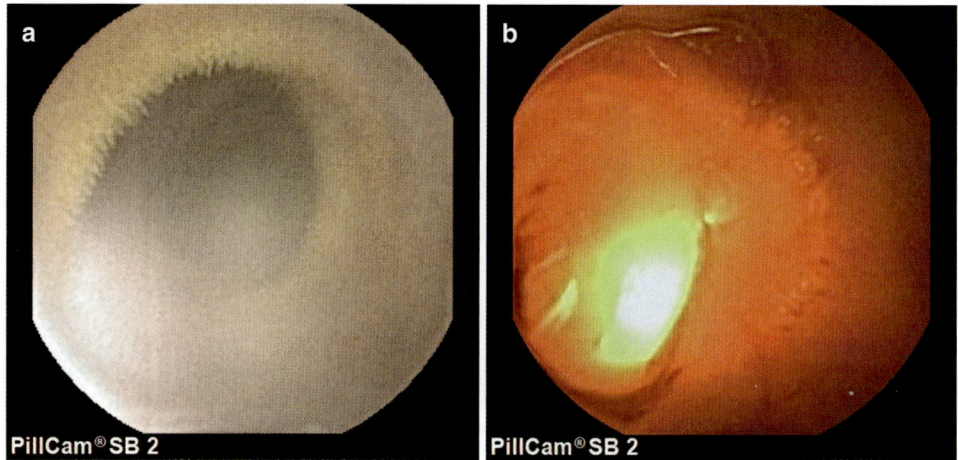

Fig. 5.18 Limitations of visualization: dark bile (**a**), coffee grounds (**b**), dark blood (**c**), fresh blood (**d**)

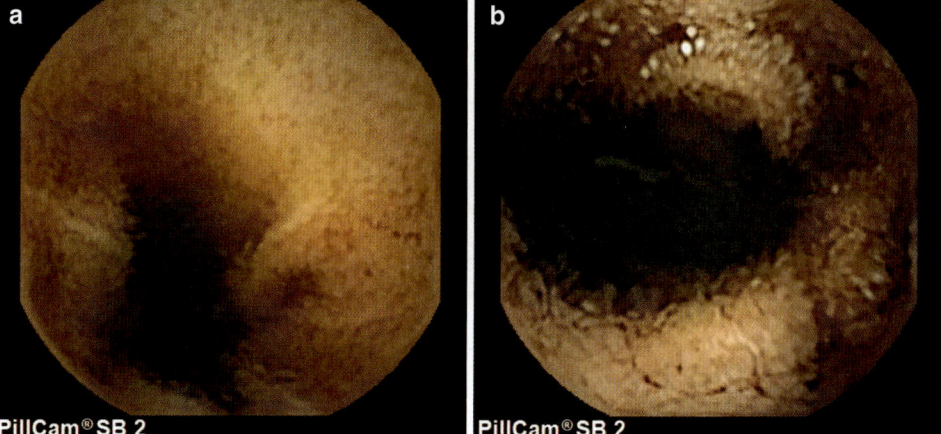

Fig. 5.18 (continued)

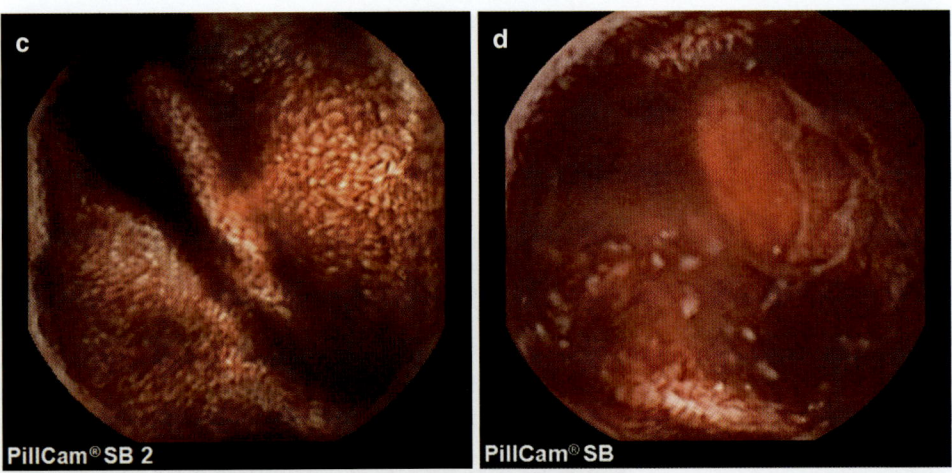

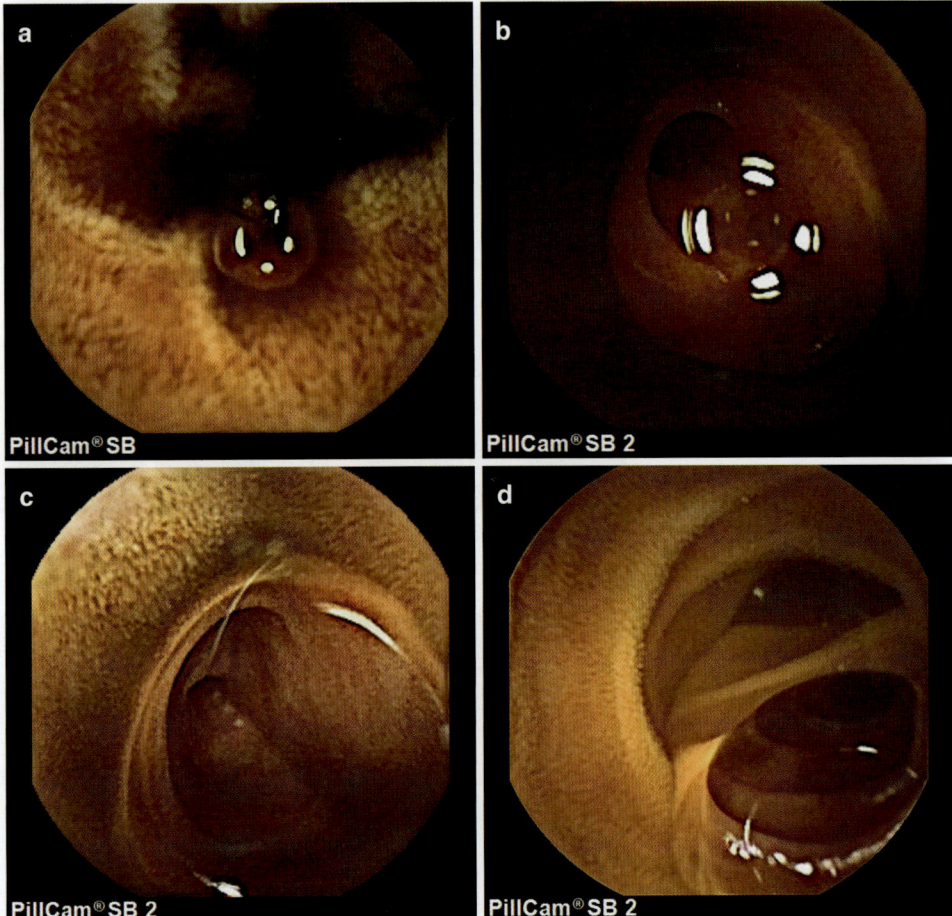

Fig. 5.19 Air bubbles create light reflection and can give a false impression of either a mass (**a**), discoloration of the mucosa (**b**), absent villi (**c**), or a second lumen (**d**). Reflection of the LEDs of the video capsule at the surface of an air bubble is seen in various shapes and sizes

Fig. 5.20 (**a**) Possible ulcer? (**b**) Floating debris, normal mucosa

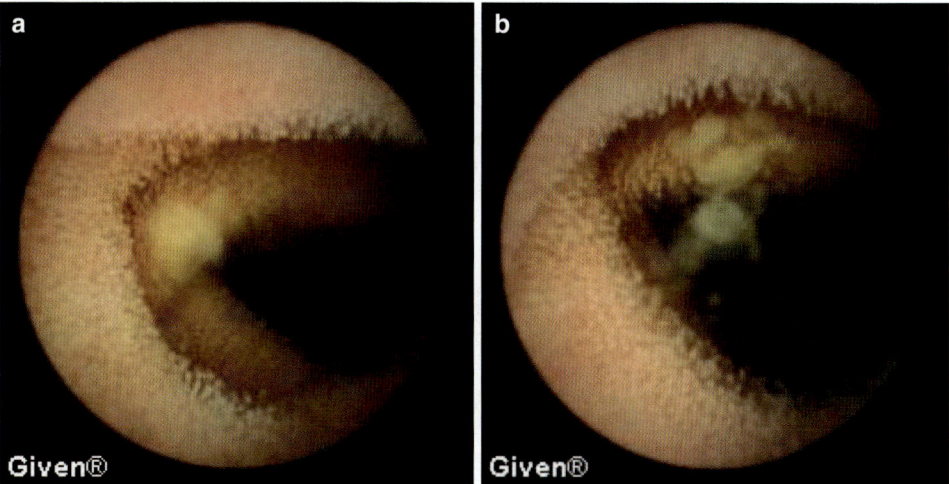

Fig. 5.21 (**a**, **b**) White lines are a normal finding

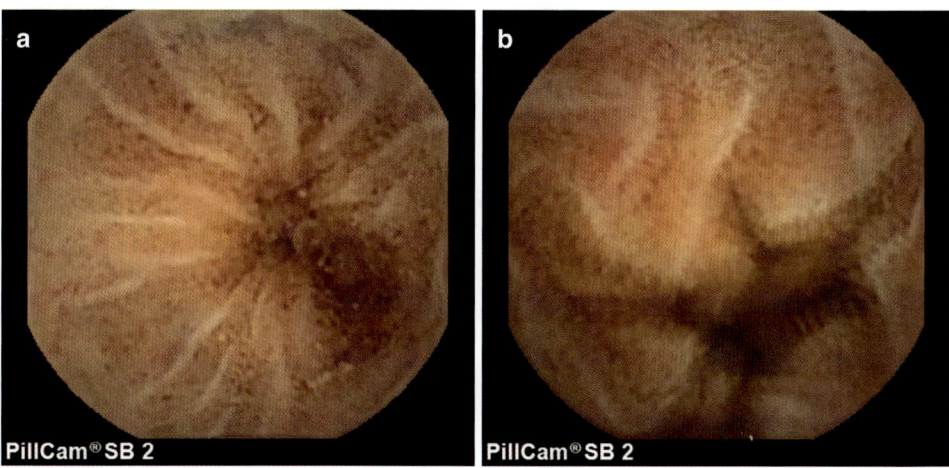

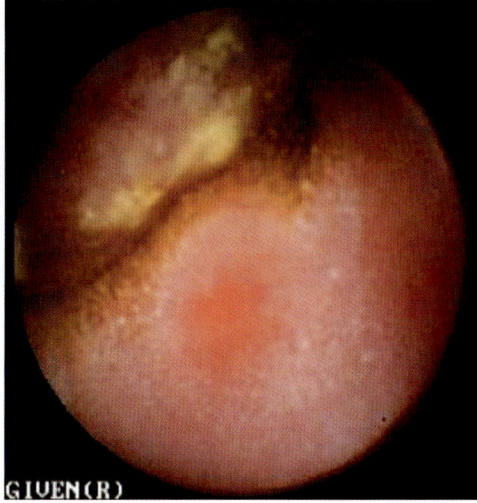

Fig. 5.22 Mucosa touching the optical dome of the capsule endoscope resembles a red spot. The finding—a tumor—is in the left top corner

Mucosa touching the optical dome of the capsule endoscope can resemble a red spot (Fig. 5.22). Red lesions are easily diagnosed as angiectasias, if they are sharply demarcated and of bright red color (Fig. 5.23a). Other red spots can be diffuse, multiple, shallow, or petechia-like (Fig. 5.23). In these patients, additional findings at VCE, such as ulcers, masses, and fibrosis (along with knowledge of clinical history), may be necessary to make a presumptive diagnosis. Definitive diagnosis may warrant histological confirmation.

White lesions are mainly related to villi. Hence, characterization of white lesions should consider the morphology of villi, as enlarged in lymphangiectasia (Fig. 5.24b) or totally or partially absent in villous atrophy (Fig. 5.24c). Duodenal adenomas are typically whitish and resemble a villous structure, but no single villus can be differentiated (Fig. 5.24d).

Capsule endoscopy is a new field of endoscopy, but it is nevertheless endoscopy. Experience gained through standard endoscopy is invaluable in the identification and interpretation of abnormalities. This image atlas is intended to aid in this interpretation.

Fig. 5.23 Red spots. (**a**) Sharply demarcated angiectasia with bright red color. (**b**) Shallow reddening with discrete mucosal fibrosis in radiation enteritis. (**c**) Infiltrating carcinoid with multiple petechial red spots. (**d**) Diffuse shallow reddening in enteropathy related to the use of nonsteroidal anti-inflammatory drugs (NSAIDs)

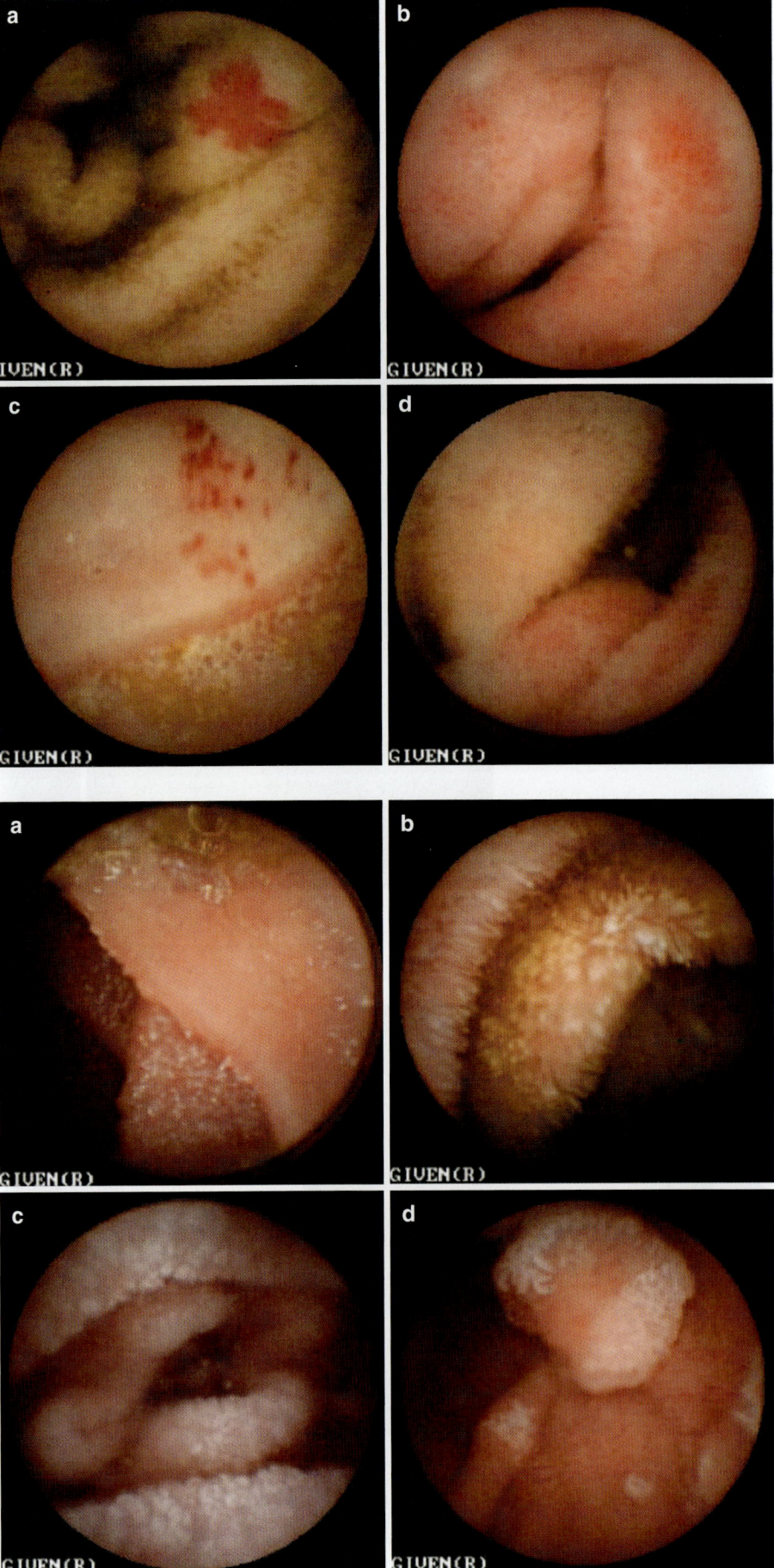

Fig. 5.24 White spots. (**a**) Dry mucosa with reflection artifacts. (**b**) White villi in genuine lymphangiectasia. (**c**) Villous atrophy with whitish remnants of villi. (**d**) Slightly elevated multifocal duodenal adenoma with gyriform appearance

References

1. Ben-Soussan E, Lecleire S, Ramirez S. Is there a way to improve reading performance of wireless capsule by the Multi-view System using maximal speed? Gastrointest Endosc. 2004;59:AB174.
2. Lewis B, Swain P. Capsule endoscopy in the evaluation of patients with suspected small intestinal bleeding: results of a pilot study. Gastrointest Endosc. 2002;56:39–43.
3. Ell C, Remke S, May A, et al. The first prospective controlled trial comparing wireless capsule endoscopy with push enteroscopy in chronic gastrointestinal bleeding. Endoscopy. 2002;34:685–9.
4. Costamagna G, Shah S, Riccioni M, et al. A prospective trial comparing small bowel radiographs and video capsule endoscopy for suspected small bowel disease. Gastroenterology. 2002;123:999–1005.
5. Fleischer D. Capsule endoscopy: the voyage is fantastic–will it change what we do? Gastrointest Endosc. 2002;56:452–6.
6. Kyriakos N, Karagiannis S, Galanis P, et al. Evaluation of four time-saving methods of reading capsule endoscopy videos. Eur J Gastroenterol Hepatol. 2012;24:1276–80.
7. Saurin JC, Lapalus MG, Cholet F, et al. Can we shorten the small-bowel capsule reading time with the "Quick-view" image detection system? Dig Liver Dis. 2012;44:477–81.
8. Subramanian V, Mannath J, Telakis E, et al. Efficacy of new playback functions at reducing small-bowel wireless capsule endoscopy reading times. Dig Dis Sci. 2012;57:1624–8.
9. Petty W, Kremer M, Biddle C. A synthesis of the Australian Patient Safety Foundation Anesthesia Incident Monitoring Study, the American Society of Anesthesiologists Closed Claims Project, and the American Association of Nurse Anesthetists Closed Claims Study. AANA J. 2002;70:193–202.
10. Lavine R, Sibert J, Gokturk M, Dickens B. Eye-tracking measures and human performance in a vigilance task. Aviat Space Environ Med. 2002;73:367–72.
11. Galinsky T, Rosa R, Warm J, Dember W. Psychophysical determinants in sustained attention. Hum Factors. 1993;35:603–14.
12. Becker A, Warm J, Dember W, Hancock P. Effects of jet engine noise and performance feedback on perceived workload in a monitoring task. Int J Aviat Psychol. 1995;5:49–62.
13. Palinkas L. Mental and cognitive performance in the cold. Int J Circumpolar Health. 2001;60:430–9.
14. Lieberman H, Falco C, Slade S. Carbohydrate administration during a day of sustained aerobic activity improves vigilance. Am J Clin Nutr. 2002;76:120–7.
15. Lane J, Phillips-Bute B. Caffeine deprivation affects vigilance performance and mood. Physiol Behav. 1998;65:171–5.
16. Lewis BS. How to read wireless capsule endoscopic images: tips of the trade. Gastrointest Endosc Clin N Am. 2004;14:11–6.
17. D'Halluin PN, Delvaux M, Lapalus MG, et al. Does the "Suspected Blood Indicator" improve the detection of bleeding lesions by capsule endoscopy? Gastrointest Endosc. 2005;61:243–9.
18. Buscaglia JM, Giday SA, Kantsevoy SV, et al. Performance characteristics of the suspected blood indicator feature in capsule endoscopy according to indication for study. Clin Gastroenterol Hepatol. 2008;6:298–301.
19. Park SC, Chun HJ, Kim ES, et al. Sensitivity of the suspected blood indicator: an experimental study. World J Gastroenterol. 2012;18:4169–74.
20. Fischer D, Schreiber R, Levi D, Eliakim R. Capsule endoscopy: the localization system. Gastrointest Endosc Clin N Am. 2004;14:25–31.
21. Li X, Chen H, Dai J, et al. Predictive role of capsule endoscopy on the insertion route of double-balloon enteroscopy. Endoscopy. 2009;41:762–6.
22. Pohl J, Aschmoneit I, Schuhmann S, Ell C. Computed image modification for enhancement of small-bowel surface structures at video capsule endoscopy. Endoscopy. 2010;42:490–2.
23. Duque G, Almeida N, Figueiredo P, et al. Virtual chromoendoscopy can be a useful software tool in capsule endoscopy. Rev Esp Enferm Dig. 2012;104:231–6.
24. Gupta T, Ibrahim M, Deviere J, Van GA. Evaluation of Fujinon intelligent chromo endoscopy-assisted capsule endoscopy in patients with obscure gastroenterology bleeding. World J Gastroenterol. 2011;17:4590–5.
25. Matsumura T, Arai M, Sato T, et al. Efficacy of computed image modification of capsule endoscopy in patients with obscure gastrointestinal bleeding. World J Gastroint Endosc. 2012;4:421–8.
26. Nakamura M, Ohmiya N, Miyahara R, et al. Usefulness of flexible spectral imaging color enhancement (FICE) for the detection of angiodysplasia in the preview of capsule endoscopy. Hepatogastroenterology. 2012;59:1474–7.
27. Kobayashi Y, Watabe H, Yamada A, et al. Efficacy of flexible spectral imaging color enhancement on the detection of small intestinal diseases by capsule endoscopy. J Dig Dis. 2012;113:614–20.
28. Krystallis C, Koulaouzidis A, Douglas S, Plevris JN. Chromoendoscopy in small bowel capsule endoscopy: blue mode or Fuji intelligent colour enhancement? Dig Liver Dis. 2011;43:953–7.
29. Gralnek IM, Defranchis R, Seidman E, et al. Development of a capsule endoscopy scoring index for small bowel mucosal inflammatory change. Aliment Pharmacol Ther. 2008;27:146–54.
30. Koulaouzidis A, Douglas S, Plevris JN. Lewis score correlates more closely with fecal calprotectin than Capsule Endoscopy Crohn's Disease Activity Index. Dig Dis Sci. 2012;57:987–93.
31. Spada C, Hassan C, Munoz-Navas M, et al. Second-generation colon capsule endoscopy compared with colonoscopy. Gastrointest Endosc. 2011;74:581–9.
32. Leighton JA, Rex DK. A grading scale to evaluate colon cleansing for the PillCam COLON capsule: a reliability study. Endoscopy. 2011;43:123–7.
33. Van Weyenberg SJ, De Leest HT, Mulder CJ. Description of a novel grading system to assess the quality of bowel preparation in video capsule endoscopy. Endoscopy. 2011;43:406–11.
34. Girelli CM, Porta P, Colombo E, et al. Development of a novel index to discriminate bulge from mass on small-bowel capsule endoscopy. Gastrointest Endosc. 2011;74:1067–74.
35. Shyung LR, Lin SC, Shih SC, et al. Proposed scoring system to determine small bowel mass lesions using capsule endoscopy. J Formos Med Assoc. 2009;108:533–8.

Education and Training in Video Capsule Endoscopy

6

Carolyn Davison and Reena Sidhu

Contents

In most countries around the world, structured training is in place for standard gastrointestinal (GI) endoscopic procedures. Despite an exponential growth worldwide in the use of video capsule endoscopy (VCE), a standardised infrastructure for training in VCE and accepted credentials for physicians who provide this service are yet to be established. With such rapid expansion in uptake of this modality comes the inherent need to develop diagnostic knowledge, skill and competence assessments [1]. In Europe, training in VCE is not a mandatory requirement of specialist training; many trainees receive no training at all in this field, and access to services and in-house training is not universal [2]. This chapter provides an overview of training issues for both the trainer and trainee, with consideration of what we need to train, how to train, whom to train and how to assess competence.

6.1   Content of Video Capsule Endoscopy Training

In contrast to standard endoscopy training, which focuses predominantly on technical competence, training in VCE requires a cognitive skill set based more on observation and interpretation of significant findings from computer images [1]. As well as understanding the indications, risks and limitations of the procedure, the competent video capsule endoscopist should be able to effectively maximise visualisation of the small bowel, accurately identify and diagnose pathology and apply appropriate management advice [3].

Assuming a sound baseline knowledge of GI anatomy and physiology, the core content of VCE training broadly covers three key areas: clinical application of VCE in practice, technical training and lesion recognition and interpretation. Recently, attempts to standardise the content of training have led to the development of core curricula. A small bowel endoscopy core curriculum recently published by the American Society of Gastrointestinal Endoscopy (ASGE) Training Committee provides recom-

The work was first published in 2006 by Springer Medizin Verlag Heidelberg with the following title: *Atlas of Video Capsule Endoscopy*.

C. Davison (✉)
Department of GI Services, South Tyneside NHS
Foundation Trust, Tyne and Wear, UK
e-mail: carolyn.davison@stft.nhs.uk

R. Sidhu
Gastroenterology and Liver Unit, Royal Hallamshire Hospital,
Sheffield, UK
e-mail: reena_sidhu@yahoo.com

Table 6.1 Overview of a core video capsule endoscopy training curriculum

Learning outcome	Content	Trainee group
Technology		
Knowledge and competent handling of the video capsule system, software functionality and accessories	Technical specifications, performance characteristics of system components:	1. VC endoscopist
	Video capsules	2. Nursing staff performing the procedure
	Sensor array/wearable antennas	
	Data recorder, real-time viewing	
	Workstation, software, network application	
	Patency capsule and scanner	
Assessment and consent		
Appropriately assess, select and consent patients for procedure, identify risk, recognise and manage special needs	Indications, fields of application, alternatives	1. VC endoscopist
	Absolute and relative contraindications	
	Capsule retention, risk reduction strategies	
	Special needs requiring modification of the procedure, including the critically ill, swallowing disorder, impaired motility	
	Endoscopic placement	
	Consent issues	
Procedure		
Understand requirements for preparation and perform procedure (video capsule and patency)	Patient preparation:	1. VC endoscopist
	Dietary/fasting, bowel purgatives, prokinetics, antifoaming agent	2. Nursing staff performing the procedure
	Management of comorbidity	
	Video capsule procedure, video download	
	Patency capsule procedure	
	Complications	
	Patient discharge	
(Pre)Reading		
Navigate software to read videos, recognise a normal study, detect and save abnormal and clinically relevant findings	Software functionality	1. VC endoscopist
	Practical methods of reading and image analysis	2. Reader extender
	Anatomical landmarks, variants of normal	
	Normal VCE mucosal appearances	
	Pathological findings, clinical relevance	
Reporting and diagnosis		
Accurately document findings, including clinical relevance, with integration of findings into management plans	Interpretation of abnormal findings	1. VC endoscopist
	Report components	
	VCE standard terminology	
	Integration of VCE findings in deriving an endoscopic diagnosis	
	Recommendations to direct patient management	

VCE video capsule endoscopy

mendations for training, intended for use by endoscopy training directors, endoscopy trainers and trainees [3]. In Europe and the United Kingdom, a similar curriculum is in the process of being formalised with European and British societies. An overview of the syllabus content of a core curriculum and relevant trainee groups is outlined in Table 6.1. This table illustrates a comprehensive training approach, but various modules can be selectively targeted to relevant trainee groups depending on their role within the capsule endoscopy pathway, including paramedical staff who also use equipment and undertake the procedure.

6.2 Methods of Training in Video Capsule Endoscopy

Numerous studies have examined different methods of training in conventional GI endoscopy [4–7]. Few studies have addressed how best to train in VCE [1]. In the past few years, however, there have been a number of advances in training methods, including the development of short courses, Web-based learning, case-based DVDs and supplemental learning resources such as clinical atlases and books.

Historically, technical training was provided by VCE suppliers, with no formal clinical training available. Systematic short courses soon followed, providing practical, computer-based training. Developed by hospital organisations and endorsed by gastroenterology societies in Europe and the United States, beginner courses were designed to provide

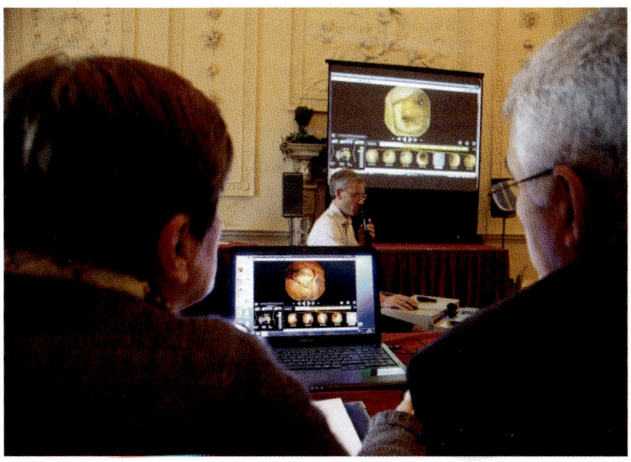

Fig. 6.1 Hands-on training at national video capsule endoscopy (VCE) course, United Kingdom

training in the application of VCE in clinical practice, use of the computer software and recognition and interpretation of small bowel pathology. The basic principles of each course include hands on training, with a significant amount of time allocated to hands-on training using a computer workstation shared between a maximum of three people to study a wide range of real cases and case sequences (Fig. 6.1). Topics covered in the beginner course include the practical use of the equipment, patient management, anatomical landmarks, normal variants and common pathology including mid-gastrointestinal bleeding and associated pathology, inflammatory lesions and tumorous lesions. Clinical cases are categorised according to pathology type. Pathology type has an important bearing on diagnostic accuracy, with agreement for inflammatory lesions or polyps being lower than for bleeding lesions [8, 9]. Polyp detection and accurate estimation of lesion size present a particular learning challenge for trainees. Larger polyps, which are the most clinically relevant, tend to be the least accurately sized even by VCE experts [10]. Another study [11] which used round discs of different sizes in an animal gut visualised by capsule endoscopy found that they were also systematically undersized by both students and experts (Fig. 6.2).

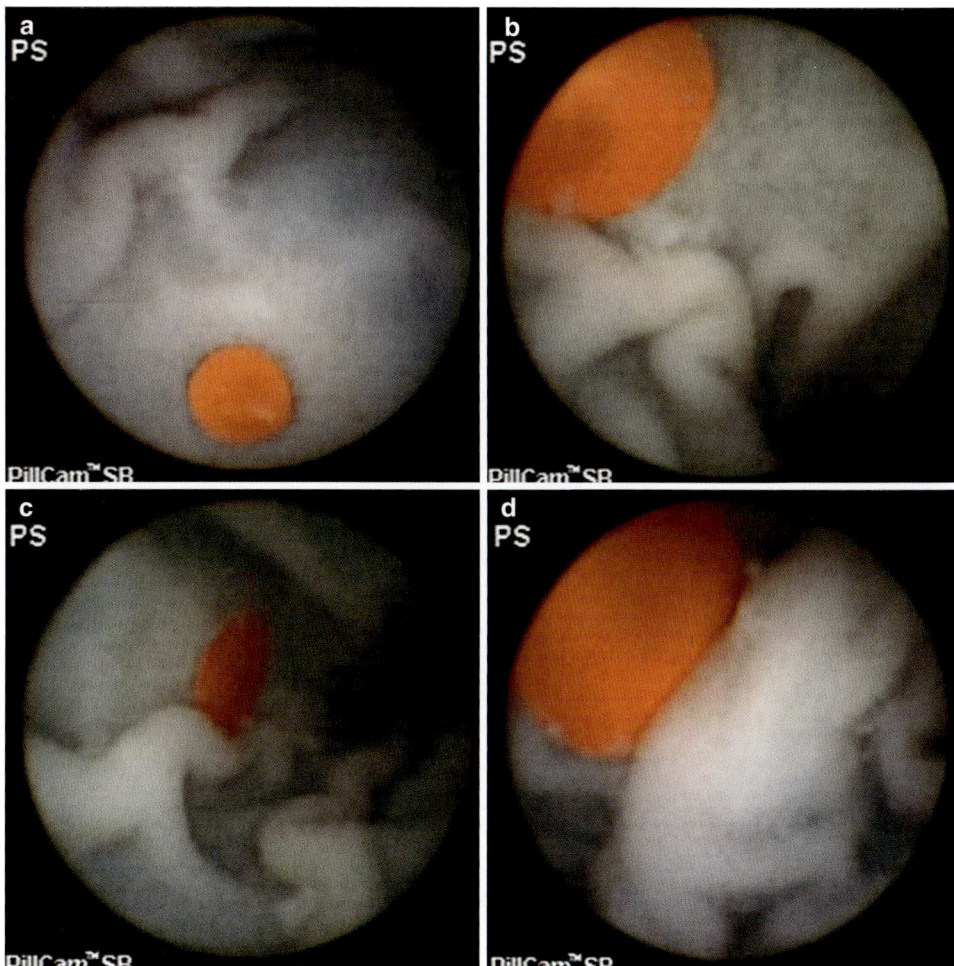

Fig. 6.2 Animal model capsule endoscopy image using red discs to estimate accuracy of lesion sizing: (**a**) 2 mm; (**b**) 8 mm; (**c**) 6 mm distant view; (**d**) 6 mm close-up view (Courtesy of Florian Graepler, MD)

However, experts with experience of more than 400 capsule endoscopy studies tended to be more precise, suggesting a learning curve even after performing many examinations. The issues raised by these studies have important implications for trainers and have helped to shape course content to address these specific skill training needs.

The positive effect of VCE courses on learning has been demonstrated in data collated from several European courses [12]. A significant improvement was shown in the ability of delegates to classify the type and relevance of small bowel findings, either pathology or variants of normal, following completion of a 1-day beginner course. Such educational benefits have been recognised by some societies, who recommend that completion of a "hands-on" course, in addition to supervised video reporting, should be a minimum requirement for those training outside a GI fellowship [3, 13, 14].

As experience with VCE has increased, so has demand for training at a higher level, resulting in the evolution of advanced short courses. Now available in several countries, these courses are designed to address the training needs of established users, with an emphasis on advancing interpretation skills and the application of these skills to improve clinical outcomes. Some European advanced programmes also include training in oesophageal and colon VCE. In the United States, advanced VCE training has moved away from the hands-on approach, eliminating the use of computer workstations. Programme content is more disease-specific, with expansion of group case-based discussion training methods.

An example of the topics covered by both beginner and advanced courses in the United Kingdom is tabulated in Table 6.2.

Web-based VCE learning is now also emerging. As a training method, Web-based learning is becoming an important addition to the medical education armoury, providing universal access to a wide range of resources that can easily be updated and enabling the learner to control the content, time and place of learning [15]. The knowledge gains of VCE Web-based interventions have been documented. A study has shown that trainees demonstrate significant improvement in lesion-recognition skills after completion of a dedicated computer-based training module (Fig. 6.3) which consisted of video clips of normal anatomical appearances, incidental and pathological findings, learning objectives and integrated feedback within multiple-choice questions [16]. In some countries where formal VCE courses are not yet established, E-learning has higher prominence as a supplemental training method. In Japan, for example, an E-learning system developed by a VCE manufacturing company has recently been licensed for physician education by the Japanese Association for Capsule Endoscopy (www.ce-learning.jp; available only in the Japanese language).

Alongside the ongoing evolution of structured electronic training programmes, the scope of E-learning has extended to

Table 6.2 Example of structured short VCE course programme in the United Kingdom

Beginner course programme (1 day)
Hands-on part 1: Using the software system
How to perform VCE
How to read and report a capsule study
Hands-on part 2: Anatomical landmarks
Patient selection and screening
Hands-on part 3: Common pathology (bleeding, inflammation, tumours)
Capsule retention and the patency system
VCE in special situations
Hands-on part 4: Grey cases, faculty and participant case studies
Advanced course programme (1 day)
Hands-on part 1: Variants of normal, look-alikes
Role of small bowel imaging in the CE era
Hands-on part 2: Unusual and rare findings, posttreatment images, incidental
Hot interpretation: faculty cases
Small bowel enteroscopy
Capsule imaging of oesophagus and colon: evidence and practicalities
Hands-on part 3: Colon capsule reading
Clinical outcomes and patient management

VCE video capsule endoscopy

other learning resources, which include online image atlases and capsule endoscopy clubs such as CapsuleEndoscopy.org (Fig. 6.4), which offer grand rounds, video webinars, discussion forums and electronic newsletter updates. Traditional study material is also available. A number of books have been published [17–20], some with accompanying DVDs with video clips [18, 19]. Published topics to date include an overview of the modality, its clinical application in practice and atlas image collections, providing the reader with a comprehensive library of common and rare pathological images, which are correlated with other imaging methods and histology.

6.3 Assessing Competence

To document competent practice, the starting point is to define measurable competency indicators and outcomes with the development of assessment processes. Currently, there are no universally accepted competency frameworks to support assessment of competence and certification of video capsule endoscopists. In the United States, the ASGE published credentialing guidelines, which recommended that training performed outside a GI fellowship should include completion of a hands-on course with a minimum of 8 h of continuing medical education, followed by a review of the first ten complete cases by a credentialed video capsule endoscopist [13]. The Korean Society of Gastrointestinal Endoscopy has

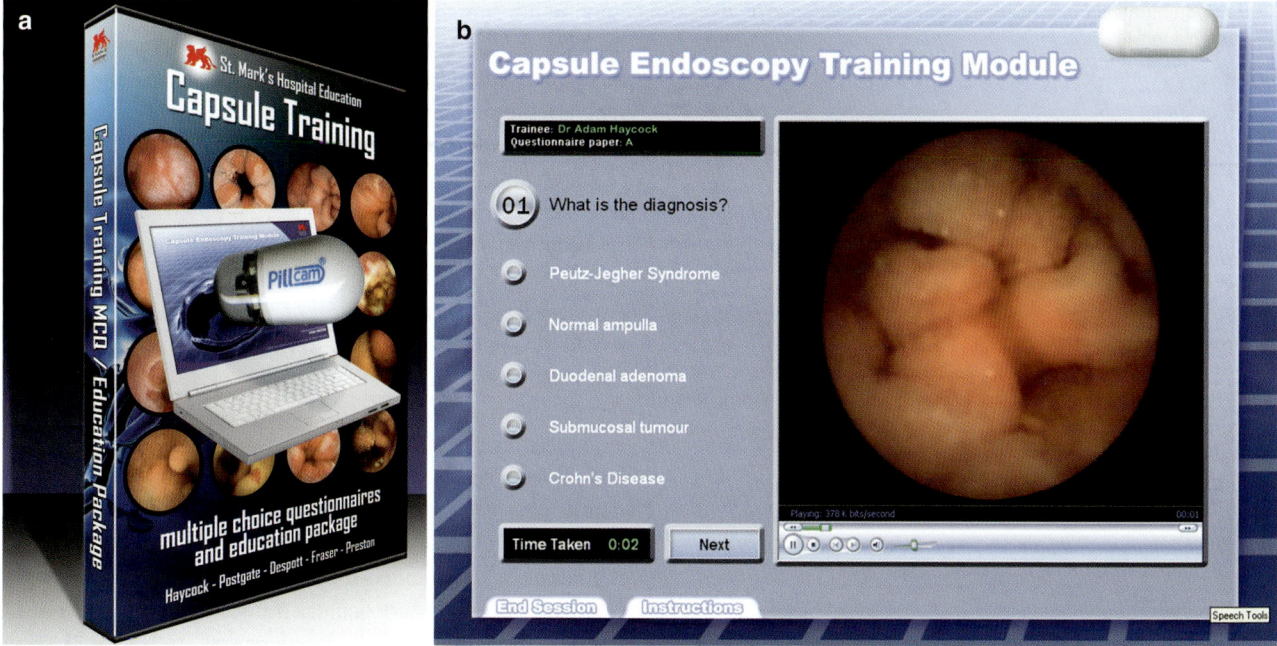

Fig. 6.3 (**a–b**) Computer-based training and evaluation module. (**a**) DVD application. (**b**) Sample assessment questions (Courtesy of Chris Fraser, MD)

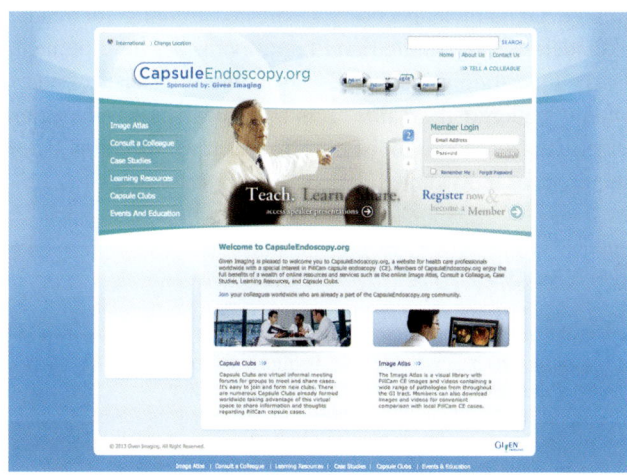

Fig. 6.4 Online learning resource www.capsuleendoscopy.org (Courtesy of Given Imaging Ltd.)

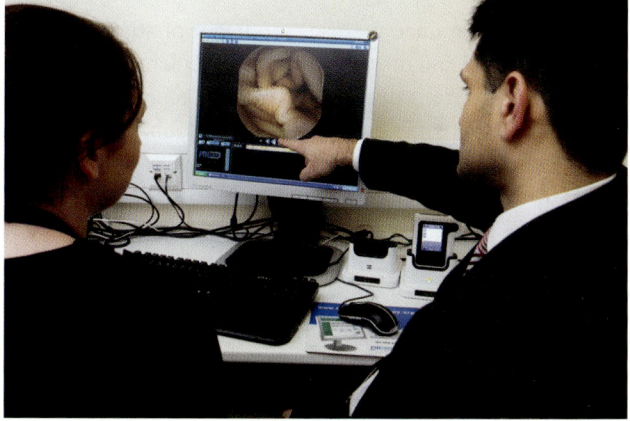

Fig. 6.5 Fellowship training in VCE

published similar guidelines with an increased threshold number of 20 studies [14]. For those training within a GI fellowship programme, the American Gastroenterology Core Curriculum Third Edition [21] defines 25 small bowel VCE studies as the minimum threshold for assessing competence. More recent recommendations provided by the ASGE Small Bowel Core Curriculum advise a minimum number of 20 supervised procedures (Fig. 6.5) to provide adequate experience for those intending to practise VCE independently [3]. There are currently no published European threshold recommendations. It is important to note, however, that proficiency

should be based on measurement of competence rather than on completion of an arbitrary number of studies.

There are currently no validated methods or tools to assess competence in VCE. Though competence in the technical aspects is readily achieved and demonstrable, assessment of cognitive competence in lesion recognition and interpretation is a more challenging process. The development of these skills and the trainee's progress should be regularly assessed during supervised video reading. This supervision process comprises three steps, with varying levels of intervention by the supervising trainer:

1. Direct: A short training period of reading studies with the trainer present, discussing findings [22]

Table 6.3 Summary of methods to assess achievement of VCE learning outcomes

Learning outcome	Assessment methods
Technology	
Knowledge and competent handling of the video capsule system, software functionality and accessories	Direct observation procedure Discussion
Assessment and consent	
Appropriately assess, select and consent patients for procedure, identify risk, recognise and manage special needs	Case-based discussion
Procedure	
Understand requirements for preparation and perform procedure (video capsule and patency capsule)	Direct observation procedure Case-based discussion
(Pre)Reading	
Navigate software to read videos, recognise a normal study, detect and save abnormal and clinically relevant findings	VCE reporting review Correlation rates (>90 %)
Reporting and diagnosis	
Accurately document findings including clinical relevance with integration of findings into management plans	Case-based discussion Formal test/examination

VCE video capsule endoscopy

2. Partial: The trainee prereads a number of studies, which are reviewed and discussed with the trainer
3. Distant: The trainee reads and reports a number of studies independently; these studies are then double-read by the trainer, with feedback provided [22]

Trainees should maintain a portfolio of their reading experience, documenting their findings and the degree of correlation of significant findings with a credentialed trainer. Tools to standardise the documentation process have been developed by some centres [23]. Once the trainee reaches a consistently high reporting correlation rate, competence may be summatively assessed. A 90 % or greater correlation rate has been advocated as a reasonable expectation [3, 22]. Assessment of competence at this stage should ideally combine a high rate of reporting correlation with a formal test of knowledge and skill. This could be an examination developed in-house [22] or using an electronic evaluation tool. A summary of assessment methods with corresponding learning outcomes is outlined in Table 6.3.

6.4 Training Needs of Nonphysician Reader Extenders

VCE reading was initially carried out only by physicians, but the increasing demand and time taken to read and report have led to the development of reader extenders [24]. Nurses are now being trained to preread capsule studies, marking thumbnails of relevant findings for further assessment by the physician. A number of published studies have demonstrated that although they are more likely to identify additional insignificant findings, nurses with different experience can reach a similar level of diagnostic accuracy to physicians in the detection of abnormal images [23, 25–31].

Within this role, different levels of skill and competence may be reached, depending on the scope of practice. At the simplest level, the acquisition of technical and basic cognitive skills enables the reader to preview the images, identify abnormalities and create nondescriptive thumbnails for physician review [24]. In the United Kingdom, some reader extenders have advanced their interpretation skills to a more advanced level of cognizance, enabling them to independently interpret the images and provide a capsule diagnosis [31]. Within other health economy models outside the United Kingdom, such extended scope of practice is unlikely.

Reader extenders are usually trained informally by physicians, with supplemental attendance at a structured short course. In the United Kingdom, 28 % of those attending short courses are nurses [32]. Many of these courses are multidisciplinary, but the content is physician-centric and does not fully meet the training needs of nurses who have a limited GI knowledge base. Dedicated training for reader extenders is very limited and requires further development. Until this training becomes available, reader extenders should undergo the same training processes as physician video capsule endoscopists, up to the level of competence required for individual practice.

References

1. Sidhu R, McAlindon ME, Davison C, et al. Training in capsule endoscopy: are we lagging behind? Gastroenterol Res Pract. 2012;2012:175248. doi:10.1155/2012/175248.
2. Sidhu R, Sakellariou P, McAlindon ME, et al. Is formal training necessary for capsule endoscopy? The largest gastroenterology trainee study with controls. Dig Liver Dis. 2008;40:298–302.
3. Rajan EA, Pais SA, Degregorio BT, et al. Small bowel endoscopy core curriculum. Gastrointest Endosc. 2013;77:1–6.
4. Shirai Y, Yoshida T, Shiraishi R, et al. Prospective randomised study on the use of a computer-based endoscopic simulator for training in esophagogastroduodenoscopy. J Gastroenterol Hepatol. 2008;23:1046–50.
5. Koch AD, Haringsma J, Schoon EJ, et al. A second-generation virtual reality simulator for colonoscopy: validation and initial experience. Endoscopy. 2008;40:735–8.
6. Rajan E, Prasad GA, Alexander JA, et al. Training in small-bowel capsule endoscopy: assessing and defining competency. Gastrointest Endosc. 2013;78:617–22.
7. Neumann M, Hahn C, Horbach T, et al. Score card endoscopy: a multicentre study to evaluate learning curves in 1 week courses using the Erlangen Endo-trainer. Endoscopy. 2003;35:515–20.
8. Pezzoli A, Cannizzaro R, Pennazio M, et al. Interobserver agreement in describing video capsule endoscopy findings: a multicentre prospective study. Dig Liver Dis. 2010;43:126–31.

9. De Leusse A, Landi B, Edery J, et al. Video capsule endoscopy for investigation of obscure gastrointestinal bleeding: feasibility, results, and interobserver agreement. Endoscopy. 2005; 37:617–21.

10. Postgate A, Tekkis P, Fitzpatrick A, et al. The impact of experience on polyp detection and sizing accuracy at capsule endoscopy: implications for training from an animal model study. Endoscopy. 2008;40:496–501.

11. Graepler F, Wolter M, Vonthein R, et al. Accuracy of the size estimation in wireless capsule endoscopy: calibrating the M2A PillCam (with video). Gastrointest Endosc. 2008;67:924–31.

12. Humbla O, McAlindon ME, Davison C, et al. Small bowel capsule endoscopy: improvement of diagnostic skills after basic hand-on training courses. Gut. 2012;61:AB266.

13. Faigel D, Baron TH, Adler DG, et al. ASGE guidelines: guidelines for credentialing and granting privileges for capsule endoscopy. Gastrointest Endosc. 2005;61:503–5.

14. Lim YJ, Moon JS, Chang DK, Gut Image Study Group. Guidelines for credentialing and granting privileges for capsule endoscopy. Korean J Gastrointest Endosc. 2008;37:393–402.

15. Chumley-Jones HS, Dobbie A, Alford CL. Web-based learning: sound educational method or hype? A review of the evaluation literature. Acad Med. 2002;77(10 Suppl):S86–93.

16. Postgate A, Haycock A, Thomas-Gibson S, et al. Computer-aided learning in capsule endoscopy leads to improvement in lesion recognition ability. Gastrointest Endosc. 2009;70:310–6.

17. Keuchel M, Hagenmüller F, Fleisher D. Atlas of video capsule endoscopy. Heidelberg: Springer; 2006.

18. Faigel D, Cave D. Capsule endoscopy. Philadelphia: Saunders, Elsevier; 2008.

19. De Franchis R, Lewis B, Mishkin D. Capsule endoscopy simplified. Thorofare: Slack; 2010.

20. Herrerias JM, Mascarenhas-Saraiva M. Atlas of capsule endoscopy 2. Sevilla: Sulime Diseño de Solutiones; 2012.

21. American Association for the Study of Liver Diseases; American College of Gastroenterology; American Gastroenterological Association (AGA) Institute; American Society for Gastrointestinal Endoscopy. The Gastroenterology Core Curriculum, Third Edition. Gastroenterology. 2007;132:2012–8.

22. Rajan E, Prasad GA, Alexander JA, et al. Teaching and assessing competence in small bowel capsule endoscopy during gastroenterology fellowship [abstract]. Gastrointest Endosc. 2011;73:AB413.

23. Brock AS, Freeman J, Roberts J, et al. A resource-efficient tool for training novices in wireless capsule endoscopy. Gastroenterol Nurs. 2012;35:317–21.

24. Davison C. Reader extender of capsule endoscopy. Tech Gastrointest Endosc. 2006;8:188–93.

25. Levinthal GN, Burke CA, Santisi JM. The accuracy of an endoscopy nurse in interpreting capsule endoscopy. Am J Gastroenterol. 2003;98:2669–71.

26. Niv Y, Niv G. Capsule endoscopy examination–preliminary review by a nurse. Dig Dis Sci. 2005;50:2121–4.

27. Bossa F, Cocomazzi G, Valvano MR, et al. Detection of abnormal lesions recorded by capsule endoscopy. A prospective study comparing endoscopist's and nurse's accuracy. Dig Liver Dis. 2006;38:599–602.

28. Caundeo Alvarez A, Garcia-Montes JM, Herrerias JM. Capsule endoscopy reviewed by a nurse: is it here to stay? Dig Liver Dis. 2006;38:603–4.

29. Sidhu R, Sanders DS, Kapur K, et al. Capsule endoscopy: is there a role for nurses as physician extenders? Gastroenterol Nurs. 2007;30:45–8.

30. Riphaus A, Richter S, Vonderach M, Wehrmann T. Capsule endoscopy interpretation by an endoscopy nurse – a comparative trial. Z Gastroenterol. 2009;47:273–6.

31. Drew K, Sidhu R, Sanders DS, et al. Blinded controlled trial comparing image recognition, diagnostic yield and management advice by doctor and nurse capsule endoscopists. Gut. 2011;60 Suppl 1:A195.

32. McAlindon M, Parker C, Hendy P, et al. Provision of service and training for small bowel endoscopy in the United Kingdom. Frontline Gastroenterol. 2012;3:98–103.

Swallowing and Motility Disorders, Pacemakers and Obesity

7

Dirk Bandorski, Martha H. Dirks, Ernest G. Seidman, and Martin Keuchel

Contents

The work was first published in 2006 by Springer Medizin Verlag Heidelberg with the following title: *Atlas of Video Capsule Endoscopy*.

D. Bandorski (✉)
Medical Clinic II, University Hospital of Giessen and Marburg, Giessen, Germany
e-mail: dirk.bandorski@hkw.med.uni-giessen.de

M.H. Dirks
Division of Gastroenterology, Hepatology and Nutrition, Hôpital Sainte-Justine, University of Montreal, Montreal, QC, Canada
e-mail: Martha.dirks.hsj@ssss.gouv.qc.ca

E.G. Seidman
McGill IBD Research Group, Digestivelab, Research Institute of McGill University Health Center, Montreal, QC, Canada
e-mail: ernest.seidman@mcgill.ca

M. Keuchel
Department of Internal Medicine, Bethesda Krankenhaus Bergedorf, Hamburg, Germany
e-mail: keuchel@bkb.info

7.1 Swallowing Disorders

Difficulties in swallowing the capsule are rarely encountered in adults. Nevertheless, any history of dysphagia or swallowing disorders should be elicited prior to capsule endoscopy [1]. Psychogenic or neurologic factors usually underlie a patient's inability or refusal to swallow the capsule. Oesophageal strictures, diverticula, webs or rings may be problematic. A history of previous surgery or radiotherapy involving the throat or oesophagus should also be elicited.

Children under the age of 8 are rarely able to swallow medication tablets, let alone the larger PillCam SB capsule (Given Imaging Ltd., Yoqneam, Israel), which measures 26.4 mm in length and 11 mm in diameter. This problem also may be encountered in older patients [2]. To preclude the loss of a capsule (the battery is activated upon removal of the capsule from its package), we recommend that patients should first be instructed to practice by swallowing candies [3]. It is worthwhile to have young patients demonstrate that they are capable of swallowing a similar-sized vitamin tablet or jelly bean before they undergo the test.

For individuals judged unable to swallow the capsule, or those with severe dysphagia or swallowing disorders, the study can be safely undertaken by introducing the capsule into the proximal duodenum endoscopically, under direct vision [3]. This goal can be accomplished by "front loading" the capsule on a gastroscope, holding it in place using a foreign-body retrieval net, a polyp retriever snare or a basket (Fig. 7.1). In our experience, the Roth net is more secure than using a snare. However, it may be difficult to open the net and release the capsule into the small space offered by the proximal duodenum in smaller children. When using a snare for such cases, it is advisable to place a variceal ligator band around the waist of the capsule, as shown in Fig. 7.1, in order to secure the capsule and prevent it from slipping off [3]. In all cases, it is advisable to employ endotracheal intubation to protect the patient's airway.

In adult patients, it has been suggested that the capsule be placed into the stomach endoscopically using an overtube (Fig. 7.2), using a polypectomy snare or a foreign-body retrieval net [4, 5]. Alternatively, others have reported simply placing the capsule into the overtube (Fig. 7.3) and pushing it forward into the stomach with the reinserted endoscope [6, 7]. However, this procedure entails the risk that the study will fail if the capsule remains in the stomach for a prolonged period, resulting in incomplete visualisation of the small bowel.

The same techniques of transferring the capsule endoscopically from the stomach into the duodenum can be

employed in patients with severe gastroparesis [3, 4]. In our experience, capsules may be retained in the stomach for prolonged periods in diabetics and in patients receiving medications that delay gastric emptying, such as narcotics. Directly preceding colonoscopy with sedation may prolong gastric transit time to several hours.

In a patient with a Zenker's diverticulum, endoscopic placement of the capsule has been described after insertion of the endoscope over a guidewire through the working channel. The capsule is held externally at the distal end by a polypectomy snare fixed on the outer surface of the endoscope [8].

More recently, a capsule delivery device (AdvanCE; US Endoscopy, Mentor, OH, USA) has been developed (Figs. 7.4 and 7.5). A special catheter containing a wire is inserted through the working channel of a standard gastroscope [9]. A plastic sheath prevents damage of the working channel by the thread at the distal end of the wire. Subsequently, the capsule holder is screwed onto the wire, and the capsule is pressed into the holder. The oesophagus can then be intubated, either blindly using this device pulled back to the scope or under direct vision if the device is pushed forward 1–2 cm. Once the duodenum is reached, the capsule is released by pulling the device's handle. Endoscopic visualisation has even been described using the capsule images displayed by a real-time viewer as guidance [10].

Endoscopic placement of the video capsule was necessary in 2 % of patients in a retrospective series [11].

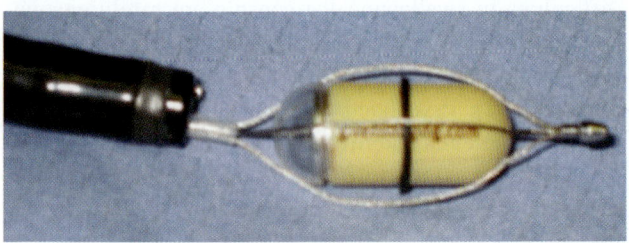

Fig. 7.1 Historic technique to "front load" a gastroscope in order to deliver the capsule endoscope directly into the duodenum in patients incapable of swallowing the device. A basket is used, with a variceal ligator placed around the waist of the capsule to secure it and prevent it from sliding out (Reprinted from Seidman et al. [3], with permission from Elsevier)

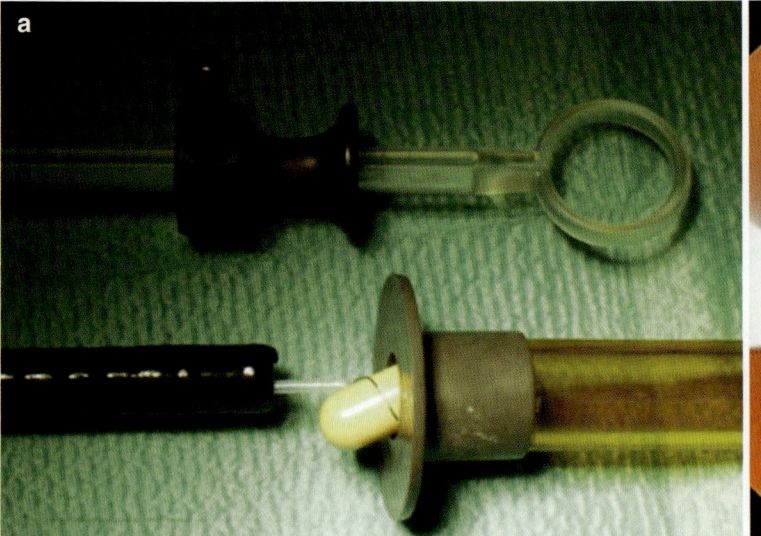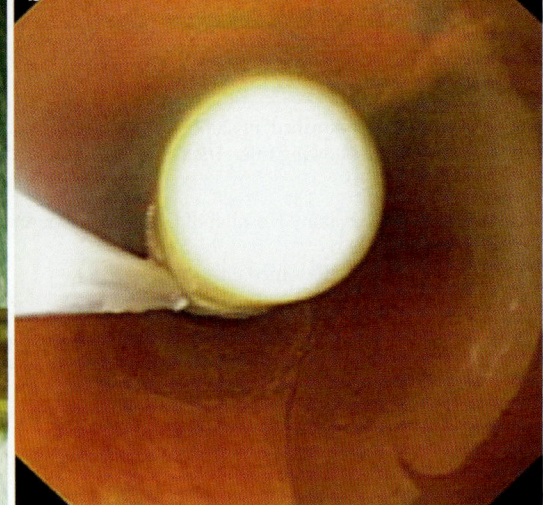

Fig. 7.2 The use of a multiuse overtube to insert the capsule into the stomach using a gastroscope. (**a**) Overtube (*right*) with inserted video capsule, held by a polypectomy snare inserted through a gastroscope (*left*) and the handle of the snare (*top*). (**b**) Endoscopic view of the capsule held by the snare at the distal end of the overtube, which is inserted into the oesophagus

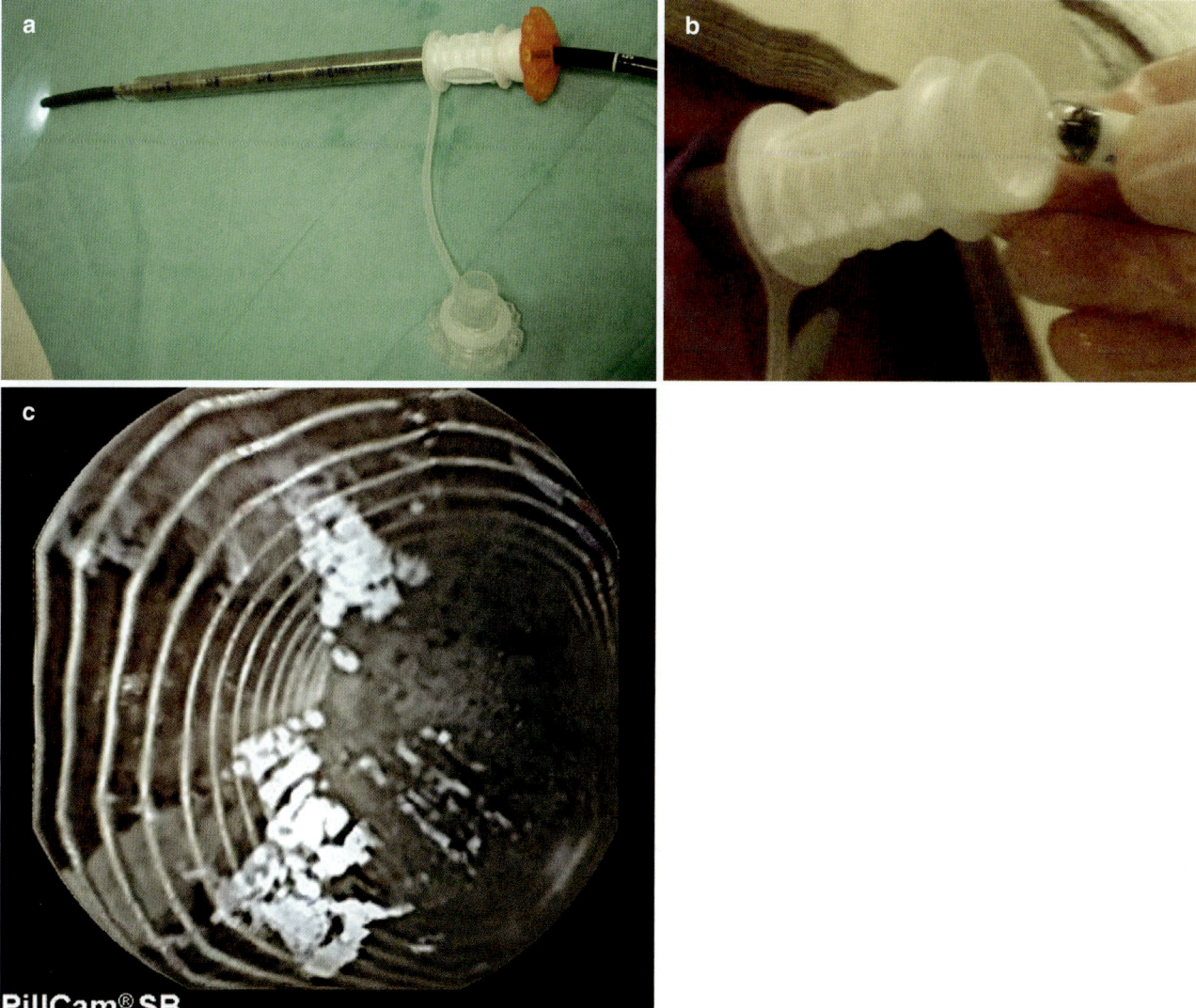

Fig. 7.3 (**a**) Single-use overtube loaded on a gastroscope. (**b**) After endoscopic positioning, the inner tube is removed to enlarge the available inner tube diameter, thus easily accommodating a capsule. (**c**) Video capsule endoscopy (VCE) view of the overtube

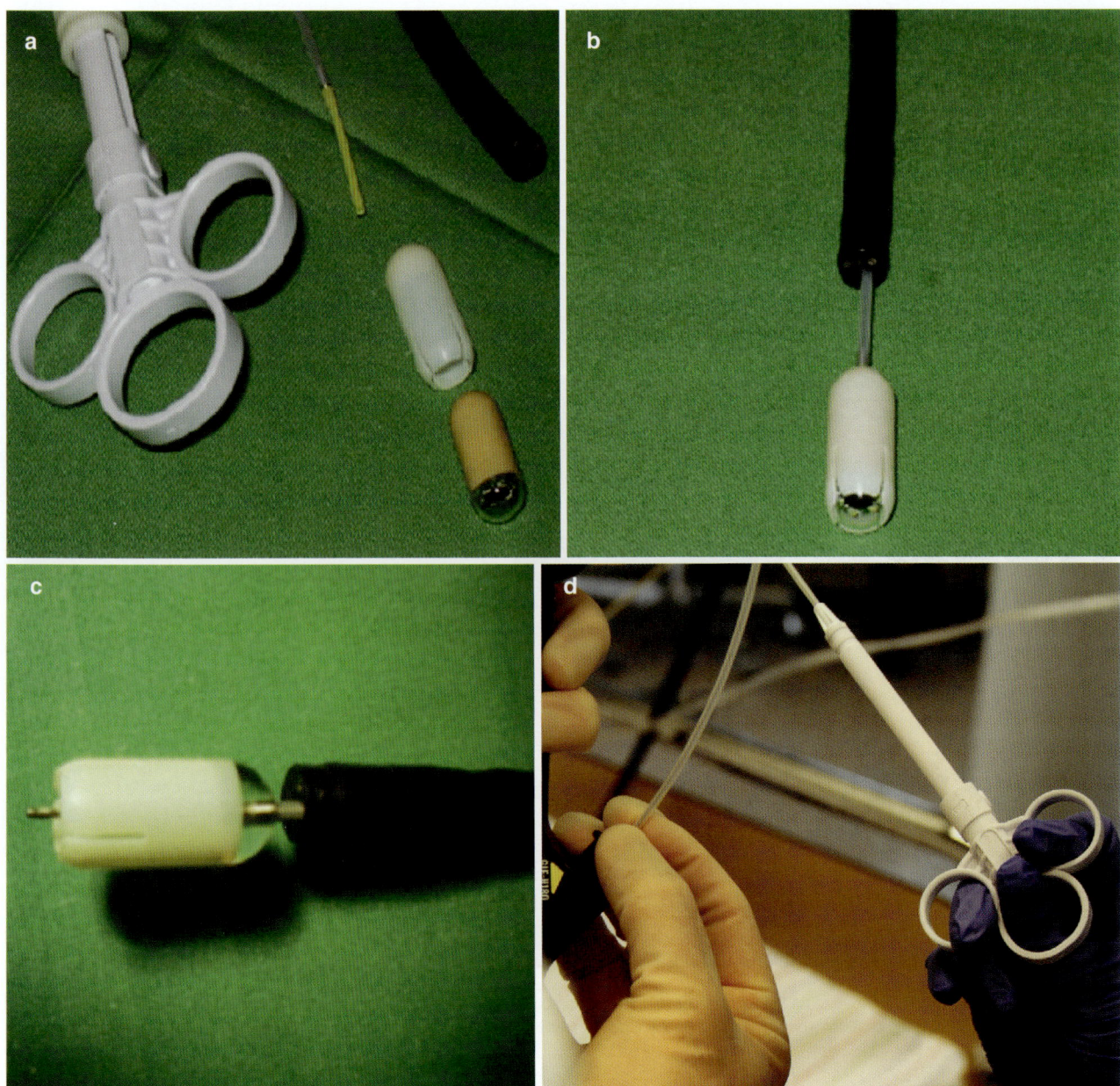

Fig. 7.4 Specific AdvanCE capsule delivery device. (**a**) Device prior to assembly. (**b**) Mounted device with capsule secured. (**c**, **d**) The capsule is released by pushing the inner wire forward using the handle

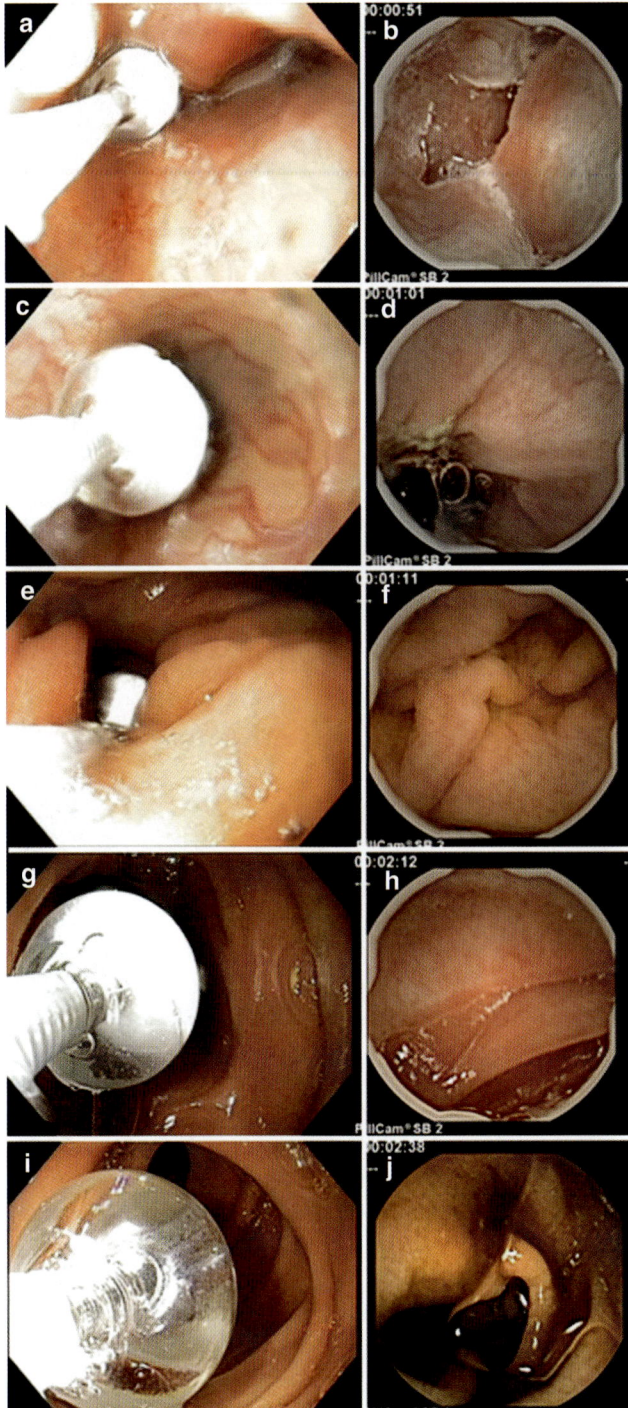

Fig. 7.5 Endoscopic placement of a capsule using the AdvanCE delivery device. Endoscopic images appear in the left column and the VCE view, in the right column. The capsule is introduced into the oesophagus under direct vision (**a, b**) and is advanced through the oesophagus (**c, d**) and the stomach to the second portion of the duodenum (**e, f**). The endoscope is straightened (**g, h**) and the capsule is released (**i, j**). Note that the white edge of the capsule holder, as seen by VCE, is no longer visible after the capsule has been released

Fig. 7.6 VCE images allowing localisation of the capsule by organ. (**a**) Small bowel. (**b**) Stomach. (**c**) Oesophagus. (**d**) Bronchi. (Courtesy of Simon Panter, MD)

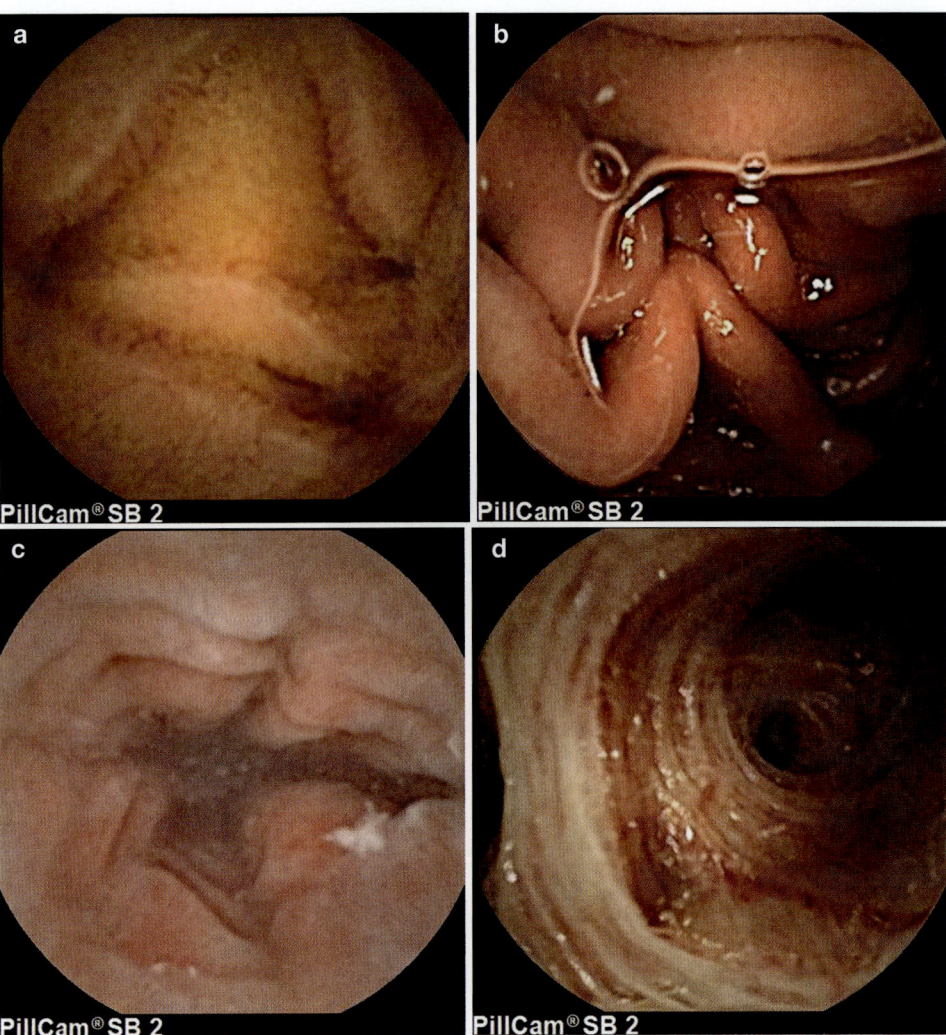

7.2 Gastric Motility Problems

All capsule systems using data transmission to an external recorder now come with a real-time viewer, which usually allows the actual position of the capsule to be localised to the oesophagus, stomach, small bowel or even bronchi by the endoscopic images (Fig. 7.6). Hence, the need for radiographs will be very limited. Capsules with data storage (Fig. 3.6) within the capsule do not provide this possibility.

A feasible approach is to watch the capsule images directly after swallowing. As oesophageal passage usually takes only seconds or a few minutes, visualisation of the stomach can easily exclude oesophageal retention or aspiration of the capsule. Because the newer capsules have markedly longer running times, some delay in gastric transit no longer necessarily influences the completeness of small bowel visualisation. Hence, it is not necessary to routinely administer prokinetic drugs to all patients before video capsule endoscopy (VCE).

Some patients, however, have extremely prolonged gastric transit time, up to several hours. Patients at risk are diabetics, those with known gastroparesis, those on narcotics, those who are immobilised and patients who swallow the capsule directly after a colonoscopy. In these patients, documentation of passage to the small bowel by real-time viewing is strongly advised. It is easy to check for passage of the capsule into the small bowel in all patients after approximately 1 h; most patients will then be able to leave the office and to drink clear liquids again.

If the capsule is still in the stomach after 1 h, a second real-time viewing can be done after another 30 min. If the capsule is still in the stomach, a prokinetic agent such as metoclopramide or domperidone can be administered. We have obtained good results by infusing erythromycin. An intravenous dose of 3 mg/kg has been proposed, based on gastric emptying studies in healthy subjects [12].

Because these approaches can result in considerable delays, however, we feel that a more effective option for

Fig. 7.7 Roth net used to grasp a swallowed capsule in the stomach in order to deposit it into the duodenum. (**a**) Capsule held securely with the Roth net. (**b**) Capsule view through the net. (**c**, **d**) Capsule has been manoeuvred into the duodenum and released there

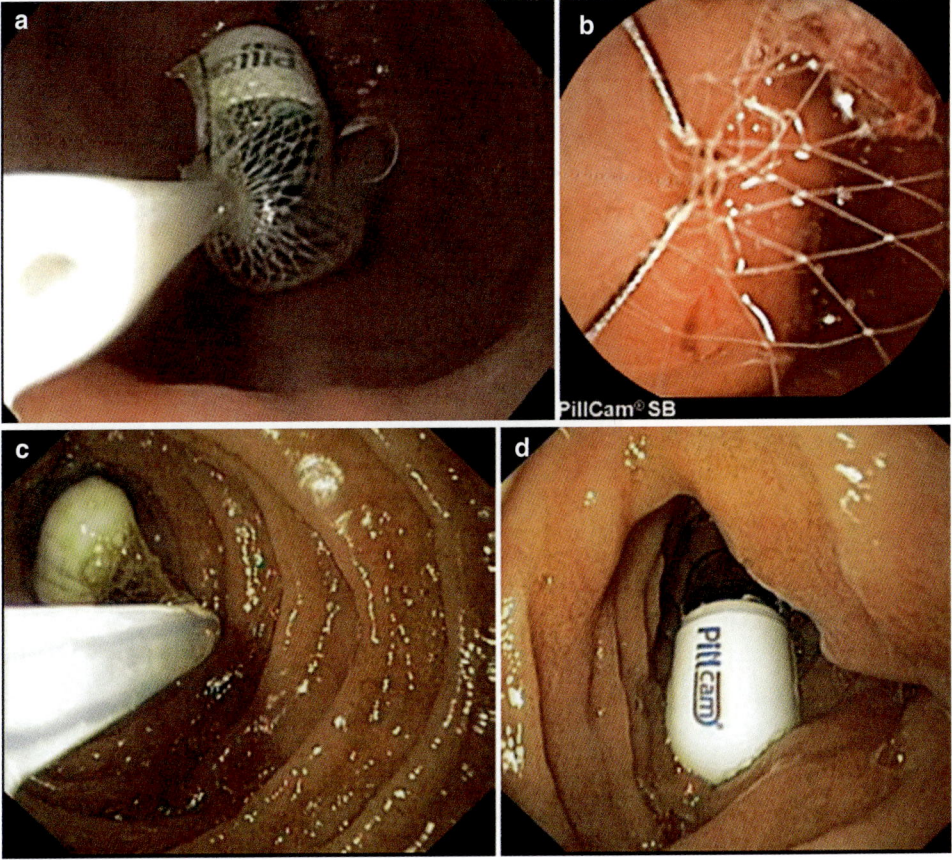

Fig. 7.8 Capsule grasped with a regular polypectomy snare. (**a**) EndoCapsule (Olympus Medical Systems, Tokyo, Japan). (**b**) PillCam Colon (Given Imaging, Yoqneam, Israel)

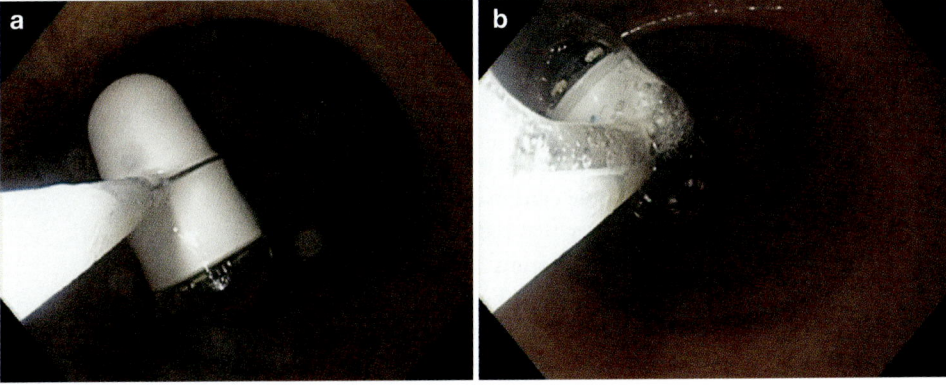

patients with known gastroparesis is endoscopic insertion of the capsule into the duodenum. Various instruments can be used to grasp and transport the swallowed capsule across the pylorus: a foreign-body grasping forceps [13], a Roth net (Fig. 7.7) [14], a polypectomy snare (Fig. 7.8) [15] or a Dormia basket (Fig. 7.9). A three-prong foreign-body grasper does not hold the capsule securely enough. The use of such insertion instruments has not yet been associated with damage to the capsule. Increases of complete small bowel visualisation from 78 to 84 % and diagnostic yield from 42 to 60 % have been demonstrated in a case-control study if capsules were placed endoscopically in patients with delayed oesophageal or gastric transit [16].

Fig. 7.9 (**a**) Capsule held in a Dormia basket. (**b**) Basket viewed from the capsule. (**c**) Capsule held lengthwise in the basket. (**d**) Capsule held crosswise in the basket

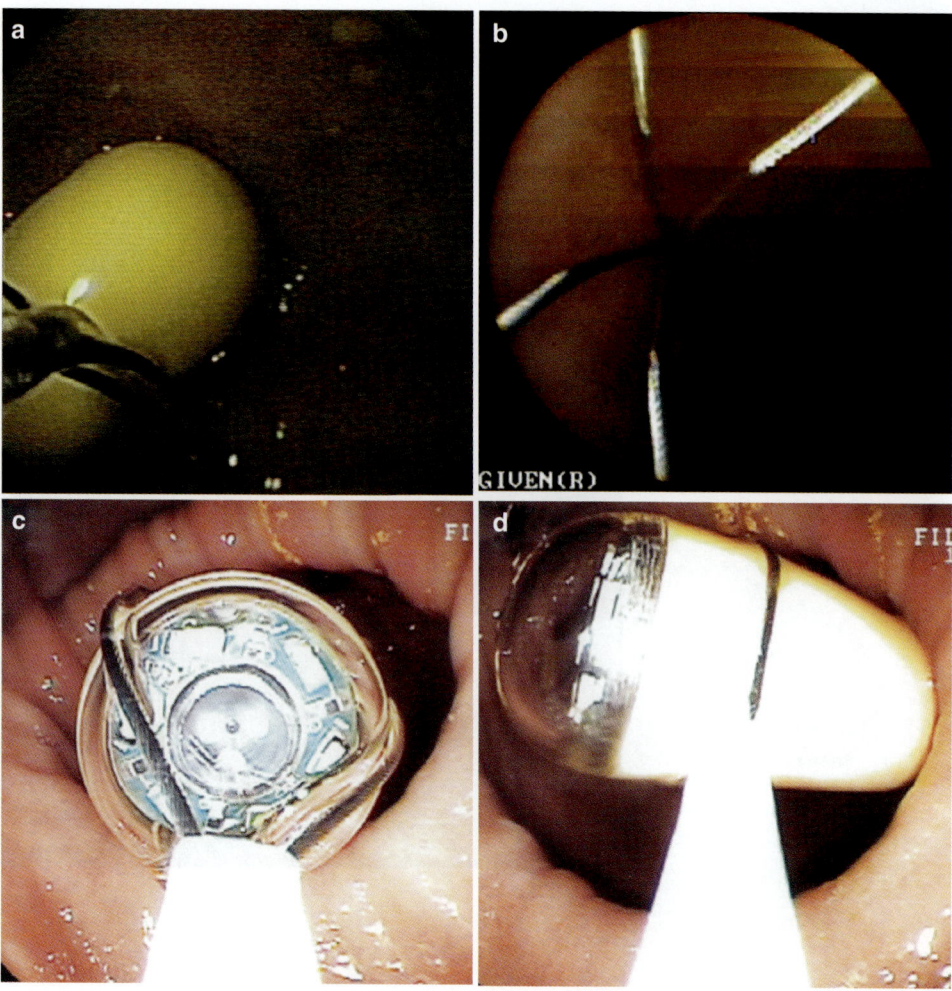

7.3   Pacemakers

7.3.1   Technical Background

Because of limited experience with VCE in patients with cardiac pacemakers and implantable cardioverter defibrillators (ICDs) and the theoretical fear that radiotransmission from the capsule might cause dangerous disturbance of these devices, the US Food and Drug Administration and the manufacturers (Given Imaging and Olympus Medical Systems) recommended not using VCE in these patients. Early reports described interference by a "test cap" (simulating video capsule transmission) that caused pacemakers to switch into interference mode (V00 or D00), but no clinically significant events resulted [17]. The same group observed in vitro interference of the test cap with ICDs, provoking a cardioverter shock, but this did not happen in patients [18]. The vast majority of published in vitro and in vivo studies have not revealed any interference between endoscopy capsules and pacemakers or ICDs [19–28]. In two in vitro studies, simulating the situation of a pacemaker or ICD inside a patient, the capsules (PillCam and EndoCapsule) were placed at different positions and finally at the closest proximity, with the capsule being placed on

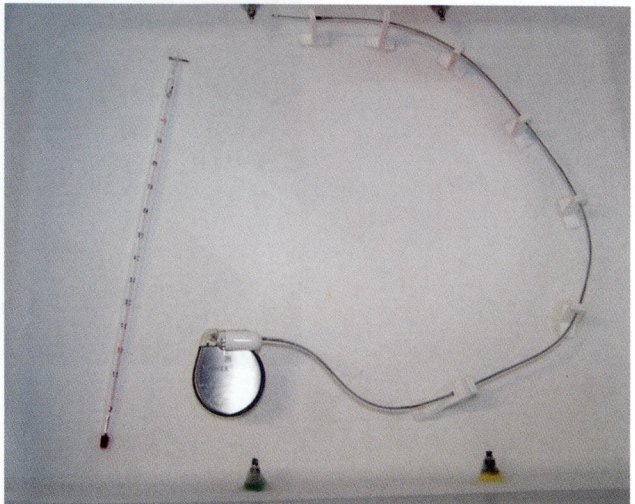

Fig. 7.10 In vitro simulation of interaction between a pacemaker and a video capsule. The pacemaker, lead and video capsule are in a bath with physiologic saline. Pin jacks that were in contact with the solution were placed low down, at the bottom of the tank. The pacemaker pulse was registered via these jacks

the case of the pacemaker or ICD for 1 min (Fig. 7.10) [22, 23]. None of the pacemakers or ICDs showed interference from a capsule. A few patients with left ventricular assist

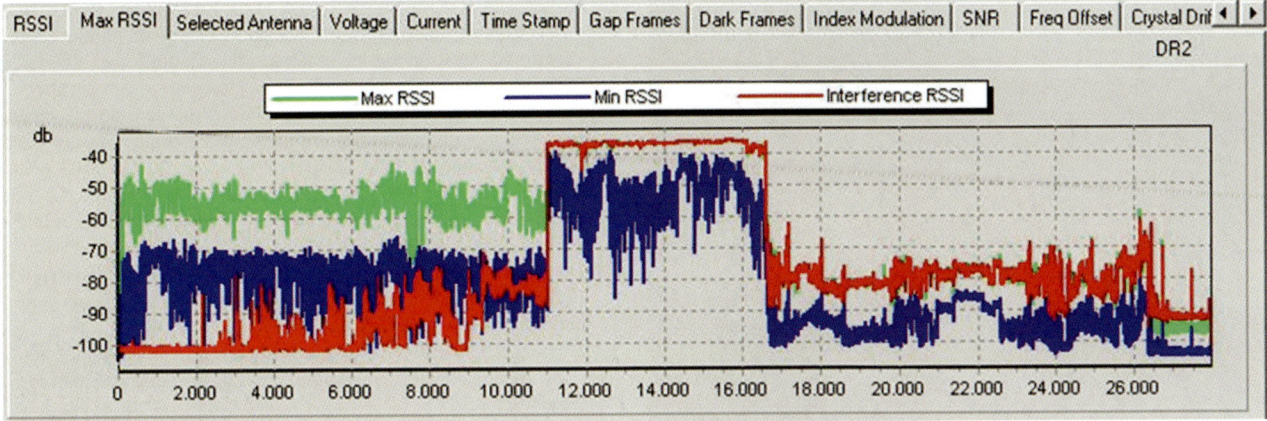

Fig. 7.11 Received signal strength indicator (RSSI) as recorded during a capsule procedure. *Green*, highest RSSI of the eight antennas and *Blue*, lowest RSSI of the eight antennas. The red curve is recorded during the transmission pauses of the capsule and represents the RSSI of external signals received by the Data Recorder. When the red curve reaches or exceeds the green curve, a loss of image data will occur. The actual graph shows the influence of a wireless monitoring device transmitting on the capsule's frequency. The resulting video had corresponding gaps (Courtesy of Konstantin Ackers, Given Imaging; reprinted from Bandorski et al. [31] with permission from the Journal of Gastrointestinal and Liver Diseases)

devices (LVADs) have undergone VCE for obscure bleeding without interference between the capsule and LVAD [29]. Additionally, based on technical data from Given Imaging concerning radiofrequency power, interference of capsules with pacemakers does not seem possible.

Chung et al. [30] investigated MiroCam (IntroMedic Co. Ltd, Seoul, Korea), in which images are transferred via 3 V current by using the human body as a conductor (Fig. 3.5), without any interference between the capsule and cardiac pacemakers or ICDs in a few patients. For the OMOM capsule system (Jinshan Science and Technology Co. Ltd., Chongqing, China), which uses similar transmission of images by radiofrequency (Fig. 3.4), studies to investigate interference are needed. Further developments of wireless capsule endoscopy systems include manual switching between image acquisition rates (OMOM) and automatic frame rate control depending on the speed of the capsule as represented by the changes of images (Fig. 3.8) (4 versus 39 images/s with PillCam Colon2 and 2 versus 6 images/s with PillCam SB3). These systems have not yet been evaluated in clinical studies, but available technical data from Given Imaging also exclude interference for PillCam Colon2 and SB3 as far as possible. Another capsule system (Fig. 3.6) stores acquired image data on an internal chip. By completely avoiding emission of current or radiofrequency waves, this system presents no possibility for potential interaction with a pacemaker or ICD.

7.3.2 Clinical Practice

For many years, VCE has been applied in patients with pacemakers or ICDs (mainly in elderly patients with mid-gastrointestinal bleeding) in spite of formal contraindication [20]. Dedicated cardiac monitoring usually has not been performed. No clinically relevant events were reported in a large series of 300 patients with pacemakers and 80 patients with ICDs [31]. Patients with 19 different pacemaker types from seven companies underwent uneventful capsule endoscopy [32]. Guidelines of the European Society for Gastrointestinal Endoscopy (ESGE) do not consider implanted cardiac devices as a contraindication at all [33]. Nevertheless, the formal contraindication that still exists should be included in the informed consent and discussed with patients who have an implanted cardiac device.

It is important to mention that telemetry can interfere with VCE, leading to loss of pictures or gaps in video (Fig. 7.11). Interference may be explained by the fact that many wireless applications (such as some telemetry systems) use the same frequency as VCE (PillCam, Given Imaging, 434.09 MHz; EndoCapsule, Olympus, 433.8 Hz). If monitoring is required, it should be performed with a wired ECG monitor.

7.4 Obesity

In patients with marked obesity, signals from the capsule's transmitter may not be powerful enough to reach sensor fields placed on the abdomen. Alternatively, it has been suggested to place the sensor field in corresponding positions on the patient's back (Fig. 7.12) in order to shorten the distance between the capsule and sensors [34]. To make the localisation software work properly, the sensor electrodes are placed inversely on the back. Systems with storage of image data inside the capsule do not require signal transmission (Fig. 3.6), which may be an advantage in severely obese patients.

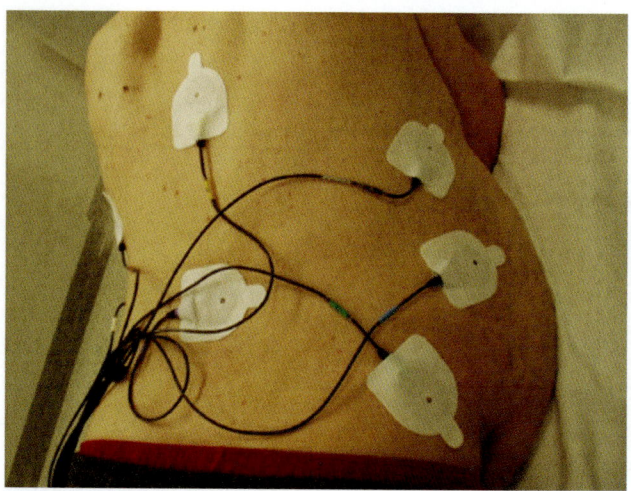

Fig. 7.12 Obese patient (140 kg) with electrodes placed inversely on his back

References

1. Barkin JS, O'Loughlin C. Capsule endoscopy contraindications: complications and how to avoid their occurrence. Gastrointest Endosc Clin N Am. 2004;14:61–5.

2. Sant'Anna AMGA, Dubois J, Miron MJ, Seidman EG. Wireless capsule endoscopy for obscure small bowel disorders: final results of the first pediatric controlled trial. Clin Gastroenterol Hepatol. 2005;3:264–70.

3. Seidman EG, Sant'Anna AMGA, Dirks MH. Potential applications of wireless capsule endoscopy in the pediatric age group. Gastrointest Endosc Clin N Am. 2004;14:207–18.

4. Carey EJ, Heigh RI, Fleischer DE. Endoscopic capsule endoscope delivery for patients with dysphagia, anatomical abnormalities, or gastroparesis. Gastrointest Endosc. 2004;59:423–6.

5. Tóth E, Fork FT, Almqvist P, Thorlacius H. Endoscopy-assisted capsule endoscopy in patients with swallowing disorders. Endoscopy. 2004;36:746–7.

6. Leung WK, Sung JJ. Endoscopically assisted video capsule endoscopy. Endoscopy. 2004;36:562–3.

7. Skogestad E, Tholfsen JK. Capsule endoscopy: in difficult cases the capsule can be ingested through an overtube. Endoscopy. 2004;36:1038.

8. Aabakken L, Blomhoff JP, Jermstad T, Lynge AB. Capsule endoscopy in a patient with Zenker's diverticulum. Endoscopy. 2003;35:799.

9. Holden JP, Dureja P, Pfau PR, et al. Endoscopic placement of the small-bowel video capsule by using a capsule endoscope delivery device. Gastrointest Endosc. 2007;65:842–7.

10. Bass LM, Misiewicz L. Use of a real-time viewer for endoscopic deployment of capsule endoscope in the pediatric population. J Pediatr Gastroenterol Nutr. 2012;55:552–5.

11. Almeida N, Figueiredo P, Lopes S, et al. Capsule endoscopy assisted by traditional upper endoscopy. Rev Esp Enferm Dig. 2008;100:758–63.

12. Boivin MA, Carey MC, Levy H. Erythromycin accelerates gastric emptying in a dose–response manner in healthy subjects. Pharmacotherapy. 2003;23:5–8.

13. Spera G, Spada C, Riccioni ME, et al. Video capsule endoscopy in a patient with a Billroth II gastrectomy and obscure bleeding. Endoscopy. 2004;36:931.

14. Fleischer DE, Heigh R, Nguyen CC, et al. Videocapsule impaction at the cricopharyngeus: first report of this complication and its successful resolution. Gastrointest Endosc. 2003;57:427–8.

15. Hollerbach S, Kraus K, Willert J, et al. Endoscopically assisted video capsule endoscopy of the small bowel in patients with functional gastric outlet obstruction. Endoscopy. 2003;35:226–9.

16. Gao YJ, Ge ZZ, Chen HY, et al. Endoscopic capsule placement improves the completion rate of small-bowel capsule endoscopy and increases diagnostic yield. Gastrointest Endosc. 2010;72:103–8.

17. Dubner S, Dubner Y, Gallino S, et al. Electromagnetic interference with implantable cardiac pacemakers by video capsule. Gastrointest Endosc. 2005;61:250–4.

18. Dubner S, Dubner Y, Rubio H, Goldin E. Electromagnetic interference from wireless video-capsule endoscopy on implantable cardioverter-defibrillators. Pacing Clin Electrophysiol. 2007;30:472–5.

19. Dirks MH, Costea F, Seidman EG. Successful videocapsule endoscopy in patients with an abdominal cardiac pacemaker. Endoscopy. 2008;40:73–5.

20. Bandorski D, Diehl KL, Jaspersen D. Kapselendoskopie bei Herzschrittmacher-Patienten: aktueller Stand in Deutschland. Z Gastroenterol. 2005;43:715–8.

21. Bandorski D, Diehl KL, Jaspersen D, Jakobs R. Kapselendoskopie und Herzschrittmacher – Ein Modellversuch zur Untersuchung möglicher Interferenzen. Endo heute. 2006;19:183–7.

22. Bandorski D, Irnich W, Brueck M, et al. Capsule endoscopy and cardiac pacemakers: investigation for possible interference. Endoscopy. 2008;40:36–9.

23. Bandorski D, Irnich W, Brück M, et al. Do endoscopy capsules interfere with implantable cardioverter-defibrillators? Endoscopy. 2009;41:457–61.

24. Payeras G, Piqueras J, Moreno VJ, et al. Effects of capsule endoscopy on cardiac pacemakers. Endoscopy. 2005;37:1181–5.

25. Guyomar Y, Vandeville L, Heuls S, et al. Interference between pacemaker and video capsule endoscopy. Pacing Clin Electrophysiol. 2004;27:1329–30.

26. Leighton JA, Sharma VK, Srivathsan K, et al. Safety of capsule endoscopy in patients with pacemakers. Gastrointest Endosc. 2004;59:567–9.

27. Leighton JA, Srivathsan K, Carey EJ, et al. Safety of wireless capsule endoscopy in patients with an implantable cardiac defibrillator. Am J Gastroenterol. 2005;100:1728–31.

28. Harris LA, Hansel SL, Rajan E, et al. Capsule endoscopy in patients with implantable electromedical devices is safe. Gastroenterol Res Pract. 2013;2013:959234.

29. Garatti A, Bruschi G, Girelli C, Vitali E. Small intestine capsule endoscopy in magnetic suspended axial left ventricular assist device patient. Interact Cardiovasc Thorac Surg. 2006;5:1–4.

30. Chung JW, Hwang HJ, Chung MJ, et al. Safety of capsule endoscopy using human body communication in patients with cardiac devices. Dig Dis Sci. 2012;57:1719–23.

31. Bandorski D, Jakobs R, Brück M, et al. Capsule Endoscopy in Patients with Cardiac Pacemakers and Implantable Cardioverter Defibrillators: (Re)evaluation of the Current State in Germany, Austria, and Switzerland 2010. Gastroenterol Res Pract. 2012; 2012:717408.

32. Bandorski D, Lotterer E, Hartmann D, et al. Capsule endoscopy in patients with cardiac pacemakers and implantable cardioverter-defibrillators - a retrospective multicenter investigation. J Gastrointestin Liver Dis. 2011;20:33–7.

33. Ladas SD, Triantafyllou K, Spada C, et al. European Society of Gastrointestinal Endoscopy (ESGE): recommendations (2009) on clinical use of video capsule endoscopy to investigate small-bowel, esophageal and colonic diseases. Endoscopy. 2010; 42:220–7.

34. Seitz U, Soehendra N. Solving the problem of video recording gaps in capsule endoscopy of overweight patients. Endoscopy. 2003;35:714.

Video Capsule Endoscopy in the Emergency Department

8

Christopher Marshall, Anupam Singh, and David R. Cave

Contents

Video capsule endoscopy (VCE) has been used extensively and effectively to detect the source of obscure gastrointestinal (GI) bleeding [1]. The possible role of capsule endoscopy in the setting of the emergency department (ED) has received scant attention, but emerging data have demonstrated that the early use of VCE in patients with obscure GI bleeding improves diagnostic and therapeutic outcomes and shortens the length of hospital stay. Studies have also demonstrated that capsule endoscopy may be useful for diagnosis of erosive esophagitis in patients with noncardiac chest pain.

We hypothesize that using video capsule endoscopy in the emergency room setting may have a role in detecting the origin of non-hematemesis GI bleeding. Hematemesis obviously implies a source of bleeding within range of the conventional gastroscope, usually in the esophagus, stomach, or duodenum. But when this population is excluded and patients with melena and hematochezia are assessed, the diagnostic yield from esophagogastroduodenoscopy (EGD) and colonoscopy (COL) is much smaller. This result is due in part to the poor predictive value of both melena and hematochezia as to the precise source of bleeding. Melena can be present in patients with pathology ranging from epistaxis to a right colonic bleed [2]. This lack of precision often results in the need to perform both EGD and COL, but because most GI bleeding stops spontaneously, many of these procedures are performed after bleeding has ceased, further reducing the reliability of the observations as to where the bleeding originated.

We also hypothesize that the use of VCE in the emergency room setting may also have a benefit for patients with noncardiac chest pain. In theory, once acute coronary syndrome has been excluded, capsule endoscopy may be able to identify esophageal lesions that could be causing symptoms. The demonstration of significant esophageal mucosal disease at the time of a negative cardiac workup could lead to the reduction of further testing, fewer repeat ED visits, and better patient management.

Contraindications to VCE as a first-line diagnostic test in the ED are presented in Table 8.1.

The work was first published in 2006 by Springer Medizin Verlag Heidelberg with the following title: *Atlas of Video Capsule Endoscopy.*

C. Marshall (✉) • A. Singh • D.R. Cave
Department of Gastroenterology,
University of Massachusetts Medical Center,
Worcester, MA, USA
e-mail: christopher.marshall@umassmemorial.org; anupam.singh@umassmemorial.org; caved@ummhc.org

Table 8.1 Contraindications to video capsule endoscopy as first-line diagnostic test in acute bleeding

Dysphagia
Gastroparesis
Gastric outlet obstruction
Known Zenker's or other large-necked diverticula in the stomach or duodenum
Uncooperative patient
Pregnancy
Prior history of radiation therapy (relative)

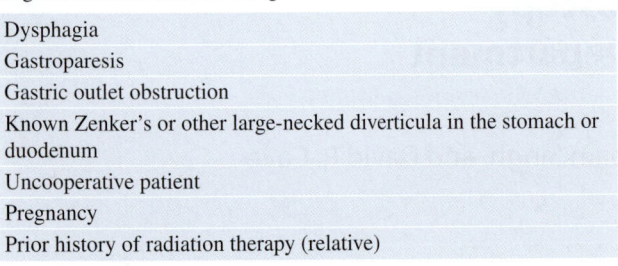

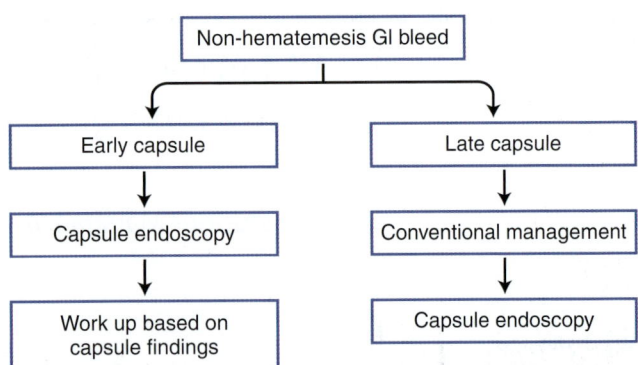

Fig. 8.1 Study design

8.1 VCE as First-Line Test in Acute Non-hematemesis Bleeding

We performed a randomized pilot study to examine the possible benefit of capsule endoscopy in the emergency setting [3]. A study was designed to determine whether early versus late use of the capsule might help in evaluating patients with non-hematemesis acute upper GI bleeding in whom the origin of bleeding was unclear (Fig. 8.1). The PillCam SB capsule (Given Imaging, Yoqneam, Israel) was allowed to traverse the intestines for 8 h. For the patients given early capsules, the data were downloaded and read as soon as possible. Results were then provided to the team taking care of the patient to facilitate workup. Results from patients who ingested the capsule before discharge but after completion of the conventional workup were provided to the patient's physician as they became available.

A total of 138 patients presented to the emergency department with GI bleeding over a 6-month period; of this number, 127 were screened and 24 had non-hematemesis acute GI bleeding and were included in the study. The early group ingested their capsule an average of 1.2 h after entry into the ED. The late group ingested their capsule a mean of 63 h after admission. Within 24 h of enrollment, 12 (75 %) of the 16 patients in the early-capsule endoscopy group had a presumptive source of bleeding detected (10 by capsule endoscopy, 1 by EGD, and 1 by COL) versus 3 (38 %) of the 8 patients in the late-capsule endoscopy group (all 3 detected by EGD) ($p = 0.099$). The median time to presumptive diagnosis by any diagnostic device was 19 h in the early-capsule endoscopy group versus 35 h in the late-capsule endoscopy group ($p = 0.06$). Overall, active bleeding was detected by capsule endoscopy in 13 (54 %) of 24 patients, by EGD in 2 (11 %) of 17 patients, and by COL in 0 of 13 patients. Capsule endoscopy provided no useful information in 4 (17 %) of 24 patients because of inability to swallow the capsule (1 patient) or because of gastric retention (3 patients). Examples of findings from this study are presented in

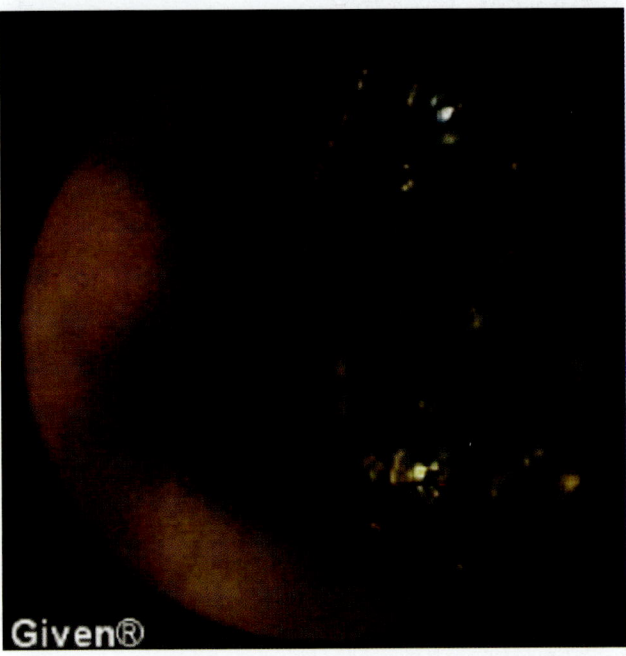

Fig. 8.2 Patient A. Late capsule shows melena in the ileum. The conventional workup was negative. Colonoscopy was refused. The precise origin of bleeding was not seen

Figs. 8.2, 8.3, 8.4, and 8.5. The anatomic site from which the bleeding originated, as determined by the video capsule, is summarized in Table 8.2.

We have demonstrated that capsule endoscopy is feasible in the ED setting. Our entry criteria for the study were clearly defined and we failed to screen only 11 of 138 patients over a 6-month period. There were no complications.

This pilot study does suggest that the use of capsule endoscopy in this selected but common scenario can accelerate the time to diagnosis, compared with conventional endoscopic intervention. The time spent in the hospital was not shortened, but this study was too small and was

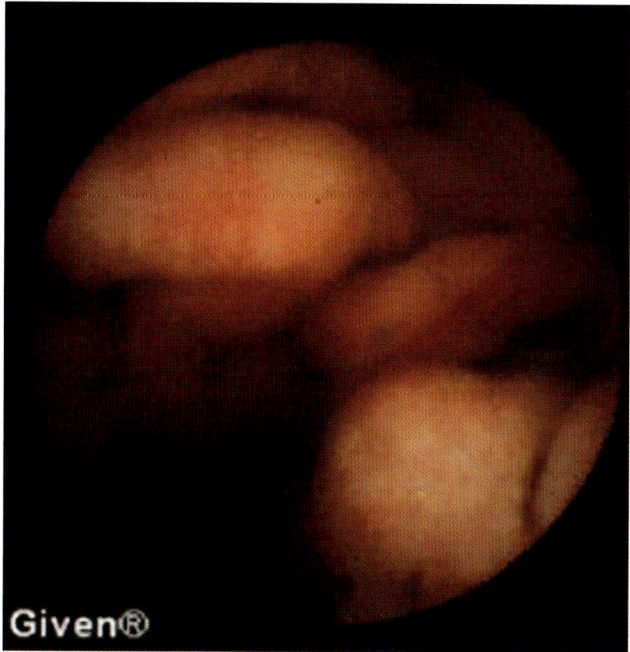

Fig. 8.3 Patient B. Early capsule shows active bleeding in the duodenum

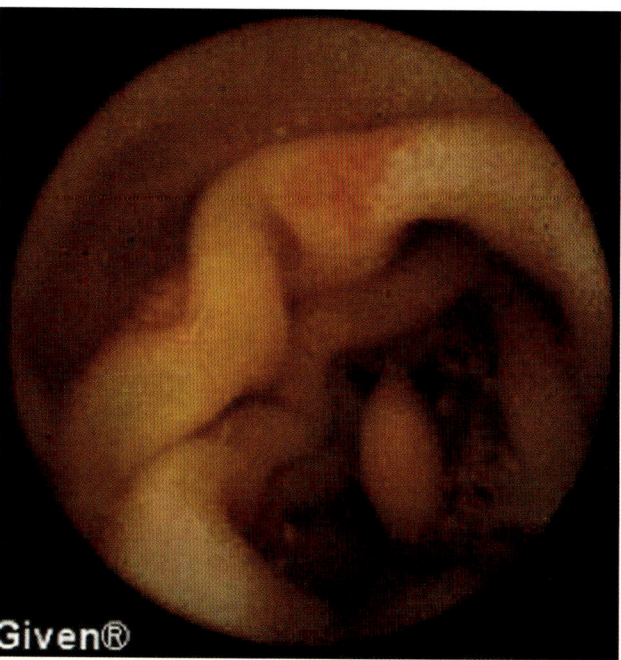

Fig. 8.5 Patient D. Early capsule shows angiectasis in the small intestine. Upper endoscopy demonstrated portal hypertensive gastropathy

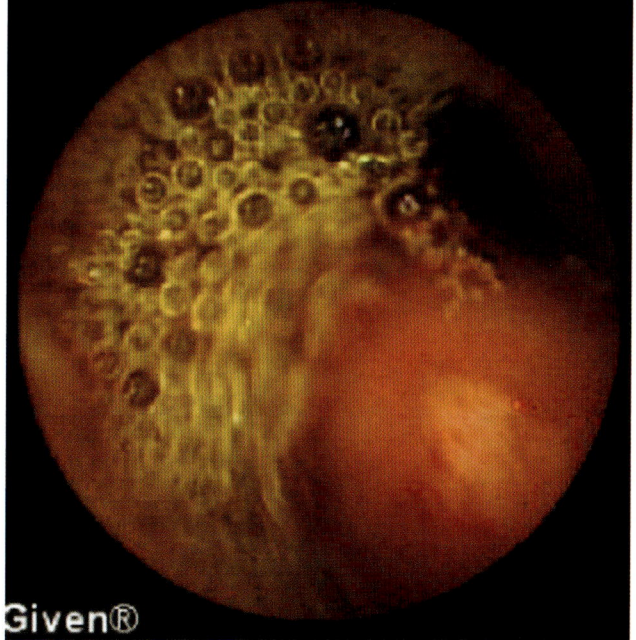

Fig. 8.4 Patient C. Late capsule shows an ulcer in the distal ileum associated with the use of nonsteroidal anti-inflammatory drugs (NSAIDs). This ulcer was the probable source of bleeding. Colonoscopy showed diverticulosis

Table 8.2 Sources of bleeding

	Early capsule ($n=13$)	Late capsule ($n=7$)
Stomach	4	2
Small bowel	4	2
Colon	1	1
Unknown	4	2

Comparative data on the exact population we studied are not available, as these patients are usually included in a more general population of GI bleeding. The number of patients studied was small, and the diagnostic yield by capsule endoscopy was numerically smaller than that reported in 2004 by Pennazio et al. [1], who noted that in their patients with obscure bleeding, if active bleeding was occurring, the diagnostic yield was 92 %.

8.2 Special Aspects of VCE in Acutely Ill Patients

Three patients retained the capsule in the stomach. This retention is not surprising, as these patients were acutely ill and probably subject to increased vagal tone that impaired gastric emptying. This problem might be reduced by the use of prokinetics (e.g., metoclopramide or erythromycin) to accelerate gastric emptying in future studies, given that this

not designed to examine this issue, which would require a much larger study. Similarly, we did not examine cost-effectiveness.

study showed a much higher gastric retention rate than previously reported. Some acceleration of the capsule should not be very important, as in this context, we are looking for bleeding more than for fine detail.

No interference was seen in our study, suggesting that monitoring equipment does not interfere with the capsule telemetry and recording. It is unlikely that the capsule endoscopy, which lasts only 8 h, will interfere with other diagnostic tests. We saw no increase in aspiration risk and would not anticipate this problem, as all patients studied were hemodynamically stable and fully conscious.

8.3 Use of PillCam ESO in Patients with Upper GI Bleeding

Real-time interrogation of the capsule is readily available and may be useful in the acute setting. A handheld computer or laptop can be connected to the capsule recording device of any of the current FDA-approved capsule systems to check at any time on the location of the video capsule in the alimentary canal and whether blood or melena is present in the lumen. A recent study looked at the use of the PillCam ESO for risk stratification in patients presenting to the emergency room with upper GI bleeding [4]. Live viewing of the capsule endoscopy accurately identified high-risk and low-risk patients in this group. The use of capsule endoscopy for risk stratification of these patients significantly reduced the time to emergent EGD and therapeutic intervention.

Another study concluded that in an ED setting, capsule endoscopy may facilitate patient triage and earlier endoscopy [5]. This study also confirmed that capsule endoscopy was feasible and safe in patients presenting with acute upper GI hemorrhage. Capsule endoscopy identified gross blood in the upper GI tract, including the duodenum, significantly more often than nasogastric tube aspiration, and it was comparable to EGD in identifying inflammatory lesions.

8.4 VCE in Severe Acute Bleeding After Negative EGD and COL

VCE is widely used in the context of obscure GI bleeding, but generally in a non-emergent manner after conventional technology has failed. This practice may be the antithesis of its eventual role in the detection of hard-to-locate, severe bleeding in the small intestine, which is often intermittent. We advocate that when conventional endoscopy fails to demonstrate a bleeding site, VCE should be used as soon as possible and appropriate (Fig. 8.6). This approach has been validated in the report by Pennazio et al. [1], who demonstrated a 92 % yield in the presence of active bleeding. We also recently demonstrated that early deployment of VCE (within 3 days of admission) results in a higher diagnostic yield and therapeutic intervention rate, associated with a hospital stay almost 4 days shorter [6]. Furthermore, in the context of recurrent bleeding, we suggest using the capsule as soon as there is evidence of renewed bleeding; further conventional endoscopy yields very little in this context and should be avoided.

8.5 Use of VCE for Noncardiac Chest Pain

The PillCam ESO has been used to determine the prevalence of esophageal mucosal disease in patients presenting to the ED with chest pain in whom acute coronary syndrome has been ruled out [7]. It was found that 38 % of the patients enrolled in the study ($n = 37$) had evidence of esophageal mucosal disease. An example of esophagitis detected in one of the patients is presented in Fig. 8.7. Early diagnosis of esophageal mucosal disease in this setting, with the ability to direct treatment, may lead to better patient management and reduce the need for further testing. This study did not have long-term follow-up; however, so it was difficult to determine whether the cause of chest pain was definitely the esophageal mucosal disease.

Fig. 8.6 Acute GI bleeding. (**a**) Normal OGD (duodenum and papilla seen with second camera of FUSE gastroscope). Colonosopy shows tarry stool in the cecum (**b**) and fresh blood in the terminal ileum (**c**). Hence, a video capsule was placed into the duodenum in the same session (**d**). As active bleeding could be observed with the real time viewer shortly after (**e**, **f**), immediate peroral single balloon enteroscopy was performed showing bleeding from jejunal diverticulosis (**g**, **h**)

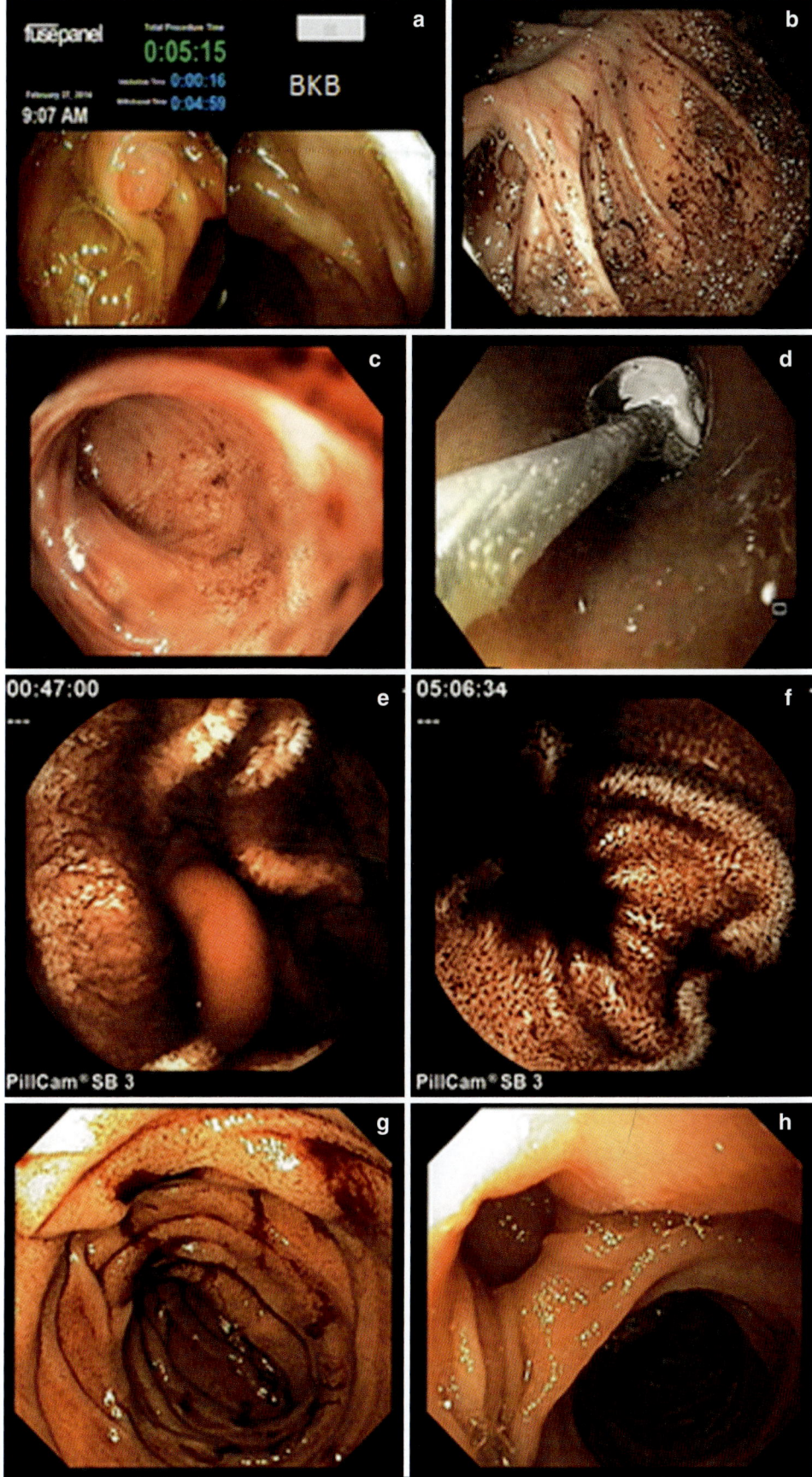

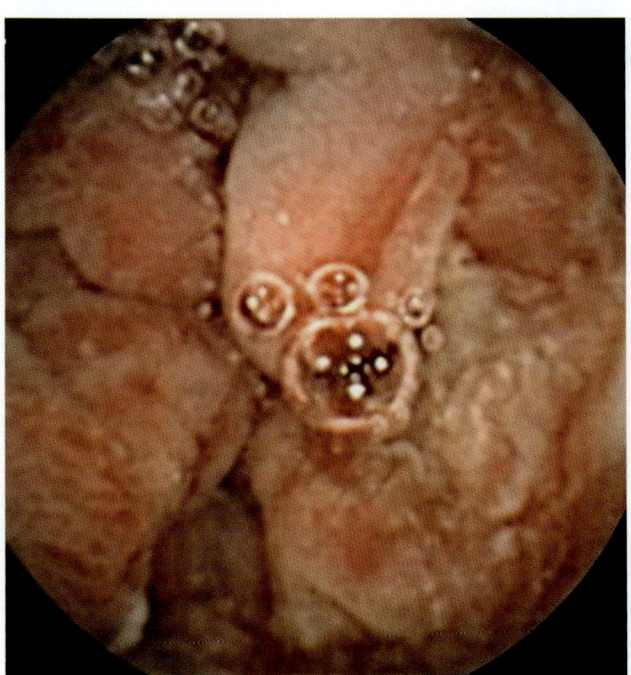

Fig. 8.7 Esophagitis seen on PillCam ESO in a patient with noncardiac chest pain

References

1. Pennazio M, Santucci R, Rondonotti E, Abbiati C, Beccari G, Rossini FP, De Franchis R. Outcome of patients with obscure gastrointestinal bleeding after capsule endoscopy: report of 100 consecutive cases. Gastroenterology. 2004;126:643–53.
2. Lee H, Cave D. Melena and its anatomic sources. Gastrointest Endosc. 2003;57:AB169.
3. Sachdev R, Hibberd P, Perlmutter M, Cave D. Capsule endoscopy in the emergency room for acute non-hematemesis gastrointestinal bleeding. Am J Gastroenterol. 2004;99:S295.
4. Rubin M, Hussain SA, Shalomov A, Cortes RA, Smith MS, Kim SH. Live view video capsule endoscopy enables risk stratification of patients with acute upper GI bleeding in the emergency room: a pilot study. Dig Dis Sci. 2011;56:786–91.
5. Gralnek IM, Ching JY, Maza I, Wu JC, Rainer TH, Israelit S, et al. Capsule endoscopy in acute upper gastrointestinal hemorrhage: a prospective cohort study. Endoscopy. 2013;45:12–9.
6. Singh A, Marshall C, Chaudhuri B, Okoli C, Foley A, Person SD, et al. Timing of video capsule endoscopy relative to overt obscure GI bleeding: implications from a retrospective study. Gastrointest Endosc. 2013;77:761–6.
7. Singh A, Lee C, Finkelberg D, Foley A, Volturo G, Gore J, et al. Use of PillCam ESO in determining the prevalence of esophageal mucosal disease in patients presenting to the emergency department with chest pain and without acute coronary syndrome [abstract]. Gastroenterology. 2010;138(5 Suppl 1):S-670.

Conclusion

The improved yield of VCE in the acute setting suggests that we should be much more aggressive in its application than is currently the case. The multidisciplinary application of VCE may have substantial payoff in terms of improved patient care and cost containment.

Patency Capsule

9

Guido Costamagna, Maria Elena Riccioni,
Riccardo Urgesi, Martin Keuchel, and Ingo Steinbrück

Contents

9.1 Principle

The PillCam patency system, an accessory to the PillCam video capsule (Given Imaging Ltd.; Yoqneam, Israel), is intended to verify adequate patency of the gastrointestinal (GI) tract in patients with known or suspected strictures prior to administration of the PillCam video capsule [1, 2].

The PillCam patency capsule (Fig. 9.1) is designed to remain intact in the GI tract for about 30–100 h (Fig. 9.2). After this time, if the capsule is still inside the body, it disintegrates spontaneously. Gastric and intestinal fluids form holes in the two plugs at both ends of the capsule over the designated period (Fig. 9.4). The fluids reach the body of the capsule through these holes and dissolve the lactose-barium mixture, leaving behind the parylene C coating and a metal radiofrequency identification (RFID) tag (Figs. 9.4 and 9.1b, c.).

Retention of the test capsule can be detected radiographically (Fig. 9.2) or with an external detector (Fig. 9.3), which responds to a small induction coil inside the capsule (Figs. 9.1c and 9.5) [3].

The work was first published in 2006 by Springer Medizin Verlag Heidelberg with the following title: *Atlas of Video Capsule Endoscopy.*

G. Costamagna (✉) • M.E. Riccioni • R. Urgesi
Department of Surgical Endoscopy,
Università Cattolica del Sacro Cuore, Rome, Italy
e-mail: gcostamagna@rm.unicatt.it;
melena.riccioni@rm.unicatt.it; riurgesi@tin.it

M. Keuchel
Department of Internal Medicine,
Bethesda Krankenhaus Bergedorf, Hamburg, Germany
e-mail: keuchel@bkb.info

I. Steinbrück
1st Medical Department, Asklepios Klinik Altona,
Hamburg, Germany
e-mail: i.steinbrueck@asklepios.com

M. Keuchel et al. (eds.), *Video Capsule Endoscopy: A Reference Guide and Atlas,*
DOI 10.1007/978-3-662-44062-9_9, © Springer-Verlag Berlin Heidelberg 2014

Fig. 9.1 Commercially available PillCam patency capsule (Given Imaging Ltd., Yoqneam, Israel). (**a**) Intact capsule. (**b, c**) Capsule after dissolving in water

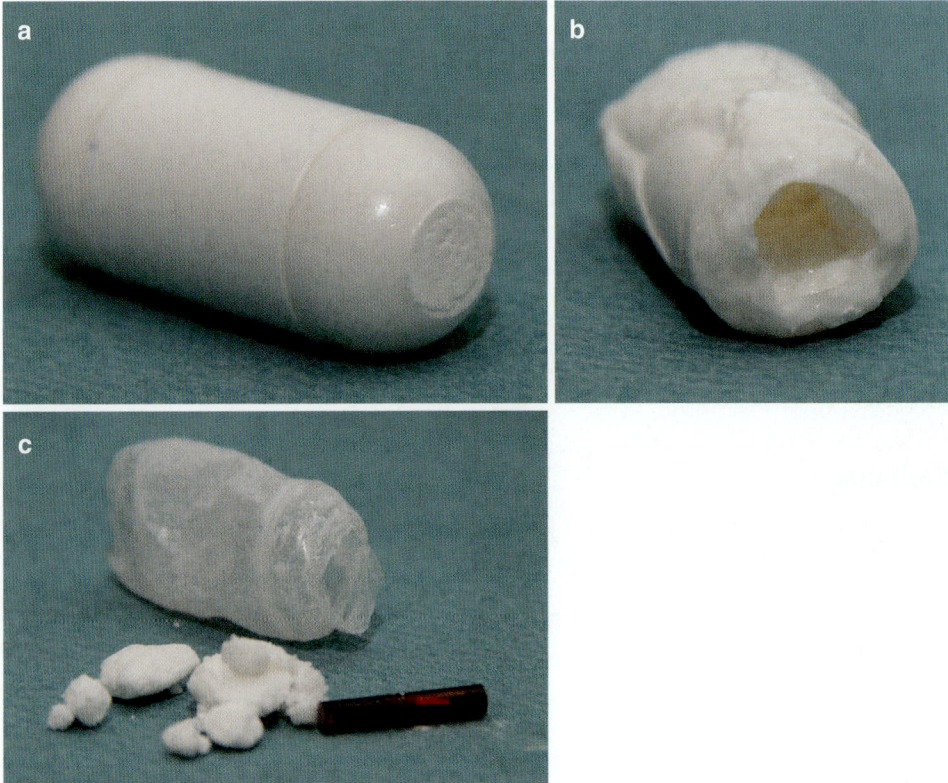

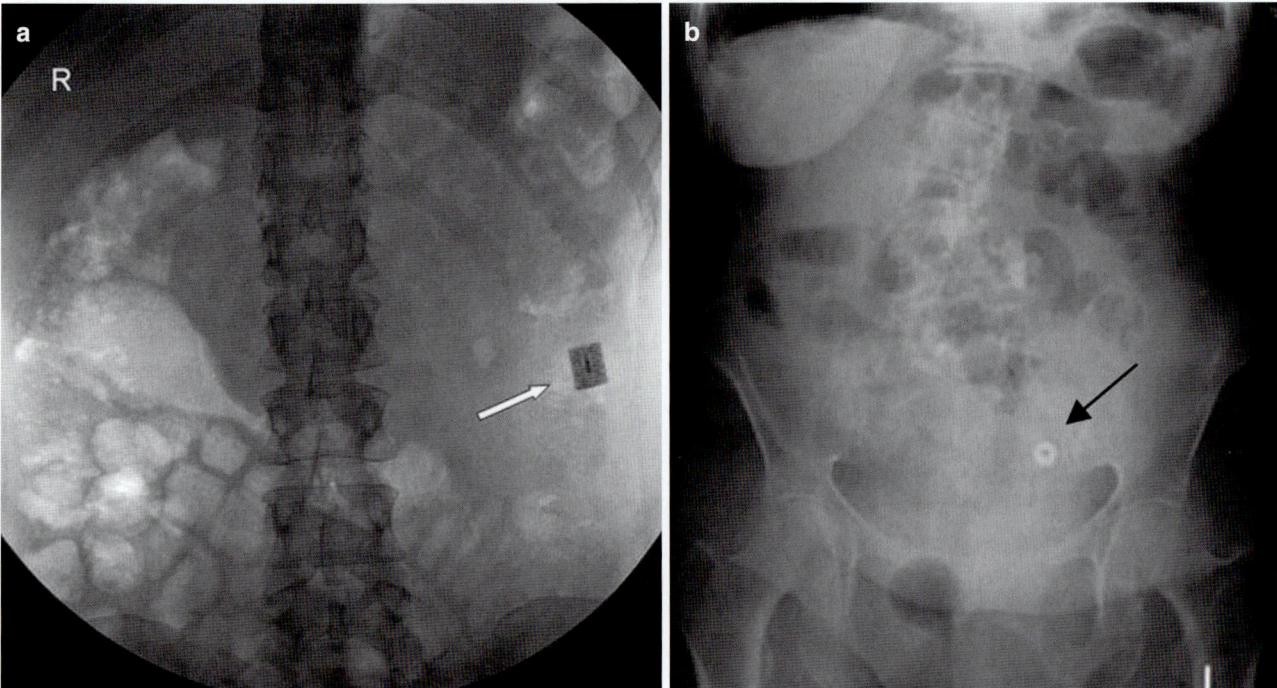

Fig. 9.2 Intact PillCam patency capsules 24 h after ingestion. (**a**) Radiograph on a longitudinal axis. (**b**) Orthograde axis in another patient

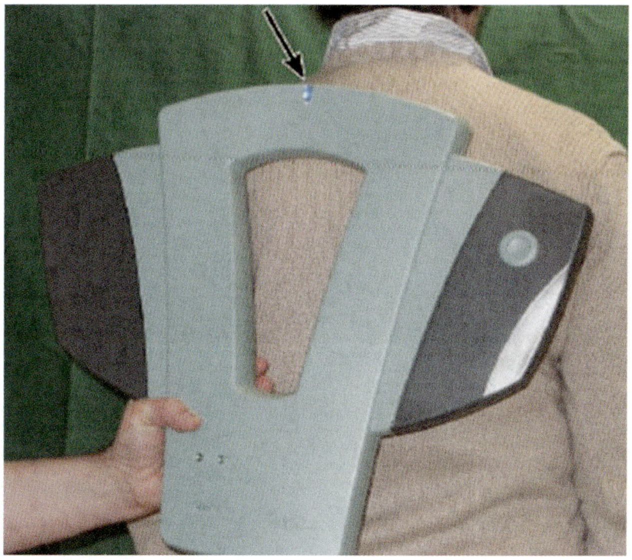

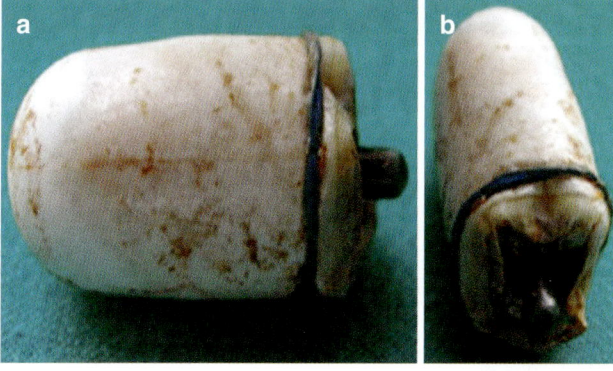

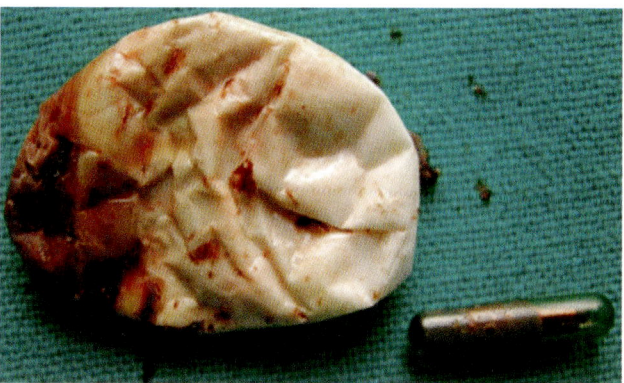

Fig. 9.5 Disintegrated M2A patency capsule, leaving coating and tag

Fig. 9.3 The blue light at the top of the detector (*arrow*) indicates the presence of the coil. It cannot be determined, however, whether the coil is still inside an intact capsule or has been released from a disintegrated capsule

9.2 Procedure

After giving informed consent, including risk of retention with need for surgery, the patient swallows the patency capsule with a glass of water. Although fasting is recommended by the manufacturer, it is not necessary to fast prior to ingestion. The patient subsequently must look carefully for the capsule with every bowel movement (Fig. 9.6).

If the capsule is not excreted the next day, the presence of the tag in the body can be proven with a detector (Fig. 9.3). This detector recognizes the tag via induction, but it cannot determine whether the capsule has dissolved or whether the tag or capsule is lodged in the small bowel or have passed into the colon. Therefore, x-ray films of the abdomen are preferable if the capsule is not excreted. Repeated x-rays or CT scans on subsequent days can document whether the capsule is lodged, has moved into the colon, or has dissolved (Figs. 9.7 and 9.8).

If only the collapsed shell of the patency capsule (Fig. 9.5) is excreted instead of the intact capsule, a significant stenosis must be assumed. In this case, video capsule endoscopy (VCE) is contraindicated unless surgery is scheduled. VCE is also contraindicated if radiography documents disintegration of the patency capsule by showing the tag without surrounding capsule (Fig. 9.7b).

Evidence of intestinal patency is the excretion of the intact patency capsule (Fig. 9.6) at any time; its disappearance, proven by the detector or x-ray or proof of its location in the colon within 30 h after ingestion, demonstrated by CT scan, colonoscopy, or fluoroscopy.

Fig. 9.4 (**a**, **b**) Beginning disintegration of the M2A patency capsule (prototype). As the maximal diameter is conserved, passing of such a capsule still indicates intestinal patency

Fig. 9.6 (**a**) Crohn's disease patient with tight ileal strictures seen on radiology. (**b**) The M2A patency capsule was excreted intact 27 h after ingestion, without adverse events. (**c–e**) The patient underwent video capsule endoscopy (VCE) using a PillCam (Given Imaging Ltd, Yoqneam, Israel), which showed ileal ulcerations and stenosis. The PillCam passed uneventfully

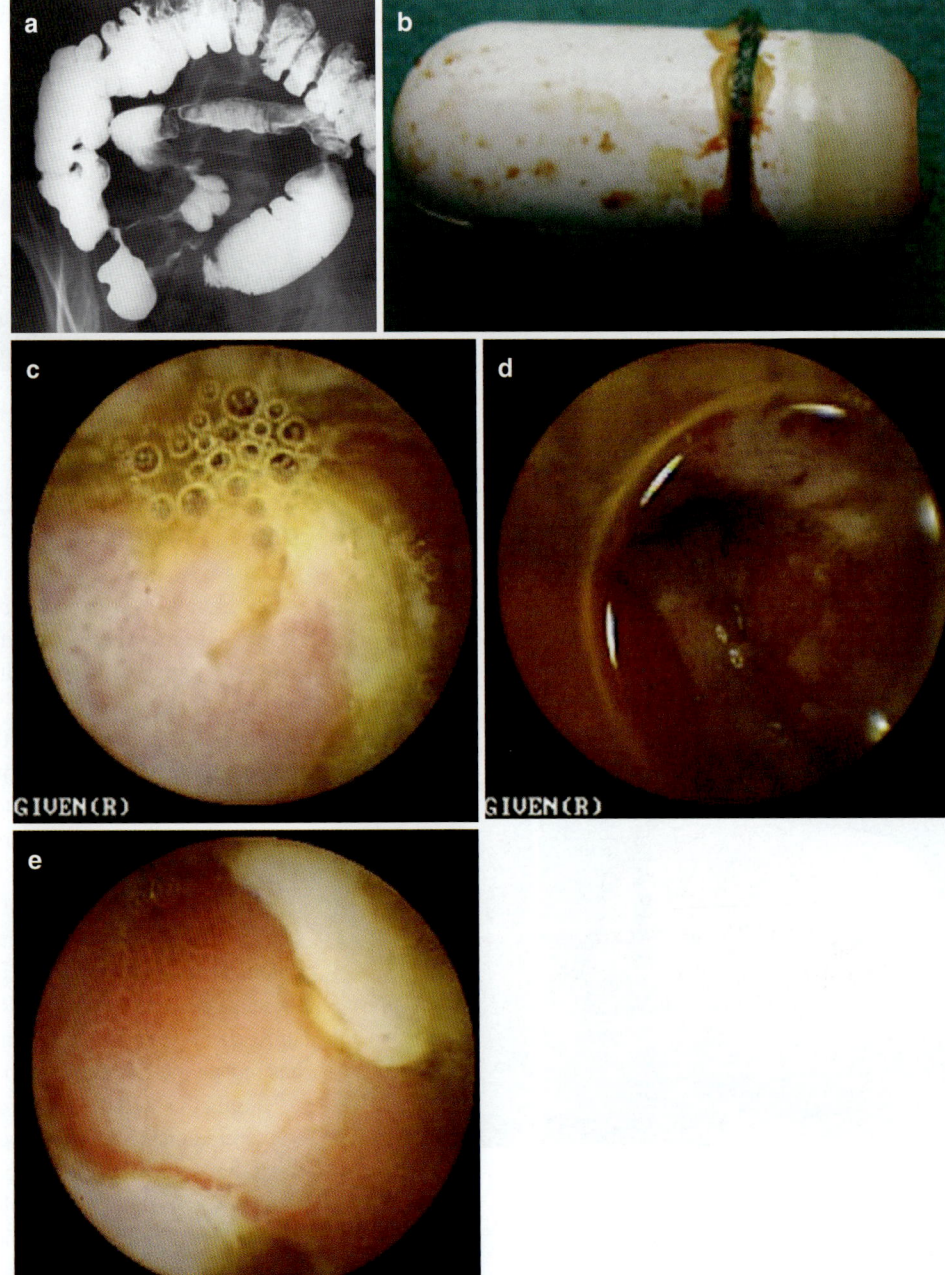

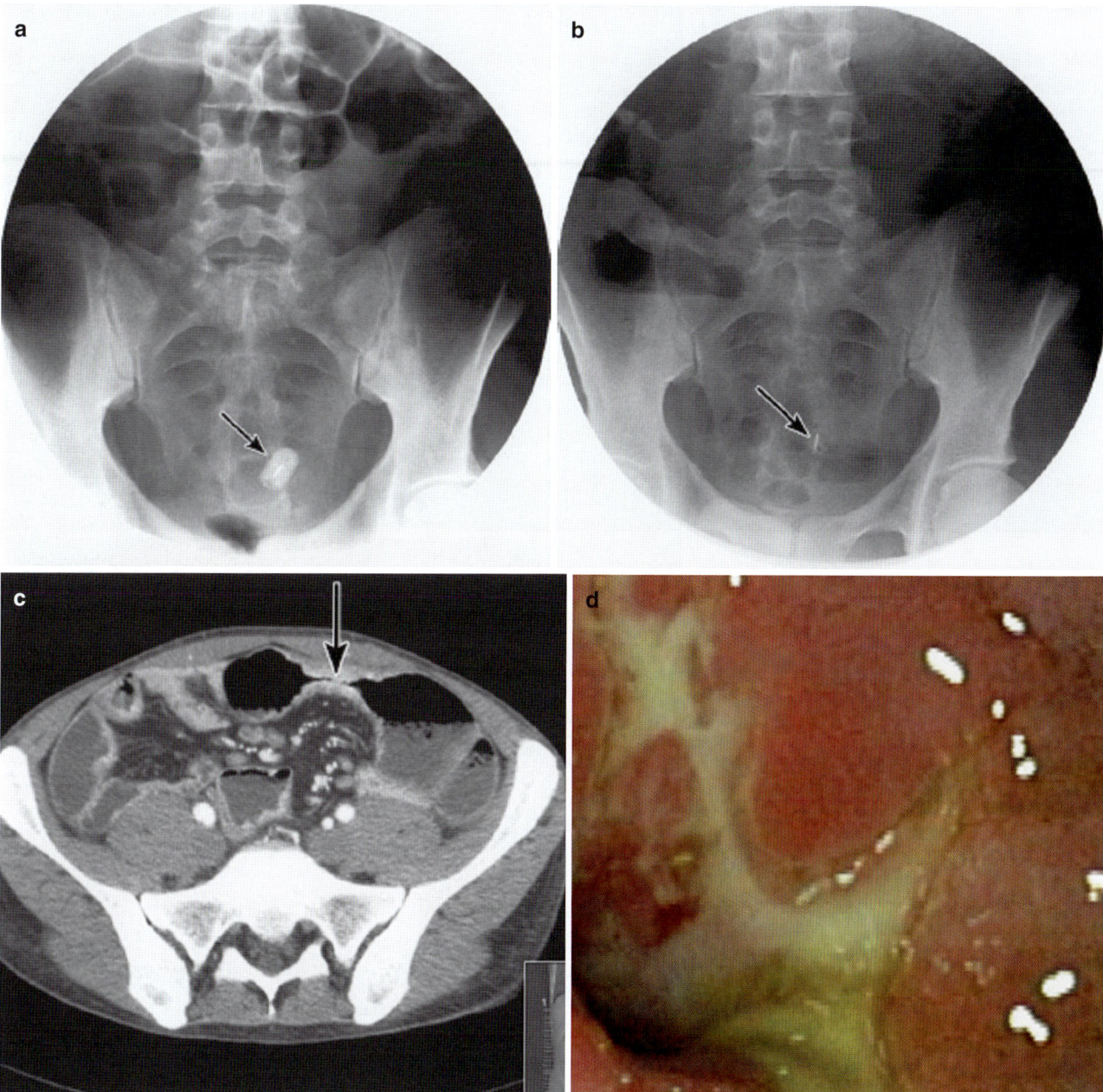

Fig. 9.7 Crohn's disease with stricture. (**a**) Intact patency capsule (*arrow*) at 24 h after ingestion. (**b**) At 50 h, only the tag (*arrow*) is visible; VCE is therefore contraindicated. (**c**) CT scanning shows circumscribed thickening with stenosis (*arrow*), dilatation, and small lymph nodes. (**d**) Enteroscopy demonstrates an impassable, ulcerated jejunal stenosis

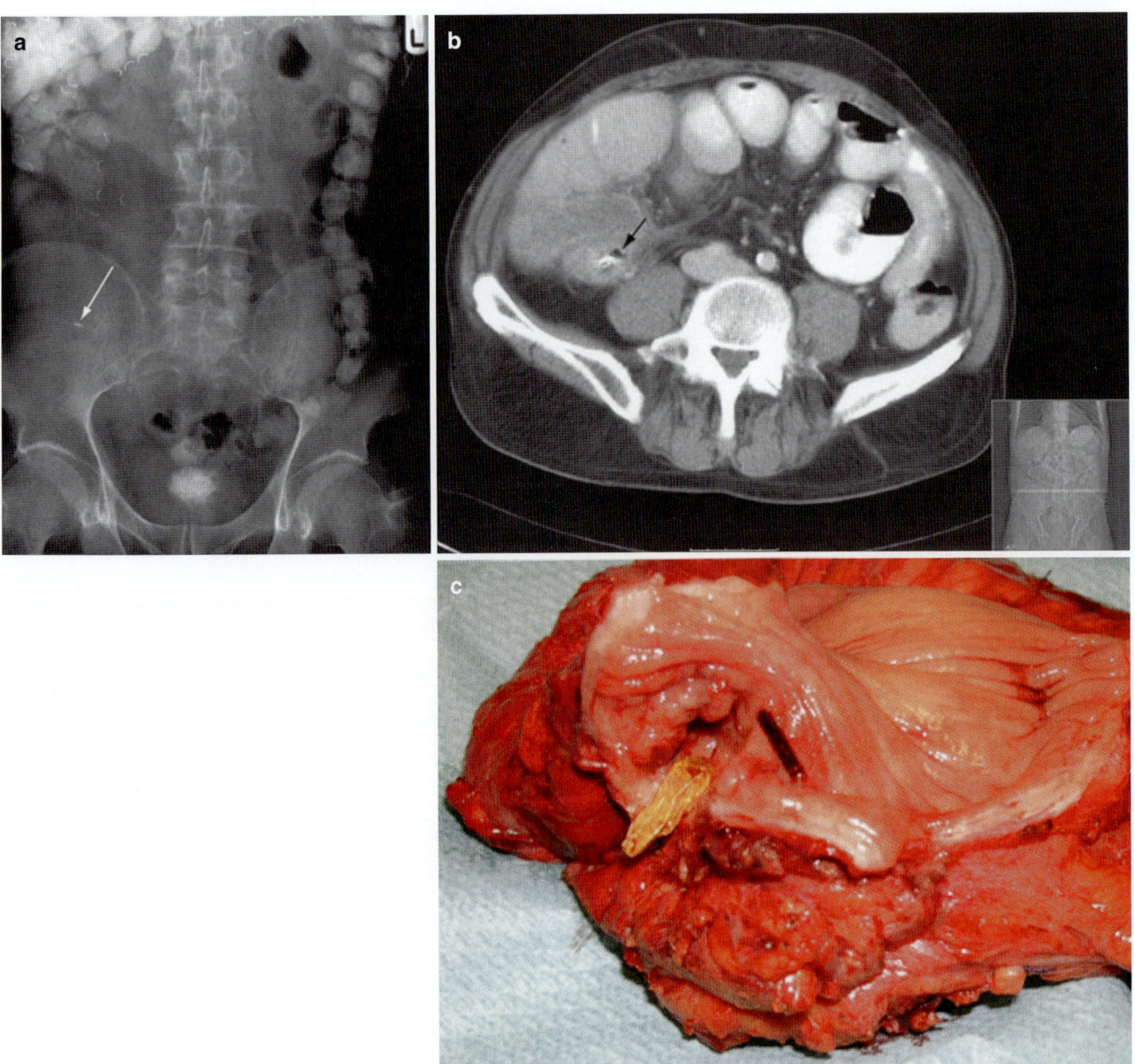

Fig. 9.8 A patient with obscure bleeding after resection of colonic carcinoma. Because of postprandial abdominal discomfort, the patency capsule was given prior to a scheduled VCE. (**a**) An abdominal x-ray shows clips after surgery and the tag of the dissolved patency capsule. (**b**) A CT scan depicts the tag in a narrow ileal lumen (Courtesy of Ernst Malzfeldt, MD.) (**c**) Surgery reveals metastatic small bowel adenocarcinoma with stenosis and remnants of the patency capsule (Courtesy of Christopher Pohland, MD). *Arrow* indicates the position of the metal tag residual of the Patency capsule dissolved

9.3   Indications

The patency capsule may offer information on functional intestinal patency and may be used as a test before VCE in patients with:

- Established diagnosis of Crohn's disease (Fig. 9.6)
- Suspicion of intestinal stenosis based on clinical, radiologic, or sonographic findings
- Prior abdominopelvic radiation
- Prior small bowel resection
- Prior major abdominal surgery with a possibility of adhesions

9.4   Clinical Applications

The patency capsule has received CE (European Conformity) certification. Several studies have assessed the clinical value of this device. As the rate of false-positive results regarding relevant strictures is significant, one study [4] suggested the use of additional radiologic tests to confirm or exclude the presence of a significant suspected stricture and to localize the capsule if its passage is delayed.

After ingestion, some patients have complained of transient abdominal pain. In a long stenosis, the patency capsule may cause obstruction requiring surgery. One patient with

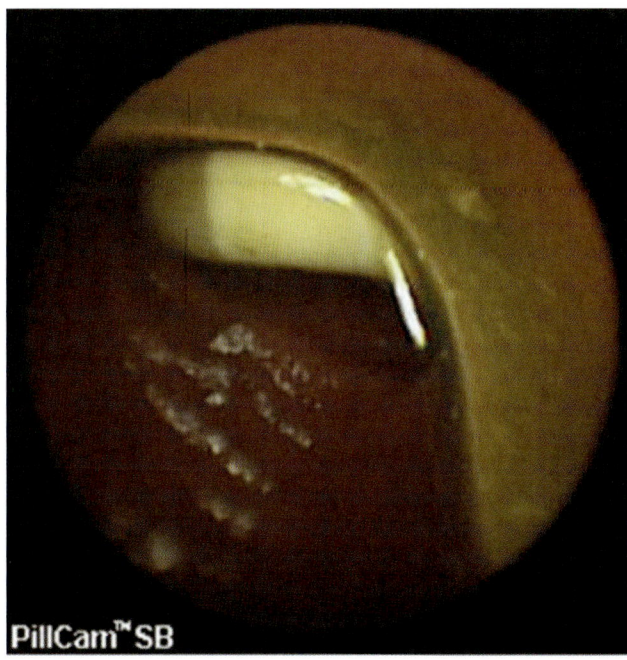

Fig. 9.9 Patency capsule seen on a video capsule image. The patient had reported the excretion of the patency capsule. Both capsules finally passed uneventfully

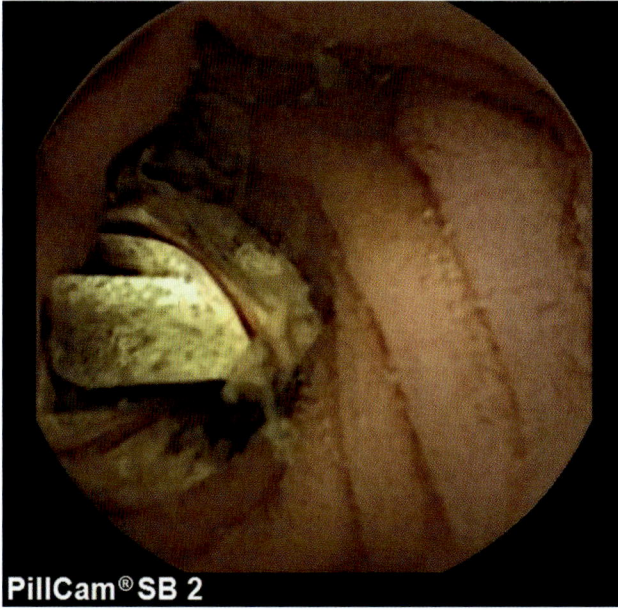

Fig. 9.10 This video capsule image shows the coating of a dissolved patency capsule in a patient with stricturing small bowel carcinoma. The video capsule was retrieved during surgery

Crohn's disease and a long stricture of the small intestine had to undergo surgery for small intestinal obstruction before the first-generation patency capsule was able to dissolve [5]. Another patient developed temporary obstruction (Fig. 40.14) [6]. This first-generation M2A patency capsule was

modified in 2006, replaced by the Agile patency capsule with two dissolvable membranes (one at each end of the capsule) rather than one, to minimize the risk that the membrane might be covered by the wall of a tight stenosis, thus preventing the capsule from dissolving in a timely manner. The Agile patency capsule is marketed today as PillCam patency capsule. In several studies in which the patency capsule showed intestinal patency [1, 2, 5, 7, 8–12], the following imaging capsule passed without incident (Fig. 9.6). If the patency capsule is presumed to be located in the colon only by x-ray, intestinal patency is not proven. In several reported cases, subsequent capsule endoscopy resulted in retention [13]. The patency capsule or its components are not visualized during VCE (Figs. 9.9 and 9.10) after a standard procedure.

References

1. Signorelli C, Rondonotti E, Villa F, et al. Use of the Given Patency System for the screening of patients at high risk of capsule retention. Dig Liver Dis. 2006;38:326–30.
2. Spada C, Shah SK, Riccioni ME, et al. Video capsule endoscopy in patients with known or suspected small bowel stricture previously tested with the dissolving patency capsule. J Clin Gastroenterol. 2007;41:576–82.
3. Caunedo-Álvarez A, Romero-Vazquez J, Herrerias-Gutierrez JM. Patency and Agile capsules. World J Gastroenterol. 2008;14: 5269–73.
4. Yadav A, Heigh RI, Hara AK, et al. Performance of the patency capsule compared with nonenteroclysis radiologic examinations in patients with known or suspected intestinal strictures. Gastrointest Endosc. 2011;74:834–9.
5. Boivin ML, Lochs H, Voderholzer WA. Does passage of a patency capsule indicate small-bowel patency? A prospective clinical trial. Endoscopy. 2005;37:808–15.
6. Gay G, Delvaux M, Laurent V, et al. Temporary intestinal occlusion induced by a patency capsule in a patient with Crohn's disease. Endoscopy. 2005;37:174–7.
7. Delvaux M, Ben Soussan E, Laurent V, et al. Clinical evaluation of the use of the M2A patency capsule system before a capsule endoscopy procedure, in patients with known or suspected intestinal stenosis. Endoscopy. 2005;37:801–7.
8. Spada C, Spera G, Riccioni M, et al. A novel diagnostic tool for detecting functional patency of the small bowel: the given patency capsule. Endoscopy. 2005;37:793–800.
9. Postgate AJ, Burling D, Gupta A, et al. Safety, reliability, and limitations of the Given Patency Capsule in patients at risk of capsule retention; a 3-year technical review. Dig Dis Sci. 2008;53:2732–8.
10. Herrerias JM, Leighton JA, Costamagna G, et al. Agile patency system eliminates risk of capsule retention in patients with known intestinal strictures who undergo capsule endoscopy. Gastrointest Endosc. 2008;67:902–9.
11. Steinbrueck I, Keuchel M, Zorn A, et al. Patency capsule reduces retention rate of small bowel video capsules in high risk patients. Endoscopy. 2009;41 Suppl 1:A529.
12. Cohen SA, Gralnek IM, Ephrath H, et al. The use of a patency capsule in pediatric Crohn's disease: a prospective evaluation. Dig Dis Sci. 2011;56:860–5.
13. Koornstra JJ, Weersma RK. Agile patency system. Gastrointest Endosc. 2009;69:602–3.

Terminology

10

Michel Delvaux, Louis Y. Korman, and Martin Keuchel

Contents

The work was first published in 2006 by Springer Medizin Verlag Heidelberg with the following title: *Atlas of Video Capsule Endoscopy*.

M. Delvaux (✉)
Department of Gastroenterology and Hepatology,
University Hospital of Strasbourg, Nouvel Hôpital Civil,
Strasbourg, France
e-mail: michel.delvaux@chru-strasbourg.fr

L.Y. Korman
Chevy Chase Clinical Research, Chevy Chase, MD, USA
e-mail: louis.korman@verizon.net

M. Keuchel
Department of Internal Medicine,
Bethesda Krankenhaus Bergedorf,
Hamburg, Germany
e-mail: keuchel@bkb.info

A standard terminology is essential if the reporting of endoscopic finding is to be reproducible, internationally uniform, and compatible with electronic data processing. A standard terminology has been developed for video capsule endoscopy (VCE) [1], following the model of the Minimal Standard Terminology (MST) created by a collaboration between the European, American, and Japanese Endoscopy Societies under the sponsorship of the Organisation Mondiale d'Endoscopie Digestive (OMED), now World Endoscopy Organisation (WEO), for the fields of esophagogastroduodenoscopy (EGD), endoscopic retrograde cholangiopancreatography (ERCP), and colonoscopy [2–4]. In 2008, the MST 3.0 version was released [5], which also includes small bowel lesions and the enteroscopy procedure. The Capsule Endoscopy Structured Terminology (CEST) has been developed following the rules established for MST and adapted to the specific needs for the reporting of findings and diagnoses in capsule endoscopy findings. The CEST has been published for an open-access use in software and scientific applications [6]. It was validated in a retrospective trial [7] showing that the majority of terms used to describe VCE findings were included in the CEST. Prospective testing resulted in a moderate interobserver agreement, with kappa values of 0.44 regardless of experience and consecutive training [8]. Others also found agreement, but with better results for experienced examiners [9, 10], suggesting a need for training as well as for regular updating of the CEST.

The CEST supports the structured reporting of all data necessary for an examination, including pathological findings. This chapter provides an overview and examples of the use of the CEST for reporting a VCE examination.

10.1 Structured Documentation of an Examination

The VCE examination report follows the general MST structure for endoscopic reporting to provide the necessary documentation of the procedure.

Documentation of a VCE examination:

- Patient data
- Procedural data (date, examiner)
- Reason (indication) for the examination
- Limitations (viewing conditions, completeness of the examination)
- Complications
- Description of findings
- Localization
- Diagnosis
- Recommendations

10.2 Findings

The "Findings" section is based on a hierarchy of descriptive levels that starts with categories of findings called "Headings" (see below). Below the headings are "Terms," followed by "Attributes" and "Attribute values."

The following headings are used for the structured description of findings in the small bowel:

- Normal
- Lumen
- Contents
- Mucosa
- Flat lesions
- Protruding lesions
- Excavated lesions

For example, fresh blood in the bowel lumen due to active bleeding is described as follows: contents (heading) – blood (term) – kind of blood (attribute) – red (attribute value). In some cases, a finding is an aggregate of different observations described under multiple headings. A stenosing tumor, for instance, is described as tumor (protruding lesion) and stenosis (lumen). Similarly, diverticulitis can be described as diverticulum (excavated lesion), ulcer (excavated lesion), and erythema (mucosa).

10.3 Localization

Localization of VCE images can be identified by time, organ, or through localization software:

- Localization by time is divided into the proximal, middle, or distal third of the small bowel. The time between the initial images of the duodenum and of the cecum is divided into three equal segments. Any delay of the capsule in the duodenum or terminal ileum and any variations in transit speed are ignored.
- Localization by organ can include the esophagus, stomach, duodenum, small bowel, terminal ileum, and colon or can be designated by anatomic landmarks such as the Z-line, pylorus, papilla, and ileocecal valve.
- Localization software shows an abdominal-wall projection of the capsule location (Fig. 10.1).

10.4 Lumen

Described under the Lumen heading are several terms, as listed in Table 10.1. Figure 10.2 illustrates various forms of stenosis and dilatation, and Fig. 10.3 shows some signs of previous surgery.

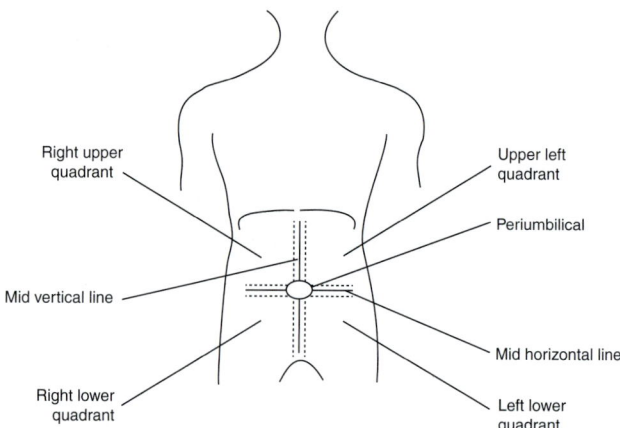

Fig. 10.1 Capsule localization based on four quadrants, the periumbilical area, a vertical line through the umbilicus (*right/left*), and a horizontal line through the umbilicus (*upper/lower*)

Table 10.1 Description of findings related to the lumen

Term	Attribute	Attribute values
Normal		
Stenosis	Type	Extrinsic compression
		Intraluminal (intrinsic) benign
		Intraluminal (intrinsic) malignant
	Traversed	Yes/no
Dilated	Longitudinal extent	Short segment/long segment/whole organ
	Wall contractions	Present/absent
Evidence of previous surgery	Type	Specify
	Suture material	Yes/no

Fig. 10.2 Stenosis/dilatation.
(**a**) Extrinsic stenosis.
(**b**) Intrinsic benign stenosis.
(**c**) Intrinsic malignant stenosis.
(**d**) Dilatation

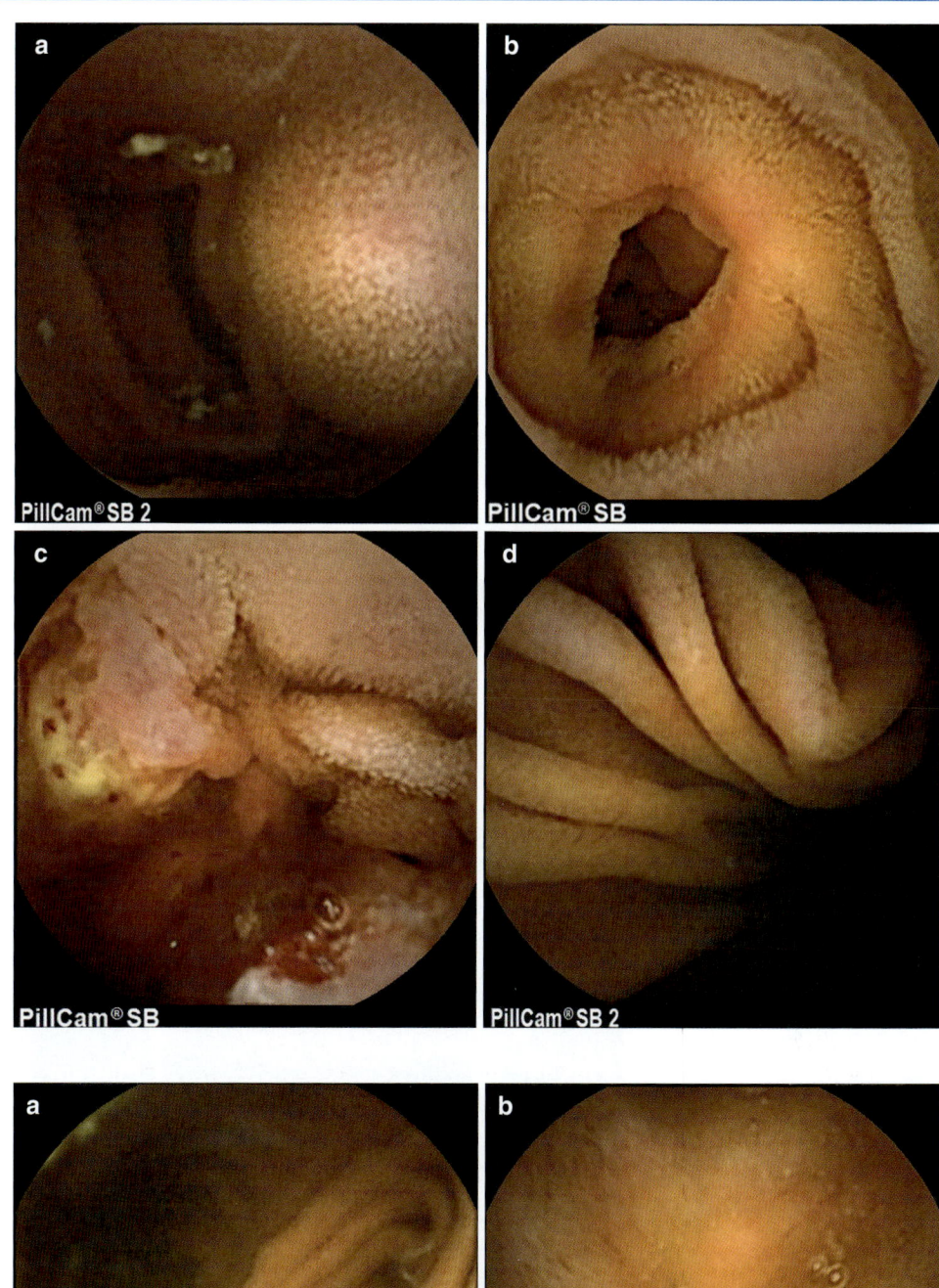

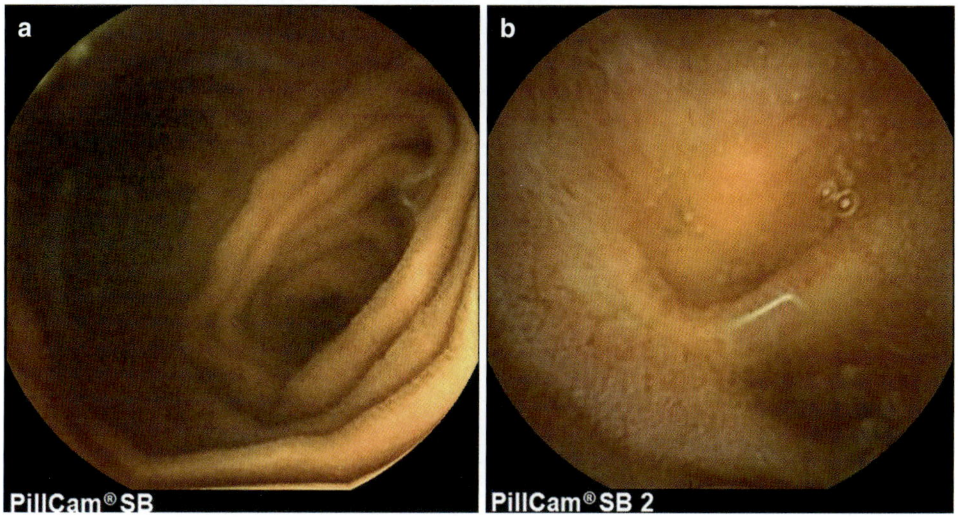

Fig. 10.3 Signs of previous surgery: anastomosis (**a**); scar and staple material (**b**)

10.5 Contents

Described under the Contents heading are several terms, as listed in Table 10.2. Figures 10.4 and 10.5 illustrate several types of these findings.

Table 10.2 Description of content findings

Term	Attribute	Attribute values
Blood	Type	Red/clot/hematin
Bile		
Parasites	Type	Specify
Foreign body	Type	Specify
Food	Type	Specify
Feces		

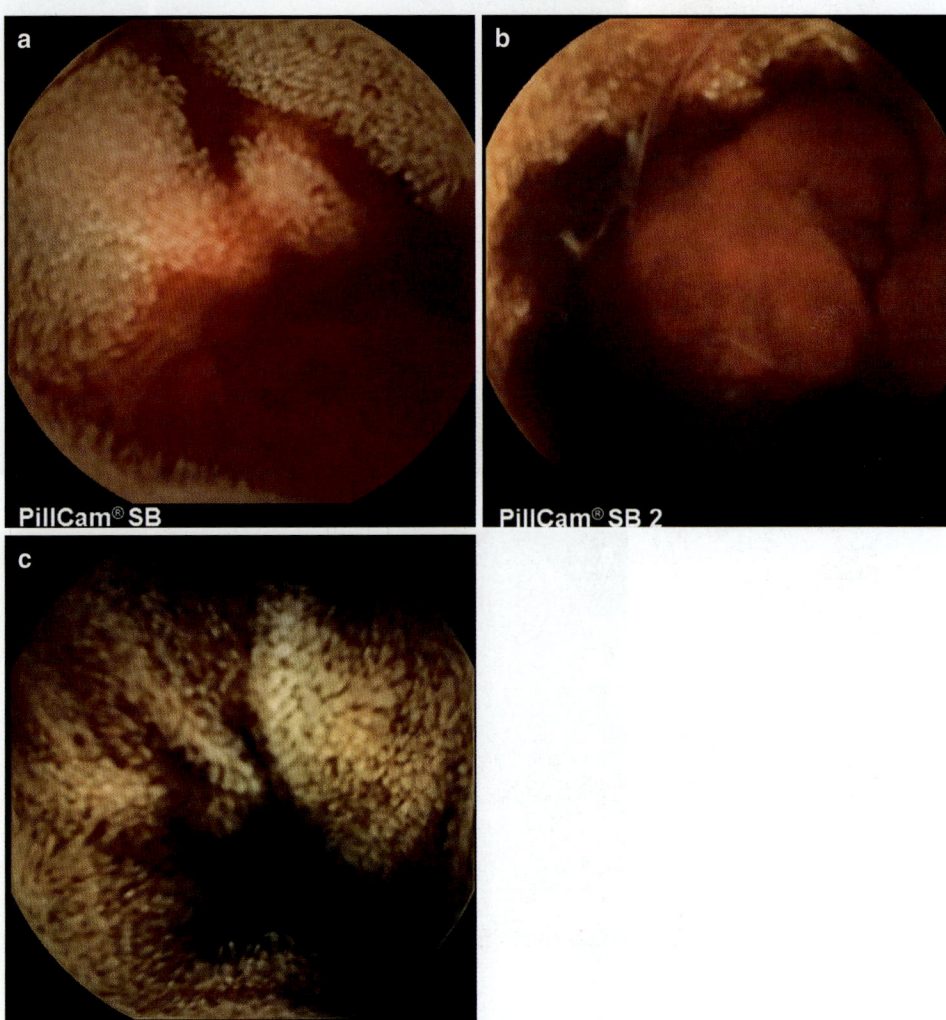

Fig. 10.4 Description of contents: (**a**) red blood. (**b**) Clot. (**c**) Hematin

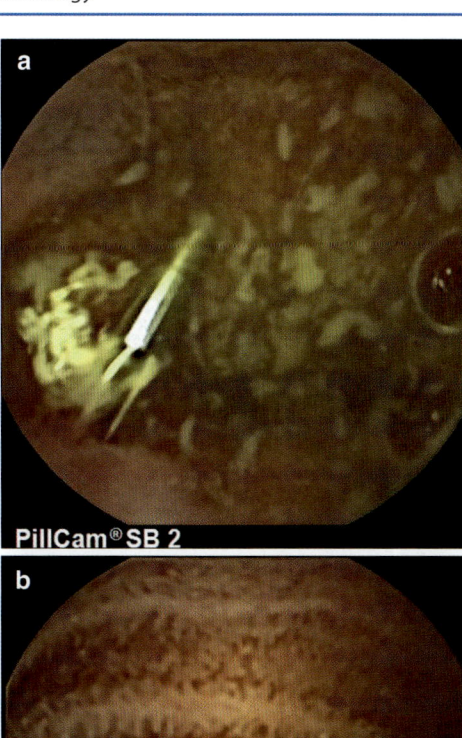

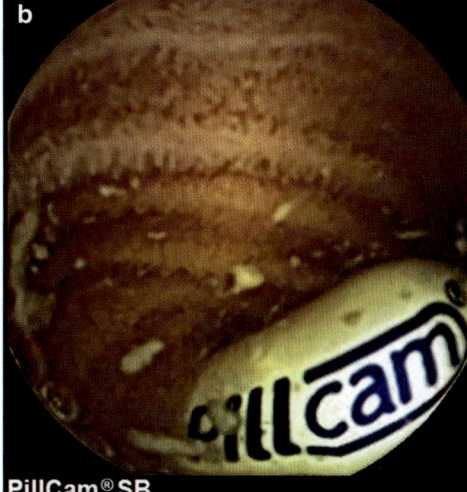

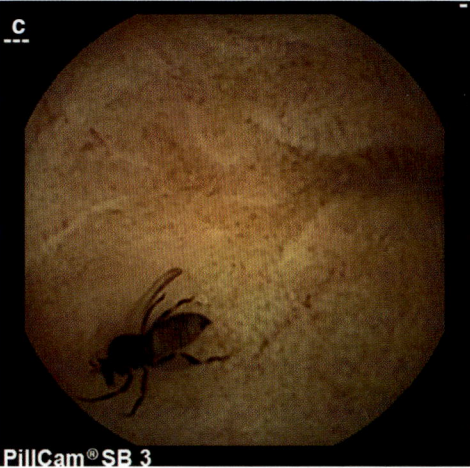

Fig. 10.5 Description of contents: (**a**) feces and foreign body (clip). (**b**) Foreign body (video capsule). (**c**) Insect (Courtesy of Thomas Teuber, MD)

10.6 Mucosa

Described under the Mucosa heading are a number of terms, as listed in Table 10.3. Figures 10.6, 10.7, and 10.8 illustrate the appearance of various types of abnormal mucosa and villi.

Table 10.3 Description of mucosa findings

Term	Attribute	Attribute values
Erythematous	Distribution pattern	Localized/patchy/diffuse
	Longitudinal extent	Short segment/long segment/whole organ
Pale	Distribution pattern	Localized/patchy/diffuse
	Longitudinal extent	Short segment/long segment/whole organ
Edematous (congested)	Distribution pattern	Localized/patchy/diffuse
	Longitudinal extent	Short segment/long segment/whole organ
Granular	Distribution pattern	Localized/patchy/diffuse
	Longitudinal extent	Short segment/long segment/whole organ
Nodular	Distribution pattern	Localized/patchy/diffuse
	Longitudinal extent	Short segment/long segment/whole organ
Atrophic	Distribution pattern	Localized/patchy/diffuse
	Longitudinal extent	Short segment/long segment/whole organ
Abnormal villi	Shape	Convoluted/swollen/blunted/absent
	Color	Whitish/yellow
	Distribution pattern	Localized/patchy/diffuse
	Longitudinal extent	Short segment/long segment/whole organ

Fig. 10.6 Abnormal mucosa:
pale (**a**), edematous (**b**),
erythematous (**c**), atrophic (**d**),
granular (**e**), nodular (**f**)

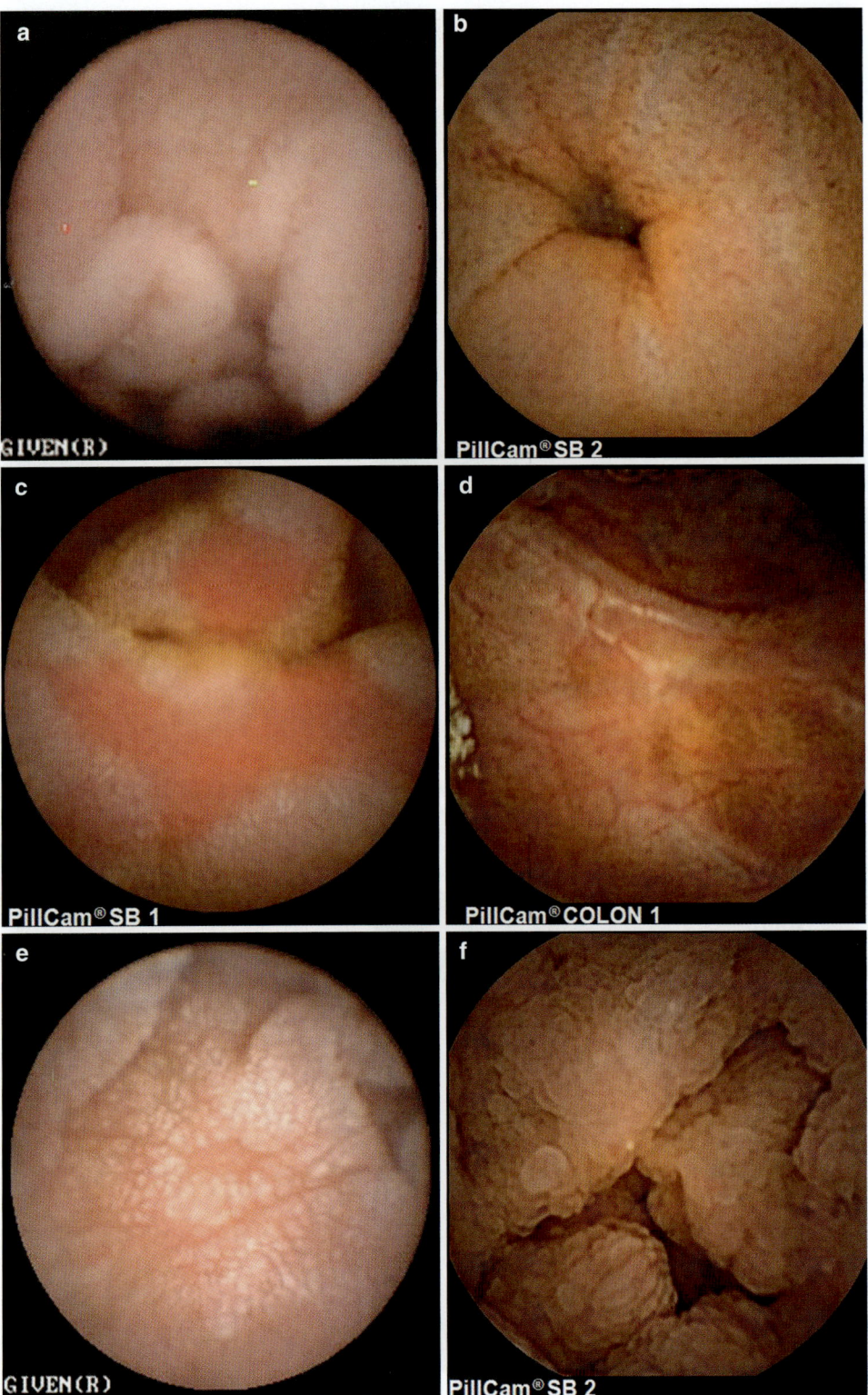

Fig. 10.7 White villi: localized and blunted (**a**), patchy (**b**), diffuse (**c**, **d**)

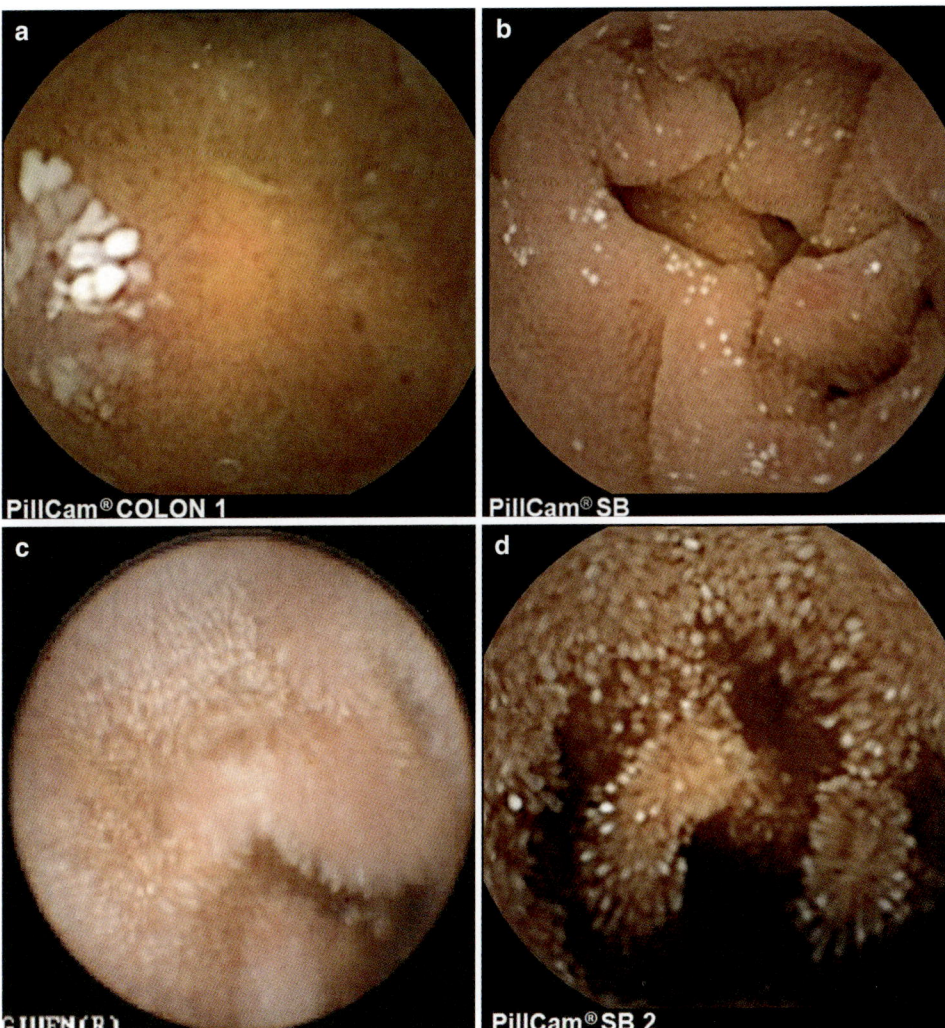

Fig. 10.8 Missing villi. Focal (**a**), patchy (**b**), diffuse (**c**)

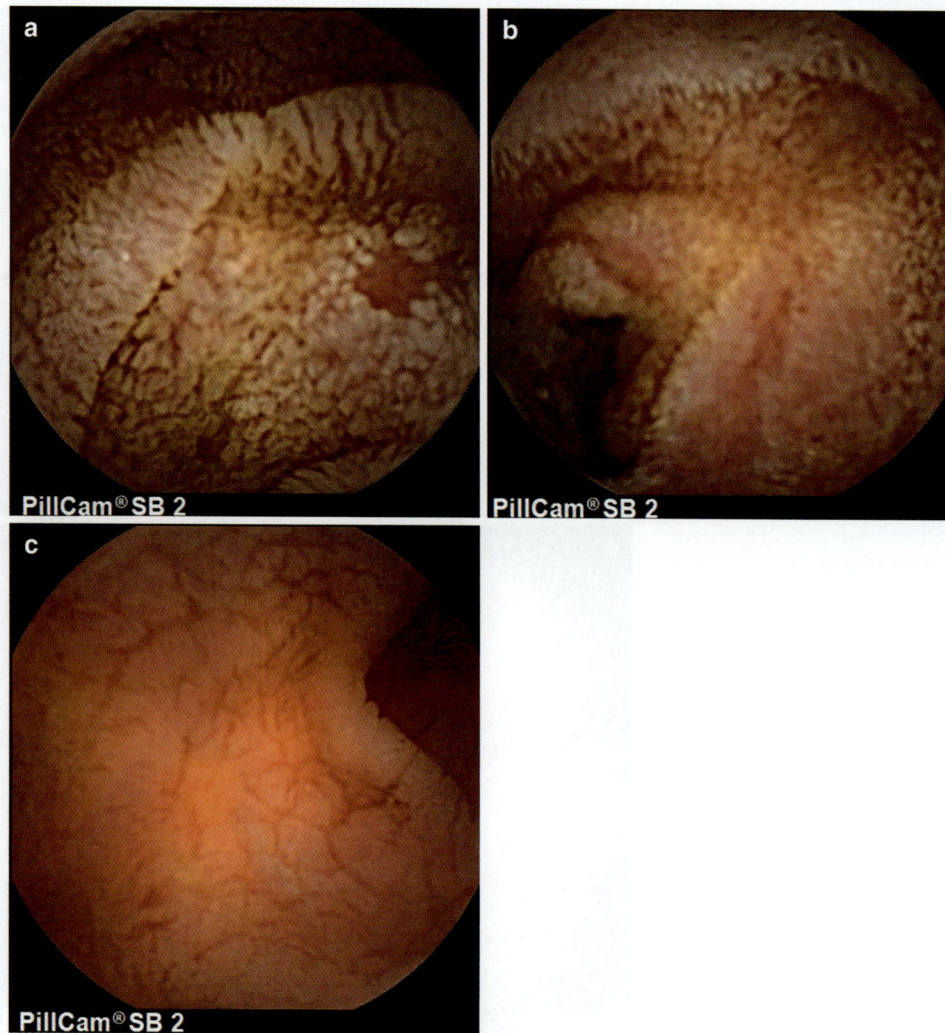

10.7 Flat Lesions

The Flat Lesions heading includes the terms *angiectasias* (Fig. 10.9), *spots* (Fig. 10.10), and *plaques*, as listed in Table 10.4.

Fig. 10.9 Angiectasias: small (**a**), medium (**b**), large (**c**), with arborization (**d**; image in blue mode)

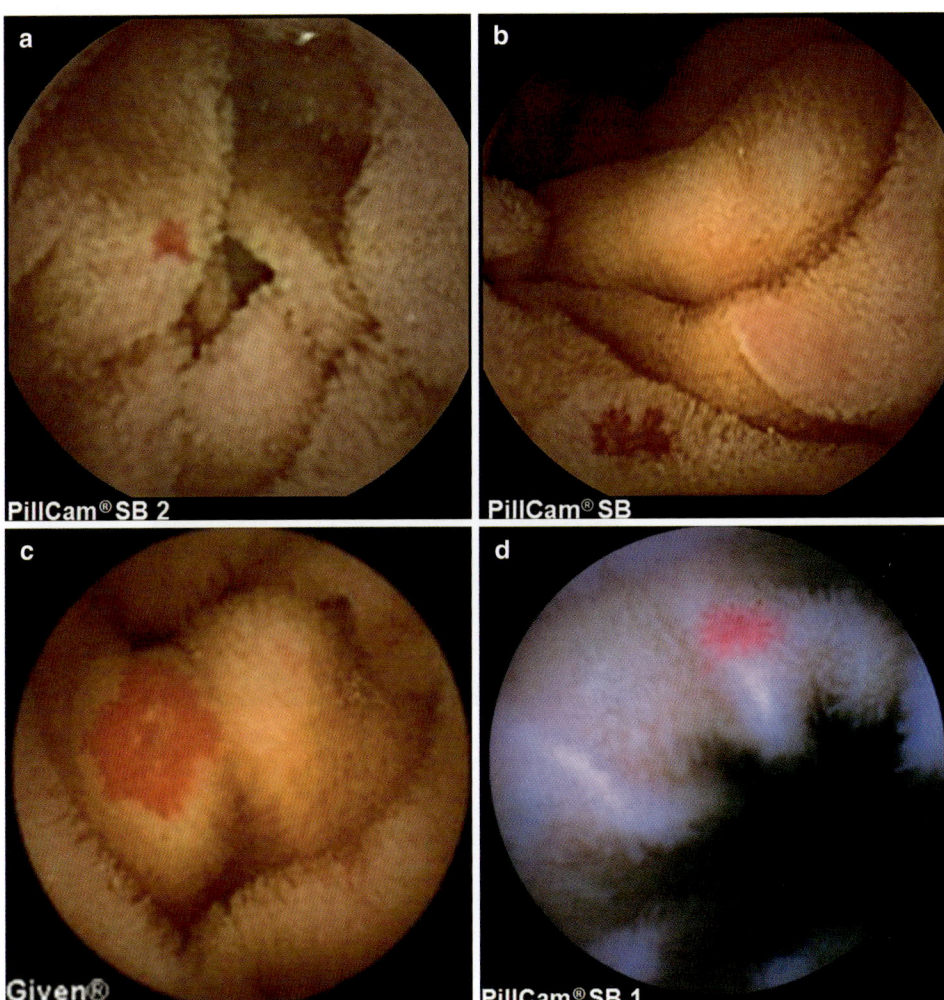

Fig. 10.10 Spots: red spot
(**a**), white spot (**b**), black spot
(**c**; ink mark)

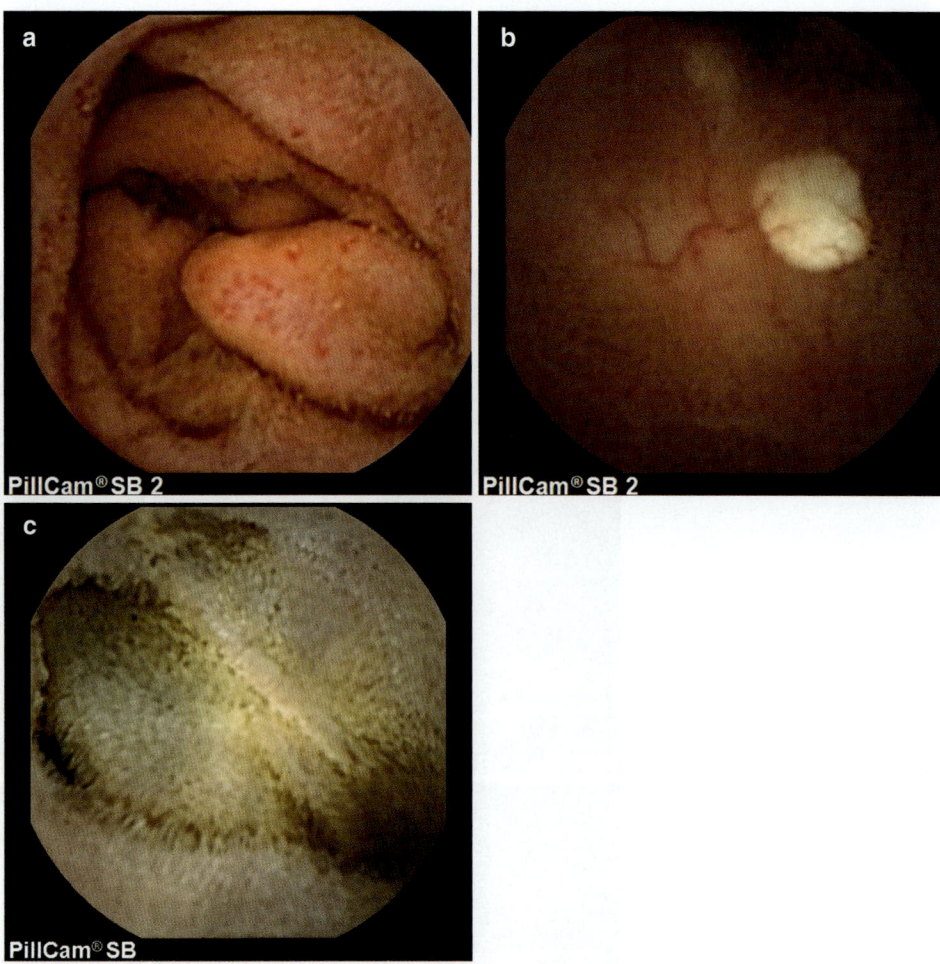

Table 10.4 Description of
flat lesions

Term	Attribute	Attribute values
Spot	Number	Single/multiple
	Type	Red/white/black
	Bleeding	Yes/no
	Distribution pattern	Localized/patchy/diffuse
	Longitudinal extent	Short segment/long segment/whole organ
Plaque	Number	Single/multiple
	Type	Red/white/black
	Distribution pattern	Localized/patchy/diffuse
	Longitudinal extent	Short segment/long segment/whole organ
Angiectasia	Number	Single/multiple
	Size	Small/medium/large
	Arborization	Yes/no
	Bleeding	Yes/no
	Stigmata of bleeding	Yes/no
	Bleeding potential	Yes/possible/no
	Distribution pattern	Localized/patchy/diffuse
	Longitudinal extent	Short segment/long segment/whole organ

10.8   Protruding Lesions

Under the Protruding Lesions heading (Table 10.5) are venous structures (Fig. 10.11), nodules and polyps (Figs. 10.12 and 10.13), and tumors (Fig. 10.14).

Table 10.5   Description of protruding lesions

Term	Attribute	Attribute values
Nodules	Number	Single/few/multiple
	Bleeding	Yes/no
	Stigmata of bleeding	Yes/no
	Distribution pattern	Localized/patchy/diffuse
	Longitudinal extent	Short segment/long segment/whole organ
Polyps	Number	Single/few/multiple
	Size	Small/medium/large
	Pedicle	Sessile/pedunculated/unknown
	Bleeding	Yes/no
Mass/tumor	Size	Small (<5 mm)/medium (5–20 mm)/large (>20 mm)
	Type	Submucosal/fungating/ulcerated/frond like/villous
	Bleeding	Yes/no
	Stigmata of bleeding	Yes/no
Venous structure	Type	Venous lake/bleb/varix
	Number bleeding	Single/few/multiple
	Bleeding	Yes/no
	Stigmata of bleeding	Yes/no
	Bleeding potential	Yes/possible/no
	Distribution pattern	Localized/patchy/diffuse
	Longitudinal extent	Short segment/long segment/whole organ

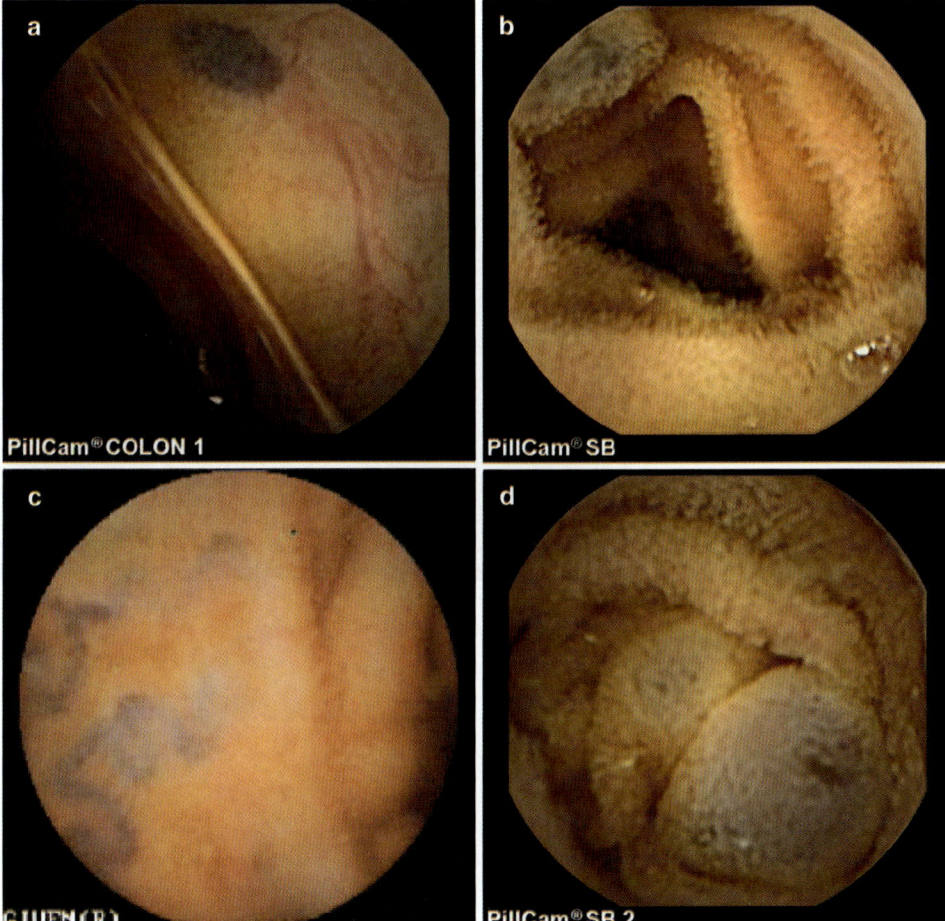

Fig. 10.11   Veins: venous lake (**a**), bleb (**b**), varix (**c**), bleeding potential present (**d**; eroded surface)

Fig. 10.12 Nodule and polyps: nodule (**a**), sessile polyp (**b**), pedunculated polyp (**c**), possibly pedunculated polyp (**d**)

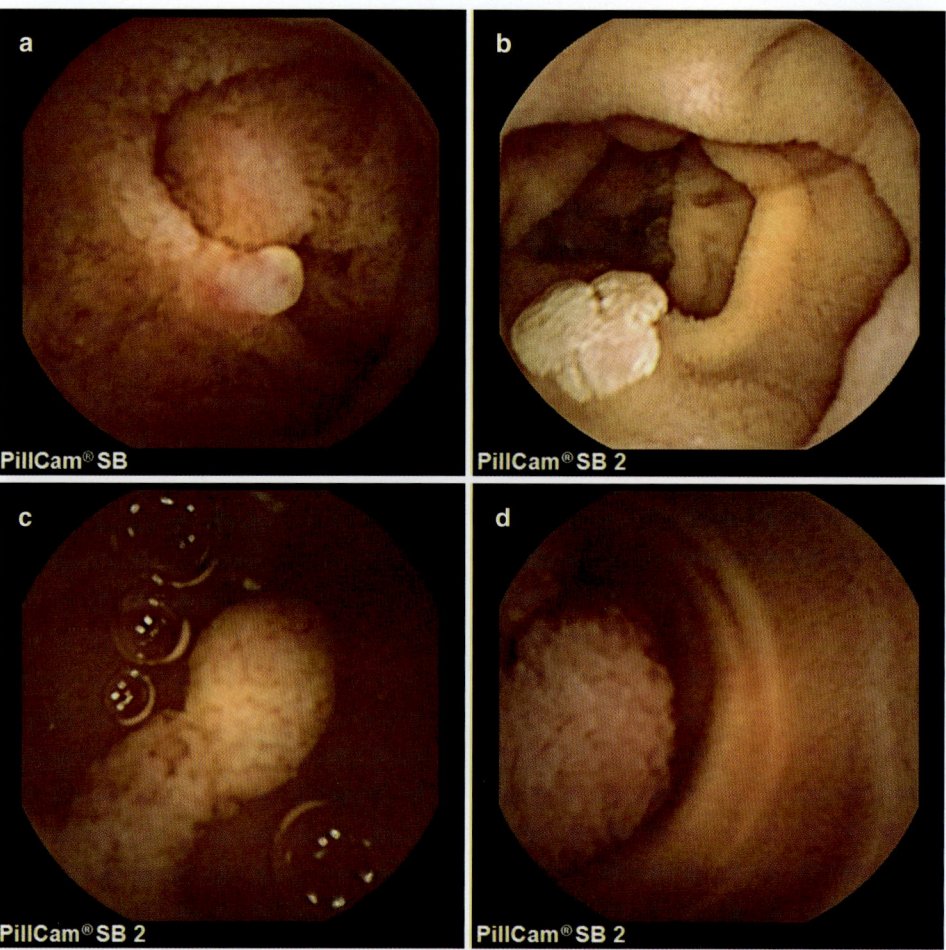

Fig. 10.13 Polyps: small (**a**), medium (**b**), large (**c**), multiple small- to medium-sized polyps (**d**)

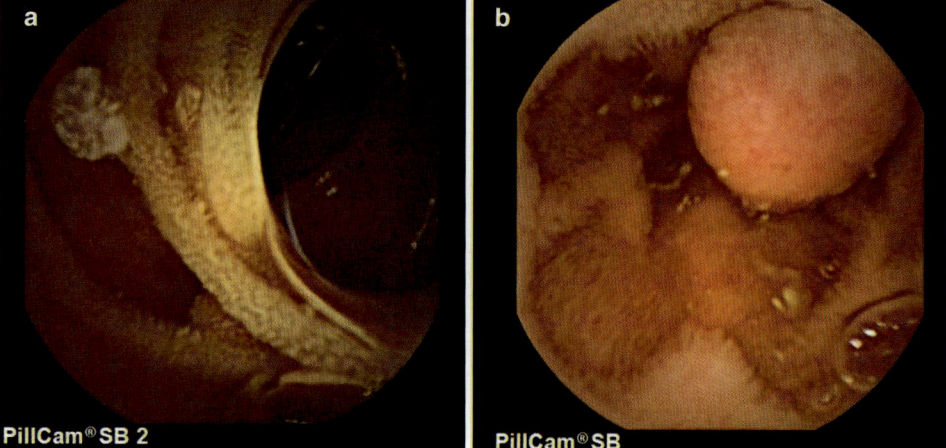

Fig. 10.13 (continued)

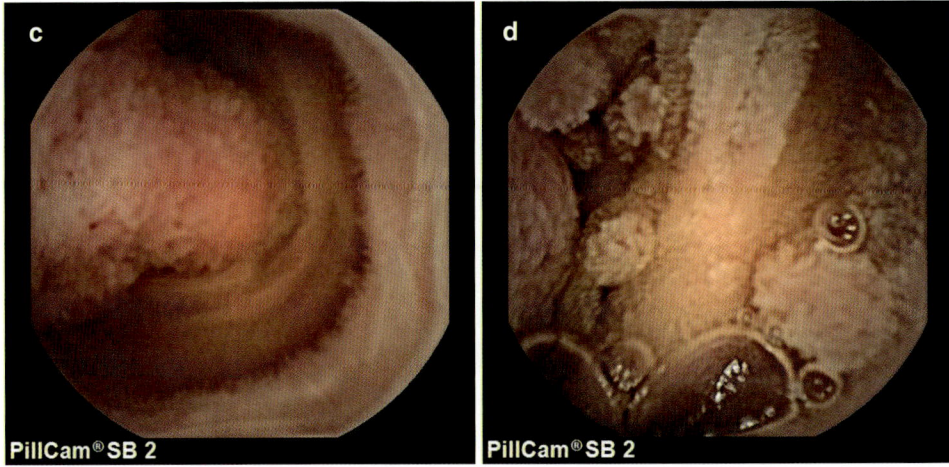

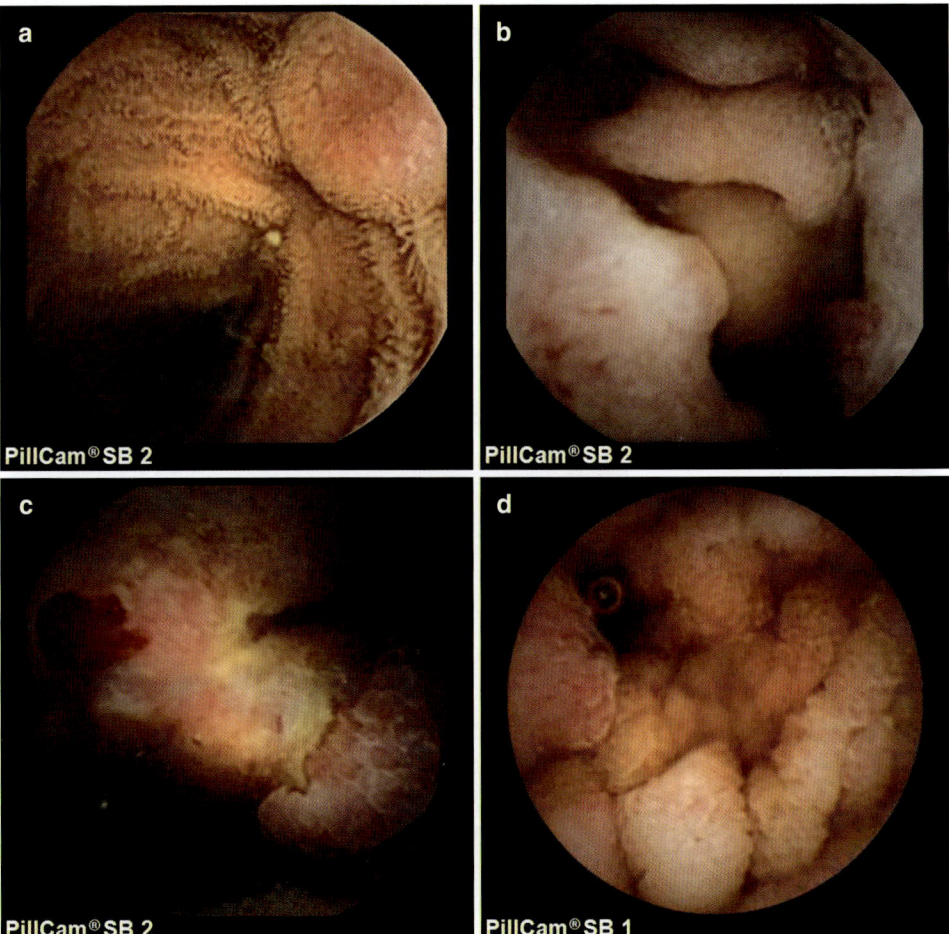

Fig. 10.14 Tumors: submucosal, medium sized (**a**); fungating, large (**b**); exulcerated, large (**c**); villous, large (**d**)

10.9   Excavated Lesions

Table 10.6 lists the various types of excavated lesions, several of which are illustrated in Fig. 10.15.

Table 10.6 Description of excavated lesions

Term	Attribute	Attribute values
Aphtha	Number	Single/few/multiple
	Distribution pattern	Localized/patchy/diffuse
	Longitudinal extent	Short segment/long segment/whole organ
Erosion	Number	Single/few/multiple
	Bleeding	Yes/no
	Stigmata of bleeding	Yes/no
	Distribution pattern	Localized/patchy/diffuse
	Longitudinal extent	Short segment/long segment/whole organ
Ulcer	Number	Single/few/multiple
	Bleeding	Yes/no
	Stigmata of bleeding	Yes/no
	Distribution pattern	Localized/patchy/diffuse
	Longitudinal extent	Short segment/long segment/whole organ
Scar		
Diverticulum		Single/multiple

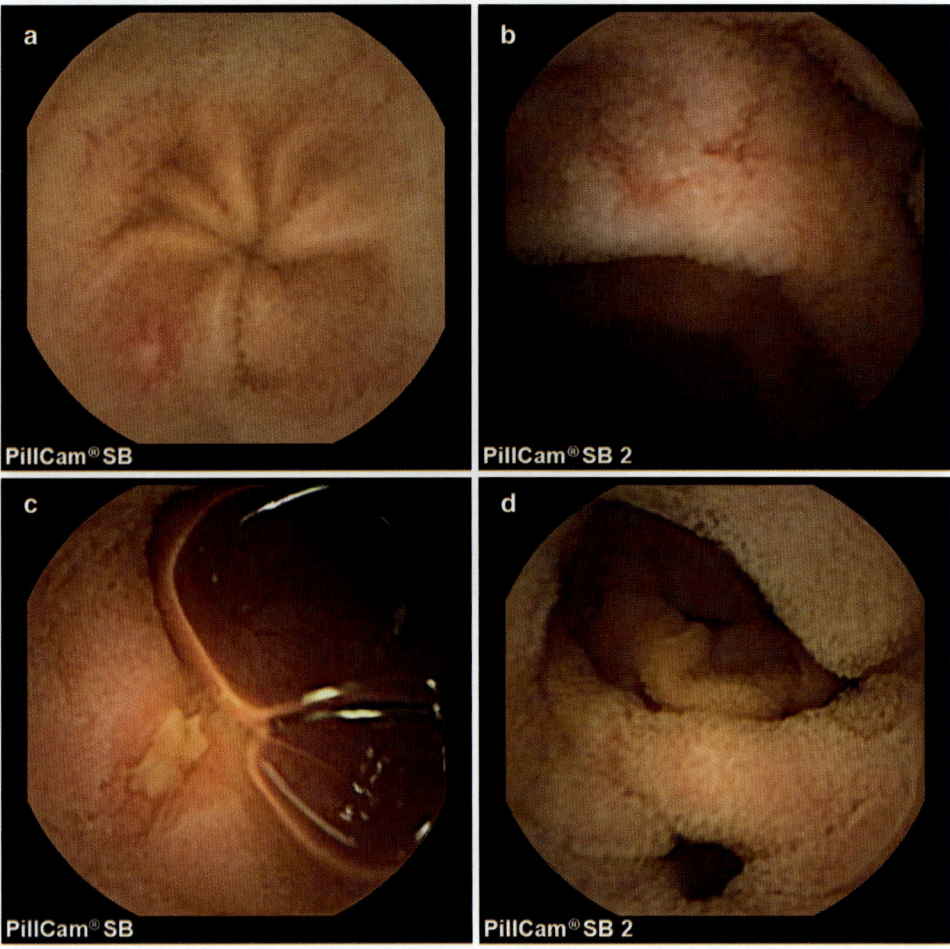

Fig. 10.15 Excavated lesions: aphtha (**a**), a few erosions (**b**), ulcer (**c**), small diverticulum (**d**)

10.10 Diagnoses

The diagnosis represents the opinion of the examiner based on clinical history and findings. The examiner should try to distinguish the diagnosis from the findings. For example, small bowel erosions can be found in both nonsteroidal anti-inflammatory drug (NSAID)-induced enteropathy and Crohn's disease. The examiner should select the diagnoses from the following list, which represents the range of common and rare small bowel diagnoses. The list of diagnoses, as proposed by the CEST, is divided into two lists of terms, the main diagnoses and other diagnoses, classified according to their frequency in clinical practice.

10.10.1 Main Diagnoses

- Normal
- Angiectasia
- Erosion
- Ulcer
- Crohn's disease
- Celiac disease
- NSAID enteritis
- Tumor
  - Benign
  - Malignant
- Bleeding of unknown origin

10.10.2 Other Diagnoses

- Diverticulum
- Tropical sprue
- Parasites
- Dieulafoy's lesion
- Hemobilia
- Phlebectasia
- Varices
- Intestinal lymphangiectasia
- Ischemic enteritis
- Vasculitis
- Radiation enteritis
- Posttransplant lymphoproliferative disorder
- Graft-versus-host disease

- Enteropathy
  - Erosive
  - Erythematous
  - Congestive
  - Hemorrhagic
- Brunner's gland hyperplasia
- Lipoma
- Xanthelasma
- Neuroendocrine tumor
- Melanoma
- GIST (gastrointestinal stromal tumor)
- Kaposi's sarcoma
- Lymphoma
- Polyp
- Juvenile polyposis
- Familial adenomatous polyposis
- Peutz-Jeghers syndrome

References

1. Korman LY. Standard terminology for capsule endoscopy. Gastrointest Endosc Clin N Am. 2004;14:33–41.
2. Maratka Z. The OMED data base: standard for nomenclature. Endoscopy. 1992;24 Suppl 2:455–6.
3. Delvaux M, Crespi M, Armengol-Miro JR, et al. Minimal standard terminology for digestive endoscopy: results of prospective testing and validation in the GASTER project. Endoscopy. 2000;32:345–55.
4. Delvaux M, Crespi M, Korman LY, Fujino MA. Minimal standard terminology for digestive endoscopy. Terms and attributes, Version 2.0. Bad Homburg: Normed Verlag; 2002.
5. Aabakken L, Rembacken B, LeMoine O, et al. Minimal standard terminology for gastrointestinal endoscopy (MST 3.0). Organization Mondiale Endoscopia Digestive (OMED). 2008. Available at: http://www.worldendo.org/mst.html.
6. Korman LY, Delvaux M, Gay G, et al. Capsule endoscopy structured terminology (CEST): proposal of a standardized and structured terminology for reporting capsule endoscopy procedures. Endoscopy. 2005;37:951–9.
7. Delvaux M, Friedman S, Keuchel M, et al. Structured terminology for capsule endoscopy: results of retrospective testing and validation in 766 small-bowel investigations. Endoscopy. 2005;37:945–50.
8. Rondonotti E, Soncini M, Girelli CM, et al. Can we improve the detection rate and interobserver agreement in capsule endoscopy? Dig Liver Dis. 2012;44:1006–11.
9. Pezzoli A, Cannizzaro R, Pennazio M, et al. Interobserver agreement in describing video capsule endoscopy findings: a multicentre prospective study. Dig Liver Dis. 2011;43:126–31.
10. Jang BI, Lee SH, Moon JS, et al. Inter-observer agreement on the interpretation of capsule endoscopy findings based on capsule endoscopy structured terminology: a multicenter study by the Korean Gut Image Study Group. Scand J Gastroenterol. 2010;45:370–4.

Duodenoscopy and Ileocolonoscopy

11

Hisao Tajiri, Friedrich Hagenmüller, and Martin Keuchel

Contents

The work was first published in 2006 by Springer Medizin Verlag Heidelberg with the following title: *Atlas of Video Capsule Endoscopy.*

H. Tajiri (✉)
Division of Gastroenterology and Hepatology,
Department of Internal Medicine, The Jikei University
School of Medicine, 3-25-8 Nishishinbashi, Tokyo 105-8461, Japan
e-mail: tajiri@jikei.ac.jp

F. Hagenmüller
1st Medical Department, Akademisches Lehrkrankenhaus der
Universität Hamburg, Paul-Ehrlich-Strasse 1, Asklepios Klinik Altona,
Hamburg 22763, Germany
e-mail: f.hagenmueller@asklepios.com

M. Keuchel
Department of Internal Medicine,
Bethesda Krankenhaus Bergedorf, Hamburg, Germany
e-mail: keuchel@bkb.info

11.1 Duodenoscopy

Before the entire small bowel is imaged by video capsule endoscopy, a careful esophagogastroduodenoscopy (EGD) should be performed. In several studies, missed sources of bleeding within the reach of a gastroscope (Fig. 11.1) were detected in a significant percentage, such as in 42 % of patients referred for push enteroscopy in one study [1].

A side-viewing duodenoscope allows a superior view of the papillary region (Fig. 11.2). In many patients, the portion of the duodenum beyond the papilla also can be visualized with a standard gastroscope. Image-enhanced endoscopy includes a variety of techniques that can be used to bring out fine details in the mucosa (Fig. 11.3) and partially also in deeper layers (Fig. 11.4) [2]. Chromoendoscopy with dye spray [3] or intravital staining [4] can be applied during endoscopy without special equipment (Fig. 11.5). Narrow band imaging (NBI) and probe-based confocal laser microscopy had 95 % sensitivity and 90 % specificity in detecting dysplasia in duodenal polyps (compared with histology) [5]. Magnification endoscopy allows detailed visualization of villi [6, 7] and vascular pattern (Fig. 11.6). Endoscopic ultrasound can also be performed to investigate protruding or infiltrating lesions, allowing the analysis of submucosa and muscularis propria (Fig. 11.4).

Duodenal biopsies are important in patients with suspected celiac sprue and other diseases such as Whipple's disease, genuine lymphangiectasia, or giardiasis suspected after negative stool tests.

Therapeutic options for hemostasis include epinephrine injection, fibrin glue, coagulation, clips, and spray of hemostatic powder. Polyps can be removed by biopsy forceps, snare resection, or endoscopic mucosa resection, depending on their size. Even en bloc endoscopic submucosal dissection (ESD) is possible in the duodenum in selected cases of endoscopic suspicion of early malignancy (Fig. 11.7).

Fig. 11.1 Small duodenal ulcer in a patient with overt gastrointestinal (GI) bleeding. (**a**) Oozing bleeding. (**b**) Visible vessel. (**c**) Narrow band imaging (NBI). The initial esophagogastroduodenoscopy (EGD) had been inconclusive, but video capsule endoscopy had shown fresh blood in the duodenum

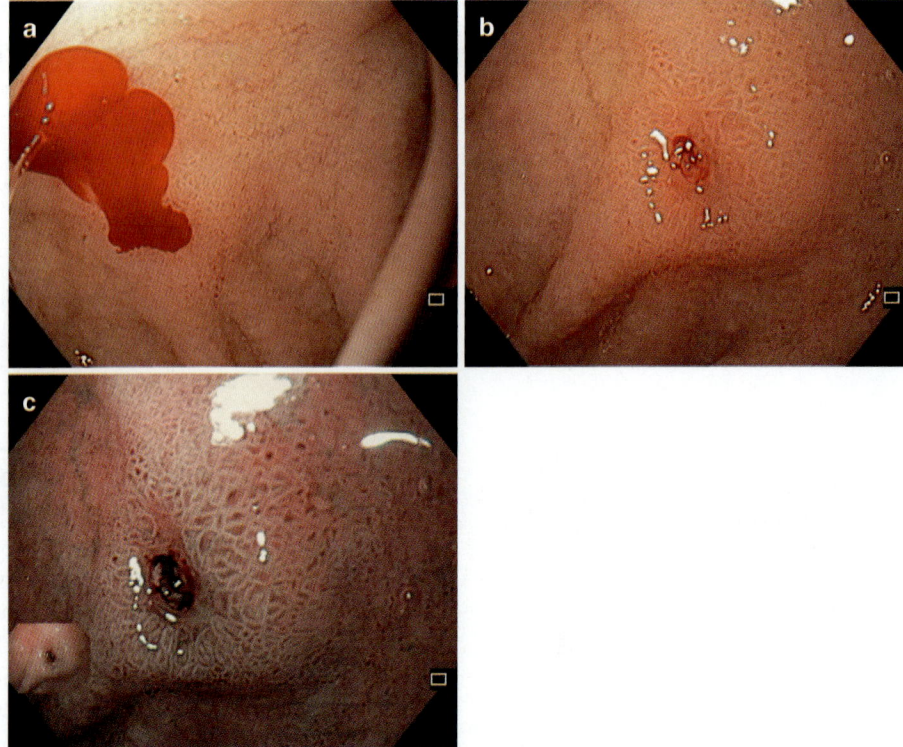

Fig. 11.2 (**a**, **b**) Side-viewing duodenoscopy clearly demonstrates the location of a submucosal tumor distal to the papilla of Vater

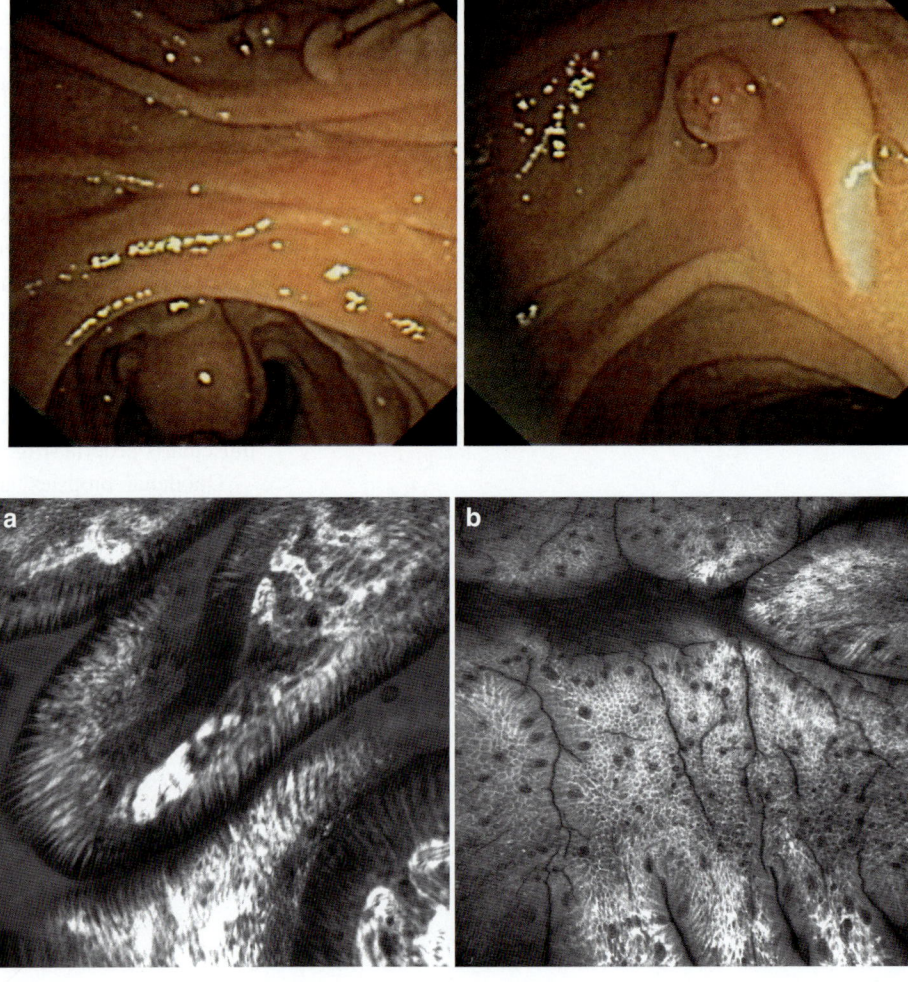

Fig. 11.3 Confocal laser microscopy. (**a**) Normal villi. (**b**) Villous atrophy

Fig. 11.4 Endoscopic ultrasound with a miniprobe (**a**) shows symmetric thickening of the mucosa (**b**) in a patient with duodenal lymphoma

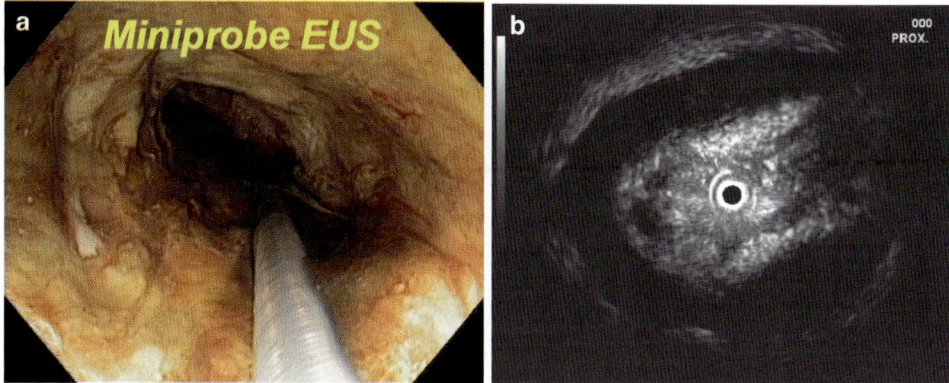

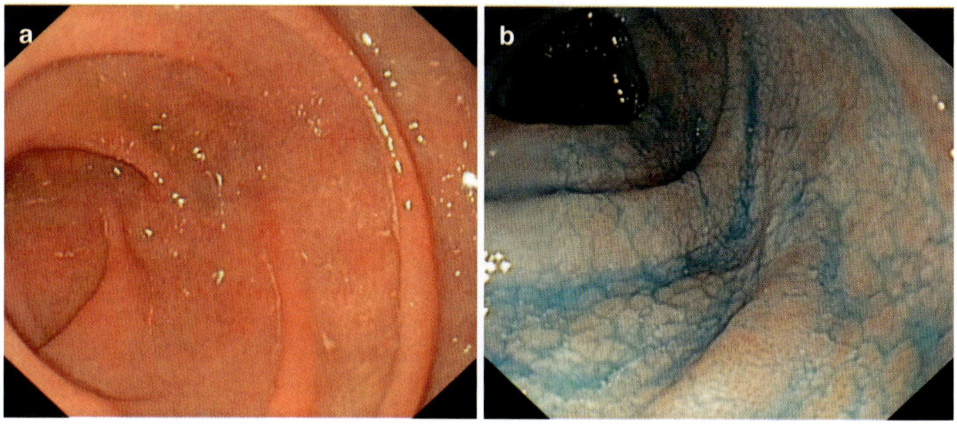

Fig. 11.5 Villous atrophy. (**a**) Native image. (**b**) Improved visualization with chromoendoscopy

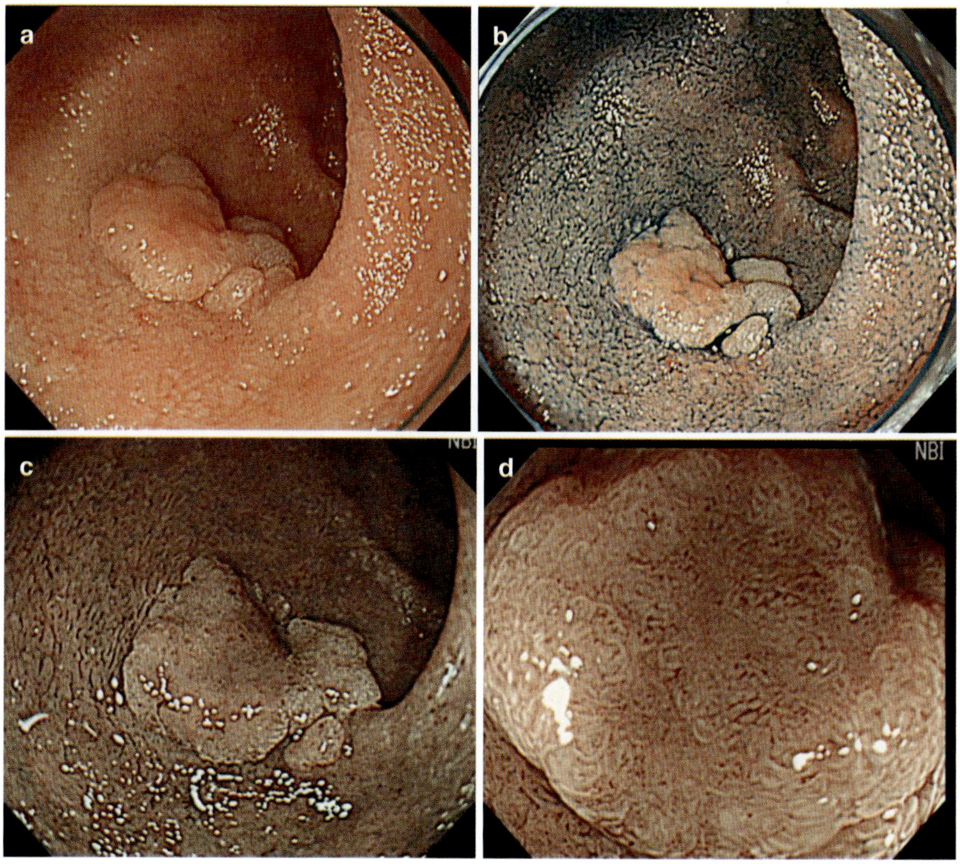

Fig. 11.6 Slightly elevated adenocarcinoma with granular surface in the duodenal bulb. (**a**) White light image. (**b**) Chromoendoscopy after indigo carmine spraying. (**c**) NBI. (**d**) NBI magnified endoscopy visualized a fine mucosal surface of minute, pitlike structure with network-pattern vasculature

Fig. 11.7 Gently elevated carcinoid tumor covered by reddish mucosa in the duodenal bulb. (**a**) White light image. (**b**) Chromoendoscopy after indigo carmine spraying. (**c**) Submucosal injection of 0.4 % sodium hyaluronate. (**d**) Circumferential isolation from surrounding normal mucosa. (**e**) Endoscopic submucosal dissection (ESD). (**f**) Mucosal defect after ESD

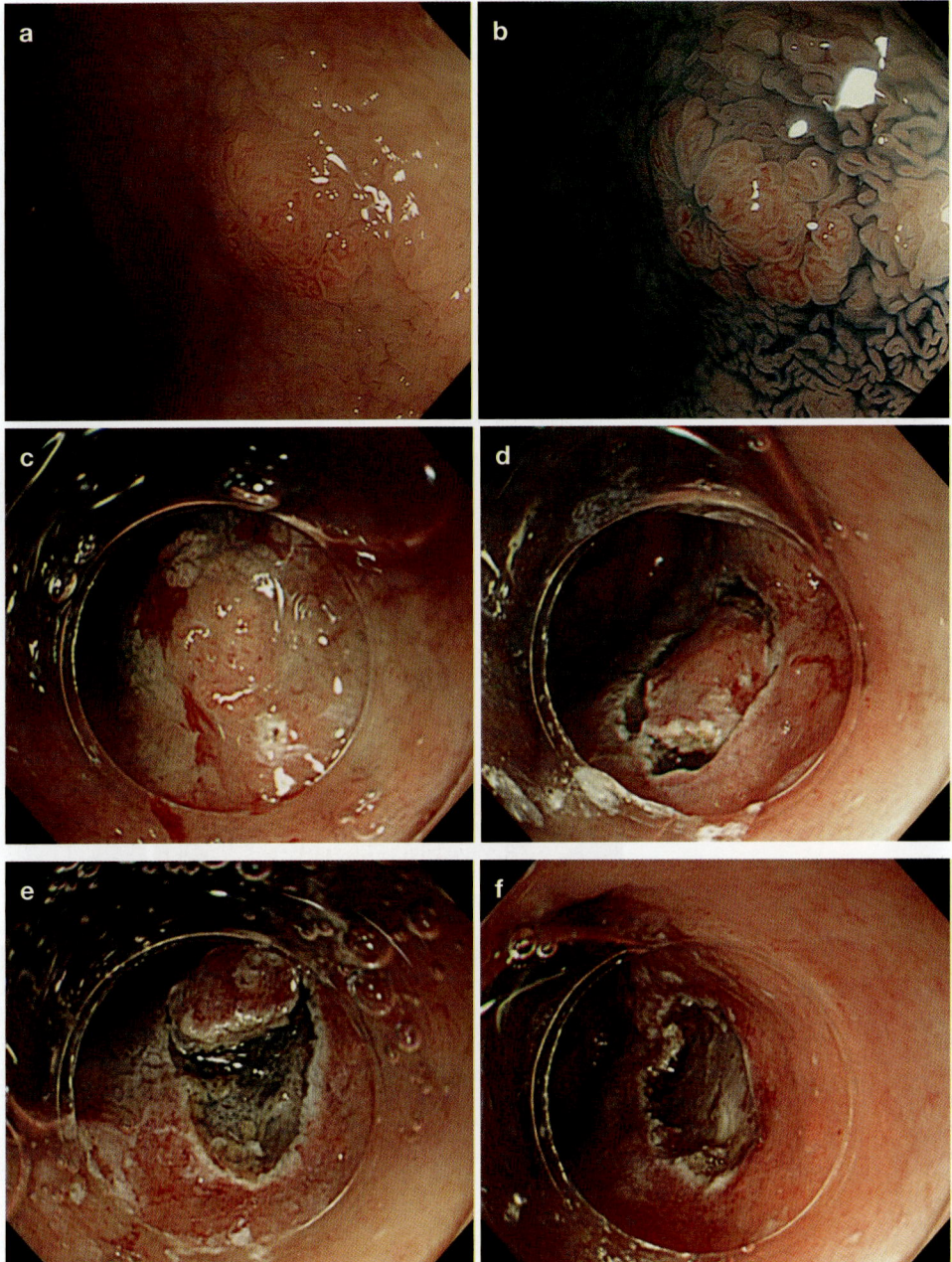

11.2   Ileocolonoscopy

Colonoscopy is the method of choice for diagnosis and treatment of lower gastrointestinal (GI) diseases [8]. Colonoscopy can provide diagnosis of the underlying disease in most patients with GI bleeding and normal EGD. Diagnoses include diverticular disease (Fig. 11.8), colonic polyps and cancer, angiectasias (especially of the cecum), inflammatory bowel disease, or infection.

Colonoscopy is the gold standard for detection of polyps and cancer. High-resolution endoscopy is helpful in also revealing flat lesions (e.g., sessile serrated adenomas, also known as sessile serrated polyps (Fig. 11.9)) and in characterizing lesions according to their pit pattern [9] (Fig. 11.10) and vascular pattern [10]. Magnifying chromoendoscopy or NBI may further increase accuracy [11].

Surveillance colonoscopy is recommended in patients with long-standing ulcerative colitis, for the prevention of colorectal carcinoma (Fig. 11.11). Detection of sometimes subtle precursor lesions as dysplasia or dysplasia-associated lesion or mass (DALM) requires multiple random biopsies or biopsies targeted by high-resolution chromoendoscopy [12].

Bowel strictures due to scarring or ulceration in patients with Crohn's disease often are accessible by ileocolonoscopy (Fig. 11.12), which can provide a diagnosis, and hydrostatic balloon dilation can treat fibrotic strictures. Video capsule endoscopy may be withheld in these patients to prevent capsule retention.

Ileocolonoscopy is still the mainstay for the diagnosis of inflammatory bowel disease [13]. Intubation of the terminal ileum is easily performed in experienced hands and adds to the management of symptomatic patients [14, 15]. Approximately 5–30 cm of the terminal ileum can be visualized after intubation of the ileocecal valve during colonoscopy. Endoscopic evaluation and optional biopsy of the terminal ileum are of particular importance in the diagnosis of Crohn's disease (Fig. 11.12a) and lymphoma. Incidental findings due to the use of nonsteroidal antiinflammatory drugs (NSAIDs) also may be seen (Fig. 11.13).

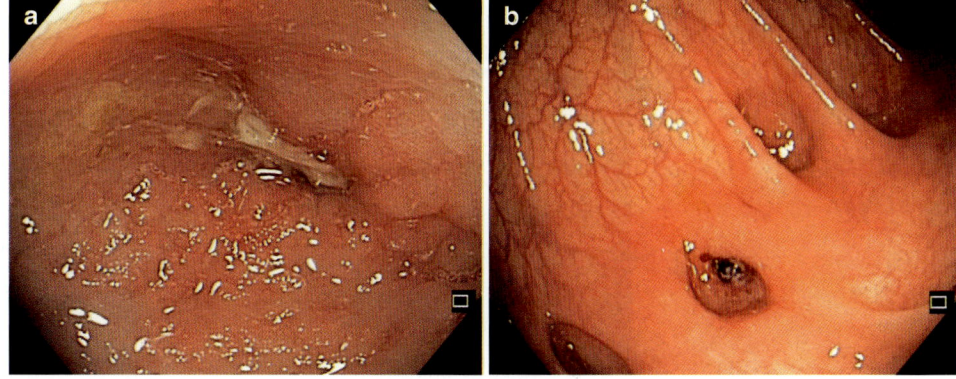

Fig. 11.8 Complications of diverticulosis. (**a**) Diverticulum with blood vessel in a patient with severe hemorrhage. (**b**) Diverticulitis

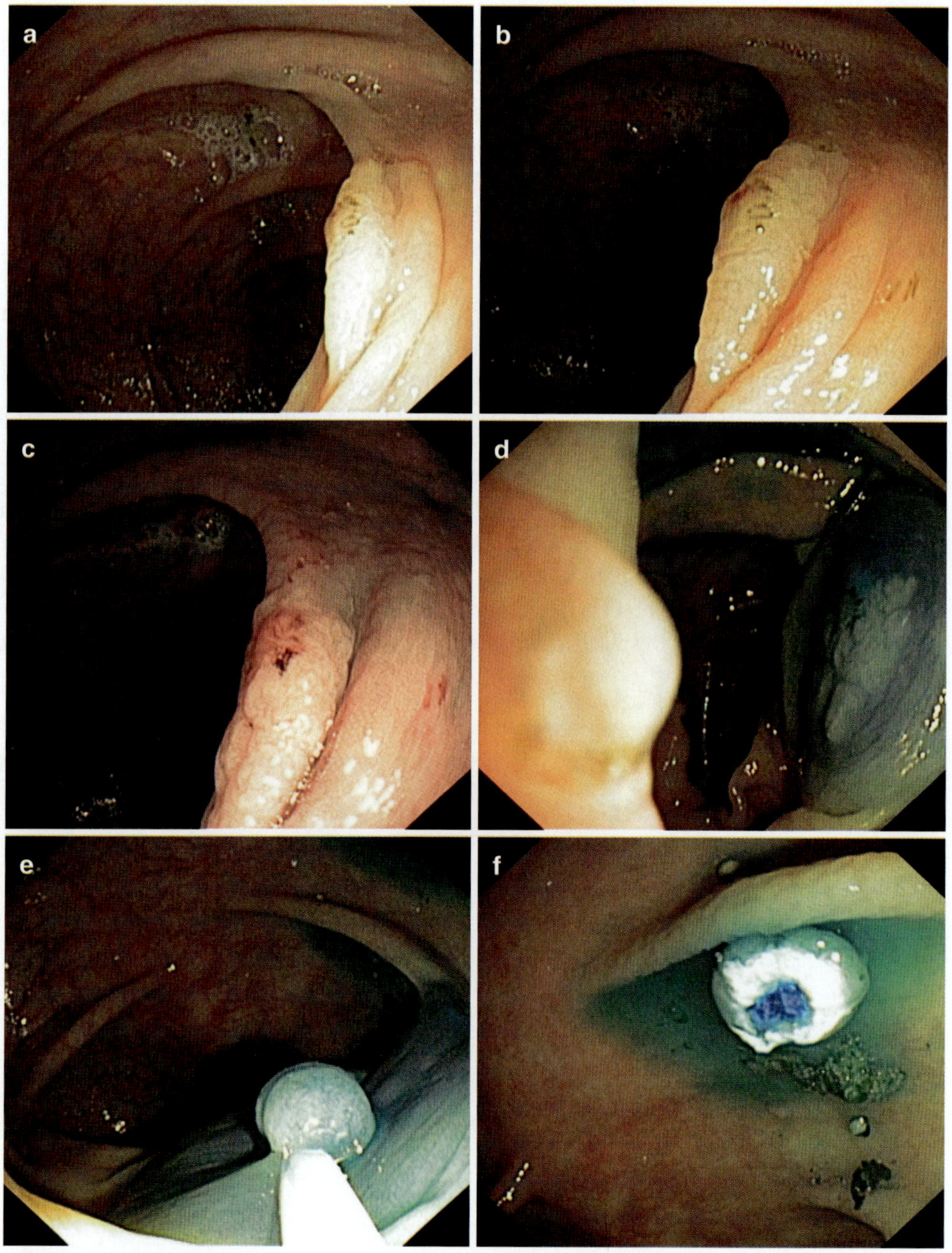

Fig. 11.9 Flat polyp (sessile serrated adenoma/polyp). (**a**, **b**) Atypical fold. (**c**) NBI. (**d**) Injection, chromoendoscopy. (**e–f**) Mucosectomy allowing histologic investigation of the polyp base

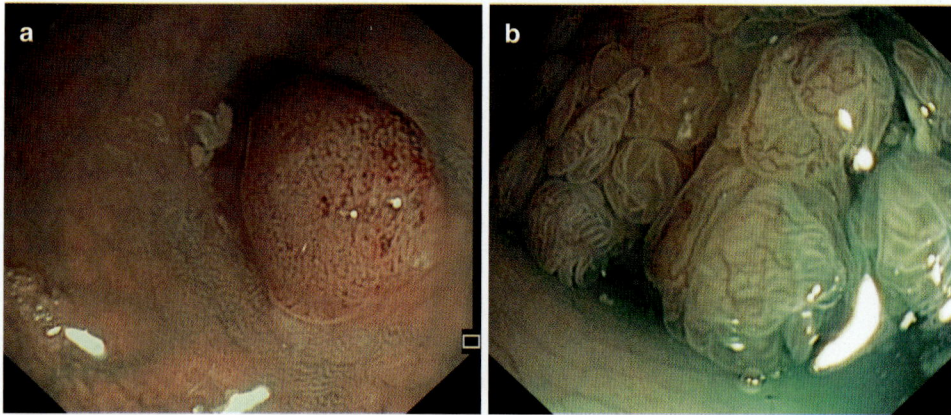

Fig. 11.10 Colon polyp (NBI observation). (**a**) Tubular adenoma with pit pattern-like appearance III$_L$. (**b**) Tubular-villous adenoma with pit pattern-like appearance IV

Fig. 11.11 Surveillance in inactive ulcerative colitis. (**a**) Scar. (**b**) Pseudopolyps (using chromoendoscopy). (**c**) Hyperplastic polyps (using NBI). (**d**) Dysplasia-associated lesion or mass (DALM)

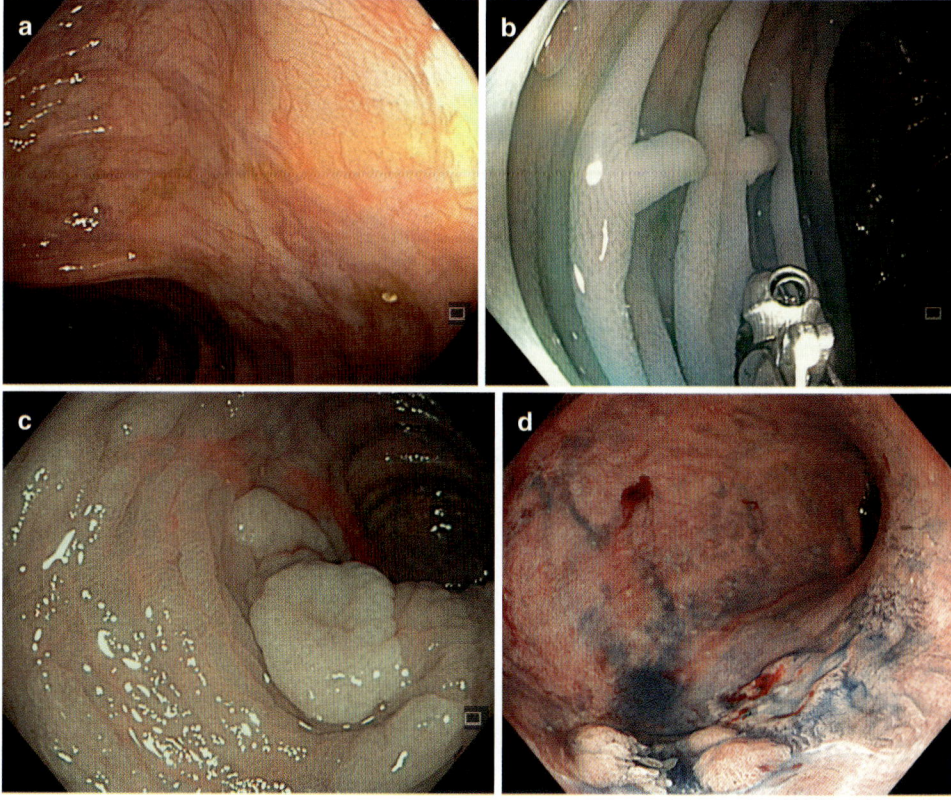

Fig. 11.12 Stenosis in Crohn's disease. (**a**) Scars with small ulcers and stenosis in the terminal ileum. (**b**) Stenosis in the sigmoid colon with active ulceration, in a different patient

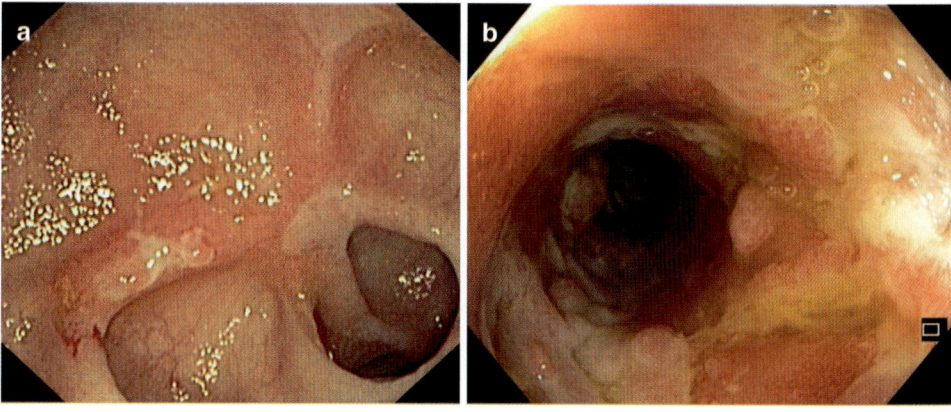

Fig. 11.13 (**a**) Subtle aphthous erosion in the terminal ileum of a patient with NSAID use, as seen during surveillance colonoscopy for colon carcinoma. (**b**) Close-up view in NBI

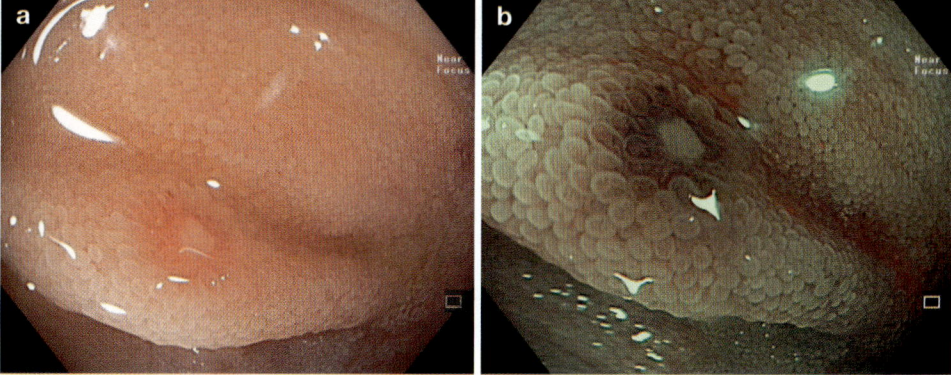

References

1. Hayat M, Axon AT, O'Mahony S. Diagnostic yield and effect on clinical outcomes of push enteroscopy in suspected small-bowel bleeding. Endoscopy. 2000;32:369–72.
2. Tajiri H, Niwa H. Recent advances in electronic endoscopes: image-enhanced endoscopy. JMAJ. 2008;51:199–203.
3. Picasso M, Filiberti R, Blanchi S, Conio M. The role of chromoendoscopy in the surveillance of the duodenum of patients with familial adenomatous polyposis. Dig Dis Sci. 2007;52:1906–9.
4. Kiesslich R, Mergener K, Naumann C, et al. Value of chromoendoscopy and magnification endoscopy in the evaluation of duodenal abnormalities: a prospective, randomized comparison. Endoscopy. 2003;35:559–63.
5. Shahid MW, Buchner A, Gomez V, et al. Diagnostic accuracy of probe-based confocal laser endomicroscopy and narrow band imaging in detection of dysplasia in duodenal polyps. J Clin Gastroenterol. 2012;46:382–9.
6. Cammarota G, Cianci R, Gasbarrini G. High-resolution magnifying video endoscopy in primary intestinal lymphangiectasia: a new role for endoscopy? Endoscopy. 2005;37:607.
7. Cammarota G, Fedeli P, Gasbarrini A. Emerging technologies in upper gastrointestinal endoscopy and celiac disease. Nat Clin Pract Gastroenterol Hepatol. 2009;6:47–56.
8. Cappell MS, Friedel D. The role of sigmoidoscopy and colonoscopy in the diagnosis and management of lower gastrointestinal disorders: endoscopic findings, therapy, and complications. Med Clin North Am. 2002;86:1253–88.
9. Kudo S, Hirota S, Nakajima T, et al. Colorectal tumours and pit pattern. J Clin Pathol. 1994;47:880–5.
10. Saito S, Tajiri H, Ohya T, et al. Imaging by magnifying endoscopy with NBI implicates the remnant capillary network as an indication for endoscopic resection in early colon cancer. Int J Surg Oncol. 2011;6:242608.
11. Choi HJ, Lee BI, Choi H, et al. Diagnostic accuracy and interobserver agreement in predicting the submucosal invasion of colorectal tumors using gross findings, pit patterns, and microvasculatures. Clin Endosc. 2013;46:168–71.
12. Van Assche G, Dignass A, Bokemeyer B, et al. Second European evidence-based consensus on the diagnosis and management of ulcerative colitis. Part 3: special situations. J Crohns Colitis. 2013;7:1–33.
13. Hommes DW, van Deventer SJ. Endoscopy in inflammatory bowel diseases. Gastroenterology. 2004;126:1561–73.
14. Cherian S, Singh P. Is routine ileoscopy useful? An observational study of procedure times, diagnostic yield, and learning curve. Am J Gastroenterol. 2004;99:2324–9.
15. Emami MH, Behbahan IS, Zade HD, Daneshgar H. New interpretation for diagnostic yield of ileoscopy: a prospective study and a brief review. J Res Med Sci. 2009;14:157–63.

Push Enteroscopy

12

Ilja Tachecí and Jan Bureš

Contents

12.1 History

For many years, the small bowel was considered to be a rare location for any pathology. This conviction, together with problems relating to construction of an endoscope dedicated to small bowel investigation, led endoscopists to be relatively uninterested in enteroscopy [1, 2]. This situation changed dramatically at the end of the twentieth century.

Three main lines of enteroscope development started in the 1970s: the ropeway type, the sonde type, and the push type. Ropeway enteroscopy was the first technique that allowed complete investigation of the small bowel [3, 4]. This method was based on insertion of the enteroscope over a Teflon tube (instead of a guide string) initially passed through the whole gastrointestinal tract up to the anus. This technique was time consuming and traumatic for the patient. In sonde enteroscopy, a balloon fixed on the endoscope tip was dragged by peristalsis through the small bowel; examination was performed during withdrawal of the instrument [5, 6]. Sonde enteroscopy was also a lengthy procedure, with no possibility of controlling insertion of the instrument. The disadvantages of both methods led to their abandonment. A push enteroscopy prototype was developed at the same time [7, 8]. The instrument was 162 cm in length. The tip was 1 cm in diameter and was inserted under fluoroscopy control. Intubation of 30 cm beyond the ligament of Treitz was presented in the first 250 cases.

Enteroscopy was initially a method with little application. Presentation of the idea that a colonoscope could be used instead of special, dedicated devices was a very important moment in the evolution of enteroscopy [9]. This approach opened the method for every endoscopy unit, and enteroscopy-controlled biopsies then gradually ousted blind biopsies obtained by means of a Rubin tube. Endoscopy allowed direct visual examination of the small bowel mucosa and biopsy sampling during one procedure, as well as repeated biopsies without removing the device. Technical developments continued, with the introduction in the 1990s of longer push enteroscopes (up to 250 cm) with

The work was first published in 2006 by Springer Medizin Verlag Heidelberg with the following title: *Atlas of Video Capsule Endoscopy*.

I. Tachecí (✉) J. Bureš
2nd Department of Internal Medicine–Gastroenterology,
University Hospital and Charles University Faculty of Medicine,
Hradec Králové, Czech Republic
e-mail: tacheci@gmail.com; bures@lfhk.cuni.cz

video technology, allowing high-quality images from the oesophagus to the jejunum. For this reason, push enteroscopy was sometimes also called deep upper endoscopy or extended esophagogastroduodenoscopy.

12.2   Methods

The latest generation of push enteroscopes have a working length of 220–250 cm, external diameters of 10.5–11.7 mm, and channel diameters of 2.2–3.8 mm (Fig. 12.1). According to the published studies, a longer instrument does not always correlate with deeper insertion or higher diagnostic yield [10]. Compared with a standard endoscope, the bending section of a push enteroscope is longer, to allow increased angulation in all directions.

No specific preparation is administered before push enteroscopy. The patient fasts for 8 h before the investigation. Examination is carried out with the patient under conscious analgosedation; general anaesthesia is usually not required. Pulse, blood pressure, and arterial oxygen saturation should be monitored during the investigation.

Because of the flexibility of the enteroscope and the winding character of the small bowel, panenteroscopy is not possible. Advancement techniques similar to those used in colonoscopy (instrument progress by pushing, rotation, shortening, and straightening of the endoscope) have a limited effect inside the small bowel. The pushing force results in stretching of the small bowel, precluding further progress and causing patient discomfort. The duodenal tight curve from the duodenal bulb around the head of the pancreas, and its relatively fixed retroperitoneal posterior position also make transmission of propelling force difficult. The enteroscope is usually passed with the patient in the left lateral or

semiprone position. If insertion is difficult, the patient may be moved to a supine, right lateral, or prone position. As in colonoscopy, abdominal pressure may be helpful.

Some prospective studies have confirmed a significant increase in insertion depth by using a semi-rigid overtube [11, 12]. This tube has an outer diameter of 14.4 mm, a flexible segment at the distal end, and a radiopaque ring at the tip. The overtube reduces looping of the scope in the stomach and is placed before the pylorus or is inserted into the duodenum after the scope straightening inside the second or third duodenal section. However, published results are mixed, and overtubes are not always used because of the risk of complications. The use of a variable stiffness enteroscope has also been tested [13]. Sometimes the investigation can be performed under fluoroscopy control, in which the position of the enteroscope is checked and looping can be avoided. Use of these techniques usually enables examination of about 40–100 cm of the small intestine beyond the ligament of Treitz [14]. Mucosal examination should be carried out during insertion as well as retraction, because minor mucosal damage can mimic vascular or inflammatory lesions. Because a hypotonic small bowel precludes enteroscope insertion, it may be necessary to use antispasmodic drugs (glucagon or hyoscine i.v.) during the withdrawal phase only.

12.3   Advantages and Diagnostic Yield

The main advantages of push enteroscopy are the short investigation time (20–45 min); full control over the device, allowing repetitive pathology visualisation; and the possibility of biopsy sampling and therapy. Therapeutic options during push enteroscopy include thermocoagulation, treatment with haemoclips, polypectomy, dilation of stenosis, removal of foreign bodies, and placement of enteral feeding tubes [15]. Complications of the procedure (present in about 1 %) are more frequent than for standard upper endoscopy and are always associated with use of an overtube. These complications include mucosal stripping, pharyngeal tear, Mallory-Weiss tear, perforation, and pancreatitis after insertion of the overtube into the small bowel [16, 17].

The diagnostic yield of push enteroscopy ranges from 13 to 78 % and depends on the indication, being highest in patients with obscure gastrointestinal bleeding and abnormal findings localised in the distal duodenum or proximal jejunum (Figs. 12.2, 12.3, 12.4, 12.5, 12.6, 12.7, 12.8, 12.9 and 12.10) [18–21]. Many studies and meta-analysis have proven the superiority of wireless capsule endoscopy over push enteroscopy for the diagnosis of small bowel pathology, with a 35–40 % incremental yield [22–27]. The published diagnostic yield of push enteroscopy in these patients is artificially increased by the identification of lesions overlooked during

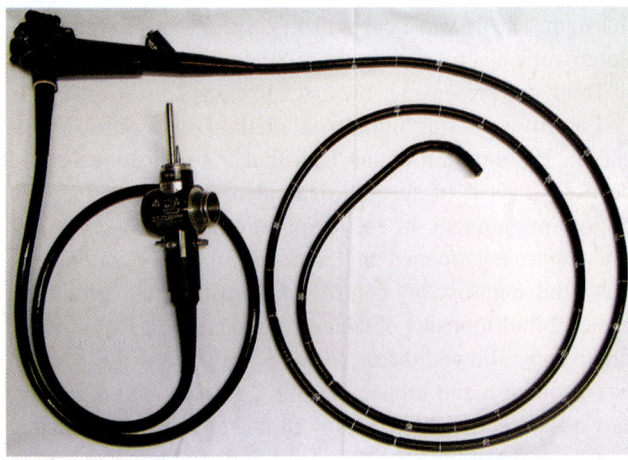

Fig. 12.1 Olympus SIF-Q140 push enteroscope (Olympus Corporation, Tokyo, Japan). The working length is 250 cm; the instrument channel diameter is 2.8 mm

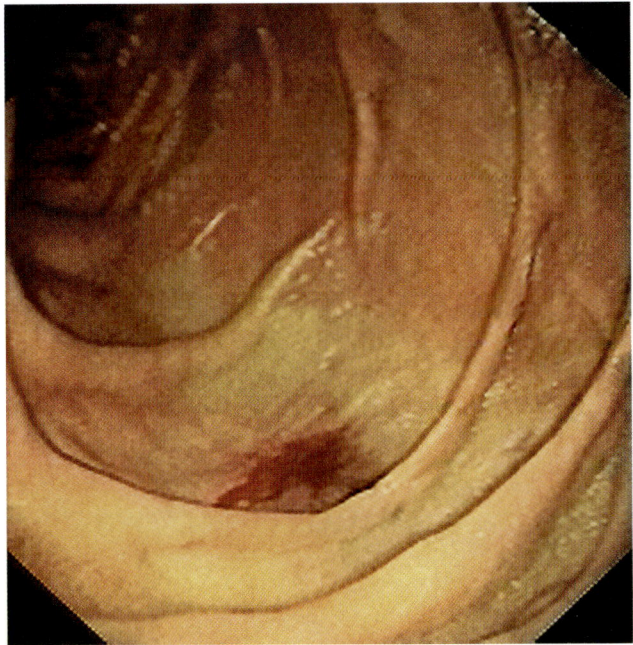

Fig. 12.2 Jejunal angiectasia with oozing bleeding in a patient with obscure overt gastrointestinal bleeding. The lesion was treated by means of bipolar electrocoagulation

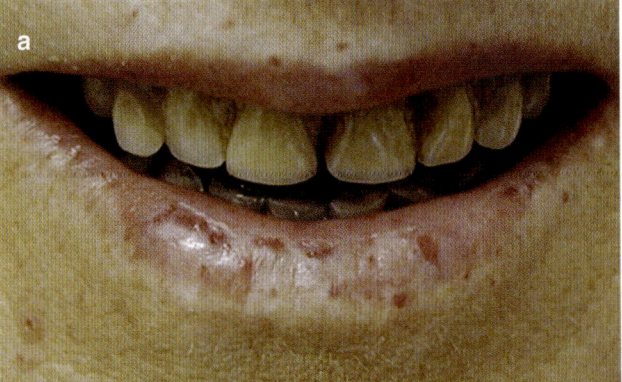

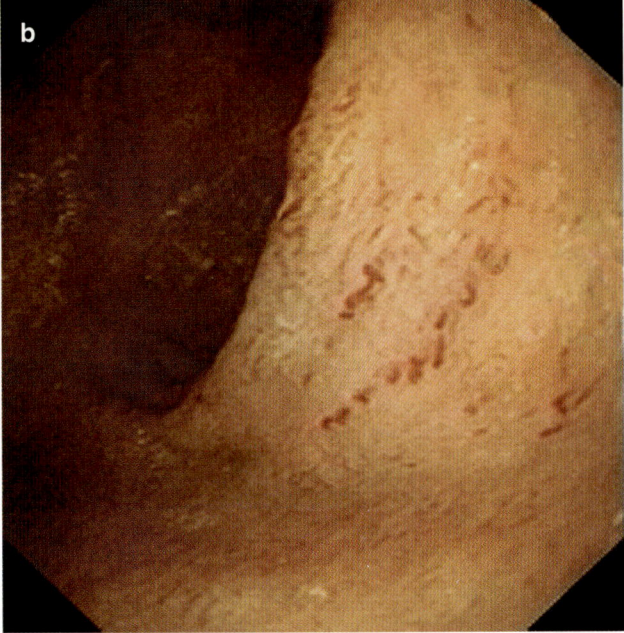

Fig. 12.3 Rendu-Osler-Weber syndrome (hereditary haemorrhagic telangiectasia, HHT). (**a**) Characteristic small red-to-violet telangiectatic lesions on the lips. (**b**) Patient was referred for push enteroscopy because of severe gastrointestinal bleeding. Typical multiple telangiectasias were diagnosed in the duodenum

initial gastroscopy [28]. The main limiting factor of push enteroscopy lies in the inability to perform panenteroscopy.

A very interesting experimental study by Appleyard et al. compared capsule endoscopy versus push enteroscopy in dogs [29]. Radiopaque coloured beads (3–6 mm) were surgically implanted into the small bowel of nine dogs (half placed within 100 cm of the pylorus, within reach of the push enteroscope), and all the animals underwent push and capsule enteroscopy. The sensitivity and specificity of push enteroscopy for detecting focal lesions within the entire small bowel were 37 and 97 %, respectively, compared with 64 and 92 % for capsule endoscopy. The higher sensitivity for capsule endoscopy was caused especially by the large number of beads found out of reach of the push enteroscope. On the other hand, the sensitivity of push enteroscopy within 100 cm of the pylorus (94 %) was superior to the sensitivity of capsule endoscopy (53 %), as capsule endoscopy missed lesions in the proximal duodenum because of the endoscopy-assisted delivery of the capsule endoscope inside the small bowel.

Although most endoscopy units (including our centre) indicate video capsule endoscopy followed by one of the deep enteroscopy methods in the majority of patients with small bowel pathology, push enteroscopy can be beneficial in some special situations, such as when a focal upper small intestinal lesion requires biopsy or endoscopy treatment and deep enteroscopy is unavailable [30]. Another role for push enteroscopy can be in patients with malabsorption. In most patients, coeliac disease can be diagnosed by means of duodenoscopy using a conventional gastroscope, carefully assessing the sec-

ond part of the duodenum and taking biopsy specimens for histology. In some patients, however, the appearance of the duodenum may be abnormal but nonspecific; push enteroscopy is then a substantial tool for proper recognition, uncovering the typical mosaic pattern in the jejunum after getting past the duodenojejunal junction at the ligament of Treitz. If coeliac disease is suspected but both endoscopic and histologic duodenal findings are normal or nonspecific, we recommend enteroscopy to assess jejunal appearance and obtain several biopsy specimens of the jejunal mucosa [31]. According to another study, duodenal biopsies are sufficient to diagnose coeliac disease of Marsh III grade, but Marsh I or II lesions may be missed in some patients [32]. Push enteroscopy improves diagnostic yield in refractory sprue and makes it possible to take several jejunal biopsies for phenotyping of intraepithelial lymphocytes [31].

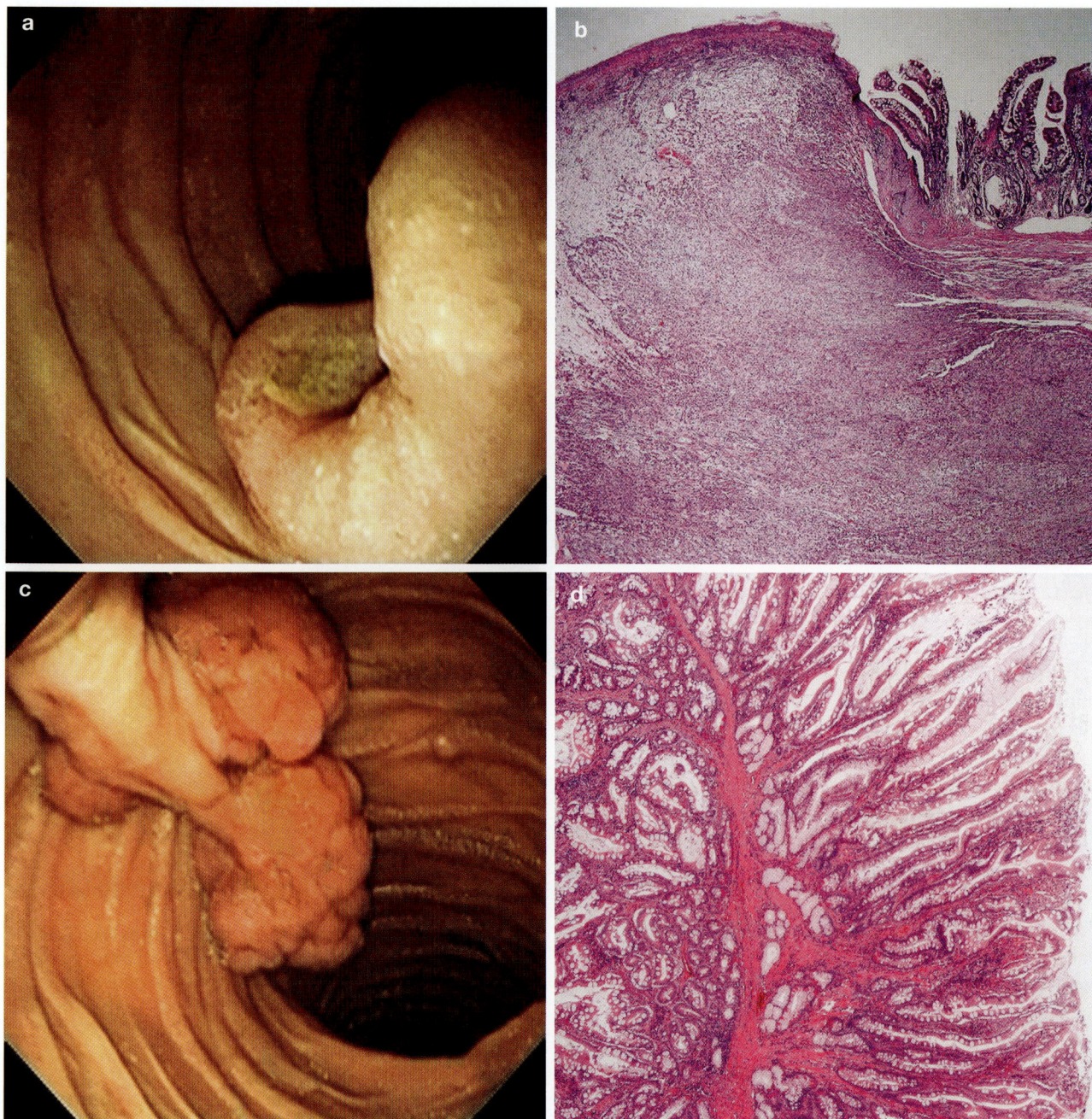

Fig. 12.4 Small bowel tumours. (**a**) Gastrointestinal stromal tumour. A large, polypoid, ulcerated, submucosal tumour in the proximal jejunum presented with occult bleeding. (**b**) Gastrointestinal stromal tumour. Histology showing a spindle-cell neoplasm localised within the submucosa, growing infiltratively into the mucosa with a superficial ulceration (haematoxylin-eosin [H&E], magnification 40×). (**c**) Peutz-Jeghers syndrome. Large stalked, lobated hamartoma in proximal jejunum. (**d**) Peutz-Jeghers syndrome. Histology of a hamartoma proving smooth-muscle bundles of the muscularis mucosae in the axial portion of the polyp, with overlying cystically dilated mucosal glands (H&E, magnification 100x)

Fig. 12.5 Jejunal adenocarcinoma; tumour created circular stenosis with fragile polypoid margins

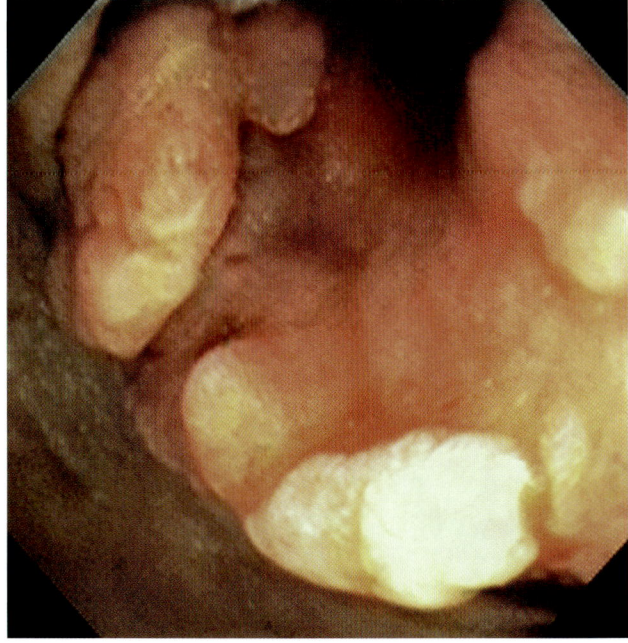

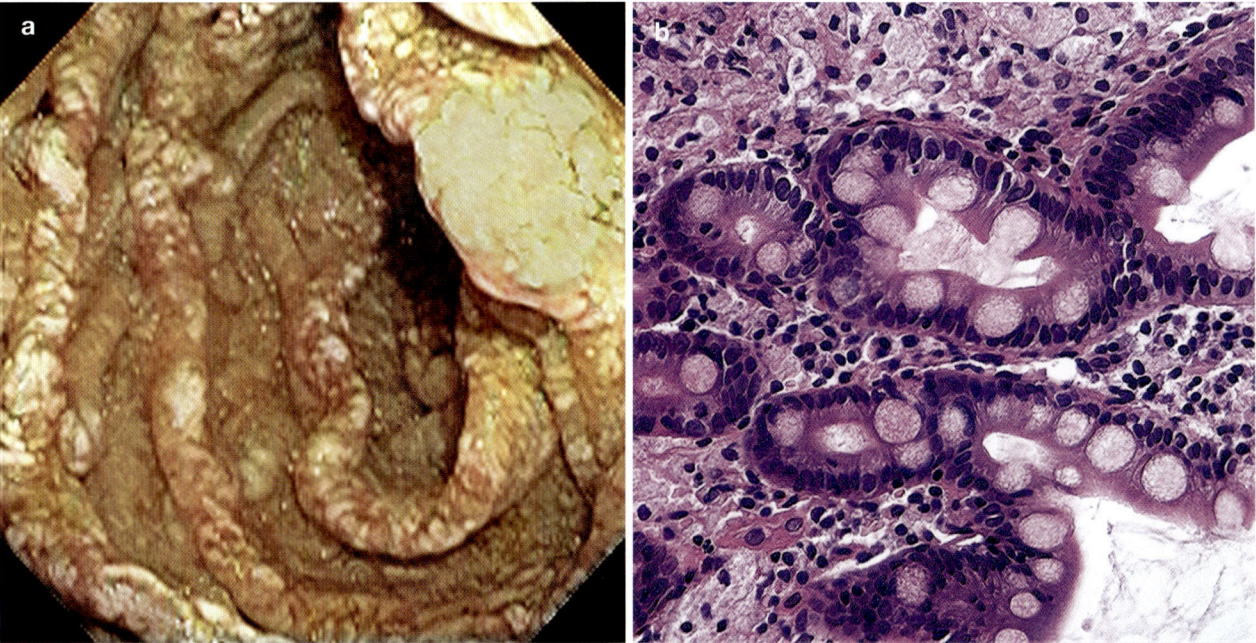

Fig. 12.6 Whipple's disease. (**a**) Oedema, focal erythema, and multiple lymphangiectasias in the jejunum. Characteristic whitish spots protrude a little above surrounding relief. Focally, the mucosa has a dusted-flour appearance. (**b**) Histology shows macrophages within the lamina propria mucosae, with strong positivity on periodic acid-Schiff (PAS) staining (magnification 100×)

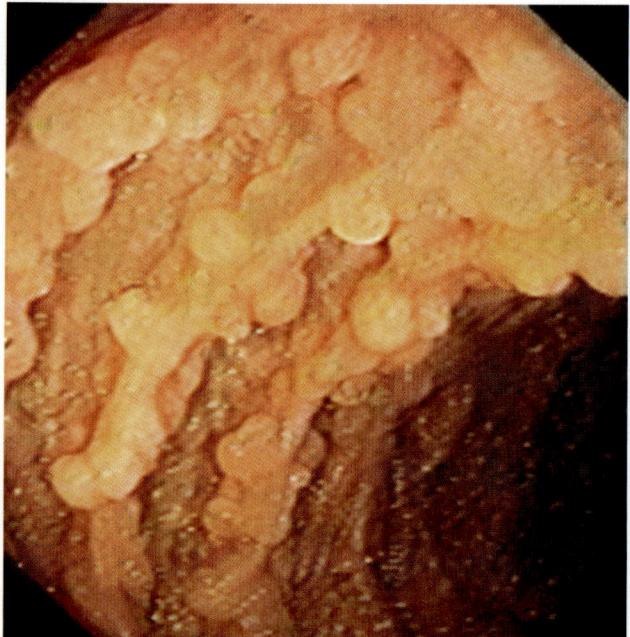

Fig. 12.7 Giardiasis of the jejunum. Lymphoid hyperplasia creates the nodular pattern of the mucosa

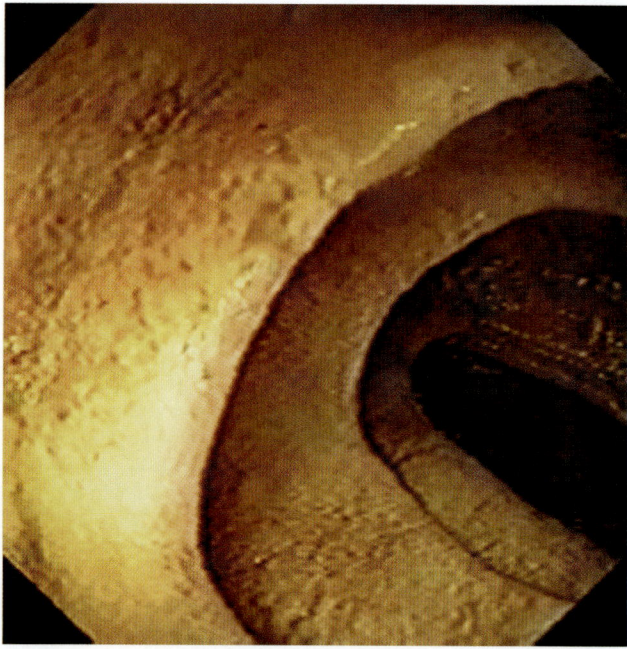

Fig. 12.8 Abetalipoproteinaemia. The proximal jejunum in this 29-year-old man was investigated because of chronic diarrhoea. Endoscopy showed swollen mucosa with grey-yellowish colour and fine granular pattern

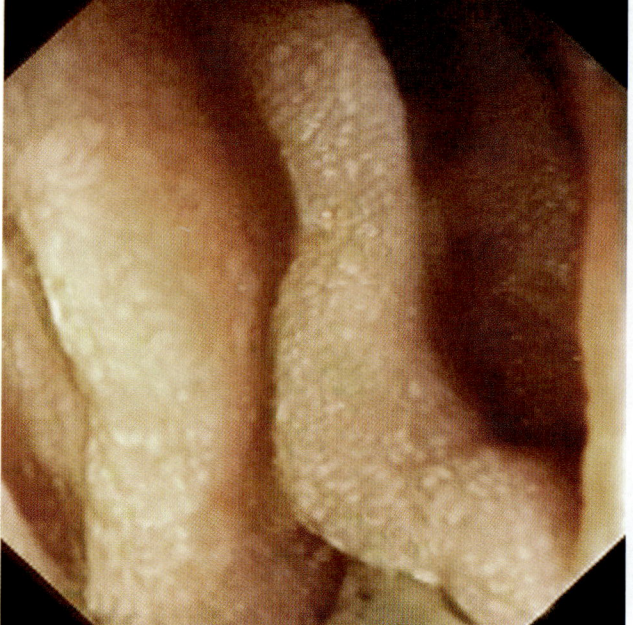

Fig. 12.9 Primary intestinal lymphangiectasia (Waldmann's disease). Jejunal folds are swollen and the mucosa of the jejunum has a fine, granular pattern. Multiple small, whitish granular spots are seen, which are caused by dilated lymphatic vessels

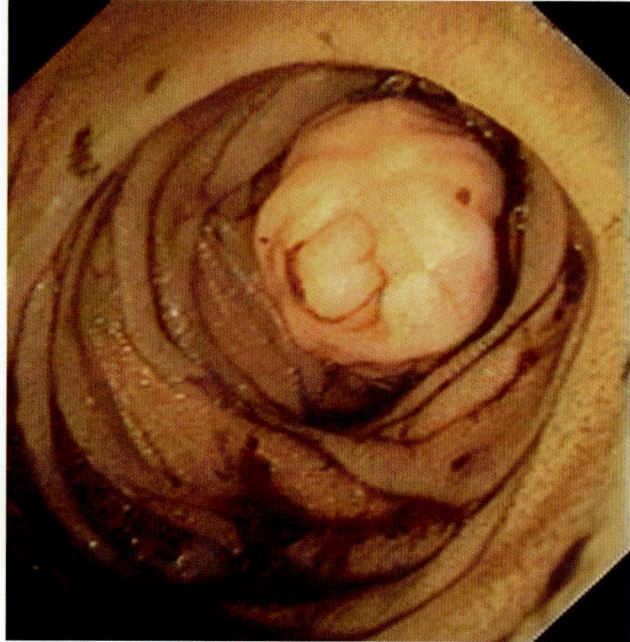

Fig. 12.10 Jejunal intussusception in a 79-year-old man with previous subtotal gastric resection because of adenocarcinoma. Ten centimetres distal to the anastomosis, a jejunal loop moves back into an efferent loop and causes mechanical ileus

References

1. Lewis BS. The history of enteroscopy. Gastrointest Endosc Clin N Am. 1999;9:1–11.
2. Vilardell F. Digestive endoscopy in the second millennium. From the lichtleiter to echoendoscopy. Stuttgart: Georg Thieme Verlag; 2006.
3. Hiratsuka H, Hasegawa M, Ushiromachi K, Endo T, Suzuki S, Nishikawa F. Endoscopic diagnosis in the small intestine. Stomach Intest. 1972;7:1679–85.
4. Classen M, Frühmorgen P, Koch H, Demling L. Peroral enteroscopy of the small and the large intestine. Endoscopy. 1972;4:157–62.
5. Tada M, Akasaka Y, Misaki F, Kawai K. Clinical evaluation of a sonde-type small intestinal fiberscope. Endoscopy. 1977;9:33–8.
6. Seensalu R. The sonde exam. Gastrointest Endosc Clin N Am. 1999;9:37–59.
7. Ogoshi K, Hara Y, Ashizawa S. New technique for small intestinal fiberoscopy. Gastrointest Endosc. 1973;20:64–5.
8. MacKenzie JF. The push exam. Gastrointest Endosc Clin N Am. 1999;9:29–30.
9. Parker H, Agayoff J. Enteroscopy and small bowel biopsy utilizing a peroral colonoscope. Gastrointest Endosc. 1983;29:139.
10. Benz C, Jakobs R, Riemann JF. Does the insertion depth in push enteroscopy depend on the working length of the enteroscope? Endoscopy. 2002;34:543–5.
11. Benz C, Jakobs R, Riemann JF. Do we need the overtube for push enteroscopy? Endoscopy. 2001;33:658–61.
12. Taylor AC, Chen RY, Desmond PV. Use of an overtube for enteroscopy: does it increase depth of insertion? A prospective study of enteroscopy with and without an overtube. Endoscopy. 2001;33:227–30.
13. Harewood GC, Gostout CJ, Farrell MA, Knipschield MA. Prospective controlled assessment of variable stiffness enteroscopy. Gastrointest Endosc. 2003;58:267–71.
14. Bureš J, Kopacova M, Tacheci I, Rejchrt S. Enteroscopy: will it achieve the complete journey? Acta Endoscopic. 2005;35:171–7.
15. Bureš J, Rejchrt S, et al. Small bowel investigation & atlas of enteroscopy. Praha: Grada Publishing; 2001.
16. Landi B, Cellier C, Fayemendy L, Cugnenc PH, Barbier JP. Duodenal perforation occurring during push enteroscopy [letter]. Gastrointest Endosc. 1996;43:631.
17. Barkin JS, Lewis BS, Reiner DK, Wave JD, Goldberg RI, Phillips RS. Diagnostic and therapeutic jejunostomy with a new, longer enteroscope. Gastrointest Endosc. 1992;38:55–8.
18. Chak A, Koehler MK, Sundaram SN, Cooper GS, Canto MI, Sivak Jr MV. Diagnostic and therapeutic impact of push enteroscopy: analysis of factors associated with positive findings. Gastrointest Endosc. 1998;47:18–22.
19. Landi B, Tkoub M, Gaudric M, Gimbaud R, Cervoni JP, Chaussade S, et al. Diagnostic yield of push type enteroscopy in relation to indication. Gut. 1998;42:421–5.
20. Descamps C, Schmit A, Van Gossum A. "Missed" upper gastrointestinal tract lesions may explain "occult" bleeding. Endoscopy. 1999;31:452–5.
21. Lin S, Branch MS, Shetzline M. The importance of indication in the diagnostic value of push enteroscopy. Endoscopy. 2003;35:315–21.
22. Saurin JC, Delvaux M, Gaudin JL, Fassler I, Villarejo J, Vahedi K, et al. Diagnostic value of endoscopic capsule in patients with obscure digestive bleeding: blinded comparison with video push-enteroscopy. Endoscopy. 2003;35:576–84.
23. Adler DG, Knipschield M, Gostout C. A prospective comparison of capsule endoscopy and push enteroscopy in patients with GI bleeding of obscure origin. Gastrointest Endosc. 2004;59:492–8.
24. Triester SL, Leighton JA, Leontiadis GI, Fleischer DE, Hara AK, Heigh RI, et al. A meta-analysis of the yield of capsule endoscopy compared to other diagnostic modalities in patients with obscure gastrointestinal bleeding. Am J Gastroenterol. 2005;100:2407–18.
25. Leighton JA, Sharma VK, Hentz JG, Musil D, Malikowski MJ, McWane TL, Fleischer DE. Capsule endoscopy versus push enteroscopy for evaluation of obscure gastrointestinal bleeding with 1-year outcomes. Dig Dis Sci. 2006;51:891–9.
26. Triester SL, Leighton JA, Leontaidis GI, Gurudu SR, Fleischer DE, Hara AK, et al. A meta-analysis of the yield of capsule endoscopy compared to other diagnostic modalities in patients with non-stricturing small bowel Crohn's disease. Am J Gastroenterol. 2006;101:954–64.
27. de Leusse A, Vahedi K, Edery J, Tiah D, Fery-Lemonnier E, Cellier C, et al. Capsule endoscopy or push enteroscopy for first-line exploration of obscure gastrointestinal bleeding? Gastroenterology. 2007;132:855–62.
28. Nguyen NQ, Rayner CK, Schoeman MN. Push enteroscopy alters management in a majority of patients with obscure gastrointestinal bleeding. J Gastroenterol Hepatol. 2005;20:716–21.
29. Appleyard M, Fireman Z, Glukhovsky A, Jacob H, Shreiver R, Kadirkamanathan S, et al. A randomized trial comparing wireless capsule endoscopy with push enteroscopy for the detection of small-bowel lesions. Gastroenterology. 2000;119:1431–8.
30. De Palma GD, Patrone F, Rega M, Simeoli I, Masone S, Persico G. Actively bleeding Dieulafoy's lesion of the small bowel identified by capsule endoscopy and treated by push enteroscopy. World J Gastroenterol. 2006;12:3936–7.
31. Bureš J, Rejchrt S, Kopacova M, Tacheci I, Papik Z, Siroky M, Pozler O. Endoscopic features of coeliac disease. Folia Gastroenterol Hepatol. 2005;3:32–41.
32. Thijs WJ, van Baarlen J, Kleibeuker JH, Kolkman JJ. Duodenal versus jejunal biopsies in suspected celiac disease. Endoscopy. 2004;36:993–6.

Double-Balloon Endoscopy

13

Hironori Yamamoto, Christian Ell, Hirito Kita, and Andrea May

Contents

The work was first published in 2006 by Springer Medizin Verlag Heidelberg with the following title: *Atlas of Video Capsule Endoscopy.*

H. Yamamoto (✉)
Department of Medicine, Division of Gastroenterology,
Jichi Medical University, Tochigi, Japan
e-mail: ireef@jichi.ac.jp

C. Ell • A. May
Medical Clinic II, Sana Klinikum Offenbach, Offenbach, Germany
e-mail: christian.ell@sana.de; andrea.may@sana.de

H. Kita
Department of Medicine, Teikyo University School of Medicine,
Tokyo, Japan
e-mail: hkita@med.teikyo-u.ac.jp

13.1 Double-Balloon Endoscopy Procedure

The method of double-balloon endoscopy (DBE) introduced by Yamamoto [1] permits noninvasive endoscopic evaluation of the small bowel while also providing therapeutic access [2–6]. Figure 13.1a shows the specifically designed video endoscopes, Fujinon EN-450P5 (regular type) and Fujinon EN-450 T5 (therapeutic type) from Fujifilm Corporation, Tokyo, Japan. The endoscope, with an attachable balloon at the tip, is used together with a soft overtube (length 145 cm) with another balloon at the distal end. To make insertion procedures safe and effective, soft latex balloons are used for both the endoscope and the overtube, and a specifically designed pump has been developed to inflate and deflate the balloons with one touch while accurately monitoring the balloon pressure (Fig. 13.1b).

First the overtube balloon is inflated in the duodenum to fix its position, and the endoscope is advanced deeper into the bowel through the stationary outer tube. Next, the balloon at the distal end of the endoscope is inflated to fix the position of the scope, and the overtube balloon is deflated and advanced. If the endoscope and overtube are now withdrawn with both balloons inflated, the small bowel will invaginate over the overtube, shortening and pleating like an accordion. The endoscope balloon can then be deflated and advanced even farther distally. This process is repeated, aided by intermittent fluoroscopy, until all relevant portions of the small bowel have been examined (Fig. 13.2). This technique can be used from the anal side as well (Fig. 13.3) [7]. A combination of oral and anal approaches can be used in the same patient to examine the entire small bowel if necessary. Total enteroscopy can be confirmed by reaching from the opposite approach an ink or clip mark that was placed during the initial examination. The success rate of total enteroscopy using DBE is reported to be over 80 % by combining both approaches [8]. A model using porcine organs for training purposes has been developed [9].

Fig. 13.1 (**a**) Double-balloon endoscopes (Fujinon EN-450P5/20 and Fujinon EN-450 T5). The working length of these endoscopes is 200 cm, with outer diameters of 8.5 and 9.4 mm and working channels of 2.2 and 2.8 mm, respectively. (**b**) Balloon controller. (Fujinon PB-20) for inflating both balloons (Fujifilm Corporation, Tokyo, Japan)

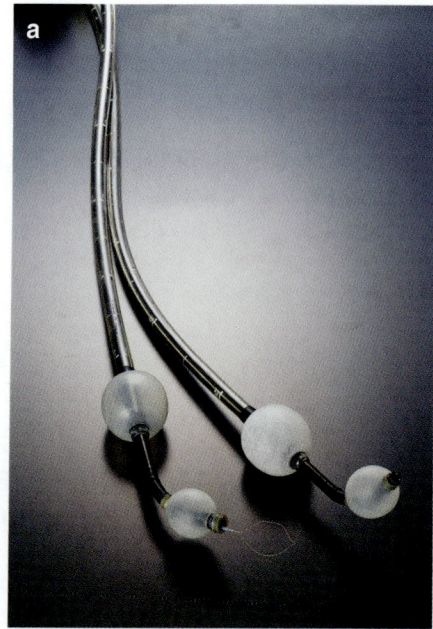
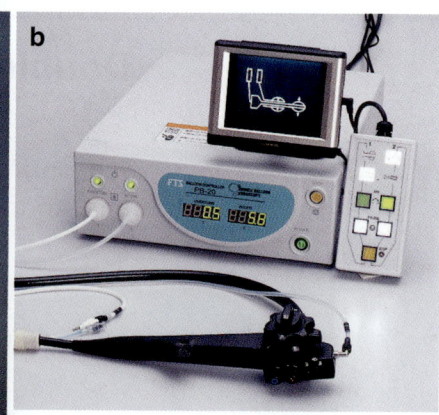

Fig. 13.2 (**a**) Illustrations demonstrate the sequential maneuvers of the instruments in the oral insertion of the double-balloon endoscope (From Yamamoto [10]; with permission from the American Gastroenterological Association). (**b**) X-ray image of enteroscope inserted from the mouth to the ascending colon. (From Yamamoto et al. [11] with permission from the American Gastroenterological Association)

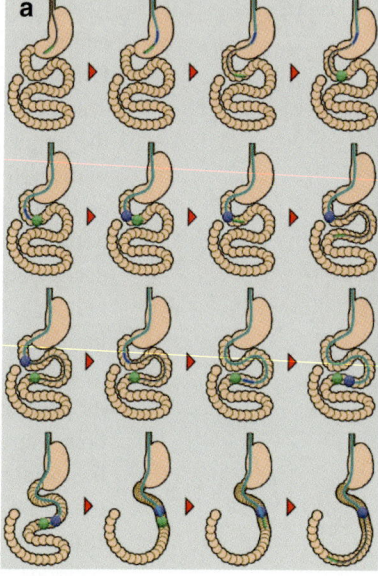
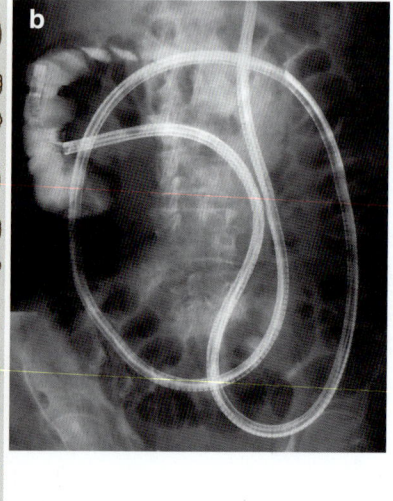

Fig. 13.3 (**a**) Illustrations demonstrate the sequential maneuvers of the instruments in the anal insertion of the double-balloon endoscope (From Yamamoto [10]; with permission from the American Gastroenterological Association). (**b**) X-ray image of enteroscope with anal approach. (From Yamamoto et al. [11]; with permission from the American Gastroenterological Association)

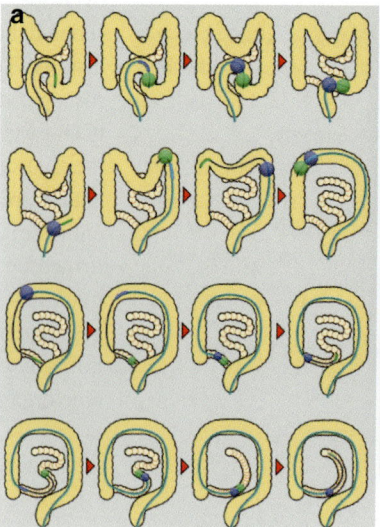
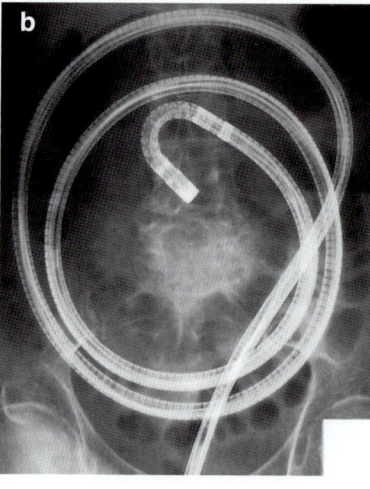

13.2 Applications

DBE also enables endoscopic observation of a blind loop or afferent loop [12], and it is also applicable for the evaluation of strictures of the small bowel [13]. To-and-fro observation of an affected area with controlled movement of the endoscope with an accessory channel enables interventions, including biopsies, hemostasis (Figs. 13.4 and 13.5) [15], balloon dilation (Fig. 13.6), stent placement, foreign body retrieval (Fig. 13.7), polypectomy (Fig. 13.8) [16, 17], and endoscopic mucosal resection (Fig. 13.9). Thus, DBE has distinct advantages that can complement the limitations of capsule endoscopy.

DBE may eliminate the need for intraoperative enteroscopy in many patients.

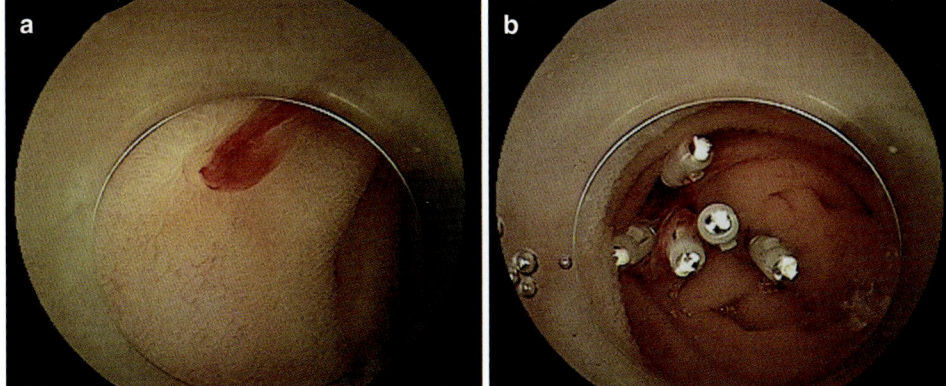

Fig. 13.4 Endoscopic hemostasis using clip placement for bleeding from jejunal type 2a vascular lesion. (**a**) Endoscopic observation of bleeding Dieulafoy's lesion in water. (**b**) Endoscopic image of the region after hemostasis with clip placement (From Yano et al. [14])

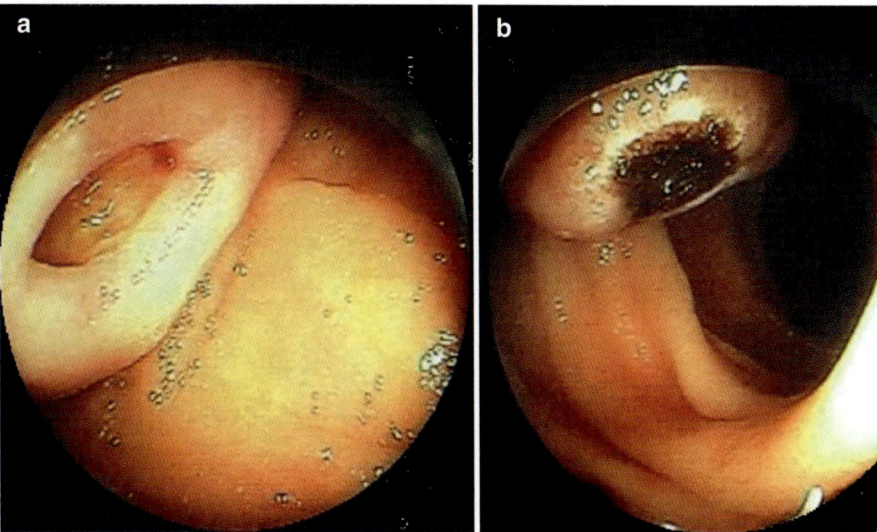

Fig. 13.5 Endoscopic hemostasis using electrosurgical coagulation for bleeding from jejunal gastrointestinal stromal tumor. (**a**) Tumor with central ulceration. (**b**) Endoscopic image of the region after hemostasis (From Nishimura et al. [15])

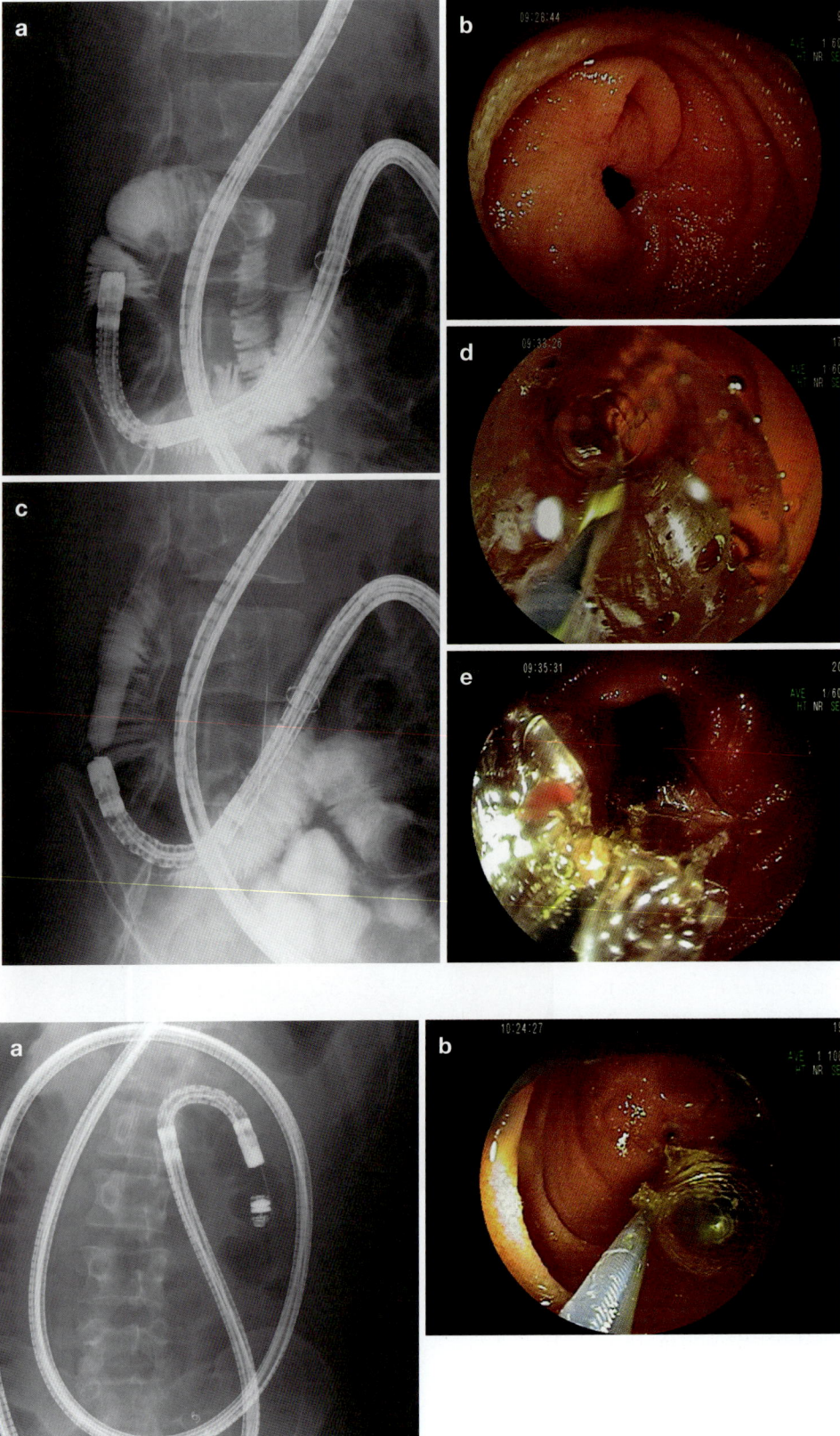

Fig. 13.6 (**a**) Fluoroscopic image of a water-soluble contrast study of the small bowel; inflating the balloon on the tip of the endoscope shows a stricture. (**b**) Endoscopic view of the fibrotic stricture in the small bowel before dilation. (**c**) Insertion of the balloon catheter into the stricture through the double-balloon endoscope. (**d**) Endoscopic view of balloon dilation. (**e**) Endoscopic view after dilation

Fig. 13.7 (**a**) Fluoroscopic image of a double-balloon endoscope retrieving a capsule, with a net catheter. (**b**) Endoscopic view of the retrieval of the capsule

Fig. 13.8 (**a**) Endoscopic view of Peutz-Jeghers polyp in the jejunum. (**b**) Endoscopic view showing the polypectomy site

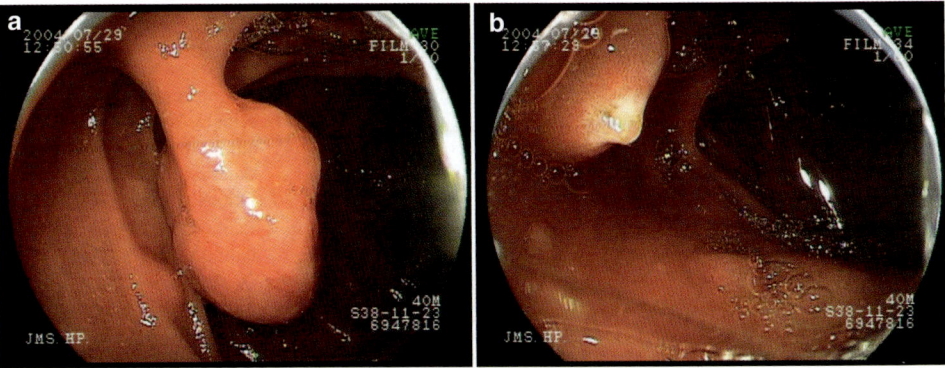

Fig. 13.9 (**a**) Endoscopic view of a tumor (*arrow*) near closed end of the duodenal afferent loop. (**b**) Endoscopic view showing the endoscopic mucosal resection site and the tumor in the forceps (From Kuno et al. [12]; with permission from the American Society for Gastrointestinal Endoscopy)

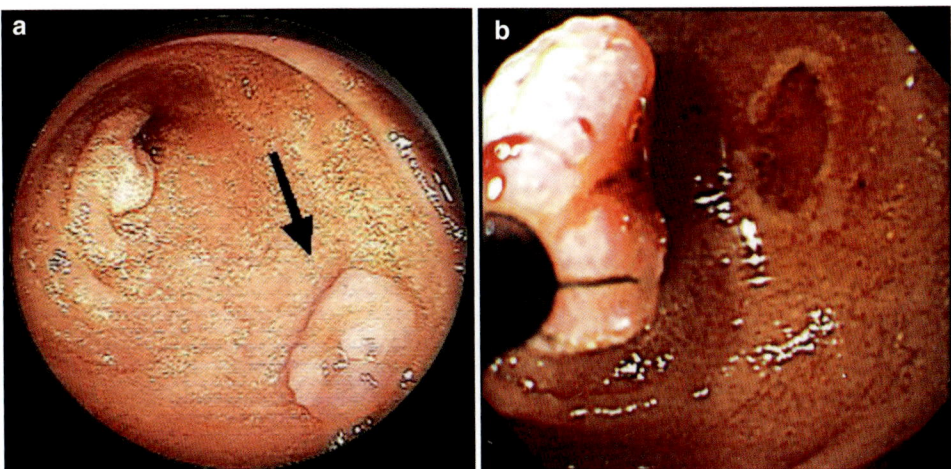

13.3 Comparison of the Most Common Flexible Enteroscopy Techniques

Three published prospective randomized studies have compared DBE with single-balloon endoscopy (SBE) [18–20]. One prospective, multicenter trial comparing the DBE and SBE techniques using the Fujinon device showed that the DBE technique was clearly superior to the SBE technique [18]. The rate of complete enteroscopy was three times higher in the DBE group (66 % versus 22 % with SBE), and DBE was associated with a higher overall diagnostic and therapeutic yield (72 % versus 48 %). These results were confirmed by a prospective single-center trial in Japan that compared the Fujinon DBE device with the Olympus SBE device, demonstrating a complete enteroscopy rate for DBE of 57 %, versus 0 % for SBE [19]. In contrast, the third multicenter trial found no differences between the two systems, but for several reasons, the conclusions must be read with caution [20, 21].

No prospective randomized studies have been published so far comparing spiral enteroscopy (SE) with SBE, but two prospective, randomized trials comparing SE with DBE have been reported [22, 23]. It was demonstrated that the average investigation time could be significantly decreased with SE. On the other hand, deeper insertion was achieved with the DBE device, comparing either the oral approach alone or the rate of complete enteroscopy, which was possible in only 8 % of patients with SE, compared with 92 % using DBE. The very low rate of complete enteroscopy is also found in the literature in the form of case reports [24]. The main problem is the uncertain effectiveness of anal spiral enteroscopy, because the passage through the colon is generally easy, but insertion of the enteroscope and the overtube through the ileocecal valve is difficult, so insertion depths into the distal small bowel are limited [25]. Also, concerns have been expressed about potentially higher risks with the use of SE in an intestine that is fragile and diseased, dilated, or stenotic [26].

References

1. Yamamoto H, Sekine Y, Sato Y, et al. Total enteroscopy with a nonsurgical steerable double-balloon method. Gastrointest Endosc. 2001;53:216–20.
2. May A, Nachbar L, Wardak A, et al. Double-balloon enteroscopy: preliminary experience in patients with obscure gastrointestinal bleeding or chronic abdominal pain. Endoscopy. 2003;35: 985–91.

3. May A, Nachbar L, Ell C. Double-balloon enteroscopy (push-and-pull enteroscopy) of the small bowel: feasibility and diagnostic and therapeutic yield in patients with suspected small bowel disease. Gastrointest Endosc. 2005;62:62–70.

4. Yamamoto H, Sugano K. A new method of enteroscopy – the double-balloon method. Can J Gastroenterol. 2003;17:273–4.

5. Ell C, May A, Nachbar L, et al. Push-and-pull enteroscopy in the small bowel using the double-balloon technique: results of a prospective European multicenter study. Endoscopy. 2005;37:613–6.

6. Di Caro S, May A, Heine DG, et al. The European experience with double balloon enteroscopy: indications, methodology, safety and clinical impact. Gastrointest Endosc. 2005;62:545–50.

7. Miyata T, Yamamoto H, Kita H, et al. A case of inflammatory fibroid polyp causing small bowel intussusception in which retrograde double-balloon enteroscopy was useful for the preoperative diagnosis. Endoscopy. 2004;36:344–7.

8. Yamamoto H, Kita H, Sunada K, et al. Clinical outcomes of double-balloon endoscopy for the diagnosis and treatment of small-intestinal diseases. Clin Gastroenterol Hepatol. 2004;2:1010–6.

9. May A, Nachbar L, Schneider M, et al. Push-and-pull enteroscopy using the double-balloon technique: method of assessing depth of insertion and training of the enteroscopy technique using the Erlangen Endo-Trainer. Endoscopy. 2005;37:66–70.

10. Yamamoto H. Double balloon endoscopy. Clin Gastroenterol Hepatol. 2005;3 Suppl 1:S27–9.

11. Yamamoto H, Yano T, Kita H, et al. New system of double-balloon enteroscopy for diagnosis and treatment of small intestinal disorders. Gastroenterology. 2003;125:1556; author reply 1556–7.

12. Kuno A, Yamamoto H, Kita H, et al. Application of double-balloon enteroscopy through Roux-en-Y anastomosis for the endoscopic mucosal resection of an early carcinoma in the duodenal afferent limb. Gastrointest Endosc. 2004;60:1032–4.

13. Sunada K, Yamamoto H, Kita H, et al. Case report: successful treatment with balloon dilatation in combination with double-balloon enteroscopy of a stricture in the small bowel of a patient with Crohn's disease. Dig Endosc. 2004;16:237–40.

14. Yano T, Yamamoto H, Sunada K, et al. Endoscopic classification of vascular lesions of the small intestine (with videos). Gastrointest Endosc. 2008;67:169–72.

15. Nishimura M, Yamamoto H, Kita H, et al. Gastrointestinal stromal tumor in the jejunum: diagnosis and control of bleeding with electrocoagulation by using double-balloon enteroscopy. J Gastroenterol. 2004;39:1001–4.

16. Kita H, Yamamoto H, Nakamura T, et al. Bleeding polyp in the mid small intestine identified by capsule endoscopy and treated by double-balloon endoscopy. Gastrointest Endosc. 2005;61:628–9.

17. Ohmiya N, Taguchi A, Shirai K, et al. Endoscopic resection of Peutz-Jeghers polyps throughout the small intestine at double-balloon enteroscopy without laparotomy. Gastrointest Endosc. 2005;61:140–7.

18. May A, Färber M, Aschmoneit I, et al. Prospective multicenter trial comparing push-and-pull enteroscopy with single- and double-balloon techniques in patients with small-bowel disorders. Am J Gastroenterol. 2010;105:575–81.

19. Takano N, Yamada A, Watabe H, et al. Single-balloon versus double-balloon endoscopy for achieving total enteroscopy: a randomized, controlled trial. Gastrointest Endosc. 2011;73:734–9.

20. Domagk D, Mensink P, Aktas H, et al. Single- vs double-balloon enteroscopy in small-bowel diagnostics: a randomized multicenter trial. Endoscopy. 2011;43:472–6.

21. May A. Small bowel endoscopy. Endoscopy. 2012;44:375–7.

22. May A, Manner H, Aschmoneit I, et al. Prospective, cross-over, single-center trial comparing oral double-balloon enteroscopy and oral spiral enteroscopy in patients with suspected small-bowel vascular malformations. Endoscopy. 2011;43:477–83.

23. Messer I, May A, Manner H, et al. Prospective, randomized single-center trial comparing double-balloon enteroscopy and spiral enteroscopy in patients with suspected small-bowel disorders. Gastrointest Endosc. 2013;77:241–9.

24. Despott EJ, Hughes S, Marden P, et al. First cases of spiral enteroscopy in the UK: let's "torque" about it! [Letter to the Editor]. Endoscopy. 2010;42:517.

25. Lara LF, Singh S, Sreenarasimhaiah J. Initial experience with retrograde overtube-assisted enteroscopy using a spiral tip overtube. Proc (Bayl Univ Med Cent). 2010;23:130–3.

26. Yamamoto H. Is double-balloon enteroscopy superior to spiral enteroscopy? Gastrointest Endosc. 2013;77:250–1.

Single-Balloon Enteroscopy

14

Kiyonori Kobayashi and Torsten Kucharzik

Contents

14.1 Procedure

After the establishment of the method of double-balloon enteroscopy, other endoscopic methods have been used to view the small intestine. In 2007, Olympus introduced a new technique, single-balloon enteroscopy (SBE), as an alternative to double-balloon enteroscopy (DBE) (Olympus Medical Systems Corp., Tokyo, Japan). The goal was to establish a simplified balloon-assisted endoscopic system that retains the effectiveness of DBE but is less time consuming. The SBE system and the technique of insertion in the small bowel are comparable to DBE, but because SBE does not have a balloon at the tip of the endoscope, the time-consuming procedure of installing the distal balloon at the beginning of the procedure is missing. A second advantage is that the technique of insertion is simplified by eliminating the need to inflate and deflate two different balloons in various steps.

The SBE system has a flexible overtube with a balloon as the distal part and a control unit that inflates and deflates the balloon (Fig. 14.1). Technical specifications of the Olympus endoscope (SIF-Q180 or SIF-Q260) are comparable to those of the therapeutic double-balloon enteroscope. It has a working

The work was first published in 2006 by Springer Medizin Verlag Heidelberg with the following title: *Atlas of Video Capsule Endoscopy.*

K. Kobayashi (✉)
Department of Gastroenterology, Klinikum Lüneburg,
Kitasato University East Hospital, Sagamihara-City,
Kanagawa Prefecture, Japan
e-mail: koba-eus@kitasato-u.ac.jp

T. Kucharzik
Department of Gastroenterology,
Klinikum Lüneburg, Lüneburg, Germany
e-mail: torsten.Kucharzik@klinikum-lueneburg.de

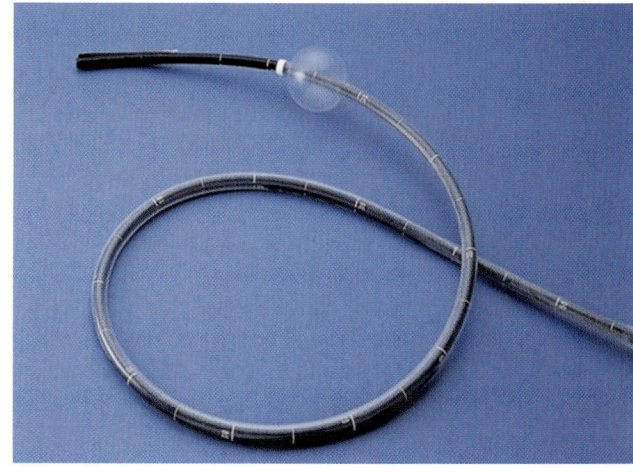

Fig. 14.1 Single-balloon enteroscope

M. Keuchel et al. (eds.), *Video Capsule Endoscopy: A Reference Guide and Atlas,*
DOI 10.1007/978-3-662-44062-9_14, © Springer-Verlag Berlin Heidelberg 2014

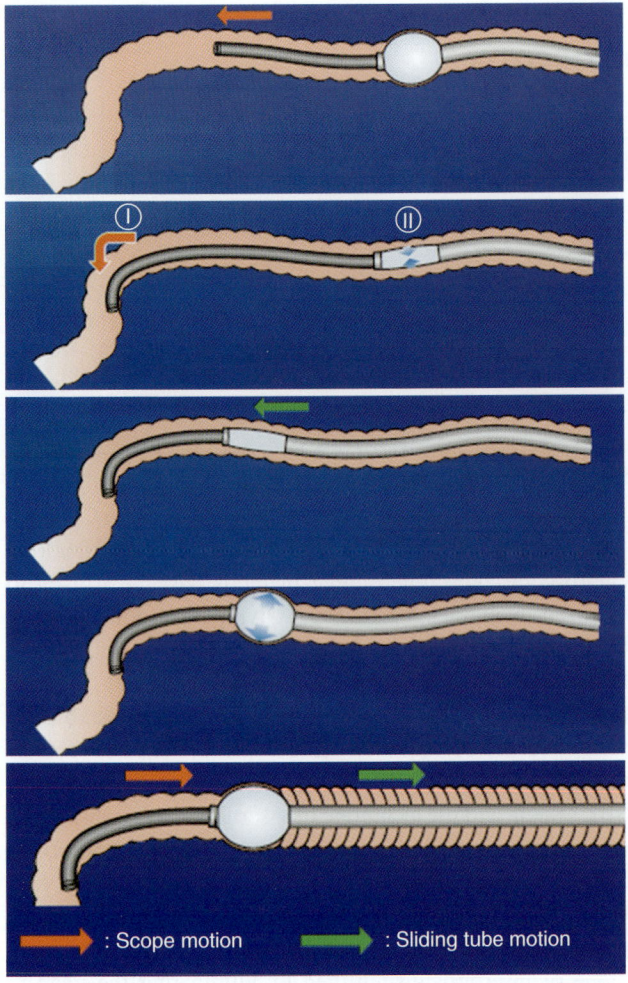

: Scope motion   : Sliding tube motion

Fig. 14.2 Technique of the single-balloon enteroscopy procedure

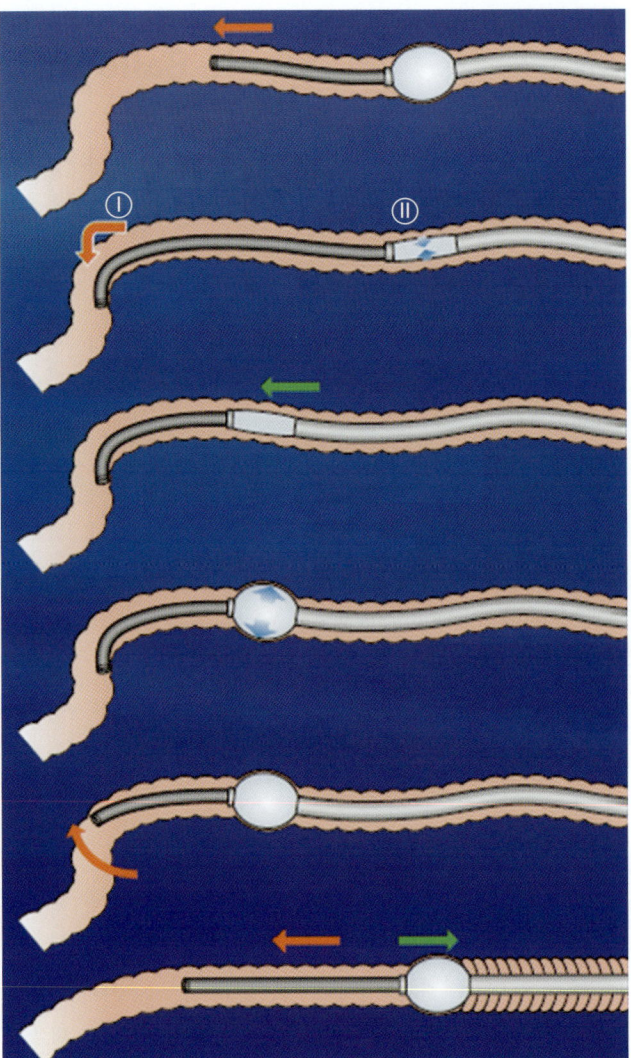

Fig. 14.3 Simultaneous pull-and-push procedure

length of 200 cm, an outer diameter of 9.2 mm, and a working channel of 2.8 mm. By using the Exera or Lucera processor of Olympus, the system can use all technical features of high-resolution endoscopy, including narrow band imaging (NBI). The splinting tube is an overtube with an inflatable balloon fixed to the distal, radiopaque tip, both made of latex-free silicone. The inner diameter of the tube is 11 mm, the outer diameter is 13.2 mm, the working length is 1,320 mm, and the total length is 1,400 mm. Inflation and deflation of the balloon (made of 0.1 mm silicon) is operated through the Olympus Balloon Control Unit (OBCU). Maximum inflation up to 42 mmHg provides stability of the system inside the intestine, avoiding damage to the intestinal mucosa.

The SBE method uses a push-and-pull method after insertion into the deep duodenum or the terminal ileum. As SBE does not have a second balloon at the tip of the endoscope, fixation of the endoscope within the intestine during advancement of the overtube is done by angulating the tip of the endoscope (Fig. 14.2). After advancing the overtube, the balloon of the overtube is inflated to ensure its position within

the small intestine. The endoscope and overtube can now be retracted through external pulling in order to shorten the small intestine and to thread the small intestine on the overtube. An advantage of SBE compared with DBE is that (parallel to the retraction) the endoscope can be further advanced into the small intestine under constant endoscopic view. This "simultaneous pull-and-push procedure" accelerates the advance into the small intestine (Fig. 14.3). The position in the intestine is ensured through angulation of the endoscopic tip and through pushing the overtube again. These steps are repeated until further advance of the endoscope into the intestine is not possible. As with DBE, the method can be performed under fluoroscopic guidance. Fluoroscopy can be helpful during initial SBE procedures to observe advancement and reduction of the enteroscope and as an aid in the detection and resolution of looping. After more expertise with this method is attained, however, the use of fluoroscopy is usually not required in clinical practice, except in patients with surgically modified anatomy or when therapeutic procedures such as dilations are required.

SBE can be performed through an antegrade (oral) or retrograde (anal) approach. The retrograde approach is usually more difficult, and the learning curve is longer. Ileocecal valve intubation is commonly easier when the patient is in the left lateral position, in order to achieve an ideal location of the ileocecal valve between 3 and 9 o'clock. If intubation of the ileocecal valve fails, it is useful to change the patient's position. If complete enteroscopy is required, it is recommended to mark the area of deepest advancement on the first approach with a tattoo of India ink, which is injected with a sclerotherapy needle. The marked area can then be visualized during enteroscopy performed with the opposite approach.

14.2   Applications

Therapeutic interventions within the intestine are comparable to interventions performed using DBE, as the diameter of the working channel and the length of the endoscope are the same. Endoscopic devices are available to perform interventions that include polypectomy, mucosectomy, hemostasis (e.g., by positioning of clips or injection), or extraction of foreign bodies (Figs. 14.4, 14.5, and 14.6).

Preparation of the patient before the endoscopy and the preparation of the endoscope do not differ from preparations for DBE. In addition to the simplification of the insertion procedure, a main advantage of SBE compared with DBE is that preparation is shorter because there is no need to fix the balloon at the tip of the endoscope [1]. Another advantage of SBE is the possibility of removing material such as polyps or foreign bodies through the overtube without extracting the whole system. This is especially useful during deep intubation of the small intestine, to avoid losing the position of the enteroscope. While leaving the overtube with the inflated balloon in the desired position, material can be extracted with the enteroscope through the overtube. After removal, the enteroscope can be inserted again into the small bowel to continue the procedure. This technique allows the removal of large polyps, for example, that can be extracted in a piecemeal manner (Fig. 14.4).

The indications for SBE do not differ from the indications for DBE. The main indication remains obscure bleeding in the small intestine (Figs. 14.5 and 14.6). Another major indication is the need for a diagnostic workup of patients with unknown inflammation of the small intestine, as in those with suspected small bowel Crohn's disease (Fig. 14.7). Other indications include the removal of polyps or the detection of tumors with biopsies (Figs. 14.8 and 14.9). Even though MRI and capsule endoscopy are usually first-line

Fig. 14.4 Large Peutz-Jeghers polyp, before (**a**) and after (**b**) polypectomy and clipping (**c**) during single-balloon enteroscopy

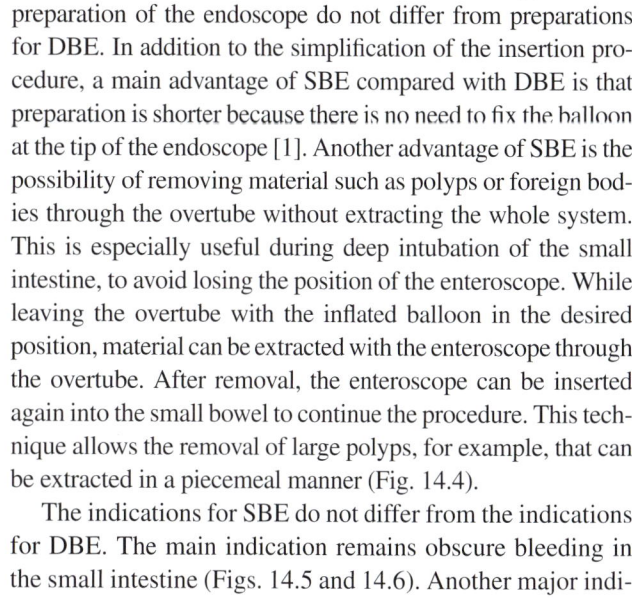
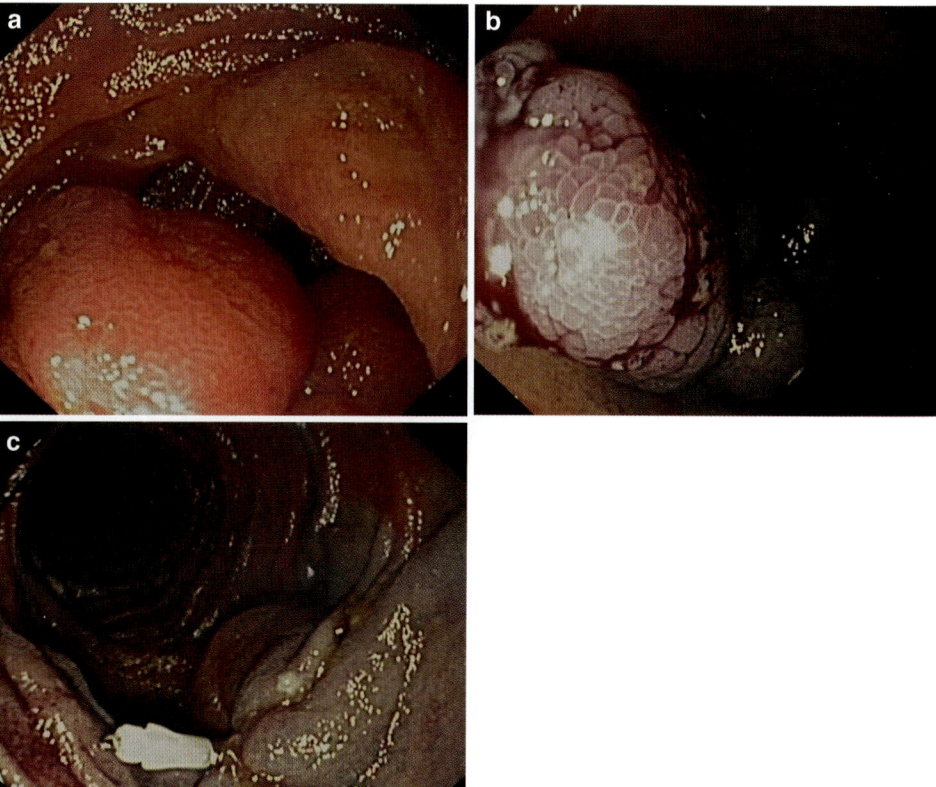

Fig. 14.5 Bleeding associated with angiectasia in the small intestine. (**a**) Enteroscopic findings showing dilated blood vessels with oozing bleeding in the ileum. (**b**) Endoscopic findings after treatment by argon plasma coagulation

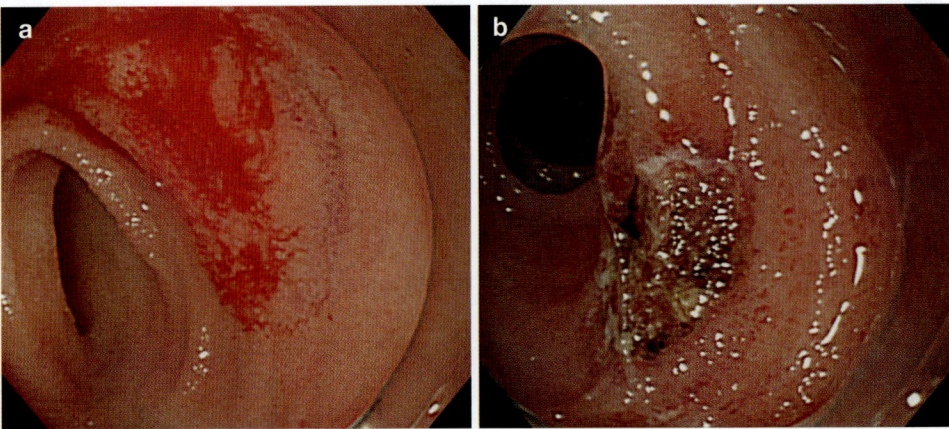

Fig 14.6 Bleeding from an erosion in the small intestine. (**a**) Enteroscopic findings showing erosions with oozing bleeding in the jejunum. (**b**) Endoscopic findings after achieving hemostasis with a clip

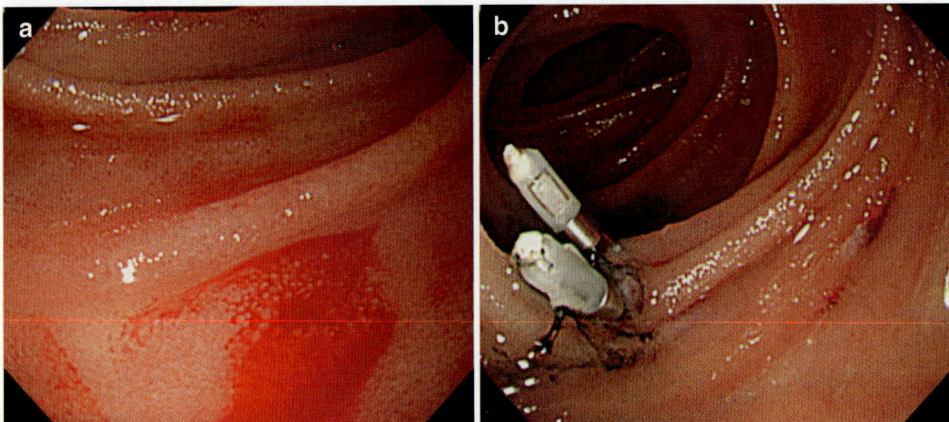

Fig. 14.7 Lesions in the small intestine of a patient with Crohn's disease. (**a**) Enteroscopic findings showing multiple, irregular-shaped ulcers and longitudinal ulcers in the ileum. (**b**) The use of indigo carmine spray allows the border of longitudinal ulcers to be clearly identified

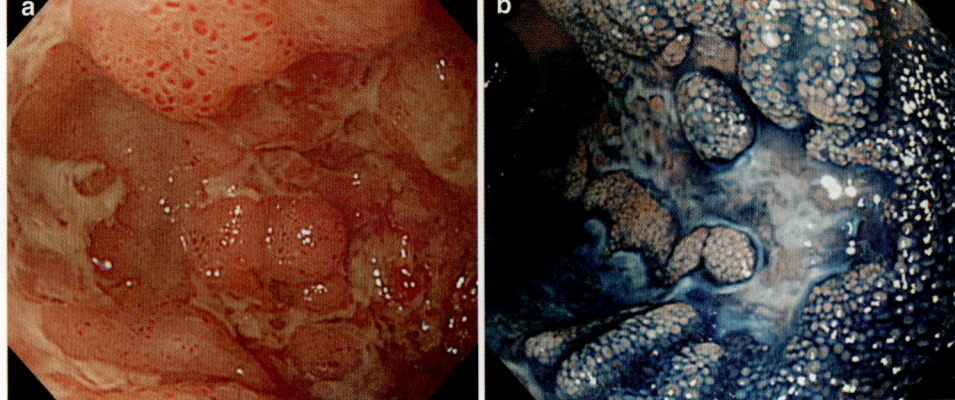

Fig. 14.8 Gastrointestinal stromal tumor (GIST) in the small intestine. (**a**) Enteroscopic findings showing a submucosal tumor in the jejunum. (**b**) Endoscopic ultrasonography (echogenic miniprobe that was placed through the working channel of the enteroscope) showing a hypoechoic mass contiguous with the muscularis propria in the wall of the small intestine. GIST was suspected. (**c**) A whitish, solid tumor was found on examination of the cut surface of the resected specimen. (**d**) Histopathologic findings showing a bundle-like proliferation of spindle-shaped tumor cells (H&E stain). (**e**, **f**) Immunohistochemical staining showed positive results for c-kit and CD34, respectively, and negative results for a-SMA and S-100. GIST was thus diagnosed

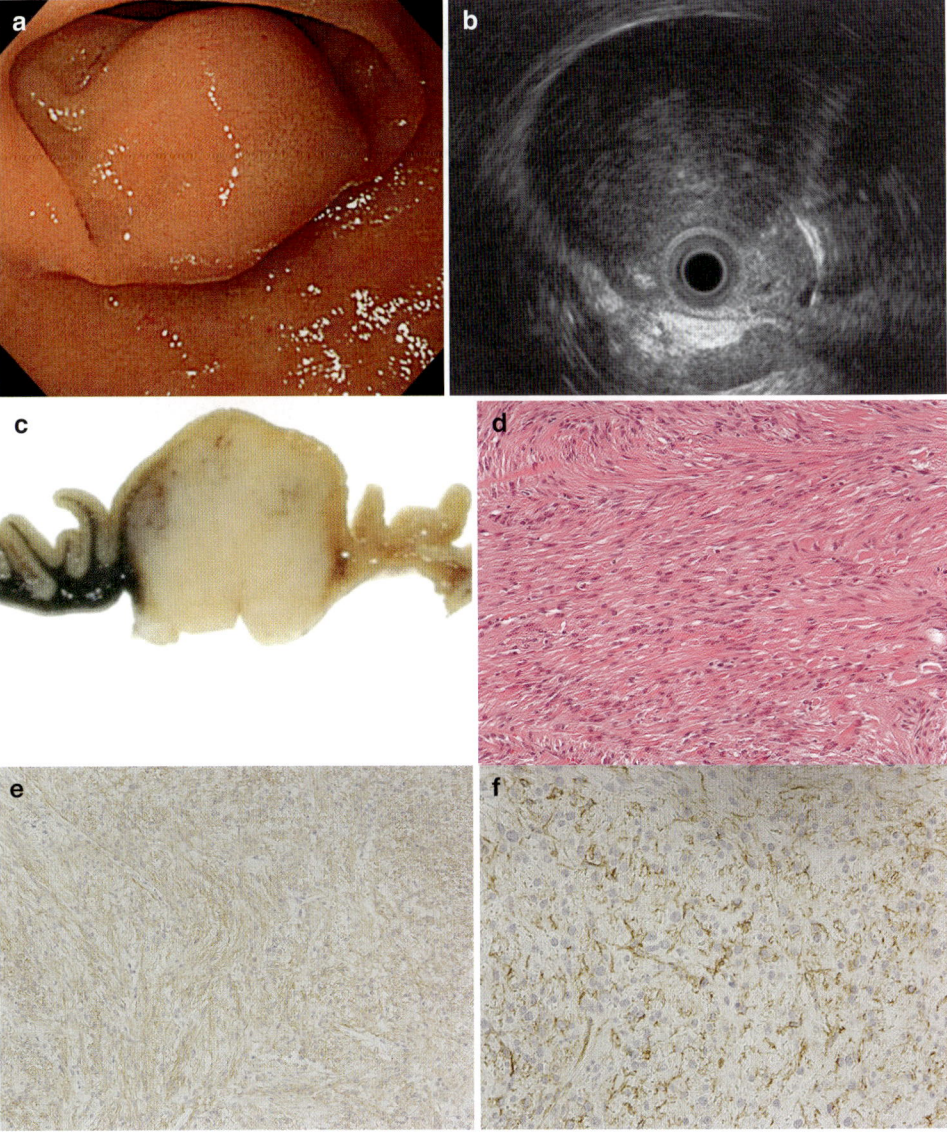

procedures in patients with suspected Crohn's disease, results frequently conflict and require endoscopic visualization and histology [2]. In addition, dilation of strictures and extraction of foreign bodies are useful indications for SBE in patients with established Crohn's disease (Fig. 14.10) [3].

In addition to diagnostic and therapeutic procedures within the small intestine, the SBE system could also be used for atypical procedures within the large intestine (e.g., difficult mucosectomies within the cecum) [4] or after failed colonoscopies [5]. SBE has also been shown to be useful for diagnostic and therapeutic procedures within the pancreaticobiliary system, such as after gastric resection or after resection of the pancreatic head [6–8].

Fig. 14.9 Follicular lymphoma in the small intestine. (**a**) Enteroscopic findings showing multiple, white, granular small protrusions in the region from the duodenum to the jejunum. (**b**) On narrow band imaging, the surrounding mucosa became brownish, allowing the lesion site to be clearly identified. (**c**) Histologic findings of a biopsy specimen, showing a typical lymphoid follicle structure with a germinal center in the lamina propria mucosa (H&E stain). (**d**) Medium-sized lymphocytes were seen in lymphoid follicles. (**e**, **f**) Immunohistochemical staining showed positive results for CD10 and Bcl-2, respectively

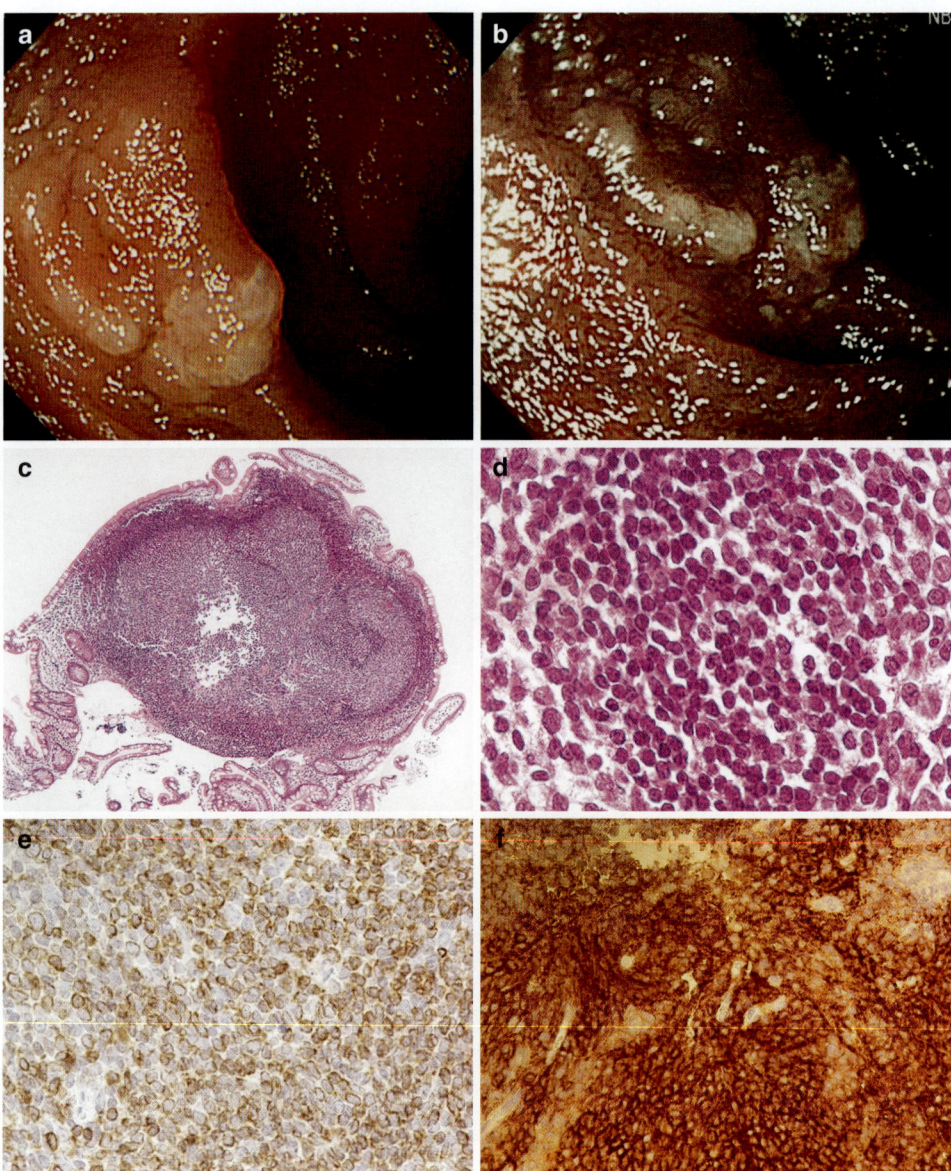

Fig. 14.10 A stricture of the small intestine associated with Crohn's disease. (**a**) Enteroscopic findings showing a severe stricture in the ileum. (**b**) Shallow ulcers were present at the stricture site. (**c**) Endoscopic balloon dilation allowed insertion of an endoscope. (**d**) Endoscopic findings after dilation

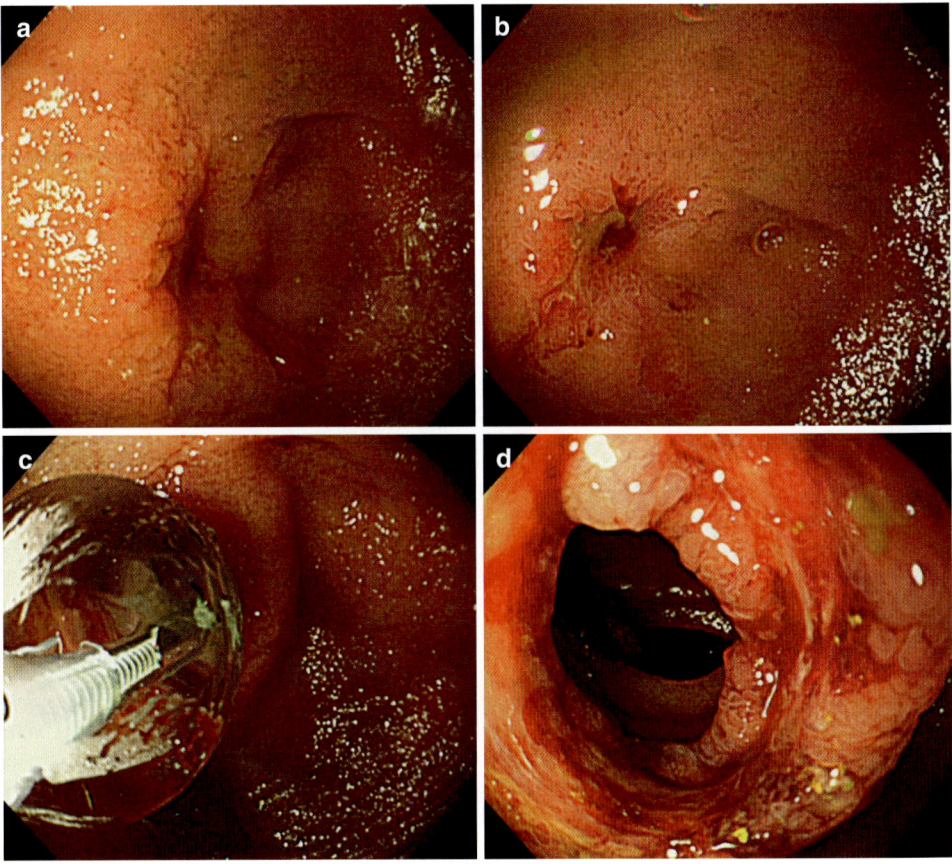

14.3 Complications

Complications during SBE are comparable to those during DBE, with a rate of complication of about 1 % during diagnostic balloon enteroscopy and up to 3–4 % using therapeutic balloon enteroscopy. Mortality of balloon enteroscopy is about 0.05 % [9–11]. To reduce adverse effects such as postendoscopic pain, SBE is more and more performed with carbon dioxide insufflation, which also increases insertion depths [12].

14.4 Clinical Results

The clinical usefulness of SBE has been determined in various studies. In an early study, SBE was used in 60 patients with suspected small bowel disease [13]. All patients underwent antegrade examinations, and 10 also received retrograde examinations. The mean procedure time was 63 min, and the mean insertion depth was 260 cm. Total enteroscopy was possible in 5 (50 %) of 10 patients. The diagnostic yields were 77 % for cases of obscure gastrointestinal bleeding, 61 % for chronic abdominal pain, and 63 % for malabsorption

syndrome. Several other authors with larger series of patients have demonstrated that SBE has a high diagnostic yield with the capability of useful therapeutic interventions [14, 15].

Studies comparing SBE versus DBE reveal conflicting results. One trial compared DBE with SBE by eliminating the distal balloon of the double-balloon enteroscope [16]. The rate of complete enteroscopy was higher in the DBE group than with the single-balloon enteroscope (DBE, 66 %, $n=33$; SBE, 22 %, $n=11$; $P<0.00001$). The yield of relevant pathologic features within the intestine was higher in the DBE group (50 %) than in the SBE group (42 %). The results were confirmed by a trial from Japan [17]. More recent trials have shown similar results for DBE and SBE regarding insertion depth and the rate of complete enteroscopy [18–20]. In a trial by Domagk and colleagues [18], the mean oral intubation depth was 253 cm with DBE and 258 cm with SBE, showing noninferiority of SBE versus DBE. Complete visualization of the small bowel was achieved in 18 % of the DBE group and 11 % of the SBE groups. Mean anal intubation depth was 107 cm in the DBE group and 118 cm in the SBE group. The diagnostic yield and mean pain scores during and after the procedures were similar in both groups. No adverse events were observed during or after the examinations.

Another trial compared SBE with spiral enteroscopy [21]. Even though the insertion depth was higher for spiral enteroscopy than for SBE, there were no significant differences in diagnostic yield or procedure time. Currently, it appears that no enteroscopic system has a major advantage. The experience of the endoscopist appears to be more relevant for a successful examination than the enteroscope that is used.

In summary, SBE is an effective endoscopic tool for the evaluation of the small bowel. Technically, it is easy and safe to perform, and it is similar to DBE in diagnostic and therapeutic yield.

References

1. Kobayashi K, Haruki S, Sada M, et al. Single-balloon enteroscopy. Nihon Rinsho. 2008;66:1371–8.
2. de Ridder L, Mensink PB, Lequin MH, et al. Single-balloon enteroscopy, magnetic resonance enterography, and abdominal US useful for evaluation of small-bowel disease in children with (suspected) Crohn's disease. Gastrointest Endosc. 2012;75:87–94.
3. Bourreille A, Ignjatovic A, Aabakken L, et al. Role of small-bowel endoscopy in the management of patients with inflammatory bowel disease: an international OMED-ECCO consensus. Endoscopy. 2009;41:618–37.
4. Arai Y, Kato T, Arihiro S, et al. Utility of single balloon enteroscopy (SBE) for difficult cases of total colonoscopy. J Interv Gastroenterol. 2012;2:12–4.
5. Teshima CW, Aktas H, Haringsma J, et al. Single-balloon-assisted colonoscopy in patients with previously failed colonoscopy. Gastrointest Endosc. 2010;71:1319–23.
6. Maaser C, Lenze F, Bokemeyer M, et al. Double balloon enteroscopy: a useful tool for diagnostic and therapeutic procedures in the pancreaticobiliary system. Am J Gastroenterol. 2008;103:894–900.
7. Shah RJ, Smolkin M, Yen R, et al. A multicenter, U.S. experience of single-balloon, double-balloon, and rotational overtube-assisted enteroscopy ERCP in patients with surgically altered pancreaticobiliary anatomy (with video). Gastrointest Endosc. 2013;77:593–600.
8. Moreels TG, Pelckmans PA. Comparison between double-balloon and single-balloon enteroscopy in therapeutic ERC after Roux-en-Y enteric-enteric anastomosis. World J Gastrointest Endosc. 2010;2:314–7.
9. Mensink PB, Haringsma J, Kucharzik T, et al. Complications of double balloon enteroscopy: a multicenter survey. Endoscopy. 2007;39:613–5.
10. Möschler O, May A, Muller MK, et al. Complications in and performance of double-balloon enteroscopy (DBE): results from a large prospective DBE database in Germany. Endoscopy. 2011;43:484–9.
11. Aktas H, de Ridder L, Haringsma J, et al. Complications of single-balloon enteroscopy: a prospective evaluation of 166 procedures. Endoscopy. 2010;42:365–8.
12. Domagk D, Bretthauer M, Lenz P, et al. Carbon dioxide insufflation improves intubation depth in double-balloon enteroscopy: a randomized, controlled, double-blind trial. Endoscopy. 2007;39:1064–7.
13. Ramchandani M, Reddy DN, Gupta R, et al. Diagnostic yield and therapeutic impact of single-balloon enteroscopy: series of 106 cases. J Gastroenterol Hepatol. 2009;24:1631–8.
14. Frantz DJ, Dellon ES, Grimm IS, et al. Single-balloon enteroscopy: results from an initial experience at a U.S. tertiary-care center. Gastrointest Endosc. 2010;72:422–6.
15. Upchurch BR, Sanaka MR, Lopez AR, et al. The clinical utility of single-balloon enteroscopy: a single-center experience of 172 procedures. Gastrointest Endosc. 2010;71:1218–23.
16. May A, Farber M, Aschmoneit I, et al. Prospective multicenter trial comparing push-and-pull enteroscopy with the single- and double-balloon techniques in patients with small-bowel disorders. Am J Gastroenterol. 2010;105:575–81.
17. Takano N, Yamada A, Watabe H, et al. Single-balloon versus double-balloon endoscopy for achieving total enteroscopy: a randomized, controlled trial. Gastrointest Endosc. 2011;73:734–9.
18. Domagk D, Mensink P, Aktas H, et al. Single- vs. double-balloon enteroscopy in small-bowel diagnostics: a randomized multicenter trial. Endoscopy. 2011;43:472–6.
19. Efthymiou M, Desmond PV, Brown G, et al. SINGLE-01: a randomized, controlled trial comparing the efficacy and depth of insertion of single- and double-balloon enteroscopy by using a novel method to determine insertion depth. Gastrointest Endosc. 2012;76:972–80.
20. Lenz P, Domagk D. Double- vs. single-balloon vs. spiral enteroscopy. Best Pract Res Clin Gastroenterol. 2012;26:303–13.
21. Khashab MA, Lennon AM, Dunbar KB, et al. A comparative evaluation of single-balloon enteroscopy and spiral enteroscopy for patients with mid-gut disorders. Gastrointest Endosc. 2010;72:766–72.

Spiral Enteroscopy and Balloon-Guided Enteroscopy

15

Peter Draganov and Martin Keuchel

Contents

15.1   Spiral Enteroscopy

15.1.1 Principle

Spiral enteroscopy (SE) uses a unique principle of deep enteroscopy. Rotational movement is translated via a soft spiral attached at the outside of an overtube into longitudinal movement. By clockwise rotation of the spiral, the small intestine is continually pleated over the overtube. The bowel and the adherent mesentery are not torqued by this procedure [1, 2].

15.1.2 Spiral Overtube

The Endo-Ease Discovery SB spiral overtube (SyncMedical, Stoughton, MA, USA) (Fig. 15.1) was approved by the US Food and Drug Administration (FDA) in 2008. It has a length of 118 cm and an inner diameter of 9.8 mm, accommodating either a Fujinon EN450-T5 or an Olympus SIFQ180 enteroscope. The distal segment of the overtube (approximately 22 cm) carries a 5.5-mm soft helix summing up to an outer diameter of 16 mm (Fig. 15.2). An Endo-Ease Vista spiral for the rectal approach is also available (Fig. 15.3).

Two handles are attached at the proximal end of the overtube. A gentle lock fixes the proximal end of the overtube to the endoscope while still allowing rotation of the handles and the overtube with the attached helix. After unlocking, the endoscope can be advanced further through the overtube. Additional lubricant can be installed through a port near the lock. The polyvinyl material makes the spiral overtube more stable than the overtubes for single-balloon or double-balloon enteroscopy. Besides the single-use spiral, there is no need for further equipment like air pumps with control units.

15.1.3 Procedure

After thorough lubrication, the endoscope is inserted into the overtube and locked at about 140–150 cm, allowing the distal end of the endoscope with the bending section to move freely.

The work was first published in 2006 by Springer Medizin Verlag Heidelberg with the following title: *Atlas of Video Capsule Endoscopy*.

P. Draganov (✉)
Division of Gastroenterology, Hepatology, and Nutrition,
University of Florida College of Medicine, Gainesville, FL, USA
e-mail: peter.draganov@medicine.ufl.edu

M. Keuchel
Department of Internal Medicine,
Bethesda Krankenhaus Bergedorf,
Hamburg, Germany
e-mail: keuchel@bkb.info

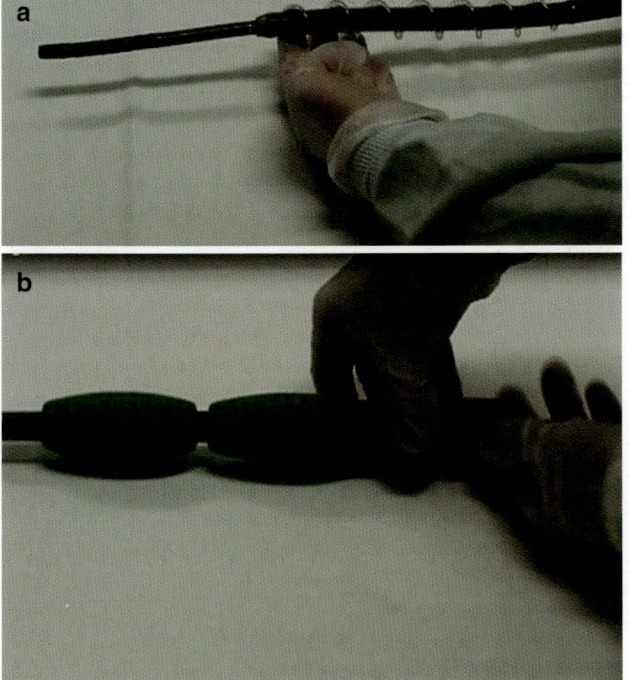

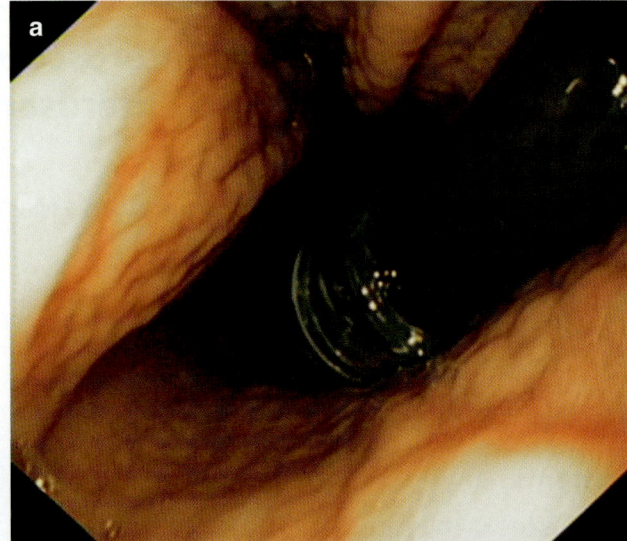

Fig. 15.1 Endo-Ease Discovery SB spiral overtube for the oral approach. (**a**) Distal end of the overtube with segment carrying the soft spiral and free part of the endoscope tip. (**b**) Green handles and black soft lock at the proximal end of the overtube

A dedicated mouthpiece must be used in order to accommodate the spiral. The free endoscope tip is advanced into the esophagus. As soon as the spiral reaches the oral cavity, rotational movements are initiated while taking care for sufficient lubrication of the overtube. Once the spiral has entered the duodenum, the endoscope is straightened to reduce gastric looping while clockwise rotation continues. Gentle pressure during further rotation helps to advance the spiral beyond the ligament of Treitz. Now the small intestine can be pleated over the overtube by continuously rotating the spiral (Fig. 15.4).

Push-and-pull maneuvers while the spiral is introduced into the gastrointestinal tract must be avoided to prevent mucosal damage. One operator controls the spiral movements while a second operator steers the endoscope, taking care for correct positioning with a minimum of air insufflation (Fig. 15.5). If the force needed to torque the handle increases, counterclockwise rotation is applied to release pressure. When further rotation is not possible, the lock is opened and the endoscope can be advanced further into the small intestine. Gently pulling the endoscope back while rotating the spiral clockwise and using the endoscope as a guide may further increase insertion depth. Fluoroscopic control (Fig. 15.6) is optional in difficult cases, but generally is not necessary.

Counterclockwise rotation of the spiral allows controlled withdrawal. The stable position of the spiral and endoscope

Fig. 15.2 Retroflexion of the endoscope in the stomach shows the tip of the spiral overtube (**a**) and the middle of the spiral section (**b**)

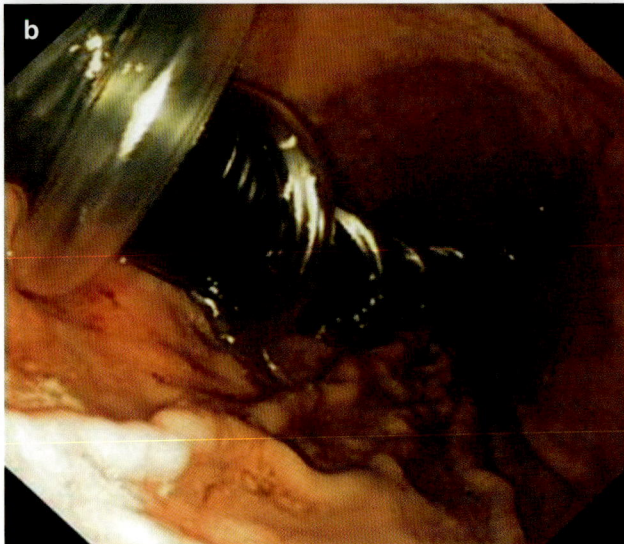

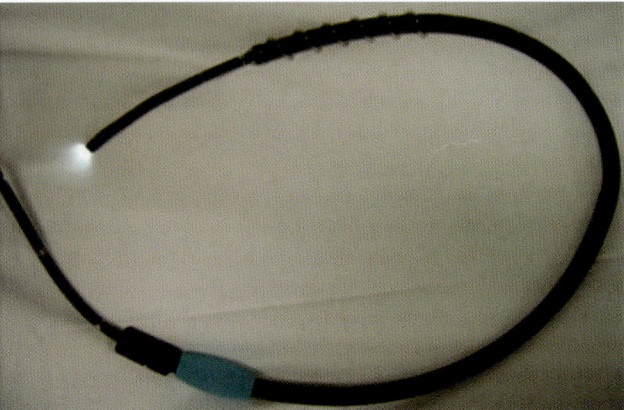

Fig. 15.3 Endo-Ease Vista spiral overtube for the rectal approach

Fig. 15.4 Principle of spiral enteroscopy. Once the spiral has reached the duodenum (**a**), the endoscope is straightened to reduce gastric looping with clockwise rotation (**b**). Gentle pressure during further rotation helps to advance the spiral beyond the ligament of Treitz (**c**). Now the small intestine can be pleated over the overtube by continuously rotating the spiral (**d**)

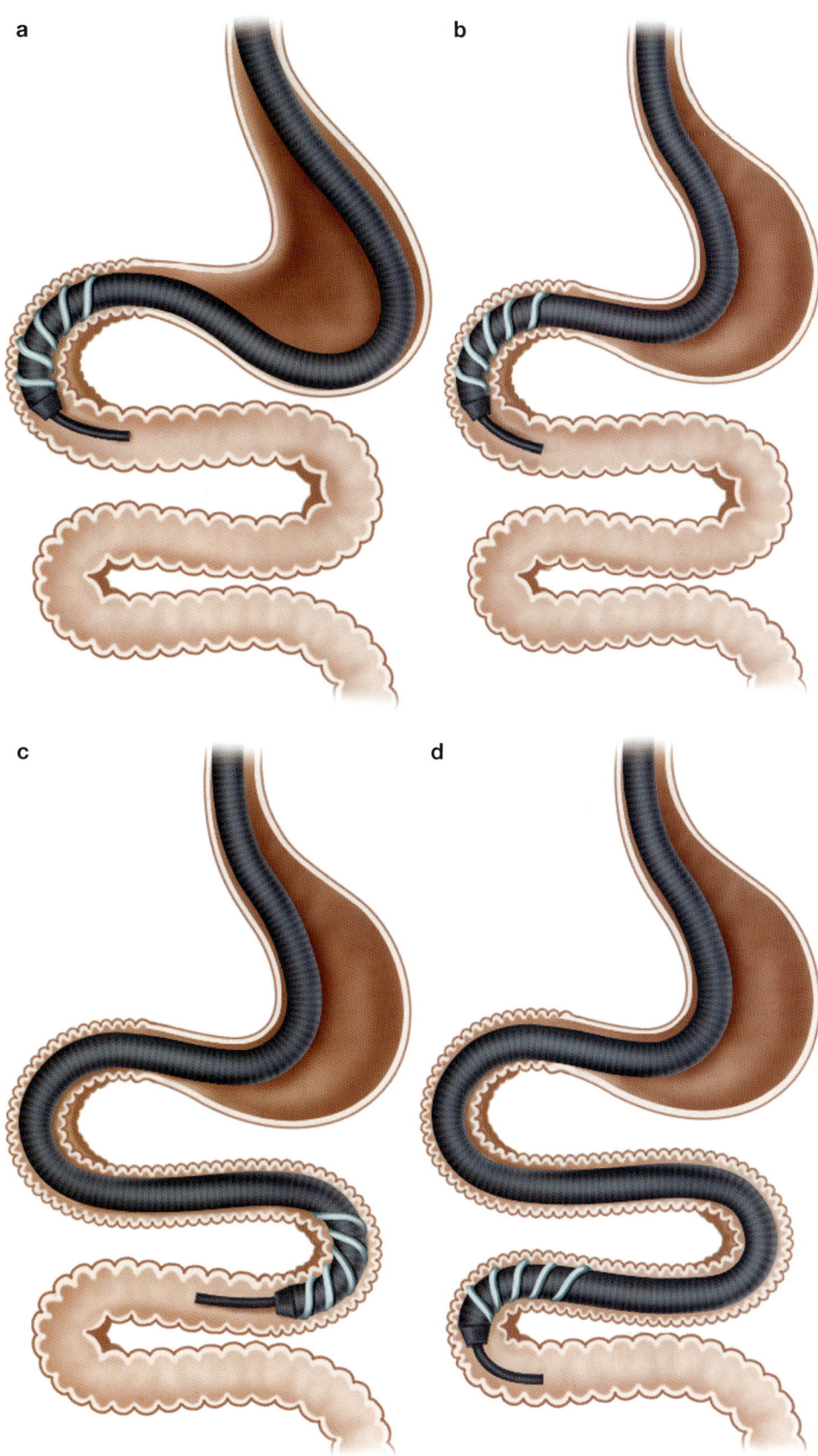

Fig. 15.5 Procedure of spiral enteroscopy. One physician rotates the spiral overtube; the other operates the endoscope (**a**). During the procedure, additional lubricant can be installed through a port into the overtube if needed (**b**)

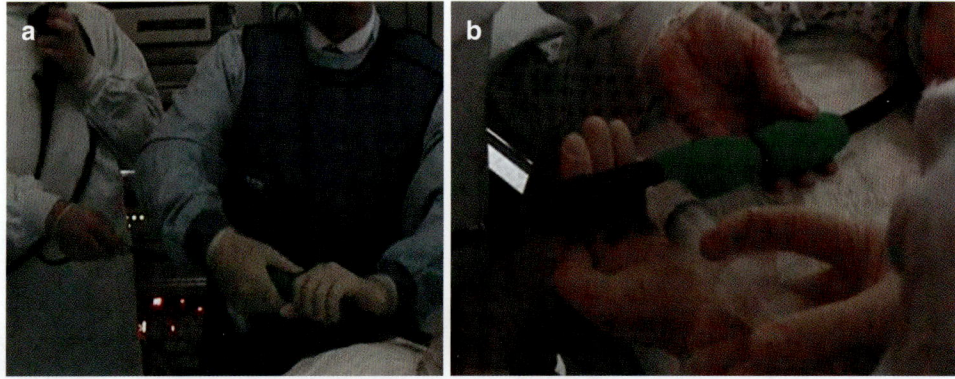

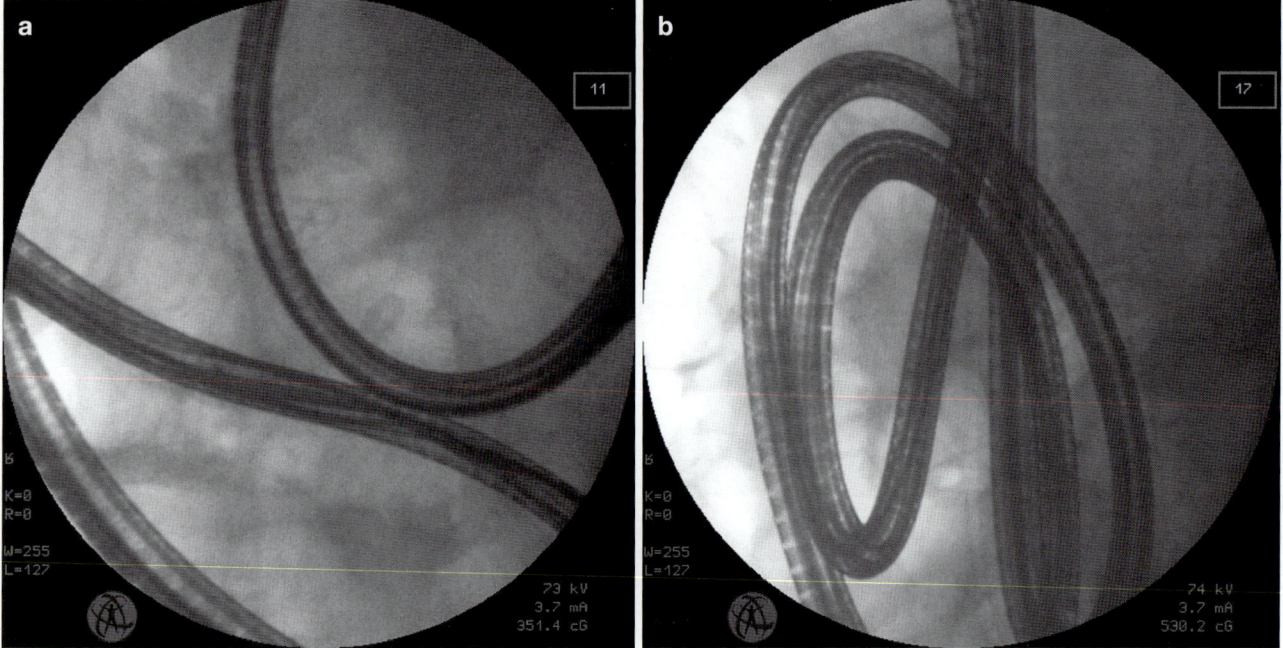

Fig. 15.6 Optional fluoroscopy during spiral enteroscopy. (**a**) In the upper loop, the overtube with spiral is visible. (**b**) Once the spiral cannot be advanced deeper, the endoscope is unlocked and pushed forward, leaving the overtube in place

is especially helpful during therapeutic procedures such as argon plasma coagulation (Fig. 15.7) or polypectomy (Fig. 15.8). A resected polyp can be easily retrieved by grasping it with the snare and withdrawing the endoscope through the spiral (Fig. 15.8d). Reinsertion allows for repeated polypectomy without changing the spiral position.

An evaluation of a training campaign showed that endoscopists experienced in enteroscopy could acquire the method confidently in a 2-day training, performing five cases under intensive supervision [3]. SE was feasible also in a small cohort of patients with surgically altered small intestinal anatomy [4].

15.1.4 Clinical Application

In a multicenter study in the United States, antegrade SE was successfully performed up to the jejunum in 93 % of patients

[5]. During a mean diagnostic procedure time of 34 min, an insertion depth of 250 cm beyond the ligament of Treitz could be achieved. Fluoroscopy was used in only 11 %. Diagnostic yield was 65 %, and most of the patients underwent endoscopic intervention (including argon plasma coagulation in 64 %).

In general, SE is applied with an antegrade approach. The retrograde approach is also feasible, mainly using the small bowel overtube primarily intended for the antegrade route. This technique is more challenging, and advancement of the spiral into the terminal ileum is not possible in all cases [6]. A study in the United States found that various enteroscopy methods were more effective using the antegrade approach than the retrograde one in terms of insertion depth and diagnostic and therapeutic yield [7]. Hence, antegrade SE will allow effective diagnosis and treatment in a short procedural time in most cases. Time for per oral insertion was as short as 28 min in a small cohort [8].

Fig. 15.7 Spiral enteroscopy with treatment of jejunal angiectasia. (**a**) Angiectasia detected by small bowel capsule endoscopy (SBCE) (PillCamSB2). (**b**) Lesion reached by spiral enteroscopy with Fujinon EN450T enteroscope. (**c**, **d**) Argon plasma coagulation

Fig. 15.8 Spiral enteroscopy with polypectomy. (**a**) Polyp detected at small bowel capsule endoscopy (OMOM capsule). (**b**) Polyp of the jejunum reached by spiral enteroscopy with Olympus enteroscope SIF 180. (**c**) Polypectomy after saline injection. (**d**) Polyp retrieval with the snare through the spiral overtube

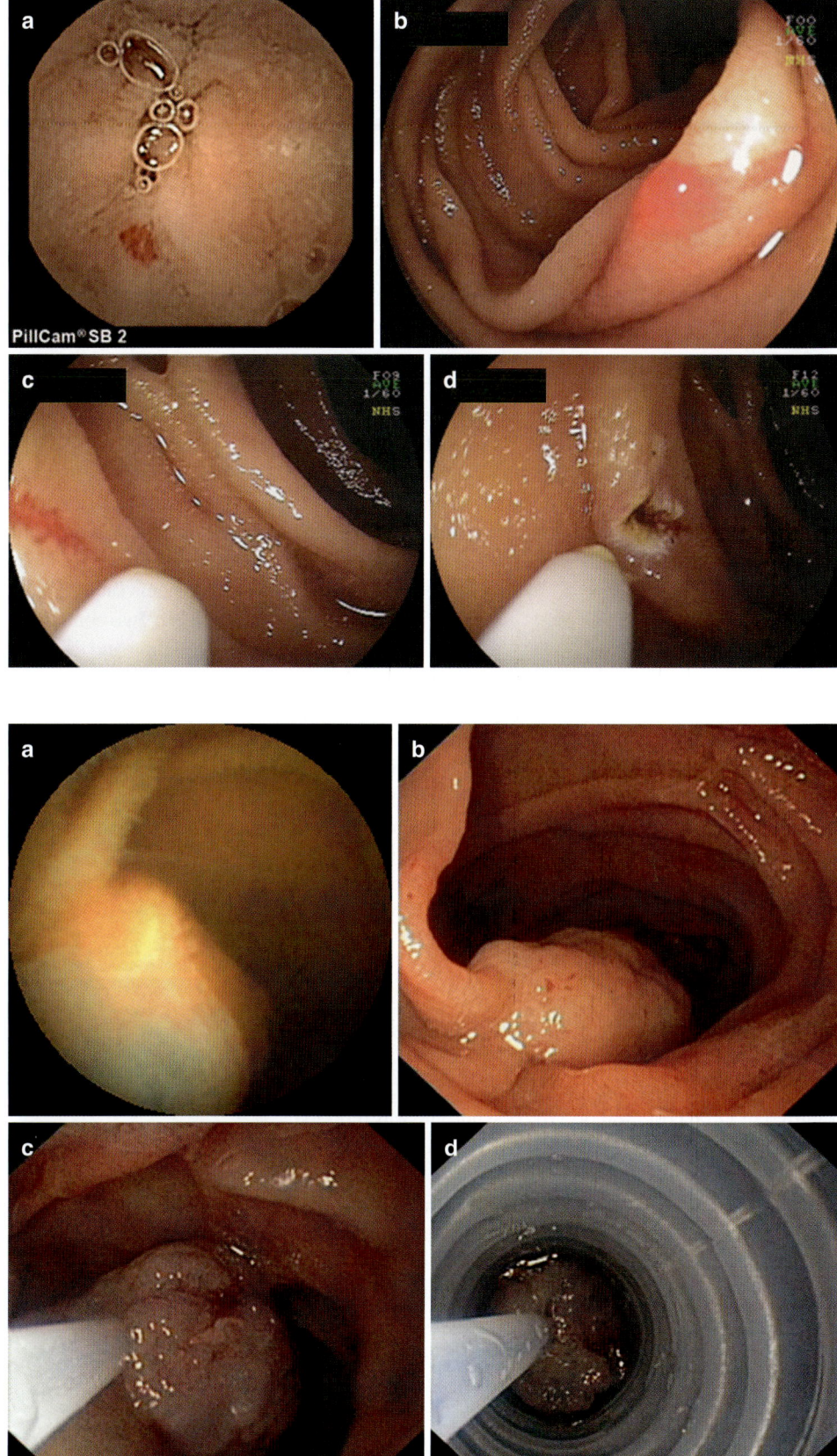

15.1.5 Comparison with Balloon-Assisted Enteroscopy

In a randomized trial, double-balloon enteroscopy (DBE) and SE had a similar diagnostic and therapeutic yield. Insertion time for SE was significantly shorter than for DBE. However, complete enteroscopy in a bidirectional approach with SE could be achieved in only 8 % of patients, versus 92 % with DBE procedures ($P = 0.002$). One perforation occurred during retrograde SE [9]. A crossover study found significantly shorter insertion times for SE and deeper insertion to the small intestine for DBE [10].

A small prospective study [11] and a multicenter, nonrandomized trial of DBE and SE following diagnostic capsule endoscopy [12] found no significant difference in therapeutic yield, insertion depth, and procedural time. In a retrospective, nonrandomized trial, single-balloon enteroscopy (SBE) and SE had a similar diagnostic yield and procedural time. SE reached deeper to the small intestine [13]. One perforation was observed during SBE.

15.1.6 Outcome

Positive findings on small bowel capsule endoscopy were reproduced by oral SE in only 54 % of patients [14], because of either false-positive findings on the capsule endoscopy or insufficient insertion depth of SE. In a study of long-term outcome 2 years after SE for obscure gastrointestinal bleeding, events of overt bleeding and number of transfusions were reduced significantly, and mean hemoglobin was higher [15].

15.1.7 Complications

Severe complications, such as perforation of the small intestine, are rare, with 0.4 % in the first 1,750 cases. Sore throat occurred in 28 % of patients, and superficial mucosal trauma occurred in 22 % [16]. Mallory-Weiss syndrome was reported in one patient (3 % of a small series) [17]. Intussusception may occur in the small bowel, especially when pulling too much backward. These cases could be resolved during the procedure. However, a case of gastroesophageal intussusception has been reported that required surgical repair [18]. Hyperamylasemia was observed in 20 % of patients after SE, but no clinical signs of pancreatitis [19]. SE has been shown to be safe as well in patients with comorbidities [20].

15.1.8 Future Developments

A newly developed enteroscope prototype with an integrated segment proximal to the bending section carrying a motor-driven spiral has been applied successfully. In all of 27 patients, a total enteroscopy could be achieved, either via a bidirectional approach (in a mean time of 58 min) or, in the last three patients of this series, by an oral approach alone. No severe complications were observed [21].

15.2 Balloon-Guided Enteroscopy

Balloon-guided enteroscopy uses a standard endoscope that is advanced into the small intestine either via the oral (antegrade) or the rectal (retrograde) approach. An advancing balloon with a very soft tip is further advanced into the small bowel and finally inflated. By pulling the advancing balloon back and pushing the endoscope forward, the small intestine is pleated over the endoscope. There is no overtube. The initial system included two balloons. Besides the advancing balloon, another balloon was fixed at the endoscope tip to stabilize the position. Air lines to both balloon and the catheter of the advancing balloon are attached alongside the endoscope (Fig. 15.9). Thus, the working channel is spared for instruments such as biopsy forceps or coagulation probes (Fig. 15.10). Two connected air pumps allow separately controlled inflation and deflation of the two balloons. Feasibility has been shown in a small series [22]. However, balloon-guided enteroscopy has not yet found wide acceptance.

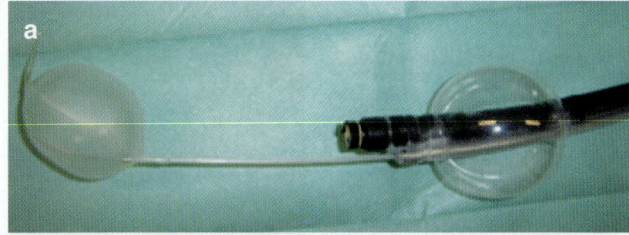

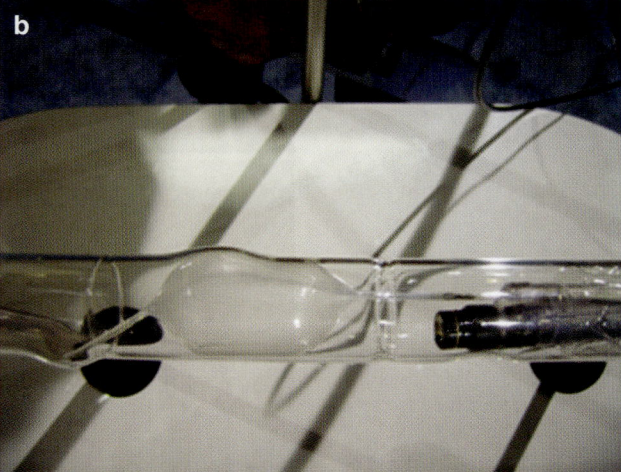

Fig. 15.9 Balloon-guided enteroscopy system (NaviAid, SMART Medical Systems, Israel). (**a**) A stabilizing balloon is attached near the tip of a standard endoscope. The advancing balloon is forwarded through a channel mounted together with the line for air insufflation of the stabilizing balloon at the outside of the endoscope. (**b**) NaviAid System in a glass model of the small intestine

Fig. 15.10 (**a**) Angiectasia in the jejunum, seen at video capsule endoscopy (PillCam SB2). (**b**) Consecutive balloon-guided enteroscopy with Pentax colonoscope and NaviAid advancing balloon ahead. (**c**) Angiectasia is reached. (**d**) Argon plasma coagulation is performed with the advancing balloon in place

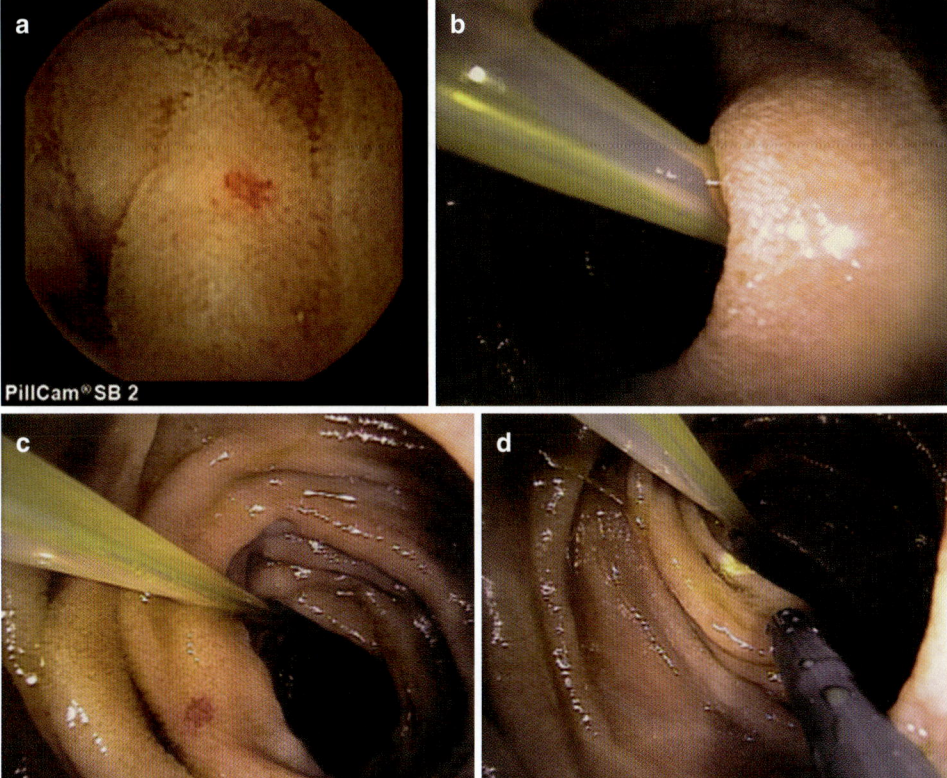

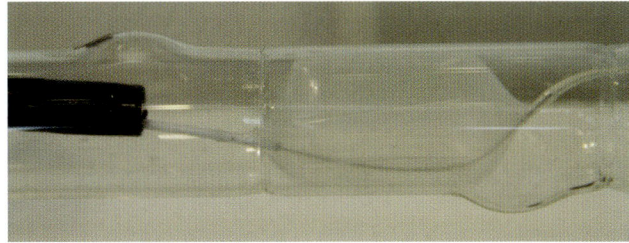

Fig. 15.11 Balloon-guided enteroscopy with single balloon advanced through the working channel

A new version of the system using only a single-balloon technique avoids cumbersome attachment of the system on the outside of the endoscope. The advancing balloon is simply introduced through the working channel and exchanged for instruments when needed (Fig. 15.11). The required minimum diameter for the accessory channel of 3.7 mm restricts use of this system to standard colonoscopes. Clinical data on performance and safety are still warranted, however.

References

1. Akerman PA, Agrawal D, Chen W, et al. Spiral enteroscopy: a novel method of enteroscopy by using the Endo-Ease Discovery SB overtube and a pediatric colonoscope. Gastrointest Endosc. 2009;69:327–32.

2. Akerman PA, Agrawal D, Cantero D, Pangtay J. Spiral enteroscopy with the new DSB overtube: a novel technique for deep peroral small-bowel intubation. Endoscopy. 2008;40:974–8.

3. Buscaglia JM, Dunbar KB, Okolo 3rd PI, et al. The spiral enteroscopy training initiative: results of a prospective study evaluating the Discovery SB overtube device during small bowel enteroscopy (with video). Endoscopy. 2009;41:194–9.

4. Buxbaum J, Kline M, Selby R. Prospective study of therapeutic spiral enteroscopy in patients with surgically altered anatomy. Surg Endosc. 2013;27:671–8.

5. Morgan D, Upchurch B, Draganov P, et al. Spiral enteroscopy: prospective U.S. multicenter study in patients with small-bowel disorders. Gastrointest Endosc. 2010;72:992–8.

6. Nagula S, Gaidos J, Draganov PV, et al. Retrograde spiral enteroscopy: feasibility, success, and safety in a series of 22 patients. Gastrointest Endosc. 2011;74:699–702.

7. Sanaka MR, Navaneethan U, Kosuru B, et al. Antegrade is more effective than retrograde enteroscopy for evaluation and management of suspected small-bowel disease. Clin Gastroenterol Hepatol. 2012;10:910–6.

8. Ramchandani M, Reddy DN, Gupta R, et al. Spiral enteroscopy: a preliminary experience in Asian population. J Gastroenterol Hepatol. 2010;25:1754–7.

9. Messer I, May A, Manner H, Ell C. Prospective, randomized, single-center trial comparing double-balloon enteroscopy and spiral enteroscopy in patients with suspected small-bowel disorders. Gastrointest Endosc. 2013;77:241–9.

10. May A, Manner H, Aschmoneit I, Ell C. Prospective, cross-over, single-center trial comparing oral double-balloon enteroscopy and oral spiral enteroscopy in patients with suspected small-bowel vascular malformations. Endoscopy. 2011;43:477–83.

11. Frieling T, Heise J, Sassenrath W, et al. Prospective comparison between double-balloon enteroscopy and spiral enteroscopy. Endoscopy. 2010;42:885–8.

12. Rahmi G, Samaha E, Vahedi K, et al. Multicenter comparison of double-balloon enteroscopy and spiral enteroscopy. J Gastroenterol Hepatol. 2013;28:992–8.

13. Khashab MA, Lennon AM, Dunbar KB, et al. A comparative evaluation of single-balloon enteroscopy and spiral enteroscopy for patients with mid-gut disorders. Gastrointest Endosc. 2010;72:766–72.

14. Buscaglia JM, Richards R, Wilkinson MN, et al. Diagnostic yield of spiral enteroscopy when performed for the evaluation of abnormal capsule endoscopy findings. J Clin Gastroenterol. 2011;45:342–6.

15. Williamson JB, Judah JR, Gaidos JK, et al. Prospective evaluation of the long-term outcomes after deep small-bowel spiral enteroscopy in patients with obscure GI bleeding. Gastrointest Endosc. 2012;76:771–8.

16. Akerman PA, Cantero D. Severe complications of spiral endoscopy in the first 1750 patients. Gastrointest Endosc. 2009;69:AB127.

17. Yamada A, Watabe H, Oka S, et al. Feasibility of spiral enteroscopy in Japanese patients: study in two tertiary hospitals. Dig Endosc. 2013;25:406–11.

18. Chaze I, Gincul R, Lepilliez V, et al. Gastroesophageal intussusception and multivisceral failure after per oral spiral enteroscopy. VJGIEN. 2013;1:230–2.

19. Teshima CW, Aktas H, Kuipers EJ, Mensink PB. Hyperamylasemia and pancreatitis following spiral enteroscopy. Can J Gastroenterol. 2012;26:603–6.

20. Judah JR, Draganov PV, Lam Y, et al. Spiral enteroscopy is safe and effective for an elderly United States population of patients with numerous comorbidities. Clin Gastroenterol Hepatol. 2010;8:572–6.

21. Akerman PA, Demarco DC, Battacharya K, et al. Endoscopic visualization of the entire small intestine in 27 consecutive patients using novel motorized spiral endoscope. Gastrointest Endosc. 2012;75:AB134.

22. Adler SN, Bjarnason I, Metzger YC. New balloon-guided technique for deep small-intestine endoscopy using standard endoscopes. Endoscopy. 2008;40:502–5.

Intraoperative Enteroscopy

16

Dirk Hartmann, Hans-Joachim Schulz,
Evgeny D. Fedorov, and Jürgen F. Riemann

Contents

The work was first published in 2006 by Springer Medizin Verlag Heidelberg with the following title: *Atlas of Video Capsule Endoscopy.*

D. Hartmann • H.-J. Schulz
Department of Internal Medicine,
Sana Klinikum Lichtenberg,
Berlin, Germany
e-mail: d.hartmann@sana-kl.de; hj.schulz@sana-kl.de

E.D. Fedorov
Digestive Endoscopy, Russia State Medical University,
Moscow University Hospital No. 31, Moscow, Russia
e-mail: efedo@mail.ru

J.F. Riemann (✉)
LebensBlicke Foundation for Prevention of Colorectal Cancer,
Ludwigshafen, Germany
e-mail: riemannj@garps.de

16.1 Indications

Intraoperative enteroscopy (IOE) is accepted as the ultimate procedure for complete evaluation of the small bowel. However, improvements in imaging modalities such as ultrasound, CT scans, and MRI, as well as the introduction of video capsule endoscopy (VCE) and balloon enteroscopy (BE) have restricted the indications for intraoperative enteroscopy to situations in which less invasive procedures have failed to yield a full diagnosis or to safely perform endoscopic therapy:

- Obscure gastrointestinal bleeding
    - "Midgut" bleeding that is massive or occurs in urgent situations when VCE or BE are not available
    - Lesions not accessible by BE
    - Lesions difficult or impossible to treat by BE
- Difficult gastrointestinal problems, such as suspected lymphoma, suspected active small bowel endocrine tumor, or suspected malignant tumors
- Crohn's disease, to identify mucosal changes and the degree of strictures that require surgical intervention
- Peutz-Jeghers syndrome, to improve polyp clearance without the need for additional enterotomies or to help reduce the frequency of laparotomies

16.2 Technique

The technique of IOE varies in several important aspects, such as the approach (laparotomy versus laparoscopy), the type of endoscopes used (pediatric colonoscope, video enteroscope, balloon enteroscope), and the technique of endoscope insertion (peroral, peranal, enterotomy).

16.2.1 Standard Procedure

The standard procedure consists of a laparotomy followed by one enterotomy (usually in the middle of the small bowel). After standard explorative laparotomy, the bowel is inspected for external changes (e.g., vascular malformation or tumors).

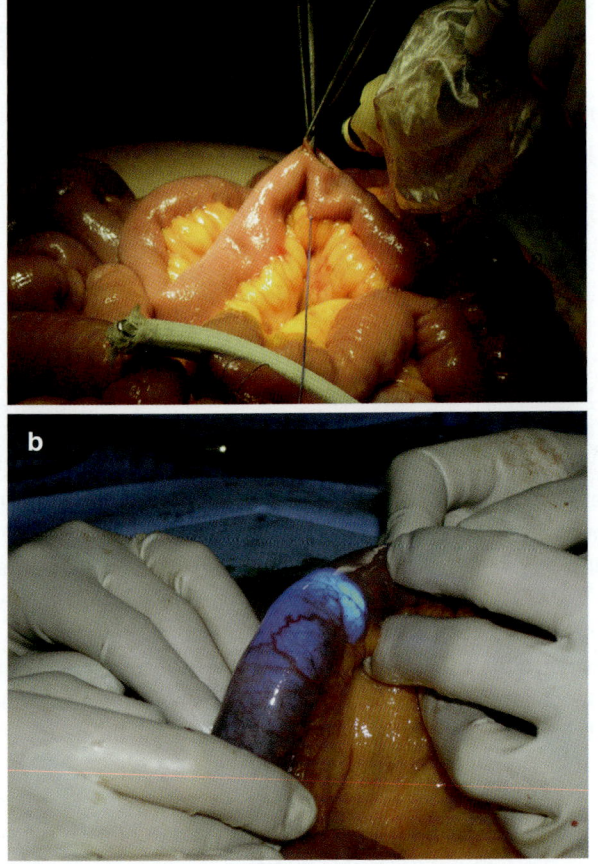

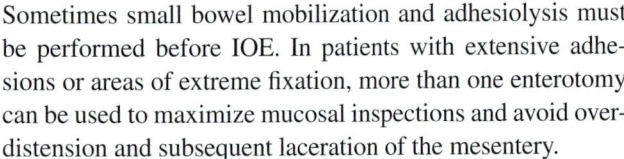

Fig. 16.1 Intraoperative enteroscopy via laparotomy. (**a**) The endoscope is inserted through an enterostomy. (**b**) Transillumination at the tip of the endoscope

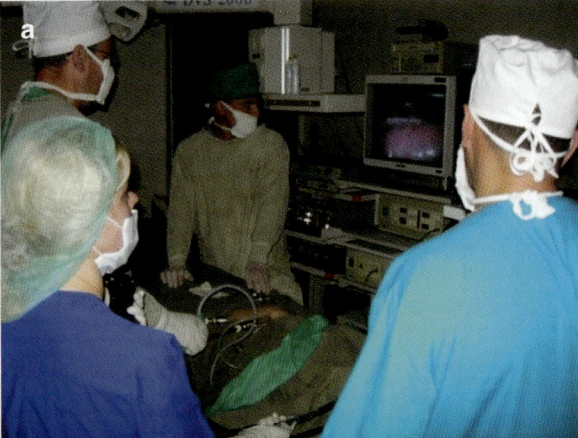

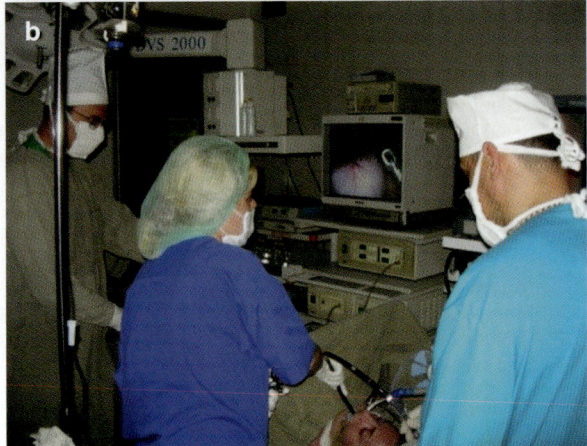

Fig. 16.2 (**a, b**) Setting of laparoscopically assisted intraoperative oral single-balloon enteroscopy

Sometimes small bowel mobilization and adhesiolysis must be performed before IOE. In patients with extensive adhesions or areas of extreme fixation, more than one enterotomy can be used to maximize mucosal inspections and avoid overdistension and subsequent laceration of the mesentery.

Usually a pediatric video colonoscope or a video enteroscope is used to perform IOE. To avoid infections in the surgical field, the cleaned and disinfected endoscope is prepared with gas sterilization, or a nonsterilized endoscope can be covered with a sterile plastic sleeve before insertion through the enterotomy (Fig. 16.1a). All patients should be given perioperative antibiotic therapy.

After insertion of the endoscope, the small bowel is examined segmentally. With an occlusion clamp lightly applied at fixed distances, overdistension of the stomach or the more distal bowel can be prevented. Noncrushing occluding clamps can also be positioned at the ileocecal valve and distal to the duodenojejunal junction. First, the proximal parts of the small bowel should be examined in the direction toward the duodenojejunal junction or up to the duodenum. Then the distal parts of the jejunum and the ileum should be inspected down to the ileocecal valve. At this point, it is very important to examine the mucosa when the endoscope is being advanced and to aspirate the inflated segment thoroughly but gently before progressing with the examination.

The endoscopic view is supplemented by simultaneously viewing the mucosa from the outside of the transilluminated bowel wall to detect pathologic lesions (Fig. 16.1b). Abnormalities seen on transillumination are also assessed internally to distinguish vascular lesions from any traumatic lesions.

16.2.2 Peroral or Peranal Techniques

Transoral and transanal methods are less likely to achieve full visualization of the small bowel. Before the method of balloon-assisted enteroscopy was adopted, many reports described failure to reach the terminal ileum in a significant number of patients [1–4]. The limited working length of endoscopes prevents the entire small bowel from being visualized by the peroral approach. Another difficulty with this technique has been looping of the endoscope in the stomach, which can be avoided by the use of an overtube. Compared with the standard procedure, the method is more time consuming and is sometimes difficult to perform.

Laparoscopically assisted total enteroscopy has been described, as well as a laparoscopically assisted balloon

Fig. 16.3 Multiple neuroendocrine tumors of the midgut. (**a**, **b**) Capsule endoscopy imaging. (**c**, **d**) Laparoscopically assisted transanal single-balloon enteroscopy. (Laparoscopic assistance with 10 mm clamps allowed the intervention to be performed safely.) (**e**, **f**) Several subtle lesions in the mid part of the small bowel. (**g**, **h**) Images of intraoperative enteroscopy

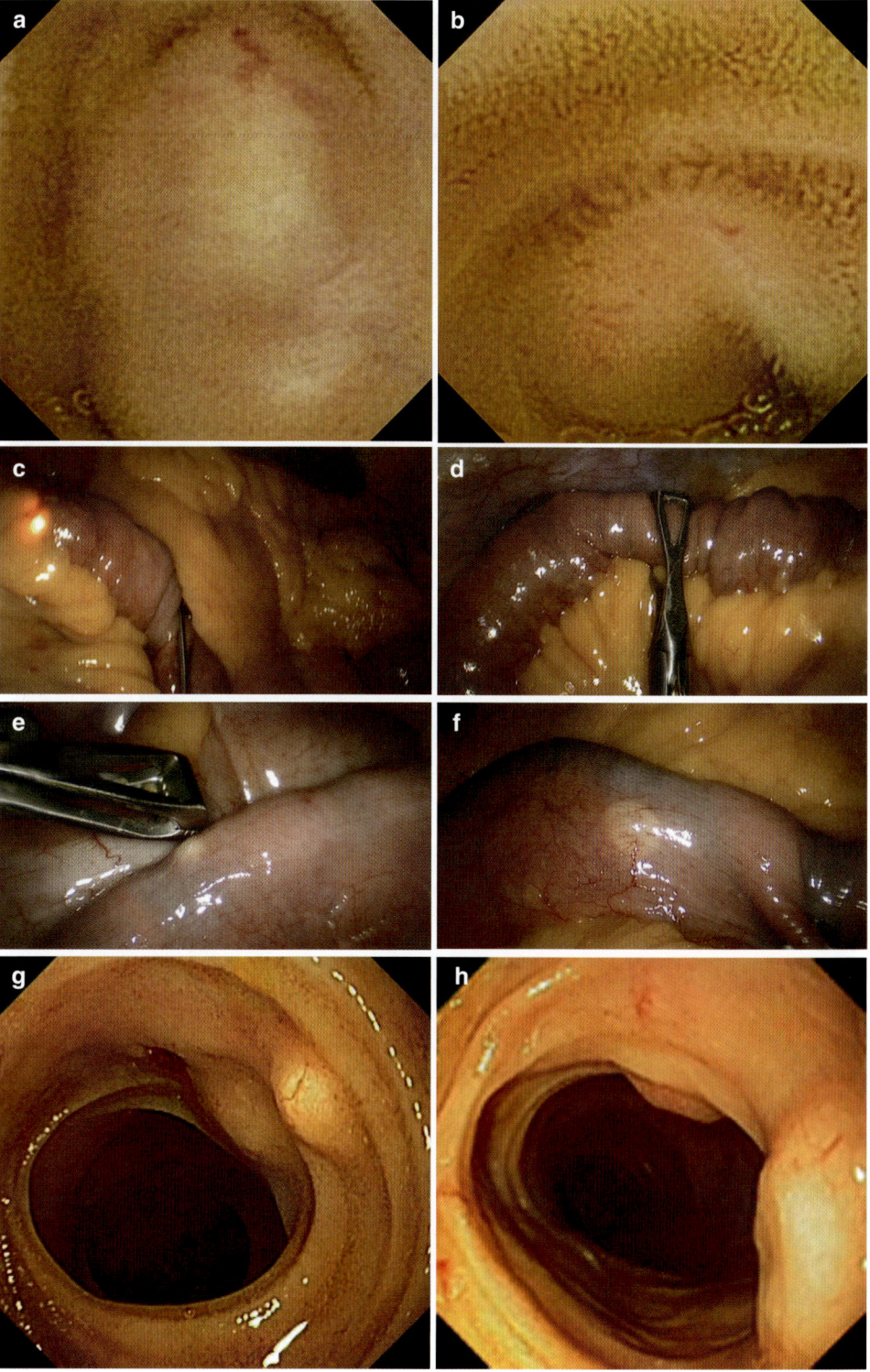

enteroscopy (Figs. 16.2 and 16.3) [5–8]. For this technique, the endoscope is inserted perorally as far as possible into the small bowel. Then the intestine is gently grasped with two Endo Babcock clamps to allow the endoscope to slide more easily. Agarwal described a special technique of laparo-enteroscopy using the laparoscope to perform IOE [9].

16.3 Treatment

Treatment (e.g., argon plasma coagulation, polypectomy, resection of submucosal tumor, removal of foreign body, dilation) may be performed endoscopically, or the affected small bowel segments may be identified endoscopically,

Fig. 16.4 Bleeding hemangioma in the mid part of the small bowel. (**a**) Capsule endoscopy imaging. (**b**) Intraoperative enteroscopy with needle. (**c**) Resected specimen. (Courtesy of Jörg Caselitz, MD) (**d**) Histology (hematoxylin-eosin). (Courtesy of Jörg Caselitz, MD)

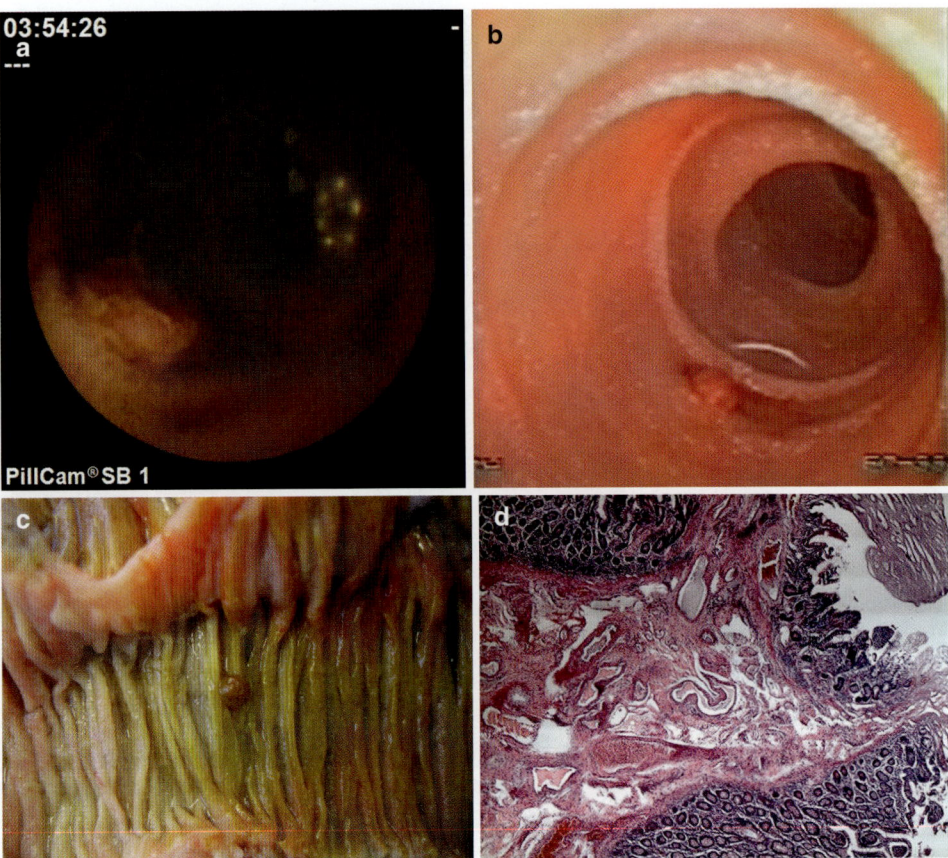

correspondingly marked, and then treated surgically, usually in the form of a segmental resection (Fig. 16.4).

16.4 Limiting Factors and Complications

Limiting factors for IOE are comorbidities and the need for general anesthesia. Adhesions with a shortened mesentery and massive hemorrhage with blood clots obscuring the intestinal lumen may limit the full use of the endoscope during IOE.

A number of complications of IOE have been reported:

- Mucosal or serosal laceration
- Intramural hematomas
- Mesenteric hemorrhage
- Perforation or miniperforation after adhesiolysis
- Paralytic ileus
- Intestinal ischemia
- Intestinal obstruction
- Wound infection
- Postoperative intra-abdominal or pulmonary infection

Complication rates vary widely, with reports ranging from 0 to 52 % [1, 2, 10–14]. Significant intraoperative complications are reported in 3 %, postoperative complications in 26 %, and 30-day mortality in 6 % [10, 14]. When a transoral or transanal method of insertion is used, the incidence of complications such as mucosal or serosal tears due to the excessive pleating or telescoping of the small bowel on to the endoscope is reported to be as high as 52 % [3].

16.5 Diagnostic Yield

16.5.1 Suspected Small Bowel Bleeding

Intraoperative enteroscopy is typically used as the last option in patients with obscure gastrointestinal bleeding requiring multiple transfusions, repeated hospitalizations, or both. In contrast to less invasive procedures, including enteroclysis and various forms of small bowel endoscopy, the ability of IOE to identify a bleeding source has been impressive, ranging from 70 to 100 % (Tables 16.1 and 16.2).

In a prospective two-center trial comparing video capsule endoscopy with IOE in 47 patients with obscure gastrointestinal bleeding, the diagnostic yield of both methods varied with the type of bleeding [10]. In patients with ongoing bleeding at the time of examination, the diagnostic yield was high (positive findings in all patients) and was greater than in

Table 16.1 Diagnostic yield of intraoperative enteroscopy in patients with obscure gastrointestinal bleeding

Study	Patients, n	Diagnostic yield, %
Bowden et al. (1980) [15]	18	89
Lau (1990) [16]	15	80
Flickinger et al. (1989) [17]	14	93
Lewis et al. (1991) [2]	23	87
Ress et al. (1992) [18]	44	70
Szold et al. (1992) [19]	30	93
Lopez et al. (1996) [20]	16	88
Douard et al. (2000) [21]	20	80
Kendrick et al. (2001) [3]	70	74
Jakobs et al. (2006) [22]	81	84
Kopácová et al. (2007) [23]	41	90
Schulz and Schmidt (2009) [14]	123	83

Table 16.2 Details of the largest series of intraoperative enteroscopy in patients with obscure gastrointestinal bleeding

Value/finding	Data
Patients, N	123
Median age, y	65
Complete enteroscopy, n	123 (100 %)
Severe complications, n	2/123 (1.6 %)
Mortality, n	1/123 (0.8 %)
Pathologic findings, n	102/123 (83 %)
Angiectasia	64/102
Ulcers	14/102
Tumor/polyp	11/102
Diverticula (Meckel/multiple)	9/102
Others (anastomotic vessels, fistula)	4/102

patients with previous overt bleeding (positive findings in 70.8 %) or with occult bleeding (positive findings in 50 %).

16.5.2 Crohn's Disease

Surgical strategies can be optimized based on IOE findings. Findings regarding the luminal status, including the degree of stricture and ulcer activity, may be helpful for therapeutic decisions during surgery in patients with Crohn's disease [24].

16.5.3 Peutz-Jeghers Syndrome

Intraoperative evaluation of the small bowel has become standard in several hospitals [25, 26]. IOE improves polyp clearance without the need for additional enterotomies and may help to reduce the frequency of laparotomies. Balloon enteroscopy and laparoscopically assisted balloon enteroscopy are minimally invasive, and single-step procedures can be used for small bowel polyp surveillance and treatment of patients with Peutz-Jeghers syndrome.

16.6 Summary

The indications for IOE have diminished in recent years owing to the development of video capsule endoscopy and balloon enteroscopy. IOE is reserved for patients with massive midgut bleeding, lesions not accessible by balloon enteroscopy, or lesions difficult or impossible to treat by balloon enteroscopy.

References

1. Desa LA, Ohri SK, Hutton KA, Lee H, Spencer J. Role of intraoperative enteroscopy in obscure gastrointestinal bleeding of small bowel origin. Br J Surg. 1991;78:192–5.
2. Lewis BS, Wenger JS, Waye JD. Small bowel enteroscopy and intraoperative enteroscopy for obscure gastrointestinal bleeding. Am J Gastroenterol. 1991;86:171–4.
3. Kendrick ML, Buttar NS, Anderson MA, Lutzke LS, Peia D, Wang KK, Sarr MG. Contribution of intraoperative enteroscopy in the management of obscure gastrointestinal bleeding. J Gastrointest Surg. 2001;5:162–7.
4. Zaman A, Sheppard B, Katon RM. Total peroral intraoperative enteroscopy for obscure GI bleeding using a dedicated push enteroscope: diagnostic yield and patient outcome. Gastrointest Endosc. 1999;50:506–10.
5. Reddy ND, Rao VG. Laparoscopically assisted panenteroscopy for snare excision. Gastrointest Endosc. 1996;44:208–9.
6. Ingrosso M, Prete F, Pisani A, Carbonara R, Azzarone A, Francavilla A. Laparoscopically assisted total enteroscopy: a new approach to small intestinal diseases. Gastrointest Endosc. 1999;49:651–3.
7. Sriram PV, Rao GV, Reddy DN. Laparoscopically assisted panenteroscopy. Gastrointest Endosc. 2001;54:805–6.
8. Ross AS, Dye C, Prachand VN. Laparoscopic-assisted double-balloon enteroscopy for small-bowel polyp surveillance and treatment in patients with Peutz-Jeghers syndrome. Gastrointest Endosc. 2006;64:984–8.
9. Agarwal A. Use of the laparoscope to perform intraoperative enteroscopy. Surg Endosc. 1999;13:1143–4.
10. Hartmann D, Schmidt H, Bolz G, Schilling D, Kinzel F, Eickhoff A, et al. A prospective two-center study comparing wireless capsule endoscopy with intraoperative enteroscopy in patients with obscure GI bleeding. Gastrointest Endosc. 2005;61:826–32.
11. Whelan RL, Buls JG, Goldberg SM, Rothenberger DA. Intraoperative endoscopy. University of Minnesota experience. Am Surg. 1989;55:281–6.
12. Krishnan RS, Kent 3rd RB. Enterovaginal fistula as a complication of intraoperative small bowel endoscopy. Surg Laparosc Endosc. 1998;8:388–9.
13. Hartmann D, Schmidt H, Schilling D, Kinze F, Eickhoff A, Weickert U, et al. Follow-up of patients with obscure gastrointestinal bleeding after capsule endoscopy and intraoperative enteroscopy. Hepatogastroenterology. 2007;54:780–3.
14. Schulz HJ, Schmidt H. Intraoperative enteroscopy. Gastrointest Endosc Clin N Am. 2009;19:371–9.
15. Bowden Jr TA, Hooks 3rd VH, Mansberger Jr AR. Intraoperative gastrointestinal endoscopy. Ann Surg. 1980;191:680–7.
16. Lau WY. Intraoperative enteroscopy–indications and limitations. Gastrointest Endosc. 1990;36:268–71.
17. Flickinger EG, Stanforth AC, Sinar DR, MacDonald KG, Lannin DR, Gibson JH. Intraoperative video panendoscopy for diagnosing sites of chronic intestinal bleeding. Am J Surg. 1989;157:137–44.

18. Ress AM, Benacci JC, Sarr MG. Efficacy of intraoperative enteroscopy in diagnosis and prevention of recurrent, occult gastrointestinal bleeding. Am J Surg. 1992;163:94–8.

19. Szold A, Katz LB, Lewis BS. Surgical approach to occult gastrointestinal bleeding. Am J Surg. 1992;163:90–2.

20. Lopez MJ, Cooley JS, Petros JG, Sullivan JG, Cave DR. Complete intraoperative small-bowel endoscopy in the evaluation of occult gastrointestinal bleeding using the sonde enteroscope. Arch Surg. 1996;131:272–7.

21. Douard R, Wind P, Panis Y, Marteau P, Bouhnik Y, Cellier C, et al. Intraoperative enteroscopy for diagnosis and management of unexplained gastrointestinal bleeding. Am J Surg. 2000;180:181–4.

22. Jakobs R, Hartmann D, Benz C, Schilling D, Weickert U, Eickhoff A, et al. Diagnosis of obscure gastrointestinal bleeding by intra-operative enteroscopy in 81 consecutive patients. World J Gastroenterol. 2006;12:313–6.

23. Kopácová M, Bureš J, Vykouřil L, Hladík P, Simkovic D, Jon B, et al. Intraoperative enteroscopy: ten years' experience at a single tertiary center. Surg Endosc. 2007;21:1111–6.

24. Almer S, Granerus G, Ström M, Olaison G, Bonnet J, Lémann M, et al. Leukocyte scintigraphy compared to intraoperative small bowel enteroscopy and laparotomy findings in Crohn's disease. Inflamm Bowel Dis. 2007;13:164–74.

25. Edwards DP, Khosraviani K, Stafferton R, Phillips RK. Long-term results of polyp clearance by intraoperative enteroscopy in the Peutz-Jeghers syndrome. Dis Colon Rectum. 2003;46:48–50.

26. Pennazio M, Rossini FP. Small bowel polyps in Peutz-Jeghers syndrome: management by combined push enteroscopy and intraoperative enteroscopy. Gastrointest Endosc. 2000;51:304–8.

Nonendoscopic Imaging Studies

17

James N.S. Hampton and Ernst J. Malzfeldt

Contents

The work was first published in 2006 by Springer Medizin Verlag Heidelberg with the following title: *Atlas of Video Capsule Endoscopy*.

J.N.S. Hampton (✉)
Radiology Department, Northern General Hospital,
Sheffield Teaching Hospitals NHS Foundation Trust,
Sheffield, UK
e-mail: james.hampton@sth.nhs.uk

E.J. Malzfeldt
Department of Radiology/Neuroradiology,
Asklepios Klinik Nord, Hamburg, Germany
e-mail: e.malzfeldt@asklepios.com

17.1 Radiographic Methods

17.1.1 Plain Abdominal Radiograph

The plain abdominal radiograph is a simple and readily accessible but nonspecific examination for the diagnosis of abdominal diseases. Interpretation of the abdominal X-ray is based on the distribution of fluid, calcification and gas. Interpretation of the diameter of the bowel loops, bowel wall thickening and the presence of gas in the bowel wall, blood vessels, biliary tree, and peritoneal cavity can help to establish a diagnosis. Erect abdominal X-rays are now rarely performed in clinical practice, but the interpretation of the number and length of fluid levels on an erect film can still be useful in the diagnosis of obstruction. Bowel obstruction can be identified on an abdominal X-ray and perforation can be seen on a supine abdominal X-ray and an erect chest X-ray (Fig. 17.1), but generally the cause of the perforation cannot be determined and further cross-sectional imaging is often performed.

17.1.2 Upper Gastrointestinal Series

The upper gastrointestinal (GI) series after the administration of oral contrast provides information on the dynamics and disturbances of intestinal transit. A detailed evaluation of the entire small bowel requires a small bowel follow through (SBFT) examination. The method used for this examination varies between different departments; after administration of an oral barium suspension, the contrast is followed through the small bowel until it reaches the caecum by intermittent abdominal films or fluoroscopic images. Once the barium has reached the colon, detailed views of the small bowel with or without palpation are taken to fully evaluate the entire small bowel. Ha et al. [1] showed that there is a wide variation in the way this examination is performed and who performs it, varying from general radiologists to those with a specialist GI interest. The SBFT examination can depict the mucosal lesions seen

Fig. 17.1 Supine abdominal
X-ray showing small bowel
obstruction (**a**) and free
intraperitoneal gas (*arrow*) (**b**).
Erect chest X-ray with free
intraperitoneal gas (*arrow*) (**c**)

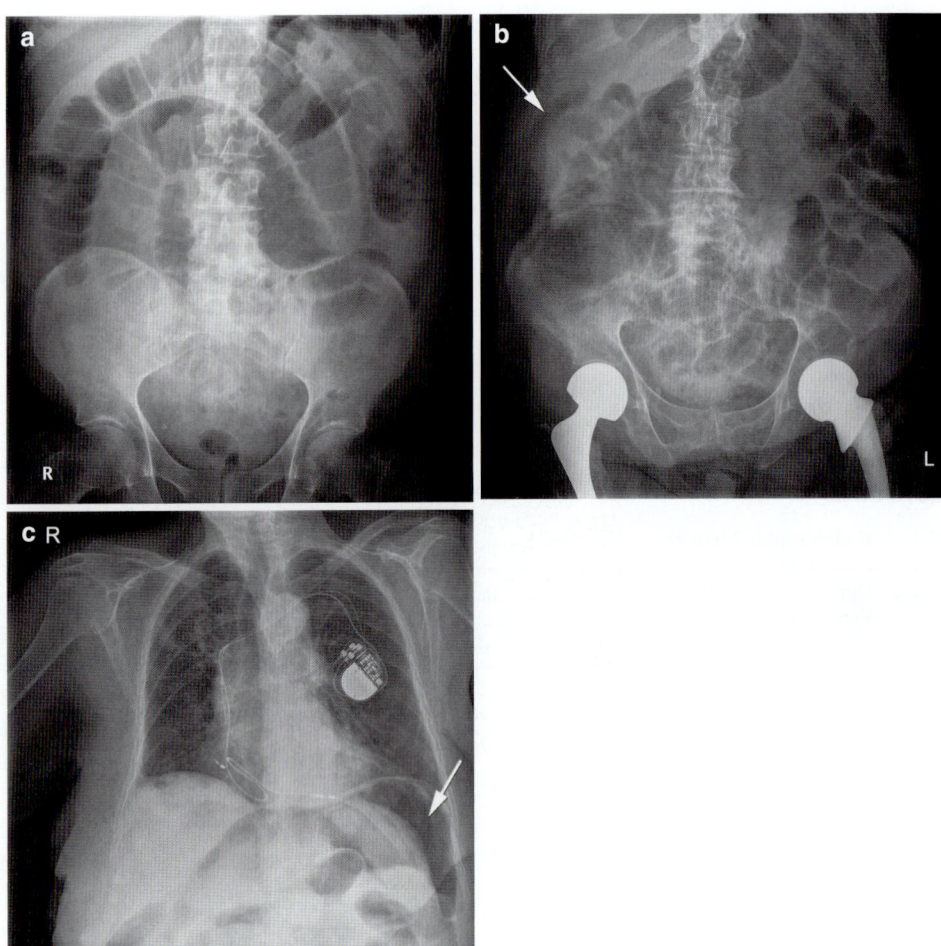

with small bowel tumours and Crohn's disease and define their position in the small bowel. It can also demonstrate some of the complications of Crohn's disease, such as fistulae and strictures and can localize the position of strictures and diverticula [2] (Fig. 17.2). The unpredictable nature of small bowel transit can make this a prolonged procedure and pathology can be difficult to detect in the multiple overlapping loops of small bowel.

17.1.3 Enteroclysis

Small bowel enteroclysis or a small bowel enema (SBE) is a contrast study of the small bowel following naso-duodenal or naso-jejunal intubation. It can be performed as a single-contrast examination with a dilute barium suspension (Sellink method) or as a double-contrast examination with barium and methylcellulose or barium and carbon dioxide. A large volume of fluid is infused into the small bowel, which

distends and volume challenges it, helping to distinguish whether strictures are due to spasm secondary to acute inflammatory disease or to fibrostenotic disease in Crohn's. SBE is performed less often than the SBFT examination [1], as it is technically more difficult and is less popular with patients because of the need for naso-duodenal or naso-jejunal intubation and the associated discomfort. An increased radiation dose is also associated with SBE, which is relevant in Crohn's disease patients who may require multiple episodes of imaging during the course of their disease; an associated increased risk of malignancy has been identified in a subgroup of patients [3].

Barium studies of the small bowel are now performed less frequently because of the increased use of cross-sectional imaging, but when performed by experienced radiologists, they still have a role to play in looking for stenoses (Fig. 17.2) and in the differential diagnosis of mucosal and submucosal abnormalities. Their ability to detect abnormalities that cause obscure GI bleeding has been shown to be as low as 11 % [4–7].

Fig. 17.2 (**a**) Small bowel follow through (SBFT) showing active Crohn's disease of the terminal ileum with ulceration, cobblestoning, and stricturing due to inflammatory disease. (**b**) SBFT with stricturing of the terminal ileum, which is causing some obstruction as the proximal bowel is dilated, and pseudosacculation (*arrow*) in keeping with chronic Crohn's disease. (**c**) Chronic Crohn's disease at the ileocolic anastomosis in a patient with a previous limited right hemicolectomy

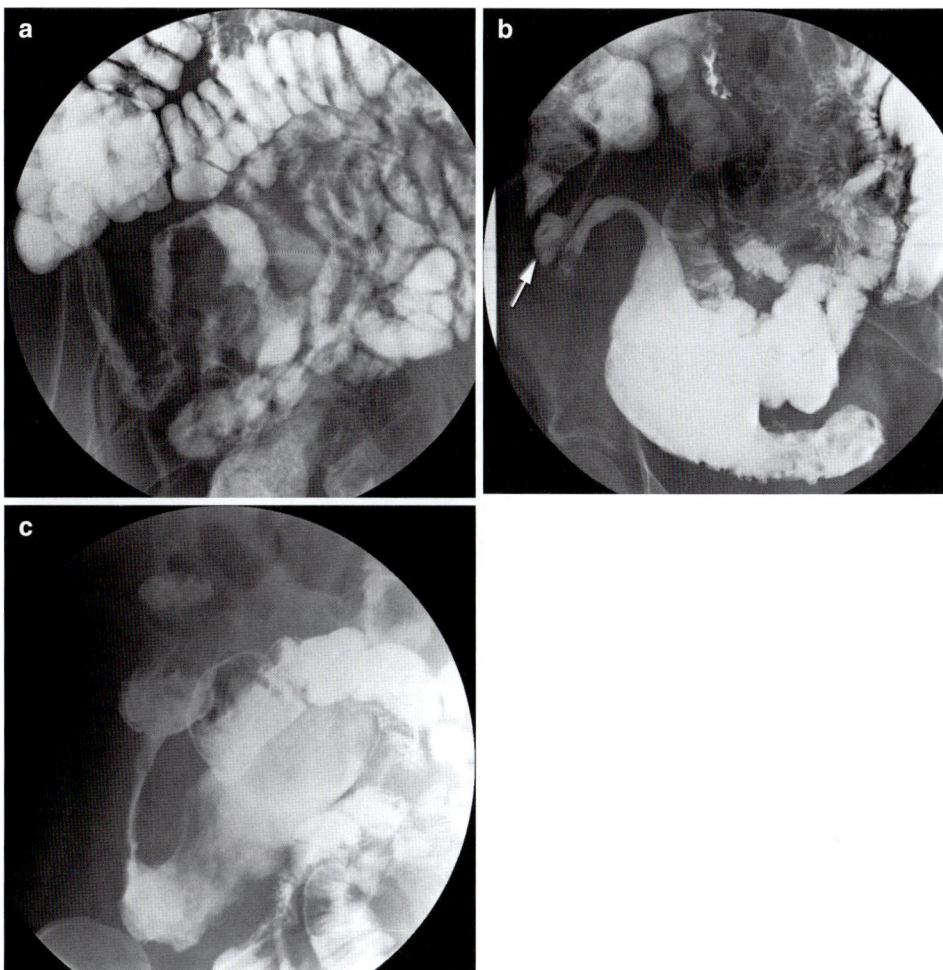

17.2 Cross-Sectional Imaging Modalities

17.2.1 CT Enterography and Enteroclysis

CT enterography and CT enteroclysis have become an established alternative to more traditional imaging modalities for the evaluation of the small bowel. The rapid developments in multi-detector CT technology allow the whole of the abdomen and pelvis to be imaged in seconds, thereby reducing motion artefacts. Excellent visualization of the small bowel wall and lumen can be achieved when the bowel is well distended with low-attenuation enteric contrast, and intravenous (IV) contrast is administered to show wall enhancement. These methods of examining the small bowel, along with MRI of the small bowel, are complementary to the use of capsule endoscopy. Capsule endoscopy has a higher detection rate for mucosal abnormalities that can be missed by other forms of imaging [8, 9], but it is limited to evaluation of the mucosa and gives no information on small bowel wall thickness and enhancement, submucosal and extraluminal masses and the complications of small bowel disease [10].

CT enterography is performed following the administration of large volumes of oral enteric contrast, usually 1,500–2,000 mL over the 30–60 min prior to the scan. Polyethylene glycol and low-contrast barium solution can be used as oral contrast agents. These are preferred to water, as they contain additives that reduce absorption from the small bowel and increasing distension [11]. The scan is typically performed at 45–50 s after the administration of IV contrast, when peak small bowel enhancement is achieved [12], but diagnostic scans also can be obtained in the portal venous phase at 65–70 s [13].

The main indications for CT enterography include the investigation of suspected and confirmed Crohn's disease, the investigation of obscure GI bleeding (OGIB) and the evaluation of suspected small bowel tumours and other small bowel disease [14]. It has been shown to be useful in evaluating Crohn's disease and other small bowel disorders [15] and OGIB [16] and in clinical management of patients with Crohn's disease [17].

CT enteroclysis is performed after naso-duodenal or naso-jejunal intubation and infusion of luminal contrast to distend the small bowel, to increase the detection of intraluminal and mural masses. It has been shown to have a high sensitivity and specificity for detecting small bowel abnormalities [18, 19].

The typical CT features of active small bowel Crohn's disease include mucosal hyperenhancement, wall thickening of more than 3 mm, mural stratification with dilated vasa recta (the comb sign) (Fig. 17.3a, b) and mesenteric fat stranding, all of which are well demonstrated on CT enterography [14, 20]. CT enterography and enteroclysis are also used to determine the cause of occult or overt OGIB; these findings can be used to decide on further management of the patient, such as surgery or the approach for enteroscopy (Fig. 17.3c–f). These modalities can also evaluate

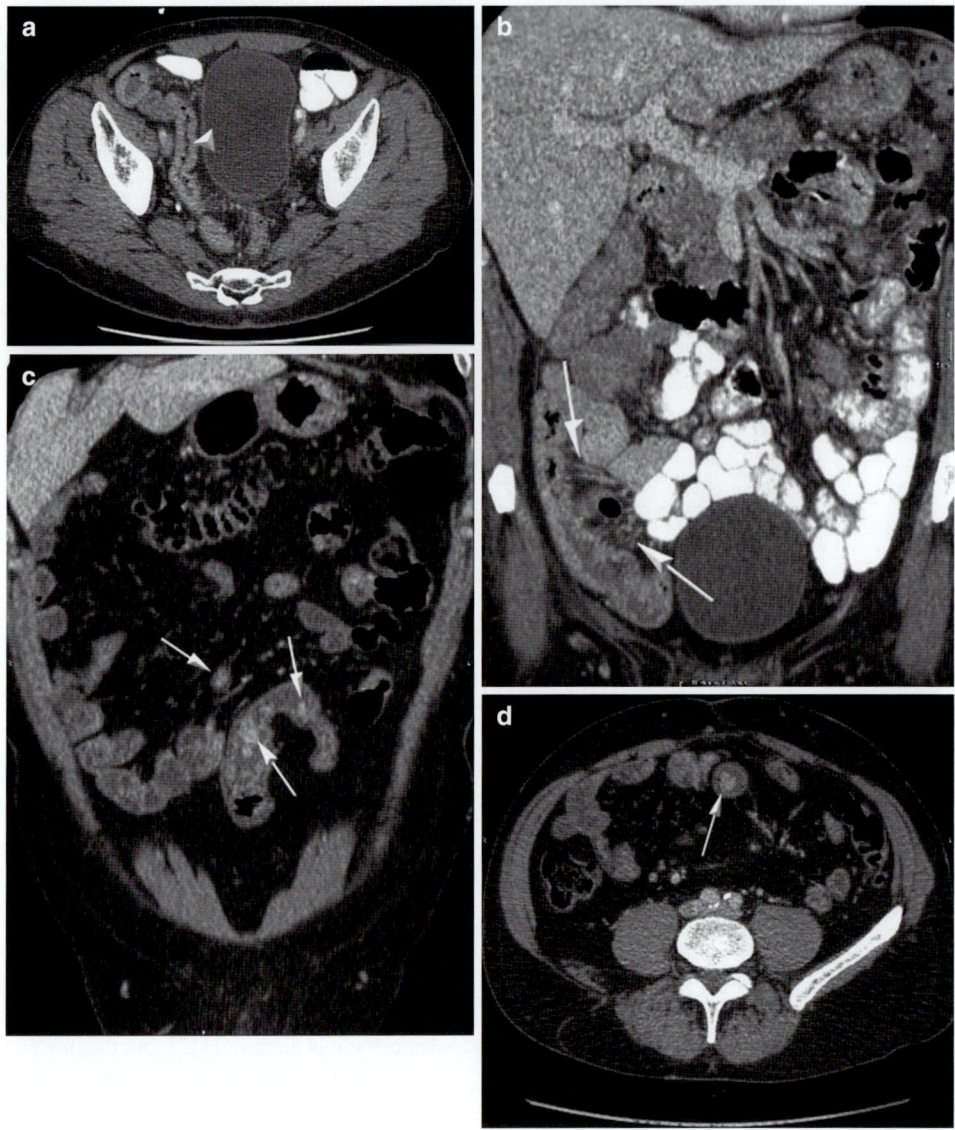

Fig. 17.3 CT scan showing acute Crohn's disease of the distal small bowel with wall thickening (*arrowhead*) (**a**), enhancement, and dilated vasa recta (*arrows*) (**b**). CT enterography with multiple polyps in the small bowel in a male patient with overt obscure gastrointestinal bleeding (OGIB) (*arrows*) (**c, d**). CT enteroclysis in a patient with episodic overt OGIB and a possible abnormality on capsule endoscopy. CT confirmed two neuroendocrine tumours of the ileum (*arrows*) (**e**) with nodal metastases (*arrowheads*) (**e, f**). CT enterography examination in a patient in whom capsule endoscopy had shown a possible vascular abnormality in the mid to distal small bowel; this was shown to be a

6-cm gastrointestinal stromal tumour (GIST), which had prominent vessels in the small bowel wall in the arterial phase scan (*arrow*) (**g**), and a largely extraluminal mass (*arrowheads*) (**g, h**). A calcified metastatic mesenteric mass from a primary small bowel neuroendocrine tumour, with typical tethering of the adjacent small bowel (*arrow*) (**i**). Multiple liver metastases from a small bowel neuroendocrine tumour, some of which are hypervascular and better visualized in the arterial phase (**j**) rather than the venous phase (**k**). A hypervascular jejunal metastasis (*arrow*) (**l**) from a primary renal tumour (*arrow*) (**m**)

Fig. 17.3 (continued)

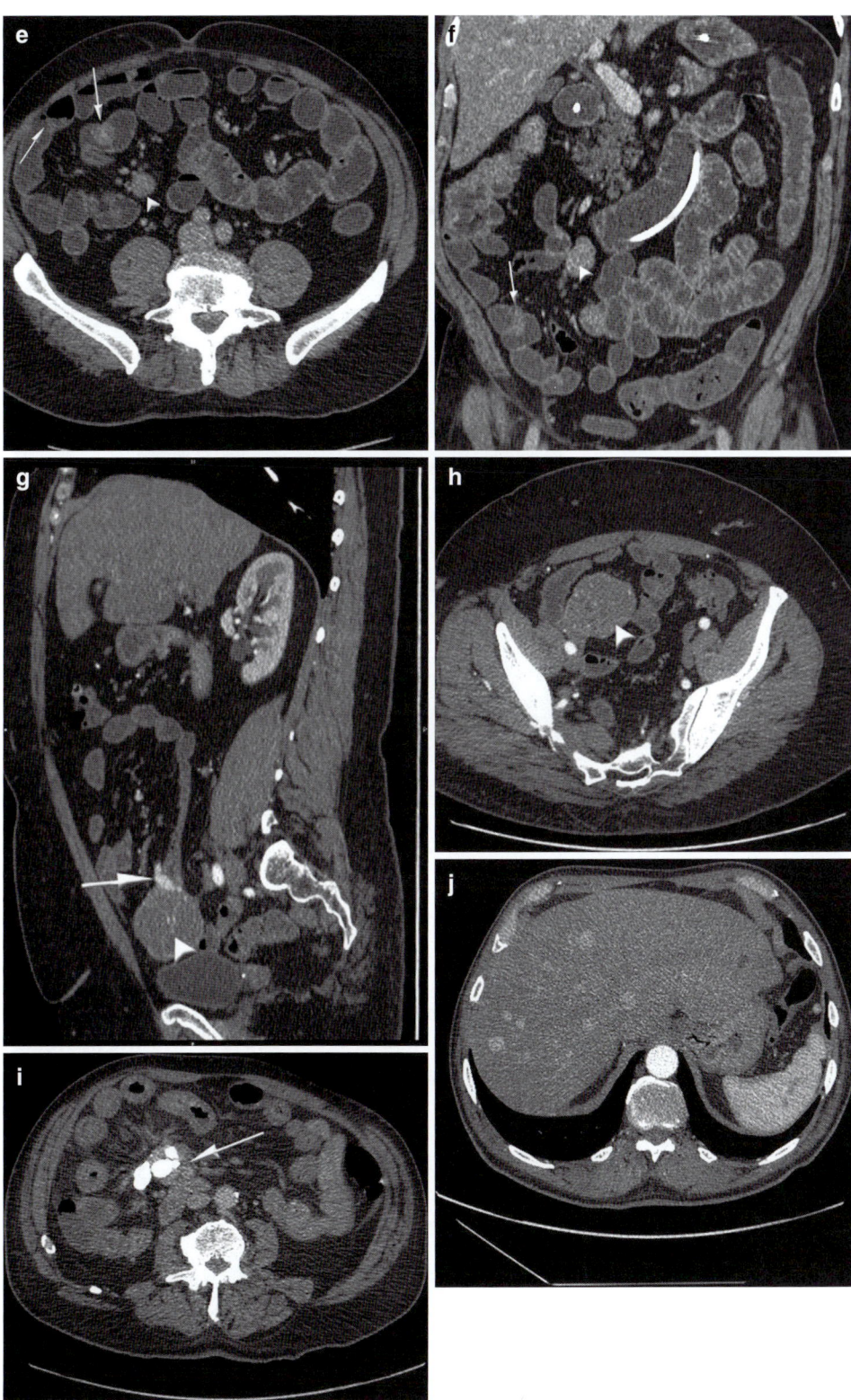

Fig. 17.3 (continued)

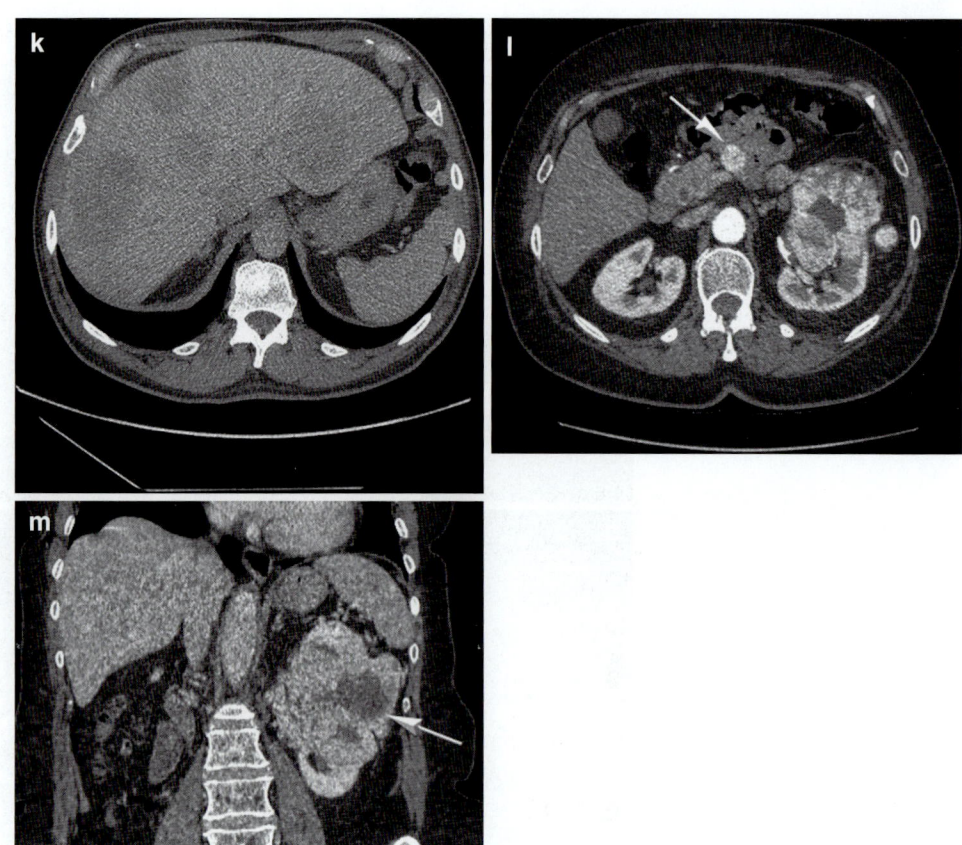

extraluminal findings in some patients with OGIB, such as gastrointestinal stromal tumours (GISTs) and can show metastatic disease associated with small bowel neuroendocrine tumours, as well as the primary tumour associated with small bowel metastases (Fig. 17.3g–m).

Conventional barium imaging of the small bowel with SBFT or enteroclysis and CT enterography or enteroclysis uses ionizing radiation to obtain diagnostic images, so there is an increased risk of radiation-induced cancers associated with the use of these techniques [21]. Some patients will require repeated investigation over the course of their disease. Some Crohn's disease patients, for instance, can receive a cumulative effective dose of radiation greater than 75 mSv, the equivalent of 3,750 chest X-rays or 34 years of background radiation, with an associated 7.3 % increased risk of all cancers [3, 21]. Some authors feel that the radiation risk from CT examinations has been overemphasized in the press, causing some patients to refuse radiologic examinations that would have benefitted their management [22]. Nevertheless, it must be remembered that all CT examinations expose the patient to ionizing radiation, so the benefit of the examination should always outweigh these risks, no matter how

small. This situation needs to be made clear to the patient and referring clinicians in justifying the examination.

17.2.2 Magnetic Resonance Enterography and Enteroclysis

Magnetic resonance (MR) enterography and MR enteroclysis are other cross-sectional imaging modalities that can be used to evaluate the small bowel. The main indications for MR imaging of the small bowel are suspected or established Crohn's disease, the detection of small bowel tumours and polyposis syndromes.

MR enterography requires the ingestion of a large volume of oral contrast to distend the small bowel, so a similar loading technique to that used in CT enterography is employed, with some local variation in the oral contrast agent used. The aim is to obtain the best small bowel distension possible, to reduce the chance of missing subtle pathology. The best small bowel distension has been demonstrated with a combination of mannitol and locust bean gum [23], but any of the hyperosmolar agents will help to reduce intestinal absorption and thus improve distension

Fig. 17.4 (**a**, **b**) MR enteroclysis demonstrating excellent distension of the small bowel. (**c**, **d**) MR enterography showing good mid and distal small bowel distension. The jejunum is not as well distended, which is sometimes a problem with MR enterography

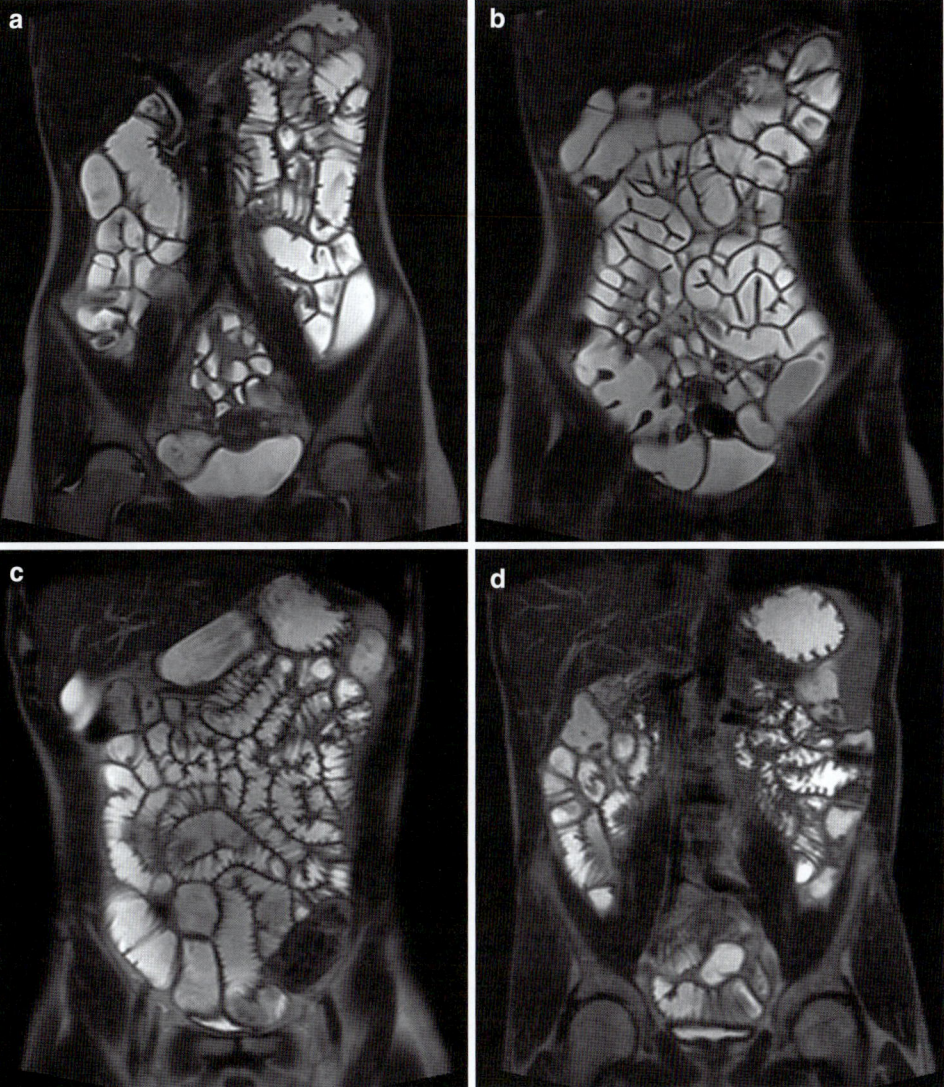

[24]. Once adequate distension has been achieved, the whole of the small bowel is imaged using a combination of T1-weighted images before and after IV contrast and T2-weighted images, some with fat suppression. The pulse sequences used vary between different institutions depending on the MRI scanner and radiologists' preference. In our practice, we routinely used a spasmolytic agent to reduce bowel wall motion artefact.

MR enteroclysis requires naso-duodenal or naso-jejunal intubation followed by infusion of the enteric contrast medium using a pump to distend the small bowel. The degree of distension is monitored in the scanner and once adequate distension is achieved, the entire small bowel is imaged. The advantage of MR enteroclysis is that it achieves better distension of the small bowel than enterography, particularly in the proximal small bowel and thus increases the detection of subtle pathology. This technique does require the placement of a naso-enteric tube, which is performed under fluoroscopic

control, thus adding some radiation dose to the procedure and increasing its complexity and patient discomfort (Fig. 17.4).

The typical findings in Crohn's disease on MR enterography or enteroclysis are bowel wall thickening, bowel wall and mesenteric oedema, bowel wall enhancement after IV contrast, increased mesenteric vascularity (the comb sign), fat wrapping and abnormal lymph nodes (Fig. 17.5).

Thickness of the small bowel wall greater than 3 mm is abnormal and typically it measures 5–10 mm in patients with Crohn's disease [25]. Submucosal oedema in the bowel wall and mesenteric oedema appear as increased signal on T2-weighted, fat-suppressed images and can be seen in patients with active inflammatory disease [26, 27]. Active inflammatory disease is seen as a layered appearance of the bowel wall on T1 fat-suppressed, postcontrast images due to mucosal and serosal hyperenhancement and submucosal oedema, as well as transmural enhancement (Fig. 17.6) [26, 28]. Increased mesenteric vascularity or the comb sign is best

Fig. 17.5 Crohn's disease of the terminal ileum with bowel wall thickening (*arrow*) (**a**) and increased enhancement with the use of intravenous contrast (**b**)

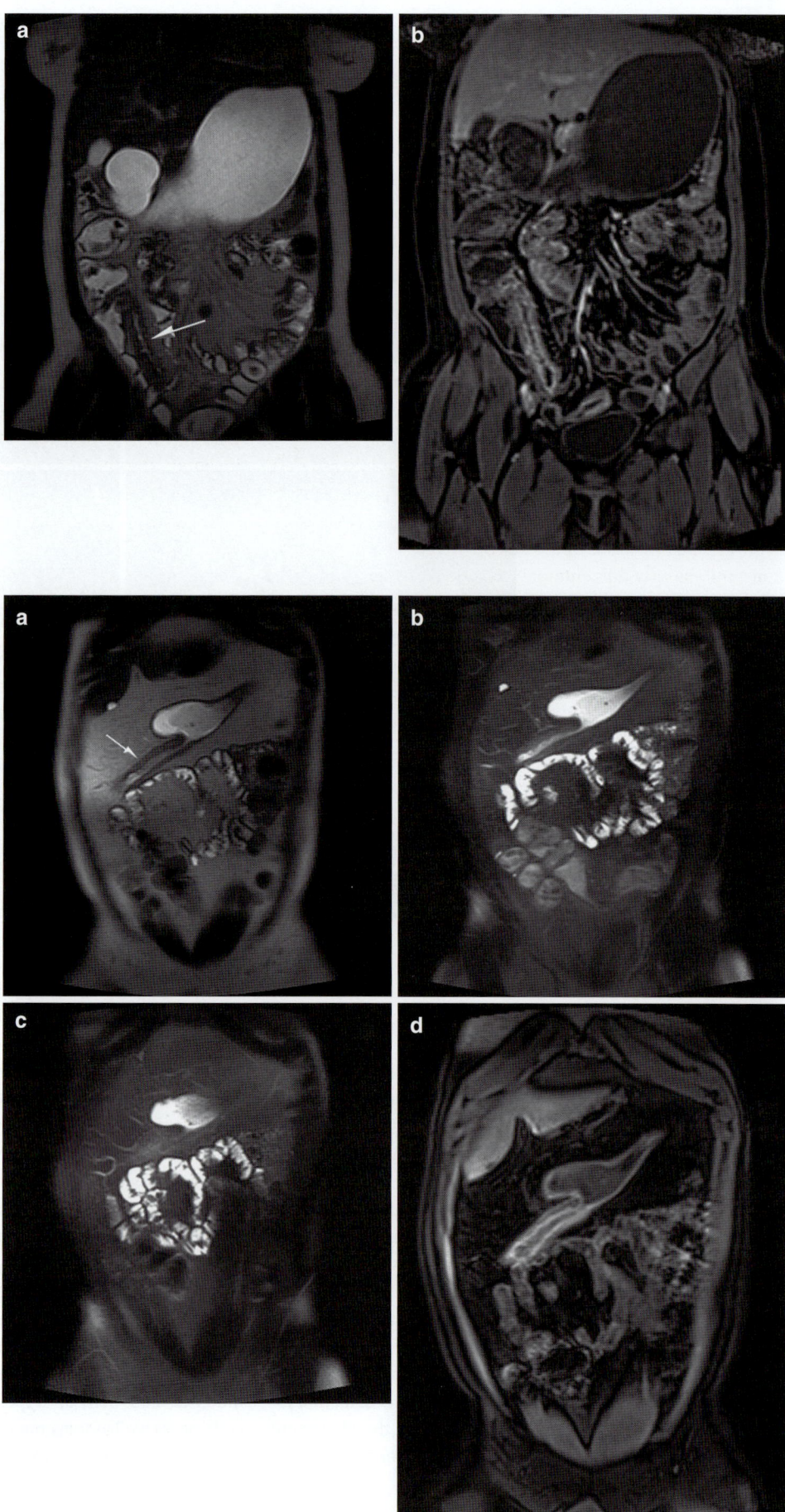

Fig. 17.6 Crohn's disease of the neo-terminal ileum in a patient who has had a previous right hemicolectomy. There is bowel wall thickening (*arrow*) (**a**), increased signal in the bowel wall (**b**) and surrounding fat (**c**), and postcontrast enhancement (**d**) in keeping with active inflammatory disease

appreciated on the postcontrast T1-weighted images as multiple parallel lines of high signal intensity, running at 90° to the bowel wall in the mesenteric fat, or as low-signal lines on true fast imaging with steady-state precession (FISP images); these signs are due to the increased blood flow in the vasa recta and suggest active disease [29, 30]. These sequences, along with fat-saturated T2-weighted images, can also detect reactive lymph nodes in the mesentery, which are often associated with active disease [31]. In addition, deep ulcers can be detected when the bowel is well distended; these are seen as thin lines of high signal intensity extending into the low-signal bowel wall (or through it, in the case of fistulating disease) (Fig. 17.7) [32]. The extramural manifestations and complications of Crohn's disease, such as fistulas and abscesses (Fig. 17.7), can also be accurately evaluated on MRI [26, 32, 33].

MR and CT examinations of the small bowel do not have a high-enough resolution to depict the early changes of Crohn's disease, such as aphthous and superficial ulceration, even when the bowel is optimally distended. In this situation, conventional barium enteroclysis and capsule endoscopy have a diagnostic advantage [32, 34, 35].

Small bowel neoplasms are rare, comprising 3–6 % of all GI tract tumours, and they often present with nonspecific symptoms, making them difficult to diagnose for the gastroenterologist and radiologist [36, 37]. MR enteroclysis has been shown to have a sensitivity and specificity of over 90 % in the detection of small bowel neoplasms [38, 39] (Fig. 17.8).

MR imaging has also been shown to be a useful test in the detection and follow-up of small bowel polyps in patients with Peutz-Jeghers syndrome and familial adenomatous polyposis. An early study showed that polyps bigger than 15 mm could be detected similarly with MR imaging and capsule endoscopy; smaller polyps were more often seen with capsule endoscopy and 5-mm polyps were detected only with capsule endoscopy. The location of the detected polyps and their exact size were more accurately determined on MRI [40]. A more recent study using MR enterography in patients with Peutz-Jeghers syndrome has shown it to be a useful alternative to capsule endoscopy. There was no difference in the detection rates of polyps larger than 10 mm between the two techniques, with MR enterography more likely to detect large polyps. The size assessment of large polyps (>15 mm) was more reproducible on MR enterography, but patients found capsule endoscopy more comfortable [41] (Fig. 17.9).

17.2.3 Catheter and CT Angiography

GI bleeding can present in many different ways, ranging from acute massive haemorrhage to occult OGIB. Catheter angiography and CT angiography can be used to attempt to identify the source of bleeding in patients who have had negative or inconclusive endoscopic examinations. Active extravasation of contrast material into the lumen of the bowel is required for either test to be positive, so they are used to investigate GI bleeding in haemodynamically unstable patients and overt OGIB and are of limited value in occult OGIB. A bleeding rate of 1 mL per minute has been shown to be required for catheter angiography to be positive in experimental studies [42, 43], and the location of the bleeding source is more likely to be demonstrated when the rate of bleeding is greater than 0.5 mL per minute [44]. If a bleeding source is identified at catheter angiography, then the cause can be treated by embolization if appropriate. A variety of different agents (e.g. microcoils, polyvinyl alcohol particles, and Gelfoam) have been used with high clinical success rates [45, 46]. Even if catheter angiography is negative for active bleeding, it may still identify possible bleeding sources by their appearance (Fig. 17.10a–c).

Experimental in vitro studies have shown that multidetector CT (MDCT) is a more sensitive test than first-order aortic branch-selective digital subtraction angiography (DSA) in detecting active haemorrhage, with a threshold for detecting bleeding of 0.35 mL per minute [47]. Active bleeding is demonstrated on CT angiography when high-density contrast material is seen to accumulate in the lumen of the bowel on the postcontrast images. A precontrast scan must be performed to ensure that the high-density material seen in the bowel was not present before the IV contrast was administered. Several studies have demonstrated the value of MDCT in detecting a cause for acute GI bleeding that had not been found by other investigations (Fig. 17.10d, e) [48–52].

Triphasic CT enterography has also been used in patients with OGIB. An initial study found a positive cause for bleeding in 45 % of patients; capsule endoscopy missed the source of bleeding in a small number of these patients. Of the patients with positive findings, 70 % had overt OGIB [53]. Subsequent studies have also shown CT enterography to be useful in patients with overt and occult OGIB. One study showed a possible sensitivity of 52 % and specificity of 89 % for detecting a cause of suspected GI bleeding in haemodynamically stable patients, with the sensitivity and specificity being higher in those patients with a first GI bleed than in those with OGIB [54]. Another study showed that multiphase CT enterography had a higher sensitivity (88 %) for detecting a source for OGIB than did capsule endoscopy (38 %) in patients with overt and obscure OGIB, largely because it detected more small bowel masses [55]. In all of these multiphase CT enterography studies, the patients received a very high radiation dose, but most were over 60 years of age, and the diagnostic information obtained may have prevented them from having other invasive investigations, with the associated morbidity and mortality.

Fig. 17.7 (**a**–**c**) Crohn's disease of the terminal ileum with bowel wall thickening and a deep penetrating ulcer (*arrow*). (**d**) Postcontrast enhancement in the same patient. (**e**, **f**) Another patient with Crohn's disease with ileoileal and ileocolic fistulas (*arrows*). (**g**) Pelvic abscesses associated with Crohn's disease. There is abnormally thickened distal small bowel in the pelvis with a high-signal abscess on a T2-weighted image (*arrow*). (**h**) With intravenous contrast, the abscess (*arrow*) is low signal with peripheral enhancement on a T1 fat-saturated image

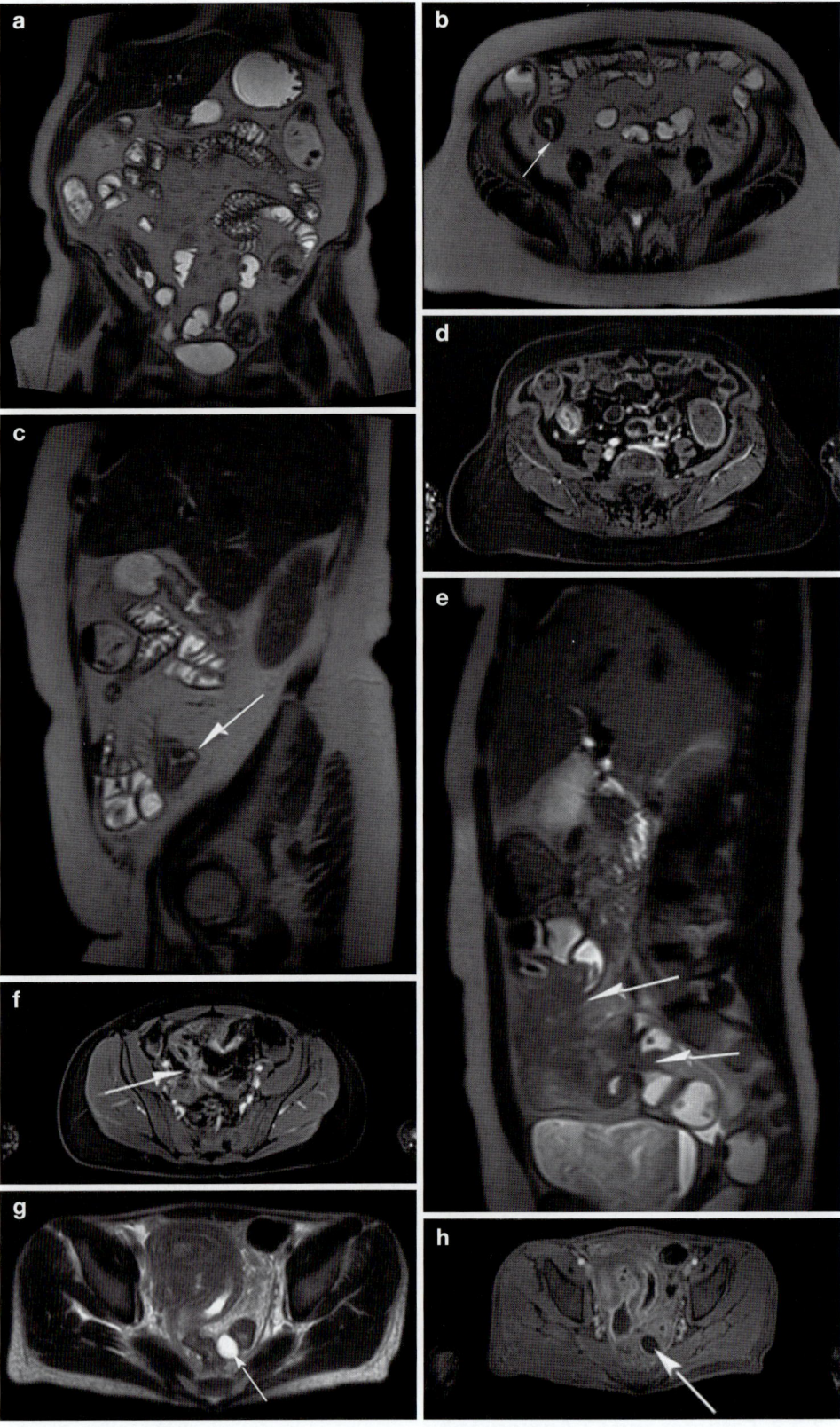

Fig. 17.8 A duodenal tumour in a patient with occult OGIB. The tumour is seen distally in the fourth part of the duodenum as a polypoid mass (*arrow*) (**a**) with more circumferential wall thickening (*arrow*) (**b**). These appearances correspond well with those seen at enteroscopy (**c, d**)

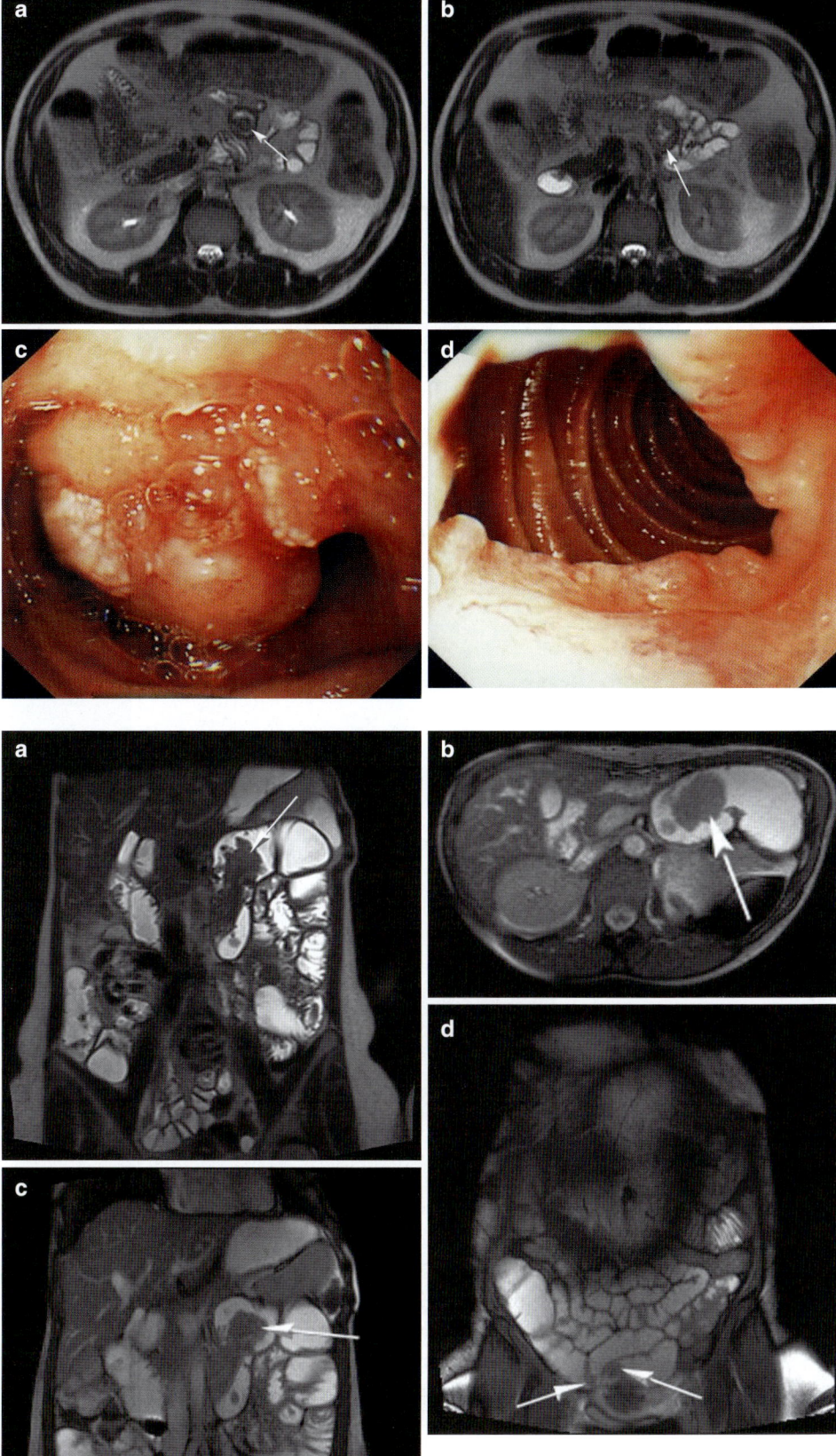

Fig. 17.9 A large polyp on a stalk in the fourth part of the duodenum in a patient with Peutz-Jeghers syndrome on a T2-weighted coronal image (*arrow*) (**a**), on axial true fast imaging with steady-state precession (FISP) image (*arrow*) (**b**), and on coronal FISP (*arrow*) (**c**). Other polyps in the ileum on a coronal true FISP (*arrow*) (**d**)

Fig. 17.10 (**a**) Catheter angiography demonstrates a bleeding point from a vessel supplying the distal ileum (*arrow*). (**b**) The bleeding has been stopped following placement of a coil in the feeding vessel (*arrow*). (**c**) Abnormal vessels supplying a large duodenal GIST, which had been bleeding: no active bleeding was seen at the time of angiography. The tumour blood supply was electively coiled prior to surgical resection. (**d**) Active bleeding on a CT angiogram in a patient with overt OGIB, the same patient as in images (**a, b**). High-density contrast is seen in the lumen of the distal small bowel (*arrow*), which is not seen on the precontrast scan (**e**), from a bleeding angioectasia

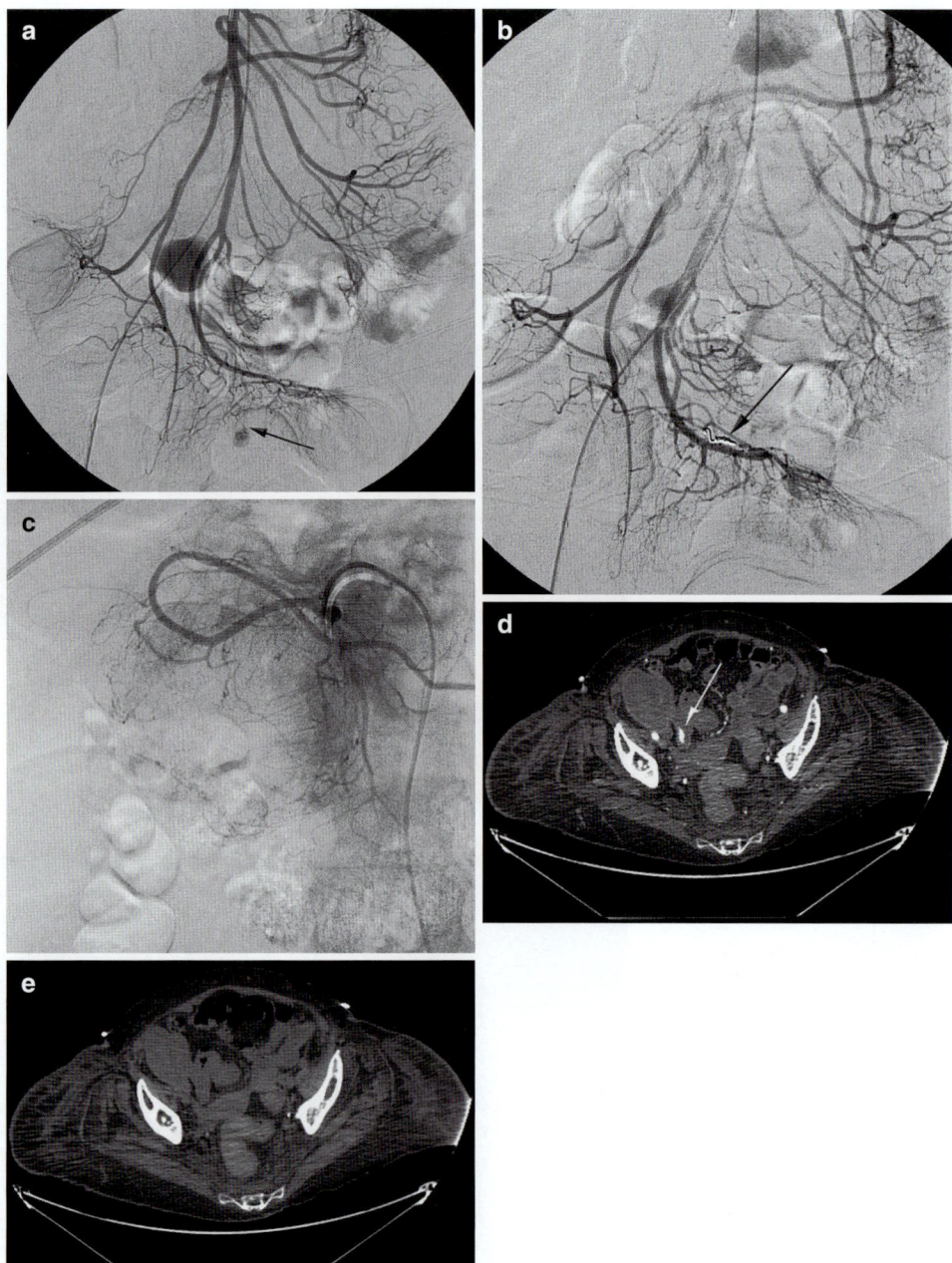

17.2.4 Nuclear Medicine Studies

Scintigraphy can detect GI bleeding at a lower bleeding rate than other diagnostic tests, being able to detect active bleeding at a rate of 0.1 mL per minute with a sensitivity and specificity of over 90 % for localization of the bleeding site [56]. Imaging is performed after tagging of red blood cells (RBC) with technetium 99 m (^{99m}TC). The other advantages of this technique are that it is noninvasive, no patient preparation is required, it can detect both arterial and venous bleeding and (because the tracer remains in the blood for a prolonged period) it is possible to detect

intermittent bleeding (Fig. 17.11a). The drawbacks to ^{99m}TC-labelled RBC scanning are that it is not routinely available out of hours in many centres, it is not therapeutic and it has been shown that its ability to localize the bleeding site can be inaccurate [57].

About 2–3 % of the general population has a Meckel's diverticulum, which is usually in the distal ileum about 50–80 cm from the ileocaecal valve. The diverticulum can contain ectopic gastric mucosa that secretes gastric acid and enzymes, which can cause local ulceration and bleeding. The ^{99m}TC-pertechnetate accumulates in gastric and ectopic gastric mucosa and can be used to demonstrate the presence of ectopic gastric mucosa that may be the cause of OGIB, with a specificity and positive predictive value of close to 100 % in children and adults (Fig. 17.11b) [58, 59].

Radionuclide imaging/scintigraphy can also be used to evaluate the bowel in inflammatory bowel disease. Leucocytes are labelled with indium-111 (^{111}In) or technetium-99 m hexamethylpropyleneamine oxime (^{99m}TC HMPAO). The labelled white cells then accumulate in the regions of inflammation. Early imaging at 30–60 min is performed when ^{99m}TC HMPAO is used, as it may be excreted into the bowel lumen. Imaging is also performed 3–4 h after the injection. If increased activity is due to inflamed bowel, it should remain constant on the two sets of images, whereas if the activity is due to excretion of the tracer into the bowel, the distribution will differ on the two sets of images

(Fig. 17.11c). Imaging with ^{111}In-labelled white cells is performed at 4 h and also sometimes at 24 h. It is not excreted into the GI tract, so any bowel activity indicates the presence of inflammatory bowel disease. A meta-analysis of 33 studies between 1993 and 2005 comparing the diagnosis of inflammatory bowel disease on ultrasound, MR, scintigraphy, and CT prospectively showed scintigraphy to have a sensitivity of 88 % and specificity of 85 % [60]. A second meta-analysis, which included 49 studies that were published between 1984 and 2004 and included nearly 4,400 patients, also showed a sensitivity and specificity around 90 % for the diagnosis of inflammatory bowel disease with either ^{111}In or ^{99m}TC-HMPAO labelled leucocyte scintigraphy [61]. Scintigraphy also exposes the patient to a lower radiation dose than barium examinations and CT, which is relevant in patients who may require repeated examinations.

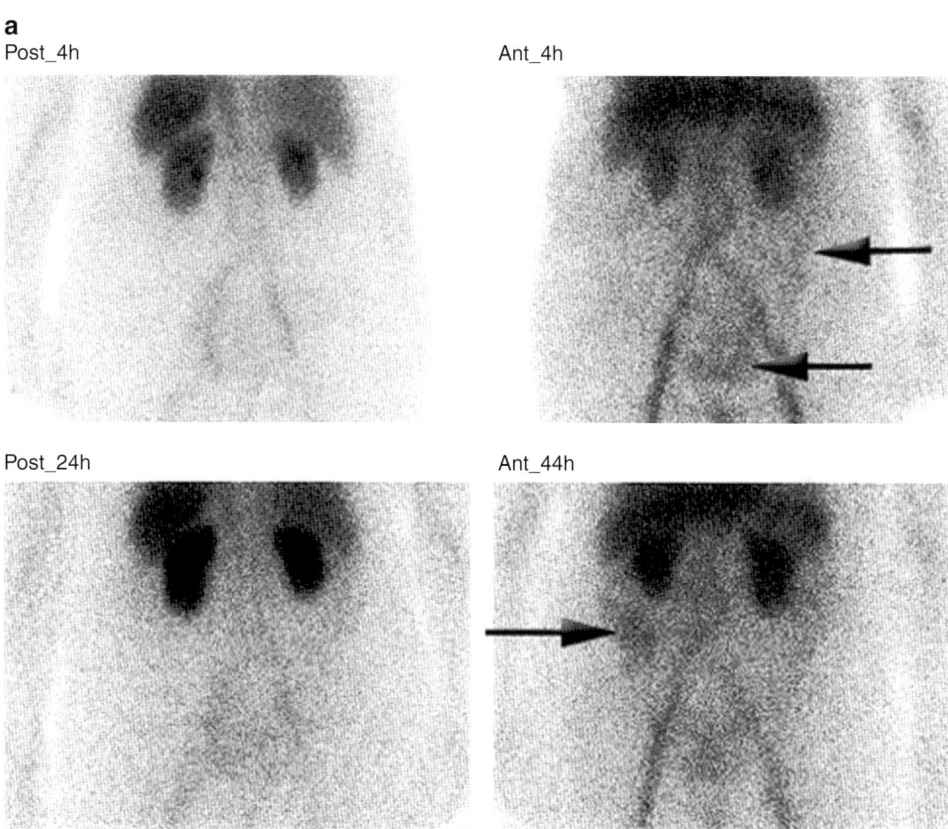

Fig. 17.11 (**a**) Increased activity is seen in the left flank and pelvis (*arrows*) on the 4-h images, and further activity is seen in the region of the ascending colon (*arrow*) on the 24-h images on a ^{99m}TC-labelled red blood cell scan in a patient with overt OGIB. The bleeding point, which had not been seen on CT or catheter angiography, was found to be from a jejunal anastomosis. (**b**) Increased activity on a ^{99m}TC-pertechnetate scan due to ectopic gastric mucosa in a Meckel's diverticulum (*arrow*), which was the cause of overt OGIB. (**c**) Increased activity on a ^{99m}TC hexamethylpropyleneamine oxime (HMPAO)-labelled white cell scan in the right iliac fossa (*arrow*) confirming Crohn's disease in a patient suspected to have Crohn's disease clinically, previous colonoscopy, terminal ileal biopsies, and MRI had been negative

Fig. 17.11 (continued)

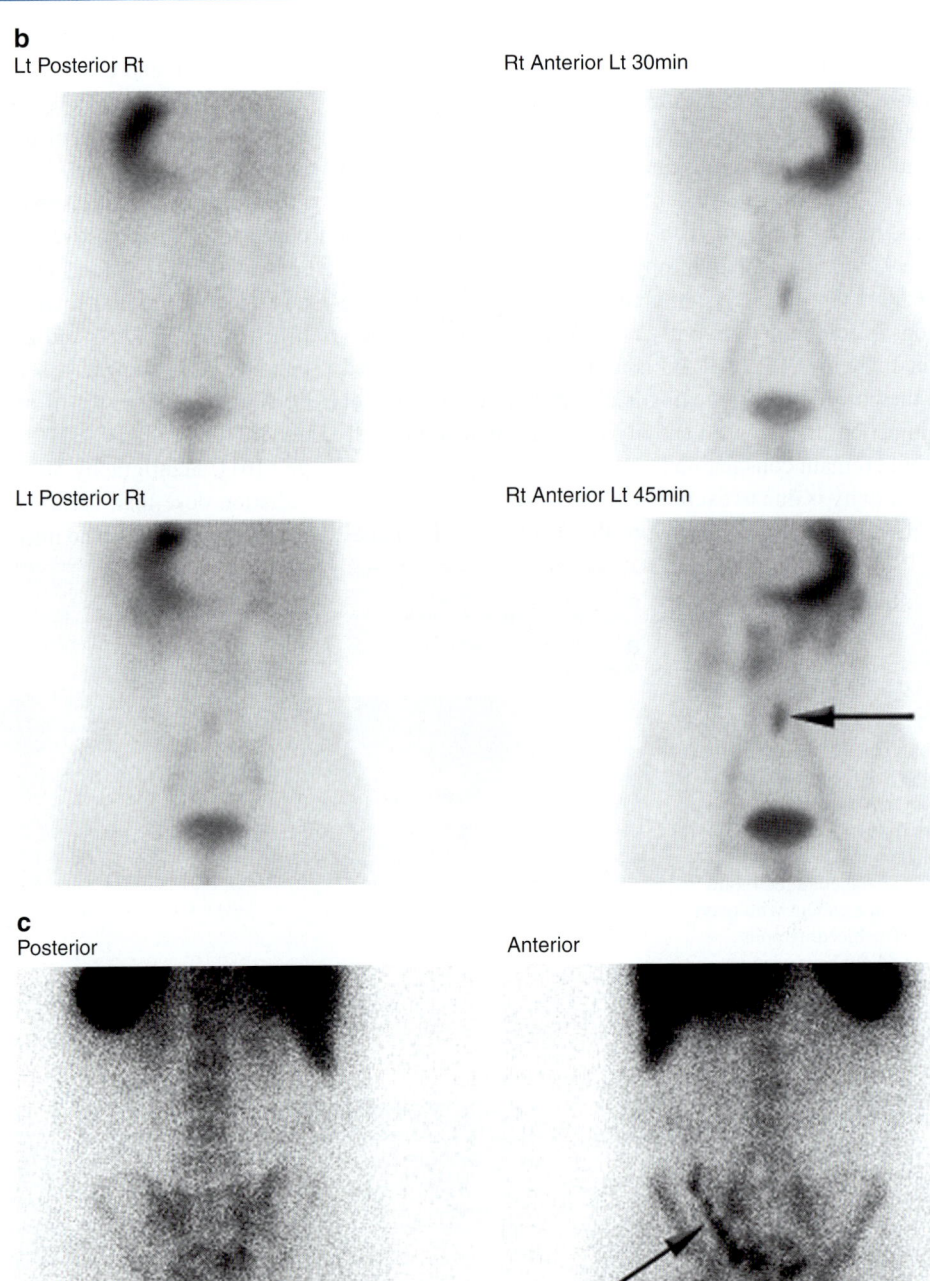

b
Lt Posterior Rt   Rt Anterior Lt 30min

Lt Posterior Rt   Rt Anterior Lt 45min

c
Posterior   Anterior

References

1. Ha A, Levine MS, Rubesin SE, et al. Radiographic examination of the small bowel: survey of practice patterns in the United States. Radiology. 2004;231:407–12.
2. Levine MS, Rubesin SE, Laufer I. Barium studies in modern radiology: do they have a role? Radiology. 2009;250:18–22.
3. Desmond AN, O'Regan K, Curran C, et al. Crohn's disease: factors associated with exposure to high levels of diagnostic radiation. Gut. 2008;57:1524–9.
4. Antes G, Neher M, Heimeyer V, Burger A. Gastrointestinal bleeding of obscure origin: role of enteroclysis. Eur Radiol. 1996;6: 851–4.
5. Antes G. Barium examinations of the small intestine and the colon in inflammatory bowel disease. Radiologie. 2003;43:9–16.
6. Nolan DJ, Traill ZC. The current role of the barium examination of the small intestine. Radiology. 1997;52:809–20.
7. Levine MS, Rubesin SE, Laufer I. Pattern approach for diseases of mesenteric small bowel on barium studies. Radiology. 2008;249: 445–60.
8. Dionisio PM, Gurudu SR, Leighton JA, et al. Capsule endoscopy has a significantly higher diagnostic yield in patients with suspected and established small-bowel Crohn's disease: a meta-analysis. Am J Gastroenterol. 2009;713:1–9.
9. Triester SL, Leighton JA, Leontiadis GI, et al. A meta-analysis of the yield of capsule endoscopy compared to other diagnostic

modalities in patients with obscure gastrointestinal bleeding. Am J Gastroenterol. 2005;100:2407–18.

10. Maglinte DDT, Sandrasegaran K, Chiorean M, et al. Radiologic investigations complement and add diagnostic information to capsule endoscopy of small bowel diseases. AJR Am J Roentgenol. 2007;189:306–12.

11. Young BM, Fletcher JG, Booya F, et al. Head-to-head comparison of oral contrast agents. J Comput Assist Tomogr. 2008;32:32–8.

12. Schindera ST, Nelson RC, DeLong DM, et al. Multi detector row CT of the small bowel: peak enhancement. Radiology. 2007;243:438–44.

13. Vandenbroucke F, Mortelé KJ, Tatli S, et al. Noninvasive multidetector computed tomography enterography in patients with small-bowel Crohn's disease: is a 40-second delay better than 70 seconds? Acta Radiol. 2007;48:1052–60.

14. Elsayes KM, Al-Hawary MM, Jagdish J, et al. CT enterography: principles, trends and interpretation of findings. Radiographics. 2010;30:1955–74.

15. Paulsen SR, Huprich JE, Fletcher JG, et al. CT enterography as a diagnostic tool. Radiographics. 2006;26:641–57.

16. Huprich JE. Multiphase CT, enterography in OGIB. Abdom Imaging. 2009;34:303–9.

17. Higgins PD, Caoili E, Zimmermann M, et al. Computed tomographic enterography adds info to clinical management in small bowel Crohn's disease. Inflamm Bowel Dis. 2007;13:262–8.

18. Boudiaf M, Jaff A, Soyer P, et al. Small bowel diseases: prospective evaluation of multi-detector row helical CT enteroclysis in 107 consecutive patients. Radiology. 2004;233:338–44.

19. Romano S, Lutio ED, Rallandi GA, et al. Multidetector computed tomography enteroclysis (MDCT-E) with neutral enteral and IV contrast enhancement in tumour detection. Eur Radiol. 2005;15:1178–83.

20. Meyers MA, McGuire PV. Spiral CT demonstration of hypervascularity in Crohn disease: "vascular jejunization of the ileum" or the "comb sign". Abdom Imaging. 1995;20:327–32.

21. Health Protection Agency. www.hpa.org.uk.

22. McCollough CH, Guimaraes L, Fletcher JG. In defence of body CT. AJR Am J Roentgenol. 2009;193:29–39.

23. Launstein TC, Schneemann H, Vogt FM, et al. Optimisation of oral contrast agents for MRI of the small bowel. Radiology. 2003;228:279–83.

24. Borthne AS, Abdelnoor M, Storaas T, et al. Osmolarity: a decisive parameter of bowel agents in intestinal magnetic resonance imaging. Eur Radiol. 2006;16:1331–6.

25. Sempere GA, Martinez Sanjuan V, Medina Chulia E, et al. MRI evaluation of inflammatory activity in Crohn's disease. AJR Am J Roentgenol. 2005;184:1829–35.

26. Maccioni F, Bruni A, Viscido A, et al. MR imaging in patients with Crohn disease: value of T2- versus T1-weighted gadolinium-enhanced MR sequences with use of an oral superparamagnetic contrast agent. Radiology. 2006;238:517–30.

27. Udayasankar UK, Martin D, Lauenstein T, et al. Role of spectral presaturation attenuated inversion-recovery fat-suppressed T2-weighted MR imaging in active inflammatory bowel disease. J Magn Reson Imaging. 2008;28:1133–40.

28. Punwani S, Rodriguez-Justo M, Bainbridge A, et al. Mural inflammation in Crohn disease: location-matched histologic validation of MR imaging features. Radiology. 2009;252:712–20.

29. Malagò R, Manfredi R, Benini L, et al. Assessment of Crohn's disease activity in the small bowel with MR-enteroclysis: clinico-radiological correlations. Abdom Imaging. 2008;33:669–75.

30. Tolan DJ, Greenhalgh R, Zeally IA, et al. MR enterographic manifestations of small bowel Crohn disease. Radiographics. 2010;30:367–84.

31. Gourtsoyianni S, Papanikolaou N, Amanakis E, et al. Crohn's disease lymphadenopathy: MR imaging findings. Eur J Radiol. 2009;69:425–8.

32. Prassopoulos P, Papanikolaou N, Grammatikakis J, et al. MR enteroclysis imaging of Crohn disease. Radiographics. 2001;21:S161–72.

33. Schmidt S, Chevallier P, Bessoud B, et al. Diagnostic performance of MRI for detection of intestinal fistulas in patients with complicated inflammatory bowel conditions. Eur Radiol. 2007;17:2957–63.

34. Golder SK, Schreyer AG, Endlicher E, et al. Comparison of capsule endoscopy and magnetic resonance (MR) enteroclysis in suspected small bowel disease. Int J Colorectal Dis. 2006;21.97–104.

35. Tillack C, Seiderer J, Brand S, et al. Correlation of magnetic resonance enteroclysis (MRE) and wireless capsule endoscopy (CE) in the diagnosis of small bowel lesions in Crohn's disease. Inflamm Bowel Dis. 2008;14:1219–28.

36. North JH, Pack MS. Malignant tumors of the small intestine: a review of 144 cases. Am Surg. 2000;66:46–51.

37. Martin RG. Malignant tumors of the small intestine. Surg Clin North Am. 1986;66:779–85.

38. Masselli G, Polettini E, Casciani E, et al. Small-bowel neoplasms: prospective evaluation of MR enteroclysis. Radiology. 2009;251:743–50.

39. Van Weyenberg SJ, Meijerink MR, Jacobs MA, et al. MR enteroclysis in the diagnosis of small-bowel neoplasms. Radiology. 2010;254:765–73.

40. Caspari R, von Falkenhausen M, Krautmacher C, et al. Comparison of capsule endoscopy and magnetic resonance imaging for the detection of polyps of the small intestine in patients with familial adenomatous polyposis or with Peutz-Jeghers' syndrome. Endoscopy. 2004;36:1054–9.

41. Gupta A, Postgate AJ, Burling D, et al. A prospective study of MR enterography and capsule endoscopy for the surveillance of adult patients with Peutz-Jegher's syndrome. AJR Am J Roentgenol. 2010;195:108–16.

42. Nusbaum M, Baum S. Demonstration of unknown sites of gastrointestinal bleeding. Surg Forum. 1963;14:374–5.

43. Nusbaum M, Baum S, Blakemore WS, Finklestein AK. Demonstration of intra-abdominal bleeding by selective arteriography: visualization of celiac and superior mesenteric arteries. JAMA. 1965;191:389–90.

44. Nusbaum M, Baum S, Blakemore WS. Clinical experience with the diagnosis and management of gastrointestinal hemorrhage by selective mesenteric catheterization. Ann Surg. 1969;170:506–14.

45. Schenker MP, Duszak Jr R, Soulen MC, et al. Upper gastrointestinal hemorrhage and transcatheter embolotherapy: clinical and technical factors impacting success and survival. J Vasc Interv Radiol. 2001;12:1263–71.

46. Funaki B. Superselective embolization of lower gastrointestinal hemorrhage: a new paradigm. Abdom Imaging. 2004;29:434–8.

47. Roy-Choudry SH, Gallagher DJ, Pilmer J, et al. Relative threshold of detection of active arterial bleeding: In vitro comparison of MDCT and digital subtraction angiography. AJR Am J Roentgenol. 2007;189:W238–46.

48. Yoon W, Jeong YY, Shin SS, et al. Acute massive gastrointestinal bleeding: detection and localization with arterial phase multi-detector row helical CT. Radiology. 2006;239:160–7.

49. Laing CJ, Tobias T, Rosenblum DI, et al. Acute gastrointestinal bleeding: emerging role of multidetector CT angiography and review of current imaging techniques. Radiographics. 2007;27:1055–70.

50. Yamaguchi T, Yoshikawa K. Enhanced CT for initial localization of active lower gastrointestinal bleeding. Abdom Imaging. 2003;28:634–6.

51. Miller FH, Hwang CM. An initial experience: using helical CT imaging to detect obscure gastrointestinal bleeding. Clin Imaging. 2004;28:245–51.

52. Junquera F, Quiroga S, Saperas E, et al. Accuracy of helical computed tomographic angiography for the diagnosis of colonic angiodysplasia. Gastroenterology. 2000;119:293–9.

53. Huprich JE, Fletcher JG, Alexander JA, et al. Obscure gastrointestinal bleeding: evaluation with 64-section multiphase CT enterography – initial experience. Radiology. 2008;246:562–71.

54. Hara AK, Blake Walker F, Silva AC, Leighton JA. Preliminary estimate of triphasic CT enterography performance in haemodynamically stable patients with suspected gastrointestinal bleeding. AJR Am J Roentgenol. 2009;193:1252–60.

55. Huprich JE, Fletcher JG, Fidler JL, et al. Prospective blinded comparison of wireless capsule endoscopy and multiphase CT enterography in obscure gastrointestinal bleeding. Radiology. 2011;260:744–51.

56. Zuckier LS. Acute gastrointestinal bleeding. Semin Nucl Med. 2003;33:297–311.

57. Howarth DM, Tang K, Lees W. The clinical utility of nuclear medicine imaging for the detection of occult gastrointestinal haemorrhage. Nucl Med Commun. 2002;23:591–4.

58. Sfakianakis GN, Haase GM. Abdominal scintigraphy for ectopic gastric mucosa: a retrospective analysis of 143 studies. AJR Am J Roentgenol. 1982;138:7–12.

59. Kong MS, Chen CY, Tzen KY, et al. Technetium-99m pertechnetate scan for ectopic gastric mucosa in children with gastrointestinal bleeding. J Formos Med Assoc. 1993;92:717–20.

60. Horsthuis K, Bipat S, Bennink RJ, Stoker J. Inflammatory bowel disease diagnosed with US, MR, scintigraphy, and CT: meta-analysis of prospective studies. Radiology. 2008;247:64–79.

61. Annovazzi A, Bagni B, Burroni L, et al. Nuclear medicine imaging of inflammatory/infective disorders of the abdomen. Nucl Med Commun. 2005;26:657–64.

Sonography

18

Guntram Lock and Uwe Matsui

Contents

In the past 30–40 years, abdominal ultrasound has become the most important tool of imaging for acute and chronic gastroenterologic diseases. There are significant differences in different countries in the use of ultrasound and in the experience with ultrasonography of the gastrointestinal tract, but there is no doubt that ultrasonography in skilled hands (as an easily accessible and rapidly available method) will provide deep and reliable insights into pathology of the abdomen, including the stomach and the small and large intestines. Often enough, abdominal ultrasonography, together with clinical presentation and laboratory values, will be sufficient to come to a definitive diagnosis and to initiate medical or operative treatment. In many other patients, ultrasonography can be used as the first imaging procedure, which will guide further diagnostic efforts in the correct direction and may determine which further diagnostic modality—upper or lower gastrointestinal endoscopy, CT or MRI scans, laparoscopy, capsule endoscopy, or other endoscopic procedures for the evaluation of the small intestine—is likely to be the most successful in coming to a diagnosis. Furthermore, intestinal ultrasonography is the imaging method of choice to control the response to treatment after a definitive diagnosis [1–3].

Abdominal ultrasound of the gastrointestinal tract may be hampered by difficult conditions such as adiposity, superimposed air, or postoperative conditions with large dressings. The storage and availability of pictures are less standardized than for radiologic procedures, and the inexperienced interpreter of ultrasound pictures may find it difficult to get an anatomic overview from the pictures alone. In addition, ultrasonography is always said to be highly dependent on the examiner's experience. This statement is true, of course, but which diagnostic method is not? The same applies to the performance and interpretation of CT or MRI scans, for instance, though probably to a lesser degree.

On the other hand, ultrasound is cheap, has no adverse effects, causes only minimal discomfort to the patient, offers the possibility of real-time examination (which is of special importance in the whole gut), and is an easy way to correlate

The work was first published in 2006 by Springer Medizin Verlag Heidelberg with the following title: *Atlas of Video Capsule Endoscopy*.

G. Lock (✉)
Clinic for Internal Medicine, Albertinenkrankenhaus,
Hamburg, Germany
e-mail: guntram.lock@albertinen.de

U. Matsui
Department of Internal Medicine,
Bethesda Krankenhaus Bergedorf, Hamburg, Germany
e-mail: matsui@bkb.info

M. Keuchel et al. (eds.), *Video Capsule Endoscopy: A Reference Guide and Atlas*,
DOI 10.1007/978-3-662-44062-9_18, © Springer-Verlag Berlin Heidelberg 2014

the location of pain or discomfort with a certain anatomic region. Overall, it may deliver fascinating and brilliant pictures with very high spatial resolution. Even if performed together with other radiologic or endoscopic methods, it may deliver important complementary information, either by direct correlation with the clinical presentation or by the possibility of extending the endoscopic luminal view to intramural or extramural processes. Paralleling the advances in information and computing technology, the continuous development of ultrasound techniques such as harmonic imaging, 3-D and panoramic imaging, probes with higher frequencies, and the introduction of contrast-enhanced ultrasonography (CEUS) has further improved the validity of ultrasonography in the past two decades [4].

18.1 Technique

Ultrasonography of the gastrointestinal tract is usually started with a standard curved array probe with a frequency of 1–5 MHz, to get an overall impression of the abdominal status and possible pathology. Specific evaluation of intestinal structures is performed with parallel scanners with a frequency of 5–15 MHz. Usually, a fasting period of some hours allows better visualization of the intestine, reducing the amount of air. On the other hand, filling the intestine with fluid (water, tea, or even a bowel cleansing preparation) can improve contrast between the lumen and bowel wall and may

help in the interpretation of certain bowel wall processes or in the assessment of intestinal motility (e.g., when looking for a stenosis or pseudo-obstruction).

With sensitive ultrasound transducers, the typical five layers of the intestinal wall well known from endoscopic ultrasound may as well be visualized in transabdominal ultrasonography. Coming from the lumen, the first hyperechoic inner layer is interpreted as the mucosal entrance echo, followed by the darker, hypoechoic mucosa, then the echogenic submucosa, the darker muscularis propria, and the echogenic exit echo (serosa) (Fig. 18.1). These phenomena are most easily seen in a fluid-filled stomach or in the colon. Any disruption of these regular layers may relate to a pathologic condition such as a tumor or inflammation.

18.2 Sonography of the Stomach

Larger carcinomas of the stomach may be seen sonographically as a hypoechoic thickening of the stomach wall with disruption of the normal wall texture (Fig. 18.2). Stomach motility may be impaired. Gastric outlet stenosis may lead to a grossly dilated stomach. Gastrointestinal stromal tumors usually present as hypoechoic, round tumors in the stomach wall, with hypervascularization in color-coded or contrast-enhanced ultrasound (Fig. 18.3). Ultrasound is not a suitable method for the detection and differentiation of gastric ulcers.

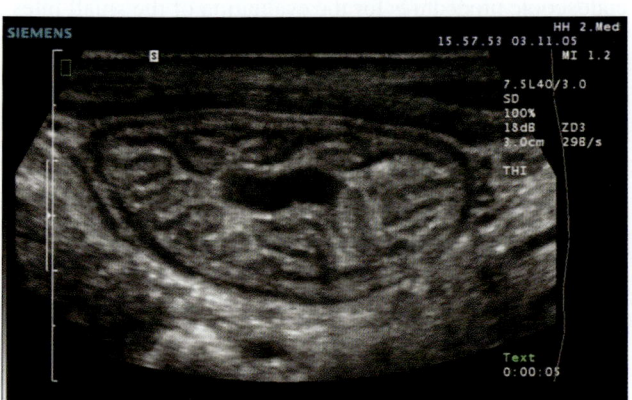

Fig. 18.1 The different sonographic layers of the stomach (here, the corpus)

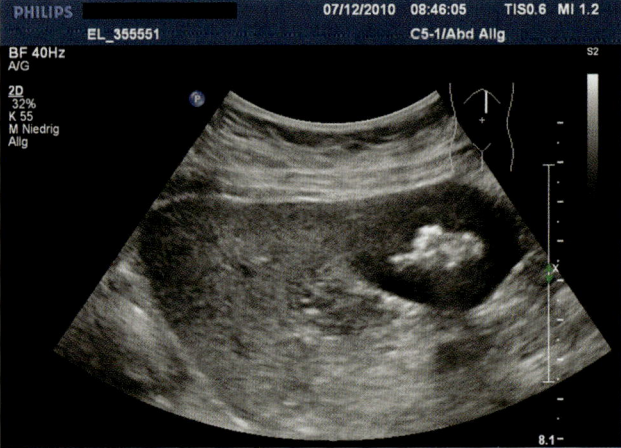

Fig. 18.2 Scirrhous carcinoma in the antrum. Note the diffuse, hypoechoic thickening of the antral wall around the hyperechoic luminal air

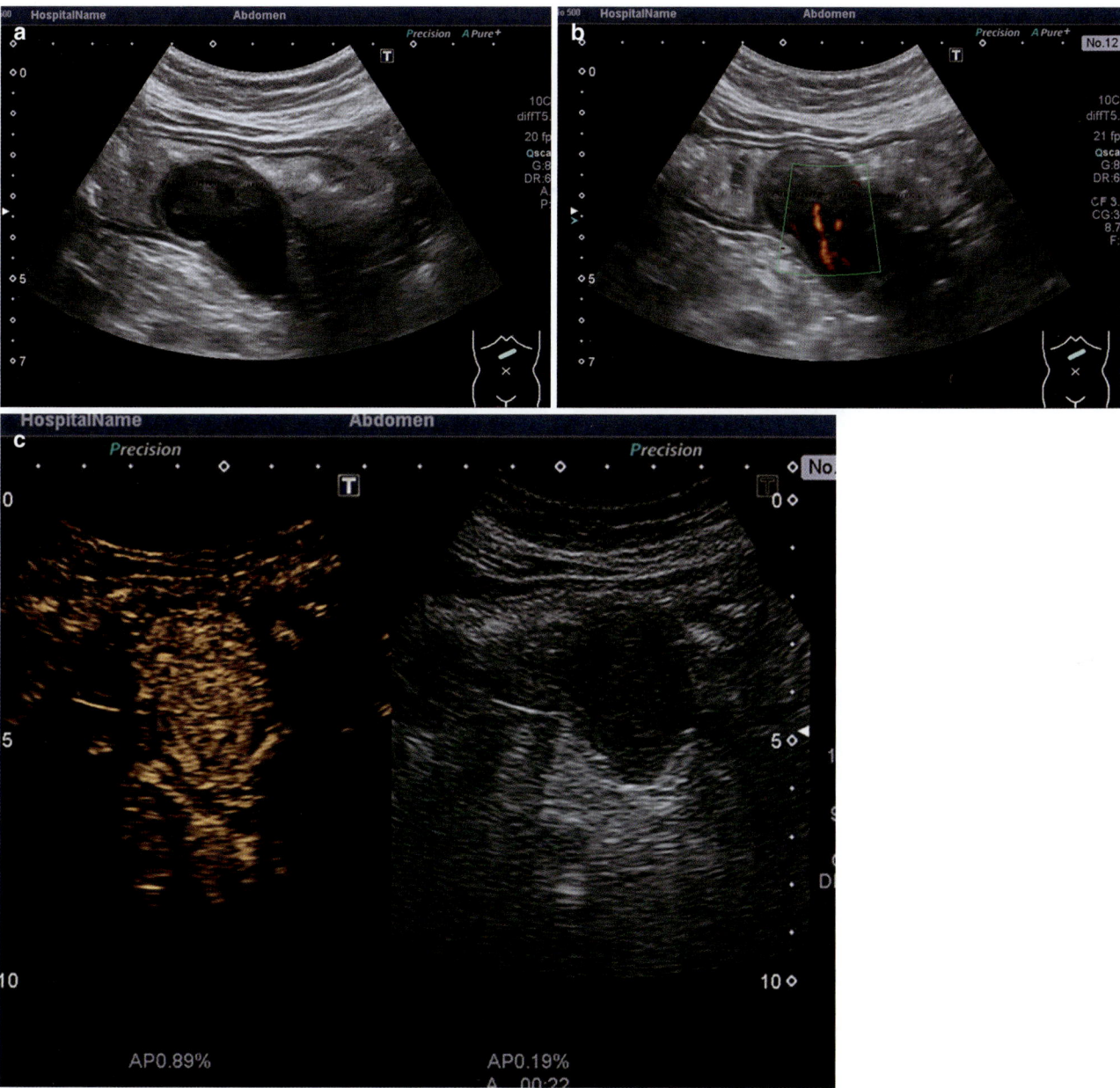

Fig. 18.3 Gastrointestinal stromal tumor of the stomach, presenting with upper gastrointestinal bleeding. (**a**, **b**) Hypoechoic, well-demarcated, and vascularized tumor within the gastric wall. (**c**) Contrast-enhanced ultrasound (*left*) and simultaneous grayscale picture (*right*), showing the hypervascularization of the tumor. (**d**, **e**) Endosonographic and endoscopic views. (**f**) Operative specimen (Courtesy of D. Boessow, Albertinen Hospital)

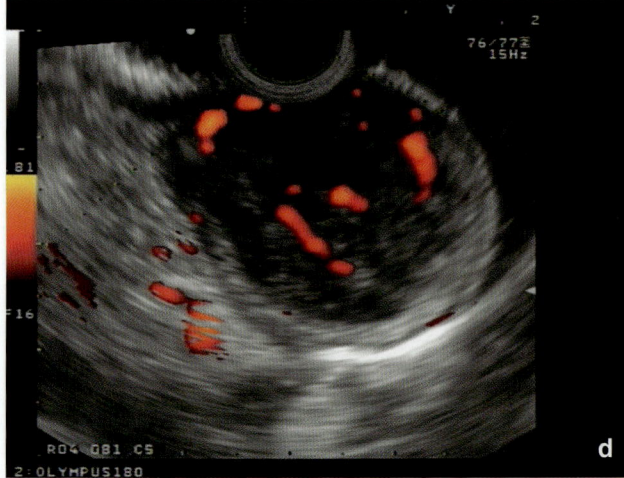

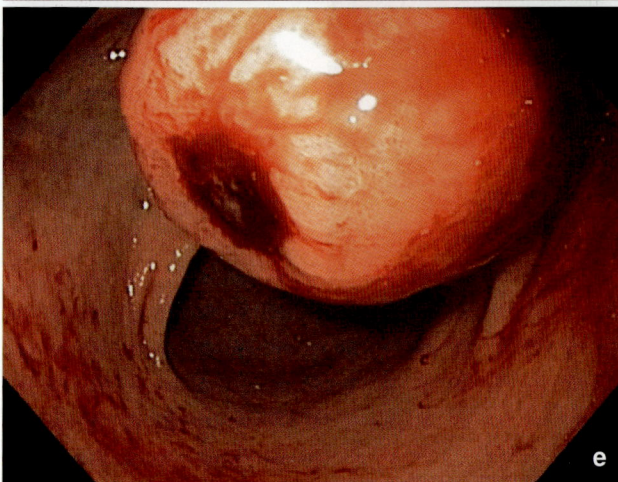

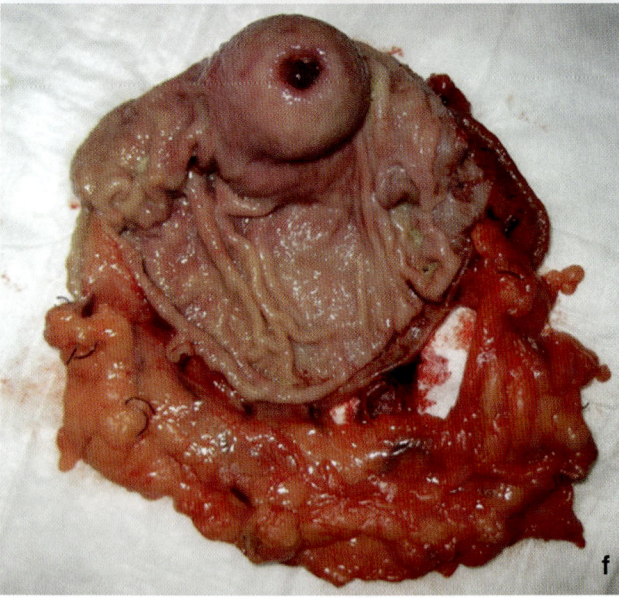

Fig. 18.3 (continued)

18.3　Sonography of the Small Intestine

Ultrasonography is an easily accessible and easily performed method to diagnose occlusive or paralytic small bowel ileus [5]. Small bowel loops are dilated and typically filled with fluid, providing good contrast to the Kerckring folds of the small intestine, one of the main criteria to differentiate small and large bowel (Figs. 18.4 and 18.5). Different amounts of free fluid may be visible. In later stages of small bowel obstruction, the intestinal wall may appear thickened by

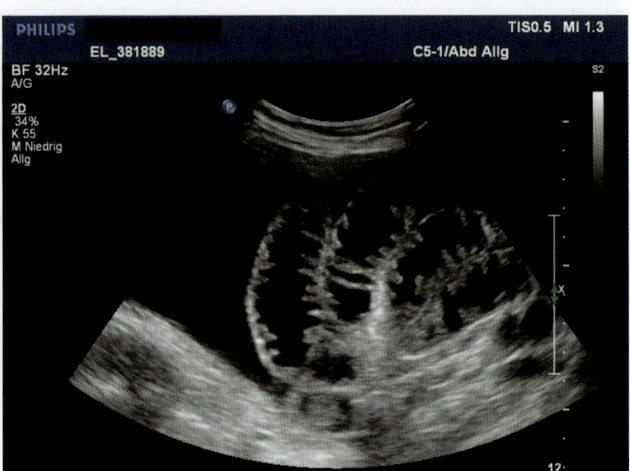

Fig. 18.4 Ileus of the small intestine. Note the dilatation of the intestinal loops, with marked Kerckring folds and free fluid

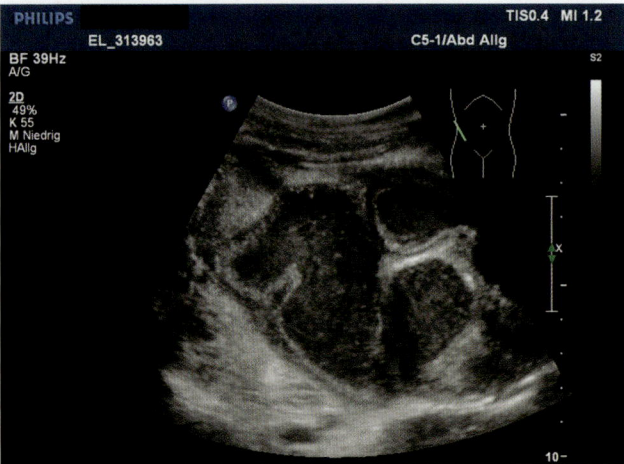

Fig. 18.5 Colonic obstruction in a patient with ovarian cancer. The absence of Kerckring folds and the presence of colonic haustra facilitate the correct anatomic classification

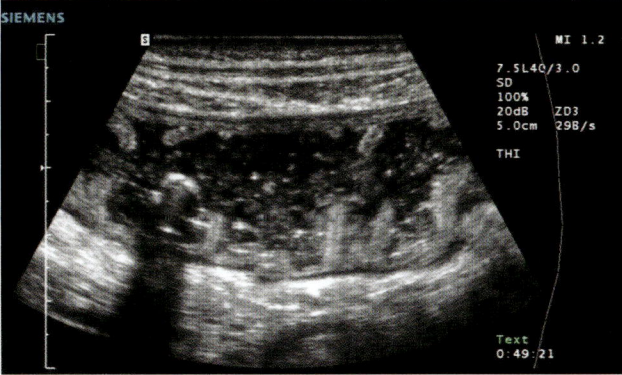

Fig. 18.6 Sonography of a patient with celiac disease showing fluid-filled intestinal lumen

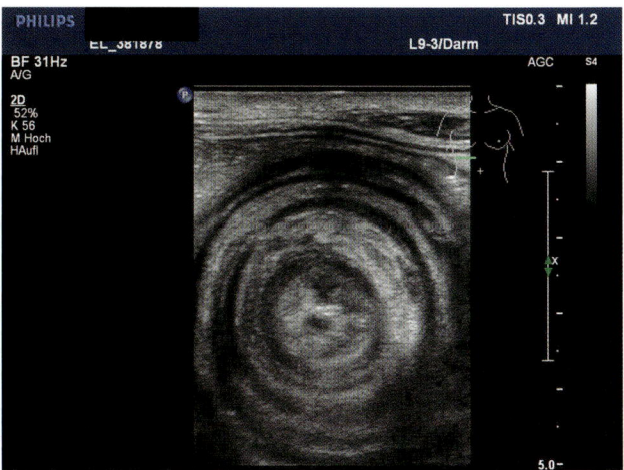

Fig. 18.7 Sonography of ileoileal invagination

Fig. 18.8 Tumors of the terminal ileum. (**a, b**) Sonographic and corresponding endoscopic pictures of two patients with a neuroendocrine tumor and (**c, d**) a small bowel carcinoma

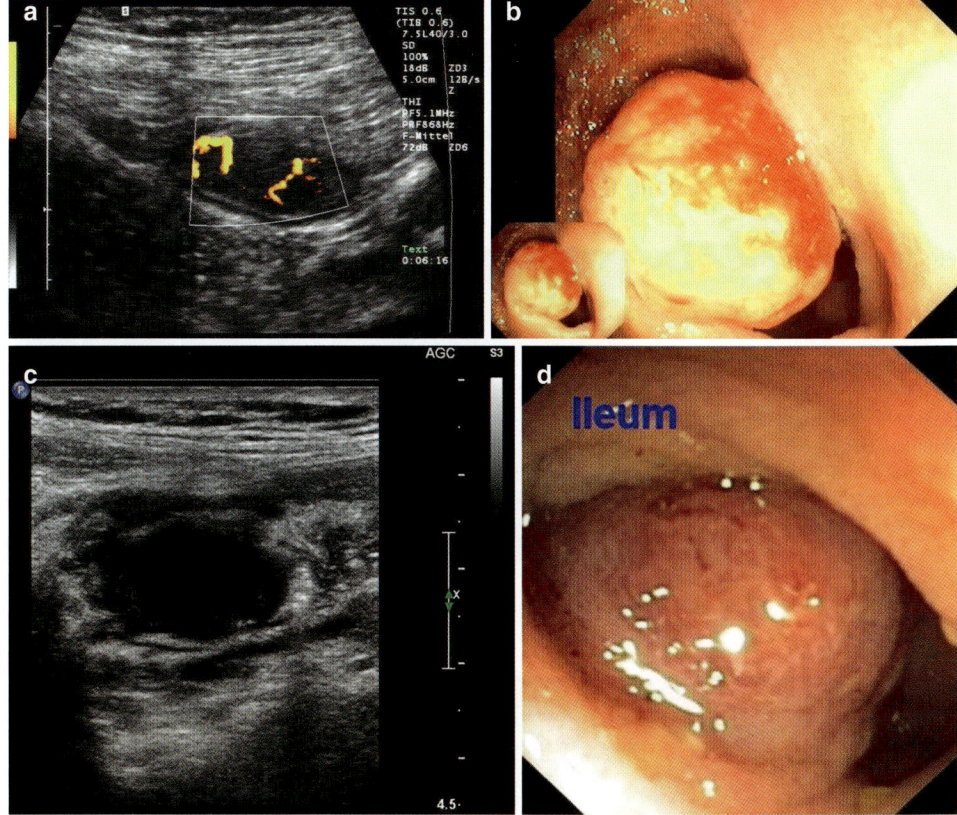

edema, and peristaltic waves may not be detectable even in an initially obstructive ileus. Distal to a stenosis, the intestine will be markedly smaller or even collapsed, thus giving hints to the localization of the obstruction. Celiac disease may show a similar picture, with fluid-filled loops of the small intestine and a typical peristalsis ("washing machine phenomenon"), but, of course, the clinical presentation will be different (Fig. 18.6).

Invagination (most often ileocolic, but also ileoileal or colocolic) is most frequent in pediatric patients, but may also occur in adults. Sonography shows the typical picture of "gut in gut," also referred to as a "bull's-eye sign" (Fig. 18.7). With a high degree of suspicion, ultrasonographic examination may lead to the detection of small bowel malignancy such as small bowel carcinoma, neuroendocrine tumors (Fig. 18.8), lymphoma, or gastrointestinal stromal tumor.

Fig. 18.9 Sonography in Crohn's disease. (**a**) Marked thickening of the terminal ileum. (**b**) An enteroenteral fistula. (**c**) Hypervascularization as a sign of ongoing inflammation

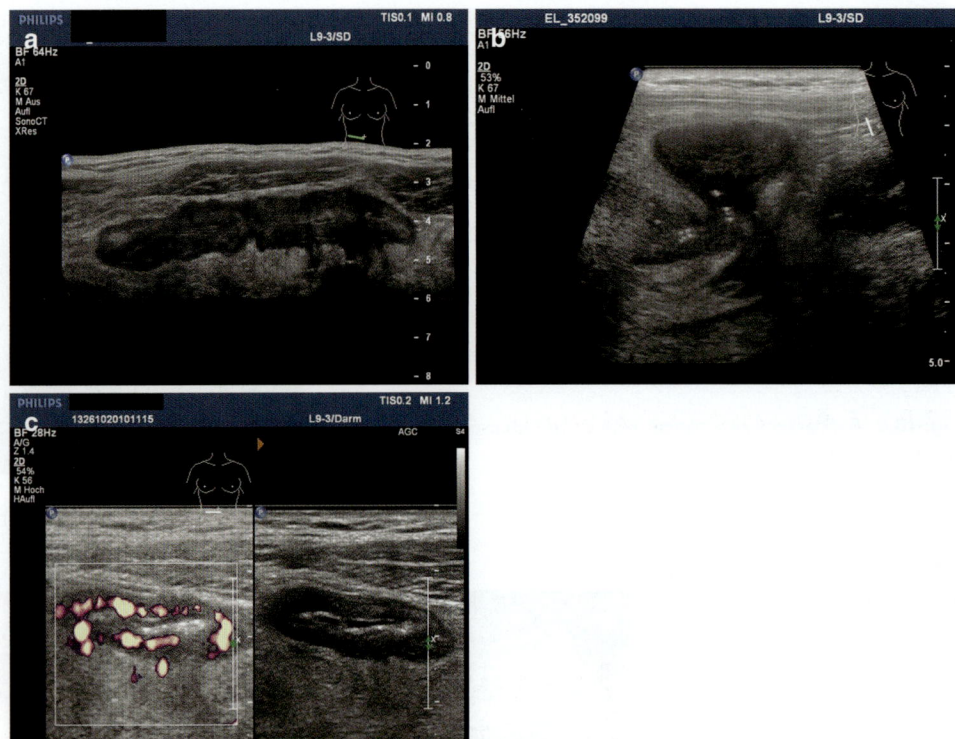

Fig. 18.10 Inflammatory stenosis in a patient with established Crohn's disease. (**a**) Power Doppler shows hyperperfusion, prestenotic dilatation, and adherent abscess. A video capsule had been retained. (**b**) Fibrotic Crohn's stenosis with marked dilatation of the small bowel lumen

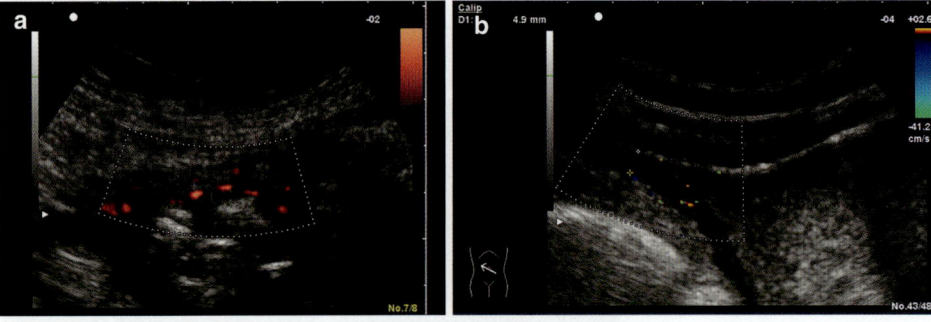

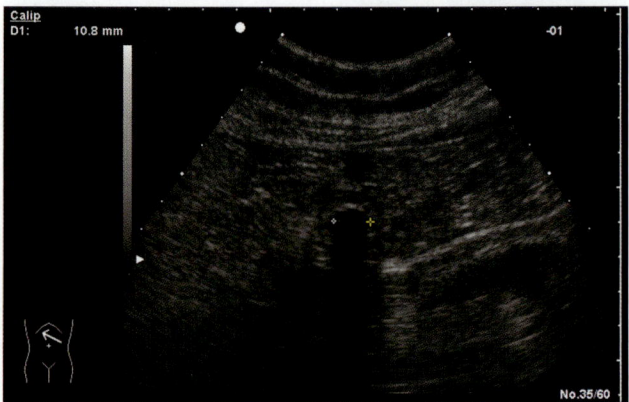

Fig. 18.11 Retained video capsule with shadow. The measured diameter was 10.8 mm, and diameter specified by manufacturer is 11 mm

In Crohn's disease, sonography is a valuable noninvasive method to determine the location and grade of inflammation in the small intestine, which most often is localized in the terminal ileum. In acute inflammation, the terminal ileum is thickened, hypoechoic, and hypervascularized. Ultrasound may detect fistula and abscesses (Fig. 18.9). Sonography plays an important role in the search for intestinal stenosis prior to scheduled video capsule endoscopy in patients with established Crohn's disease. In cases of inflammatory stenosis (Fig. 18.10a), therapy might rather be medical or surgical, whereas short fibrotic stenosis (Fig. 18.10b) may be eligible for balloon dilation during device-assisted enteroscopy (see Figs. 13.6 and 14.10). Retained capsules may be detected sonographically (Fig. 18.11), although this method is not sensitive enough to exclude retention.

18.4 Sonography of the Appendix

Acute appendicitis presents as a markedly thickened and round appendix, often with a hypoechoic wall, free fluid around the appendix, and marked tenderness on ultrasonographic palpation. A perityphlitic abscess may present as an onion-shaped thickening of the appendiceal region, and it may be difficult or impossible to identify the appendix itself in this abscess. Sonography also may detect rare conditions such as a mucinous neoplasia of the appendix (Fig. 18.12).

18.5 Sonography of the Large Intestine

Ultrasonography is also a valuable tool to detect and to stage inflammatory conditions of the colon [6].

Diverticulitis as a common cause of lower left abdominal pain is diagnosed by the echogenic diverticula and a segmental, hypoechoic thickening of the colon wall, often together with an abscess or even with gas bubbles as a sign of perforation (Fig. 18.13).

Different forms of colitis may present as bowel wall thickening with or without loss of the sonographic layers (Fig. 18.14).

Colonic carcinomas usually appear as hypoechoic thickenings of the colonic wall. For larger, clearly visible tumors, local T staging may be done by ultrasonography. It sometimes can be difficult, however, to differentiate between inflammatory and neoplastic lesions (Fig. 18.15), and ultrasound is not a suitable tool to rule out colonic polyps or carcinomas.

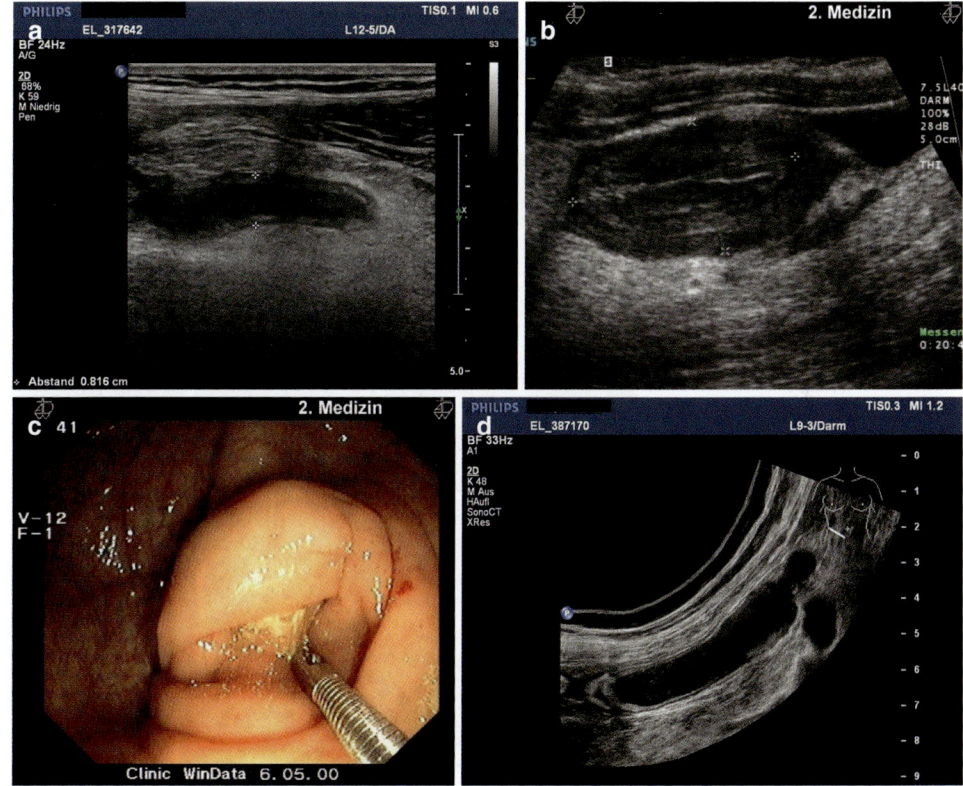

Fig 18.12 Sonography of the appendix. (**a**) Acute appendicitis. (**b**, **c**) Sonographic and endoscopic appearance of the appendix in a patient with chronic perityphlitic abscess. (**d**) Mucinous neoplasia of the appendix

Fig. 18.13 Sonography in diverticulitis. (**a**) Hypoechoic segmental wall thickening around a diverticulum. (**b**) Small abscess in diverticulitis. (**c**) Small amounts of air outside the colon (*arrow*) as asign of perforation

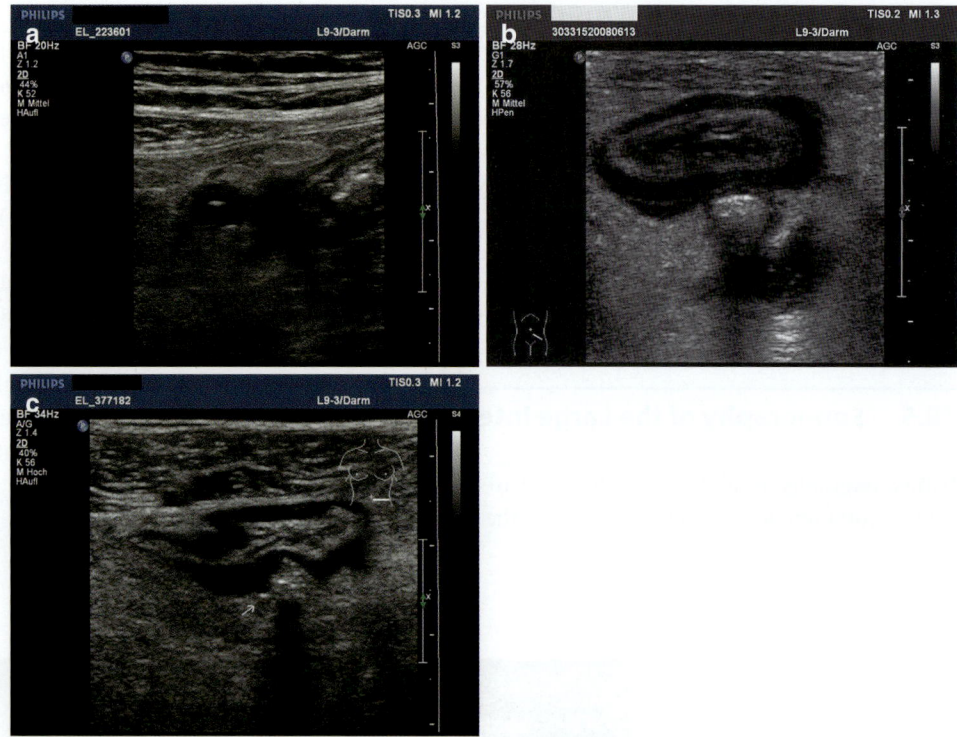

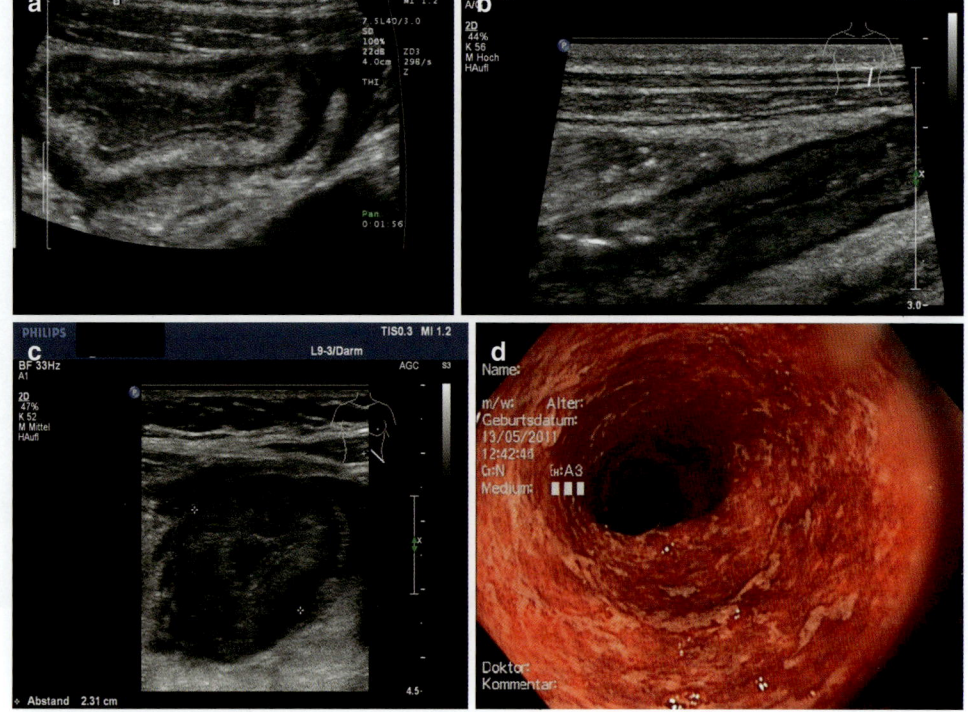

Fig. 18.14 Acute colitis. (**a**) Ulcerative colitis. (**b**) Cytomegalovirus (CMV) colitis in a patient with HIV infection. (**c**, **d**) Sonographic and endoscopic pictures of a patient with severe enterohemorrhagic *E. coli* (EHEC) colitis

Fig. 18.15 Sonographic images of colonic carcinoma. (**a**) Sigmoid carcinoma with destruction of normal sonographic layers. (**b**) Relatively flat carcinoma, which is difficult to differentiate from segmental colitis

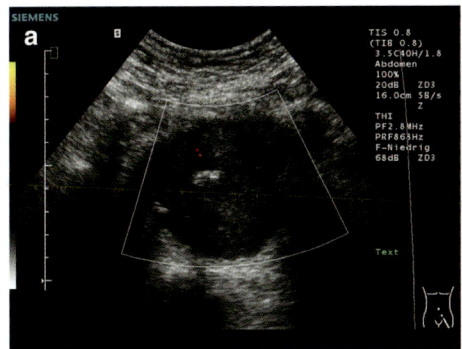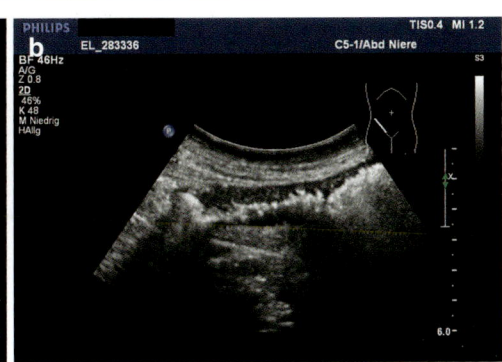

References

1. Lock G, Hirschbühl K, Jechart G. Sonografie. In: Messmann H, editor. Klinische Gastroenterologie. Stuttgart: Georg Thieme; 2012. p. 96–107.
2. Nuernberg D, Ignee A, Dietrich CF. Current status of ultrasound in gastroenterology–bowel and upper gastrointestinal tract--part 1 [in German]. Z Gastroenterol. 2007;45:629–40.
3. Nuernberg D, Ignee A, Dietrich CF. Current status of ultrasound in gastroenterology–bowel and upper gastrointestinal tract--part 2 [in German]. Z Gastroenterol. 2008;46:355–66.
4. Braden B, Ignee A, Hocke M, et al. Diagnostic value and clinical utility of contrast enhanced ultrasound in intestinal diseases. Dig Liver Dis. 2010;42:667–74.
5. Nylund K, Odegaard S, Hausken T, et al. Sonography of the small intestine. World J Gastroenterol. 2009;15:1319–30.
6. Hollerweger A. Colonic diseases: the value of US examination. Eur J Radiol. 2007;64:239–49.

Normal Small Intestine

19

Ingo Steinbrück, Martin Keuchel, Friedrich Hagenmüller, and Axel von Herbay

Contents

The work was first published in 2006 by Springer Medizin Verlag Heidelberg with the following title: *Atlas of Video Capsule Endoscopy*.

I. Steinbrück (✉) • F. Hagenmüller
1st Medical Department, Asklepios Klinik Altona,
Hamburg, Germany
e-mail: i.steinbrueck@asklepios.com;
f.hagenmueller@asklepios.com

M. Keuchel
Department of Internal Medicine, Bethesda Krankenhaus Bergedorf,
Hamburg, Germany
e-mail: keuchel@bkb.info

A. von Herbay
Hansepathologie, Hamburg, Germany
e-mail: pathologe@vonHerbay.de

19.1 Macroscopic Anatomy

The small bowel is a tubular organ 3–4 m in length, which starts at the pylorus and terminates at the ileocecal valve [1]. In a recent study, the small bowel length measured from the ligament of Treitz to the ileocecal valve was 2.83–3.45 m [2]. It is usually subdivided into the duodenum, jejunum, and ileum. The most proximal portion is the C-shaped duodenum, approximately 25 cm long, which is almost a fixed retroperitoneal structure. Four subdivisions of the duodenum are recognized: the first or superior portion (bulb, D1); the second or descending portion, which includes the papilla of Vater (D2); the third or horizontal portion (D3); and the fourth or ascending portion (D4). At the duodenojejunal flexure (the so-called ligament of Treitz), which is left of the midline at the level of the second lumbar vertebra, the duodenum becomes continuous with the intra-abdominal small intestine. Just by convention, the jejunum comprises the upper two-fifths of the intraperitoneal small intestine, and the distal three-fifths are designated as the ileum. The multiple intra-abdominal coils are mobile; they are attached to the mesentery (Fig. 19.1). The diameter decreases from about 25 mm in the duodenum to 19 mm in the distal ileum [3].

The lumen of the small bowel is ringed by circular mucosal folds with a thickness of 1.8 mm (duodenum) to 2.1 mm (distal ileum), the so-called valvulae conniventes (Kerckring's folds), which gradually decrease distally from 4.6 (duodenum) to 1.5 (distal ileum) per 2.5 cm [3].

The arterial blood is supplied to the jejunum and ileum by anastomosing branches of the superior mesenteric artery. The duodenum additionally receives blood from the celiac trunk. Venous drainage is towards the portal venous system via the superior mesenteric veins and is parallel to the arteries. Lymphatic drainage starts in the villi with lymphatic capillaries, which become confluent to form a central chylous vessel; this vessel passes through a submucosal network into mesenteric lymphatic vessels and lymph nodes, finally entering via the thoracic duct into the venous circulation.

Fig. 19.1 Small bowel. (**a**) Intraoperative view (Courtesy of Marco Sailer, MD). (**b**) Selective digital subtraction angiography of the superior mesenteric artery, demonstrating blood supply of the small bowel (Courtesy of Doris Welger, MD). (**c**) Contrast radiograph of the normal small bowel. (**d**) Three-dimensional localization software (EndoCapsule EC-S10, Olympus), showing passage of the video capsule through the small bowel (*pink* stomach, *green* small intestine, *violet* right colon)

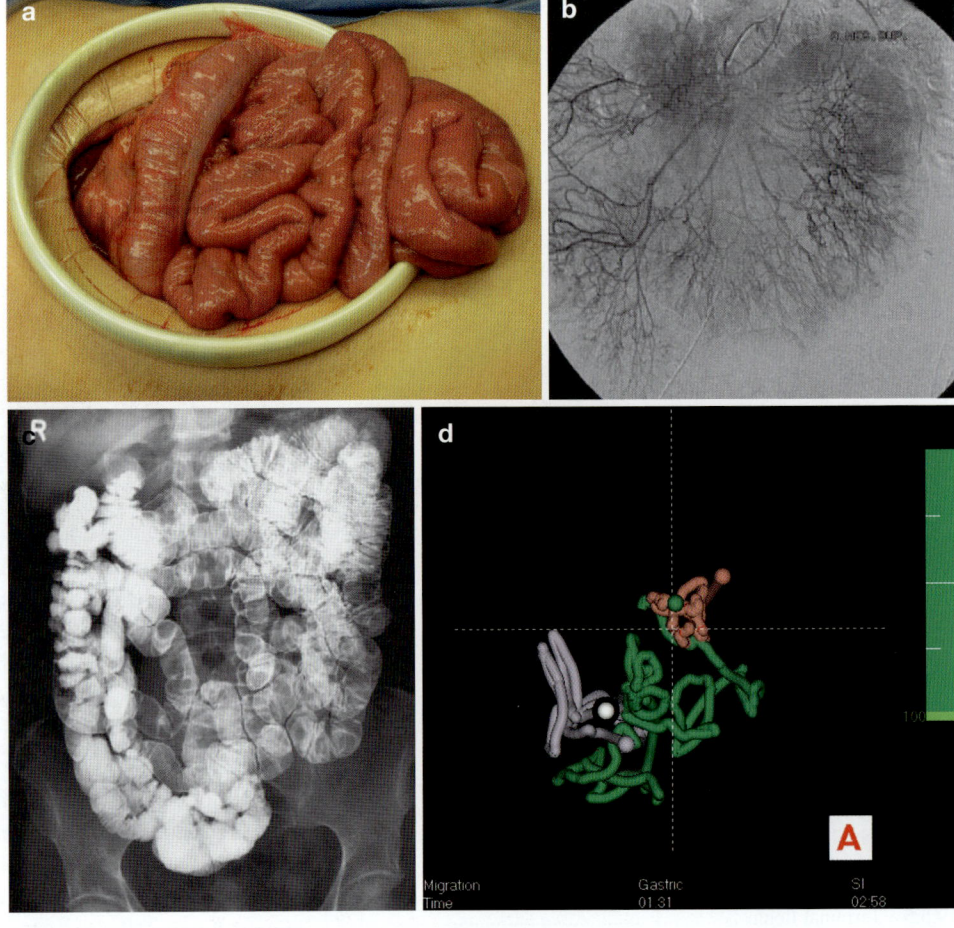

19.2 Microscopic Anatomy

The anatomic layers of the small bowel wall are (from the inside out) the mucosa, submucosa, muscularis propria, and serosa. The mucosal surface is characterized by leaflike and fingerlike extensions, the villi. Intervening and beneath the villi are short tubular glands, the crypts of Lieberkühn. The epithelium is composed of specialized columnar cells, or enterocytes; mucus-producing goblet cells; secretory Paneth's cells; and diverse endocrine cells. A distinctive feature of the duodenum is the presence of mucoid Brunner's glands [4]. Multiple disseminated lymphoid follicles are present along the duodenum, jejunum, and ileum, but the terminal ileum contains aggregates of lymphoid follicles known as Peyer's patches. They are covered by a specialized immunocompetent epithelium (microfold [M] cells). Together they form the mucosa-associated lymphatic tissue (MALT).

19.3 Function

Two of the major functions of the small bowel are to break down and absorb nutrients and to absorb water and electrolytes. The absorption of vitamin B_{12} and bile acid occurs exclusively in the terminal ileum. Further functions are secretion, endocrine activity, motility, and immunologic defense.

19.4 Normal Video Capsule Endoscopy of the Small Intestine

The resolution of video capsule endoscopy (VCE) provides a detailed view of the bowel mucosa, including the villi. As in flexible endoscopy, the type of capsule endoscope (Chap. 4), as well as the settings for the monitor, affect the appearance of the image (Fig. 19.2).

Fig. 19.2 Visualization of the small bowel with various video capsules. (**a**) PillCam SB3 (Given Imaging, Yoqneam, Israel). (**b**) EndoCapsule EC-S10 (Olympus Medical Systems, Tokyo, Japan) (**c**) Mirocam (IntroMedic, Seoul, Korea). (**d**) OMOM capsule (Jinshan Science and Technology, Chongqing, China). (**e**) Capsocam (CapsoVision, Saratoga, CA, USA)

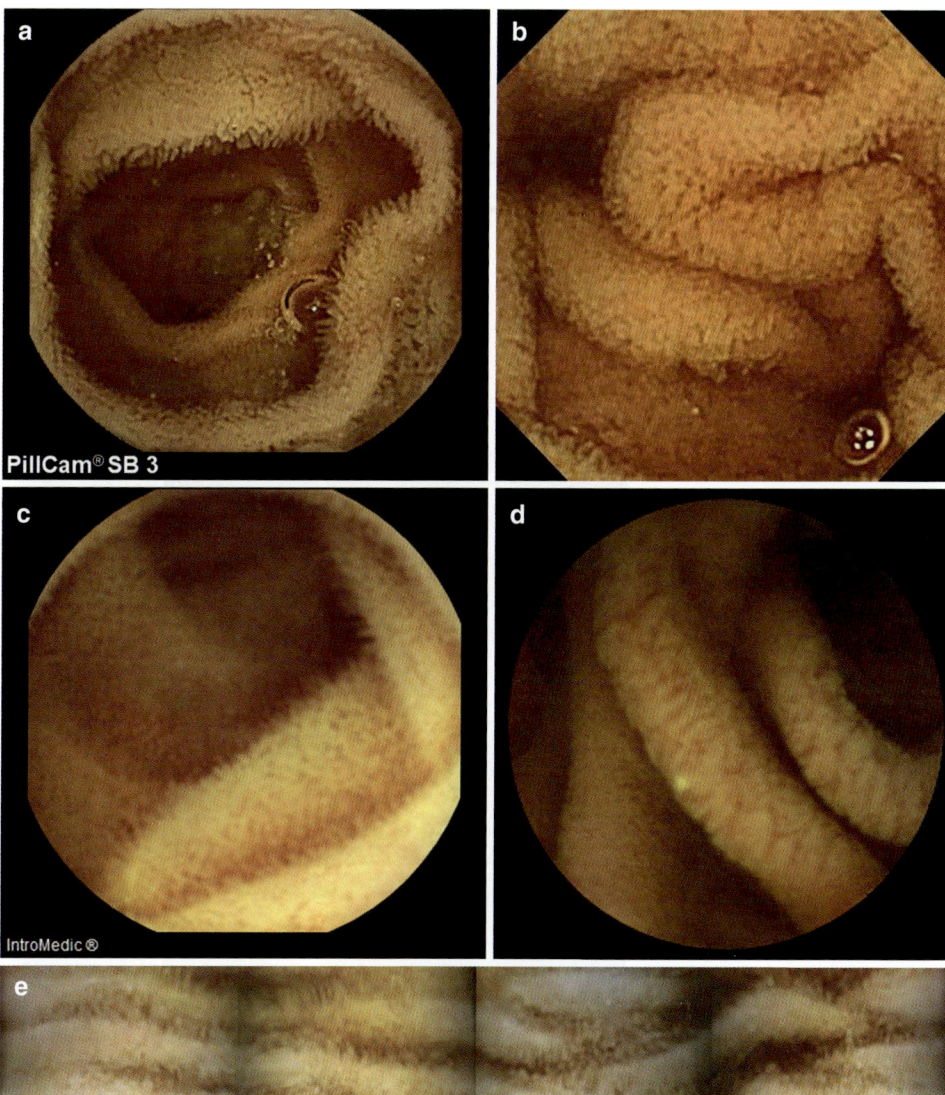

VCE shows various characteristics of the normal small bowel:

- Yellow-orange-colored mucosa
- Circular folds
- Villi
- Small vessels and occasional larger veins
- Peristalsis: propulsive and occasional retropulsive contractions
- Bile, air bubbles, and debris in secretions
- Peyer's patches in the terminal ileum

Quite often yellow or white submucosal plaques can be observed in the entire small bowel. These are most likely to be lymphangiectasias and can be regarded as an anatomic variant [5].

19.4.1 Villi

The villi in the fluid-filled small bowel can be very clearly seen and evaluated when viewed at a tangential angle (Fig. 19.3a, b). The high resolution of modern video endoscopy and VCE has substituted reflected light microscopy (Fig. 19.3c). The villi in the duodenal bulb (see Fig. 19.9a) are broader and flatter than in the more distal small bowel. The villous architecture of the jejunum and ileum, on the other hand, can hardly be distinguished by endoscopic inspection (Fig. 19.4).

Fig. 19.3 Villi in close-up, in a fluid-filled small bowel. (**a**) Video capsule endoscopy (VCE). (**b**) Reflected light microscopy. (**c**) High-definition endoscopy. (**d**) Histology. (**e**) Probe-based confocal laser microscopy. (**f**) Electron microscopy of the small intestine, showing cells with microvilli and intracellular mitochondria (Courtesy of Soumitra Ghoshroy, PhD)

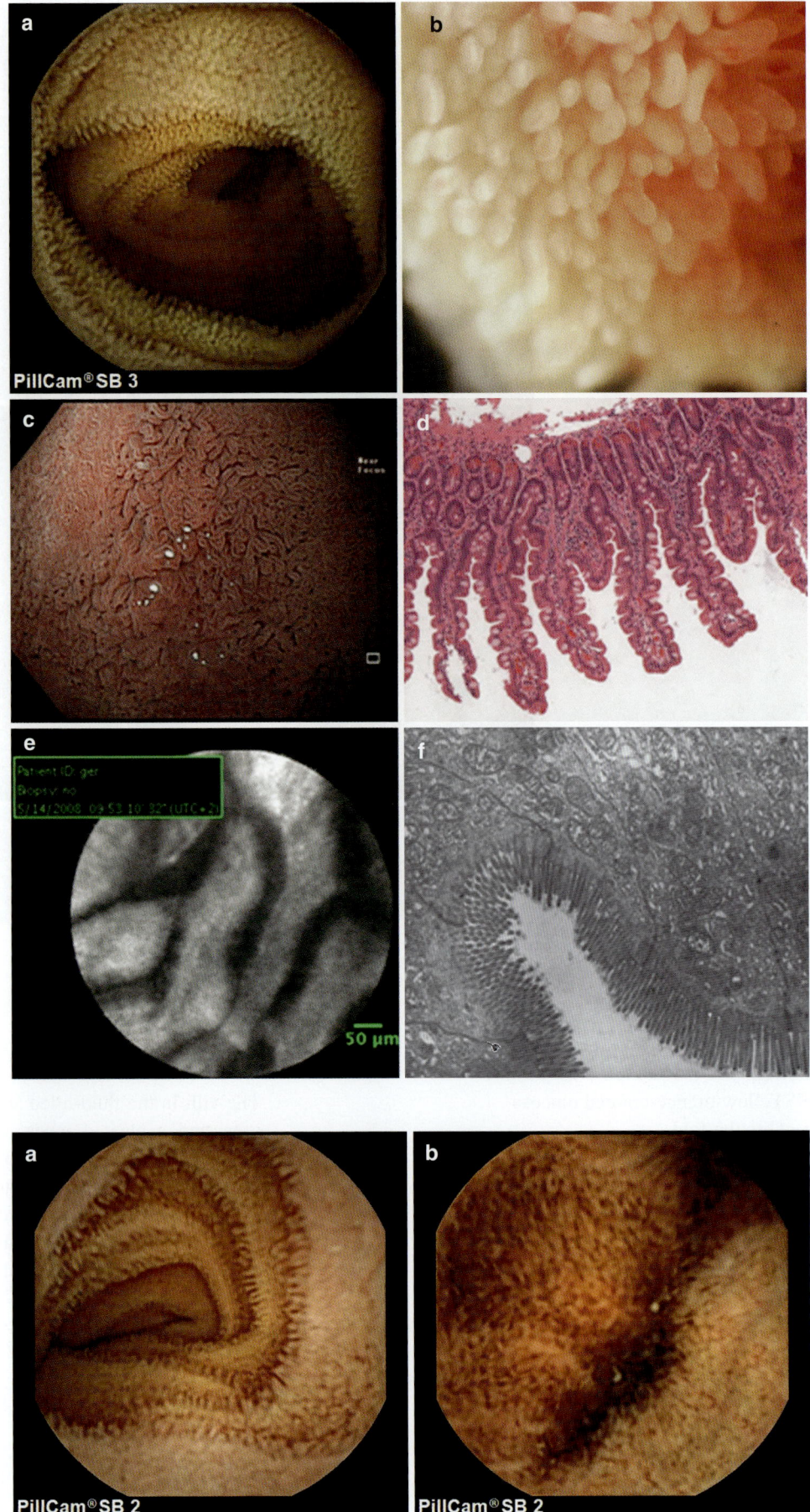

Fig. 19.4 The jejunum (**a**) and ileum (**b**) cannot be reliably distinguished by endoscopy just by the appearance of their villi

Fig. 19.5 Vessels have a smaller caliber in the jejunum (**a** VCE; **b** flexible spectral imaging color enhancement (FICE)–1 mode) than in the ileum (**c** VCE; **d** FICE1)

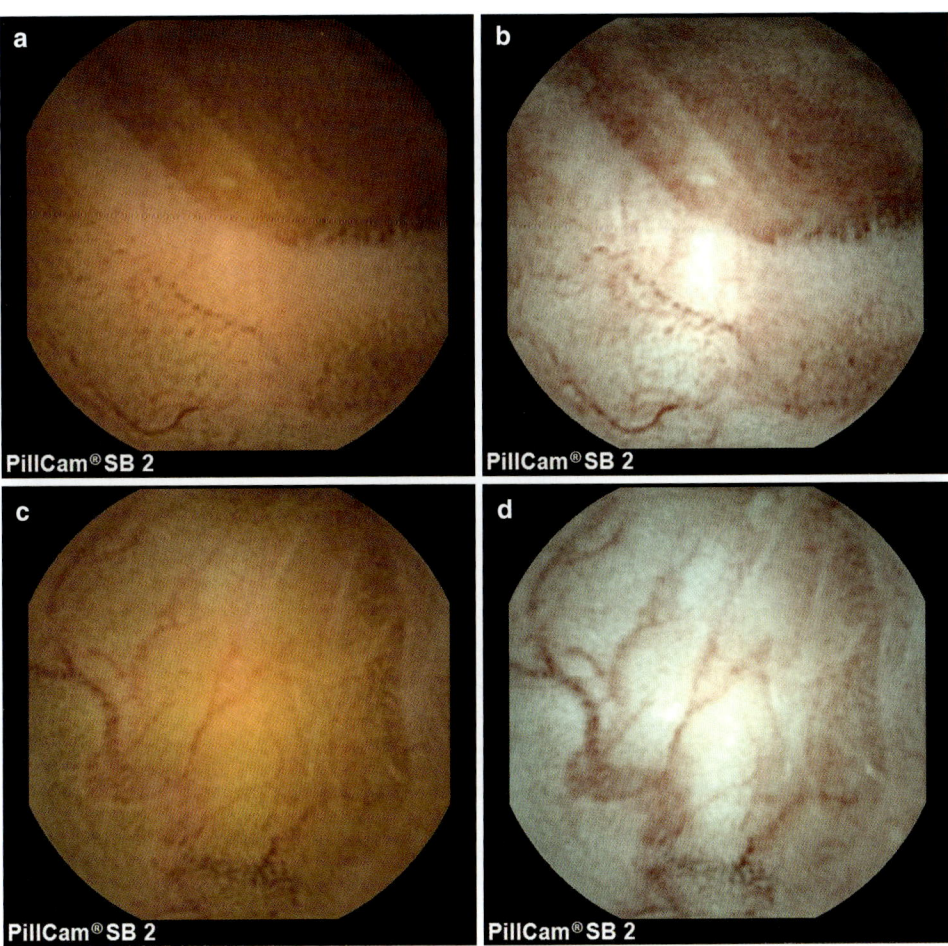

19.4.2 Vessels

Blood vessels are most clearly visualized when viewed directly from above. The vascular pattern in the ileum is more distinct than in the other segments (Fig. 19.5).

19.4.3 Motility

The small bowel shows brisk peristaltic activity, recognized by the contraction and migration of the valvulae conniventes and small superimposed folds. The contractions show varying temporal patterns, with smaller bidirectional movements and intermittent forceful, propulsive contractions (Fig. 19.6). This pattern may temporarily arrest the movement of the capsule, propel it quickly forward, or occasionally cause it to move backward. In contrast to flexible endoscopy, bowel motility can be observed during VCE with no effects from air insufflation or sedatives.

However, the use of prokinetic drugs to hasten the gastric passage of the capsule, as well as bowel preparation before VCE, may have a significant influence on small intestinal transit time. Transit times have been measured in patients, whereas data on healthy subjects are sparse. (Small intestinal transit in a small number of healthy volunteers was found to be 143 min [6].) So far, experience in interpreting motility observations is limited. Variations in speed are demonstrated by a speed/time bar in RAPID software (Given Imaging, Yoqneam, Israel) (Fig. 19.7). Software algorithms are under investigation to analyze motion patterns from VCE images [7]. A new capsule type, measuring pH, temperature, and pressure (SmartPill, Given Imaging), has been developed, able to investigate transit times of the stomach, small bowel, and colon [8]. Intermittent pressure waves can be seen during the small bowel passage (Fig. 19.8). The capsule may move past the same lesion several times because of bidirectional peristalsis, mimicking the presence of multiple lesions.

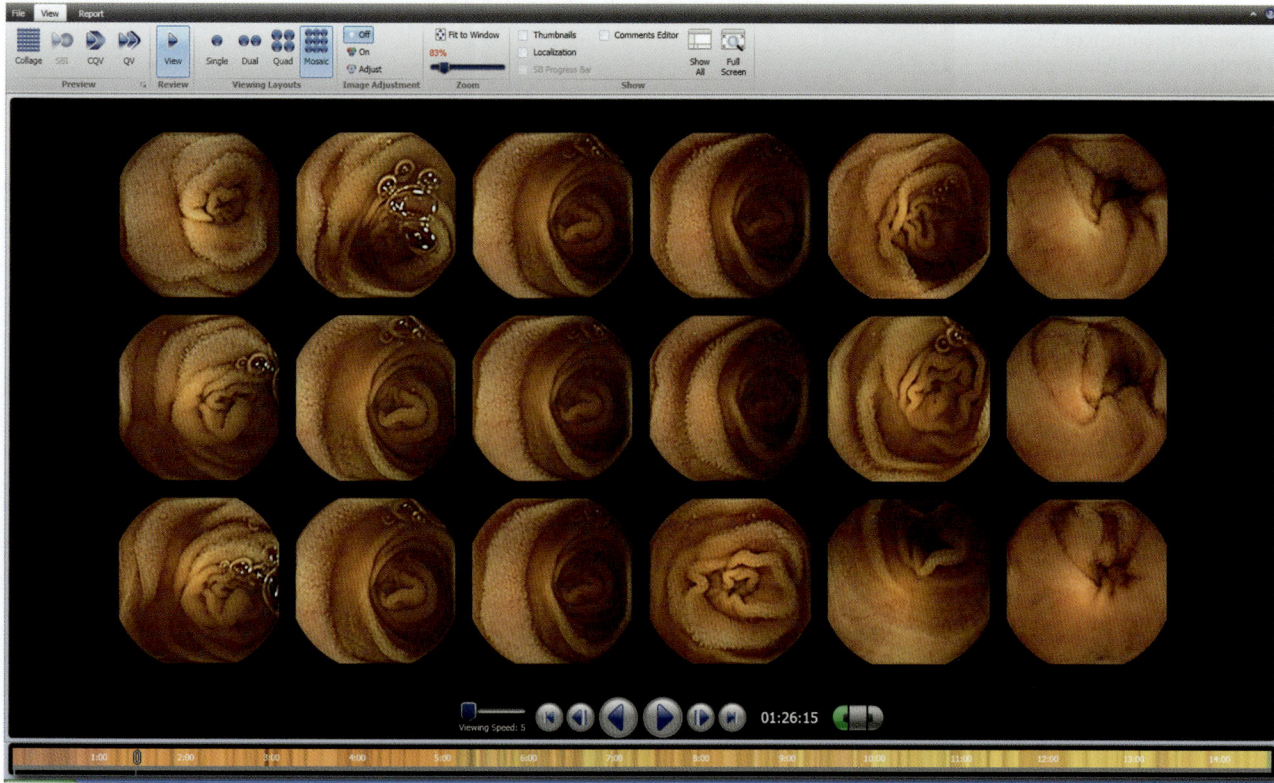

Fig. 19.6 Different phases of small bowel contractions displayed in overview mode

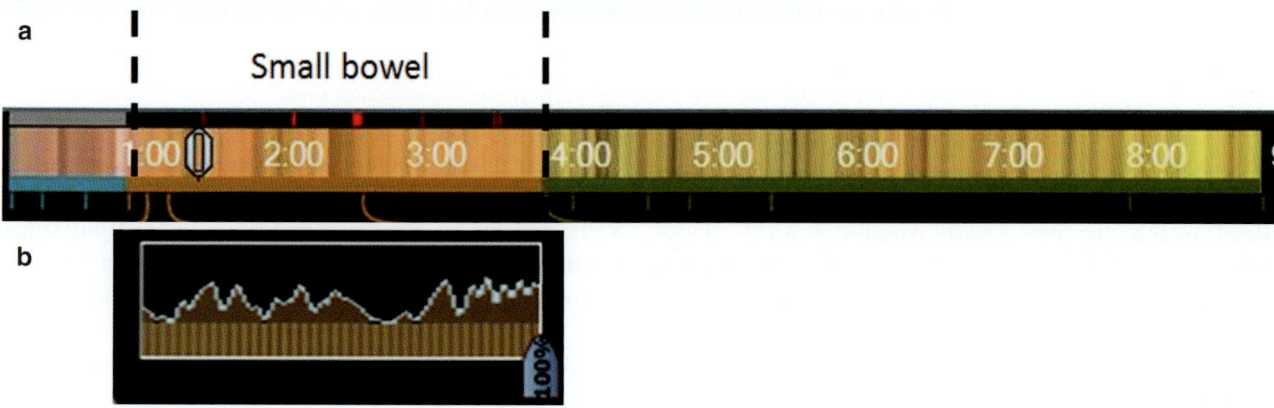

Fig. 19.7 (**a**) Time bar with mean image color. (**b**) After defining the landmarks for start and end of small bowel transit, Rapid 8 software displays another bar showing variation of capsule speed during small bowel passage

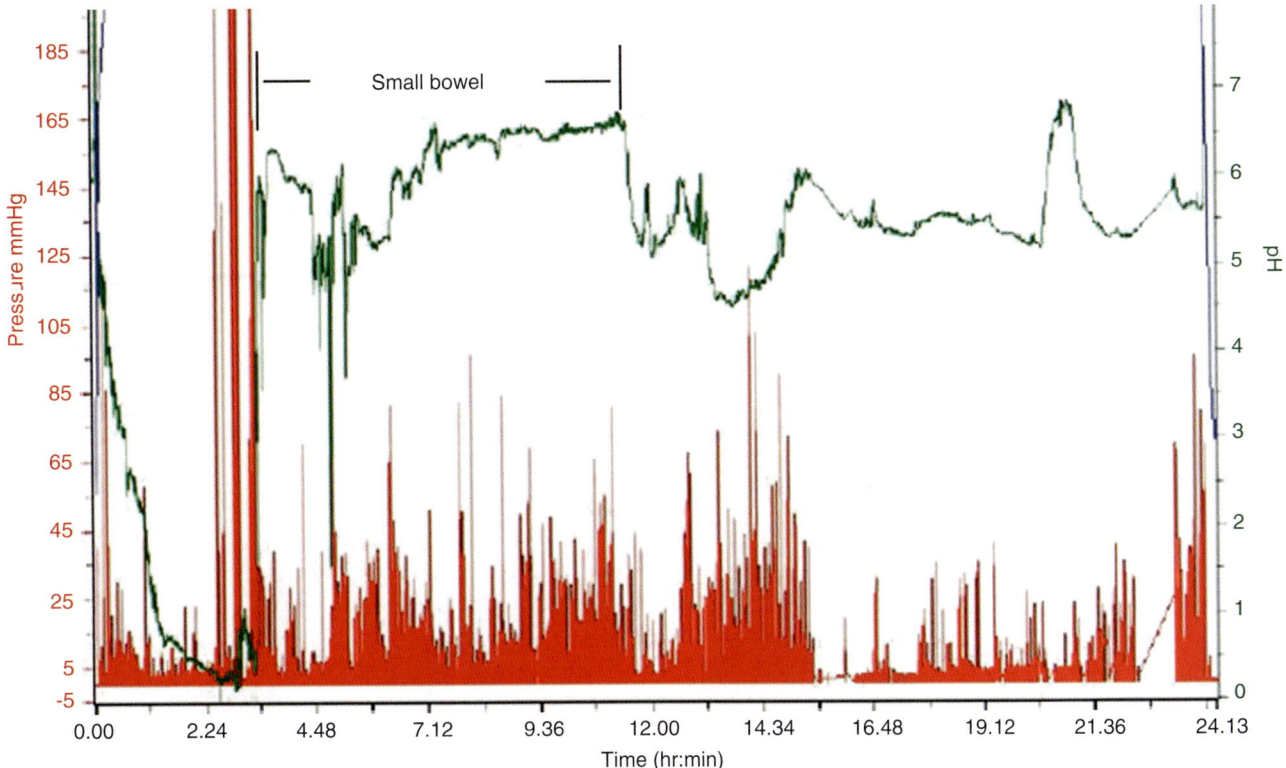

Fig. 19.8 Wireless SmartPill study. Small bowel motility as measured by pressure (*red curve*) is seen as intermittent peristalsis. Before passage from the stomach to the duodenum, there are strong contractions followed by a rapid increase of pH (*green curve*). A slight drop in pH signals passage to the colon

19.5 Subdivision of the Small Intestine

As no anatomic landmarks are available, the subdivision of the small bowel in VCE interpretation is based purely on pragmatic considerations. The time that elapses between the reference points of the pylorus and the first cecal image is divided into three equal parts. Thus, the small bowel segments in VCE may be listed in this way:

- Duodenum
- Proximal third of the small bowel
- Middle third of the small bowel
- Distal third of the small bowel
- Terminal ileum

The jejunum and ileum are hardly distinguishable by their endoscopic features, but the duodenum and terminal ileum can be identified. Localization software is occasionally helpful in distinguishing the distal duodenum from the jejunum and the terminal ileum from the mid ileum. These boundaries cannot be precisely defined, however.

19.5.1 Duodenum

While the capsule is still in the stomach, it is occasionally possible to get a transpyloric view into the duodenal bulb (Fig. 19.9a). If the capsule is pointing in a favorable direction, the distal aspect of the pylorus may be visible from within the bulb as a circular ridge (Fig. 19.9b-d). This happens in about one-third of all examinations [9] and should not be mistaken for abnormal folds or tumors, especially as this view may reappear after some time because of retrograde movement of the capsule. Brunner's glands may produce a nodular mucosal pattern (Fig. 19.10). Folds are first seen past the apex of the bulb (Fig. 19.11a), and circular folds first appear in the descending duodenum (Fig. 19.11b). Bile is usually visible in the bowel lumen at this level.

Fig. 19.9 (**a**) View through the pylorus into the duodenal bulb. (**b**) Retrograde view of the pylorus from within the duodenal bulb in the same patient. (**c, d**) VCE showing retrograde view of the pylorus in other patients

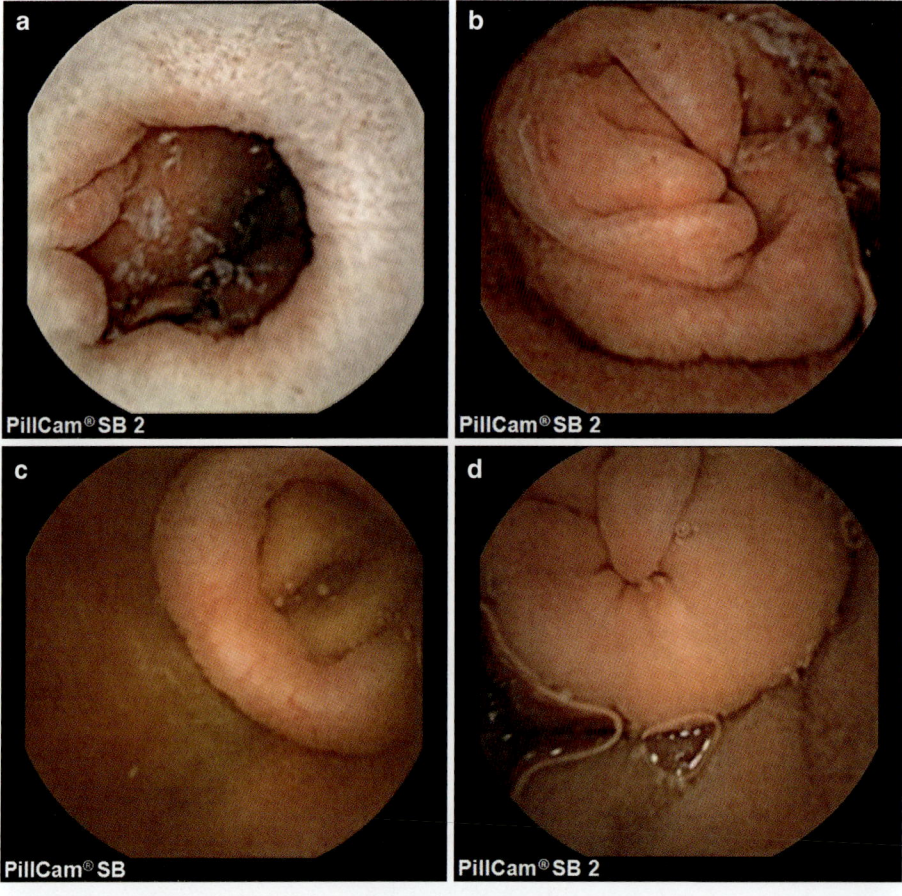

Fig. 19.10 (**a**) Micronodular hyperplasia of Brunner's glands in the duodenal bulb. (**b**) Small nodules of ectopic gastric mucosa close to the pylorus

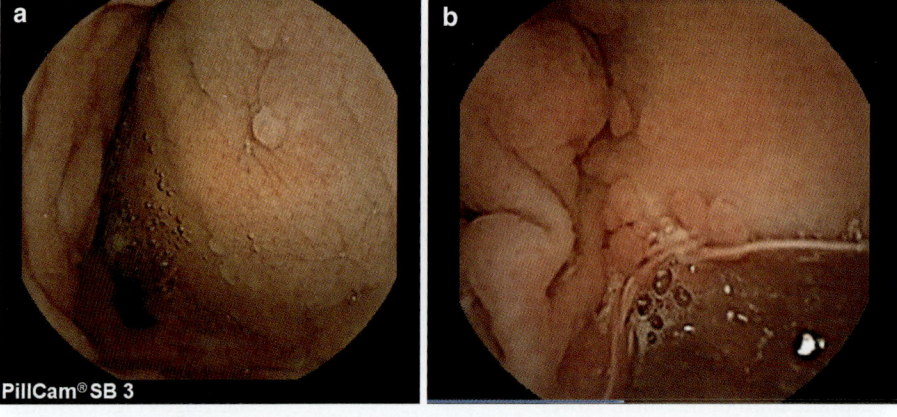

Fig. 19.11 (**a**) Duodenum, distal bulb. (**b**) Duodenum, descending portion

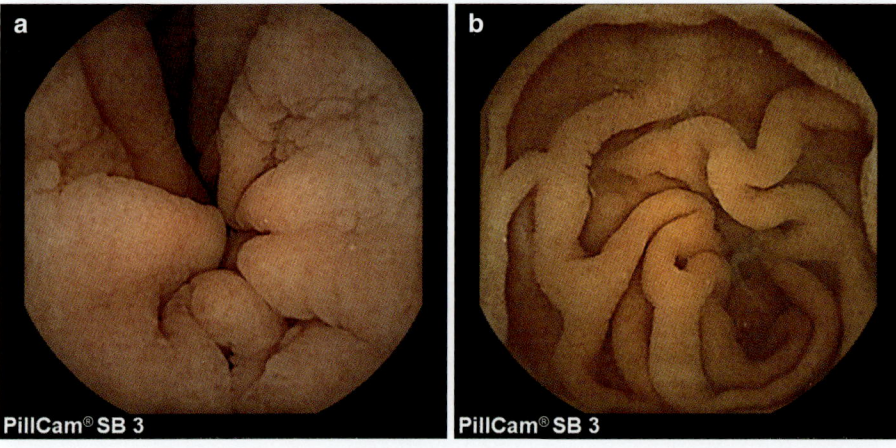

19.5.2 Papilla of Vater

The papilla of Vater (Fig. 19.12) is imaged in only about 18 % of patients by small bowel capsule endoscopy [9], but in 60 % with a double-headed colon capsule [10]. The minor papilla is very rarely seen (Fig. 44.26). Time after ingestion to reach the papilla is quite variable, as is the time interval between passage through the pylorus to the papilla. Usually this takes only seconds to a few minutes, but rarely, prolonged stay of the capsule in the duodenum or retroperistalsis may cause visualization of the papilla up to 1 or 2 h after it passes the pylorus.

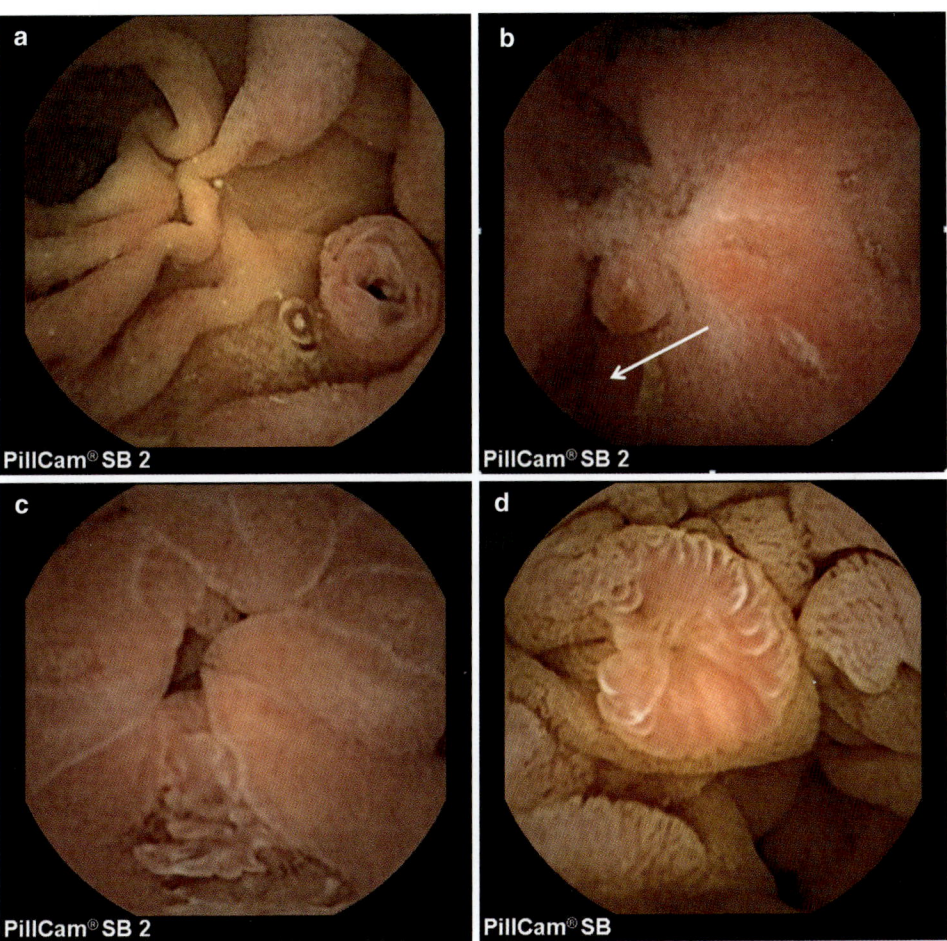

Fig. 19.12 (**a–d**) Variants of the papilla of Vater; (**b**) shows flow of bile (*arrow*)

19.5.3 Jejunum and Ileum

Kerckring's folds or valvulae conniventes are a typical endoscopic feature of the small bowel (Fig. 19.13). They appear in the descending duodenum, sparing the duodenal bulb. Kerckring's folds are more dense and prominent in the jejunum than in the ileum, although there is no clear boarder (Fig. 19.14).

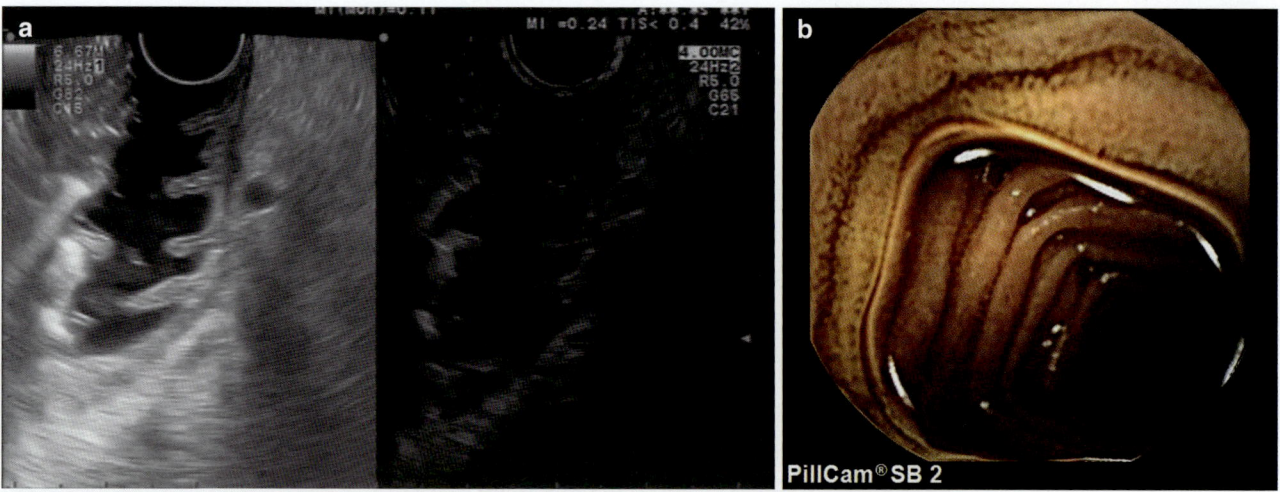

Fig. 19.13 Kerckring's folds. (**a**) Endoscopic ultrasound. (**b**) VCE

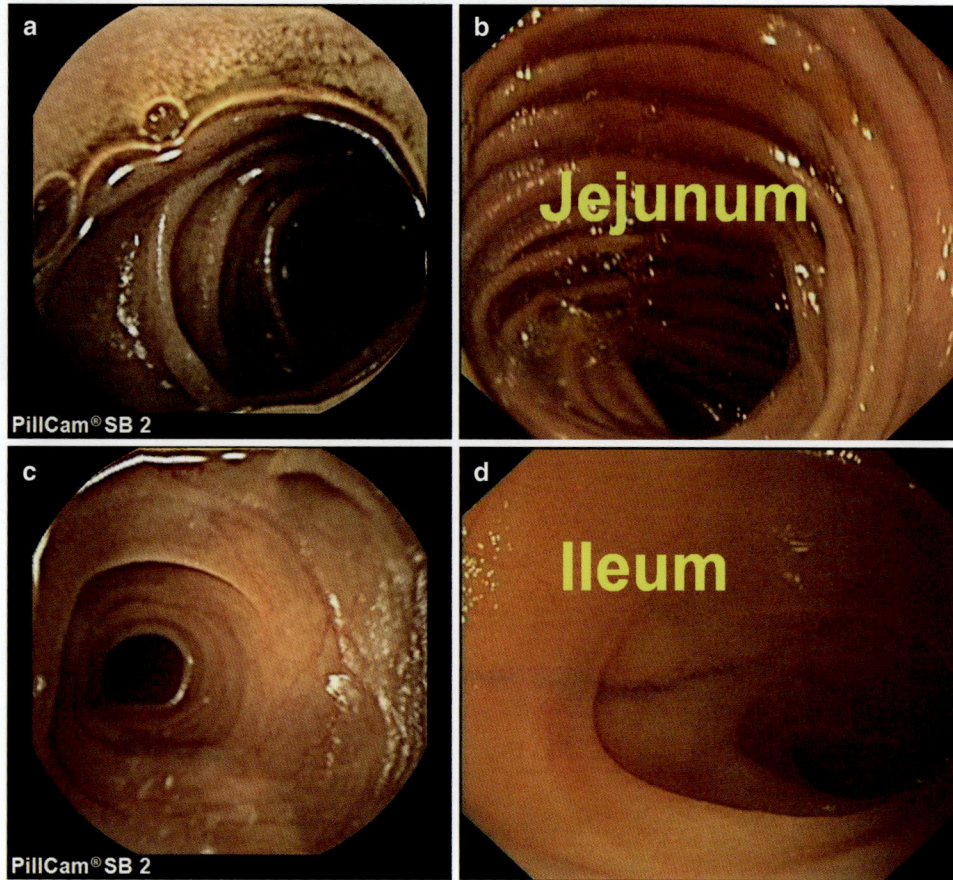

Fig. 19.14 Kerckring's folds are more dense and prominent in the jejunum (**a** VCE; **b** spiral enteroscopy) than in the ileum (**c** VCE; **d** spiral enteroscopy)

19.5.4 Common Findings

In the duodenal bulb, small Brunner's glands (Fig. 19.10a) and islets of heterotopic gastric mucosa (Fig. 19.10b) are frequent findings. White lines are a normal feature of small intestinal mucosa when the capsule is looking at the edge of a fold (Figs. 19.13 and 19.14), with the villi bent to both sides (Fig. 19.15). Small foci of white villi and flat or protruding lymphatic cysts are harmless lesions (Fig. 19.16). Occasionally adjacent organs, such as the liver or spleen, may produce a blue shadow (Fig. 19.17). Impressions from other small intestinal loops present as bulges (Chap. 5).

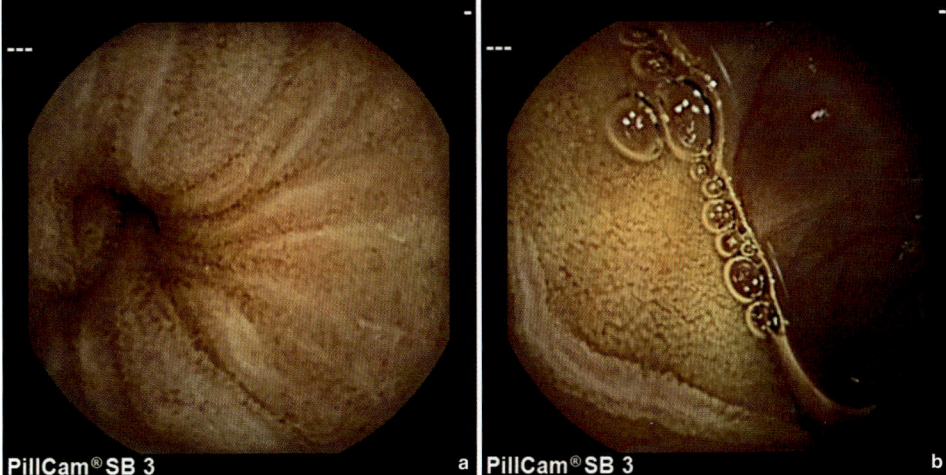

Fig. 19.15 (**a**, **b**) White lines are a normal feature of small bowel at VCE

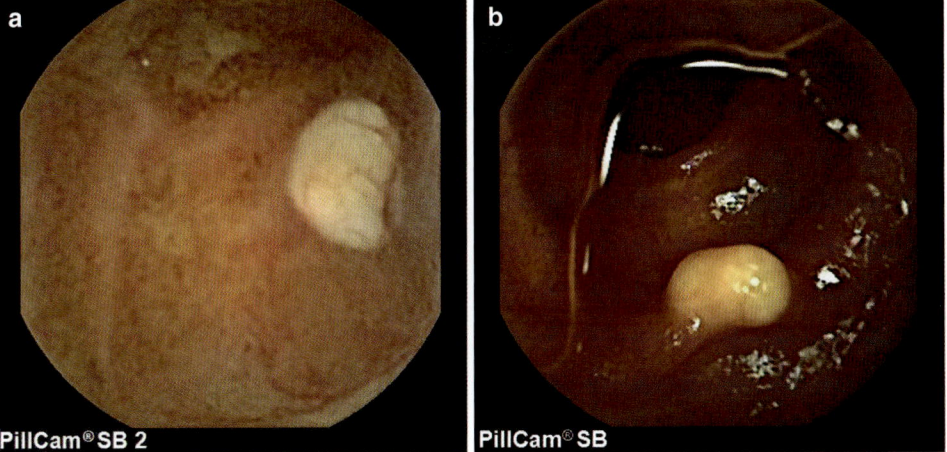

Fig. 19.16 Variants of normal: flat (**a**) and elevated (**b**) small lymphatic cysts

Fig. 19.17 (**a**, **b**) *Blue shadow* behind the small intestinal wall; localization in the right upper quadrant is suggestive for liver

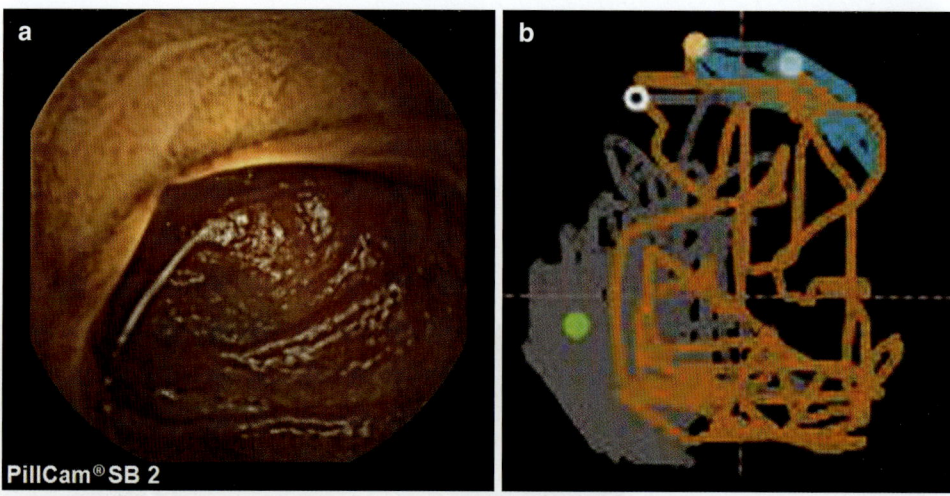

19.5.5 Terminal Ileum

A characteristic feature of the terminal ileum is the presence of multiple small lymph follicles (Figs. 19.18 and 19.19).

The vascular markings are more conspicuous than in the proximal small bowel. Sometimes vision is obscured due to inspissated bile, air bubbles, or feces.

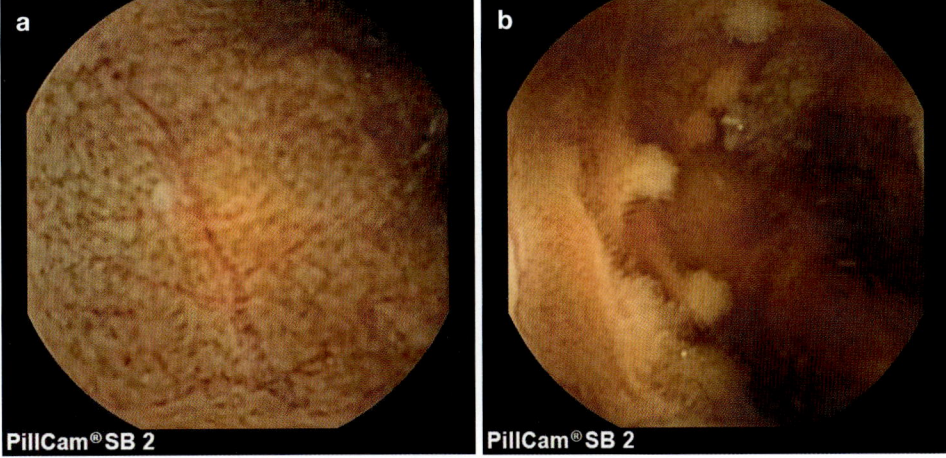

Fig. 19.18 Lymph follicles in the terminal ileum. (**a**) Diminutive, white nodule. (**b**) Medium-sized, pedunculated nodules

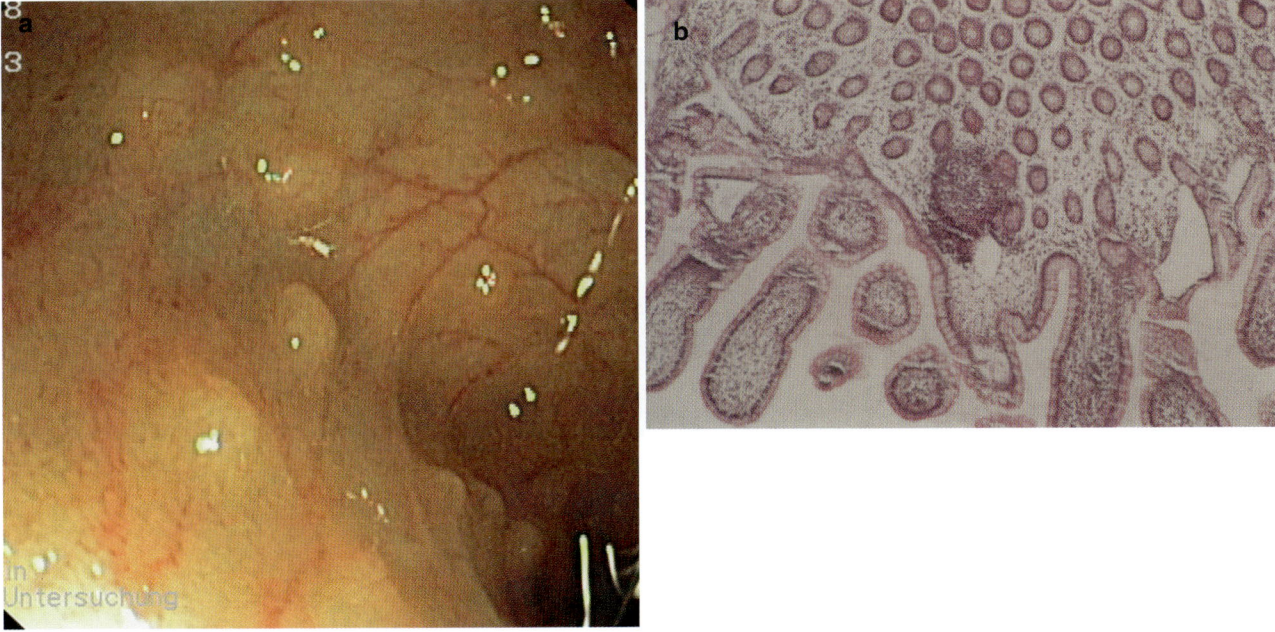

Fig. 19.19 (**a**) Small lymph follicles at flexible ileoscopy. (**b**) Histology showing small lymph follicle, hematoxylin and eosin stain (Courtesy of Jörg Caselitz, MD)

19.5.6 Ileocecal Valve

At the ileocecal valve, sometimes longitudinal, stretched vessels are seen (Fig. 19.20a), and villi may become scattered at this transition zone between the small and large intestines (Fig. 19.20b). The ileocecal valve is visualized (from the cecum, Fig. 19.21) in about 20 % of all patients [9]. The capsule may move back and forth in the terminal ileum for some time. Passage of the capsule through the valve itself is usually very abrupt, yielding only an initial image of the colon.

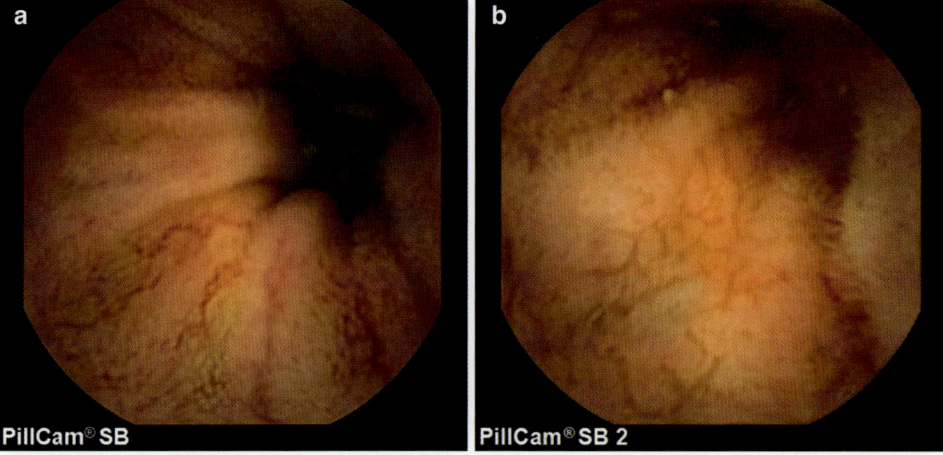

Fig. 19.20 (**a**) Longitudinal vessel at the ileocecal valve. (**b**) Villous alterations are normal directly before the opening of the ileocecal valve, including mosaic pattern and focal atrophy

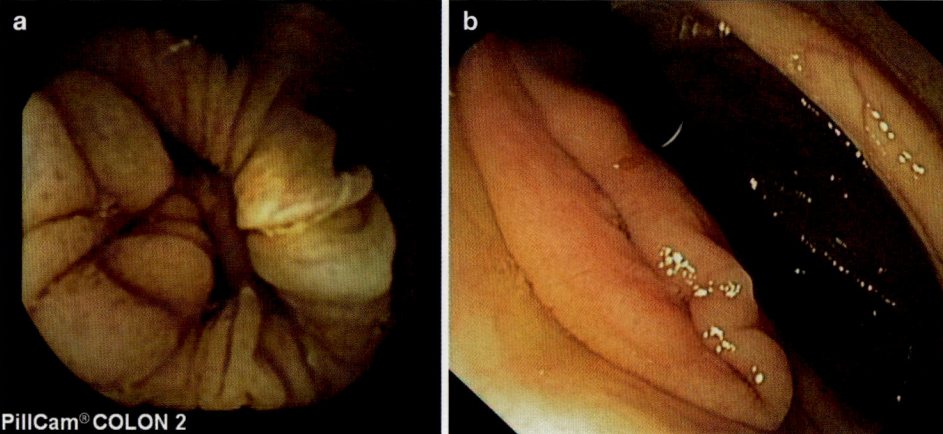

Fig. 19.21 Ileocecal valve visible from the cecum at VCE (**a**) and at endoscopic retroflexion (**b**)

References

1. von Herbay A. Anatomie, Entwicklung und Fehlbildungen von Dünn- und Dickdarm. In: Caspary WF, Stein J, editors. Darmkrankheiten. Klinik, Diagnostik und Therapie. Berlin/Heidelberg/New York: Springer; 1999. p. 3–16.
2. Gondolesi G, Ramisch D, Padin J, et al. What is the normal small bowel length in humans? First donor-based cohort analysis. Am J Transplant. 2012;12 Suppl 4:S49–54.
3. Cronin CG, Delappe E, Lohan DG, et al. Normal small bowel wall characteristics on MR enterography. Eur J Radiol. 2010;75:207–11.
4. Dobbins 3rd WO. Diagnostic pathology of the intestinal mucosa. An atlas and review of biopsy interpretation. Berlin/Heidelberg/New York: Springer; 1990.
5. Bellutti M, Mönkemüller K, Fry LC, et al. Characterization of yellow plaques found in the small bowel during double-balloon enteroscopy. Endoscopy. 2007;39:1059–63.
6. Gat D, Fireman Z, Scapa E, et al. Transit times for the capsule endoscop--ffect of colon prep on small bowel transit time of the capsule. Endoscopy. 2001;33(Suppl I):A2004.
7. Drozdzal M, Segui S, Vitria J, et al. Adaptable image cuts for motility inspection using WCE. Comput Med Imaging Graph. 2013;37:72–80.
8. Iida H, Endo H, Sekino Y, et al. A new non-invasive modality for recording sequential images and the pH of the small bowel. Hepatogastroentcrology. 2012;59:413–4.
9. Nakamura M, Ohmiya N, Shirai O. Advance of video capsule endoscopy and the detection of anatomic landmarks. Hepatogastroenterology. 2009;56:1600–5.
10. Karagiannis S, Ducker C, Dautel P, et al. Identification of the duodenal papilla by colon capsule endoscope. Z Gastroenterol. 2010;48:753–5.

Diverticula

20

André Van Gossum, Martin Keuchel, and Ervin Tóth

Contents

The work was first published in 2006 by Springer Medizin Verlag Heidelberg with the following title: *Atlas of Video Capsule Endoscopy*.

A. Van Gossum (✉)
Department of Hepato-Gastroenterology,
Erasme Hospital—Free University of Brussels, Brussels, Belgium
e-mail: andre.vangossum@erasme.ulb.ac.be

M. Keuchel
Department of Internal Medicine,
Bethesda Krankenhaus Bergedorf, Hamburg, Germany
e-mail: keuchel@bkb.info

E. Tóth
Department of Gastroenterology,
Skåne University Hospital, Malmö, Sweden
e-mail: ervin.toth@med.lu.se

20.1 Acquired Diverticula of the Small Intestine

20.1.1 Definition

Acquired diverticula of the small bowel are pseudodiverticula that protrude through muscular gaps in the mesenteric side of the bowel wall.

20.1.2 Epidemiology

Small bowel diverticula are most commonly located in the duodenum (Figs. 20.1 and 20.2), followed by the jejunum; they are very rarely found in the ileum [1]. Diverticula in the jejunum or ileum occur in 1–5 % of the population [2].

20.1.3 Clinical Features

Acquired diverticula are usually asymptomatic. They occasionally present with abdominal pain, intestinal bleeding [3], perforation [4], and less commonly with bowel obstruction [5, 6] or bacterial overgrowth [7].

20.1.4 Endoscopy

A small diverticular opening is easy to identify by video capsule endoscopy (VCE) (Fig. 20.3). With a larger opening, it is very common to find a septum between the mouth of the diverticulum and the bowel lumen (Fig. 20.2), an apparent double lumen, and folds radiating into the neck of the diverticulum. These features are difficult to distinguish from an acute bend in a normal loop of small bowel. The capsule may linger for some time in the area of the diverticulum or may enter a larger diverticular pouch (Fig. 20.1). Capsule entrapment in small bowel diverticulosis has been reported [8]. In small intestinal diverticulosis, multiple

Fig. 20.1 PillCam Colon capsule (Given Imaging, Yoqneam, Israel) entrapped in a large duodenal diverticulum with the typical trabecular aspect. (**a**) Localization trace shows lack of progression. The capsule was excreted spontaneously later. (**b**) Side-viewing duodenoscopy. (**c**) CT scan with large diverticulum (*arrow*)

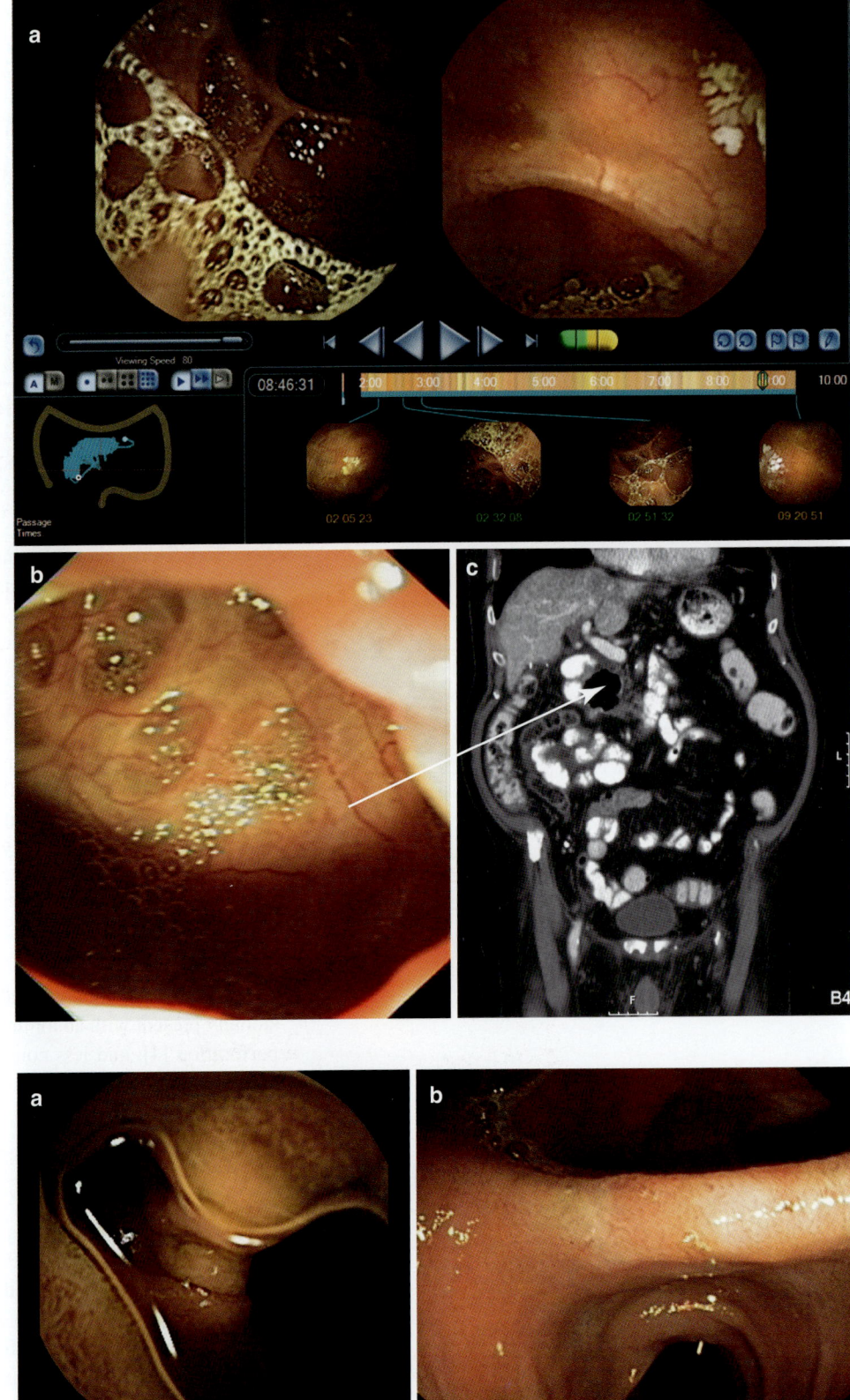

Fig. 20.2 Duodenal diverticulum as seen using video capsule endoscopy (VCE) (**a**) and a side-viewing duodenoscope (**b**)

Fig. 20.3 Medium- and small-sized diverticula of the small bowel, as seen with VCE (**a, c**) and single-balloon enteroscopy (**b, d**). Incidental findings in a patient with Peutz-Jeghers syndrome

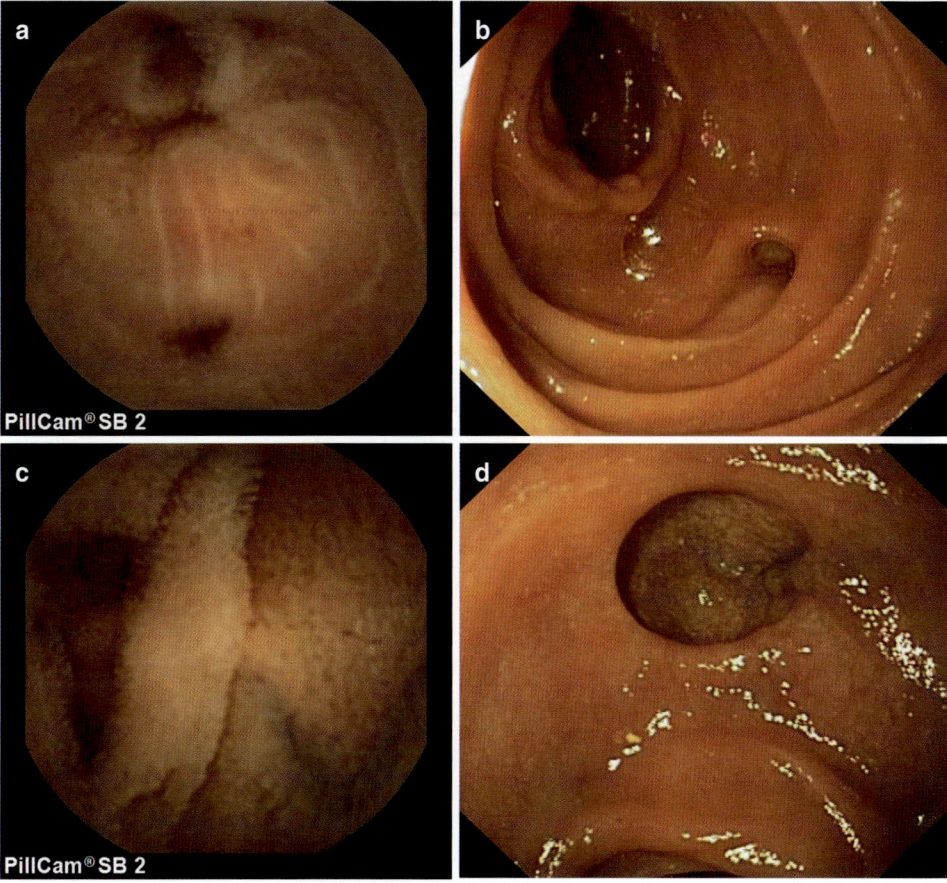

Fig. 20.4 (**a, b**) Diverticulosis of the small intestine

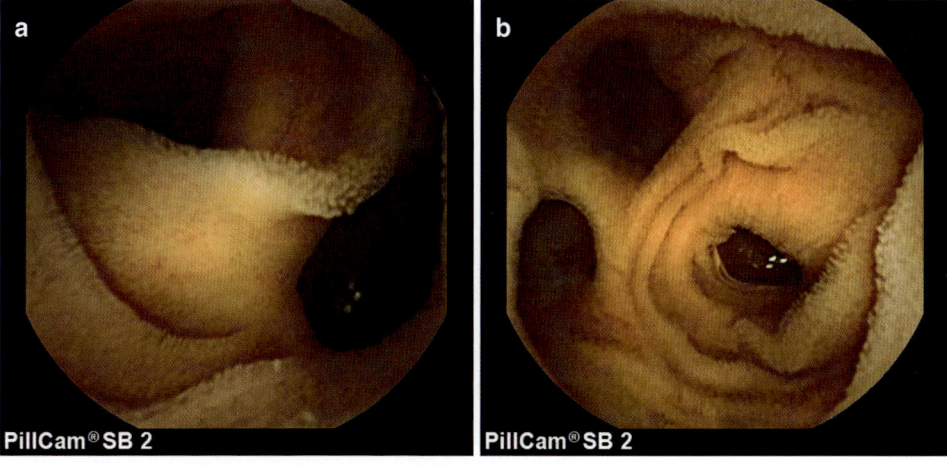

diverticula are seen (Fig. 20.4). Occasionally large vessels within a diverticulum, a potential source of bleeding, can be visualized (Fig. 20.5). Fresh blood in a small bowel segment with diverticula can help in localization of the origin of bleeding (Fig. 20.6). Peridiverticular redness and ulceration are endoscopic signs of diverticulitis (Fig. 20.7). Detection by double-balloon enteroscopy of diverticula missed by VCE has been reported [9]; probably the rapid passage of the capsule and lack of luminal distension were responsible for the failure of VCE.

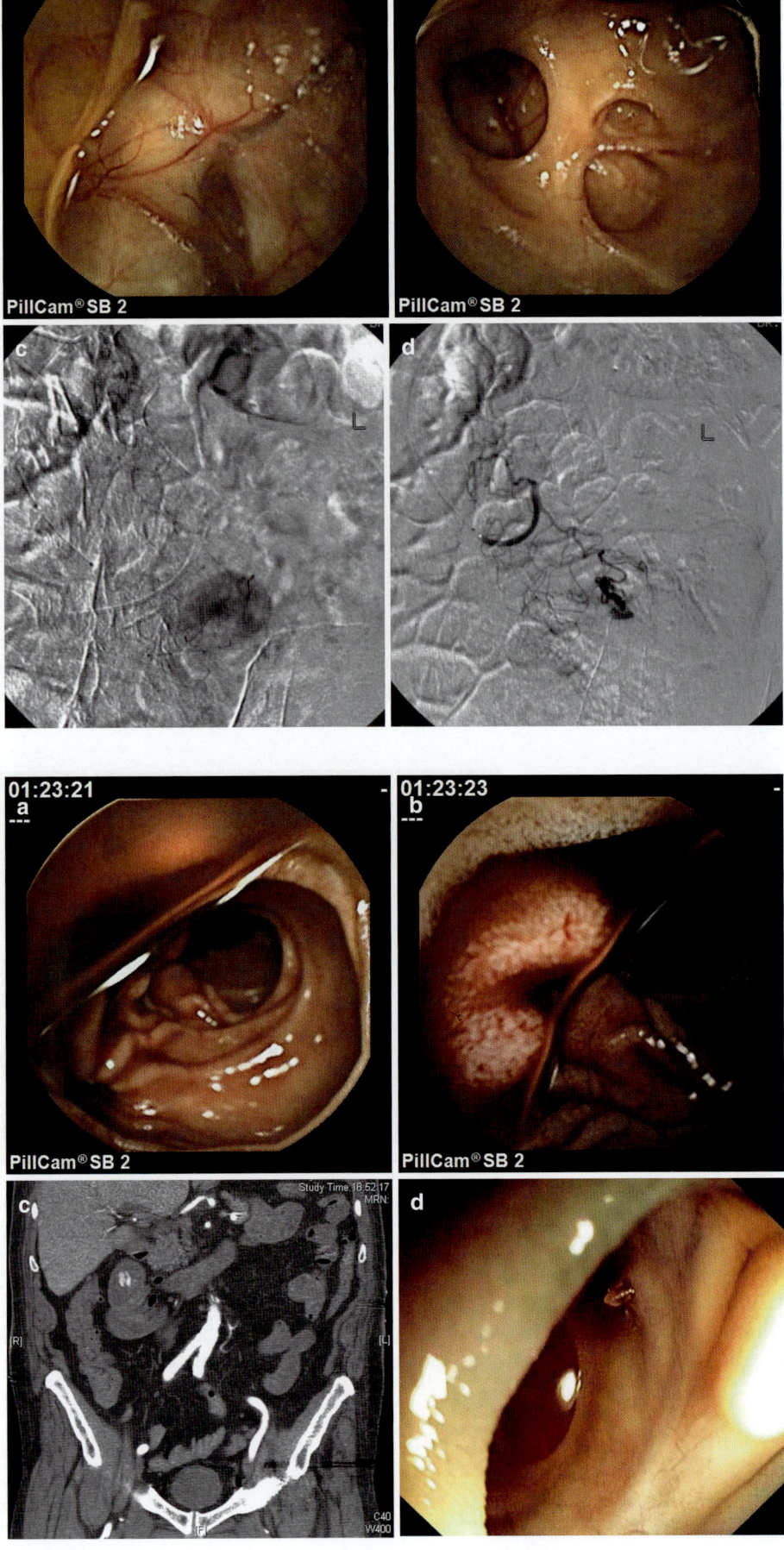

Fig. 20.5 Small bowel diverticulum. This elderly patient had recurrent transfusion-dependent bleeding initially considered to be from known colonic diverticula. A large vessel at the bottom of the diverticulum was seen by VCE (**a**, **b**) and selective angiography (**c**, **d**). No rebleeding occurred after coiling (Courtesy of Matthias Joanowitsch, MD)

Fig. 20.6 Active bleeding from jejunal diverticulosis, as seen with VCE (**a**, **b**), urgent CT angiography (**c**) (Courtesy of Jörg Sievers, MD). Urgent push enteroscopy (**d**) shows a blood vessel in one of the diverticula

20.1.5 Treatment

Most diverticula of the small intestine do not require treatment [10]. Antibiotics may be indicated for patients with diverticulitis or bacterial overgrowth in the diverticular pouch. Surgical treatment is necessary in cases of perforation, bowel obstruction due to volvulus or intussusception, and massive bleeding [11, 12].

20.2 Meckel's Diverticulum

20.2.1 Definition

A Meckel's diverticulum results from an abnormal persistence of the embryonic vitelline (omphalomesenteric) duct. It is the most common gastrointestinal anomaly, with a prev-

alence of up to 3 %. In adults, it is typically located on the antimesenteric side of the bowel 60–90 cm oral to the ileocecal valve (Fig. 20.8). In approximately 50 % of patients, the diverticulum contains ectopic mucosa, usually gastric mucosa (Figs. 20.9 and 20.10), which may ulcerate (Figs. 20.11 and 20.12) and bleed. Ectopic gastric mucosa can be detected by technetium scanning, but sensitivity in adults is rather low (Fig. 20.10).

20.2.2 Clinical Features

Meckel's diverticula usually are asymptomatic. If clinical manifestations are present, they typically consist of painless intestinal bleeding [13]. Abdominal pain is less common. Diverticulitis, perforation, intussusception, bowel obstruction, and associated tumors are rare.

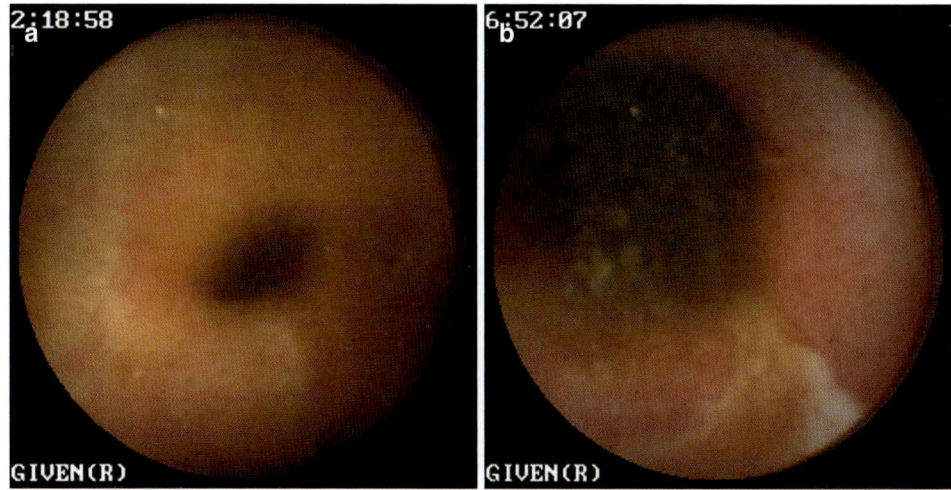

Fig. 20.7 Diverticulitis. (**a**) Multiple diverticula in the small bowel, showing no sign of irritation proximally. (**b**) Distal diverticula showed redness and shallow ulcerations. This patient presented clinically with iron deficiency anemia, and iron kinetics indicated occult gastrointestinal bleeding. Enteroclysis was normal

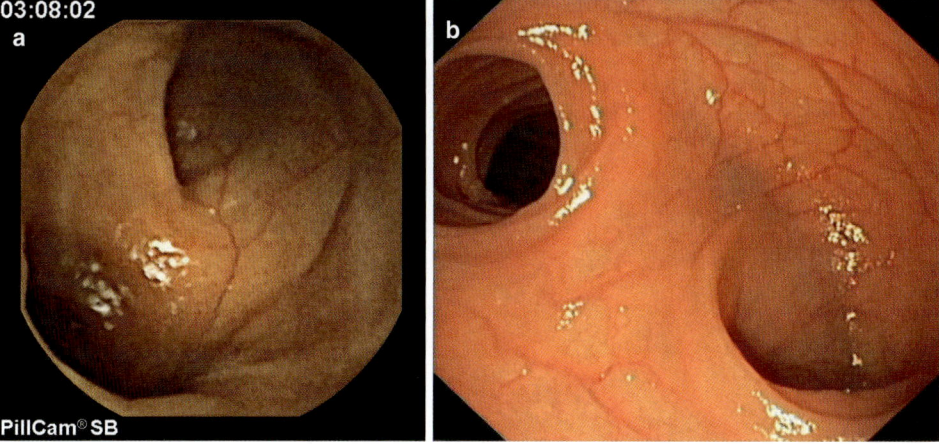

Fig. 20.8 Large entrance of a Meckel's diverticulum without ulceration, on VCE (**a**) and retrograde single-balloon enteroscopy (**b**)

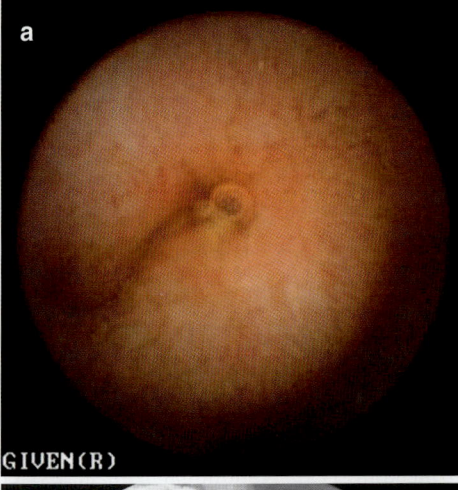

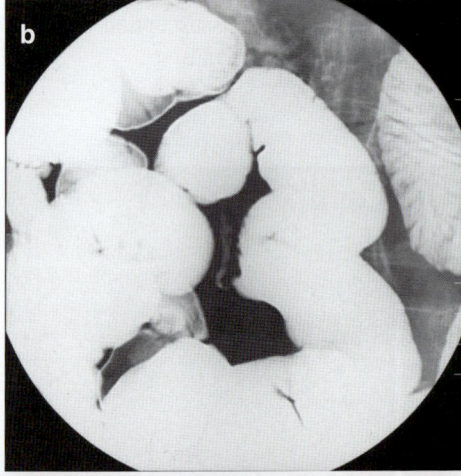

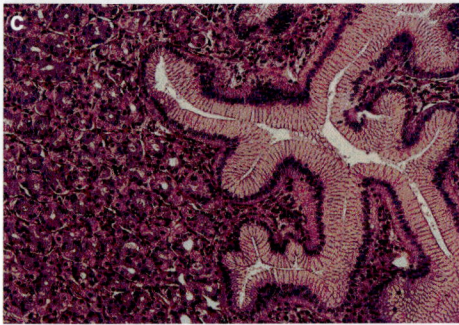

Fig. 20.9 Meckel's diverticulum. (**a**) Small, noninflamed diverticular orifice. (**b**) Enteroclysis shows a very narrow diverticulum. (**c**) Histology shows Meckel's diverticulum with ectopic gastric tissue

20.2.3 Endoscopy

Video capsule endoscopy can detect diverticula of the middle or lower small bowel, possibly with an associated ulcer (Figs. 20.11 and 20.12), ectopic gastric mucosa (Figs. 20.9 and 20.10), or both [14]. Larger diverticula may cause a visible indentation of adjacent small bowel loops. There are isolated cases that can be diagnosed only by VCE [15]. Often it is difficult to distinguish a diverticular septum from a normal fold in an angled loop of small bowel. An everted diverticulum can mimic a tumor [16] or a polyp (Fig. 20.13) [17]. Seldom, active bleeding is observed with a Meckel's diverticulum [18]. A capsule can enter a large Meckel's diverticulum, causing delayed transit or even retention [19]. The capsule may pause at a diverticulum for some time, causing the same pouch to be imaged more than once. No data are currently available on the sensitivity and specificity of VCE in the diagnosis of Meckel's diverticulum. However, detection of Meckel's diverticulum by retrograde double-balloon enteroscopy after inconclusive VCE has been reported [20].

20.2.4 Treatment

Treatment consists of surgical resection in symptomatic patients. Asymptomatic Meckel's diverticula often are removed as a precautionary measure during a surgical procedure for some other indication, although doing so is not routinely recommended for adults [21].

20.3 Small Intestinal Duplication Cysts

Duplication cysts are very rare congenital abnormalities. Like Meckel's diverticulum, they manifest predominantly in childhood. They can occur anywhere in the gastrointestinal tract. When affecting the small intestine, they are located on the mesenteric side, whereas Meckel's diverticulum is found at the antimesenteric side. VCE may show a diverticulum, which can be ulcerated [22] (Fig. 20.14).

Fig. 20.10 (**a**) Polypoid mass of ectopic gastric mucosa in a Meckel's diverticulum. (**b**) Specimen cut open to show portions of the ectopic gastric mucosa (*asterisk*) (Courtesy of Hanns-Olof Wintzer, MD). The patient presented clinically with intestinal bleeding requiring transfusion. Technetium scanning was negative

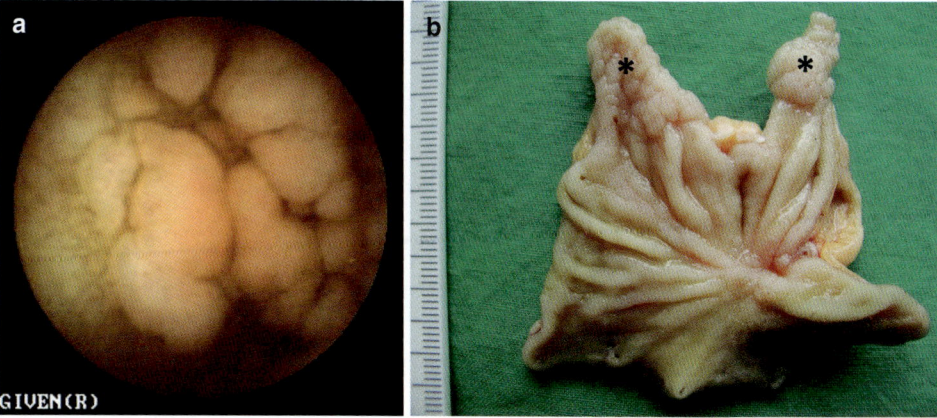

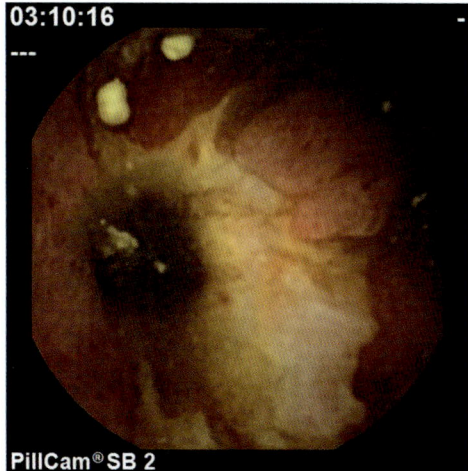

Fig. 20.11 Medium-sized entrance of a Meckel's diverticulum with circular ulceration

Fig. 20.12 Meckel's diverticulum in a 75-year-old patient with transfusion-dependent anemia under thrombocyte aggregation inhibition. (**a, b**) VCE shows two lumina and the edge of an ulcer. Note delayed capsule passage at the diverticulum. (**c, d**) Double-balloon enteroscopy with selective enterography demonstrates the diverticulum and an ulcer of the mucosa opposite the opening of the diverticulum. (**e, f**) Resected specimen (Courtesy of Curosh Taylessani, MD)

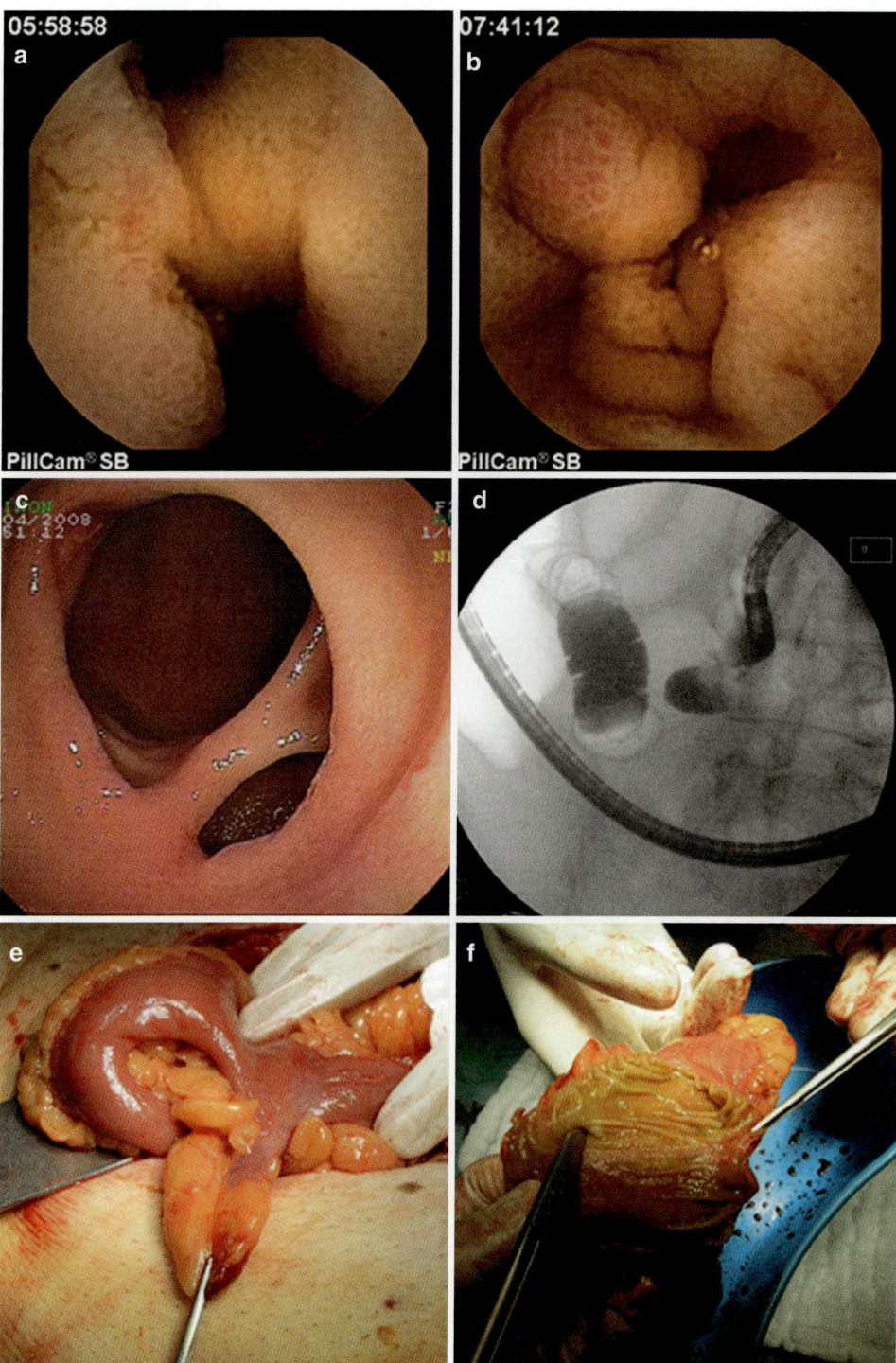

Fig. 20.13 Everted Meckel's diverticulum. (**a**, **c**) Polyp-like tumor with erosion seen in the ileum by VCE. (**b**, **d**) Double-balloon enteroscopy showed a fingerlike polypoid lesion with erosion 80 cm proximal to the ileocecal valve. A biopsy specimen from the lesion showed gastric mucosa (Courtesy of Gabrielle Wurm Johansson MD, Artur Nemeth MD, and Jörgen Nielsen, MD) (From Wurm Johansson et al. [17]; with permission)

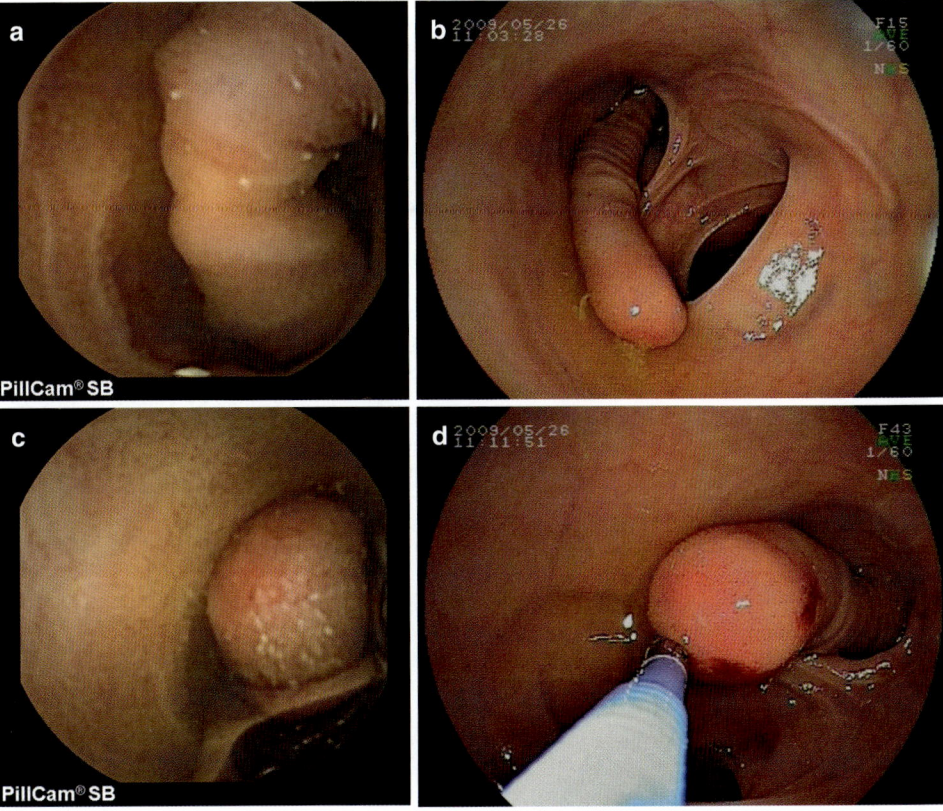

Fig. 20.14 Ileal duplication cyst in an adult with anemia. (**a**, **b**) VCE shows an ulcerated diverticulum. (**c**) Enteroclysis with retained capsule in an ileal diverticulum. (**d**) Mesenteric duplication cyst before resection (From Toth et al. [22]; with permission)

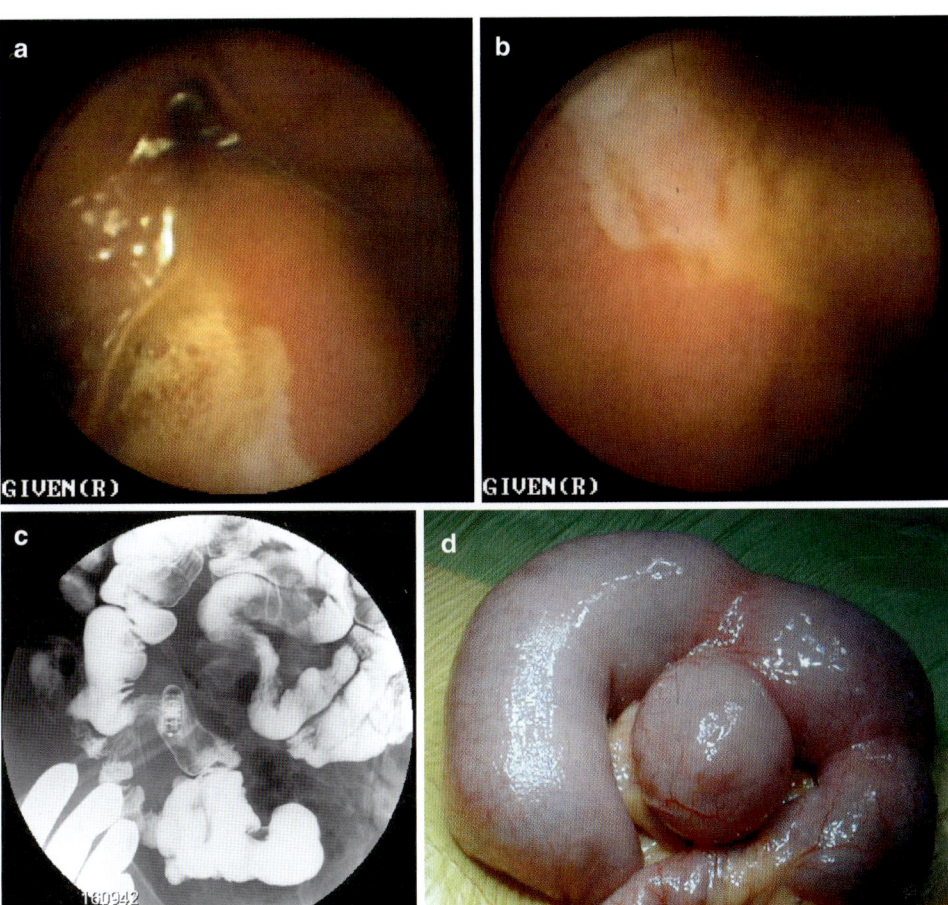

References

1. Akhrass R, Yaffe MB, Fischer C, et al. Small-bowel diverticulosis: perceptions and reality. J Am Coll Surg. 1997;184:383–8.
2. Chow DC, Babaian M, Taubin HL. Jejunoileal diverticula. Gastroenterologist. 1997;5:78–84.
3. Baltes P, Matsui U, Sievers J, Keuchel M. Jejunal diverticulum with active bleeding. Video J Encyclopedia GI Endosc. 2013;1: 248–9.
4. Butler JS, Collins CG, McEntee GP. Perforated jejunal diverticula: a case report. J Med Case Rep. 2010;4:172.
5. Agnifili A, Gola P, Gianfelice F, et al. Rare digestive hemorrhage caused by diverticular pathology of the small intestine. Minerva Chir. 1990;45:721–4.
6. Kouraklis G, Mantas D, Glivanou A, et al. Diverticular disease of the small bowel: report of 27 cases. Int Surg. 2001;86:235–9.
7. Choung RS, Ruff KC, Malhotra A, et al. Clinical predictors of small intestinal bacterial overgrowth by duodenal aspirate culture. Aliment Pharmacol Ther. 2011;33:1059–67.
8. Gaba RC, Schlesinger PK, Wilbur AC. Endoscopic video capsules: radiologic findings of spontaneous entrapment in small intestinal diverticula. AJR Am J Roentgenol. 2005;185:1048–50.
9. Hussain SA, Esposito SP, Rubin M. Identification of small bowel diverticula with double-balloon enteroscopy following non-diagnostic capsule endoscopy. Dig Dis Sci. 2009;54:2296–7.
10. Wilcox RD, Shatney CH. Surgical implications of jejunal diverticula. South Med J. 1988;81:1386–91.
11. Wilcox RD, Shatney CH. Surgical significance of acquired ileal diverticulosis. Am Surg. 1990;56:222–5.
12. Nightingale S, Nikfarjam M, Iles L, Djeric M. Small bowel diverticular disease complicated by perforation. Aust N Z J Surg. 2003;73:867–9.
13. Chiu EJ, Shyr YM, Su CH, et al. Diverticular disease of the small bowel. Hepatogastroenterology. 2000;47:181–4.
14. Baltes P, Steinbrück I, Stövesand-Ruge B, et al. Endoscopic appearance of Meckel's diverticulum. Video J Encyclopedia GI Endosc. 2013;1:223–5.
15. Mylonaki M, MacLean D, Fritscher-Ravens A, Swain P. Wireless capsule endoscopic detection of Meckel's diverticulum after nondiagnostic surgery. Endoscopy. 2002;34:1018–20.
16. Dubcenco E, Tang SJ, Streutker CJ, et al. Meckel's diverticulum mimicking small bowel tumor. Gastrointest Endosc. 2004;60:263.
17. Wurm Johansson G, Nemeth A, Nielsen J, et al. An unusual case of chronic blood loss in the small intestine. Gut. 2011;60:773.
18. Tang SJ, Dubcenco E, Kortan P. Bleeding Meckel's diverticulum. Gastrointest Endosc. 2004;60:264.
19. Courcoutsakis N, Pitiakoudis M, Mimidis K, et al. Capsule retention in a giant Meckel's diverticulum containing multiple enteroliths. Endoscopy. 2011;43 Suppl 2:E308–9.
20. Manner H, May A, Nachbar L, Ell C. Push-and-pull enteroscopy using the double-balloon technique (double-balloon enteroscopy) for the diagnosis of Meckel's diverticulum in adult patients with GI bleeding of obscure origin. Am J Gastroenterol. 2006;101:1152–4.
21. Stone PA, Hofeldt MJ, Campbell JE, et al. Meckel diverticulum: ten-year experience in adults. South Med J. 2004;97:1038–41.
22. Toth E, Lillienau J, Ekelund M, et al. Ulcerated small intestine duplication cyst: unusual source of gastrointestinal bleeding revealed by wireless capsule. Gastrointest Endosc. 2006;63:192–4.

Arteriovenous Diseases

21

Marco Pennazio, Martin Keuchel, Dennis M. Jensen, and Gareth S. Dulai

Contents

The work was first published in 2006 by Springer Medizin Verlag Heidelberg with the following title: *Atlas of Video Capsule Endoscopy.*

M. Pennazio (✉)
Division of Gastroenterology,
San Giovanni Battista University Teaching Hospital,
Turin, Italy
e-mail: pennazio.marco@gmail.com

M. Keuchel
Department of Internal Medicine,
Bethesda Krankenhaus Bergedorf,
Hamburg, Germany
e-mail: keuchel@bkb.info

D.M. Jensen • G.S. Dulai
UCLA Digestive Disease Center,
Los Angeles, CA, USA
e-mail: djensen@mednet.ucla.edu;
gdulai@mednet.ucla.edu

21.1   Angiectasias

21.1.1 Definition

Angiectasia (synonyms: vascular ectasia, angiodysplasia, telangiectasia, arteriovenous malformation, or AVM) is a circumscribed dilatation of the capillary vessels in the mucosa or submucosa of the gastrointestinal (GI) tract.

21.1.2 Clinical Features

Angiectasias are the most common lesions identified in the small bowel of patients with obscure GI bleeding, yet they can be missed by capsule endoscopy—especially in the stomach, duodenum, and colon. It should be understood that though angiectasias are commonly seen, they may or may not bleed (Fig. 21.1). Clinical correlation and exclusion of other lesions are therefore required. Certain hereditary, iatrogenic, and acquired conditions can predispose to bleeding from angiectasias, most notably the use of aspirin, nonsteroidal anti-inflammatory drugs (NSAIDs), and anticoagulants.

The acquired form of angiectasia is the most common pathologic finding in patients with obscure GI bleeding. An increased incidence is seen in association with aging, hemodialysis, heart failure, aortic stenosis (Heyde's syndrome) [1], radiation therapy, and von Willebrand's syndrome [2]. Gastric antral vascular ectasia or watermelon stomach is a special case, which may be associated with autoimmune disorders (Figs. 29.14b–d and 44.16), liver cirrhosis, or end-stage renal disease.

The hereditary form is known as hereditary hemorrhagic telangiectasia (HHT) or Osler–Weber–Rendu disease (Fig. 21.2) [3]. HHT, inherited as an autosomal dominant trait, affects approximately 1 in 5,000 people. To date, three of the genes mutated in HHT have been identified. A clinical diagnosis can be made when three of the four Curaçao criteria (epistaxis, telangiectasias, visceral vascular lesions,

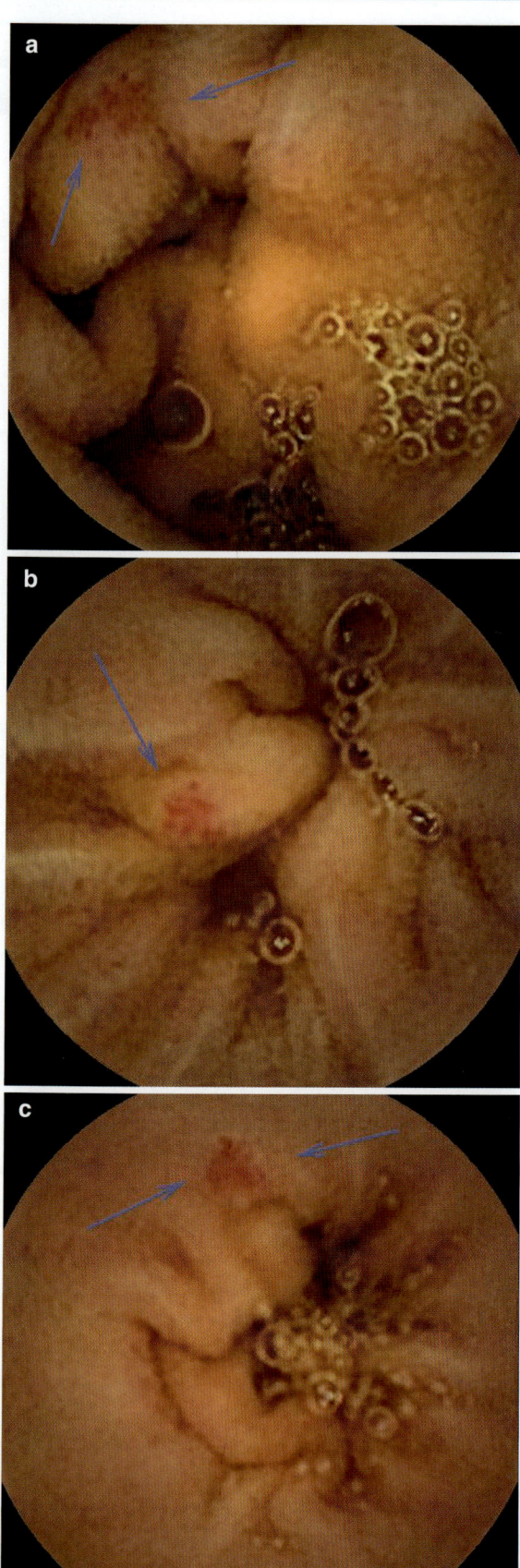

Fig. 21.1 (**a-c**) Jejunal angiectasias (*arrows*)

and/or positive family history) are present [4]. Although significant GI hemorrhage occurs in about one fifth of patients with HHT, VCE studies have found GI angiectasia in more than two thirds of cases. VCE makes possible precise mapping of lesions and has a considerable impact on the management of these patients [5].

21.1.3 Diagnosis

Diagnostic criteria for the endoscopic appearance of angiectasias are not uniform and have not been validated. For example, a small, flat, clearly demarcated red spot (as in Fig. 21.3a) may be an angiectasia, petechia, effect of bowel preparation, erosion, or inflammation. These red spots should be distinguished from the more characteristic fernlike appearance of an angioma with central vessel (Fig. 21.2). Active bleeding in the vicinity of an angiectasia is helpful in confirming the source of bleeding (Fig. 21.3).

Recently, a classification of vascular lesions of the small intestine useful for therapeutic decision-making was proposed [6], as shown in Table 21.1.

Radiographic imaging studies are usually unrewarding, but angiography may be diagnostic in rare cases when severe active bleeding is present. Biopsy is not recommended for clearly identifiable lesions because of the risk of bleeding, but it can be used to differentiate an atypical-appearing

Fig. 21.2 (**a–c**) Multiple fernlike angiectasias in a patient with hereditary hemorrhagic telangiectasia (HHT) on small bowel capsule endoscopy (SBCE). (**d**) Intrahepatic shunt seen at duplex sonography. (**e**, **f**) Telangiectasias of the lips and tongue in HHT patients

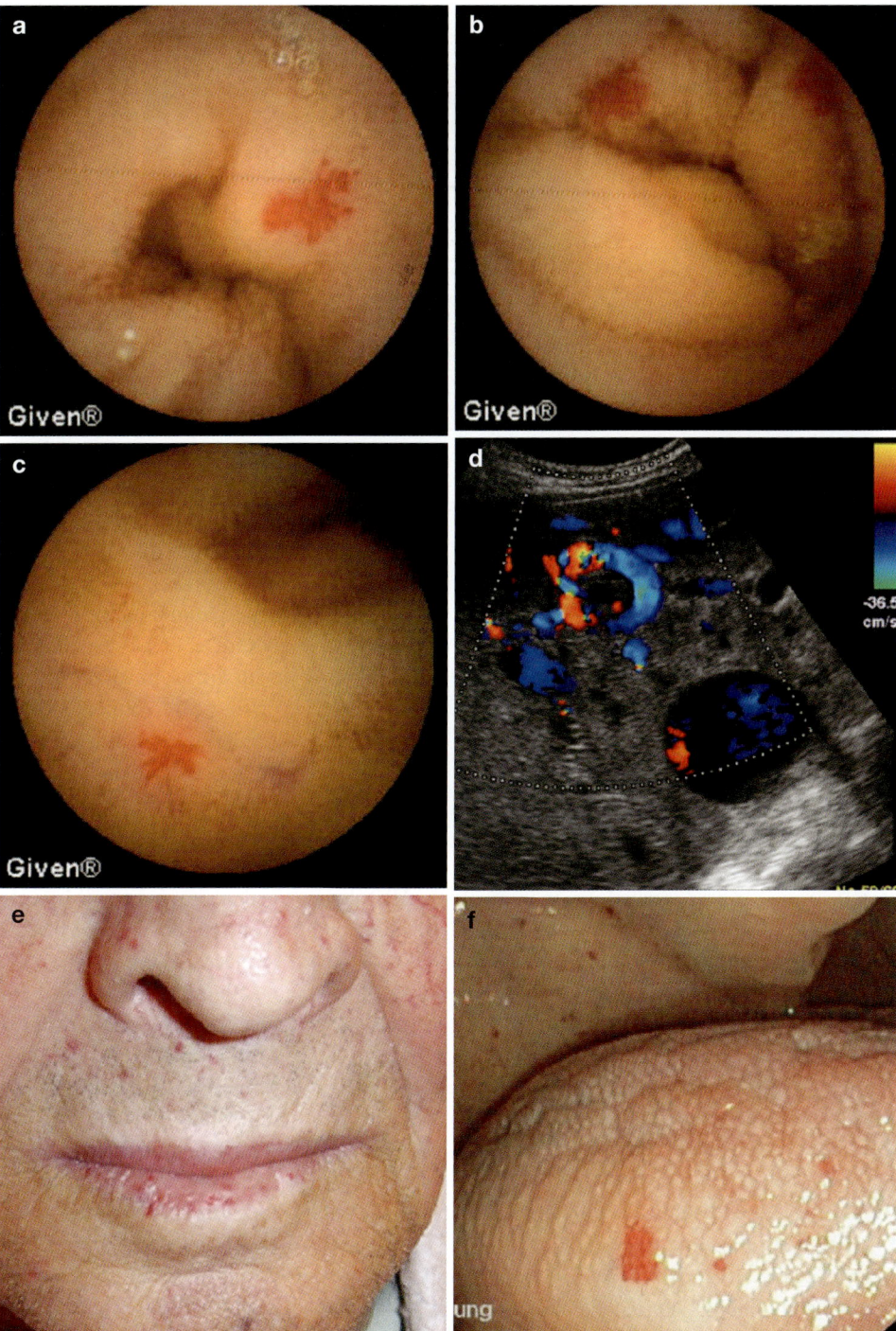

Fig. 21.3 (**a**, **b**) In patients with end-stage renal disease and recurrent transfusion-requiring gastrointestinal (GI) bleeding, VCE revealed minute jejunal angiectasias with active bleeding

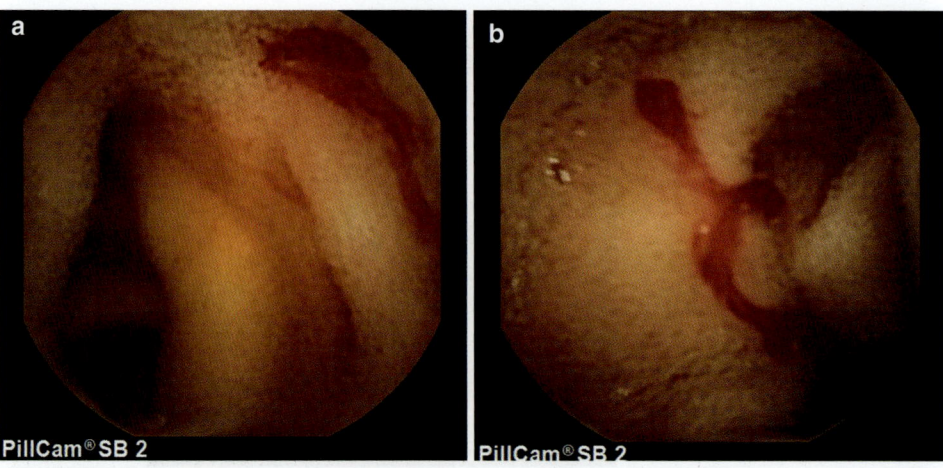

Table 21.1 Vascular lesions of the small intestine (Yano–Yamamoto classification)

Type	Description
Type 1a	Punctuate erythema (<1 mm), with or without oozing
Type 1b	Patchy erythema (a few mm), with or without oozing
Type 2a	Punctuate lesions (<1 mm), with pulsatile bleeding
Type 2b	Pulsatile red protrusion, without surrounding venous dilatation
Type 3	Pulsatile red protrusion, with surrounding venous dilatation
Type 4	Not classified by above categories

lesion from redness related to inflammation. Histologic examination of larger lesions can show small, distended, lacuna-like vessels with intraluminal red cells (Fig. 21.4b), but most lesions defy histologic diagnosis because of their small size (shrinkage with processing of the specimen, error in targeting the biopsy, etc.).

21.1.4 Treatment

Treatment should be considered when angiectasias are seen to be actively bleeding or when they are the only potential sources of bleeding identified. New medical and endoscopic treatment modalities are clearly needed. At present, endoscopic coagulation (Fig. 21.5) may be done with electrocautery (bipolar, argon plasma), heater probe, or laser [7]. Large,

focal lesions can be treated surgically by a segmental resection of the small bowel [8]. Empiric treatment (iron replacement, epoetin alfa, transfusion, and avoidance of platelet aggregation inhibitors such as aspirin or clopidogrel, NSAIDs, or anticoagulants) may be considered for patients with diffuse involvement or for rebleeding after endoscopic or surgical treatment [9]. Intraoperative treatment of diffuse small bowel lesions is usually ineffective. With the advent of device-assisted enteroscopy (Chap. 13, 14, and 15), it is possible to reach more intestinal lesions without the need for surgery. Although prospective studies are still lacking, recent data show that endoscopic therapy using double-balloon endoscopy for small bowel vascular lesions in patients with recurrent obscure GI bleeding allows a long-term remission in more than half of the patients [10]. Hormonal therapy may be administered, but its benefit has not been confirmed [11]. Anecdotal reports have been published on the use of somatostatin analogues [12, 13]. Although the evidence is still limited and the cost-efficacy and long-term tolerance of octreotide has yet to be tested, somatostatin analogues are clearly an option for patients presenting with obscure bleeding from GI angiectasia. The monthly administration of long-acting octreotide makes this formulation a convenient option for long-term therapy [14]. Data from a recent randomized study suggest that thalidomide also may be an effective and relatively safe treatment for patients with refractory bleeding from small bowel angiectasia if pregnancy is reliably excluded [15].

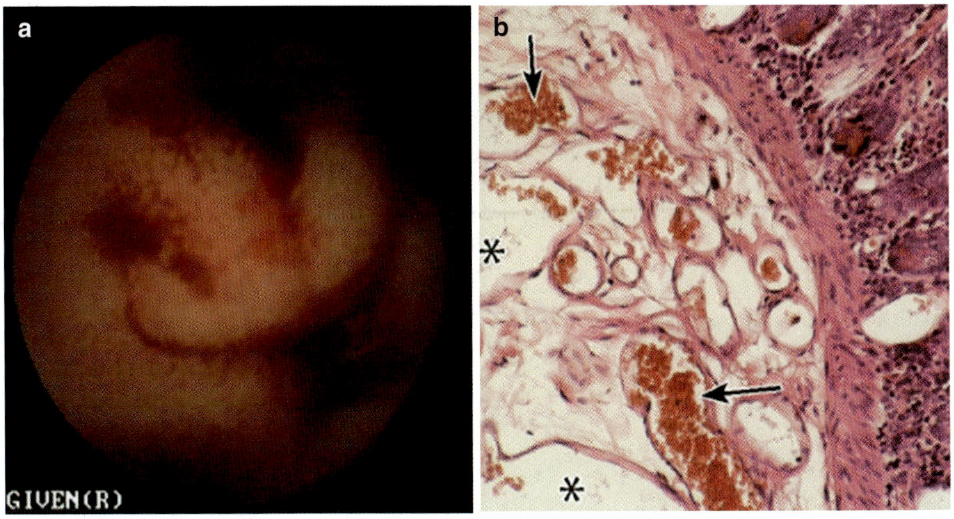

Fig. 21.4 Images from an 83-year-old man with transfusion-requiring intestinal blood loss. (**a**) An angiectasia in the middle of the VCE image is poorly visible because of dark blood. Active bleeding was observed more distally. Intraoperatively, multiple angiectasias of the jejunum were treated by segmental resection. (**b**) Histology of resected segment from the small intestine, with angiectasias (*asterisk*) and intraluminal erythrocytes (*arrow*). (hematoxylin–eosin [H&E] stain; courtesy of Jörg Caselitz, MD)

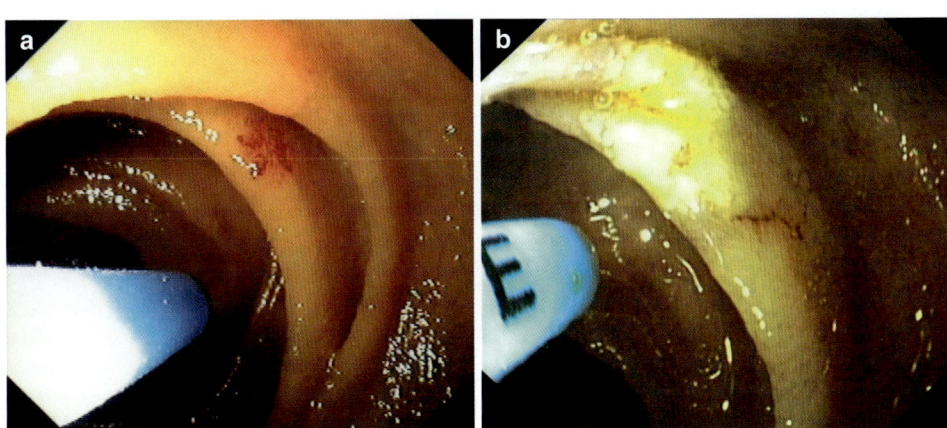

Fig. 21.5 Single-balloon enteroscopy: angiectasia before (**a**) and after (**b**) electrocoagulation

21.2 Dieulafoy's Lesion

21.2.1 Definition

A Dieulafoy's lesion is a protruding, large-caliber submucosal artery without macroscopic ulceration. The lesion may bleed profusely, and rebleeding is common. Arteries may be more than 2 mm in size. These lesions most commonly occur in the stomach [16]. Bleeding from Dieulafoy's lesions of the small bowel seems to be much more frequent than previously estimated, with most of these lesions being located in the proximal jejunum [17].

21.2.2 Treatment

Endoscopic hemostasis can be achieved by injection, coagulation, clipping, rubber band ligation, or a combination of these techniques. If endoscopic treatment is ineffectual, a segmental bowel resection is indicated.

21.2.3 Endoscopy

Without active (arterial-type) bleeding or other stigmata such as a nonbleeding visible vessel, Dieulafoy's lesions are often difficult to identify. When active bleeding is present, the source may be obscured by blood (Fig. 21.6). Even when the bleeding stops, the lesion may be missed because of its small size.

21.3   Blue Rubber Bleb Nevus Syndrome

This is a very rare hereditary syndrome characterized by multiple hemangiomas involving the GI tract (Figs. 21.7 and 21.8a) and the skin (Fig. 21.8b). At endoscopy, soft, blue, rubbery hemangiomas may be seen throughout the GI tract [18].

Treatment can be difficult because the distribution of lesions is often diffuse. The principal options are endoscopic coagulation and surgical resection [19].

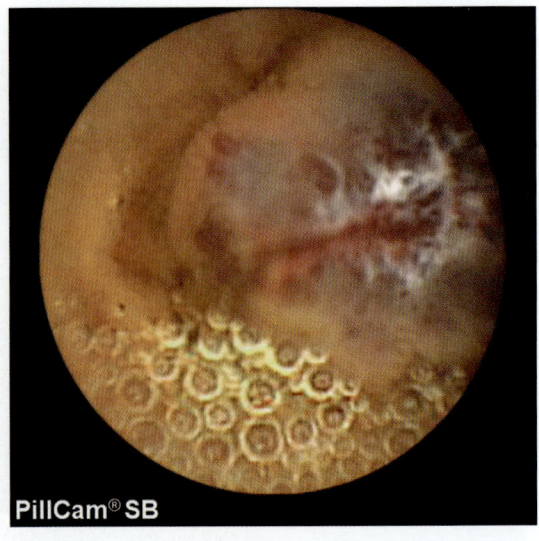

Fig. 21.7 Blue rubber bleb nevus syndrome: hemangiomas of the small bowel

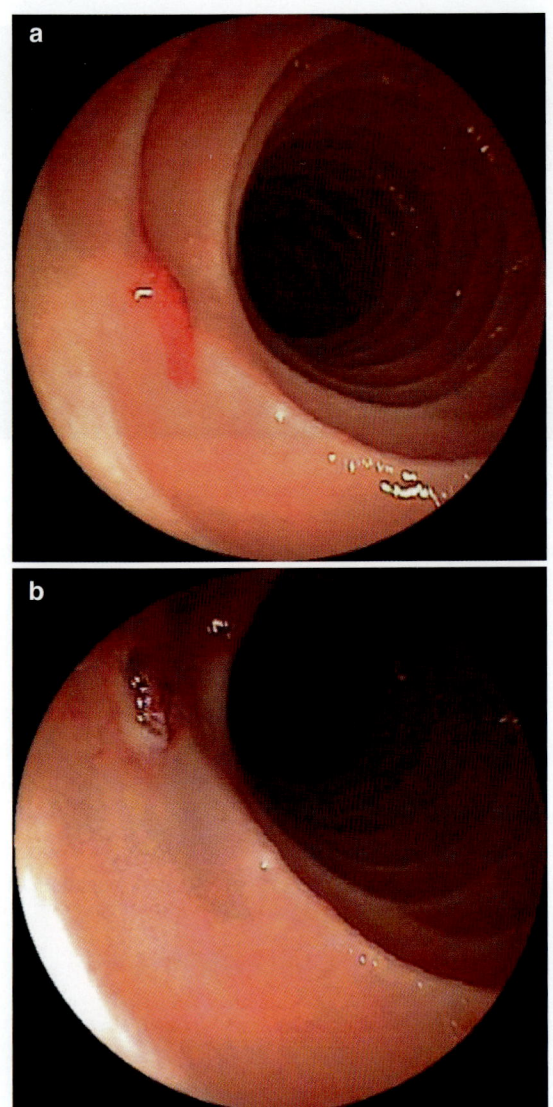

Fig. 21.6 (**a**) Bleeding jejunal Dieulafoy's lesion at double-balloon enteroscopy. (**b**) After argon plasma coagulation

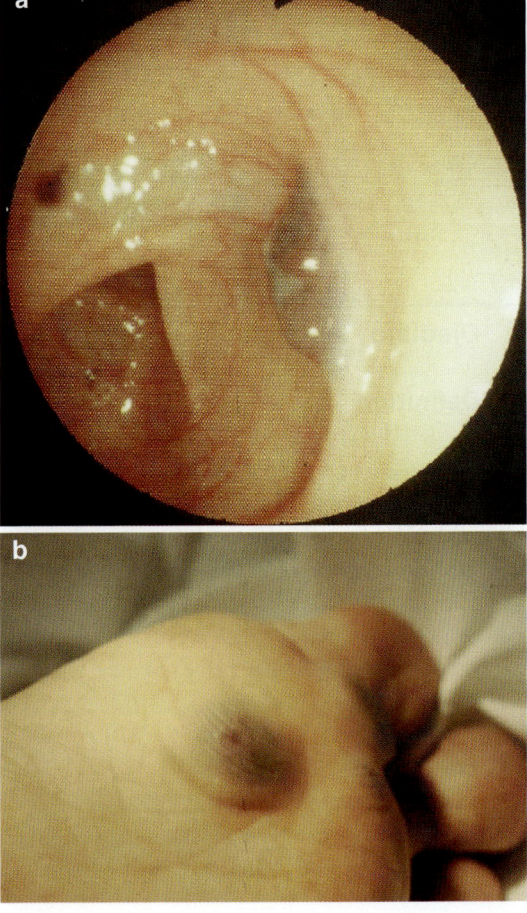

Fig. 21.8 Blue rubber bleb nevus syndrome: hemangioma of the colon (**a**) and skin (**b**)

21.4 Venous Ectasias and Varices

Large veins are frequently seen during capsule endoscopy of the normal small bowel. It is not unusual to find small venous ectasias (Fig. 21.9), which generally do not bleed. However, if varices (Figs. 21.10, 21.11, and 21.12) or venous ectasias with an eroded surface are found, they should be considered a potential bleeding source [20, 21].

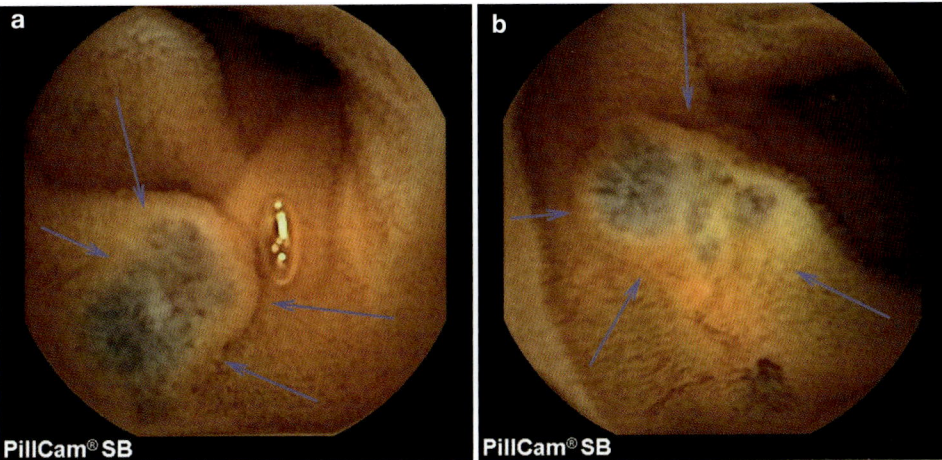

Fig. 21.9 (**a**, **b**) Venectasias (arrows): nonbleeding, incidental findings on VCE

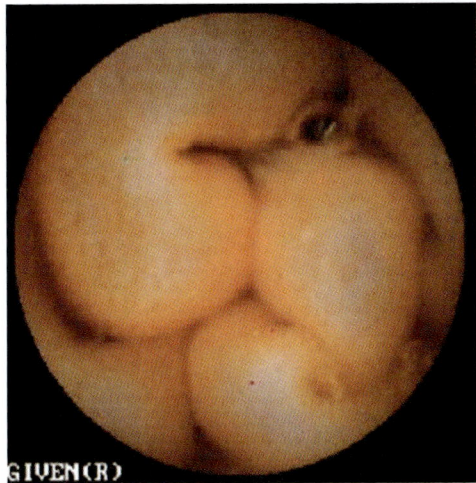

Fig. 21.10 Duodenal varices in a patient with liver cirrhosis who had recurrent transfusion-requiring bleeding episodes

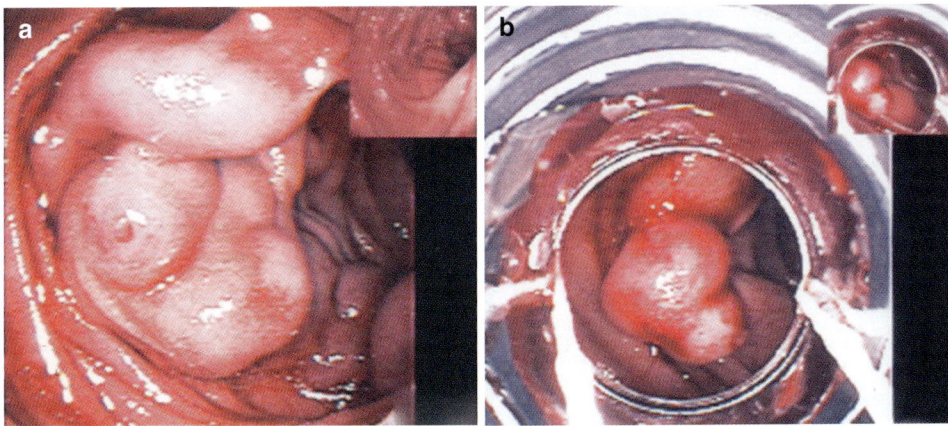

Fig. 21.11 Large convolution of varices in the deep duodenum with hematocystic spot (**a**) due to liver cirrhosis in a patient who experienced hemorrhagic shock. After rubber band ligation (**b**), no further bleeding occurred

Fig. 21.12 Ileal varix with large mucosal defect causing severe mid-GI bleeding, seen at VCE (**a**) (Courtesy of Jörg Albert, MD). With double-balloon enteroscopy, an injection of histoacryl and lipiodol was performed (**b**). The varix was obliterated, as seen in an endoscopic image (**c**) and a CT scan (**d**)

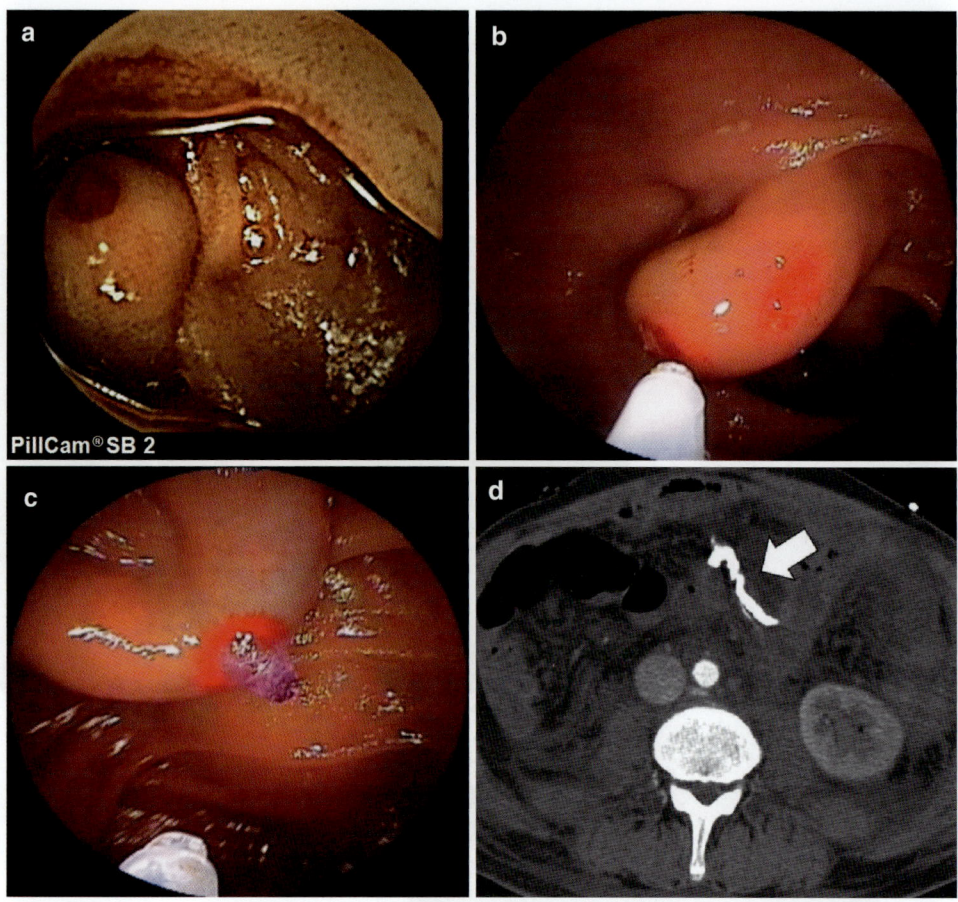

21.5   Portal Hypertensive Enteropathy

Enteropathic lesions develop secondarily to portal hypertension caused by hepatic cirrhosis or portal vein thrombosis with congestion of the mesenteric veins (Fig. 21.13a). The clinical significance of the enteropathic lesions is difficult to assess [22, 23]; it is discussed in Chap. 23.

On endoscopy, patchy redness of the mucosa (Fig. 21.13b) [24] and diffuse venous ectasias, possibly accompanied by small, superficial mucosal defects, are nonspecific findings. Small bowel varices [21] or red bumps/polyps [25] may be found in rare cases.

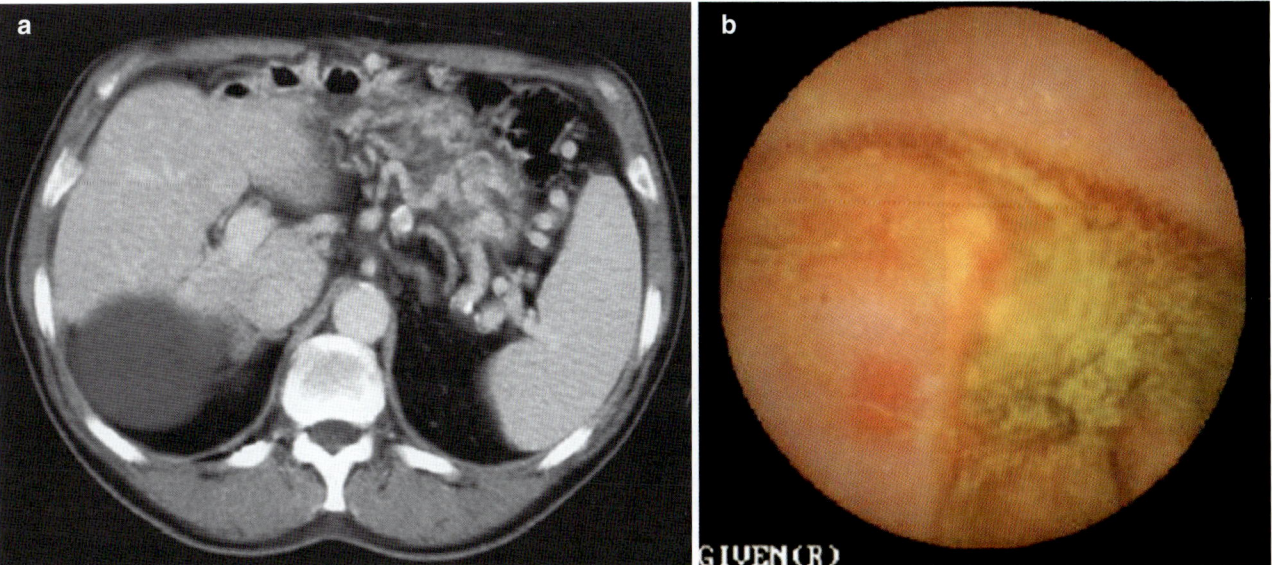

Fig. 21.13 Splenic vein thrombosis. (**a**) CT scan shows collaterals, state after partial liver resection. (Courtesy of Ernst Malzfeldt, MD). (**b**) VCE reveals red spots in the jejunum

21.6 Ischemic Enteropathy

21.6.1 Definition

Ischemic enteropathy represents an acute or chronic occlusion of the celiac trunk, the superior mesenteric artery, or a systemic low-flow state (e.g., shock, sepsis, bypass, etc.) with or without small-vessel disease. The chronic form is almost always related to atherosclerosis and is rarely symptomatic because of the development of a collateral supply. Acute and chronic ischemic lesions also can result from the angiographic embolization of small bowel segmental arteries done for purposes of hemostasis.

21.6.2 Clinical Features

Postprandial abdominal pain, diarrhea, and weight loss are the clinical hallmarks of chronic ischemia of the small bowel [26]. The acute form may be characterized by abdominal pain, acute abdomen, bleeding, and even rare instances of perforation, depending on the extent of the infarction.

21.6.3 Diagnosis

The mainstays in the diagnosis of ischemic enteropathy are arterial (subtraction) angiography and color Doppler sonography. Endoscopy has a confirmatory role if there is clinical suspicion of acute ischemia, and it can demonstrate the presence of residual strictures. Acute intestinal ischemia may be associated with edema and bleeding (Fig. 21.14). Ulcers of the small bowel are frequently segmental and circumferential (Fig. 21.15), whereas patchy lesions may be observed in chronic, partially compensated ischemia (Fig. 21.16).

21.6.4 Treatment

Acute mesenteric ischemia will require embolectomy or segmental resection, but in chronic ischemia, angiographic intervention can be effective (Fig. 21.16e–g) [27].

Fig. 21.14 Patient with acute mesenteric ischemia due to cardiogenic shock. (**a**) VCE revealed edematous swelling of a long segment, with dark blood. (**b**) Resection of an ischemic jejunal segment after intraoperative enteroscopy, because of hemorrhagic shock. (**c**) Histology shows ischemia (Courtesy of Michel Delvaux, MD, and Gerard Gay, MD)

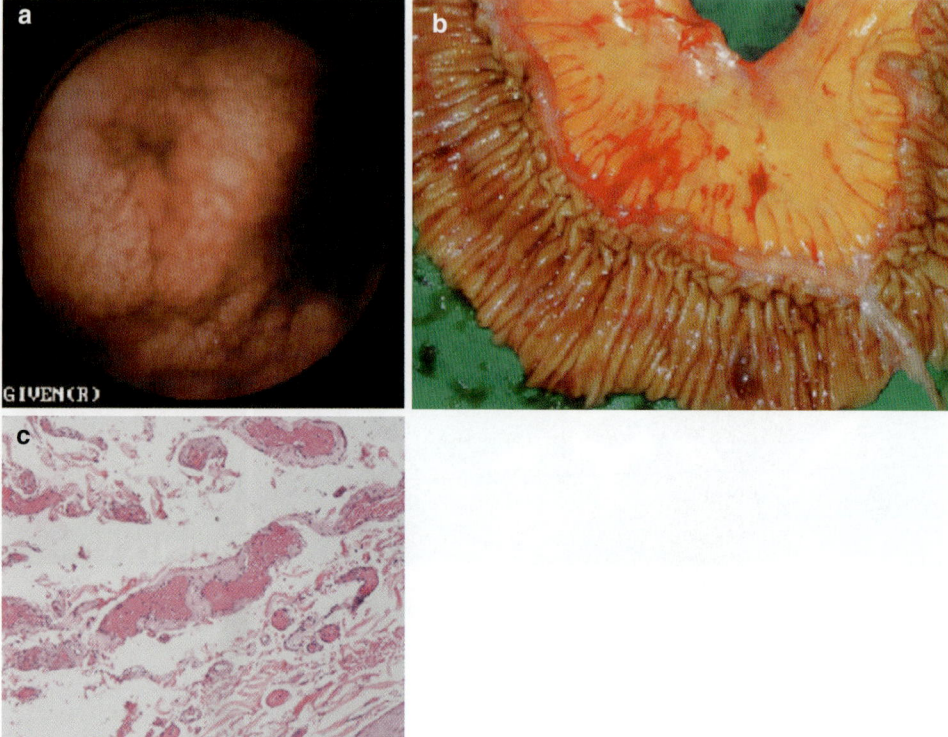

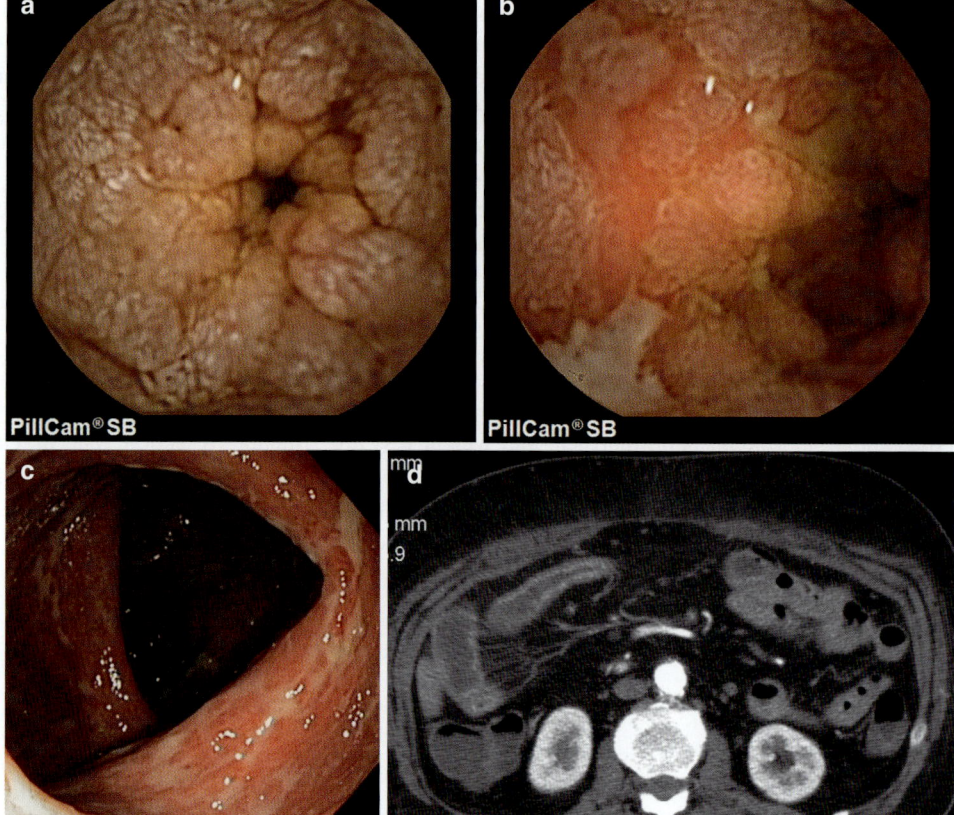

Fig. 21.15 Ischemic enteritis. Diarrhea followed embolectomy of the superior mesenteric artery for embolic occlusion. (**a**) VCE shows unspecific mosaic pattern of proximal small bowel with whitish and partially atrophic villi. (**b**) Remaining serpiginous ulcers in the distal small bowel and the ascending colon (**c**, colonoscopy). (**d**) CT scan shows thickened ileal loop (*arrow*)

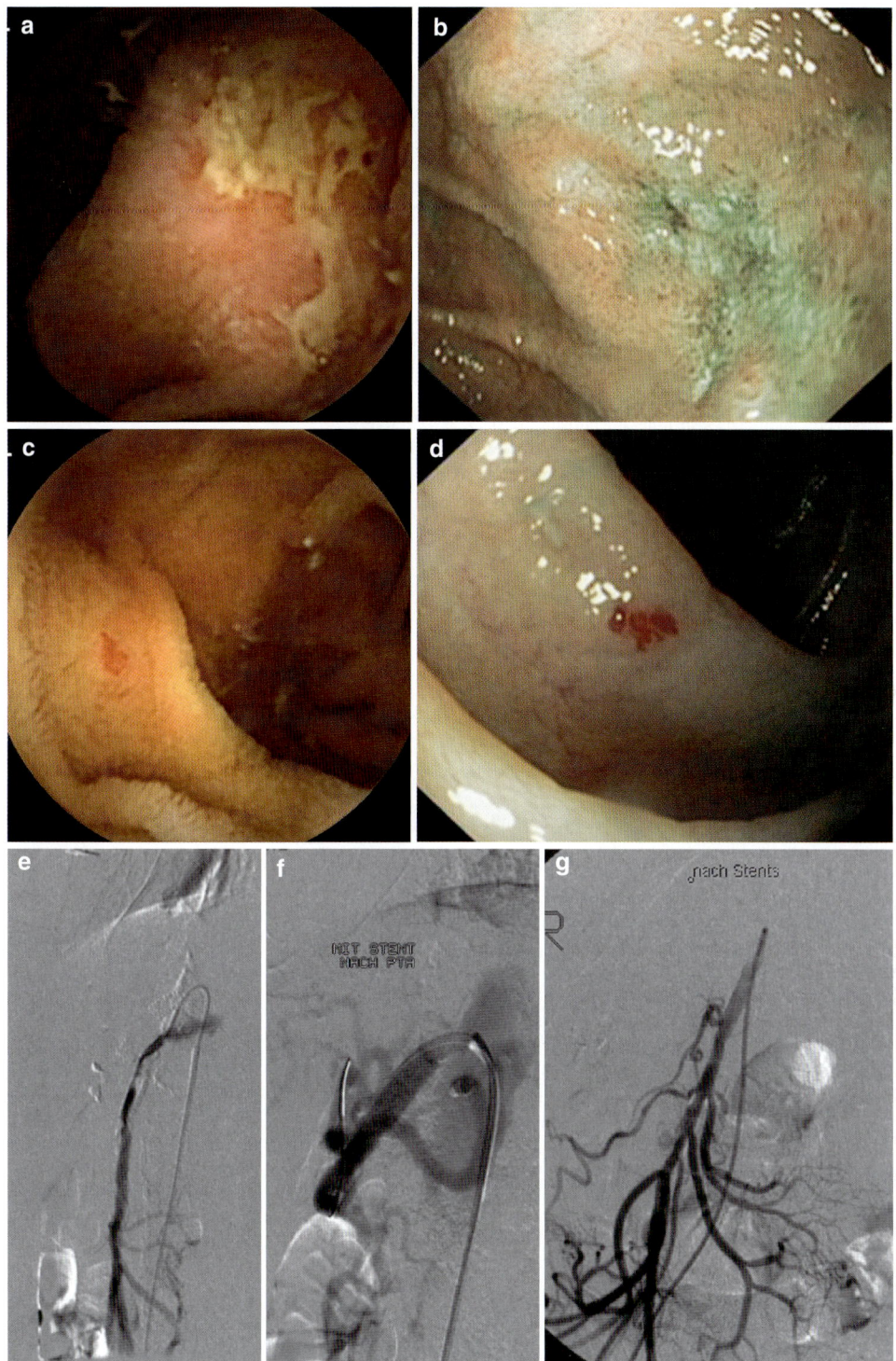

Fig. 21.16 Ischemic enteropathy, seen at VCE (**a**, **c**), and single-balloon enteroscopy (**b**, **d**). (**a**, **b**) Ulcerations. (**c**, **d**) Angiectasia-like lesions. (**e**) Selective angiography shows stenosis of the superior mesenteric artery. (**f**, **g**) Angioplasty and stent placement had a favorable result (Courtesy of Matthias Joanowitsch, MD). Repeat VCE after 8 weeks showed normal small bowel

References

1. Warkentin TE, Moore JC, Morgan DG. Gastrointestinal angiodysplasia and aortic stenosis. N Engl J Med. 2002;347:858–9.
2. Warkentin TE, Moore JC, Anand SS, et al. Gastrointestinal bleeding, angiodysplasia, cardiovascular disease, and acquired von Willebrand syndrome. Transfus Med Rev. 2003;17:272–86.
3. van den Driesche DS, Mummery CL, Westermann CJ. Hereditary hemorrhagic telangiectasia: an update on transforming growth factor beta signaling in vasculogenesis and angiogenesis. Cardiovasc Res. 2003;58:20–31.
4. Shovlin CL. Hereditary haemorrhagic telangiectasia: pathophysiology, diagnosis and treatment. Blood Rev. 2010;24:203–19.
5. Grève E, Moussata D, Gaudin JL, et al. High diagnostic and clinical impact of small-bowel capsule endoscopy in patients with hereditary hemorrhagic telangiectasia with overt digestive bleeding and/or severe anemia. Gastrointest Endosc. 2010;71: 760–7.
6. Yano T, Yamamoto H, Sunada K, et al. Endoscopic classification of vascular lesions of the small intestine (with videos). Gastrointest Endosc. 2008;67:169–72.
7. Pavey DA, Craig PI. Endoscopic therapy for upper-GI vascular ectasias. Gastrointest Endosc. 2004;59:233–8.
8. Steffani KD, Eisenberger CF, Gocht A, et al. Recurrent intestinal bleeding in a patient with arterio-venous fistulas in the small bowel, limited mesenteric varicosis without portal hypertension and malrotation type I. Z Gastroenterol. 2003;41:587–90.
9. Lewis BS. Medical and hormonal therapy in occult gastrointestinal bleeding. Semin Gastrointest Dis. 1999;10:71–7.
10. Samaha E, Rahmi G, Landi B, et al. Long-term outcome of patients treated with double balloon enteroscopy for small bowel vascular lesions. Am J Gastroenterol. 2012;107:240–6.
11. Junquera F, Feu F, Papo M, et al. A multicenter, randomized, clinical trial of hormonal therapy in the prevention of rebleeding from gastrointestinal angiodysplasia. Gastroenterology. 2001;121:1073–9.
12. Blich M, Fruchter O, Edelstein S, Edoute Y. Somatostatin therapy ameliorates chronic and refractory gastrointestinal bleeding caused by diffuse angiodysplasia in a patient on anticoagulation therapy. Scand J Gastroenterol. 2003;38:801–3.
13. Rossini FP, Arrigoni A, Pennazio M. Octreotide in the treatment of bleeding due to angiodysplasia of the small intestine. Am J Gastroenterol. 1993;88:1424–7.
14. Brown C, Subramanian V, Wilcox CM, Peter S. Somatostatin analogues in the treatment of recurrent bleeding from gastrointestinal vascular malformations: an overview and systematic review of prospective observational studies. Dig Dis Sci. 2010;55:2129–34.
15. Ge ZZ, Chen HM, Gao YJ, et al. Efficacy of thalidomide for refractory gastrointestinal bleeding from vascular malformation. Gastroenterology. 2011;141:1629–37.
16. Lee YT, Walmsley RS, Leong RWL, Sung JJS. Dieulafoy's lesion. Gastrointest Endosc. 2003;58:236–43.
17. Dulic-Lakovic E, Dulic M, Hubner D, et al. Bleeding Dieulafoy lesions of the small bowel: a systematic study on the epidemiology and efficacy of enteroscopic treatment. Gastrointest Endosc. 2011;74:573–80.
18. Fish L, Fireman Z, Kopelman Y, Sternberg A. Blue rubber bleb nevus syndrome: small-bowel lesions diagnosed by capsule endoscopy. Endoscopy. 2004;36:836.
19. Shahed M, Hagenmüller F, Rösch T, et al. A 19-year-old female with blue rubber bleb naevus syndrome. Endoscopic laser photocoagulation and surgical resection of gastrointestinal angiomata. Endoscopy. 1990;22:54–6.
20. Ostrow B, Blanchard RJ. Bleeding small-bowel varices. Can J Surg. 1984;27:88–9.
21. Tang SJ, Zanati S, Dubcenco E, et al. Diagnosis of small-bowel varices by capsule endoscopy. Gastrointest Endosc. 2004;60: 129–35.
22. Viggiano TR, Gostout CJ. Portal hypertensive intestinal vasculopathy: a review of the clinical, endoscopic, and histopathologic features. Am J Gastroenterol. 1992;87:944–54.
23. Desai N, Desai D, Pethe V. Portal hypertensive jejunopathy: a case control study. Indian J Gastroenterol. 2004;23:99–101.
24. Evrard S, Le Moine O, Devière J, et al. Unexplained digestive bleeding in a cirrhotic patient. Gut. 2004;53:1771.
25. Sawada K, Ohtake T, Ueno N, et al. Multiple portal hypertensive polyps of the jejunum accompanied by anemia of unknown origin. Gastrointest Endosc. 2011;73:179–82.
26. Brandt LJ, Boley SJ. AGA technical review on intestinal ischemia. Gastroenterology. 2000;118:954–68.
27. HHT Foundation International. http:\\curehht.org

Intestinal Lymphangiectasia

22

Ervin Tóth, Felix Wiedbrauck,
and Jürgen F. Riemann

Contents

The work was first published in 2006 by Springer Medizin Verlag Heidelberg with the following title: *Atlas of Video Capsule Endoscopy*.

E. Tóth (✉)
Department of Gastroenterology,
Skåne University Hospital, Malmö, Sweden
e-mail: ervin.toth@med.lu.se

F. Wiedbrauck
Department of Gastroenterology,
Allgemeines Krankenhaus Celle, Celle, Germany
e-mail: felix.wiedbrauck@akh-celle.de

J.F. Riemann
LebensBlicke Foundation for Prevention of Colorectal Cancer,
Ludwigshafen, Germany
e-mail: riemannj@garps.de

22.1 Clinical Features

Endoscopically, the villi of the small bowel in intestinal lymphangiectasia typically appear white and may be swollen [1, 2]. Less commonly, tiny white spots are visible in the mucosa. The whitish discoloration of the villi is caused by chylomicrons, which accumulate in and obstruct the dilated lymphatic capillaries. These changes can also be demonstrated histologically. Lymphangiectasia is characterized endoscopically as localized, patchy, or diffuse. Diffuse lymphangiectasia causes the mucosa to appear "snow covered" or "dusted with powdered sugar" at endoscopy.

Functional lymphangiectasia is dependent on food intake and appears to have no pathologic significance (Fig. 22.1) [3]. *Secondary* lymphangiectasia is an accompanying feature of many underlying intestinal and extraintestinal diseases [4]. There is also the very rare *primary* form (also called idiopathic or essential), with severe exudative enteropathy [5].

White, swollen villi are occasionally found in a localized area (*focal* lymphangiectasia); this form has not been shown to have pathologic significance (Fig. 22.2). *Cystic* lymphangiectasia is also a harmless finding unless the lesions are exceptionally large or eroded (see Chap. 33).

22.2 Secondary Lymphangiectasia

The causes of secondary lymphangiectasia (Table 22.1) should be investigated based on the history and clinical examination and, if necessary, by performing microbiologic tests and imaging studies, such as sonography, CT scans, or MRI (Figs. 22.3, 22.4, 22.5, 22.6, 22.7, 22.8, 22.9, 22.10, 22.11, 22.12, and 22.13) [6]. If the patient has concomitant diarrhea and malabsorption, it is advisable to proceed with an endoscopic biopsy of the small bowel. A correlation with the appearance of angiectasias has been observed [7].

Uncharacteristic lymphangiectasias and specific features of the underlying disease may occur in segments of the small intestine that are widely separated from each other.

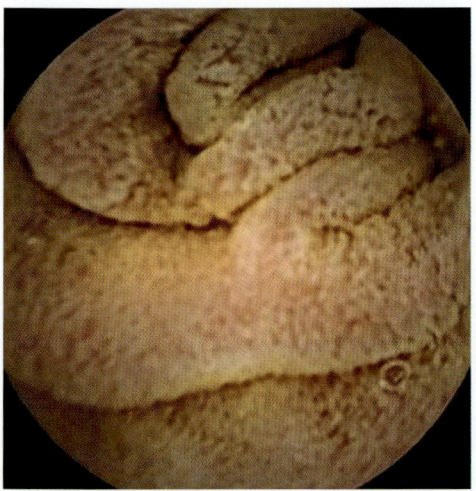

Fig. 22.1 Functional lymphangiectasia with mild diffuse edema and whitish villi

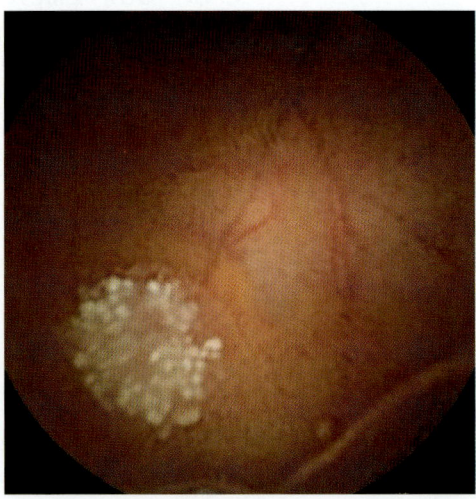

Fig. 22.2 Focal lymphangiectasia

Fig. 22.3 Unspecific lymphangiectasia with patchy white and swollen villi (**a**) accompanied by petechia-like red spots (**b**). These video capsule endoscopy (VCE) findings are sometimes seen in nonsteroidal anti-inflammatory drug (NSAID) enteropathy

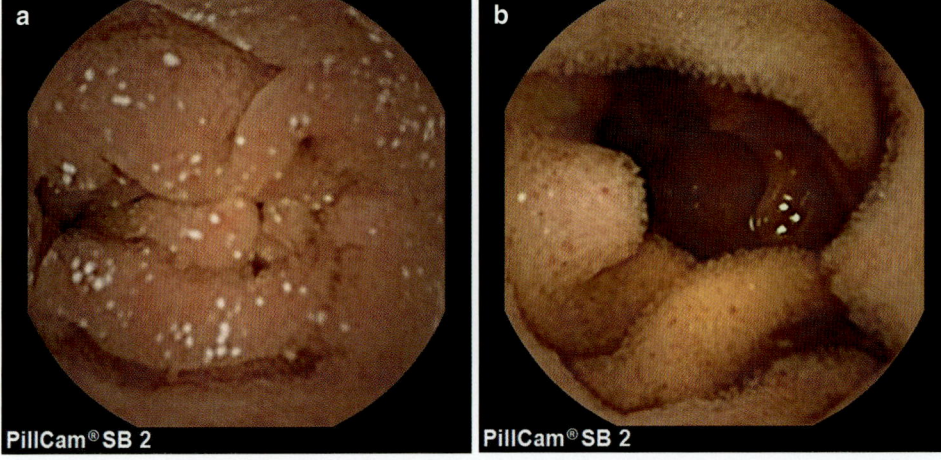

Fig. 22.4 Inflammation: lymphangiectasia secondary to Crohn's disease. (**a**) Early lesion with a few white villi surrounding a small mucosal defect in the proximal small bowel. (**b**) Diffusely swollen and white villi in the distal small bowel

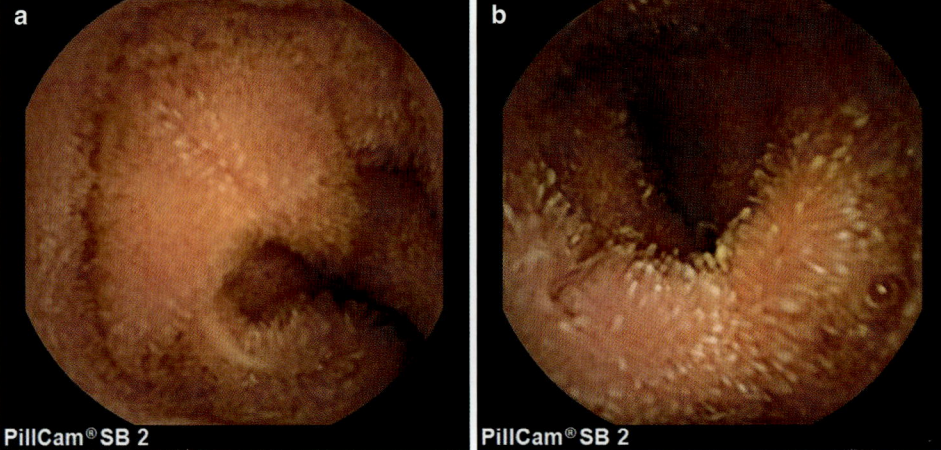

Fig. 22.5 Collagenosis: lymphangiectasia secondary to lupus erythematosus. (**a**) Diffusely swollen white villi in the distal jejunum. (**b**) Erosion surrounded by diffusely swollen white villi in the proximal jejunum

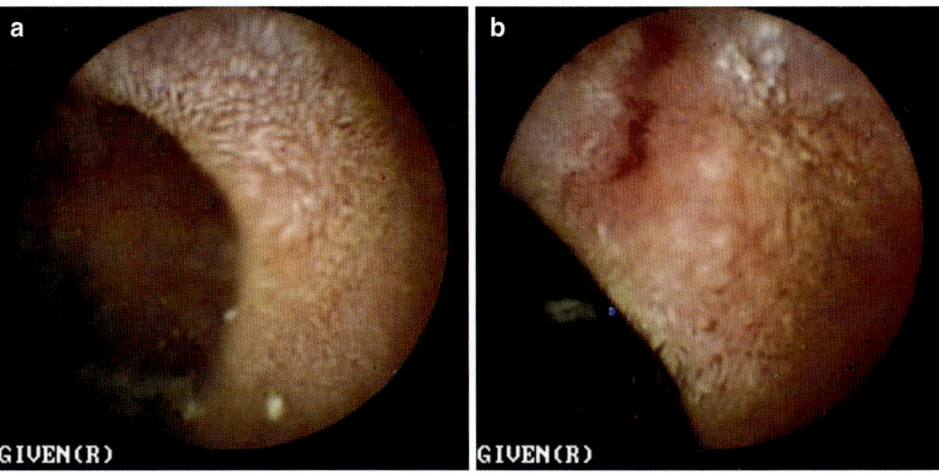

Fig. 22.6 Infection: diffuse lymphangiectasia in HIV infection (**a**) and atypical mycobacteriosis (**b**) (pseudo-Whipple's disease)

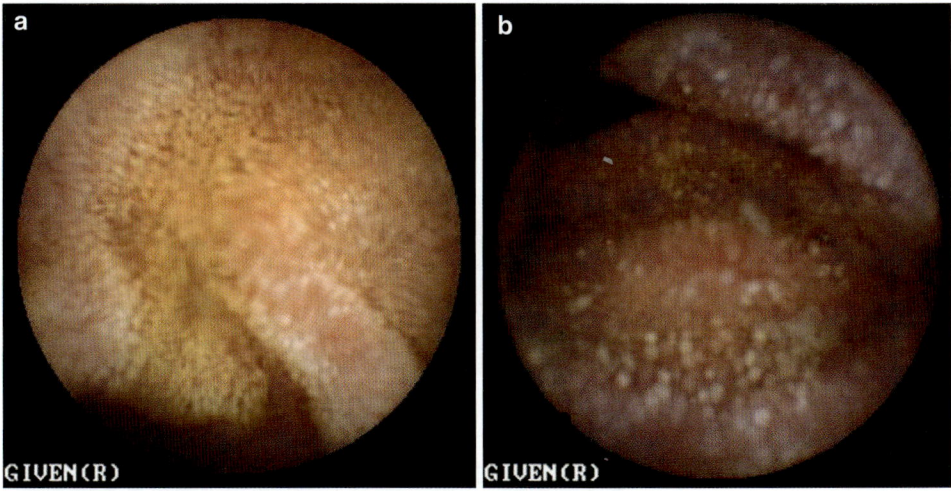

Fig. 22.7 (**a**, **b**) Infection: diffuse secondary lymphangiectasia in the proximal jejunum, due to salmonellosis

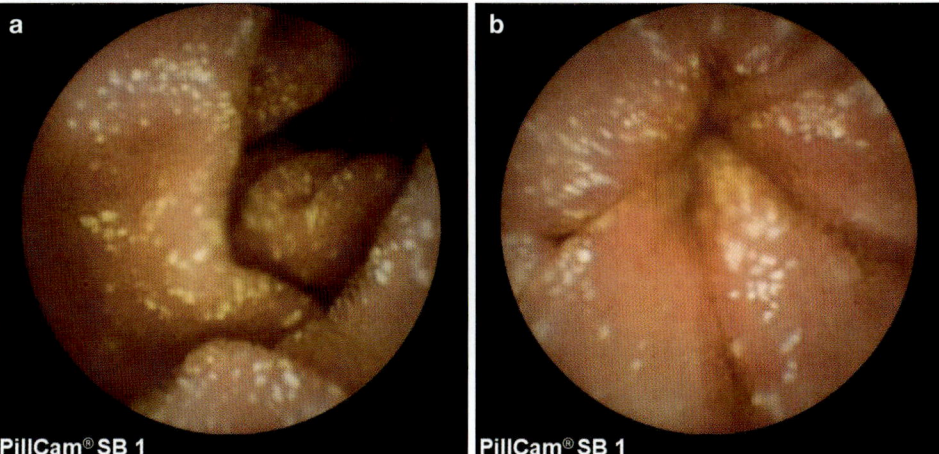

Fig. 22.8 Lymphangiectasia secondary to mantle cell lymphoma. White and distorted villi are seen on the mucosa of the infiltrated area. Note the pathologic vessel on the left side of the VCE image

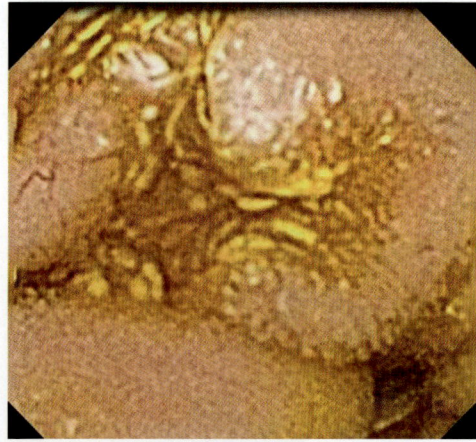

Fig. 22.9 Lymphangiectasia secondary to adenocarcinoma. The phenomenon is seen proximal to the tumor (**a**) and in the direct neighborhood (**b**)

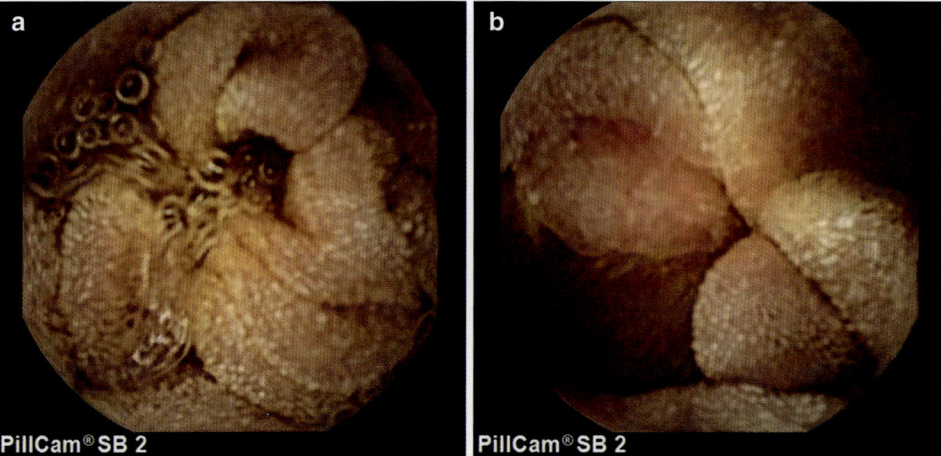

Fig. 22.10 Lymphangiectasia secondary to metastasis of endometrial carcinoma. (**a**) Diffuse lymphangiectasia due to impaired lymphatic drainage. (**b**) Necrotic bleeding metastasis on the left side of the VCE image

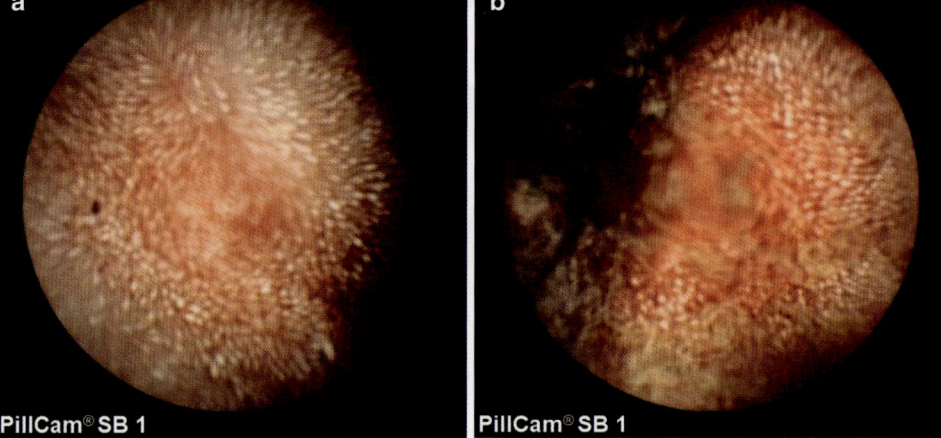

Fig. 22.11 Lymphangiectasia secondary to tumor of the mesentery and history of radiation. Edematous swelling of the mucosa and villi at VCE (**a**) and push enteroscopy (**b**). Club-shaped white villi and bleeding at VCE (**c**, **d**) and push enteroscopy (**e**). Calcified tumor of the mesentery on CT scan (**f**) (Courtesy of Jörg Sievers, MD). Sonographic image (**g**)

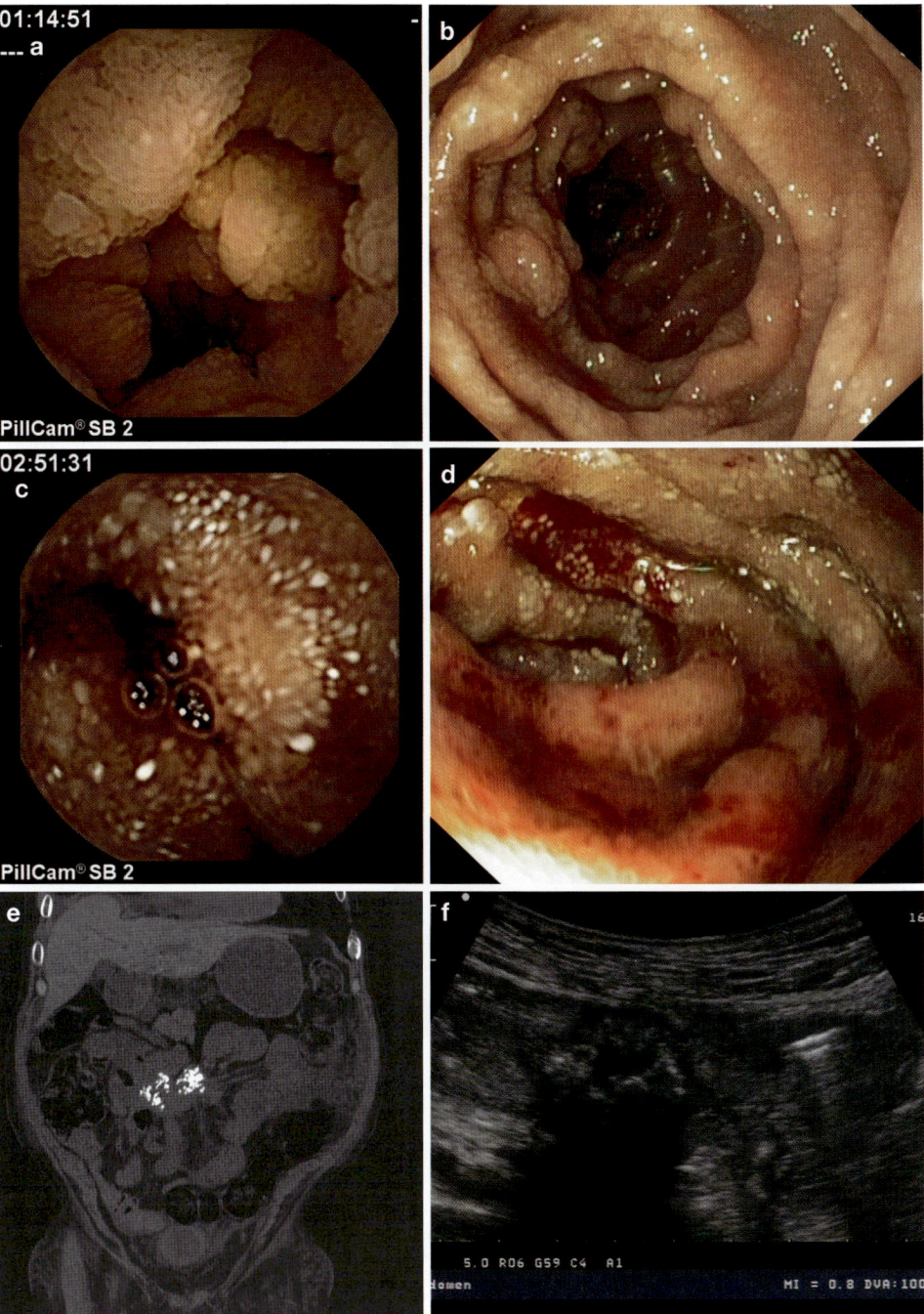

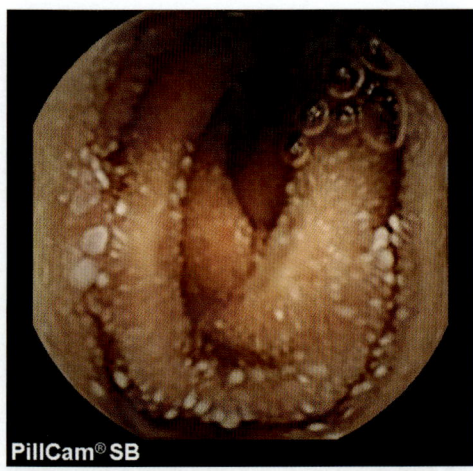

Fig. 22.12 Lymphangiectasia secondary to radiation enteropathy. Fibrosis with thickened folds and club-shaped white villi

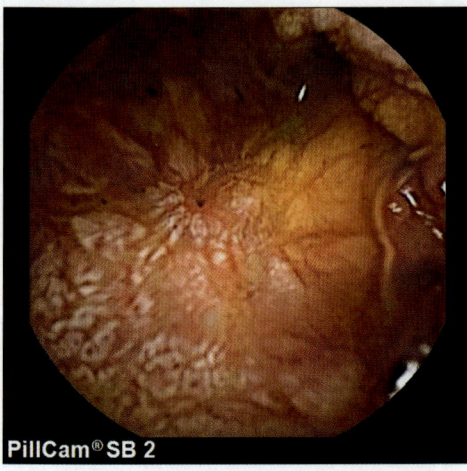

Fig. 22.13 Ischemic enteritis with partially healed ulcers and diffuse lymphangiectasia

22.3 Primary Lymphangiectasia

Primary lymphangiectasia (Waldmann disease) [8] is a very rare, presumably hereditary disease that predominantly affects children and adolescents. No other defects are described in these patients.

Typical clinical features are diarrhea, exudative enteropathy with malassimilation, protein-deficiency edema, ascites, and lymphocytopenia.

On endoscopy, primary lymphangiectasia (Fig. 22.14) may appear more pronounced and involve a longer intestinal segment than the secondary form. Additionally, the mucosa itself may have a whitish appearance [9], as if covered by a thin blanket of snow. Biopsy confirmation (Fig. 22.14f) is advised [10, 11].

The initial treatment is to place the patient on a low-fat diet with medium-chain fatty acids [12]. Albumin substitution may be helpful. Diet seems to be more effective in children than in adults [13]. Somatostatin has been tried as an experimental therapy [14].

Table 22.1 Etiology of secondary lymphangiectasia

Source	Examples
Infections	Whipple's disease (Fig. 28.1)
	Salmonellosis (Fig 22.7)
	Atypical mycobacteriosis (Fig. 22.6b)
	HIV (Fig. 22.6a)
	Tuberculosis (Fig. 28.3)
Inflammations	Crohn's disease (Fig.22.4)
	Collagenosis (Fig. 22.5)
Intra-abdominal tumors	Lymphoma (Fig. 22.8)
	Carcinoma (Fig. 22.9)
	Metastasis (Fig. 22.10)
Iatrogenic causes	Radiation enteritis (Figs. 22.11 and 22.12)
	Radical lymphadenectomy
	Cardiovascular ischemic right heart failure (Fig. 22.13)

Fig. 22.14 Primary lymphangiectasia in a 17-year-old female patient with protein-losing enteropathy, edema, lymphopenia, and weight loss. (**a**–**d**) Lymphangiectasia with extremely enlarged white villi is starting in the proximal small bowel with a patchy distribution and then becoming diffuse. (**e**) Conventional enteroscopy. (**f**) Histology showing dilated vessels without erythrocytes (hematoxylin–eosin stain). (**f** Courtesy of Peer Flemming, MD, and Axel Wellmann, MD)

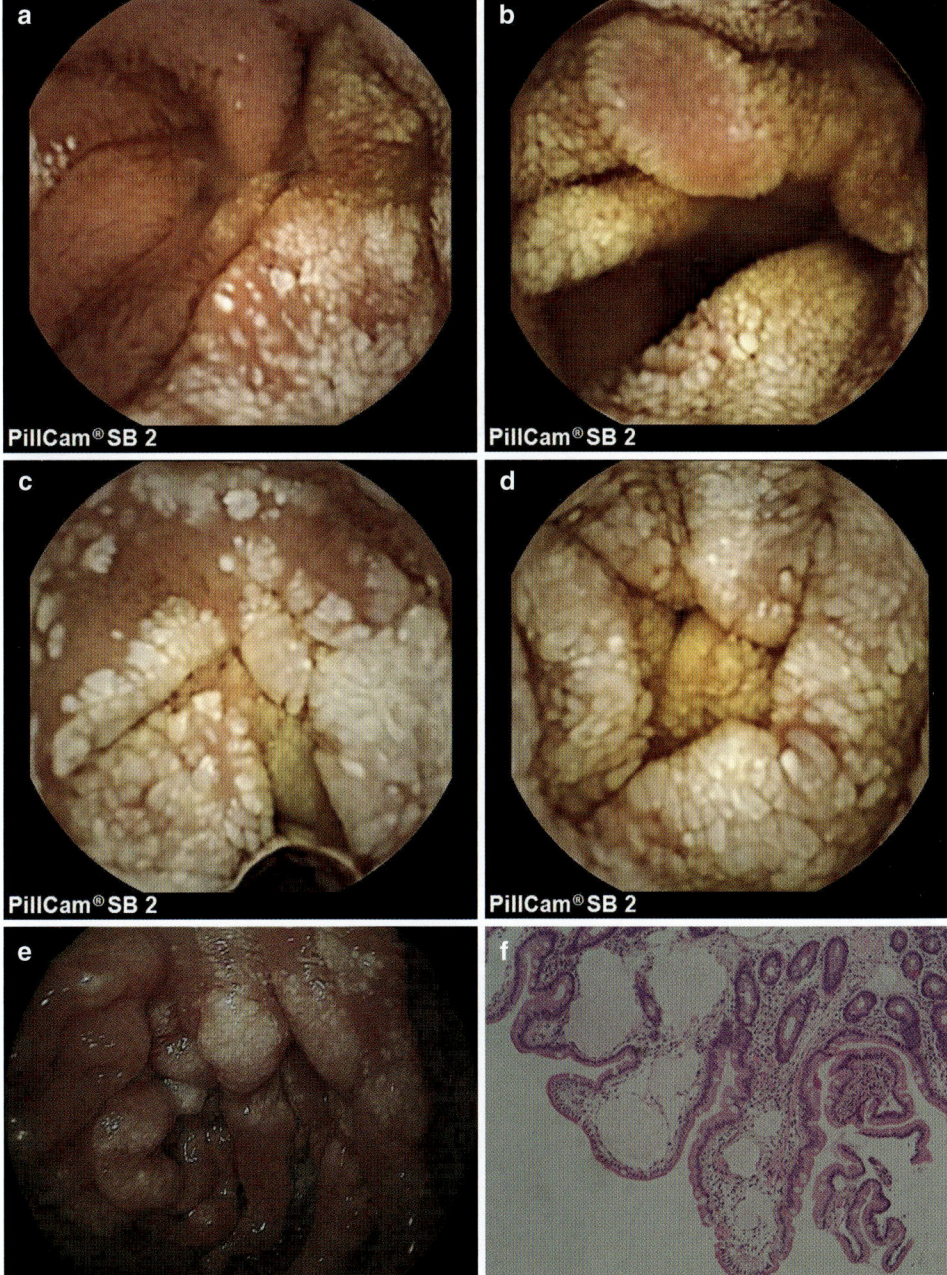

22.4 Lymphangiectasia as Part of a Syndrome

Intestinal lymphangiectasia may occur together with other syndromes:

- The yellow nail syndrome comprises dystrophic yellow nails, lymphedema, pleural effusion, and intestinal lymphangiectasia (Fig. 22.15) [15, 16].

- Hennekam syndrome, an autosomal recessive inherited disorder, includes intestinal lymphangiectasia and lymphedema, together with facial anomalies and mental retardation (Fig. 22.16) [17].

- Noonan's syndrome may occur as an autosomal dominant inherited condition or sporadically. Abnormalities of the face, neck, sternum, and heart (e.g., pulmonic stenosis) may be accompanied by intestinal lymphangiectasia (Chap. 29) [18].

Fig. 22.15 Yellow nail syndrome. VCE reveals swollen mucosa with thick and short villi covered with opalescent, milky fluid in the jejunum (**a**) and ileum (**b**). (Case of Ervin Tóth, MD, and Henrik Thorlacius, MD). Duodenal biopsy shows lymphangiectasia (**c**). This patient presented with hypoalbuminemia, bilateral lower limb edema, and slowly growing, dystrophic yellow nails (**d**) (**c, d** Courtesy of Åke Danielsson, MD)

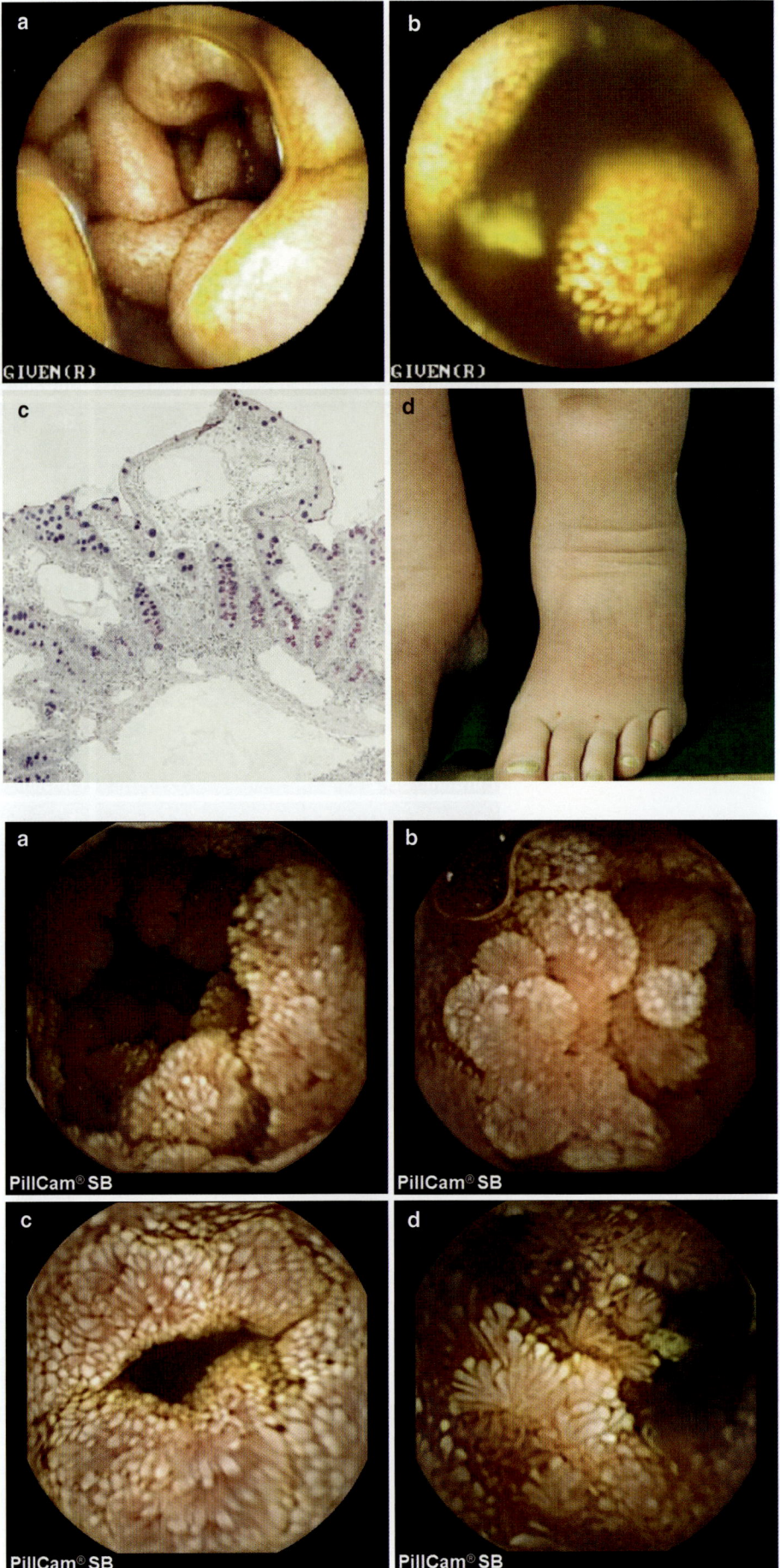

Fig. 22.16 (**a–d**) Hennekam syndrome in a 9-year-old boy. Seen are enlarged white villi with partial polypoid distribution (Courtesy of Philip Bufler, MD)

References

1. Asakura H, Miura S, Morishita T, et al. Endoscopic and histopathological study on primary and secondary intestinal lymphangiectasia. Dig Dis Sci. 1981;26:312–20.

2. Riemann JF, Schmidt H. Synopsis of endoscopic and other morphological findings in intestinal lymphangiectasia. Endoscopy. 1981;13:60–3.

3. Barnes RE, deRidder PH. Fat absorption in patients with functional intestinal lymphangiectasia and lymphangiectic cysts. Am J Gastroenterol. 1993;88:887–90.

4. Fürstenau M, Kratzsch KH, Zimmermann S, Büttner W. Fiberendoskopischer Nachweis, Häufigkeit und klinische Bedeutung der intestinalen Lymphangiektasie. Z Gesamte Inn Med. 1977;32:638–40.

5. Takenaka H, Ohmiya N, Hirooka Y, et al. Endoscopic and imaging findings in protein-losing enteropathy. J Clin Gastroenterol. 2012;46:575–80.

6. Fox U, Luciani G. Disorders of the intestinal mesenteric lymphatic system. Lymphology. 1993;26:61–6.

7. Macdonald J, Porter V, Scott NW, McNamara D. Small bowel lymphangiectasia and angiodysplasia: a positive association; novel clinical marker or shared pathophysiology? J Clin Gastroenterol. 2010;44:610–4.

8. Waldmann TA, Steinfeld JL, Dutcher TF, et al. The role of the gastrointestinal system in idiopathic hypoproteinemia. Gastroenterology. 1961;41:197–207.

9. Aoyagi K, Iida M, Yao T, et al. Characteristic endoscopic features of intestinal lymphangiectasia: correlation with histological findings. Hepatogastroenterology. 1997;44:133–8.

10. Freeman HJ, Nimmo M. Intestinal lymphangiectasia in adults. World J Gastrointest Oncol. 2011;3:19–23.

11. Oh TG, Chung JW, Kim HM, et al. Primary intestinal lymphangiectasia diagnosed by capsule endoscopy and double balloon enteroscopy. World J Gastrointest Endosc. 2011;3:235–40.

12. Munck A, Sosa VG, Faure C, et al. Suivi de long cours des lymphangiectasies intestinales primitives de l'enfant. À propos de six cas. Arch Pediatr. 2002;9:388–91.

13. Wen J, Tang Q, Wu J, et al. Primary intestinal lymphangiectasia: four case reports and a review of the literature. Dig Dis Sci. 2010;55:3466–72.

14. Kuroiwa G, Takayama T, Sato Y, et al. Primary intestinal lymphangiectasia successfully treated with octreotide. J Gastroenterol. 2001;36:129–32.

15. Danielsson A, Tóth E, Thorlacius H. Capsule endoscopy in the management of a patient with a rare syndrome – yellow nail syndrome with intestinal lymphangiectasia. Gut. 2006;55:233.

16. Malek NP, Ocran K, Tietge UJ, et al. A case of the yellow nail syndrome associated with massive chylous ascites, pleural and pericardial effusions. Z Gastroenterol. 1996;34:763–6.

17. Hennekam RC, Geerdink RA, Hamel BC, et al. Autosomal recessive intestinal lymphangiectasia and lymphedema, with facial anomalies and mental retardation. Am J Med Genet. 1989;34:593–600.

18. Keberle M, Mork H, Jenett M, et al. Computed tomography after lymphangiography in the diagnosis of intestinal lymphangiectasia with protein-losing enteropathy in Noonan's syndrome. Eur Radiol. 2000;10:1591–3.

Portal Hypertension

23

Pedro Narra Figueiredo and Shinji Tanaka

Contents

The major consequence of portal hypertension is bleeding, particularly from esophageal varices (Fig. 23.1) [1]. Digestive bleeding has also been found to occur from gastric sources (Fig. 23.2) [2] and colorectal sources [3, 4]. The recognized existence of portal hypertensive gastropathy [5] and portal hypertensive colopathy [6] suggests that the small bowel may also present endoscopic lesions related to portal hypertension. In fact, Thiruvengadam and Gostout [7] reported in 1989 on three patients presenting with blood loss, who had diffuse erythema and scattered petechiae in the stomach and in the duodenum and jejunum. Since then, the small bowel, previously considered to be the most difficult segment of the gut to study, has come to be easily explored using new endoscopic methods such as capsule endoscopy and double-balloon enteroscopy. This development in the field of small bowel endoscopy has allowed significant progress

The work was first published in 2006 by Springer Medizin Verlag Heidelberg with the following title: *Atlas of Video Capsule Endoscopy*.

P.N. Figueiredo (✉)
Department of Gastroenterology,
University of Coimbra, Coimbra, Portugal
e-mail: pnf11@sapo.pt

S. Tanaka
Department of Endoscopy,
Hiroshima University Hospital, Hiroshima, Japan
e-mail: colon@hiroshima-u.ac.jp

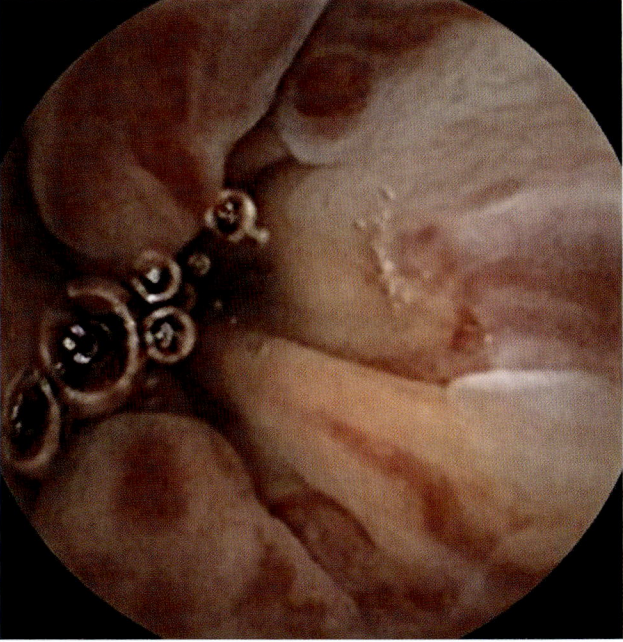

Fig. 23.1 Esophageal varices

M. Keuchel et al. (eds.), *Video Capsule Endoscopy: A Reference Guide and Atlas*,
DOI 10.1007/978-3-662-44062-9_23, © Springer-Verlag Berlin Heidelberg 2014

Fig. 23.2 Portal hypertensive
gastropathy. (**a**) Mild portal
hypertensive gastropathy.
(**b**) Severe portal hypertensive
gastropathy

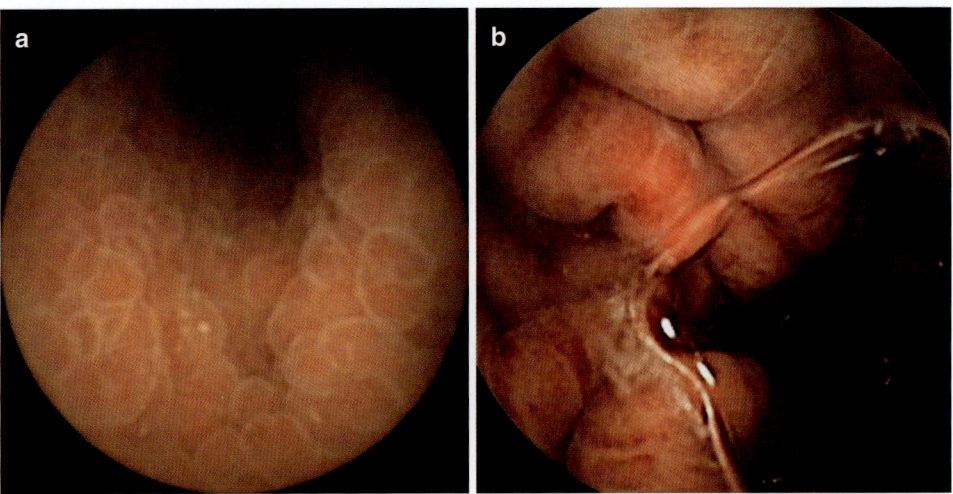

in the study of small bowel diseases, including the implications of portal hypertension.

The concept of portal hypertensive vasculopathy, including portal hypertensive gastropathy, portal hypertensive colopathy, and portal hypertensive enteropathy (PHE), proposed by Viggiano and Gostout [8] to describe the effects of portal hypertension in the gut, is not unanimously accepted, however. Although the association between portal hypertensive gastropathy and portal hypertensive colopathy is well documented in a large series of cirrhotic patients [6], the studies that address this issue and include PHE show conflicting results. A paper by De Palma et al. [9] found that PHE is significantly more common in the presence of hypertensive gastropathy and portal hypertensive colopathy, but two other studies [10, 11] found no association between the presence of PHE (documented by capsule endoscopy) and the presence of portal hypertensive gastropathy and portal hypertensive colopathy.

De Palma et al. [9] reported the changes found in the mucosa of the small bowel in patients with portal hypertension. They used capsule endoscopy to study 37 cirrhotic patients and 34 controls and considered the presence of abnormalities resembling mucosal inflammation and/or vascular lesions to be manifestations of PHE. These findings were detected in 67.5 % of the cirrhotic patients and in none of the controls. In accordance with this, the endoscopic lesions in the small bowel of patients with portal hypertension may be classified as mucosal abnormalities, which include a reticulate pattern (Fig. 23.3), sometimes with erythema (Fig. 23.4), or as vascular lesions, which include angiectasia-like lesions (Fig. 23.5) and varices (Fig. 23.6). These findings are detected in 65–69 % of patients with portal hypertension [9, 11–14], regardless of the presence of cirrhosis [11]. The same papers report the presence of varices in up to 27 % of the patients [11], but in others, only 8 % of the

patients present this finding [9]. There is also huge variability in the prevalence of angiectasia-like lesions, ranging from 63 % [15] to 22 % [14], and in abnormalities resembling mucosal inflammation, found in 13 % of patients by De Palma et al. [9] but in 63 % by Canlas et al. [16].

An important issue is whether angiectasia-like lesions detected by capsule endoscopy should be considered a small bowel manifestation of portal hypertension. Although angiectasia seems to be the main cause of acute bleeding from the small bowel in patients with portal hypertension, documented in all patients in the series presented by De Palma et al. [9] and in one of two patients in another series [11], the frequency of detection of these lesions was similar in patients with portal hypertension and in the control group [11]. In fact, in a recently published paper [17], angiectasia and red spots, which were reported as portal hypertensive lesions in previous studies, showed no correlation with the hepatic venous pressure gradient. Therefore, angiectasia-like lesions probably should not be considered a small bowel manifestation of portal hypertension. Further studies aimed at recognizing the clinical consequences of the small bowel endoscopic findings in these patients (as regards bleeding episodes or transfusion requirements, for example) should probably consider separately those who present angiectasia-like lesions.

The main question is the clinical impact of these findings, as the significance of the endoscopic lesions suggestive of PHE is uncertain. Some studies report active bleeding from the small bowel of cirrhotic patients [9, 11], but a recently published study involving 40 patients with liver cirrhosis (50 % presenting abnormal vascular findings in the small bowel), who were observed for 5–27 months (median 16.3), suggested that capsule endoscopy findings had no impact on the clinical course [18].

Two options exist when dealing with small bowel manifestations of portal hypertension. The first is to perform

Fig. 23.3 Reticulate pattern.
(**a**, **b**) Reticulate pattern.
(**c**) Reticulate pattern with a
polyp

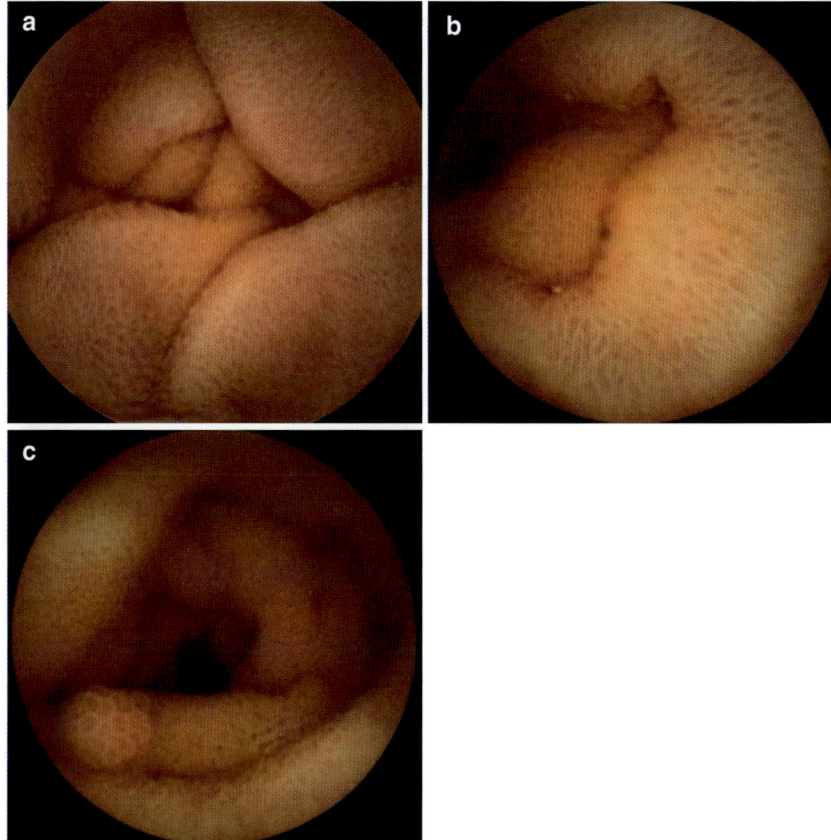

Fig. 23.4 Reticulate pattern
with erythema. (**a**, **b**)
Reticulate pattern with
erythema. (**c**) Ileocecal valve
with erythema

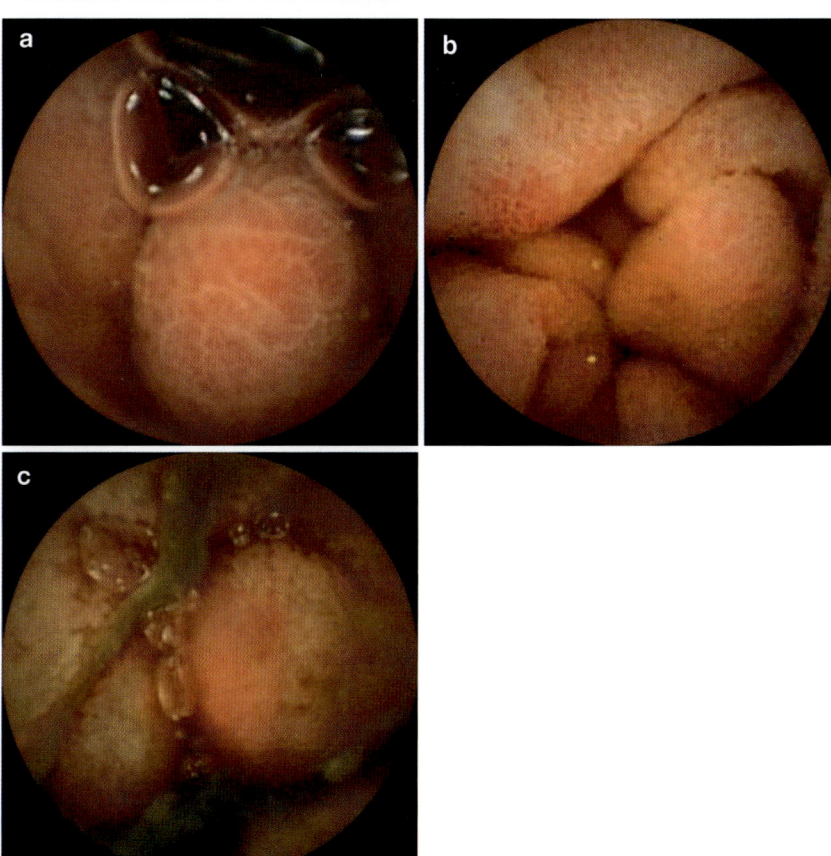

Fig. 23.5 Angiectasia-like lesions. (**a–c**) Small angiectasia-like lesions

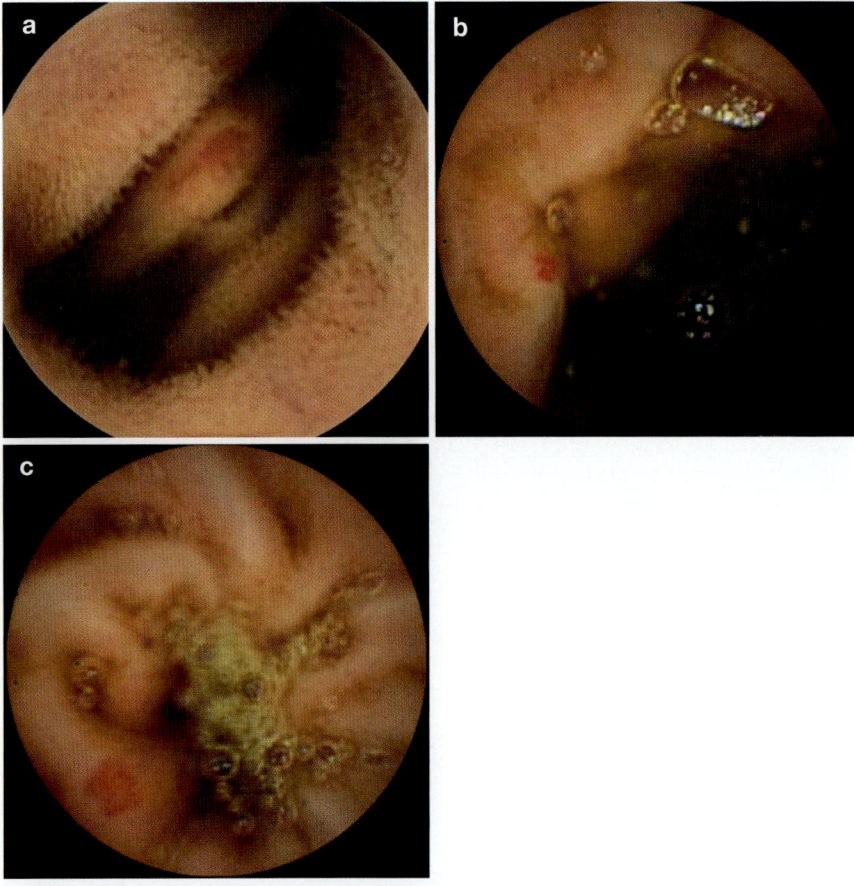

Fig. 23.6 Varices in the small bowel. (**a–d**) Blue lesions, compatible with varices

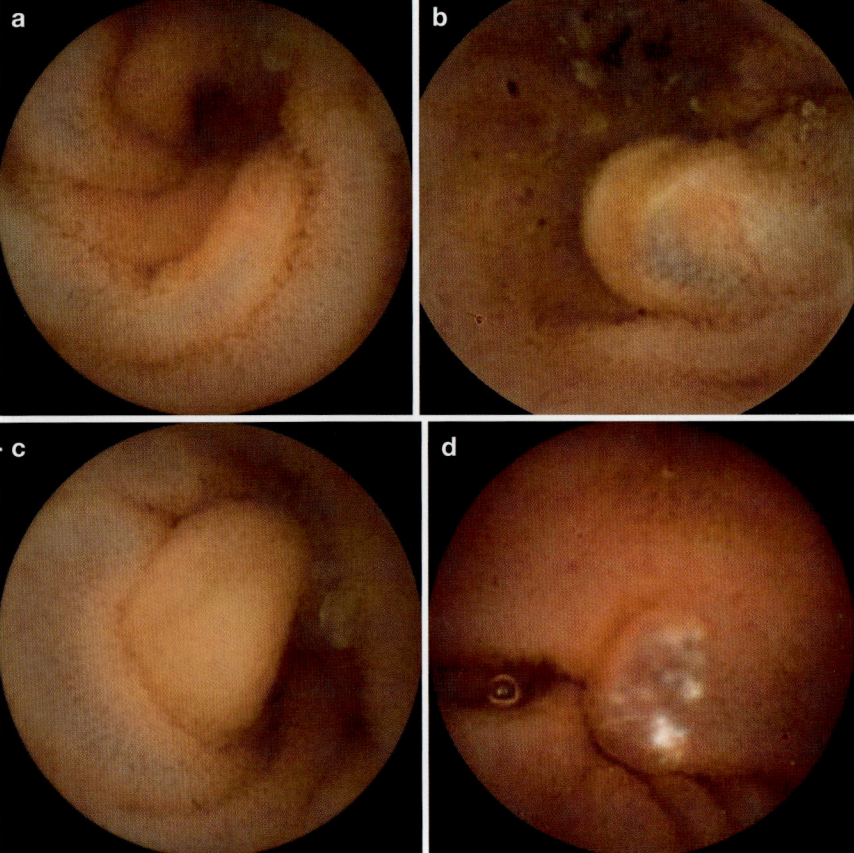

enteroscopy only in patients who present obscure digestive bleeding. This was the choice of De Palma et al. [9], who found active bleeding in four patients (10.8 %), the source being angiectasia-like lesions. The other diagnostic option is to include enteroscopy in the workup of all cirrhotic patients, regardless of the presence of hemorrhage. Not surprisingly, when including patients without a previous history of obscure digestive bleeding, fewer patients with portal hypertension present active bleeding [11]. In fact, enteroscopy probably should be used only in patients who present obscure digestive bleeding [19]. In this context, capsule endoscopy is the preferred method for two reasons: (1) It allows a complete examination of the small bowel and is obviously more efficient in detecting small bowel manifestations of portal hypertension than other diagnostic modalities, such as retrograde ileoscopy [20, 21]. (2) An accurate diagnosis may enable a therapeutic intervention. In fact, endoscopic treatments for angiectasia-like lesions, such as clipping and argon plasma coagulation (APC), can be performed in patients with portal hypertension using double-balloon enteroscopy [22].

References

1. Garcia-Tsao G. Portal hypertension. Curr Opin Gastroenterol. 2002;18:351–9.
2. Primignani M, Carpinelli L, Preatoni P, Battaglia G, Carta A, Prada A, et al. Natural history of portal hypertensive gastropathy in patients with liver cirrhosis. The New Italian Endoscopic Club for the study and treatment of esophageal varices (NIEC). Gastroenterology. 2000;119:181–7.
3. Bresci G, Parisi G, Capria A. Clinical relevance of colonic lesions in cirrhotic patients with portal hypertension. Endoscopy. 2006;38:830–5.
4. Misra SP, Dwivedi M, Misra V, Dharmani S, Kunwar BK, Arora JS. Colonic changes in patients with cirrhosis and in patients with extrahepatic portal vein obstruction. Endoscopy. 2005;37:454–9.
5. Burak KW, Beck PL. Diagnosis of portal hypertensive gastropathy. Curr Opin Gastroenterol. 2003;19:477–82.
6. Bini EJ, Lascarides CE, Micale PL, Weinshel EH. Mucosal abnormalities of the colon in patients with portal hypertension: an endoscopic study. Gastrointest Endosc. 2000;52:511–6.
7. Thiruvengadam R, Gostout CJ. Congestive gastroenteropathy–an extension of nonvariceal upper gastrointestinal bleeding in portal hypertension. Gastrointest Endosc. 1989;35:504–7.
8. Viggiano TR, Gostout CJ. Portal hypertensive intestinal vasculopathy: a review of the clinical, endoscopic, and histopathologic features. Am J Gastroenterol. 1992;87:944–54.
9. De Palma GD, Rega M, Masone S, Persico F, Siciliano S, Patrone F, et al. Mucosal abnormalities of the small bowel in patients with cirrhosis and portal hypertension: a capsule endoscopy study. Gastrointest Endosc. 2005;62:529–34.
10. Repici A, Pennazio M, Ottobrelli A, Barbon V, De Angelis C, De Lio A, et al. Endoscopic capsule in cirrhotic patients with portal hypertension: spectrum and prevalence of small bowel lesions. Endoscopy. 2005;37 Suppl 1:A72.
11. Figueiredo P, Almeida N, Lérias C, Lopes S, Gouveia H, Leitão MC, et al. Effect of portal hypertension in the small bowel: an endoscopic approach. Dig Dis Sci. 2008;53:2144–50.
12. Abdelaal UM, Morita E, Nouda S, Kuramoto T, Miyaji K, Fukui H, et al. Evaluation of portal hypertensive enteropathy by scoring with capsule endoscopy: is transient elastography of clinical impact? J Clin Biochem Nutr. 2010;47:37–44.
13. Aoyama T, Oka S, Aikata H, Nakano M, Nakano M, Watari I, et al. Small bowel abnormalities in patients with compensated liver cirrhosis. Dig Dis Sci. 2013;58:1390–6.
14. Goulas S, Triantafyllidou K, Karagiannis S, Nicolaou P, Galanis P, Vafiadis I, et al. Capsule endoscopy in the investigation of patients with portal hypertension and anemia. Can J Gastroenterol. 2008;22:469–74.
15. Kovács M, Pák P, Pák G, Fehér J, Rácz I. Small bowel alterations in portal hypertension: a capsule endoscopic study. Hepatogastroenterology. 2009;56:1069–73.
16. Canlas KR, Dobozi BM, Lin S, Smith AD, Rockey DC, Muir AJ, et al. Using capsule endoscopy to identify GI tract lesions in cirrhotic patients with portal hypertension and chronic anemia. J Clin Gastroenterol. 2008;42:844–8.
17. Takahashi Y, Fujimori S, Narahara Y, Gudis K, Ensaka Y, Kosugi Y, et al. Small intestinal edema had the strongest correlation with portal venous pressure amongst capsule endoscopy findings. Digestion. 2012;86:48–54.
18. Urbain D, Vandebosch S, Hindryckx P, Colle I, Reynaert H, Mana F, et al. Capsule endoscopy findings in cirrhosis with portal hypertension: a prospective study. Dig Liver Dis. 2008;40:392–3.
19. Jimenez-Saenz M, Romero-Vazquez J, Caunedo-Alvarez A, Herrerias-Gutierrez JM. Capsule endoscopy: a useful tool in portal hypertensive enteropathy. Gastrointest Endosc. 2006;64:152.
20. Misra SP, Dwivedi M, Misra V, Gupta M. Ileal varices and portal hypertensive ileopathy in patients with cirrhosis and portal hypertension. Gastrointest Endosc. 2004;60:778–83.
21. Rana SS, Bhasin DK, Jahagirdar S, Raja K, Nada R, Kochhar R, et al. Is there ileopathy in portal hypertension? J Gastroenterol Hepatol. 2006;21:392–7.
22. Kodama M, Uto H, Numata M, Hori T, Hori T, Murayama T, et al. Endoscopic characterization of the small bowel in patients with portal hypertension evaluated by double balloon endoscopy. J Gastroenterol. 2008;43:589–96.

Video Capsule Endoscopy in Suspected Crohn's Disease

24

Jonathan A. Leighton, Kenji Watanabe, Federico Argüelles-Arias, and Juan Manuel Herrerías Gutiérrez

Contents

The work was first published in 2006 by Springer Medizin Verlag Heidelberg with the following title: *Atlas of Video Capsule Endoscopy*.

J.A. Leighton (✉)
Division of Gastroenterology and Hepatology, Mayo Clinic, Scottsdale, AZ, USA
e-mail: leighton.jonathan@mayo.edu

K. Watanabe
Department of Gastroenterology, Graduate School of Medicine, Osaka City General Hospital, Osaka, Japan
e-mail: kenjiw@med.osaka-cu.ac.jp

F. Argüelles-Arias • J.M. Herrerías-Gutiérrez
Department of Gastroenterology,
Hospital Universitario Virgen Macarena, Seville, Spain
e-mail: farguelles@telefonica.net; jmherrerias@doctorcat.net

24.1 Introduction

Until the implementation of video capsule endoscopy (VCE), the diagnosis of small bowel Crohn's disease was usually made by small bowel radiology or ileocolonoscopy and in some cases by enteroscopy. Without doubt, VCE has emerged as a diagnostic tool able to identify lesions of the small bowel that are undetectable by conventional endoscopy and radiologic studies. Crohn's disease was first described as a chronic inflammatory disease of the terminal ileum in association with intestinal stenoses or fistulae. We now know that Crohn's disease can affect the entire gastrointestinal tract from the mouth to the anus and in particular the more proximal regions of the small bowel. According to current guidelines for suspected Crohn's disease, the first-line diagnostic procedure to establish the diagnosis is ileocolonoscopy and biopsies from the terminal ileum and the colon [1].

When Crohn's disease affects only the colon or the most distal aspect of the terminal ileum, it is relatively easy to make a diagnosis by ileocolonoscopy. When ileoscopy is not possible or the disease is more proximal, however, the diagnosis can be challenging. In addition, it is known that small bowel Crohn's disease may present as a patchy disease and may skip bowel segments, including the terminal ileum. Furthermore, endoscopy cannot reach the terminal ileum in 15 % of patients. In these cases, an endoscopic and histologic diagnosis may not be possible with ileocolonoscopy alone, and additional imaging modalities are often required [2]. Finally, there are studies suggesting that examination of the terminal ileum alone may not be predictive of disease activity in the entire small bowel [3].

Evidence suggests that the initial location of Crohn's disease does influence the natural evolution of the disease and the risk of complications and surgery. Involvement of the small bowel tends to be more severe than colonic involvement. For example, patients with ileal disease have a 69 % probability of surgery at 5 years, compared with 19 % for those with involvement of other bowel segments [4]. In addition, most patients with small bowel Crohn's disease eventually develop strictur-

Fig. 24.1 Magnetic resonance enteroscopy (MRE) shows vascular engorgement (comb sign) (*yellow arrows*) in a patient with Crohn's disease

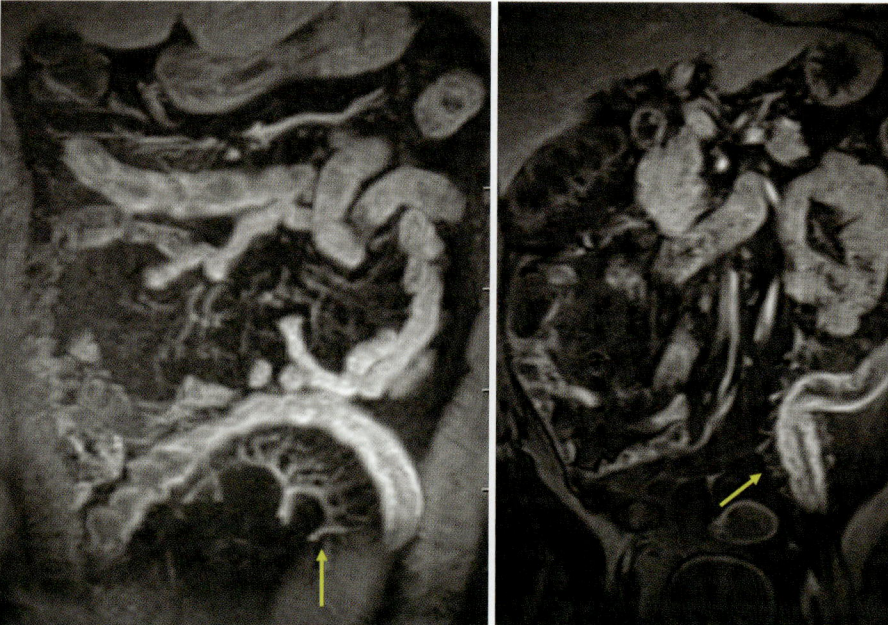

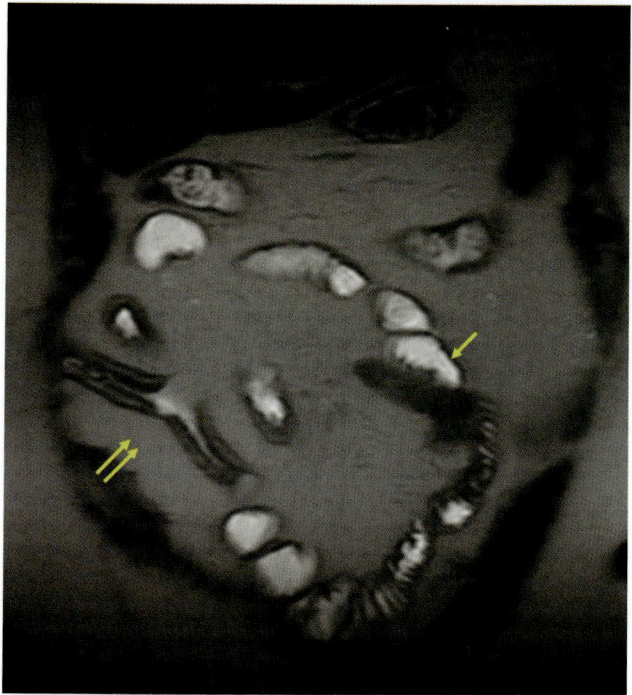

Fig. 24.2 MRE from a patient with Crohn's disease, showing ileal bowel wall thickening (*double arrow*) and normal intestinal wall (*single arrow*)

ing or perforating complications; earlier diagnosis and intervention can help to prevent these complications [5].

Therefore, imaging methods such as magnetic resonance enterography (MRE) and VCE are especially important and necessary to reach a diagnosis in this type of patient, as various radiologic methods and endoscopies sometimes make a final diagnosis only after many years. For this reason, MRE (Figs. 24.1 and 24.2) may be the preferred modality for evaluation of small bowel disease; especially in young patients suspected of having

Crohn's disease, most of whom will undergo frequent, repeated studies [6]. This technique is not available in all centers, moreover an expert radiologist is required due to the fact that superficial mucosal lesions can be overlooked [7]. When VCE is feasible (after strictures are ruled out), it shows slightly greater sensitivity for mucosal lesions than MRE [8].

24.2 Video Capsule Endoscopy in Patients with Suspicion of Crohn's Disease

At present, no test is the gold standard for the definitive diagnosis of Crohn's disease; the diagnosis results from the overall clinical, analytic, radiologic, and endoscopic findings [9]. In patients with suspected Crohn's disease, VCE has a potential role, especially for those patients with only small bowel involvement that is proximal to the terminal ileum.

The main problem reported with VCE is that although its yield is high, many of the mucosal changes detected are not specific for Crohn's disease [10]. In asymptomatic individuals and in as many as two thirds of individuals regularly using nonsteroidal anti-inflammatory drugs (NSAIDs), mucosal abnormalities can be observed and may be indistinguishable from Crohn's disease [11]. The establishment of certain criteria to identify which patients might benefit from VCE for the diagnosis of Crohn's disease is necessary, as is a score to better define whether the lesions observed signify Crohn's disease.

The first consensus declaration of the International Conference on Capsule Endoscopy (ICCE) concluded that VCE is able to identify lesions of the mucosa of the small bowel that are overlooked by other imaging techniques and also can define suspected Crohn's disease groups [12]. The ICCE later published an algorithm defining criteria suspicious for Crohn's disease [13] (Fig. 24.3). Ileocolonoscopy is the

Fig. 24.3 Criteria for suspected Crohn's disease. *CRP* C-reactive protein, *ESR* erythrocyte sedimentation rate, *MRE* MR enteroscopy, *PSC* primary sclerosing cholangitis, *SB* small bowel

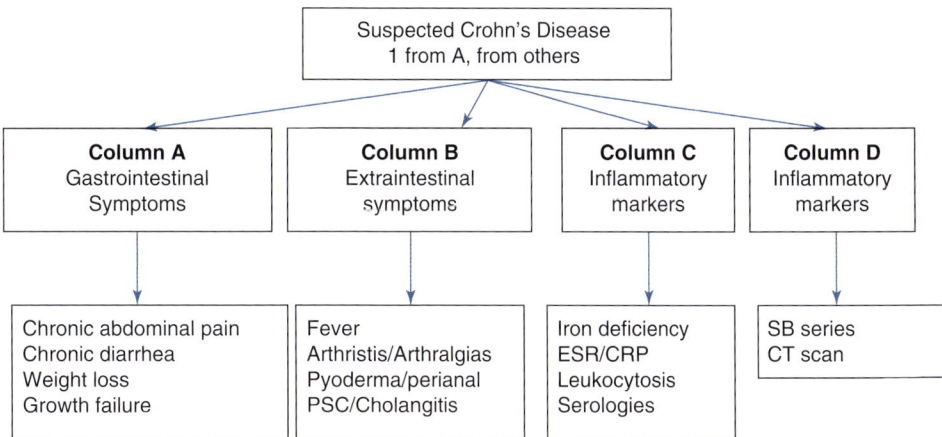

initial procedure of choice and should always be performed prior to VCE, but VCE should be considered for suspected Crohn's disease in any patient with negative ileocolonoscopy who presents with abdominal pain or diarrhea in association with extraintestinal manifestations, elevated inflammatory markers, or abnormalities on other imaging tests [14].

Initial studies assessing the use of VCE in patients with suspected Crohn's disease suggested a higher diagnostic yield with this technique than with other modalities [15]. Fireman et al. [16] evaluated the efficacy of VCE in patients with a suspicion of small bowel Crohn's disease that was undetected by other diagnostic techniques, including small bowel follow-through (SBFT), upper gastrointestinal endoscopy, and colonoscopy. This study included 17 patients: 9 with anemia, 8 with abdominal pain, 7 with diarrhea, and 3 with weight loss; the average duration of symptoms was 6.2 years. VCE confirmed the diagnosis of Crohn's disease in 71 % of these patients, in whom other methods were ineffective. Similarly, in order to assess the usefulness of VCE in these patients, Herrerías et al. [17] published another study including 21 patients with a suspicion of Crohn's disease. Compatible lesions were observed in the small bowel in 43 % of the patients, again supporting the effectiveness of VCE in the diagnosis of small bowel Crohn's disease.

More recent studies have confirmed these earlier findings and have shown that VCE can detect the presence of lesions compatible with Crohn's disease that were overlooked by conventional diagnostic techniques. These studies again suggest that VCE has a greater diagnostic potential than other techniques such as SBFT, ileocolonoscopy, or abdominal CT. These studies also confirm the high negative predictive value of a normal capsule study. Solem et al. [2] evaluated the sensitivity and specificity of ileocolonoscopy, abdominal CT, VCE, and SBFT. This study demonstrated that ileocolonoscopy in combination with abdominal CT or SBFT was more effective than VCE with abdominal CT, SBFT, or ileocolonoscopy, because of the low specificity of VCE. The largest comparative study of different imaging modalities included VCE, CT enterography (CTE), and MR enterography (MRE) performed after ileocolonoscopy [18]. The

results suggested that VCE was significantly superior to CTE or MRE in detecting Crohn's disease in the proximal small bowel. Overall, these comparative studies suggest that VCE is more sensitive than SBFT and may be more sensitive than cross-sectional imaging with CTE and MRE, especially when inflammation is more proximal.

Subsequently, a meta-analysis including nine studies with 250 patients compared VCE with other small bowel imaging techniques and concluded that VCE is superior to all other modalities in the diagnosis of nonstricturing small bowel Crohn's disease. The study showed a number needed to treat (NNT) of 3 to yield one additional diagnosis of Crohn's disease, compared with small bowel barium radiography, and an NNT of 7 compared with ileocolonoscopy [19].

As VCE has become a popular method of examining the small bowel in adults, studies on its use in pediatrics have also increased in the past few years. Several studies have assessed the diagnostic effectiveness, safety, and tolerability of VCE in pediatric patients [20–23], and they have shown that VCE is an effective method to detect lesions in the small bowel in children with suspected Crohn's disease, with results similar to those in adults.

24.3 Scoring Systems for Inflammatory Bowel Mucosa Disease Observed by VCE

To objectively grade small bowel inflammation, several scoring systems for inflammatory diseases of the small bowel mucosa detected by VCE have recently been developed. The Lewis Index [24] scores three parameters (villous edema, ulceration, and stenosis), which are weighted based on extent and severity. A score lower than 135 is classified as normal or clinically insignificant. Scores between 135 and 790 are classified as mild and scores higher than 790 as moderate to severe. Although this scoring system will help in standardizing severity, it cannot specify the etiology of the mucosal inflammatory changes observed. The Lewis score has been integrated into the PillCam software (Given Imaging, Rapid Reader), making it more accessible. Mow et al. [25] published their experience using VCE in patients with inflammatory bowel disease. Of 22 patients, 9 (40 %) were given a diagnosis of definite Crohn's disease based on findings of linear erosions and multiple ulcerations by the capsule study. Of these nine patients, five had subsequent histologic findings in agreement with the capsule findings and a clinical diagnosis of Crohn's disease. An outcome measure diagnostic of Crohn's disease was made when three or more ulcerations were present. Larger prospective studies are needed to confirm these findings.

Korman et al. [26] proposed the Capsule Endoscopy Structured Terminology (CEST), which has been adopted as the terminology to be used for lesion description. Investigators used the CEST to create a description of the VCE findings (erythema, edema, nodularity, ulcer, stenosis), number of findings, distribution pattern, longitudinal extent, shape, and size to create this scoring system. Gal et al. [27] published a similar scoring system, which they called the Capsule Endoscopy Crohn's Disease Activity Index (CECDAI); it includes evaluation of three parameters (inflammation, extent of disease, and presence of stricture), all of which are graded on a numeric

scale, with the small bowel divided into proximal and distal halves. The authors reported that the kappa for the final score for each patient between different evaluations was 0.87.

Although these scoring systems can objectively and quantitatively describe the number and severity of mucosal abnormalities detected, they have no utility in distinguishing Crohn's disease from other inflammatory disorders. In addition, none of the scoring systems have been shown to correlate with the patient's clinical status or symptom-based Crohn's Disease Activity Index (CDAI) score.

24.4 Early Crohn's Disease Lesions Observed by Video Capsule Endoscopy

In patients with Crohn's disease, conventional endoscopy typically reveals so-called skip lesions, areas of inflammation interposed with normal-appearing mucosa. It is believed that tiny aphthous erosions (Fig. 24.4) are the earliest mucosal changes endoscopically seen. When

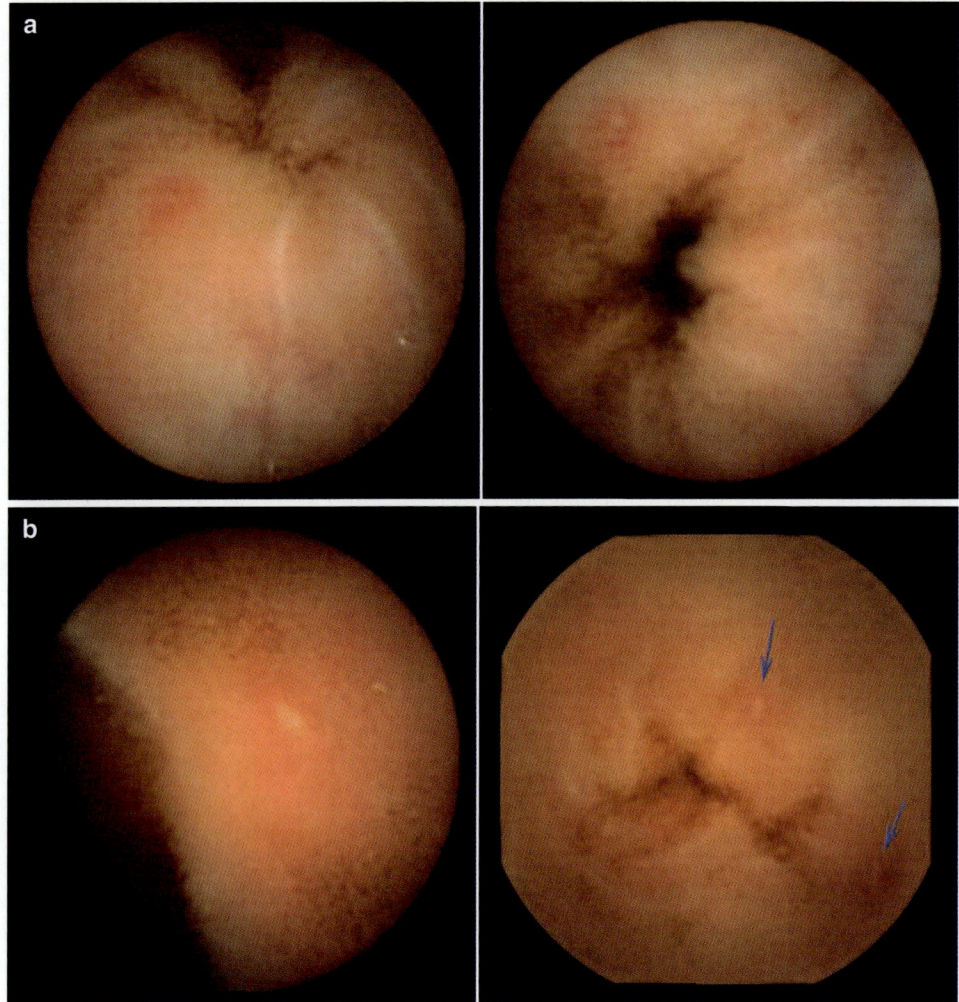

Fig. 24.4 (**a**) This 52-year-old woman was evaluated for chronic abdominal pain and occasional diarrhea. Capsule endoscopy identified tiny aphthous lesions suggesting Crohn's disease; the diagnosis was subsequently confirmed by histology. (**b**) Tiny aphthous erosion in two patients wit suspected Crohn's Disease (*arrows*)

Fig. 24.5 Deep small bowel ulcers in several patients, all with suspected Crohn's disease (*arrows*)

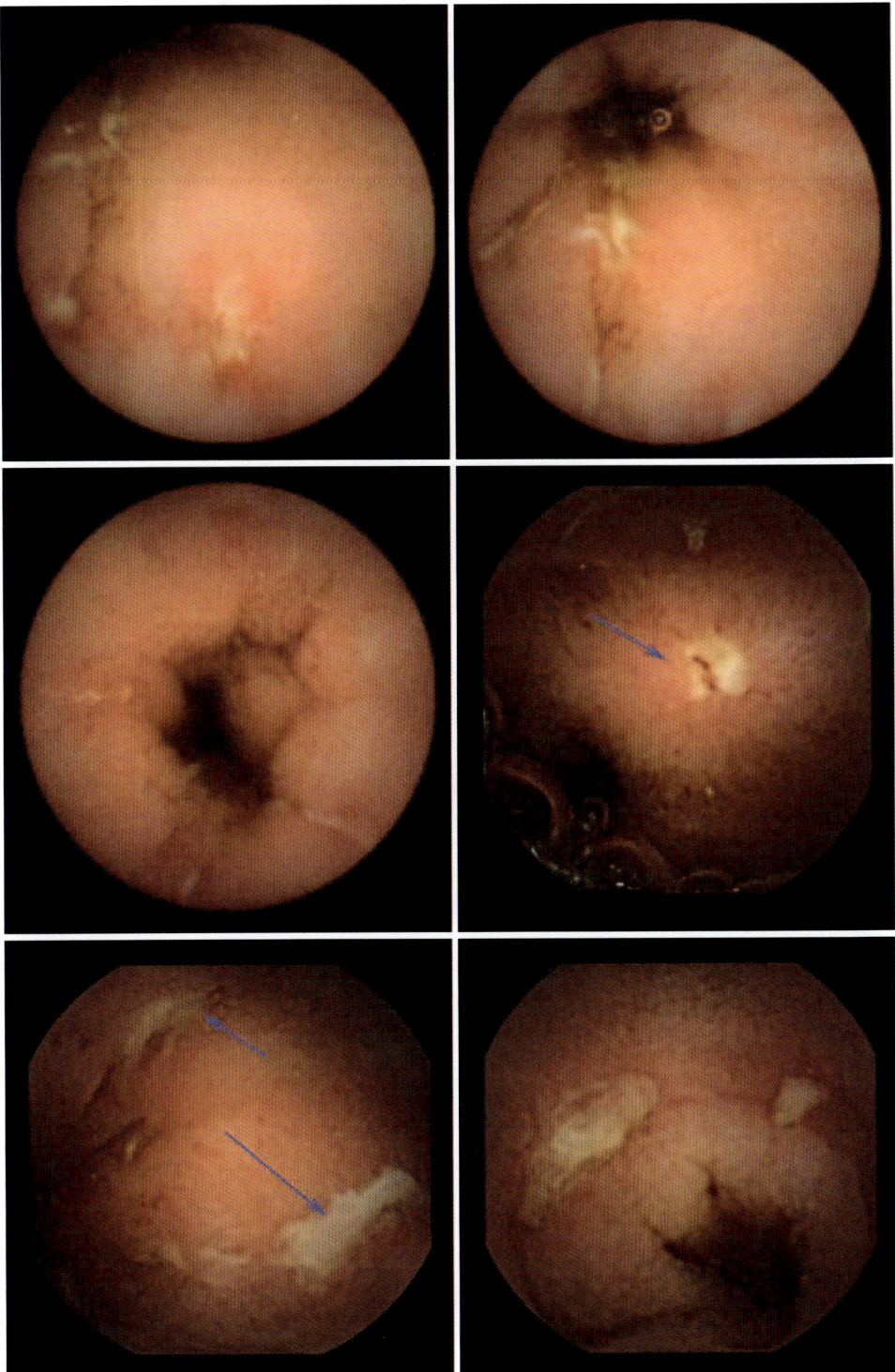

Crohn's disease progresses to a more severe state, ulcerations can enlarge and become deep [28] (Fig. 24.5). Although the presence of small ulcerations on the ileocecal valve or within the terminal ileum in a symptomatic individual is consistent with Crohn's disease, these lesions are nonspecific and can also be drug induced, as seen in individuals taking NSAIDs [29], or they can be of infectious origin, as seen with *Yersinia* infection and tuberculosis.

The spectrum of lesions seen with VCE in patients with Crohn's disease is varied; the lesions resemble those observed by conventional endoscopy. The lesions observed depend on the extent and severity of the Crohn's disease activity. Video capsule endoscopy can detect mucosal fissures (Fig. 24.6),

Fig. 24.6 Mucosal fissure in two patients with suspected Crohn's disease; gastroscopy, ileocolonoscopy, and small bowel follow-through were negative

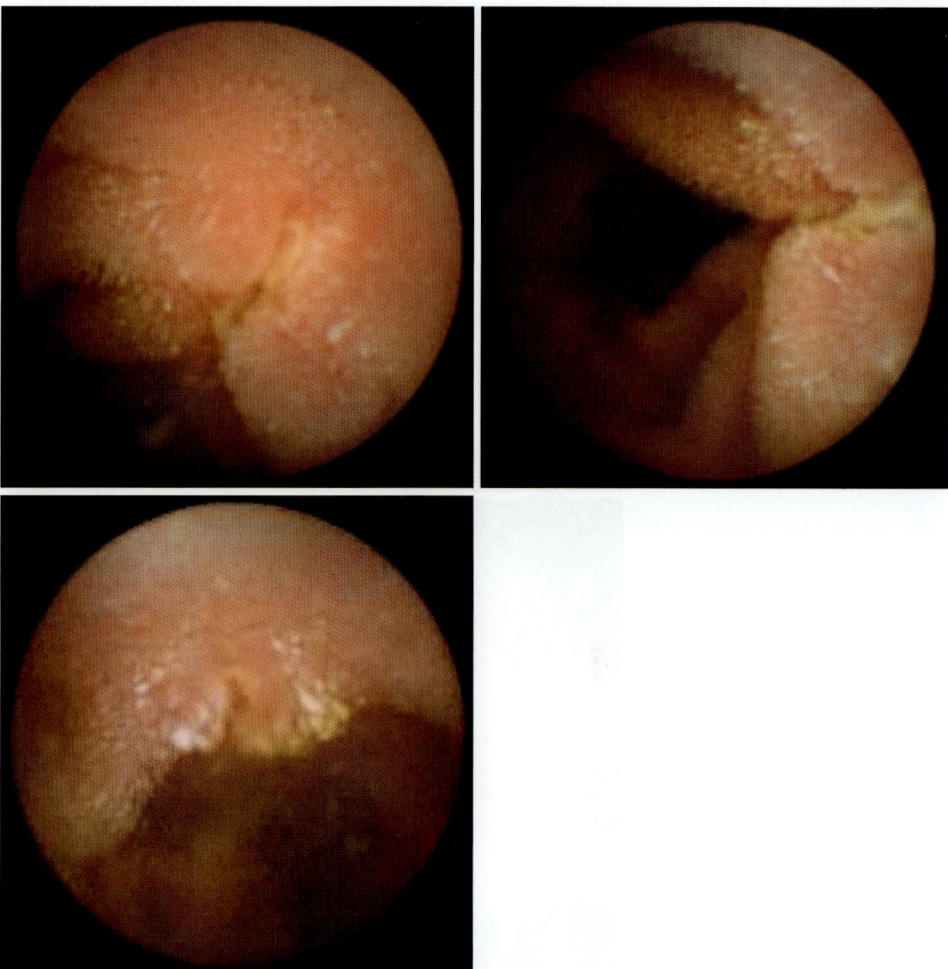

strictures, scarring, bleeding lesions, polyps, pseudopolyps, and linear, round, and irregular ulcers (Figs. 24.7, 24.8, and 24.9). In addition, cobblestoning (multiple longitudinal ulcers running parallel and hill-like elevations due to submucosal swelling), aphthous ulcerations, or stenotic ulcerated areas of mucosa can also be observed [30]. Though these lesions are considered typical of Crohn's disease, VCE may also detect more subtle lesions that often are not visualized by conventional radiologic techniques, such as erythema, edema, loss of villi and denudated areas (Fig. 24.10), and aphthous ulcers. Sometimes other small alterations such as lymphangiectasia or nodular lymphoid hyperplasia (Fig. 24.11) can be observed. These lesions, although less specific, could be considered as early manifestations of Crohn's disease [30, 31]. Aphthous ulcers, which typically have white bases with a small ring of surrounding erythema, in many cases are the initial lesions in early Crohn's disease (Fig. 24.12).

It is important to consider that several cases of Crohn's disease have been reported in which the initial aphthous lesions eventually developed into typical longitudinal ulcers. Chiba et al. [32] reported four cases of the "red ring sign" as the first early lesion of Crohn's disease. The red halo appearance surrounding lymphoid follicles seems to precede visible aphthoid ulcers and is possibly related to the follicles' physiological role as a portal of entry for potentially pathogenic agents [28]. In a study by Krauss et al. [31], the aim was to compare the morphology of lymphoid follicles in Crohn's disease, using confocal laser endomicroscopy in correlation with histologic and immunohistochemical findings of biopsies. They enrolled 46 patients with Crohn's disease and 67 control patients. They standardized images from the terminal ileum and the colon using white light video endoscopes and confocal laser endomicroscopy to analyze subsurface structure of lymphoid follicles. Targeted biopsies of lymphoid follicles were analyzed using hematoxylin and eosin (H&E) stain and immunohistochemistry. Lymphoid follicles were seen in all parts of the lower gastrointestinal tract, but mostly in the terminal ileum and cecum. Endoscopy in 15 of 17 patients with possible early Crohn's disease

Fig. 24.7 Large and small linear ulcers (*arrows*) in suspected Crohn's disease

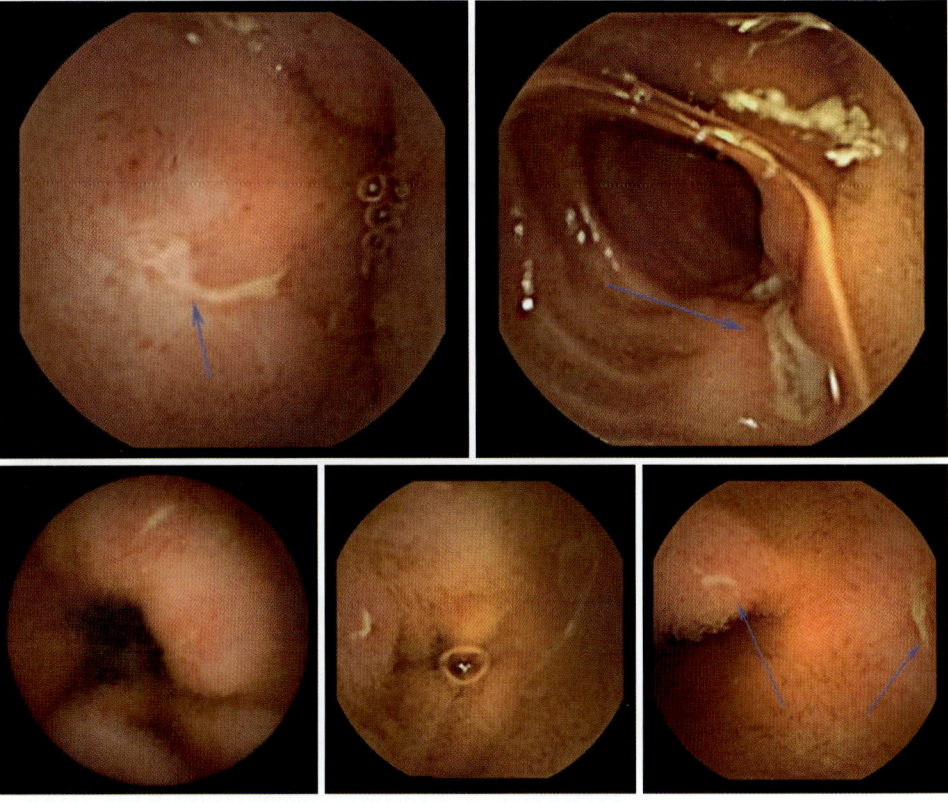

Fig. 24.8 Round ulcers in a 31-year-old man of Indian origin. Iron deficiency anemia was diagnosed about 12 years previously. When no cause could be found for abdominal pain and bloody diarrhea occurred, video capsule endoscopy was performed, leading to the diagnosis of Crohn's disease

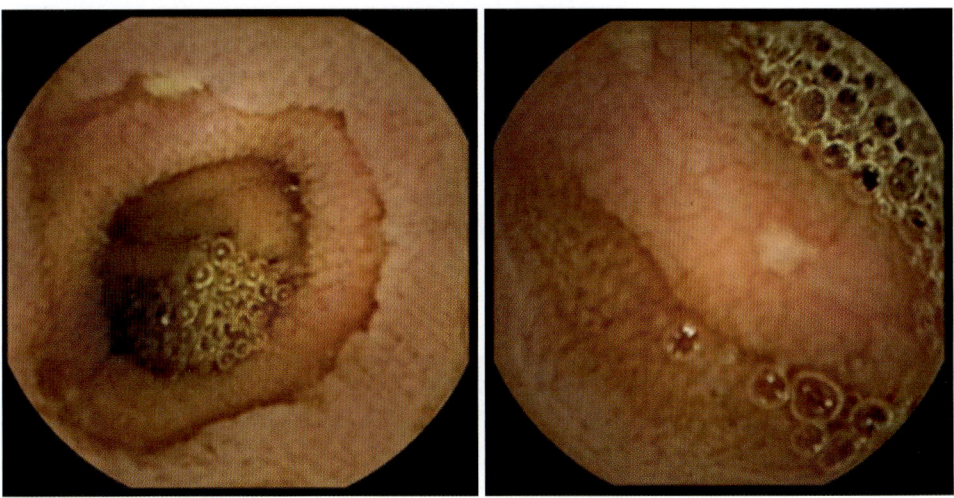

showed lymphoid follicles surrounded by a red ring; in some of them, early aphthous ulcers were also seen. These studies suggest that lymphoid follicles with red rings may represent the earliest lesion in Crohn's disease and thus may be considered as an early marker of disease. These results should be confirmed in larger, prospective studies.

Ileoscopy can miss Crohn's disease of the terminal ileum because the disease can skip the distal ileum or be confined to the intramural portion of the bowel wall and the mesentery. In a recent study [3], 153 patients with Crohn's disease

were evaluated and underwent ileal intubation during endoscopy; 67 (43.8 %) of them had a normal endoscopic appearance on ileoscopy. Despite the normal results on ileoscopy, 36 (53.7 %) of these patients had active, small bowel Crohn's disease. In 11 patients (30.6 %), the disease skipped the distal ileum; 23 patients (63.9 %) developed only intramural and mesenteric disease of the distal ileum, and 2 patients (5.6 %) had only upper gastrointestinal tract involvement. These patients had a shorter duration of disease (less than 5 years in 61.1 %) than those with a Crohn's disease diagnosis

Fig. 24.9 Irregular and stellate ulcers in suspected Crohn's disease

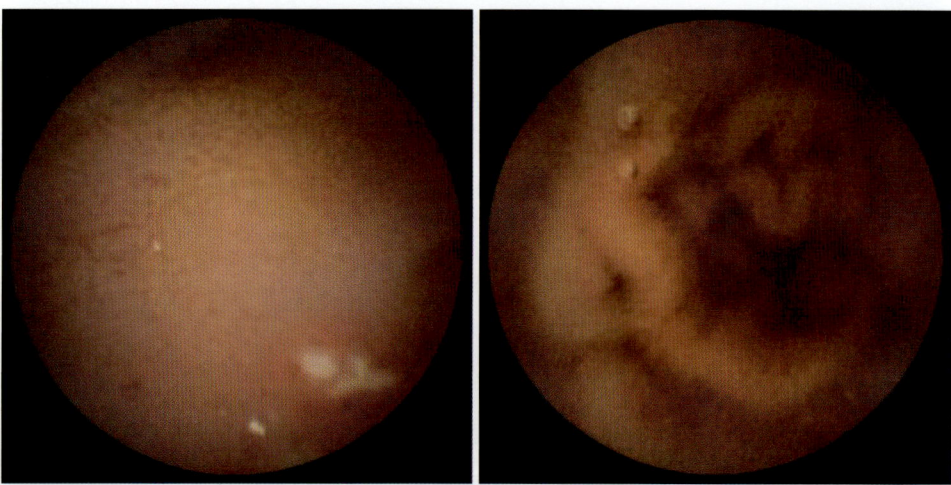

Fig. 24.10 Villi loss and denudated area in a patient with suspected Crohn's disease

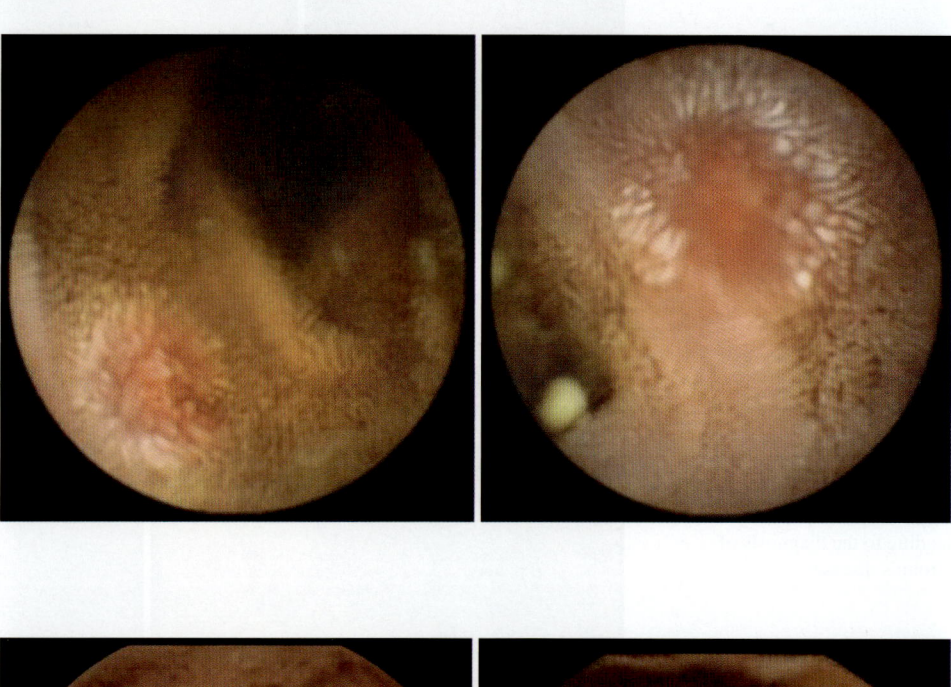

Fig. 24.11 Nodular lymphoid hyperplasia (*arrows*) in Crohn's disease

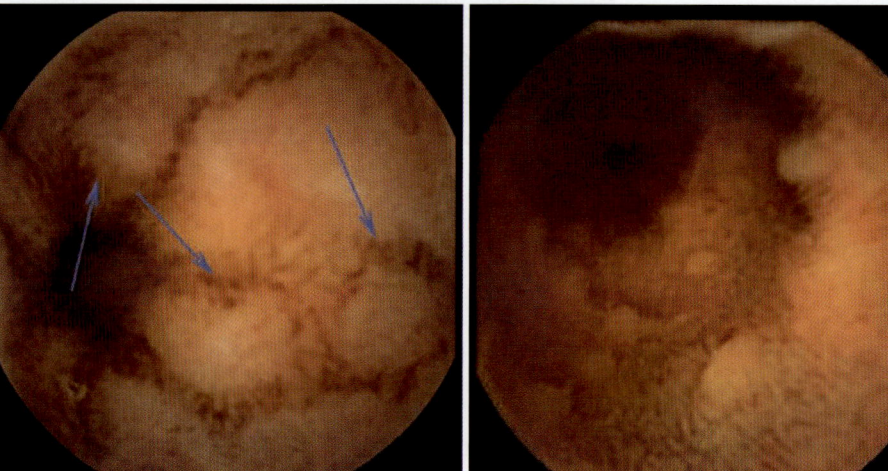

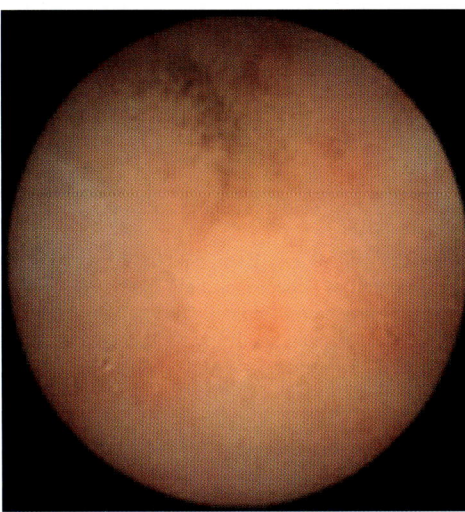

Fig. 24.12 Multiple tiny aphthous ulcers surrounded by completely normal mucosa, in the same patient as shown in Fig. 24.4a

based on ileoscopy (less than 5 years in 41.1 %). This study confirmed the fact that Crohn's disease of the small bowel can be missed with ileoscopy, and VCE can play an important role in these patients.

24.5   Patency Capsule

Capsule retention is perhaps the most feared adverse event in patients with CD due to small bowel strictures. In suspected CD, it appears that the risk of retention is low and less than 2 %. However, in patients with known CD, the risk increases to 6.7–13 % [33, 34]. Unfortunately, studies suggest that significant strictures can be missed with radiologic studies, and thus, barium small bowel X-rays and CT/MR enterography may not be adequate screening tests prior to CE [35, 36]. The use of a patency capsule prior to CE in patients with suspected obstruction has led to a significant reduction in the incidence of capsule retention [37]. In another study, 106 patients with suspected small bowel obstruction ingested the patency capsule prior to CE. The capsule was excreted intact in 56 % of patients, who subsequently underwent CE without retention. Forty percent of these patients had positive findings on CE [38]. These studies confirm the utility of the patency capsule prior to CE in patients with known CD or suspected obstruction to eliminate the risk of capsule retention. There is currently no evidence to suggest that the patency capsule is necessary in suspected CD without signs of obstruction.

Conclusions

It is well known that Crohn's disease is characterized by transmural inflammation with early lesions manifesting as aphthous ulcers that may progress to larger and deeper ulcers, which in turn may lead to fistulae or to fibrotic strictures [39]. For most patients, ileocolonoscopy is the first diagnostic test of choice, but in patients with suspected Crohn's disease who have inflammation proximal to the terminal ileum and in those where ileoscopy is unsuccessful, VCE may play an important role in the diagnosis. In these subgroups of patients, VCE may lead to a more prompt diagnosis, helping these patients to benefit from early treatment or altered management.

References

1. Van Assche G, Dignass A, Panes J, European Crohn's and Colitis Organisation (ECCO), et al. The second European evidence-based consensus on the diagnosis and management of Crohn's disease: definitions and diagnosis. J Crohns Colitis. 2010;4:7–27.
2. Solem CA, Loftus Jr EV, Fletcher JG, et al. Small-bowel imaging in Crohn's disease: a prospective, blinded, 4-way comparison trial. Gastrointest Endosc. 2008;68:255–66.
3. Samuel S, Bruining DH, Loftus Jr EV, et al. Endoscopic skipping of the distal terminal ileum in Crohn's disease can lead to negative results from ileocolonoscopy. Clin Gastroenterol Hepatol. 2012;10:1253–9.
4. Veloso FT, Ferreira JT, Barros L, Almeida S. Clinical outcome of Crohn's disease: analysis according to the Vienna classification and clinical activity. Inflamm Bowel Dis. 2001;7:306–13.
5. Cosnes J, Cattan S, Blain A, et al. Long-term evolution of disease behavior of Crohn's disease. Inflamm Bowel Dis. 2002;8:244–50.
6. Ramalho M, Herédia V, Cardoso C, et al. Magnetic resonance imaging of small bowel Crohn's disease. Acta Med Port. 2012; 25:231–40.
7. Albert JG, Martiny F, Krummenerl A, et al. Diagnosis of small bowel Crohn's disease: a prospective comparison of capsule endoscopy with magnetic resonance imaging and fluoroscopic enteroclysis. Gut. 2005;54:1721–7.
8. Crook DW, Knuesel PR, Froehlich JM, et al. Comparison of magnetic resonance enterography and video capsule endoscopy in evaluating small bowel disease. Eur J Gastroenterol Hepatol. 2009; 21:54–65.
9. Stange EF, Travis S, Vermeire S, European Crohn's and Colitis Organisation, et al. European evidence based consensus on the diagnosis and management of Crohn's disease: definitions and diagnosis. Gut. 2006;55 Suppl 1:i1–15.
10. Goldstein JL, Eisen GM, Lewis B, et al. Video capsule endoscopy to prospectively assess small bowel injury with celecoxib, naproxen plus omeprazole, and placebo. Clin Gastroenterol Hepatol. 2005;3:133–41.
11. Maiden L, Thjodleifsson B, Theodors A, et al. A quantitative analysis of NSAID-induced small bowel pathology by capsule enteroscopy. Gastroenterology. 2005;128:1172–8.
12. Kornbluth A, Colombel JF, Leighton JA, Loftus E. ICCE consensus for inflammatory bowel disease. Endoscopy. 2005;37:1051–4.
13. Mergener K, Ponchon T, Gralnek I, et al. Literature review and recommendations for clinical application of small-bowel capsule

endoscopy, based on a panel discussion by international experts. Consensus statements for small-bowel capsule endoscopy, 2006/2007. Endoscopy. 2007;39:895–909.

14. Lewis BS. Expanding role of capsule endoscopy in inflammatory bowel disease. World J Gastroenterol. 2008;14:4137–41.

15. Eliakim R, Suissa A, Yassin K, et al. Wireless capsule video endoscopy compared to barium follow-through and computerised tomography in patients with suspected Crohn's disease. Dig Liver Dis. 2004;36:519–22.

16. Fireman Z, Mahajna E, Broide E, et al. Diagnosing small bowel Crohn's disease with wireless capsule endoscopy. Gut. 2003;52:390–2.

17. Herrerías JM, Caunedo A, Rodriguez-Téllez M, et al. Capsule endoscopy in patients with suspected Crohn's disease and negative endoscopy. Endoscopy. 2003;35:564–9.

18. Jensen MD, Nathan T, Rafaelsen SR, Kjeldsen J. Diagnostic accuracy of capsule endoscopy for small bowel Crohn's disease is superior to that of MR enterography or CT enterography. Clin Gastroenterol Hepatol. 2011;9:124–9.

19. Triester SL, Leighton JA, Leontiadis GI, et al. A meta-analysis of the yield of capsule endoscopy compared to other diagnostic modalities in patients with non-stricturing small bowel Crohn's disease. Am J Gastroenterol. 2006;101:954–64.

20. Argüelles-Arias F, Caunedo A, Romero J, et al. The value of capsule endoscopy in pediatric patients with a suspicion of Crohn's disease. Endoscopy. 2004;36:869–73.

21. Ge ZZ, Chen HY, Gao YJ, et al. Clinical application of wireless capsule endoscopy in pediatric patients for suspected small bowel diseases. Eur J Pediatr. 2007;166:825–9.

22. De Angelis GL, Fornaroli F, de Angelis N, et al. Wireless capsule endoscopy for pediatric small-bowel diseases. Am J Gastroenterol. 2007;102:1749–57.

23. Cohen SA, Klevens AI. Use of capsule endoscopy in diagnosis and management of pediatric patients, based on meta-analysis. Clin Gastroenterol Hepatol. 2011;9:490–6.

24. Gralnek IM, DeFranchis R, Seidman E, et al. Development of a capsule endoscopy scoring index for small bowel mucosal inflammatory change. Aliment Pharmacol Ther. 2008;27:146–54.

25. Mow WS, Lo SK, Targan SR, et al. Initial experience with wireless capsule enteroscopy in the diagnosis and management of inflammatory bowel disease. Clin Gastroenterol Hepatol. 2004;2:31–40.

26. Korman LY, Delvaux M, Gay G, et al. Capsule endoscopy structured terminology (CEST): proposal of a standardized and structured terminology for reporting capsule endoscopy procedures. Endoscopy. 2005;37:951–9.

27. Gal E, Geller A, Fraser G, et al. Assessment and validation of the new capsule endoscopy Crohn's disease activity index (CECDAI). Dig Dis Sci. 2008;53:1933–7.

28. Fujimura Y, Kamoi R, Iida M. Pathogenesis of aphthoid ulcers in Crohn's disease: correlative findings by magnifying colonoscopy, electron microscopy, and immunohistochemistry. Gut. 1996;38:724–32.

29. Lengeling RW, Mitros FA, Brennan JA, Schulze KS. Ulcerative ileitis encountered at ileocolonoscopy: likely role of nonsteroidal agents. Clin Gastroenterol Hepatol. 2003;1:160–9.

30. Salgado M, Mascarenhas-Saraiva M. Inflammatory disease of the small bowel. In: Herrerías JM, Mascarenhas-Saraiva M, editors. Atlas of capsule endoscopy. Sevilla: Sulime; 2012. p. 194–7.

31. Krauss E, Agaimy A, Neumann H, et al. Characterization of lymphoid follicles with red ring signs as first manifestation of early Crohn's disease by conventional histopathology and confocal laser endomicroscopy. Int J Clin Exp Pathol. 2012;5:411–21.

32. Chiba M, Iizuka M, Ohtaka M, et al. Four cases of the red ring sign. Gastrointest Endosc. 1992;38:728–30.

33. Barkin JS, Friedman S. Wireless capsule endoscopy requiring surgical intervention: the world's experience. Am J Gastroenterol. 2002;97:S298.

34. Cave D, Legnani P, de Franchis R, Lewis BS. ICCE consensus for capsule retention. Endoscopy. 2005;37:1065–7.

35. Delvaux MM, Laurent V, Regent D. Should an entero-CT scanner (CT) necessarily precede capsule endoscopy (CE) recording when exploring patients with suspected small intestinal disease (SID). Gastrointest Endosc. 2004;59:AB175.

36. Fernandez-Diez S, Asteinza M, Gonzales F, et al. Capsule retention in small bowel strictures: a retrospective study. Paper presented at the Fourth International Conference on Capsule Endoscopy (ICCE 2005), Miami, 6–8 Mar 2005.

37. Signorelli C, Rondonotti E, Villa F, et al. Use of the Given Patency System for the screening of patients at high risk for capsule retention. Dig Liver Dis. 2006;38:326–30.

38. Herrerias JM, Leighton JA, Costamagna G, et al. Agile patency system eliminates risk of capsule retention in patients with known intestinal strictures who undergo capsule endoscopy. Gastrointest Endosc. 2008;67:902–9.

39. Rutgeerts PJ. From aphthous ulcer to full-blown Crohn's disease. Dig Dis. 2011;29:211–4.

Established Crohn's Disease

25

Winfried A. Voderholzer, Asher Kornbluth,
and Peter E. Legnani

Contents

The work was first published in 2006 by Springer Medizin Verlag Heidelberg with the following title: *Atlas of Video Capsule Endoscopy*.

W.A. Voderholzer (✉)
Gastroenterology Practice, Berlin, Germany
e-mail: wvoderho@googlemail.com

A. Kornbluth • P.E. Legnani
Mount Sinai Hospital, New York, NY, USA
e-mail: asher.kornbluth@mssm.edu; peter.legnani@mssm.edu

25.1 Natural History

Studies on the natural history of Crohn's disease reveal that it is a progressive disease marked by spontaneous relapses; if left untreated, it can lead over time to severe, disabling bowel damage and dysfunction. Only 10 % of patients show prolonged clinical remission. Up to one third of patients have evidence of a stricturing or penetrating intestinal complication at diagnosis, and at least half have experienced an intestinal complication within 20 years after diagnosis. The annual incidence of hospitalizations is about 20 %. Half of patients require surgery within 10 years after diagnosis [1]. Young age, immediate need for corticosteroids, perianal disease, colonic resection, repeated small bowel resection, stricturing phenotype, substantial weight loss, and specific endoscopic lesions may predict a disabling disease course [2]. Considerable evidence is accumulating that achievement of mucosal healing will not only control symptoms but also will reduce the patient's need for steroids, hospitalization, and surgery.

25.2 Treatment

There is strong evidence that patients with Crohn's disease should stop smoking. There are no strict general nutritional recommendations. Enteral nutrition may have a positive effect but is difficult for patients to tolerate beyond a short term.

Several medications can treat Crohn's disease pharmacologically. The 5-aminosalicylic acid (ASA) agents are often useful for mild to moderate disease, especially in the colon. For mild to moderate disease involving the ileum and ascending colon, budesonide (an oral, topically active corticosteroid with extensive first-pass hepatic metabolism) is effective. In patients with more severe disease, oral and intravenous corticosteroids are useful for inducing clinical remission, but they are not effective as maintenance medications and are associated with frequent and potentially serious toxicity. Antibiotics such as metronidazole, ciprofloxacin, or both may be useful for patients with mild to moderate inflammation (particularly in the colon) and for

Fig. 25.1 Endoscopic balloon dilation of a colonic stricture in a patient with Crohn's disease. The stricture is shown before (**a**) and during (**b**) dilatation. After dilatation, the prestenotic bowel segment can be visualized (**c**)

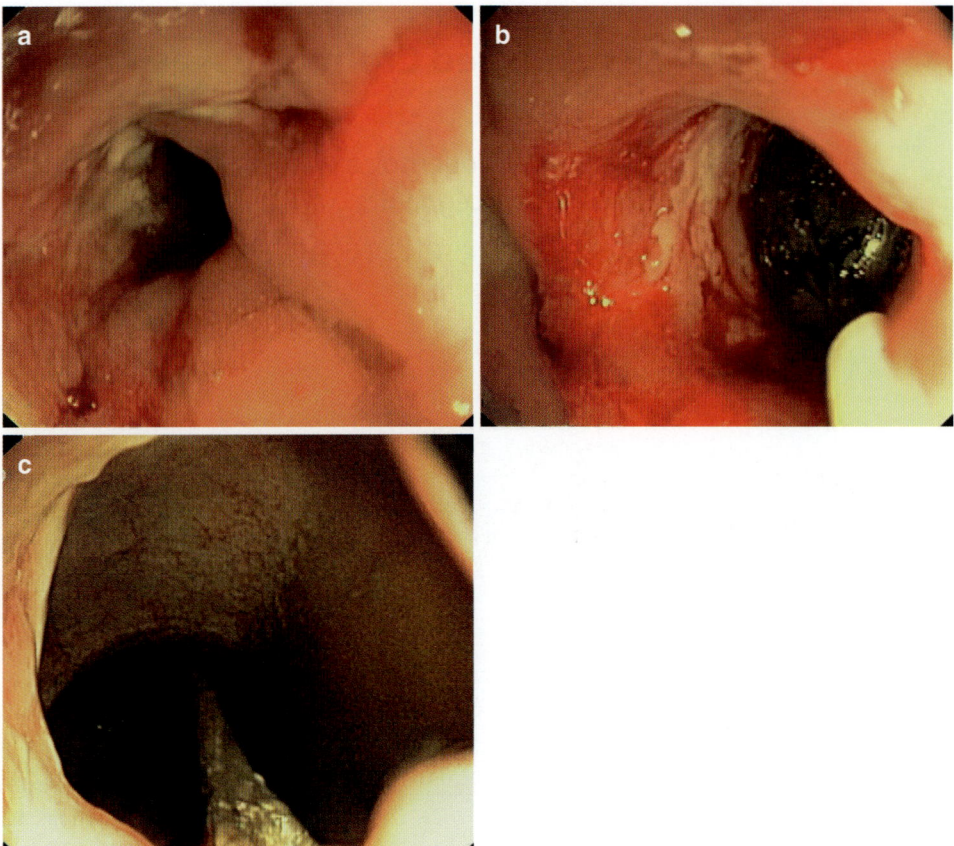

those with mild perianal disease. Immunomodulatory drugs such as 6-mercaptopurine (6-MP), azathioprine, or methotrexate should be used in chronic active cases as steroid-sparing agents, or when 5-ASA medication, antibiotics, or budesonide fail to control symptoms. The anti-tumor necrosis factor (TNF) alpha antibodies infliximab, adalimumab, or certolizumab pegol should be used in patients that do not respond to standard treatments. To maintain remission, azathioprine, 6-MP, methotrexate, infliximab, adalimumab, and certolizumab pegol have all demonstrated efficacy. Recently a small, randomized controlled trial found that infliximab introduced soon after surgery was effective in preventing endoscopic and clinical remission for more than 1 year. Metronidazole and 6-MP/azathioprine may also reduce relapse after surgical remission, but probably with less effectiveness than infliximab.

Endoscopic balloon dilation (Fig. 25.1) may be used in selected patients with strictures due to Crohn's disease. Surgery should be used restrictively for patients with abscesses, complex perianal or internal fistulas that do not respond sufficiently to medical therapy, fibrostenotic strictures with symptoms of partial or complete obstruction, high-grade dysplasia, or cancer [2].

25.3 Diagnostic Methods

Apart from clinical monitoring, several methods are useful in establishing the diagnosis, specifying the extent and activity of the disease, and monitoring disease activity at follow-up. These methods include ultrasound, CT or MR enterography, conventional endoscopy, conventional or balloon-assisted enteroscopy, and video capsule endoscopy (VCE).

25.3.1 Ultrasound

As discussed in Chap. 18, abdominal ultrasound (Fig. 25.2) is a noninvasive and generally available method. It can be performed as a native or contrast-enhanced examination. In the hand of an experienced investigator, it may provide the most useful information about disease activity, strictures, fistulas, and abscesses. In centers with expert experience, contrast-enhanced ultrasound has been shown to be comparable to CT enteroclysis [3]. In anorectal disease, transrectal ultrasound may assist the colorectal surgeon's therapeutic approach.

Fig. 25.2 Power Doppler ultrasound examination showing ileal wall thickening (**a**) and inflammatory enhanced wall perfusion of the ascending colon (**b**). (Courtesy of Jürgen Bauditz, MD)

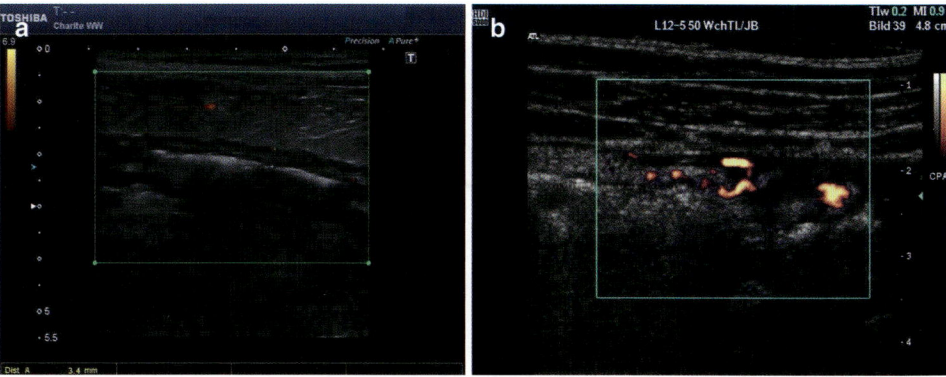

Fig. 25.3 MR enterography. (**a**) *Arrows* indicate wall thickening in the terminal ileum. (**b**) Skip lesions: *white arrows* indicate healthy bowel segments, and *red arrows* indicate inflamed bowel segments. (**c**) Interenteric abscess (*between arrows*). (Courtesy of Gerd Diederichs, MD)

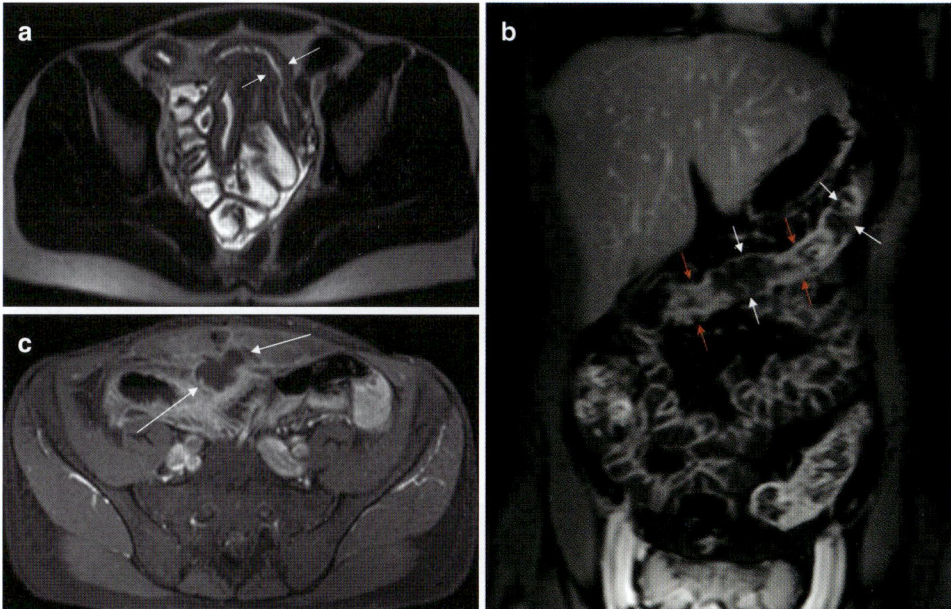

25.3.2 Radiology

Although conventional enteroclysis may be useful in selected patients, CT and/or MR enterography is usually found to be more clinically useful. To date, the most sensitive radiologic method is CT enterography, which provides the highest spatial resolution and may detect strictures, abscesses, and fistulas. Its use is limited by radiation exposure and the common use of contrast media, however. MR enterography is nonradiating and does not require iodine-containing contrast media (Fig. 25.3). Therefore, it has become the preferred method for follow-up examinations and the management of complications such as fistula or abscess. CT and MR enteroclysis are very effective in detecting intestinal pathology, but they are hampered by poor patient tolerance of intestinal tube placement, as well as the limitations mentioned above.

25.3.3 Conventional Endoscopy

Ileocolonoscopy is the most important diagnostic method for evaluating patients with terminal ileal and colonic disease and observing their responses to therapy. It also aids in obtaining mucosal biopsies (Figs. 25.4 and 25.5d), performing cancer surveillance in high-risk individuals, and examining and dilating strictures. Because of the difference in distribution and pattern of inflammation, endoscopy can also help to differentiate between ulcerative colitis and Crohn's disease.

Ileocolonoscopy may also be used as a screening tool to detect colorectal cancer. Because patients with extensive colonic involvement have an incidence of carcinoma up to 25-fold higher than normal, a yearly ileocolonoscopy is indicated for these patients after 8–10 years.

Moreover, because primary sclerosing cholangitis (PSC) is a risk factor for colon cancer, a yearly ileocolonoscopy is justified as soon as the coexistence of PSC and colitis is established [4].

Esophagogastroduodenoscopy (EGD) helps to diagnose proximal disease involvement (Fig. 25.5).

25.3.4 Conventional and Balloon-Assisted Enteroscopy

Whereas with conventional (push) enteroscopy, only the proximal small intestine can be visualized, and a total examination of the small intestine can be performed by using balloon-assisted enteroscopy (BAE), discussed in Chaps. 13 and 14. Most studies on BAE have been performed with double-balloon endoscopy.

The advantages of these examinations include the capability to take biopsy specimens and to treat strictures by using balloon dilation, but their use is somewhat limited by their invasive nature (complication rate, 1.2 % [5]) and the need for experienced endoscopists. At present, data on BAE are sparse, and it cannot be generally recommended for Crohn's disease patients, unless standard examinations have been inconclusive and tissue sampling would alter management [6].

25.3.5 Video Capsule Endoscopy

VCE is a very sensitive method to detect small bowel lesions. It is superior to conventional radiology [7, 8], to CT enteroclysis [9, 10], and to MR enterography for proximal lesions [11]. To avoid capsule retention, however, these studies have included only patients with non-stricturizing

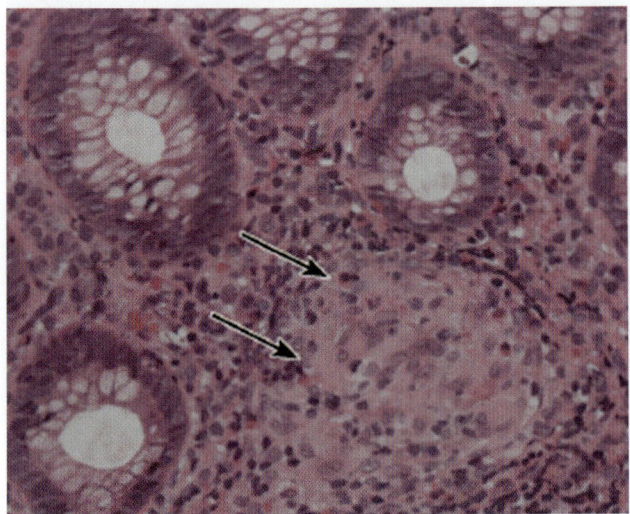

Fig. 25.4 Typical epitheloid cell granuloma (*arrows*) in Crohn's disease (Courtesy of Wilko Weichert, MD)

Fig. 25.5 Lesions of Crohn's disease seen with conventional endoscopy. (**a**) Gastric aphthae. (**b**) Duodenal aphtha. (**c**) Duodenal stricture seen with esophagogastroduodenoscopy (EGD). (**d**) Ileocolonoscopy showing cobblestone pattern in the terminal ileum (Courtesy of Christian Jürgensen, MD)

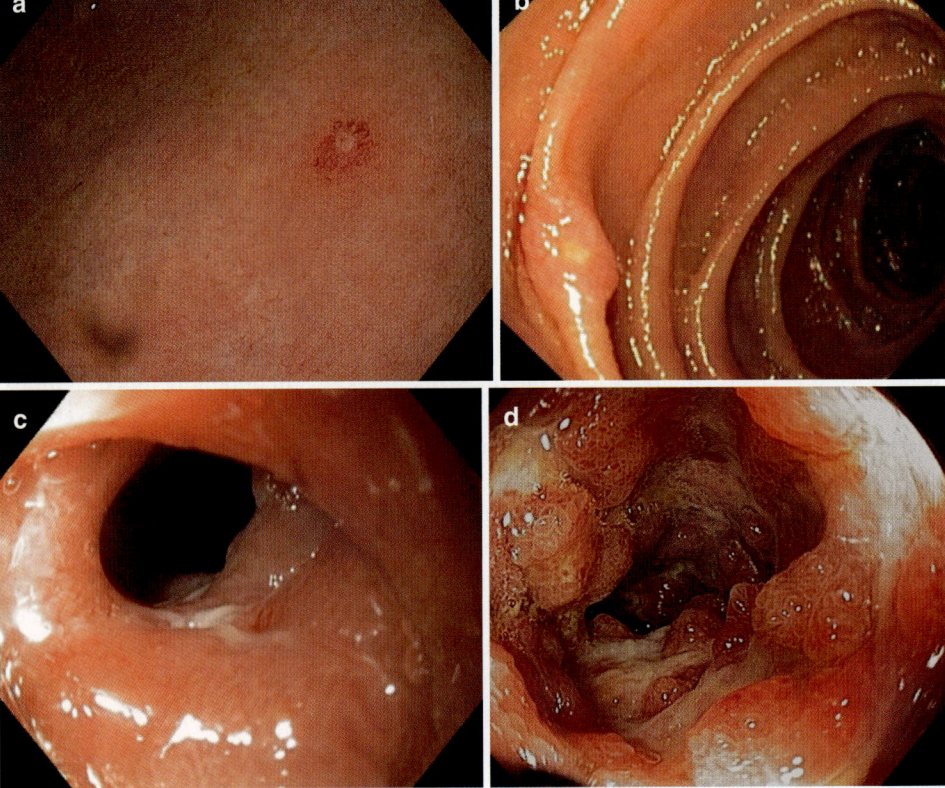

disease. Moreover, VCE cannot perform histologic sampling, and it may yield false-positive results in healthy patients. Pathologic findings (specifically "mucosal breaks") are noted in up to 14 % of healthy individuals [12].

25.4 Morphology of Lesions

Classic lesions seen are notched or shallow aphthae (Fig. 25.6), fissural ulcers (Fig. 25.7), and craterlike ulcers (Fig. 25.8a). Lesions may be hemorrhagic (Fig. 25.9) or may present as a cobblestone pattern (Figs. 25.8b and 25.5d). Progressive disease may result in peri-intestinal abscesses (Fig. 25.3c), fistulas, or both. The lesions typically show a discontinuous pattern of involvement, which may be seen best at enteroclysis, with normal mucosa intervening between diseased segments (so-called skip lesions, Fig. 25.3b). The endoscopic appearance of strictures is not a definite indicator of whether a VCE capsule can pass through (Figs. 25.10). VCE in an early stage of Crohn's disease may demonstrate circumscribed lesions such as villous denudation (Fig. 25.11), which apparently are precursors to

the typical aphthous lesions [13]. Patients with superficial lesions may present with normal findings in small bowel follow-through or CT enteroclysis.

25.5 Clinical Applications of VCE in Established Crohn's Disease

Whereas the role of VCE in "suspected Crohn's disease" has been established (see Chap. 24), its importance for patients with known Crohn's disease remains controversial. Diagnostic yield has to be weighed against a comparably high risk of capsule retention. Therefore, international guidelines state that VCE should be reserved for those patients with a high clinical suspicion of Crohn's disease despite negative investigation by ileocolonoscopy and other imaging techniques [6, 14]. Additionally, it is emphasized that small bowel strictures should be excluded before VCE is performed [4]. It seems obvious that radiologic imaging should precede VCE because of the potential for unrecognized strictures to cause small bowel obstruction requiring emergency surgery.

Fig. 25.6 Video capsule endoscopy (VCE) showing aphthae. (**a**) Multiple jejunal aphthae. (**b**) Notched jejunal aphtha. (**c**) Single aphtha in the ileum. (**d**) Single aphtha in the jejunum. (Courtesy of Robert Wentrup, MD)

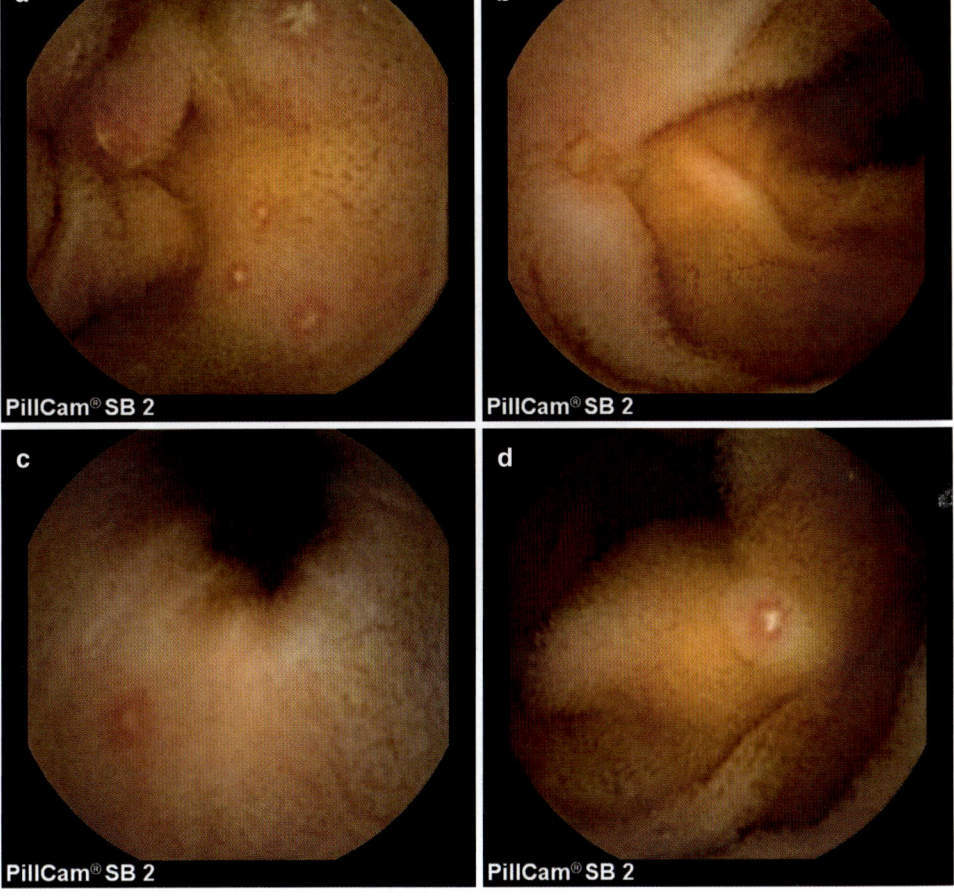

Fig. 25.7 (**a**, **b**) Fissural ulcers, viewed with VCE. (Courtesy of Robert Wentrup, MD)

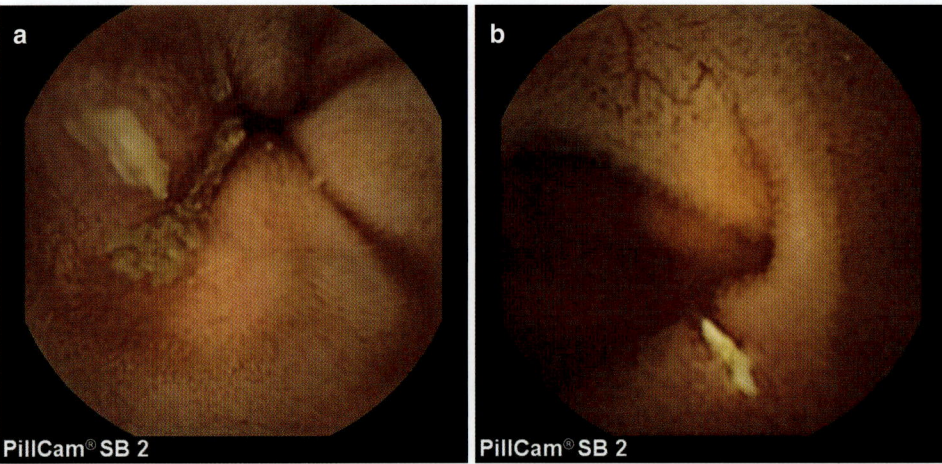

Fig. 25.8 VCE showing ileal ulcers. (**a**) A single large ulcer. (**b**) Multiple small ulcers with cobblestone mucosa

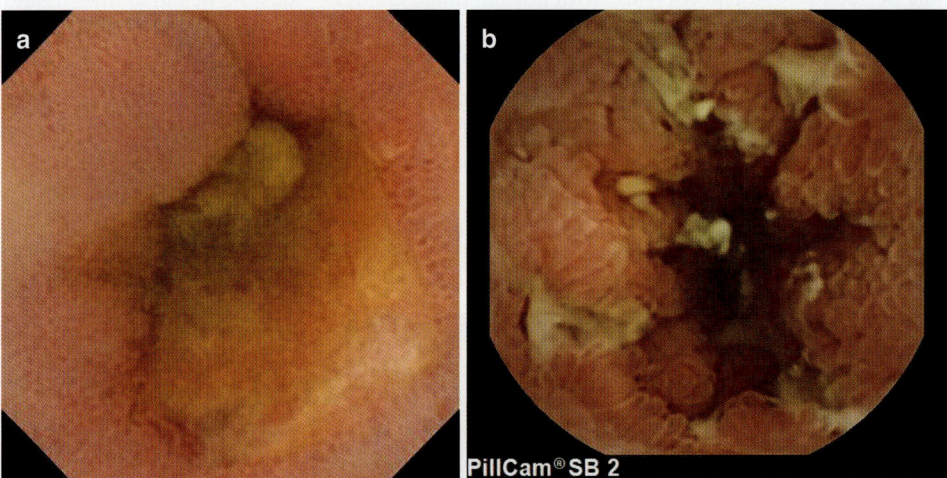

Fig. 25.9 VCE showing hemorrhagic lesions in the terminal ileum. (**a**) Petechiae. (**b**) More pronounced hemorrhagic mucosa. (Courtesy of Robert Wentrup, MD)

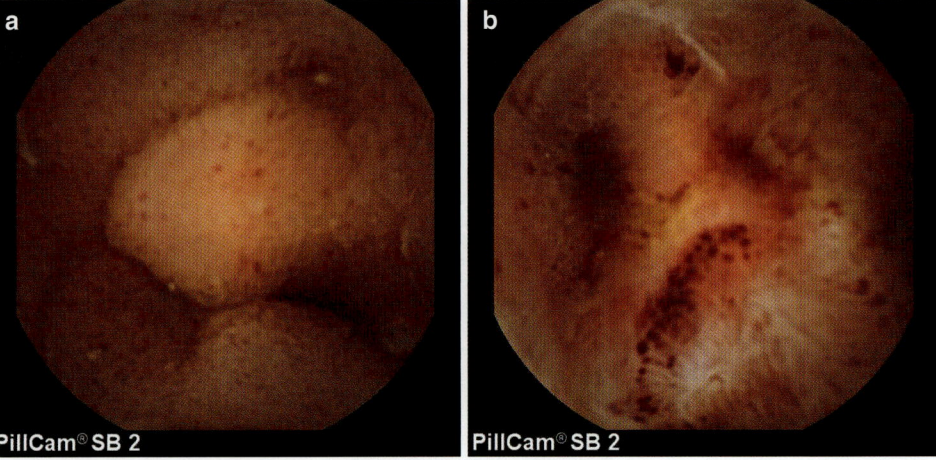

Fig. 25.10 (**a**, **b**) VCE aspect of ileal strictures in two patients. Both capsules passed the stenosis. (Courtesy of Robert Wentrup, MD)

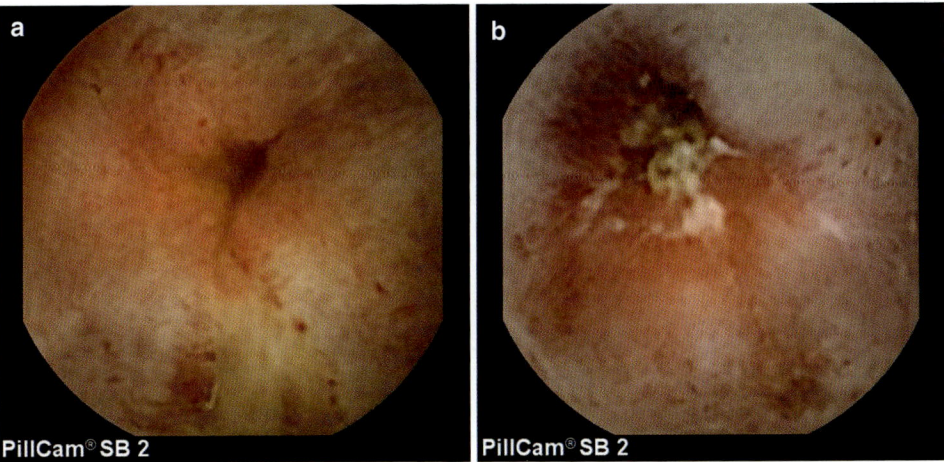

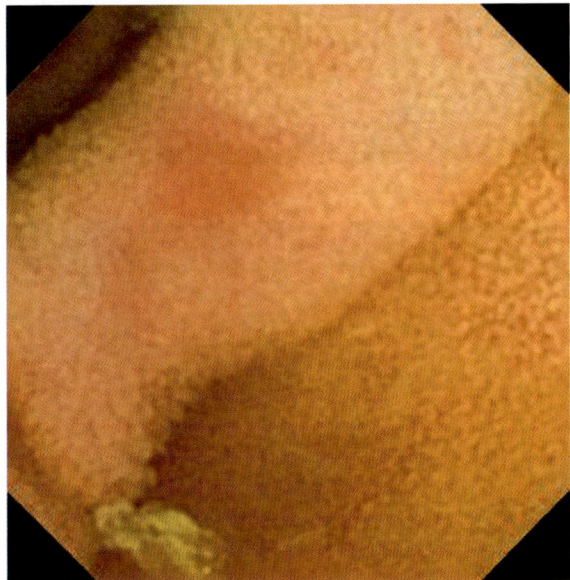

Fig. 25.11 VCE shows duodenal view of initial villous denudation

Although the clinical application of VCE is limited in Crohn's disease, its use is worth considering in some situations, as discussed below.

25.5.1 Unclear Symptoms, Unclear Diagnosis

VCE may be helpful in patients with unclear symptoms. For example, proof of involvement of the proximal small intestine supports the escalation of medical therapy, whereas a lack of inflammatory lesions may discourage escalation. In one study of 14 Crohn's disease patients with unexplained findings, the clinical outcome changed in 3 of 5 patients with iron deficiency anemia and in 2 of 3 patients with abdominal pain [15]. Altogether, Crohn's disease therapy in this small study was changed in 64 % of the patients. Another recent paper [16] studied whether symptoms represented flares in disease activity. VCE yielded negative findings in about 48 % of symptomatic patients, leading the authors to infer that the symptoms were caused by other diseases, such as bacterial overgrowth or irritable bowel syndrome. These authors concluded that the use of VCE prevented unnecessary treatments and recommended that every patient with Crohn's disease should undergo capsule endoscopy early in the evolution of the disease, in order to have an accurate estimation of disease extension. Nevertheless, this study had a retrospective design and did not describe a follow-up, so the results must be interpreted with caution [17]. Another study in patients with established Crohn's disease found a change in medication (most commonly budesonide or corticosteroids) within 3 months after VCE [18]. This study was also performed retrospectively, however, and the authors state that prospective studies are necessary in order to clarify this issue.

An interesting application of VCE may be differentiation between ulcerative colitis and Crohn's disease in patients with inflammatory bowel disease of unclassified type (indeterminate colitis). In these patients, VCE revealed mucosal changes suggestive of Crohn's disease in up to 28 % of patients [19, 20]. The largest study on such patients found lesions of the small intestine in about 15 %, especially in those with previous colectomy [21].

Therefore, although prospective studies are missing, VCE may have a role in evaluating patients with Crohn's disease who have unexplained symptoms, in order to guide appropriate therapy in some patients and prevent the use of unnecessary drugs in others.

25.5.2 Postoperative Recurrence

Capsule endoscopy may be useful to determine early postoperative recurrence of Crohn's disease [22]. In one prospective study, capsule endoscopy was more sensitive in detecting

Fig. 25.12 Ultrasound shows small bowel stricture (**a**) with massive prestenotic dilatation (**b**). MRI shows extremely dilated small bowel loops (**c**) (Courtesy of Roman Fischbach, MD). Stricture seen with double-balloon enteroscopy (**d**)

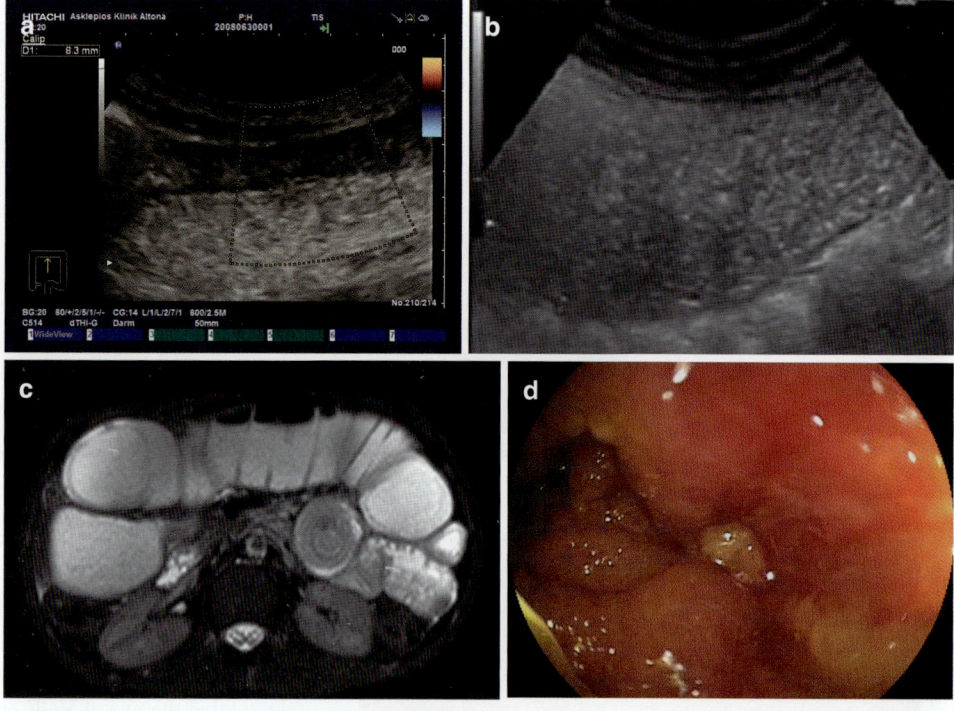

Fig. 25.13 (**a**) Patency capsule was retained and temporarily caused abdominal pain. (**b**) Jejunal stricture was seen on spiral enteroscopy

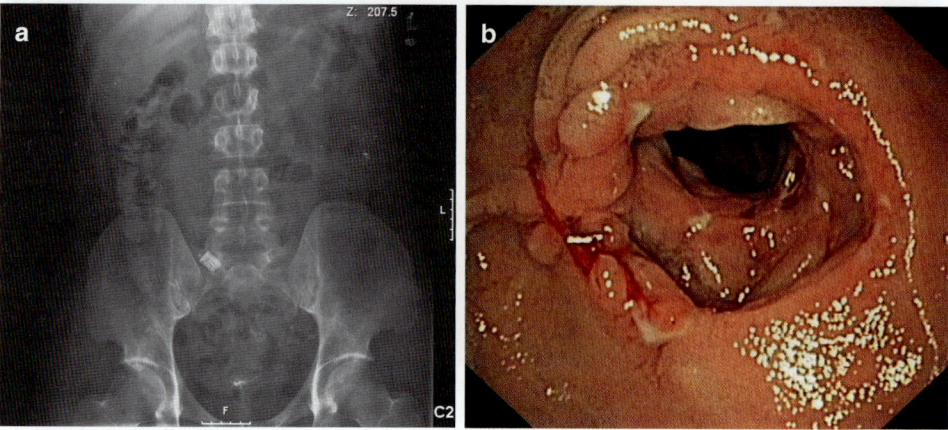

proximal lesions, but ileocolonoscopy was more sensitive overall [23]. Therefore, VCE may be a valuable tool for assessing postoperative disease activity if ileocolonoscopy is contraindicated or unsuccessful [6].

25.5.3 Capsule Indices and Mucosal Healing

Pharmacologic studies on mucosal healing may gain importance in the future. Of course, ileocolonoscopy will remain the most useful tool for evaluating mucosal healing in Crohn's disease. For instance, it showed that after 3 months of infliximab therapy, about two thirds of patients were in remission [24]. There is one report, however, of a case of bleeding due to Crohn's disease lesions of the small intestine that were

detected only by VCE. Under immunosuppressant therapy, the lesions healed and the bleeding stopped [25]. One Greek study examined 40 patients by VCE before and after therapy. Although the authors observed some improvement of Crohn's-like lesions, VCE did not find a significant correlation between clinical improvement and mucosal healing [26]. Nonetheless, if mucosal healing becomes a more frequently used parameter to determine therapeutic efficacy, VCE may become a more frequently utilized noninvasive tool.

Therefore, in analogy to the CDEIS (Crohn's Disease Endoscopic Index of Severity), validated by ileocolonoscopy, two major attempts to establish a scoring system for VCE (Figs. 25.12 and 25.13) (Tables 25.1 and 25.2) have been developed [27, 28]. Kappa values for interobserver variability have been reported to range from 0.48 to 0.87.

Table 25.1 Parameters and weightings for the capsule endoscopy scoring index ("Lewis score") [27]

Parameter	Number		Longitudinal extent		Descriptors	
First tertile						
Villous appearance	Normal	0	Short segment	8	Single	1
	Edematous	1	Long segment	12	Patchy	14
			Whole segment	20	Diffuse	17
Ulcer	None	0	Short segment	5	<¼	9
	Single	3	Long segment	10	¼–½	12
	Few	5	Whole segment	15	>½	18
	Multiple	10				
Second tertile						
Villous appearance	Normal	0	Short segment	8	Single	1
	Edematous	1	Long segment	12	Patchy	14
			Whole segment	20	Diffuse	17
Ulcer	None	0	Short segment	5	<¼	9
	Single	3	Long segment	10	¼–½	12
	Few	5	Whole segment	15	>½	18
	Multiple	10				
Third tertile						
Villous appearance	Normal	0	Short segment	8	Single	1
	Edematous	1	Long segment	12	Patchy	14
			Whole segment	20	Diffuse	17
Ulcer	None	0	Short segment	5	<¼	9
	Single	3	Long segment	10	¼–½	12
	Few	5	Whole segment	15	>½	18
	Multiple	10				
Stenosis – rated for whole study						
Stenosis	None	0	Ulcerated	24	Traversed	7
	Single	14	Non-ulcerated	2	Not traversed	10
	Multiple	20				

Table 25.2 Parameters of the capsule endoscopy Crohn's disease activity index (Niv score) [29]

Inflammation score	
None	0
Mild to moderate edema/hyperemia/denudation	1
Severe edema/hyperemia/denudation	2
Bleeding, exudate, aphthae, erosion, small ulcer (<0.5 cm)	3
Moderate ulcer (0.5–2 cm), pseudopolyp	4
Large ulcer (>2 cm)	5
Extent of disease	
No disease—normal examination	0
Focal disease (single segment is involved)	1
Patchy disease (2–3 segments are involved)	2
Diffuse disease (>3 segments are involved)	3
Stricture score	
None	0
Single passed	1
Multiple passed	2
Obstruction (no passage)	3
Segmental score $= (A \times B) + C$	
Total score $=$ proximal $([A \times B] + C) +$ distal $([A \times B] + C)$	

According to the published data, validation of the latter score seems to be more advanced [29]. However, it should be noted that neither scoring system can establish the diagnosis of Crohn's disease by itself. Moreover, scoring is limited to the small bowel alone and is useless in colonic disease. Nevertheless, scoring systems are needed in order to objectively measure the degree of mucosal inflammation in future pharmacologic studies.

25.6   Strictures

Strictures are described in one third of patients with Crohn's disease and increase with the duration of disease (Fig. 25.12). Strictures of the gastrointestinal tract may complicate Crohn's disease or may be seen postoperatively. They may be asymptomatic or cause obstructive symptoms. Strictures may be fibrotic, inflammatory, and malignant or may occur at previous anastomoses. Endoscopy, when possible, is indicated for assessment and biopsy.

Strictures are associated with an increased risk of capsule retention in VCE. Retention should be suspected when the capsule does not reach the colon in the recorded study. In this situation, it is advisable to follow up with a self-report of capsule excretion or a plain abdominal radiograph 14 days after the capsule examination [30].

Higher-grade strictures can be detected in standard radiologic studies, but most strictures that cause capsule retention or impaction are not detected radiographically prior to VCE. Capsule retention occurred in 13 % of patients with known Crohn's disease even though strictures were not seen on some radiographic studies done prior to the VCE [31].

A retained endoscopy capsule only rarely causes acute symptomatic obstruction and can remain intact for up to 4 years. However, single cases of acute obstruction have been reported, with perforation resulting in emergency surgery [32]. For this reason, if there is doubt about the possible presence of a stricture, the use of the Patency Capsule test device (Given Imaging Ltd., Yoqneam, Israel) is recommended (Chap. 9, Figs. 25.13 and 25.14). The patency capsule is a self-dissolving capsule that is the same size as the video capsule. It contains a radiofrequency identification tag that allows it to be detected by a scanning device placed on the abdominal wall. The tag can also be seen easily with a plain abdominal film. If its passage is blocked by a stricture, the capsule dissolves 40–80 h after ingestion. Unfortunately, the first generation of patency capsules, with a single opening for dissolving, resulted in small bowel obstruction with a complication rate of 3–13 %, similar to the complication rate of the wireless capsule itself. Therefore, an alternative capsule, the "Agile capsule" (Given Imaging Ltd., Yoqneam, Israel), was developed with two openings. To date, only one major study has been performed, with 106 patients being included [33]. Even in this

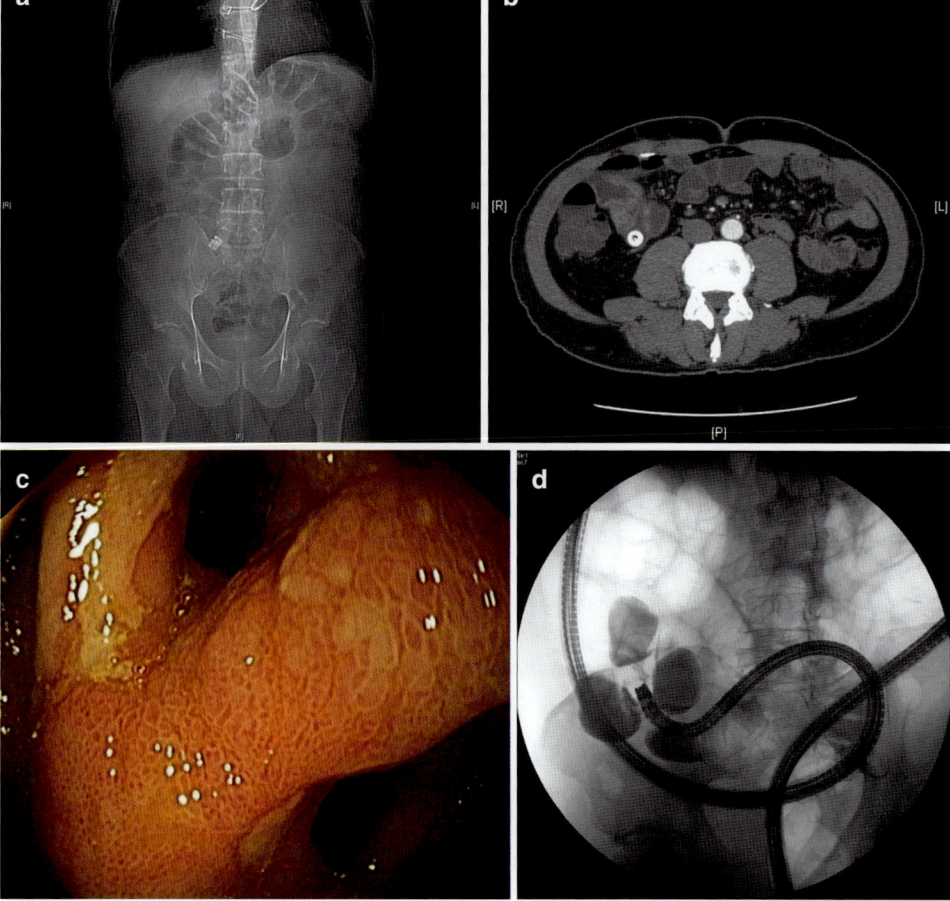

Fig. 25.14 Complex anatomy after small bowel resection. (**a**) A patency capsule was held up and excreted intact after 3 days. (**b**) A CT scan shows a thickened anastomosis with the Patency capsule (Courtesy of Jörg Sievers, MD). (**c**) Single-balloon enteroscopy reveals anastomotic ulcers as the cause of iron deficiency anemia. (**d**) Selective enterography shows a complex anastomotic situation

study, one bowel obstruction occurred, and capsule-induced symptoms may have occurred in 13 patients. The lack of an ideal capsule to prove bowel patency suggests to us that capsules should not be given in the presence of strictures longer than 15 cm [34] and radiologic exclusion of long strictures should be performed before any capsule examination.

If the capsule endoscope is retained by an inflammatory stricture, high doses of intravenous steroids administered for several days may restore passage [34]. If chronic fibrotic strictures are associated with obstructive symptoms, endoscopy with balloon dilation may relieve symptoms, as shown in an open-label series [35]. Local steroid injection along with balloon dilation may improve outcome. Surgery is indicated when there is a high suspicion of malignancy or intractable obstructive symptoms.

References

1. Peyrin-Biroulet L, Loftus Jr EV, Colombel JF, Sandborn WJ. The natural history of adult Crohn's disease in population-based cohorts. Am J Gastroenterol. 2010;105:289–97.
2. Baumgart DC, Sandborn WJ. Crohn's disease. Lancet. 2012;380:1590–605.
3. Onali S, Calabrese E, Petruzziello C, et al. Small intestine contrast ultrasonography vs computed tomography enteroclysis for assessing ileal Crohn's disease. World J Gastroenterol. 2012;18:6088–95.
4. Hoffmann JC, Preiß JC, Autschbach F, et al. Clinical practice guideline on diagnosis and treatment of Crohn's disease. Results of a German evidence-based consensus conference. Z Gastroenterol. 2008;46:1094–146.
5. Möschler O, May A, Müller MK, German EC, DBE. Study Group. Complications in and performance of double-balloon enteroscopy (DBE): results from a large prospective DBE database in Germany. Endoscopy. 2011;43:484–9.
6. Bourreille A, Ignjatovic A, Aabakken L, et al. Role of small-bowel endoscopy in the management of patients with inflammatory bowel disease: an international OMED–ECCO consensus. Endoscopy. 2009;41:618–37.
7. Liangpunsakul S, Chadalawada V, Rex DK, et al. Wireless capsule endoscopy detects small bowel ulcers in patients with normal results from state of the art enteroclysis. Am J Gastroenterol. 2003;98:1295–8.
8. Eliakim R, Fischer D, Suissa A, et al. Wireless capsule video endoscopy is a superior diagnostic tool in comparison to barium follow-through and computerized tomography in patients with suspected Crohn's disease. Eur J Gastroenterol Hepatol. 2003;15:363–7.
9. Triester SL, Leighton JA, Leontiadis GI, et al. A meta-analysis of the yield of capsule endoscopy compared to other diagnostic modalities in patients with non-stricturing small bowel Crohn's disease. Am J Gastroenterol. 2006;101:954–64.
10. Voderholzer WA, Beinhoelzl J, Rogalla P, et al. Small bowel involvement in Crohn's disease: a prospective comparison of wireless capsule endoscopy and computed tomography enteroclysis. Gut. 2005;54:369–73.
11. Albert J. Small bowel imaging in managing Crohn's disease patients. Gastroenterol Res Pract. 2012;2012:502198.
12. Goldstein JL, Eisen G, Lewis B, et al. Video capsule endoscopy to prospectively assess small bowel injury with celecoxib, naproxen plus omeprazole, and placebo. Clin Gastroenterol Hepatol. 2005;3:133–41.
13. Mitty R, Cave DR, Brighton MA. Focal villous denudation: a precursor to aphthoid ulcers in Crohn's disease as detected by video capsule endoscopy. Gastroenterology. 2002;122(Suppl):A217.
14. Sidhu R, Sanders DS, Morris AJ, et al. Guidelines on small bowel enteroscopy and capsule endoscopy in adults. Gut. 2008;57:125–36.
15. Lorenzo-Zúñiga V, de Vega VM, Domènech E, Cabré E, Mañosa M, Boix J. Impact of capsule endoscopy findings in the management of Crohn's Disease. Dig Dis Sci. 2010;55:411–4.
16. Mehdizadeh S, Chen GC, Barkodar L, Enayati PJ, Pirouz S, Yadegari M, et al. Capsule endoscopy in patients with Crohn's disease: diagnostic yield and safety. Gastrointest Endosc. 2010;71:121–7.
17. Redondo-Cerezo E. Role of wireless capsule endoscopy in inflammatory bowel disease. World J Gastrointest Endosc. 2010;16:179–85.
18. Long M, Barnes E. The impact of capsule endoscopy on management of inflammatory bowel disease: a single tertiary care center experience. Inflamm Bowel Dis. 2011;17:1855–62.
19. Maunoury V, Savoye G, Bourreille A, Bouhnik Y, Jarry M, Sacher-Huvelin S, et al. Value of wireless capsule endoscopy in patients with indeterminate colitis (inflammatory bowel disease type unclassified). Inflamm Bowel Dis. 2007;13:152–5.
20. Lopes S, Figueiredo P, Portela F, Freire P, Almeida N, Lerias C, et al. Capsule endoscopy in inflammatory bowel disease type unclassified and indeterminate colitis serologically negative. Inflamm Bowel Dis. 2010;16:1663–8.
21. Mehdizadeh S, Chen G, Enayati PJ, Cheng DW, Han NJ, Shaye OA, et al. Diagnostic yield of capsule endoscopy in ulcerative colitis and inflammatory bowel disease of unclassified type (IBDU). Endoscopy. 2008;40:30–5.
22. Pons Beltrán V, Nos P, Bastida G, Beltrán B, Argüello L, Aguas M, et al. Evaluation of postsurgical recurrence in Crohn's disease: a new indication for capsule endoscopy? Gastrointest Endosc. 2007;66:533–40.
23. Bourreille A, Jarry M, D'Halluin PN, Ben-Soussan E, Maunoury V, Bulois P, et al. Wireless capsule endoscopy versus ileocolonoscopy for the diagnosis of postoperative recurrence of Crohn's disease: a prospective study. Gut. 2006;55:978–83.
24. Björkesten CG, Nieminen U, Turunen U, Arkkila PE, Sipponen T, Färkkilä MA. Endoscopic monitoring of infliximab therapy in Crohn's disease. Inflamm Bowel Dis. 2011;17:947–53.
25. Akhtar RY, Lewis BS, Ullman T. Mucosal healing of Crohn's disease demonstrated by capsule endoscopy in a woman with obscure gastrointestinal bleeding. Am J Gastroenterol. 2009;104:1065–6.
26. Efthymiou A, Viazis N, Mantzaris G, et al. Does clinical response correlate with mucosal healing in patients with Crohn's disease of the small bowel? A prospective, case-series study using wireless capsule endoscopy. Inflamm Bowel Dis. 2008;14:1542–7.
27. Gralnek IM, Defranchis R, Seidman E, Leighton JA, Legnani P, Lewis BS. Development of a capsule endoscopy scoring index for small bowel mucosal inflammatory change. Aliment Pharmacol Ther. 2008;27:146–54.
28. Gal E, Geller A, Fraser G, Levi Z, Niv Y. Assessment and validation of the new capsule endoscopy Crohn's disease activity index (CECDAI). Dig Dis Sci. 2008;53:1933–7.
29. Niv Y, Ilani S, Levi Z, Hershkowitz M, Niv E, Fireman Z, et al. Validation of the Capsule Endoscopy Crohn's Disease Activity Index (CECDAI or Niv score): a multicenter prospective study. Endoscopy. 2012;44:21–6.
30. Swaminath A, Legnani P, Kornbluth A. Video capsule endoscopy in inflammatory bowel disease: past, present, and future. Inflamm Bowel Dis. 2012;16:1254–62.
31. Cheifetz AS, Kornbluth AA, Legnani P, Schmelkin I, Brown A, Lichtiger S, Lewis BS. The risk of retention of the capsule

endoscope in patients with known or suspected Crohn's disease. Am J Gastroenterol. 2006;101:2218–22.

32. Parikh DA, Parikh JA, Albers GC, Chandler CF. Acute small bowel perforation after wireless capsule endoscopy in a patient with Crohn's disease: a case report. Cases J. 2009;2:7607.

33. Herrerias JM, Leighton JA, Costamagna G, et al. Agile patency system eliminates risk of capsule retention in patients with known

intestinal strictures who undergo capsule endoscopy. Gastrointest Endosc. 2008;67:902–9.

34. Boivin ML, Lochs H, Voderholzer W. Does passage of the patency capsule indicate small bowel patency? A prospective clinical evaluation. Endoscopy. 2005;37:808–15.

35. Saunders BP, Brown GJ, Lemann M, Rutgeerts P. Balloon dilation of ileocolonic strictures in Crohn's disease. Endoscopy. 2004;36:1001–7.

Villous Atrophy

26

Detlef Schuppan, Chris J. Mulder, Pekka Collin,
and Joseph A. Murray

Contents

The work was first published in 2006 by Springer Medizin Verlag
Heidelberg with the following title: *Atlas of Video Capsule Endoscopy.*

D. Schuppan (✉)
1st Medical Clinic,
University Medical Center Mainz, Mainz, Germany
e-mail: detlef.schuppan@unimedizin-mainz.de

C.J. Mulder
Department of Gastroenterology,
VU University Medical Center, Amsterdam, The Netherlands
e-mail: cjmulder@vumc.nl

P. Collin
Gastroenterology Outpatient Clinic,
Tampere University Hospital, Tampere, Finland
e-mail: pekka.collin@uta.fi

J.A. Murray
Division of Gastroenterology and Hepatology,
Mayo Clinic, Rochester, MN, USA
e-mail: murray.joseph@mayo.edu

The most frequent cause of villous atrophy is celiac disease; less common etiologies are combined immunodeficiency states, drug-induced injury, radiation damage, recent chemotherapy, graft-versus-host disease, specified infections (giardiasis, Whipple's disease), and unspecified tropical disease (tropical sprue). Premalignant or malignant consequences of celiac disease include refractory celiac disease, ulcerative jejunitis, enteropathy-associated intestinal T-cell lymphoma (EATL), and small intestinal carcinoma. Video capsule endoscopy (VCE) offers a good supplementary method for detecting and managing these complications, but VCE alone generally cannot achieve a differential diagnosis for villous atrophy.

26.1 Celiac Disease

26.1.1 Definition

In celiac disease (synonyms: gluten-sensitive enteropathy, nontropical sprue, celiac sprue), the ingestion of gluten from grains (wheat, barley, and rye) results in inflammation of the small bowel mucosa, with subsequent crypt hyperplasia and villous atrophy. The mucosal damage causes a variety of gastrointestinal and nongastrointestinal symptoms and often malabsorption. The diagnosis is usually suggested by positive autoantibodies confirmed by endoscopy and duodenal biopsy. A gluten-free diet results in the resolution of symptoms and eventually the healing of the mucosa. The most well-known extraintestinal manifestation is dermatitis herpetiformis (Fig. 26.1), a blistering skin rash with different degrees of enteropathy; this rash responds to a gluten-free diet [1].

26.1.2 Etiology

Celiac disease is an immune-mediated disease with a genetic predisposition; HLA-DQ2 or HLA-DQ8 is prevalent in virtually all celiac patients, but also in 30–35 % of the population [2]. Dietary gluten induces a T-cell-

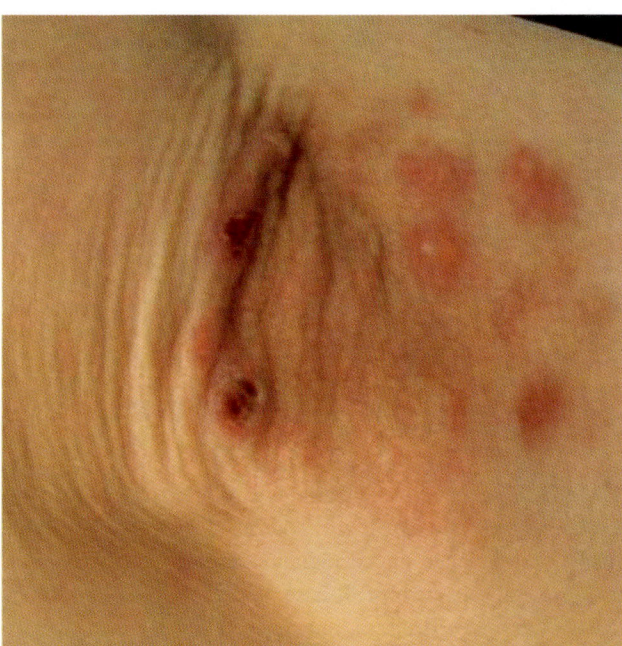

Fig. 26.1 Dermatitis herpetiformis

driven, B-cell-mediated reaction to the autoantigen tissue transglutaminase (tTG). The immune response results in mucosal inflammation and injury [3]. Mucosal atrophy is most evident in the proximal intestine [4].

26.1.3 Prevalence and Clinical Features

Autoantibody screening using IgA anti-tissue transglutaminase (tTGA) and endomysial antibodies (EMA) [5] confirmed by biopsy have shown that celiac disease is common, with a prevalence of 1 % or more in Caucasian populations [6–8]. The prevalence of clinically detected celiac disease is much lower, probably because symptoms may be subtle and unspecific [8]. Symptoms of classic celiac disease are diarrhea, loss of weight, and anemia due to iron or folic acid deficiency, but most patients have minor or atypical symptoms. Family history, osteoporosis, or associated autoimmune diseases such as autoimmune thyroiditis, type I diabetes, or Sjögren's syndrome increase the likelihood of celiac disease [6, 9]. Many patients have no symptoms whatsoever.

26.1.4 Histology

The histologic hallmarks of celiac disease are lymphocytic infiltration of the small bowel, crypt hyperplasia, and mucosa villous atrophy. A modified version of the Marsh classification (Table 26.1) is used to describe findings, with partial, subtotal, and total villous atrophy (Marsh lesions III a, b, and c, respectively). Lesions of Marsh types I (intraepithelial lymphocytosis) and II (with the addition of crypt

Table 26.1 Modified Marsh classification of celiac disease pathology [10–12]

0	Normal (refers only to patients with celiac sprue treated by diet)
I	Infiltrative type (>40 IEL/100 epithelial cells)
II	Hyperplastic type (>40 IEL/100 epithelial cells and crypt hyperplasia)
III	Destructive type (villous atrophy)
IIIa	Mild
IIIb	Subtotal
IIIc	Total

IEL intraepithelial lymphocytes

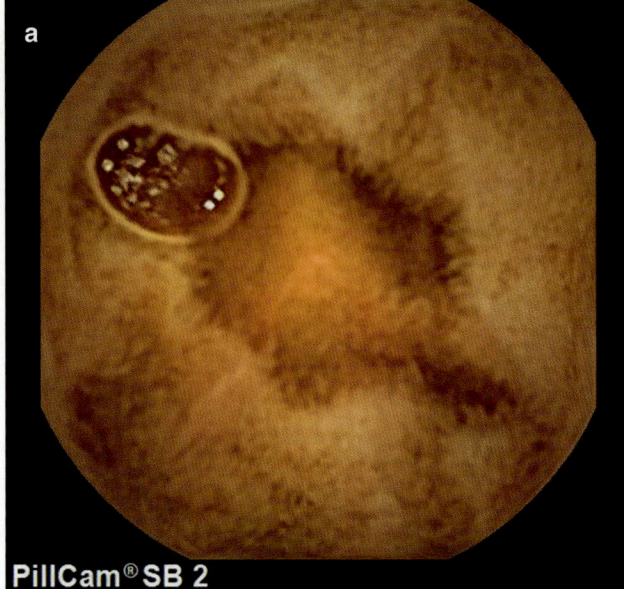

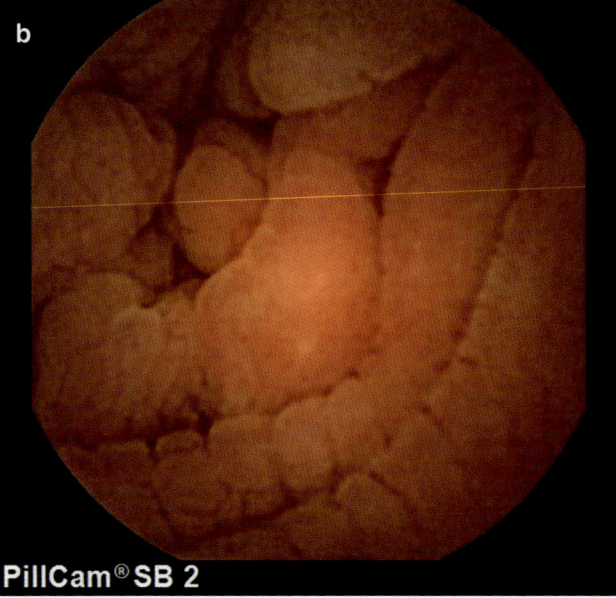

Fig. 26.2 Video capsule endoscopy (VCE) images of normal villi (**a**) and villous atrophy (**b**)

Fig. 26.3 Villous atrophy, decreasing from proximal to distal. (**a**) Subtotal to total atrophy (corresponding to Marsh IIIb to IIIc). (**b**) Mild atrophy (corresponding to Marsh IIIa). (**c**, **d**) Fairly normal villi

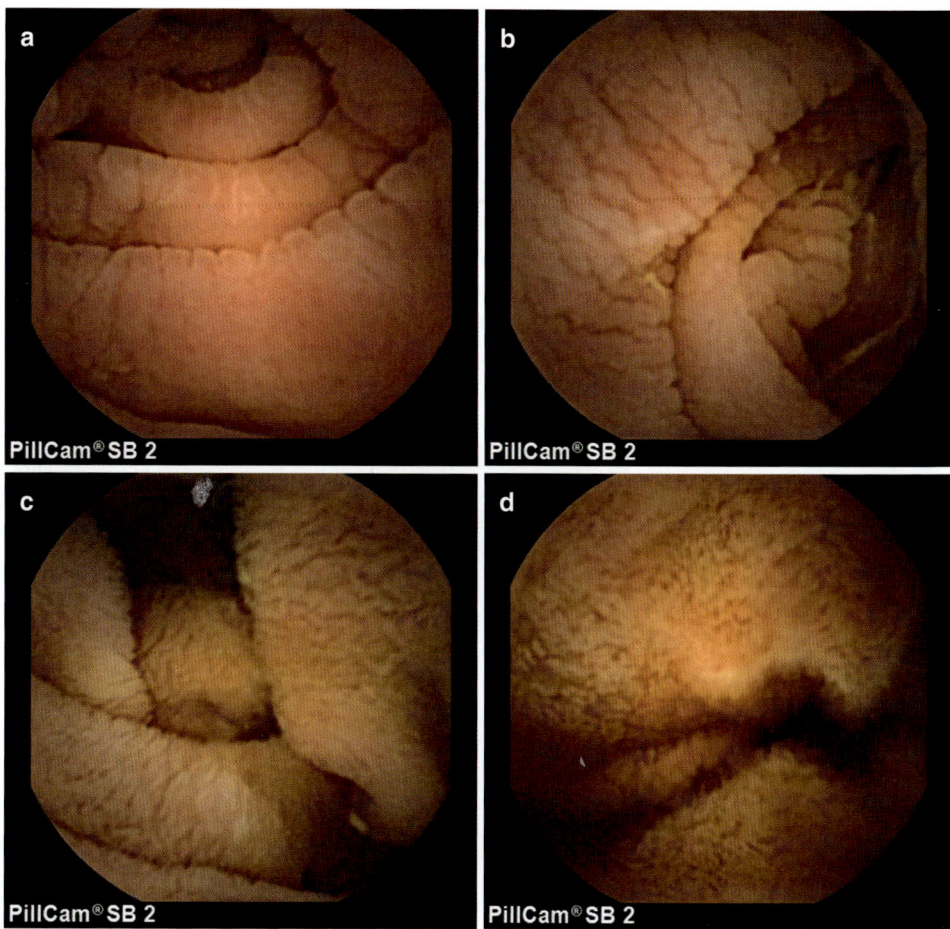

Fig. 26.4 Scalloped valvulae, fissures, and a mosaic mucosal pattern, as viewed using VCE (**a**) and enteroscopy (**b**)

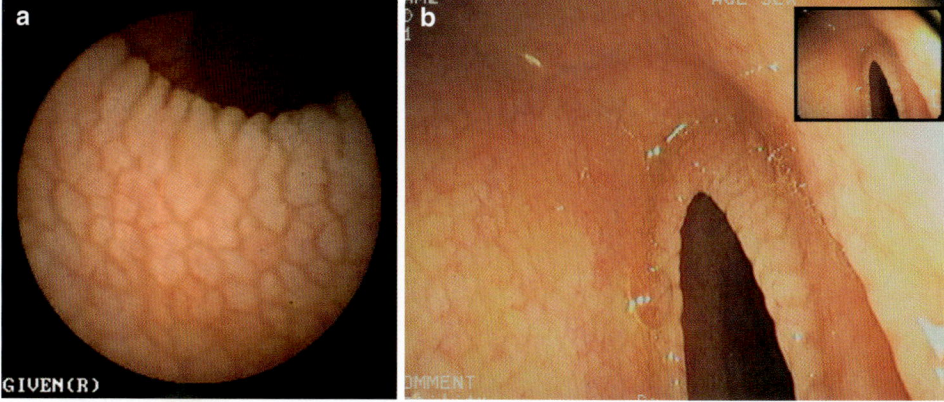

hyperplasia) are unspecific signs of early celiac disease [10, 11]. VCE can distinguish a lesion of Marsh type III lesion (Fig. 26.2) from Marsh types 0, I, or II, but a more specific differentiation is not possible. VCE is better than histology at assessing the extent of atrophy (Fig. 26.3), however, and is better at detecting patchy atrophic changes. Reduced visibility of villi or absent villi on several successive folds, scalloping and loss of circular folds, fissuring, and mosaic pattern and nodularity of the mucosa are typical VCE findings in celiac disease (Fig. 26.4).

26.1.5 Treatment

To date, the only management of celiac disease is a lifelong gluten-free diet. Symptoms improve in about 70 % of patients within 2 weeks after the introduction of the diet. The mucosal healing takes usually longer, 1–2 years, and often remains incomplete [13, 14]. The prognosis of celiac disease is good, and in well-treated patients the occurrence of malignancies and the mortality rate do not differ from those in the population in general. Possible late complications of untreated celiac disease include osteoporosis and apparently the development of refractory celiac disease and EATL or small intestinal carcinoma [15].

26.2 Refractory Celiac Disease

Sometimes, patients on a strictly gluten-free diet do not respond or relapse. Persistent villous atrophy and manifest symptoms with the maintenance of a gluten-free diet for 1–2 years is called refractory celiac disease (RCD) [16, 17]. RCD is less common than previously thought, appearing in less than 1 % of celiac disease patients. Small bowel atrophy is often extensive (Fig. 26.5). There are two subtypes of RCD: RCD type I with normal polyclonal T cells in mucosa is responsive to steroids and immunosuppressants. In premalignant (type II) RCD, there is growth of an aberrant monoclonal intestinal T-cell population, which can be detected histologically by abnormal mucosal cells (CD8 negative, cytoplasmic CD3 positive) and by polymerase chain reaction for T-cell receptors from intestinal lymphocytes. RCD type II often evolves into overt T-cell lymphoma (see below) [18]. Ulcerative jejunitis (Fig. 26.6), intestinal

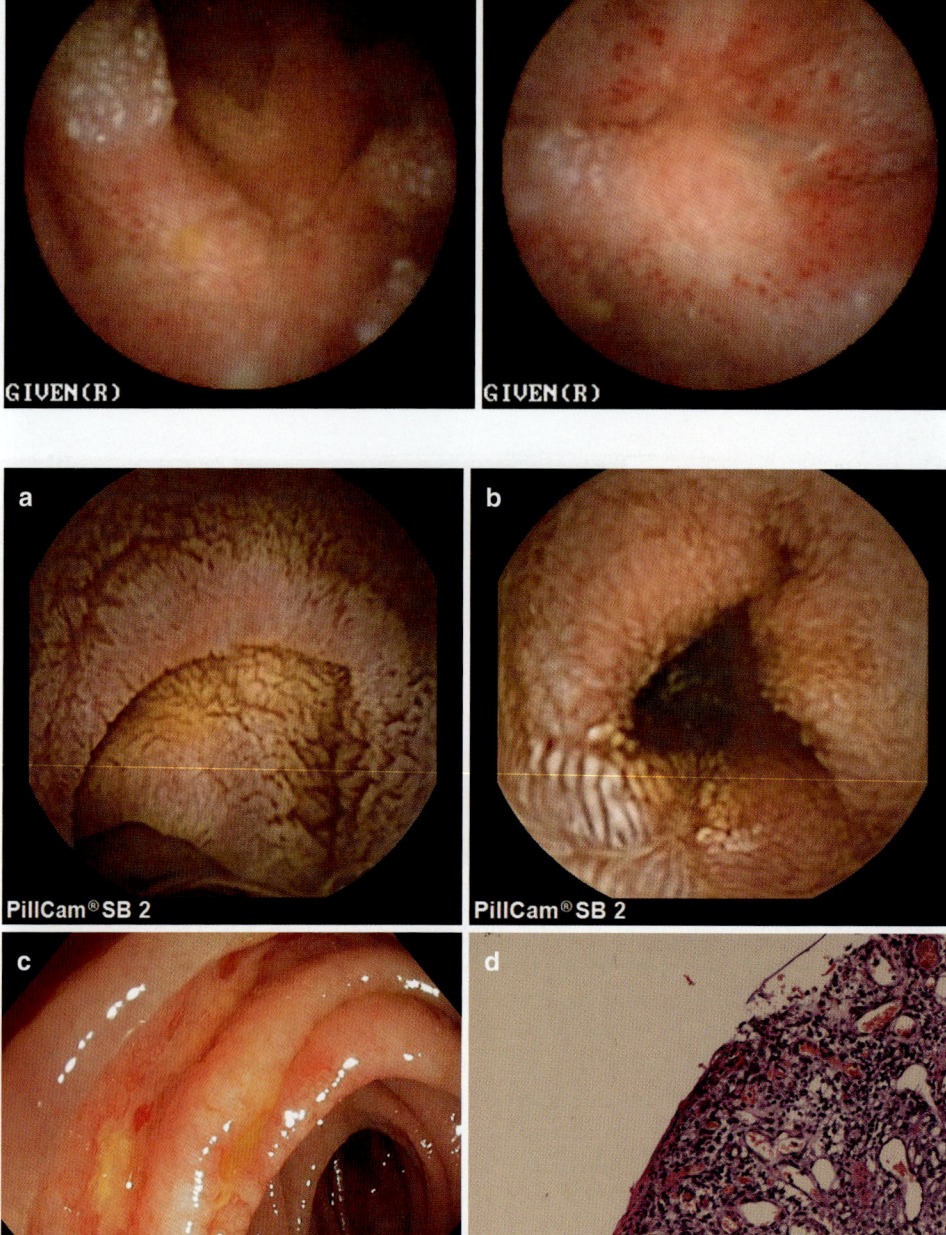

Fig. 26.5 Refractory sprue type II. (**a**) Lymphangiectatic changes. (**b**) Mucosal hemorrhage in the distal small bowel

Fig. 26.6 Ulcerative jejunoileitis in an elderly patient with weight loss, diarrhea, and malabsorption. VCE showing fissures, partial villous atrophy (**a**), and partially healed ulcer with surrounding lymphangiectasia (white villi) (**b**). (**c**) Enteroscopy. (**d**) Histology (H&E stain; Courtesy of Jörg Caselitz, MD)

stricture, and mass lesions are indicative of malignant development of EATL (Fig. 26.7) or, less often, small intestinal adenocarcinoma (Fig. 26.8).

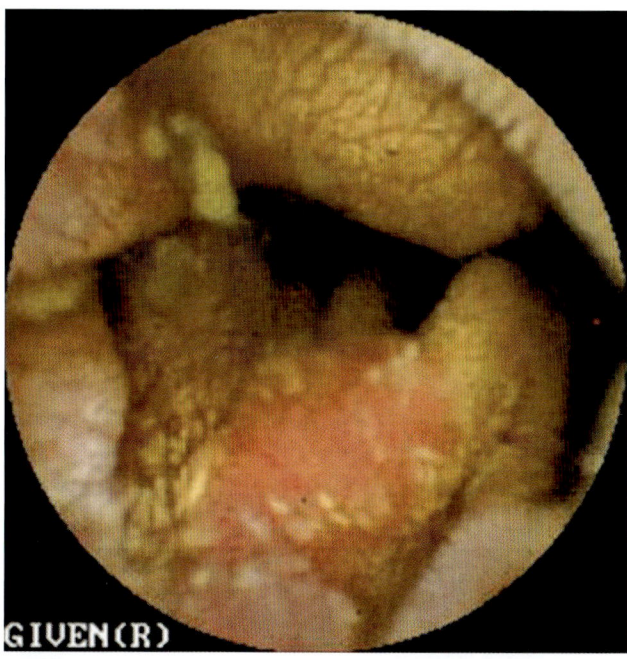

Fig. 26.7 Celiac disease and enteropathy-associated T-cell lymphoma (EATL)

26.3 Indications of Video Capsule Endoscopy in Celiac Disease

VCE is not recommended as a primary diagnostic study, because of its high cost and inability to furnish a biopsy sample [19]. The specificity of EMA and tTGA usually makes VCE unnecessary in antibody-positive patients. VCE may be considered if endoscopy and small intestinal biopsy are not possible and serology is negative. It also may be helpful in assessing the extent and severity of small bowel involvement [4].

The lack of mucosal response in 1–2 years is usually an indication for VCE, regardless of symptoms. New, recurrent, or even persistent alarm symptoms (loss of weight, diarrhea, fever, abdominal pain, loss of appetite) while a celiac patient is adhering to a gluten-free diet may indicate VCE, in addition to small bowel histology, radiologic examinations, and endoscopies [20]. VCE should be carried out in all patients with established RCD. Atrophy is the most common finding in VCE used to study symptomatic, treated celiac disease. This finding has specificity, as incidental changes such as erosions are more likely to be associated with the use of nonsteroidal anti-inflammatory drugs (NSAIDs) than with celiac disease [21]. VCE may alter the management of these patients [22], and a vigorous search

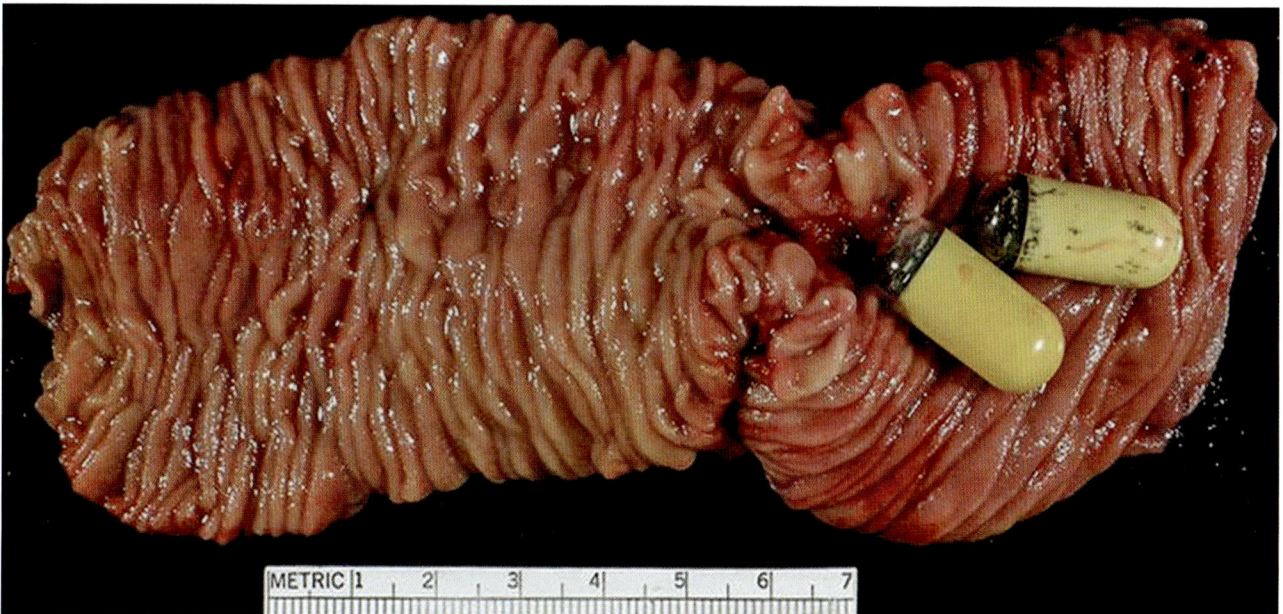

Fig. 26.8 Celiac disease and adenocarcinoma. Resected specimen showing stenosis and two retained video capsules

for small intestinal lymphoma is necessary, especially in patients with RCD type II. Knowing the extent of mucosal atrophy (only proximal or more advanced) may also have some prognostic significance. In follow-up or management (immunosuppression), VCE can also be used to verify the mucosal response.

26.4 Autoimmune Enteropathy

Autoimmune enteropathy is a very rare disorder of unknown etiology, characterized by extensive villous atrophy in the small intestine (Fig. 26.9). Anti-enterocyte antibodies are found in 75 % of patients [23]. Gluten is not the trigger, and no antibodies to tTG are found. Treatment with steroids and immunosuppressants is of variable efficacy [24]. VCE can be applied in the diagnosis and follow-up of the disorder.

26.5 Other Causes of Villous Atrophy

It has long been recognized that diarrhea is a common side effect of many drugs. Recently, two drugs have been shown to be associated with a severe chronic enteropathy that is similar to celiac disease in morphology but lacks tTG antibodies and a response to the gluten-free diet. These drugs are mycophenolate mofetil (MMF), most often seen in the context of transplantation, and olmesartan, an angiotensin 2 receptor blocker used to treat hypertension [25, 26].

Collagenous sprue is another entity characterized by severe malabsorption, villous atrophy, and thick band of collagen deposited under the surface epithelial layer (Fig. 26.10) [17]. This entity can be multifactorial (celiac disease, drugs, autoimmune, tropical sprue), and it can be associated with failure to respond to appropriate treatment. The VCE appearance is similar to celiac disease, but there may be a whitish discoloration of the mucosa (Fig. 26.11).

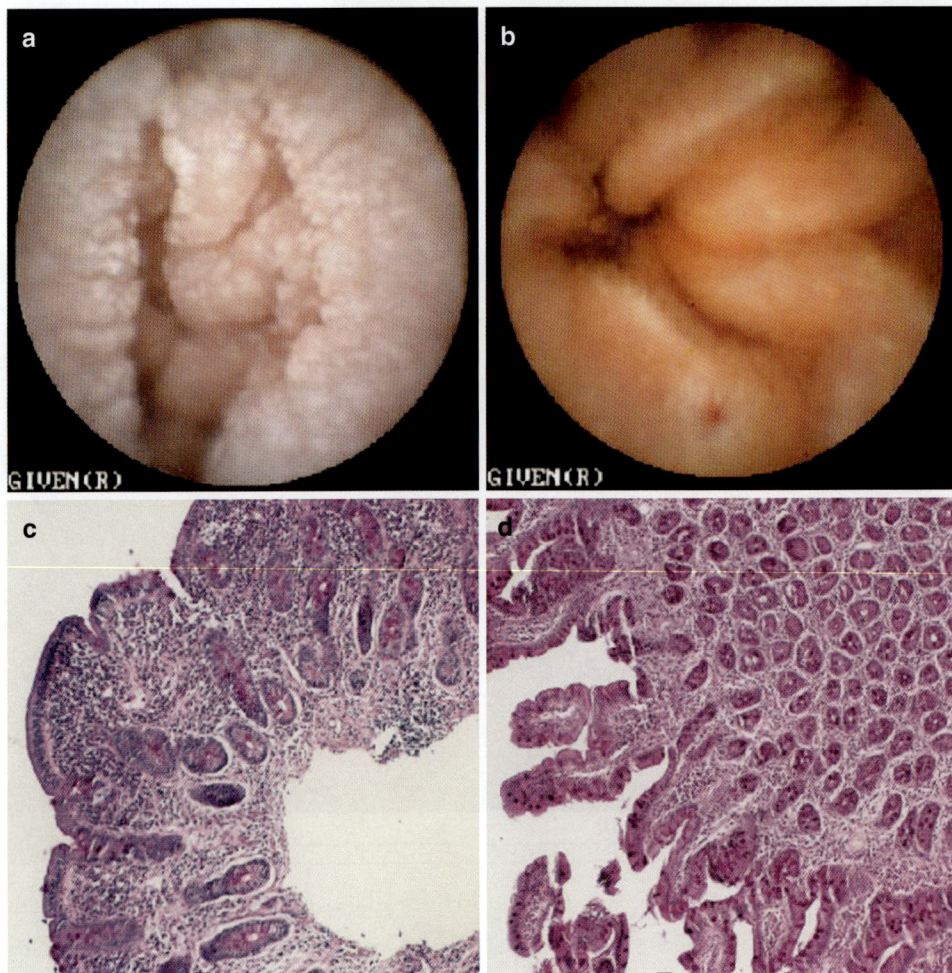

Fig. 26.9 Villous atrophy in autoimmune enteropathy. (**a**) Initial finding of VCE. (**b**) After 20 months of low-dose steroids, the villi appear normal with small erosions. (**c**) Initial histology (H&E stain) showed villous atrophy, crypt hyperplasia, and (polyclonal) lymphocytic infiltration. (**d**) Essentially normal findings after treatment (Courtesy of Jörg Caselitz, MD)

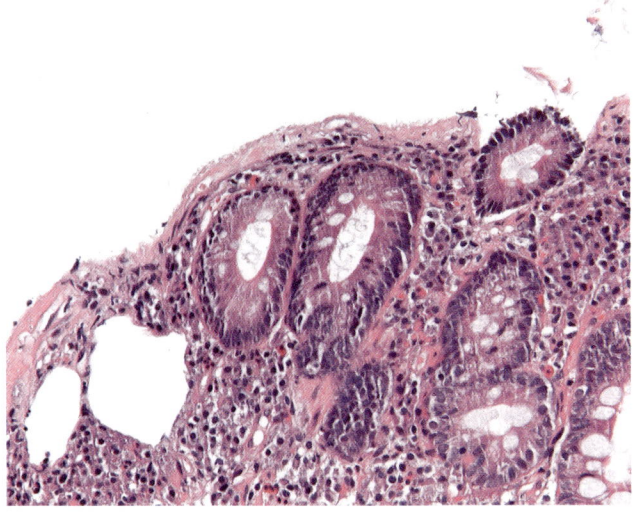

Fig. 26.10 Collagenous sprue, histology (H&E stain)

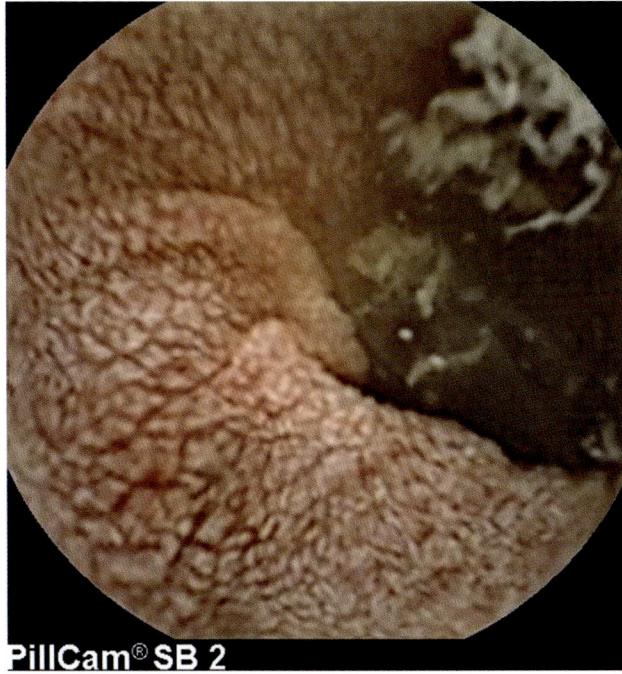

Fig. 26.11 Collagenous sprue, viewed using VCE

References

1. Collin P, Reunala T. Recognition and management of the cutaneous manifestations of celiac disease: a guide for dermatologists. Am J Clin Dermatol. 2003;4:13–20.
2. Karell K, Louka AS, Moodie SJ, et al. HLA types in celiac disease patients not carrying the DQA1*05-DQB1*02 (DQ2) heterodimer: results from the European genetics cluster on celiac disease. Hum Immunol. 2003;64:469–77.
3. Schuppan D, Junker Y, Barisani D. Celiac disease: from pathogenesis to novel therapies. Gastroenterology. 2009;137:1912–33.
4. Murray JA, Rubio-Tapia A, Van Dyke CT, et al. Mucosal atrophy in celiac disease: extent of involvement, correlation with clinical presentation, and response to treatment. Clin Gastroenterol Hepatol. 2008;6:186–93.
5. Leffler DA, Schuppan D. Update on serologic testing in celiac disease. Am J Gastroenterol. 2010;105:2520–4.
6. Fasano A, Berti I, Gerarduzzi T, et al. Prevalence of celiac disease in at-risk and not-at-risk groups in the United States: a large multicenter study. Arch Intern Med. 2003;163:286–92.
7. Mäki M, Mustalahti K, Kokkonen J, et al. Prevalence of celiac disease among children in Finland. N Engl J Med. 2003;348:2517–24.
8. Rubio-Tapia A, Ludvigsson JF, Brantner TL, et al. The prevalence of celiac disease in the United States. Am J Gastroenterol. 2012; 107:1538–44.
9. Collin P, Huhtala H, Virta L, et al. Diagnosis of celiac disease in clinical practice: physician's alertness to the condition essential. J Clin Gastroenterol. 2007;41:152–6.
10. Marsh MN. Gluten, major histocompatibility complex, and the small intestine. A molecular and immunobiologic approach to the spectrum of gluten sensitivity ('celiac sprue'). Gastroenterology. 1992;102:330–54.
11. Oberhuber G, Caspary WF, Kirchner T, Borchard F, Stolte M, et al. Diagnosis of celiac disease and sprue. Recommendations of the German Society for Pathology Task Force on Gastroenterologic Pathology. Pathologe. 2001;22:72–81.
12. Oberhuber G, Granditsch G, Vogelsang H. The histopathology of coeliac disease: time for a standardized report scheme for pathologists. Eur J Gastroenterol Hepatol. 1999;11:1185–94.
13. Collin P, Mäki M, Kaukinen K. Complete small intestine mucosal recovery is obtainable in the treatment of celiac disease. Gastrointest Endosc. 2004;59:158–9.
14. Lee SK, Lo W, Memeo L, et al. Duodenal histology in patients with celiac disease after treatment with a gluten-free diet. Gastrointest Endosc. 2003;57:187–91.
15. van de Water JM, Cillessen SA, Visser OJ, et al. Enteropathy associated T-cell lymphoma and its precursor lesions. Best Pract Res Clin Gastroenterol. 2010;24:43–56.
16. Al-Toma A, Verbeek WH, Hadithi M, et al. Survival in refractory coeliac disease and enteropathy-associated T-cell lymphoma: retrospective evaluation of single-centre experience. Gut. 2007;56:1373–8.
17. Rubio-Tapia A, Murray JA. Classification and management of refractory coeliac disease. Gut. 2010;59:547–57.
18. Cellier C, Delabesse E, Helmer C, et al. Refractory sprue, coeliac disease, and enteropathy-associated T-cell lymphoma. Lancet. 2000;356:203–8.
19. Cellier C, Green PHR, Collin P, Murray J. ICCE concensus for celiac disease. Endoscopy. 2005;37:1055–9.
20. Van Weyenberg SJ, Smits F, Jacobs MA, et al. Video capsule endoscopy in patients with nonresponsive celiac disease. J Clin Gastroenterol. 2013;47:393–9.
21. Atlas DS, Rubio-Tapia A, Van Dyke CT, et al. Capsule endoscopy in nonresponsive celiac disease. Gastrointest Endosc. 2011;74:1315–22.
22. Collin P, Rondonotti E, Lundin KE, et al. Video capsule endoscopy in celiac disease: current clinical practice. J Dig Dis. 2012;13:94–9.
23. Montalto M, D'Onofrio F, Santoro L, et al. Autoimmune enteropathy in children and adults. Scand J Gastroenterol. 2009;44:1029–36.
24. Akram S, Murray JA, Pardi DS, et al. Adult autoimmune enteropathy: Mayo Clinic Rochester experience. Clin Gastroenterol Hepatol. 2007;5:1282–90.
25. Kamar N, Faure P, Dupuis E, et al. Villous atrophy induced by mycophenolate mofetil in renal-transplant patients. Transpl Int. 2004;17:463–7.
26. Rubio-Tapia A, Herman ML, Ludvigsson JF, et al. Severe spruelike enteropathy associated with olmesartan. Mayo Clin Proc. 2012;87: 732–8.

Eosinophilic Enteritis

27

Ernest G. Seidman, Martha H. Dirks,
Victoria Alejandra Jiménez-Garcia,
and Juan Manuel Herrerías-Gutiérrez

Contents

The work was first published in 2006 by Springer Medizin Verlag Heidelberg with the following title: *Atlas of Video Capsule Endoscopy.*

E.G. Seidman (✉)
McGill IBD Research Group, Digestive lab, Research Institute of McGill University Health Center, Montreal, QC, Canada
e-mail: ernest.seidman@mcgill.ca

M.H. Dirks
Division of Gastroenterology, Hepatology and Nutrition, Hôpital Sainte-Justine, University of Montreal, Montreal, QC, Canada
e-mail: Martha.dirks.hsj@ssss.gouv.qc.ca

V.A. Jiménez-Garcia • J.M. Herrerías-Gutiérrez
Department of Gastroenterology, Hospital Universitario Virgen Macarena, Seville, Spain
e-mail: jmherrerias@doctorcat.net

27.1 Definition

Eosinophilic digestive diseases are a group of rare and heterogeneous conditions characterized by patchy or diffuse eosinophilic infiltration of gastrointestinal tissue. Over the past decade, there has been a remarkable increase in the incidence of primary eosinophilic digestive diseases, as well as a vigorous increase in data linking the development of these illnesses to atopy.

Although any part of the gastrointestinal tract can be affected (such as the biliary tract in isolation [1]), these disorders mainly include eosinophilic esophagitis, eosinophilic gastritis, eosinophilic gastroenteritis, eosinophilic enteritis, and eosinophilic colitis [2]. It is debated whether the occasional patients who present with apparent eosinophilic esophagitis and marked eosinophilic inflammation extending to other segments of the gastrointestinal tract represent primary eosinophilic esophagitis or whether the eosinophilic esophagitis is part of eosinophilic gastroenteritis [3]. Eosinophilic gastroenteritis is a rare entity, the pathogenesis of which is not well known. It is characterized by intense eosinophilic infiltration in at least one layer of the stomach, small bowel, or both.

Eosinophilic esophagitis is the most common form of eosinophilic digestive diseases, followed by the stomach, the small intestine, and the colon. Eosinophilic gastroenteritis was originally described in 1937 by Kaijser [4].

Presentation may vary depending on location and on the depth and extent of bowel wall involvement; it usually runs a chronic relapsing course. To classify the disease into mucosal, muscular, and serosal types based on the depth of involvement, it is important to consider whether the patient has any other known causes of eosinophilic infiltration, such as drug reactions, parasitic infections, or cancer [5].

27.2 Etiology

The pathogenesis and etiology of the disease are not well understood. As a part of the host defense mechanism, eosinophils are normally present in gastrointestinal mucosa. The

M. Keuchel et al. (eds.), *Video Capsule Endoscopy: A Reference Guide and Atlas,*
DOI 10.1007/978-3-662-44062-9_27, © Springer-Verlag Berlin Heidelberg 2014

gastrointestinal tract is really the only nonhematopoietic organ that contains eosinophils, with the cecal and appendiceal regions being the parts with the highest concentrations [6].

Many patients with eosinophilic enteritis have a history of seasonal allergies and other allergic problems such as food sensitivities, eczema, asthma, and atopy [7]. Elevated serum IgE levels are also typical. These findings suggest that the hypersensitivity response plays a major role in pathogenesis. Eosinophils directly communicate with T cells and mast cells in a bidirectional manner, although eosinophil recruitment into inflammatory tissue is a complex process, regulated by a number of inflammatory cytokines. In the intestinal wall, IL-3, IL-5, and granulocyte-macrophage colony-stimulating factor (GM-CSF) have been included in this process of recruitment and activation [8]. Recently, eotaxin has been shown to have an integral role in regulating the homing of eosinophils into the lamina propria of the stomach and small intestine [9].

27.3 Clinical Features

No standards for the diagnosis of eosinophilic enteritis exist, but an elevated index of clinical suspicion is necessary [10]. About 80 % of patients have had symptoms for several years [11], because conventional tools are unable to make the diagnosis, which is usually difficult.

The disease is relatively uncommon. It predominantly affects males, typically young adults or children. Signs and symptoms are related to the site, extent, and layer of the gastrointestinal wall involved, so they may differ. Symptoms include abdominal pain (90 %), vomiting (60 %), nausea (50 %), and abdominal distension (50 %) [12]. Other symptoms are weight loss and diarrhea [13].

The disease is classified histopathologically into three major types:

1. Predominantly mucosal (in 60 % of the patients), manifested mainly as abdominal pain, vomiting, diarrhea, weight loss, and malabsorption [14]. Patients frequently present iron deficiency anemia and may have peripheral edema due to the protein-losing enteropathy [15].
2. Predominantly muscle layer (in about 30 % of the patients), causing bowel wall thickening and variable degrees of intestinal obstruction [16]. Stenotic lesions elsewhere in the gut may mimic Crohn's strictures.
3. Predominantly serosal (in about 10 % of the patients), manifested as eosinophilic ascites and intense peripheral eosinophilia [17].

Pericardial or even pleural effusions may occur in a polyserositis-like presentation. Tissue eosinophilia also rarely may involve extraintestinal organs [18] such as the peritoneum, gallbladder [19], spleen, pancreas (Fig. 27.1) [20, 21], and urinary bladder [22].

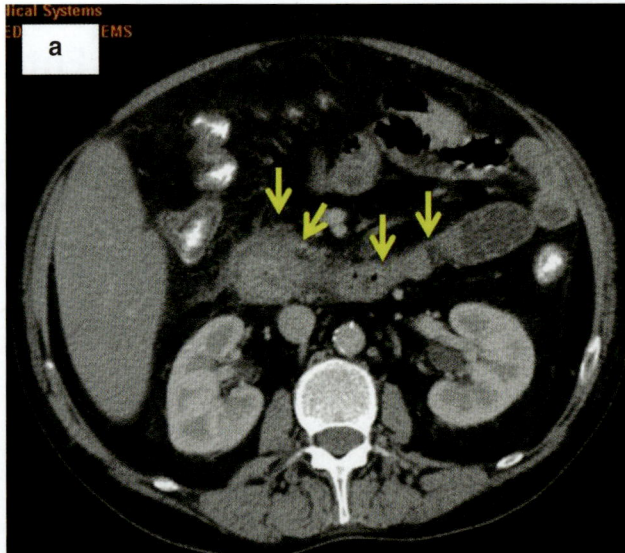
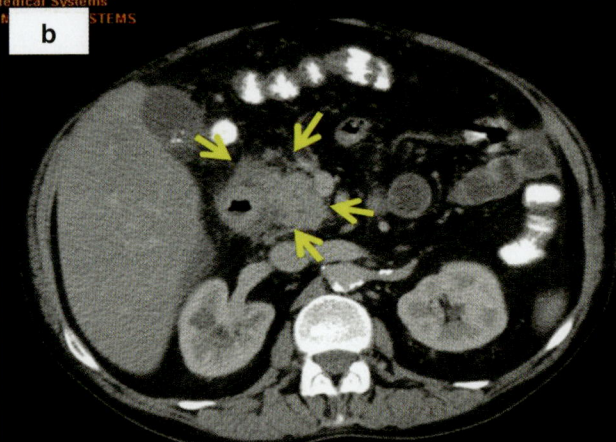
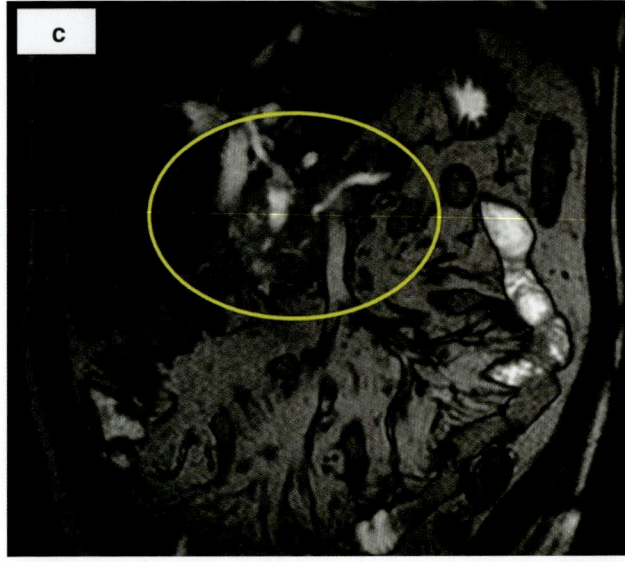

Fig. 27.1 Patient with eosinophilic gastroenteritis and pancreatitis, manifested as a pancreatic head mass visible on abdominal CT scans. (*arrow*) Pancreatic head infiltration by eosinophile (**a, b**) and MRI of the abdomen. (*oval*) Infiltration by eosinophile of pancreatic head (**c**)

27.4 Diagnosis

The diagnosis is based on the histologic demonstration of tissue eosinophilia, in the absence of other causes. The number of eosinophils per high-power field required to diagnose eosinophilic enteritis has not been uniformly agreed upon. For this reason, an experienced, knowledgeable pathologist is essential for interpreting biopsy specimens in patients with suspected eosinophilic enteritis. It has been reported that peripheral eosinophilia is uniformly associated with eosinophilic gastroenteritis.

Intestinal involvement can be determined only by performing enteroscopy (push, double-balloon, or single-balloon) to identify the affected area and take samples (Fig. 27.2.)

Talley et al. [23] have identified three main diagnostic criteria:

1. The presence of gastrointestinal symptoms
2. Biopsies demonstrating eosinophilic infiltration of one or more areas of the gastrointestinal tract
3. No evidence of parasitic or extraintestinal disease

It is now known that the small bowel lesions are focal and often inaccessible to endoscopic biopsy. In addition, if subserosal disease involves the small bowel, biopsy of the mucosal layer taken during endoscopy (gastroscopy, enteroscopy, or colonoscopy) usually fails to diagnose eosinophilic gastroenteritis. In these patients, a laparotomy or laparoscopic biopsy is required to make a diagnosis. It is also necessary to consider in the differential diagnosis of eosinophilic gastroenteritis other entities that could induce

the same symptoms [5]. Occasionally, when there is ascites, a cytologic study can help to diagnose predominant serosal eosinophilic gastroenteritis.

27.5 Video Capsule Endoscopy

The endoscopic appearance in eosinophilic gastroenteritis is nonspecific. Though no articles have been published exclusively about capsule endoscopy and eosinophilic enteritis, some cases have been reported that are greatly clarifying. Without any doubt, capsule endoscopy now represents an essential tool for the diagnosis of eosinophilic enteritis; it can avoid surgery in some patients and can noninvasively observe the patient's treatment and condition [24].

The typical endoscopic findings in the small intestine are sharply demarcated foci of severe villous atrophy and multiple, erythematous mucosal lesions throughout the small bowel [25, 26] (Figs. 27.3 and 27.4). Other lesions observed in eosinophilic enteritis include erythematous, friable, nodular, and occasional ulcerative changes (Fig. 27.5). Gastric inflammation is found in some patients (Fig. 27.6), as are thickening of folds and inflammatory polyps (Fig. 27.7). A fair number of patients have no visible mucosal abnormalities.

In one study of 15 patients, 10 had only nonspecific gastritis or colitis, and 2 had shallow gastric or duodenal ulcers [27]. Strictures may occur (Fig. 27.8) [28], which may cause capsule retention [29]. Dark blue coloration of the deeper layers of the wall of the small bowel can be found in some patients, with normal villi and no surface erosions [30]. In others, capsule endoscopy can observe jejunal bleeding followed by ileal obstruction [31].

It is important to consider that after treatment, the patient's symptoms normally improve, and a follow-up capsule endoscopy examination usually shows the absence of mucosal lesions in the small bowel [26].

We show a case of a 70-year-old woman suffering from abdominal pain and bloating with nausea and occasional vomiting (Fig. 27.3). We also present a case of a 41-year-old man who was evaluated for chronic abdominal pain, some episodes of diarrhea, and no significant weight loss (Fig. 27.4). We also present the case of a patient recently returned from Thailand with acute abdominal pain and eosinophilia (Fig. 27.9).

27.6 Treatment

No standard treatment has been developed for eosinophilic enteritis. The factors deserving consideration when deciding on the best treatment for an individual patient include

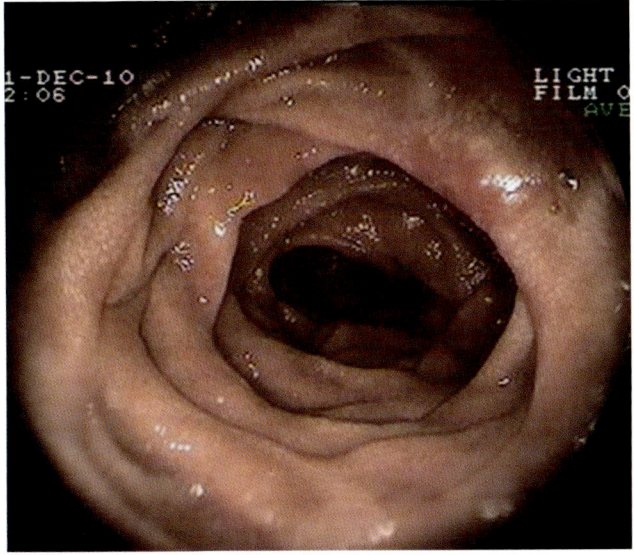

Fig. 27.2 Enteroscopy on a patient with gastroenteropathy predominantly affecting the mucosa, which is observed in certain atrophic and denuded areas. The biopsy showed intense eosinophil infiltration

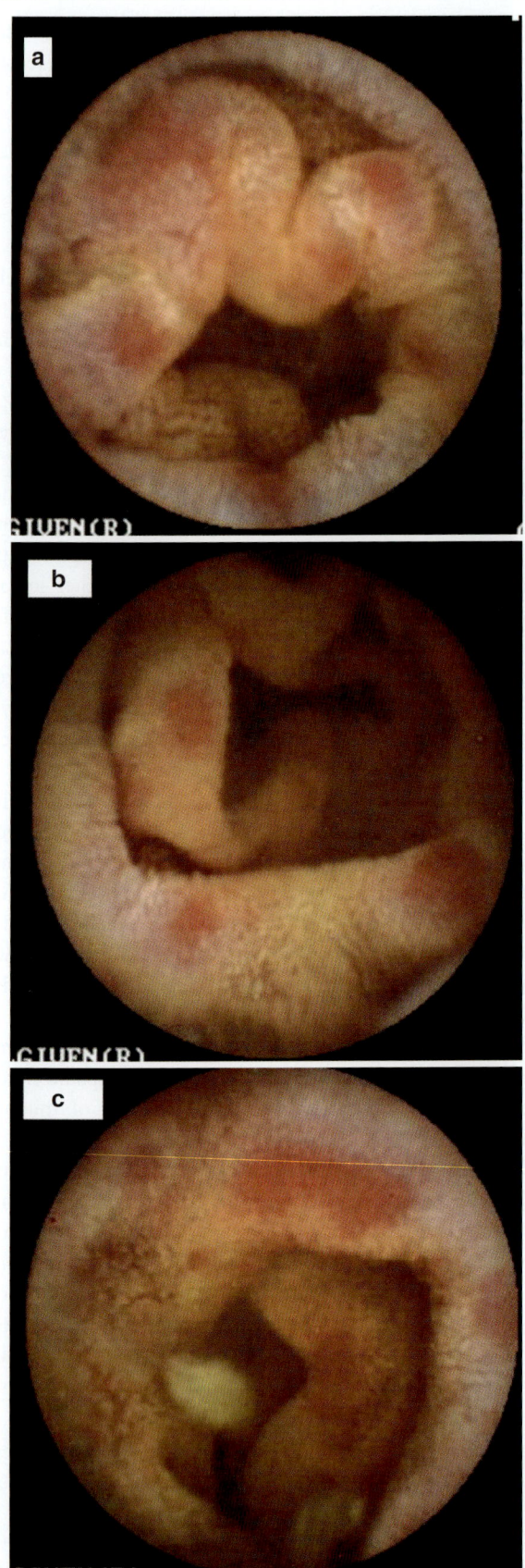

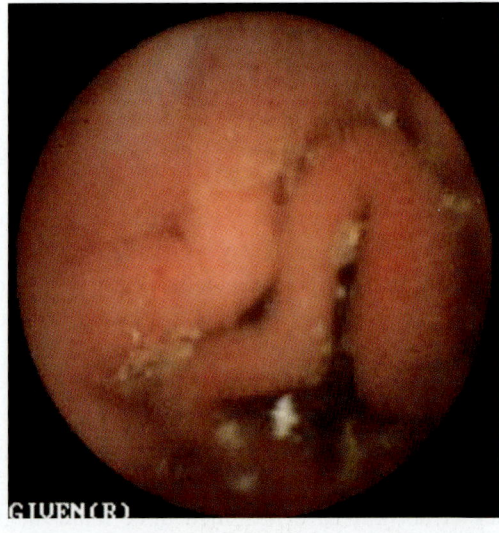

Fig. 27.4 Erythematous mucosal lesions in the small bowel in a 41-year-old man evaluated for chronic abdominal pain, some episodes of diarrhea, and no significant weight loss

the patient's age and the severity of the clinical manifestations [32]. The treatment consists of an elimination diet in cases of food allergies. For these patients, food allergy testing and elemental diets should be considered before a trial of corticosteroids. Furthermore, it has been reported that spontaneous remission may occur in up to 40 % of patients [33]. But in the majority of patients, corticosteroids are the mainstay of therapy. Symptom relief usually occurs within a few weeks of the initiation of treatment [34]. The beneficial effects of steroids in eosinophilic disorders are mediated by inhibition of eosinophil growth factors, IL-3, IL-5, and GM-CSF.

As the long-term use of systemic corticosteroids is associated with growth abnormalities, bone abnormalities, mood disturbances, and adrenal axis suppression, other treatments have been studied. These alternative treatments include topical glucocorticoids that deliver drugs to specific segments of the gastrointestinal tract and have no systemic adverse effects. Among these are budesonide, histamine H-1 receptor antagonists, and mast cell-stabilizing drugs (e.g., cromoglycate). Montelukast, a selective and competitive leukotriene receptor antagonist, also may be considered, as a corticosteroid-sparing agent [35]. Review of the literature shows that montelukast is efficient in treating eosinophilic enteritis in some patients, especially because of its low number of adverse effects, effectiveness, and low cost [36].

Fig. 27.3 (**a–c**) Demarcated foci of severe villous atrophy and multiple erythematous mucosal lesions through the small bowel in a 70-year-old woman evaluated for abdominal pain and bloating with nausea and occasional vomiting

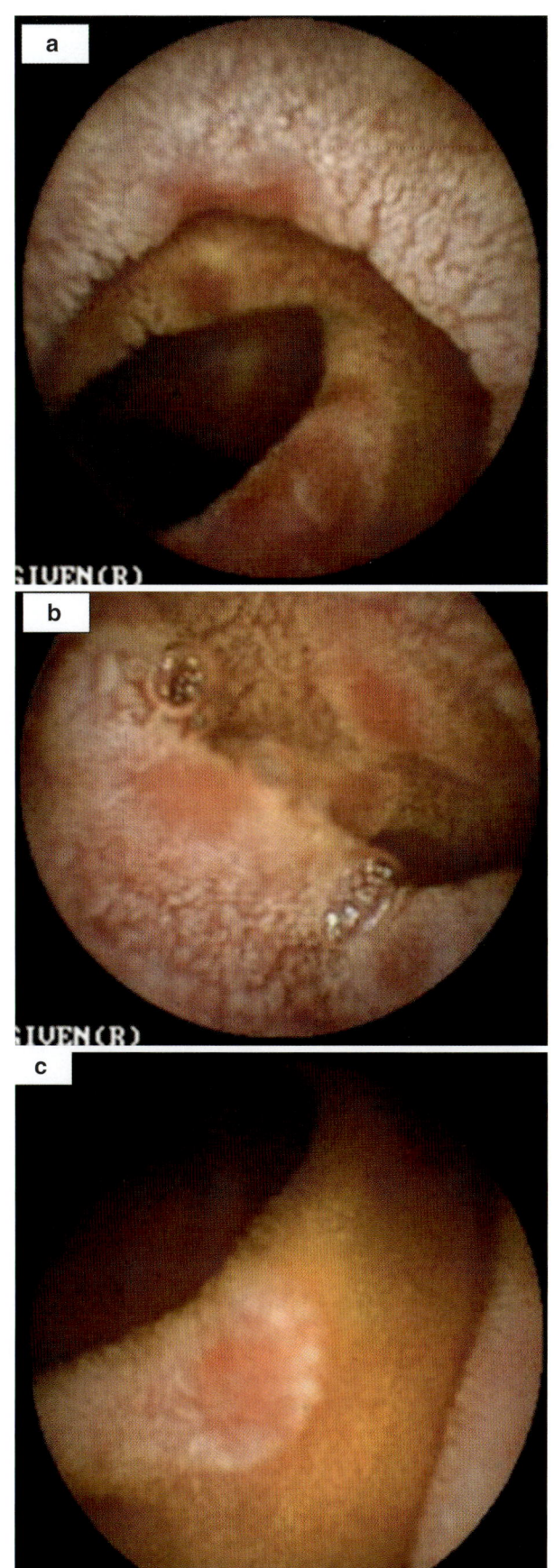

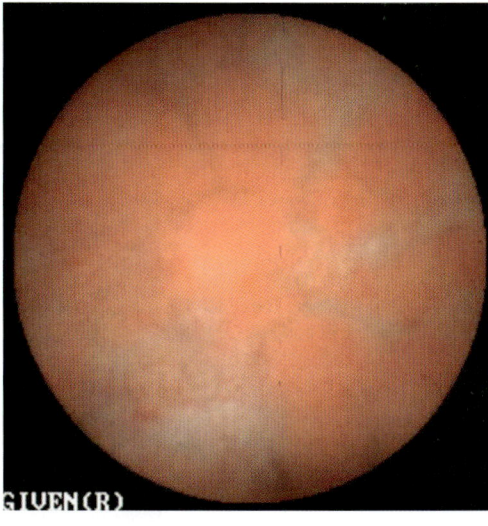

Fig. 27.6 Gastric inflammation in eosinophilic gastroenteritis

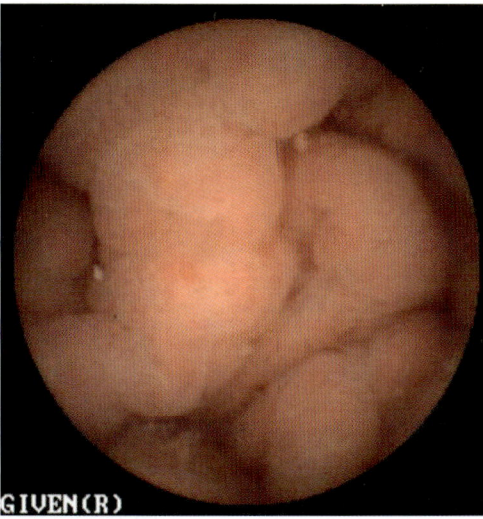

Fig. 27.7 Thickening of folds and inflammatory polyps in eosinophilic gastroenteritis

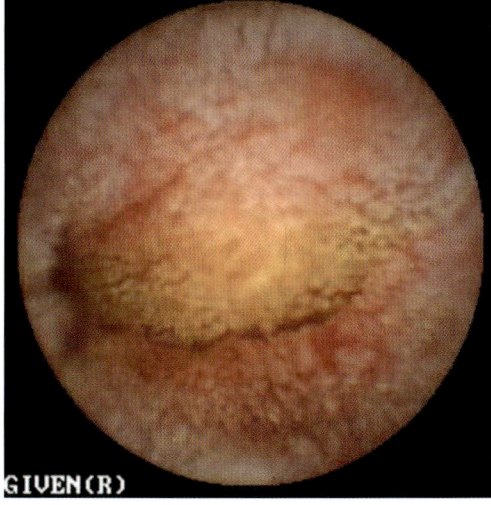

Fig. 27.5 (**a–c**) Erythematous, friable, and ulcerative changes throughout the small bowel in eosinophilic gastroenteritis

Fig. 27.8 Strictures surrounded by erythematous mucosal lesions in a case of eosinophilic gastroenteritis. The video capsule endoscopy (VCE) capsule passed the stricture

Fig. 27.9 This patient, recently returned from Thailand, had acute abdominal pain and eosinophilia. Small bowel loops were distended (**a**) and thickened (**b**) (Courtesy of Roman Fischbach, MD.) A Patency capsule (Given Imaging Ltd., Yoqneam, Israel) passed intact. VCE shows impression/invagination (**c**), intramural hemorrhage (**d**), white nodules seen at VCE (**e**), and single balloon enteroscopy (SBE) (**f**). Additionally, small ulcers were found at VCE (**g**) in a short segment and confirmed by SBE (**h**). Biopsy showed eosinophilic enteritis. No parasites or worm eggs were detectable in stool. Antibodies against *Dirofilaria immitis* were positive, probably cross-reactive with other helminths

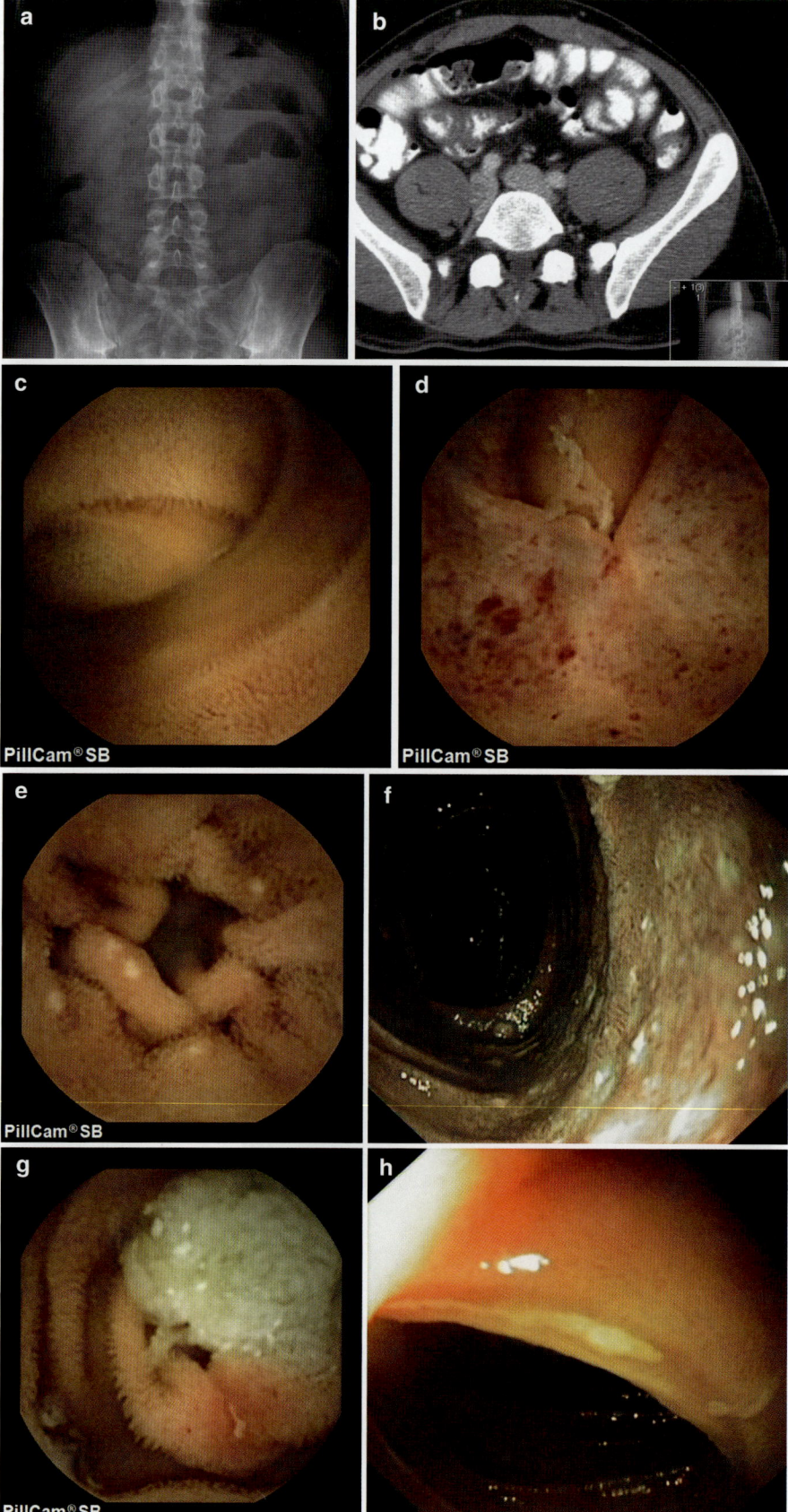

References

1. Polyak S, Smith T, Mertz H. Eosinophilic gastroenteritis causing pancreatitis and pancreaticobiliary ductal dilation. Dig Dis Sci. 2002;47:1091–5.
2. Rothenberg ME. Eosinophilic gastrointestinal disorders (EGID). J Allergy Clin Immunol. 2004;113:11–28.
3. Khan S, Orenstein SR. Eosinophilic gastroenteritis. Gastroenterol Clin North Am. 2008;37:333–48.
4. Kaijser R. Allergic disease of the gut from the point of view of the surgeon. Arch Klin Chir. 1937;188:36–64.
5. Oh HE, Chetty R. Eosinophilic gastroenteritis: a review. J Gastroenterol. 2008;43:741–50.
6. Straumann A, Simon HU. The physiological and pathophysiological roles of eosinophils in the gastrointestinal tract. Allergy. 2004;59:15–25.
7. Von Wattenwyl F, Zimmermann A, Netzer P. Synchronous first manifestation of an idiopathic gastroenteritis and bronchial asthma. Eur J Gastroenterol Hepatol. 2001;13:721–5.
8. Desreumaux P, Bloget F, Seguy D, et al. Interleukin 3, granulocyte-macrophage colony-stimulating factor, and interleukin 5 in eosinophilic gastroenteritis. Gastroenterology. 1996;110:768–74.
9. Mishra A, Hogan S, Brandt E, Rothenberg M. An etiological role for aeroallergens and eosinophils in experimental esophagitis. J Clin Invest. 2001;107:83–90.
10. Kelly KJ. Eosinophilic gastroenteritis. J Pediatr Gastroenterol Nutr. 2000;30:S28–35.
11. Christopher V, Thompson M, Hughes S. Eosinophilic gastroenteritis mimicking pancreatic cancer. Postgrad Med J. 2002;78:498–9.
12. Lucendo AJ, Arias A. Eosinophilic gastroenteritis: an update. Expert Rev Gastroenterol Hepatol. 2012;6:591–601.
13. Siewart E, Lammert F, Koppitz P, et al. Eosinophilic gastroenteritis with severe protein-losing enteropathy: successful treatment with budesonide. Dig Liver Dis. 2006;38:55–9.
14. Lee C, Changchien C, Chen P, et al. Eosinophilic gastroenteritis: 10 years experience. Am J Gastroenterol. 1993;88:70–4.
15. Pungpapong S, Stark ME, Cangemi JR. Protein-losing enteropathy from eosinophilic enteritis diagnosed by wireless capsule endoscopy and double-balloon enteroscopy. Gastrointest Endosc. 2007;65:917–8.
16. Shweiki E, West J, Klena J, et al. Eosinophilic gastroenteritis presenting as an obstructing cecal mass – a case report and review of the literature. Am J Gastroenterol. 1999;94:3644–55.
17. Miyamoto T, Shibata T, Matsuura S, et al. Eosinophilic gastroenteritis with ileus and ascites. Intern Med. 1998;35:779–82.
18. Robert F, Omura E, Durant JR. Mucosal eosinophilic gastroenteritis with systemic involvement. Am J Med. 1977;62:139–43.
19. Jimenez-Saenz M, Villar-Rodriguez JL, Torres Y, et al. Biliary tract disease: a rare manifestation of eosinophilic gastroenteritis. Dig Dis Sci. 2003;48:624–7.
20. Lyngbaek S, Adamsen S, Aru A, Bergenfeldt M. Recurrent acute pancreatitis due to eosinophilic gastroenteritis. Case report and literature review. JOP. 2006;7:211–7.
21. Caunedo-Álvarez A. Gastroenteritis eosinofílica: aspectos clínicos y terapéuticos [in Spanish]. RAPD Online. 2012;35:245–54.
22. Gregg JA, Utz DC. Eosinophilic cystitis associated with eosinophilic gastroenteritis. Mayo Clin Proc. 1974;49:185–7.
23. Talley NJ, Shorter RG, Phillips SF, Zinsmeister AR. Eosinophilic gastroenteritis: a clinicopathological study of patients with disease of the mucosa, muscle layer, and subserosal tissues. Gut. 1990;31:54–8.
24. Romero-Vázquez J, Cordero-Ruiz P, Caunedo-Álvarez A, Herrerías-Gutiérrez JM. Malabsorption syndromes and capsule endoscopy. In: Herrerías JM, Mascarenhas-Saraiva M, editors. Atlas of capsule endoscopy. 2nd ed. Sevilla: Sulime; 2012. p. 211–3.
25. Guilhon de Araujo Sant'Anna AM, Dubois J, Miron MC, Seidman EG. Wireless capsule endoscopy for obscure small-bowel disorders: final results of the first pediatric controlled trial. Clin Gastroenterol Hepatol. 2005;3:264–70.
26. Endo H, Hosono K, Inamori M, et al. Capsule endoscopic evaluation of eosinophilic enteritis before and after treatment. Digestion. 2011;83:134–5.
27. Chen MJ, Chu CH, Lin SC, et al. Eosinophilic gastroenteritis: clinical experience with 15 patients. World J Gastroenterol. 2003;9:2813–6.
28. Attar A, Cazals-Hatem D, Ponsot P. Videocapsule endoscopy identifies stenoses missed by other imaging techniques in a patient with eosinophilic gastroenteritis. Clin Gastroenterol Hepatol. 2011;9:A28.
29. Seidman EG, Sant'Anna AMGA, Dirks MH. Potential applications of wireless capsule endoscopy in the pediatric age group. Gastrointest Endosc Clin N Am. 2004;14:207–17.
30. Koumi A, Panos MZ. A new capsule endoscopy feature of serosal eosinophilic enteritis. Endoscopy. 2009;41 Suppl 2:E280.
31. Kim N, Kim JW, Hwang JH, et al. Visualization of jejunal bleeding by capsule endoscopy in a case of eosinophilic enteritis. Korean J Intern Med. 2005;20:63–7.
32. Hogan SP, Rothenberg ME. Review article: the eosinophil as a therapeutic target in gastrointestinal disease. Aliment Pharmacol Ther. 2004;20:1231–40.
33. de Chambrun GP, Gonzalez F, Canva JY, et al. Natural history of eosinophilic gastroenteritis. Clin Gastroenterol Hepatol. 2011;9:950–6.
34. Lin HH, Wu CH, Wu LS, Shyu RY. Eosinophilic gastroenteritis presenting as relapsing severe abdominal pain and enteropathy with protein loss. Emerg Med J. 2005;22:834–5.
35. Schwartz DA, Pardi DS, Murray JA. Use of montelukast as steroid-sparing agent for recurrent eosinophilic gastroenteritis. Dig Dis Sci. 2001;46:1787–90.
36. De Maeyer N, Kochuyt AM, Van Moerkercke W, Hiele M. Montelukast as a treatment modality for eosinophilic gastroenteritis. Acta Gastroenterol Belg. 2011;74:570–5.

Infectious Diseases of the Small Intestine

28

Peter Baltes, Adriana Safatle-Ribeiro, Martin Keuchel, and D. Nageshwar Reddy

Contents

The work was first published in 2006 by Springer Medizin Verlag Heidelberg with the following title: *Atlas of Video Capsule Endoscopy*.

P. Baltes (✉) • M. Keuchel
Department of Internal Medicine,
Bethesda Krankenhaus Bergedorf, Hamburg, Germany
e-mail: baltes@bkb.info; keuchel@bkb.info

A. Safatle-Ribeiro
Department of Gastroenterology, University of Sao Paulo,
Sao Paulo, Brazil
e-mail: adrisafatleribeiro@terra.com.br

D.N. Reddy
Department of Medical Gastroenterology, Asian Institute of
Gastroenterology, Hyderabad, India
e-mail: aigindia@yahoo.co.in

Most infections that involve the small bowel are self-limiting, and endoscopic examination is rarely indicated in these cases. Suspicion of microbial enteritis can be confirmed by stool cultures and, if necessary, by detection of toxins or antigens. Persistent diarrhea and associated symptoms such as weight loss, fever, arthralgia, and neurologic deficits or findings such as anemia, inflammatory signs, eosinophilia, or signs of malabsorption warrant further investigation. Besides microscopic stool examination, the main tool for this purpose is flexible endoscopy with tissue sampling from the duodenum, terminal ileum, and colon. Video capsule endoscopy (VCE) can sometimes reveal changes in the jejunum or ileum, and it has a high negative predictive value to exclude such lesions. Its usefulness is limited by its inability to obtain biopsy specimens, but it can direct the type and approach of subsequent enteroscopy by providing information on localization and extent of the detected lesions.

28.1 Whipple's Disease

28.1.1 Clinical Features

Whipple's disease is very rare. It is characterized by diarrhea, malassimilation, arthritis, neurologic deficits, and psychiatric changes.

28.1.2 Etiology

The causative organism of Whipple's disease is *Tropheryma whipplei* [1]. Affected individuals may suffer from a cellular immune defect [2].

28.1.3 Diagnosis

The diagnosis is based on a small bowel biopsy with the detection of periodic acid–Schiff (PAS)-positive macrophages. It can be confirmed by a polymerase chain reaction (PCR) assay in an intestinal biopsy.

28.1.4 Endoscopy

Endoscopy may reveal a glassy, gelatinous edema; lymphangiectasia (Fig. 28.1), [3]; erosions; ulcers; and diffuse hemorrhage [4–7]. Similar findings may be noted in intestinal histoplasmosis, atypical mycobacteriosis, or multiple myeloma [8, 9].

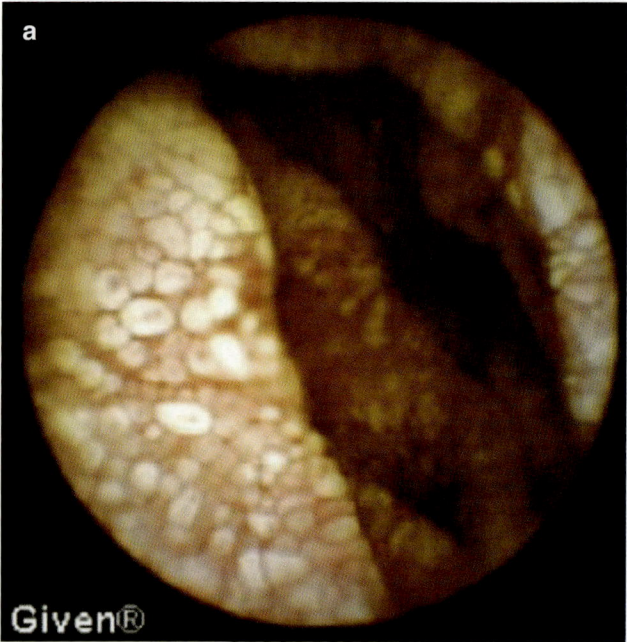

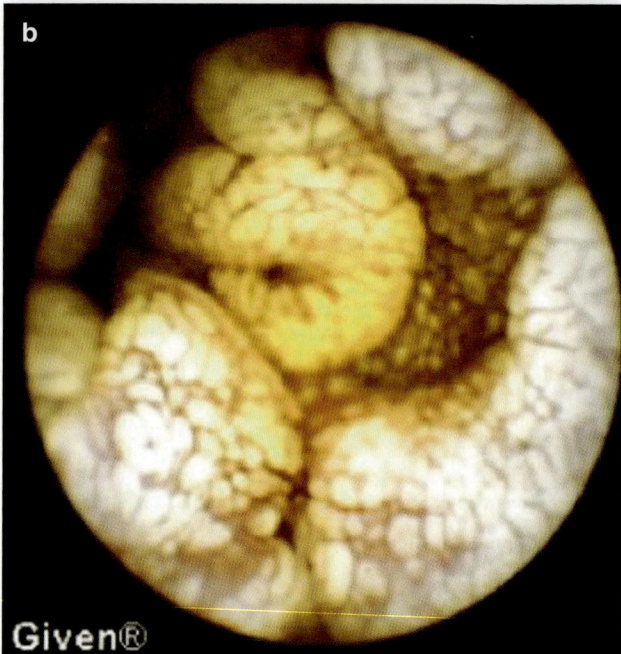

Fig. 28.1 Whipple's disease. Diffuse lymphangiectasia with swollen, whitish, club-shaped villi (**a**) and diffuse edema (**b**). (Courtesy of Ingo Franke, MD)

28.1.5 Treatment

Long-term antibiotic therapy is necessary, considering the involvement of the central nervous system. The therapeutic regimen consists of initial therapy with cephalosporin followed by a 12-month course of trimethoprim and sulfamethoxazole. Mucosal healing under this therapy has been reported, but failure of this regimen has been reported as well [10, 11].

28.2 Infection with Atypical Mycobacteria

28.2.1 Clinical Features

Intestinal involvement by atypical mycobacteria is known to occur alone or in addition to pulmonary and cutaneous involvement [12]. The infection may take an asymptomatic course or may become disseminated, especially in immuno-compromised patients [13].

28.2.2 Etiology

The infection is caused by atypical mycobacteria. Over 125 species have been described, including *Mycobacterium avium-intracellulare* (MAI) and *Mycobacterium genavense*.

28.2.3 Diagnosis

Diagnosis is based on the histologic detection of acid-fast rods in biopsy material, on PCR assay, or by culturing the organism from blood, bone marrow, biopsy specimens, or sputum. Due to the ubiquitous occurrence of MAI, detection of the organism in normally sterile materials like blood is the most accurate test. Detection of environmental mycobacteria in sputum often represents colonization.

28.2.4 Endoscopy

Infection with MAI often bears an endoscopic resemblance to Whipple's disease, giving rise to the term "pseudo-Whipple's disease" (Fig. 28.2). Infections with *M. genavense* may show edema, increased friability, or lymphangiectatic areas [14].

28.2.5 Treatment

If treatment is necessary, it consists of an antimycobacterial combination regimen based on sensitivity testing and often including classic antituberculosis substances. The course of treatment may be prolonged, depending on the patient's immune status.

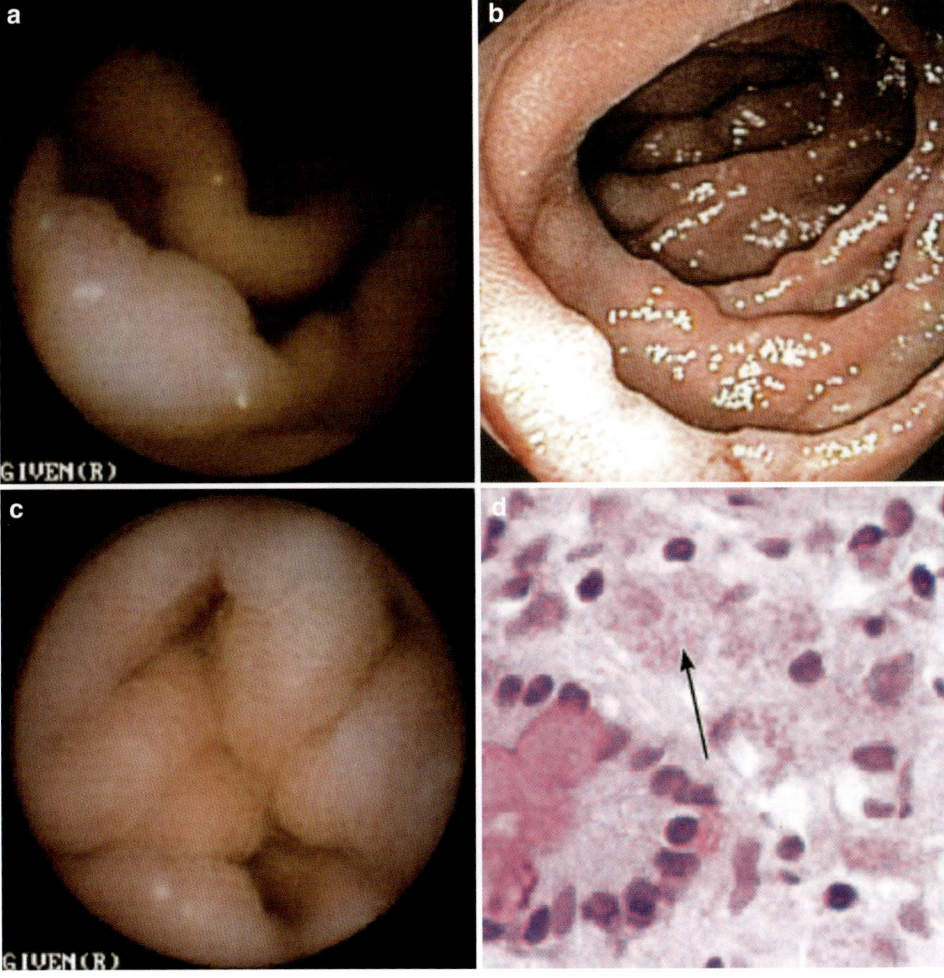

Fig. 28.2 "Pseudo-Whipple's disease" in a young man with chronic diarrhea, malassimilation, and lymphadenopathy. *Mycobacterium avium-intracellulare* was isolated from lymph nodes. The patient was HIV negative. (**a, c**) Examination of the jejunum with video capsule endoscopy (VCE) shows diffuse, glassy edema with indistinct villi and luminal narrowing. The capsule passed through the lumen without impediment. (**b**) Corresponding image from push enteroscopy (Courtesy of Wolfgang Cordruwisch, MD). (**d**) Histology revealed weakly PAS-positive macrophages (Courtesy of Axel von Herbay, MD)

28.3 Tuberculosis

28.3.1 Etiology

Gastrointestinal tuberculosis most frequently involves the small intestine and ileocecum [15, 16]. Gastrointestinal tuberculosis may occur as a primary infection with *Mycobacterium bovis* or may be secondary to pulmonary infection with *Mycobacterium tuberculosis*.

28.3.2 Diagnosis

The diagnosis can be established by the biopsy detection of caseating granulomas and acid-fast rods and also by genetic testing (PCR) and culture studies. Stool PCR has proven to be as sensitive as sputum tests in patients with pulmonary tuberculosis [17], so the detection of *M. tuberculosis* in stool samples does not prove involvement of the gastrointestinal tract. On the other hand, gastrointestinal lesions can be found in asymptomatic patients with pulmonary tuberculosis [18].

28.3.3 Endoscopy

Edematous swelling and patchy redness are typical but unspecific findings in affected mucosa (Figs. 28.3 and 28.4). Ulcers are most commonly found in the ileocecal region (Fig. 28.5); strictures and obstructions also have been described [19, 20]. Differentiating intestinal tuberculosis from other ulcerative diseases of the small intestine can be challenging, especially in countries with a high prevalence of tuberculosis and Crohn's disease. In Crohn's disease, ulcers may appear longitudinal or aphthous, whereas tuberculosis may present with oblique or transverse ulcers with

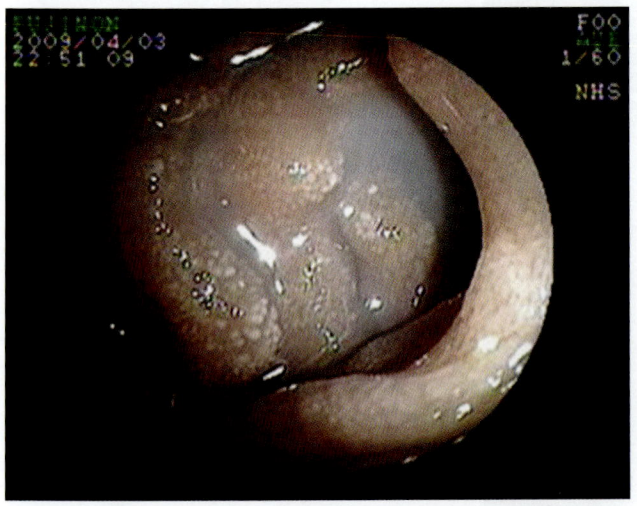

Fig. 28.3 Diffuse swelling, lymphangiectasia, and exudation in intestinal tuberculosis (double-balloon enteroscopy)

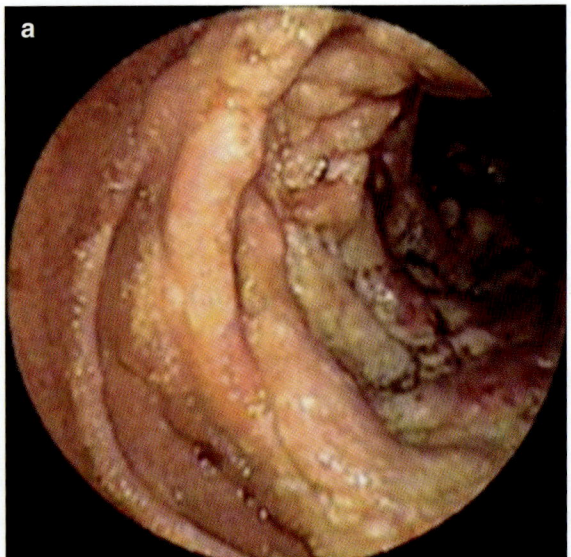

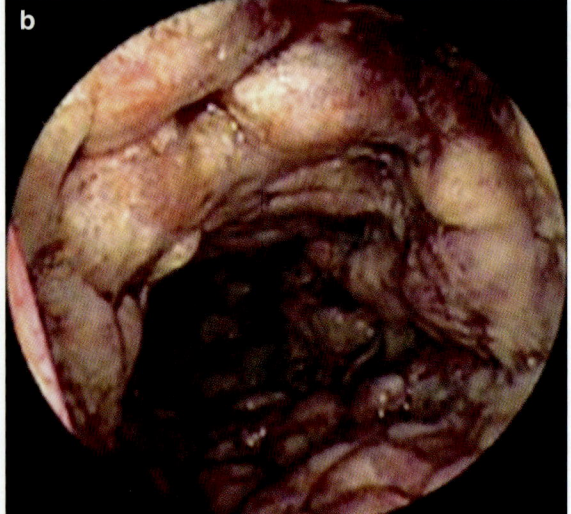

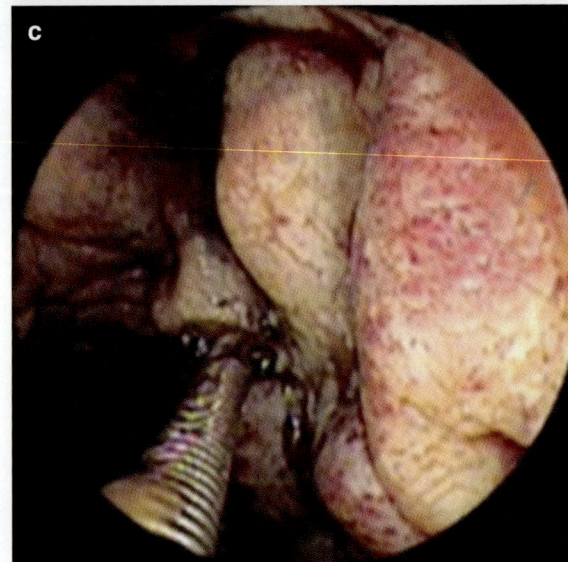

Fig. 28.4 (a–c) Diffuse infiltration of small intestinal mucosa in a patient with tuberculosis. Double-balloon enteroscopy shows diffuse swelling, erythema, and white and livid discoloration

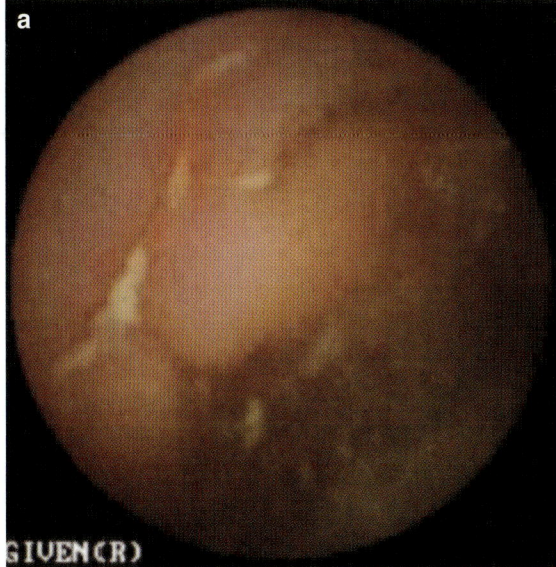

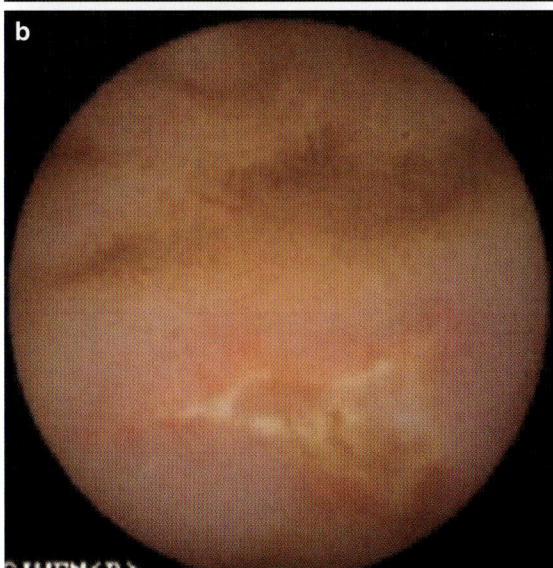

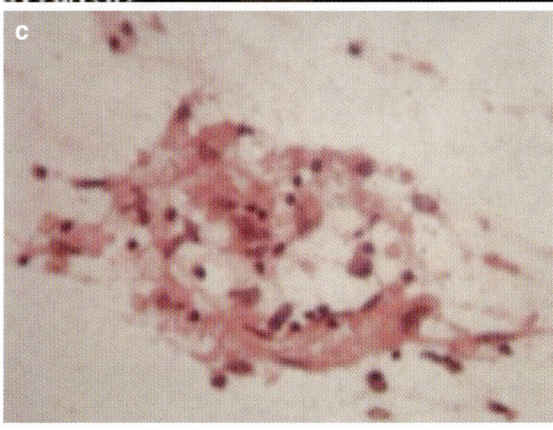

Fig. 28.5 Intestinal tuberculosis. VCE. (**a**, **b**) Edema and ulcers in the ileum (Reprinted from Reddy et al. [23], with permission from Georg Thieme Verlag). (**c**) Biopsy from the terminal ileum shows portions of a granuloma with epithelioid and giant cells, consistent with tuberculosis

a necrotic base, as well as hypertrophic or nodular lesions [21–23]. Oblique ulcers also can be found in chronic, non-specific multiple ulcers of the small intestine (CNSU) (Chap. 32), however, and lesions related to the use of nonsteroidal anti-inflammatory drugs (NSAIDs) may present with discrete ulcerations and concentric stenosis (Chap. 30) [24, 25]. Because of the morphologic resemblance, differentiation of these lesions through biopsy is warranted.

28.3.4 Treatment

Treatment consists of a combination regimen like that used for pulmonary tuberculosis. Recent studies showed similar effectiveness for 6-month and 9-month regimens [26].

28.4 Intestinal Spirochetosis

28.4.1 Etiology

The organisms causing intestinal spirochetosis are spirochetes such as *Borrelia eurygyrata*, *Brachyspira aalborgi*, *Brachyspira hyodysenteriae*, and *Serpulina pilosicoli*. There is no clinical relation to borreliosis or syphilis. The detection of intestinal spirochetosis in asymptomatic individuals may represent colonization, but it should be considered in the differential diagnosis of symptomatic patients, especially those suffering from immunodeficiency [27].

28.4.2 Clinical Features

Patients may present with abdominal pain, which sometimes resembles appendicitis. Chronic diarrhea, constipation, and weight loss also have been reported.

28.4.3 Diagnosis

Diagnosis can be established by biopsies of the colorectal or small bowel mucosa. Spirochetes can be detected in the specimens by microscopy and can be differentiated by PCR [28].

28.4.4 Endoscopy

Colonoscopic examination often shows normal mucosa. In some patients, lymphoid follicular hyperplasia or hemorrhagic lesions can be found [29]. Possible findings at small bowel capsule endoscopy are lymphoid follicular hyperplasia and aphthous ulcers (Fig. 28.6).

Fig. 28.6 Intestinal spirochetosis. Lymphoid hyperplasia in the proximal duodenum (**a**) and aphthae (*circle*) in the proximal and mid-small bowel (**b**) (VCE, courtesy of Brigitta Reinke, MD.) Single-balloon enteroscopy shows nodules (**c**) and an irregular mucosal defect without ulceration (**d**). Biopsy specimen (Giemsa stain) showed lymphoid hyperplasia (**e**) and a pathognomonic bacterial layer on the mid-small bowel mucosa (**f**), confirming intestinal spirochetosis. (Courtesy of Ilske Oschlies, MD)

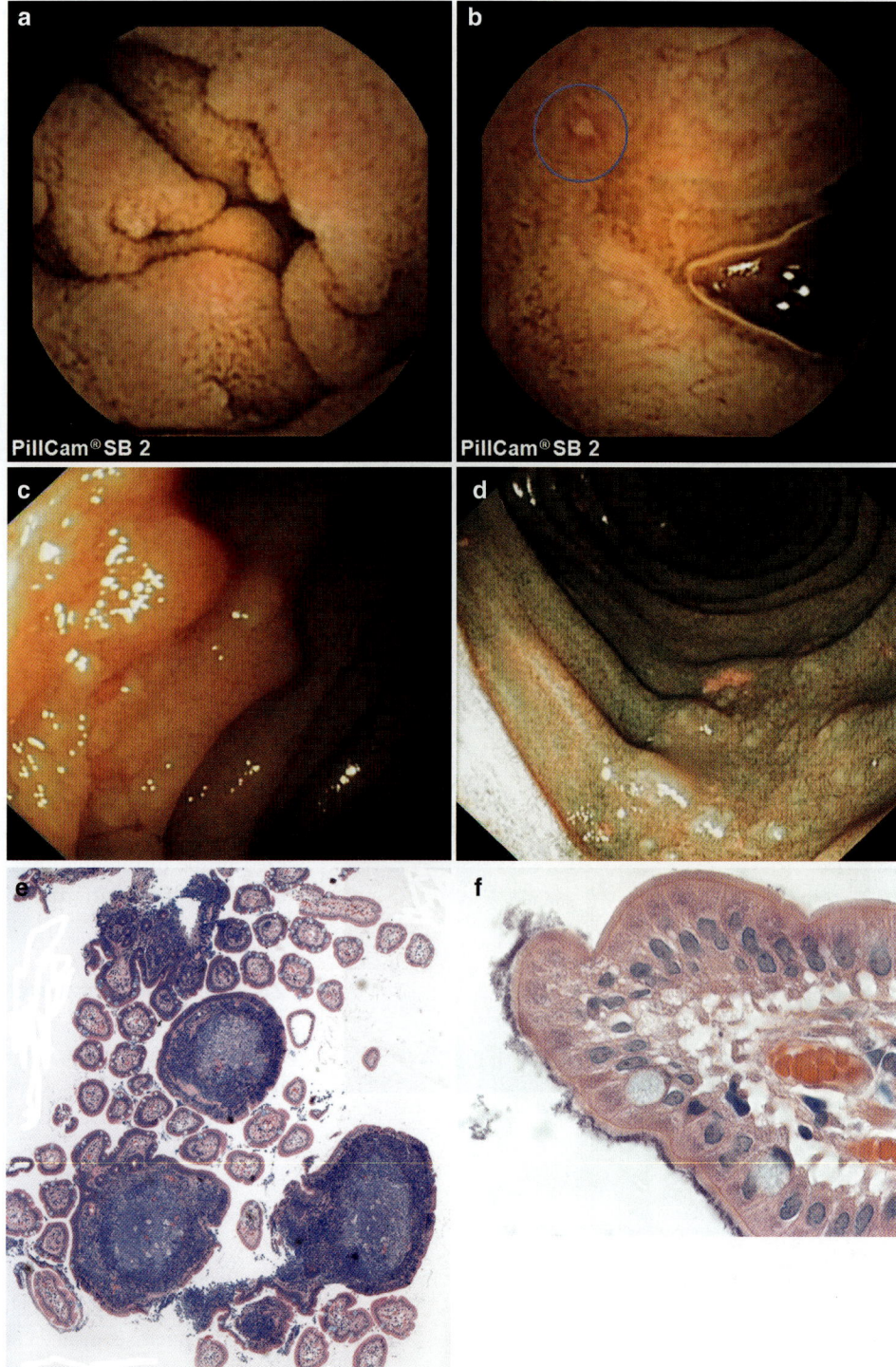

28.4.5 Treatment

Symptomatic intestinal spirochetosis can be treated with nitroimidazoles; metronidazole is the first-line drug of this type.

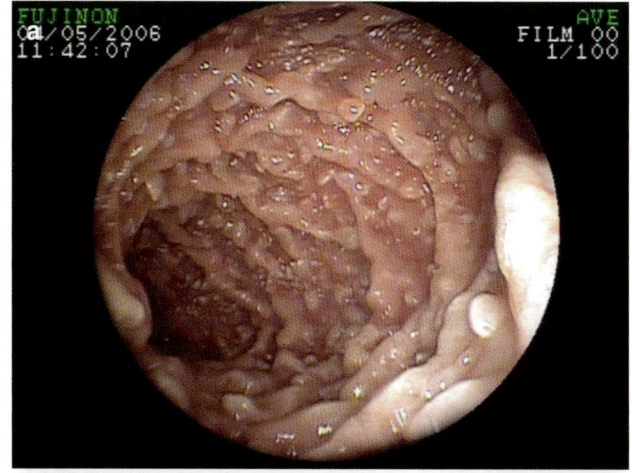

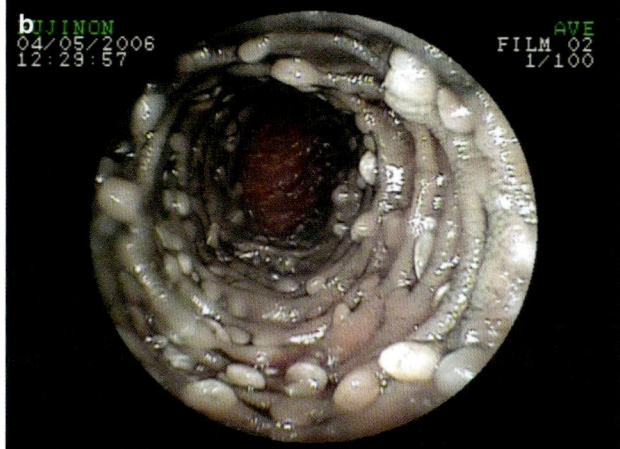

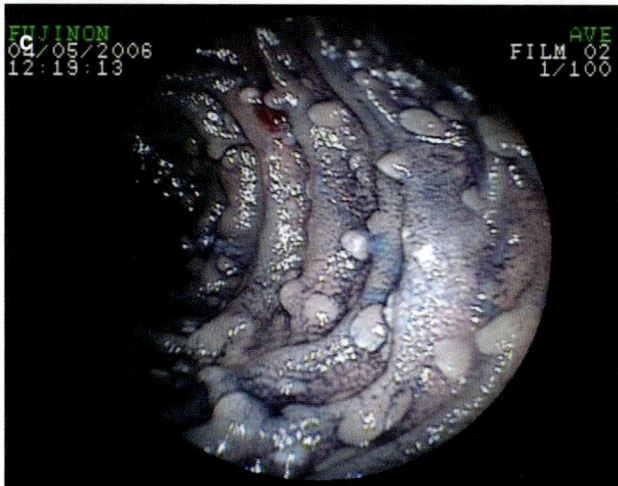

Fig. 28.7 (**a–c**) Immunoproliferative small intestinal disease (IPSID) with multiple, diffusely distributed nodules over a long segment of the small intestine. Double-balloon enteroscopy (DBE). A native image (**b**), DBE with Fujinon intelligent color enhancement (FICE), DBE chromoendoscopy with indigo carmine

28.5 Immunoproliferative Small Intestinal Disease

28.5.1 Etiology

Immunoproliferative small intestinal disease (IPSID) is a form of extranodal marginal zone lymphoma (mucosa-associated lymphoid tissue (MALT lymphoma)) involving the small intestine. The production of truncated alpha heavy chains also led to the term *alpha heavy chain disease*, and the endemic presentation in the Middle East and Africa led to the term *Mediterranean lymphoma*. Bacterial infection of the small intestine as with *Campylobacter jejuni* has been attributed to the development of IPSID [30].

28.5.2 Clinical Features

Clinical presentation includes abdominal pain, secretory diarrhea, and malabsorption [31].

28.5.3 Endoscopy

Multiple nodules of the small intestine can be observed [32–34] (Fig. 28.7).

28.6 Cytomegalovirus Enteritis

28.6.1 Etiology

Cytomegalovirus (CMV) is a DNA virus from the group of herpesviruses. After primary infection, the virus persists and may later be activated or reactivated. Severe courses of disease can be found in patients with immunosuppression due to malignant diseases, pharmacologic treatment, or AIDS.

28.6.2 Clinical Features

The infection often remains asymptomatic, but it may affect the lungs, central nervous system, retina, liver, biliary tract, and all portions of the gastrointestinal tract. Mid-gastrointestinal bleeding, ulcers, perforation, and necrosis have all been described in the small bowel [35–38].

28.6.3 Diagnosis

The diagnosis is based on the biopsy detection of typical cytomegalic cells ("owl's eye cells") (Fig. 28.8), antigen detection in biopsy samples, and PCR assay in peripheral

Fig. 28.8 Cytomegalovirus (CMV) enteritis in a 59-year-old man with cachexia and tetraparesis. The HIV-negative patient was taking methotrexate for rheumatoid arthritis. Capsule endoscopy was performed for chronic diarrhea and malassimilation. (**a, b**) VCE reveals small erosions, petechiae, and punched-out mucosal defects. (**c**) Punched-out, noninflamed ulcers on enteroscopy (Courtesy of Christoph Manegold, MD). (**d**) Histology shows typical owl's eye cells (*arrows*) (Courtesy of Andreas Gocht, MD)

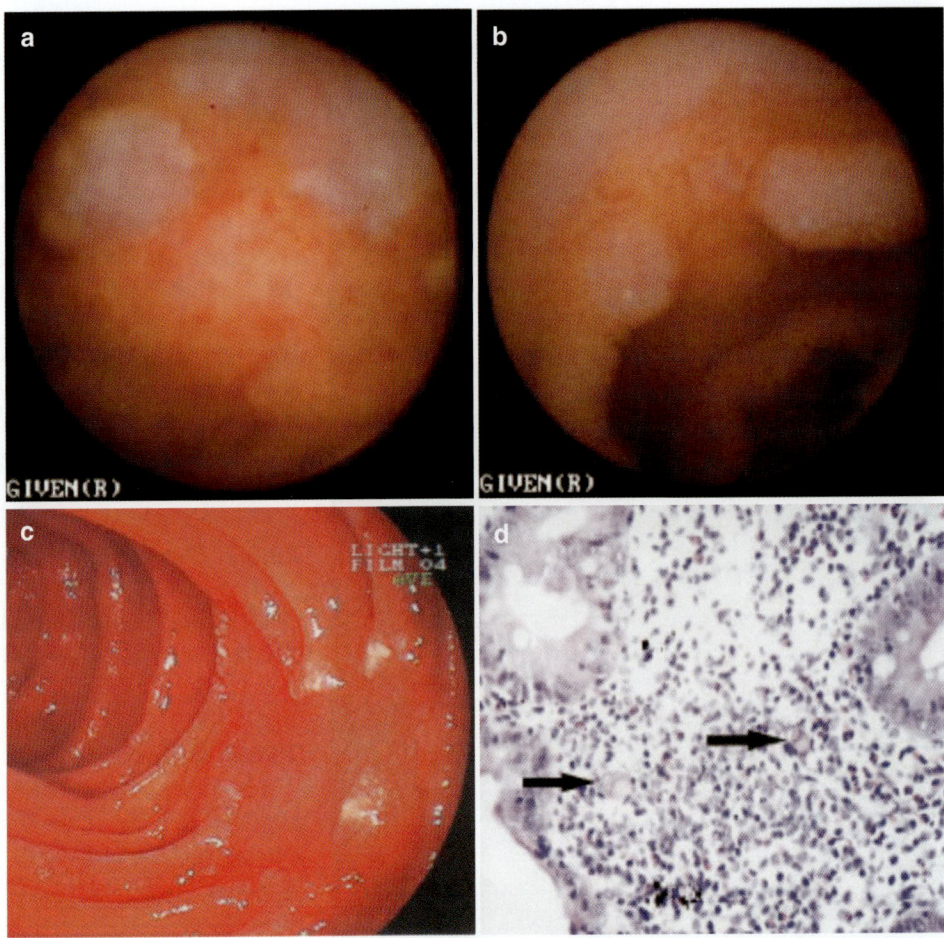

blood lymphocytes. IgM antibodies may be detectable in immunosuppressed patients.

28.6.4 Endoscopy

CMV ulcers often show no inflammatory reaction and have a punched-out appearance. Typically the ulcer base is not covered by fibrinous exudate [39] (Fig. 28.8).

28.6.5 Treatment

Most immunocompetent patients do not need treatment. Immunosuppressed patients may be treated with intravenous ganciclovir or oral valganciclovir; cidofovir or foscarnet can be used as second-line drugs.

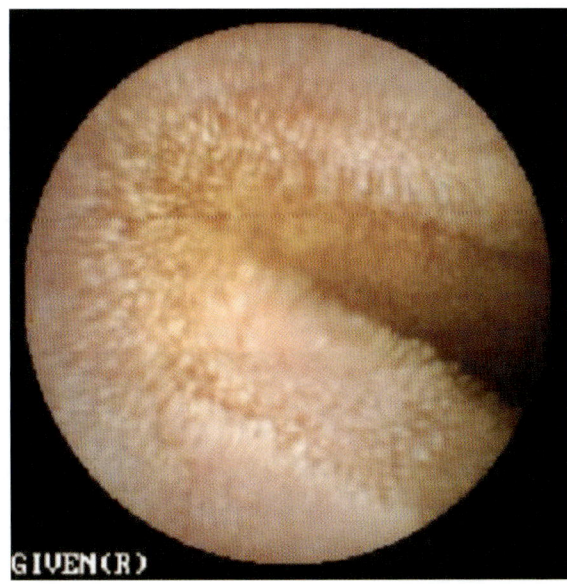

Fig. 28.9 Diffuse, nonspecific lymphangiectasia in an AIDS patient with malassimilation

28.7 AIDS

Patients with AIDS can develop enteritis due to a variety of causes [40]. These include mycobacteriosis, histoplasmosis, CMV infection, strongyloidiasis, and cryptosporidiosis [13, 41, 42]. Histologic and/or microbiologic identification of the causative organism is essential for planning a specific therapy. Malassimilation in patients suffering from AIDS may result from enteritis caused by HIV itself. HIV enteropathy is diagnosed by exclusion (Fig. 28.9). Endoscopic sign of HIV enteropathy may be diffuse, unspecific lymphangiectasia [43]. These enteropathies have become less common with the widespread use of highly active antiviral therapy, but they may be difficult to diagnose and treat [44].

Thinking the other way around, in patients with unusual findings at VCE, a detailed history is important and HIV testing might be considered.

Apart from lesions obviously of infectious origin, patients with HIV infection or AIDS may present with other rare and unusual gastrointestinal manifestations caused by inflammation, medication, or yet undiagnosed infections [45]. Examples of mesenteric panniculitis or severe gastric ulceration are shown in Figs. 28.10 and 28.11.

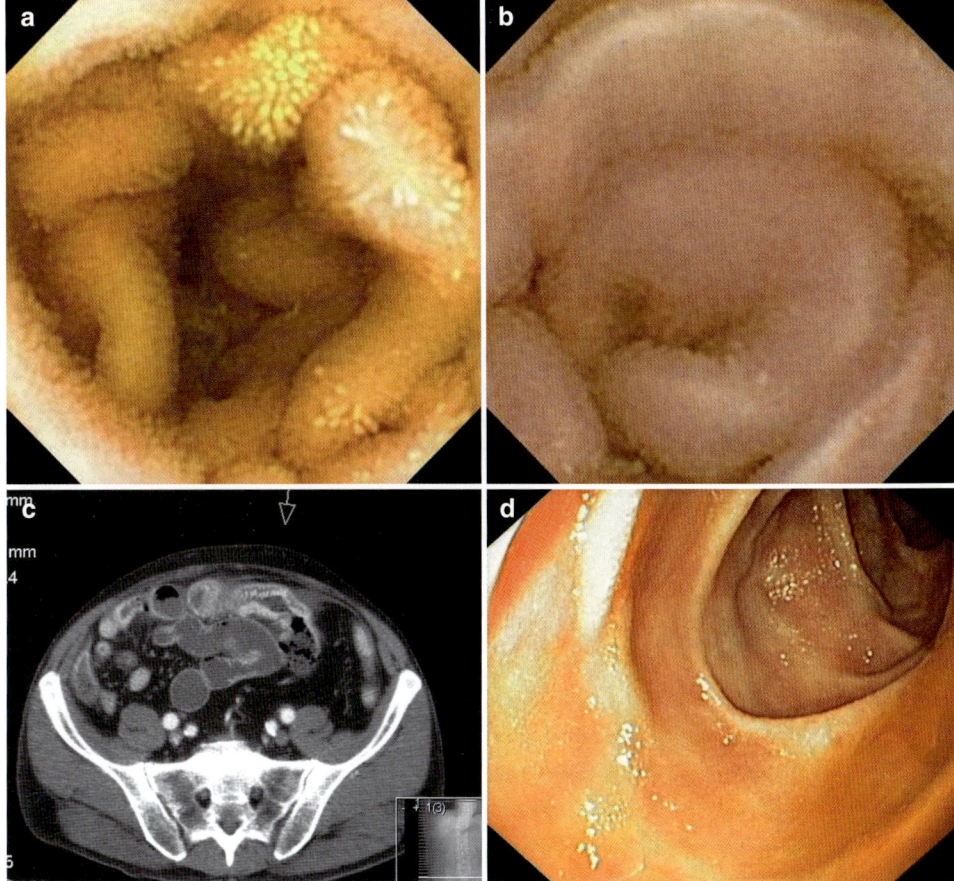

Fig. 28.10 Panniculitis in an HIV-positive patient. VCE shows lymphangiectasia (**a**) and thickened, fibrotic small bowel wall (**b**). A CT scan (**c**) shows inflammation of the visceral tissue. (Courtesy of Roman Fischbach, MD.) Single-balloon enteroscopy (**d**) demonstrates fibrosis and reduced motility of the jejunum

Panniculitis may occur as a rare complication of AIDS. This group of diseases is characterized by inflammation of adipose subcutaneous or visceral tissue. A diagnosis of panniculitis can be suggested by CT scans and verified by biopsy sampling. Further classification is made by histologic characteristics. If fat necrosis and inflammation predominate, the condition is called *mesenteric panniculitis*, whereas if fibrosis and retraction predominate, the condition is known as *retractile mesenteritis*. As the inflammatory reaction affects the mesentery and visceral fat tissue, only indirect signs, such as lymphangiectasia or mucosal fibrosis leading to hypomotility, can be observed (Fig. 28.12).

Although capsule endoscopy does not provide the possibility of biopsies, it may present an interesting possibility to investigate the entire gastrointestinal tract in HIV patients with a single-use endoscope (Fig. 28.13).

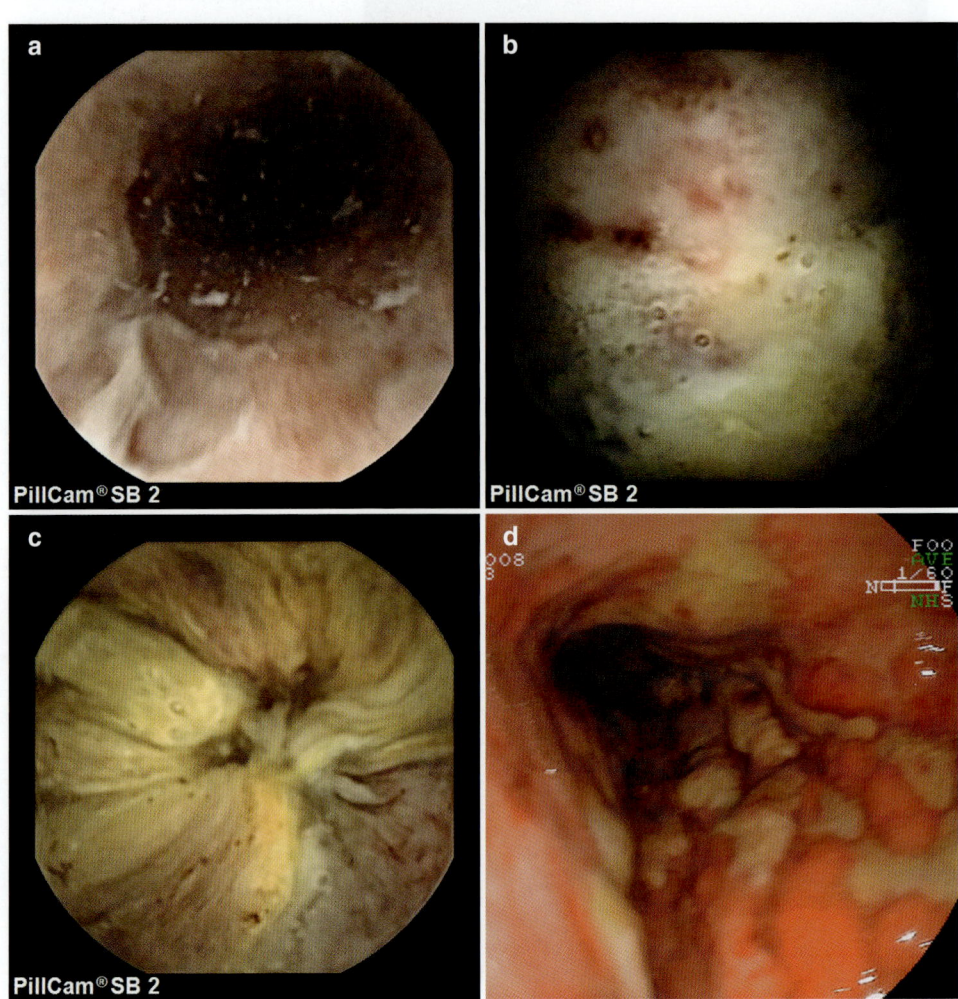

Fig. 28.11 Severe ulceration of the entire stomach in an AIDS patient with dysphagia. (**a**) Reflux esophagitis. Ulcerated stomach in VCE (**b**, **c**) and in gastroscopy (**d**). Histology was nonspecific

Fig. 28.12 PillCam COLON capsule for anemia in a patient positive with HIV and CMV serology shows monilial esophagitis (**a**), as well as erosions (*arrows*) (**b**, **c**), and lymphoid hyperplasia (**d**) of the small bowel

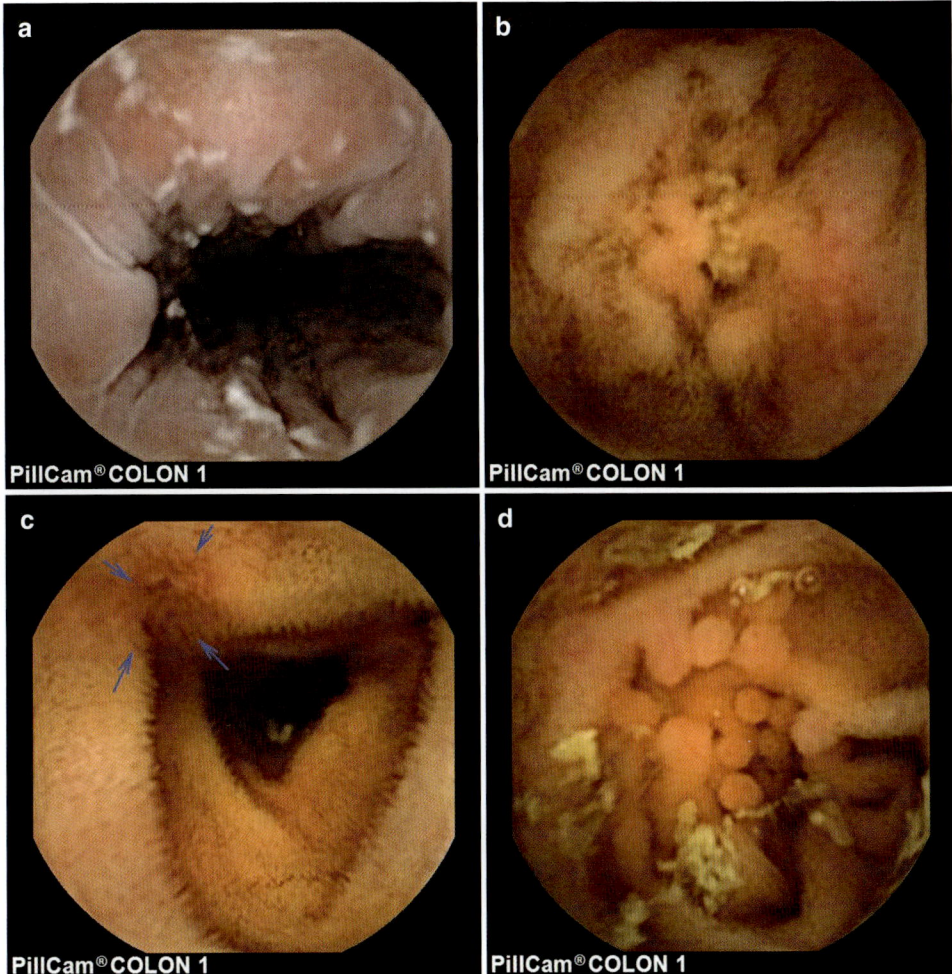

28.8 Blastomycosis

28.8.1 Etiology

South American blastomycosis is a fungal infection caused by *Paracoccidioides brasiliensis*.

28.8.2 Clinical Features

Besides sometimes mutilating cutaneous forms, visceral manifestations can affect multiple organs, including the lung, brain, and others, including the small intestine in rare cases [46]. Immunosuppression or diabetes frequently accompanies blastomycosis [47].

28.8.3 Diagnosis

Fungal cultures and antibody tests can be used for diagnosis. A characteristic feature at histology is the steering wheel-like appearance of the pathogen (Fig. 28.13).

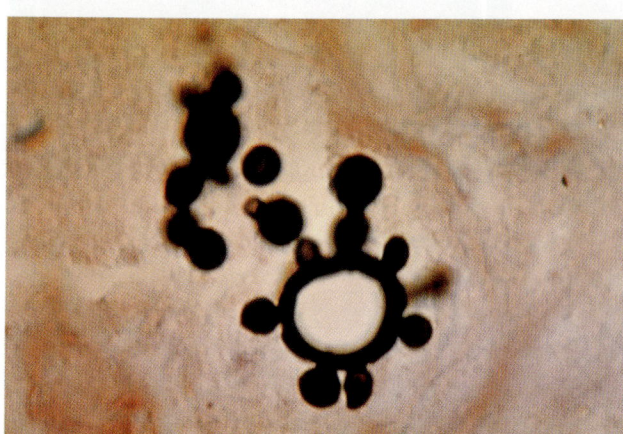

Fig. 28.13 Histopathology of *Paracoccidioidomycosis brasiliensis*. Methenamine silver stain (Courtesy of Dr. Lucille K. Georg, Centers for Disease Control and Prevention, Atlanta, GA, USA)

28.8.4 Endoscopy

Lesions may be nodular, ulcerous, or stenotic [48]. Besides nodules and ulcers, lymphangiectasia also can be seen at endoscopy [34] (Fig. 28.14).

28.8.5 Treatment

Systemic amphotericin B has been widely used for treatment.

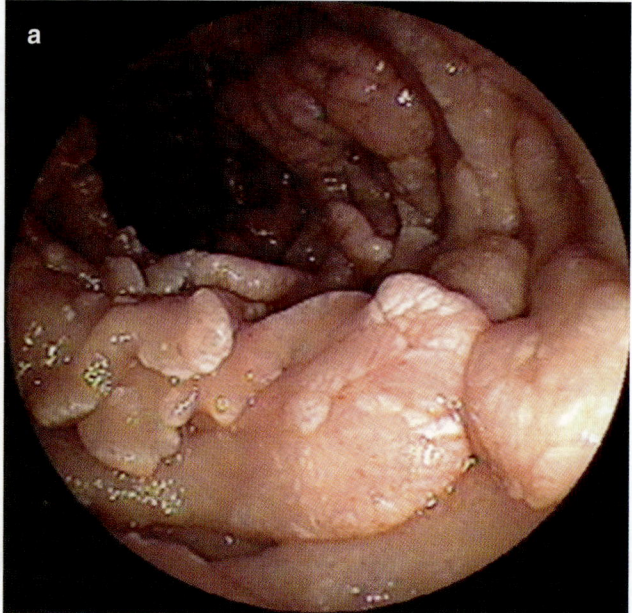

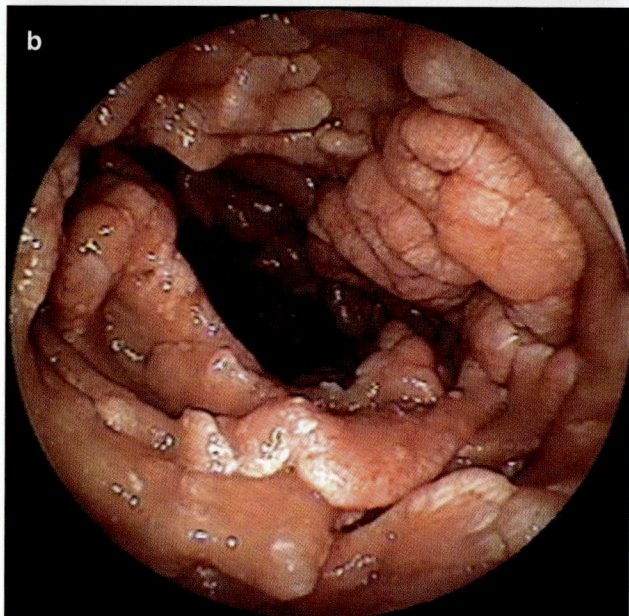

Fig. 28.14 (**a**, **b**) Small intestinal blastomycosis with diffuse, nodular, and patchy mucosal swelling and white villi seen at double-balloon enteroscopy

28.9 Giardiasis

Giardiasis is caused by the protozoon *Giardia lamblia*, which is present worldwide in varying frequency, with a higher prevalence in the tropics. *G. lamblia* preferably affects the upper gastrointestinal tract.

28.9.1 Clinical Features

The typical manifestation is diarrhea, in some cases causing severe illness. Most infected persons are asymptomatic or have only minor, nonspecific symptoms, but the course is sometimes prolonged [49]. The infection may be self-limiting. Imidazole derivates are effective in treatment [50].

28.9.2 Diagnosis

The first-line diagnostic test is stool examination. The diagnostic yield of an enzyme-linked immunoassay is superior to the previously used microscopic evaluation.

28.9.3 Endoscopy

Endoscopy is usually normal in giardiasis. Rarely, lymphoid hyperplasia of the entire small intestine (Fig. 28.15) or villous atrophy may be visible, for example, in patients with immunoglobulin A deficiency [51]. At endoscopy, it is possible to obtain duodenal aspirate for immediate microscopic examination, but histology from duodenal biopsy is preferable to duodenal aspirate. Histology usually demonstrates normal intestinal architecture with trophozoites adhering to the mucosa (Fig. 28.16).

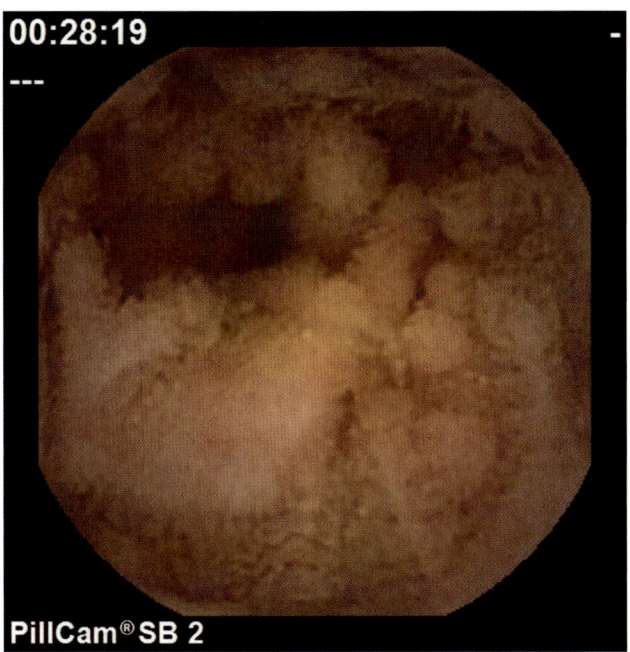

Fig. 28.15 Giardiasis. Lymphofollicular hyperplasia throughout the entire small intestine in a young patient with Giardiasis and underlying common variable immunodeficiency disease (CVID, Courtesy of Jörg Albert, MD)

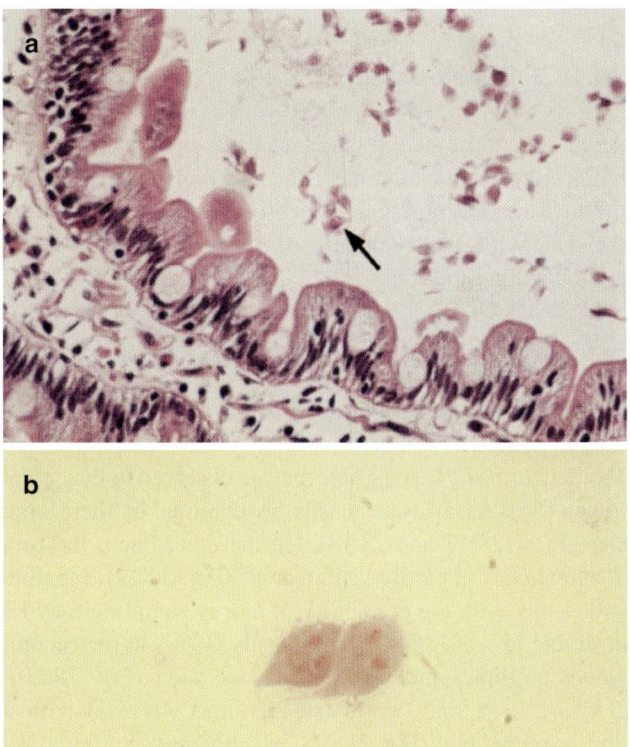

Fig. 28.16 Giardiasis. (**a**) Duodenal biopsy shows trophozoites in the overlying mucus. (**b**) Trophozoites at higher magnification

28.10 Helminthiases

28.10.1 Epidemiology

Helminth infections are more prevalent in the tropics and subtropics, so it is more common to find parasitic worms during capsule endoscopy in those regions [52]. Human pathogenic helminthes can be divided into nematodes (roundworms), cestodes (tapeworms), and trematodes (flukes). Nematodes are found most frequently in the small bowel lumen. *Ascaris lumbricoides*, the largest of these, may be up to 30 cm long. Smaller nematodes are the whipworm *Trichuris trichiura*, the pinworm *Enterobius vermicularis*, and the hookworms *Ancylostoma duodenale* and *Necator americanus* (up to 12 mm) and *Strongyloides stercoralis* (2 mm). For *Necator americanus*, occurrence of eosinophilic enteropathy has been observed by capsule endoscopy [53]. Tapeworms (*Taenia solium, Taenia saginata*, or *Diphyllobothrium latum/nihonkaiense*) may reach a length of up to several meters in the small intestine, causing malnutrition, vitamin deficiency, obstruction, and even intestinal bleeding [54, 55].

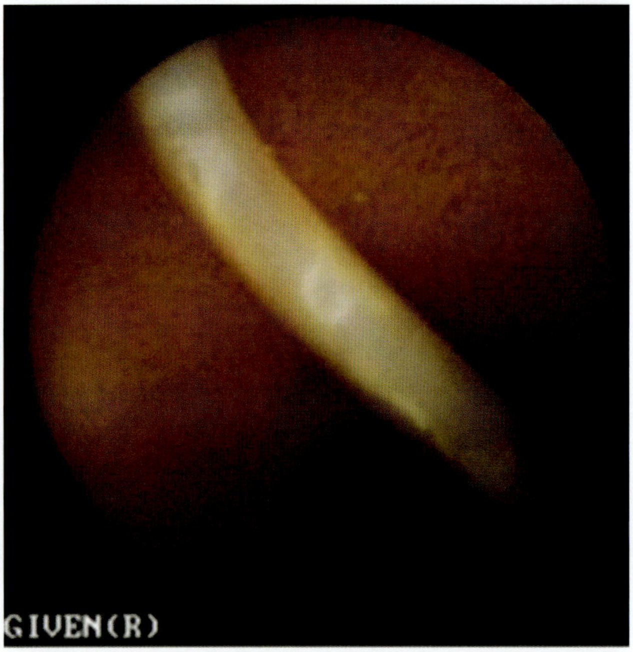

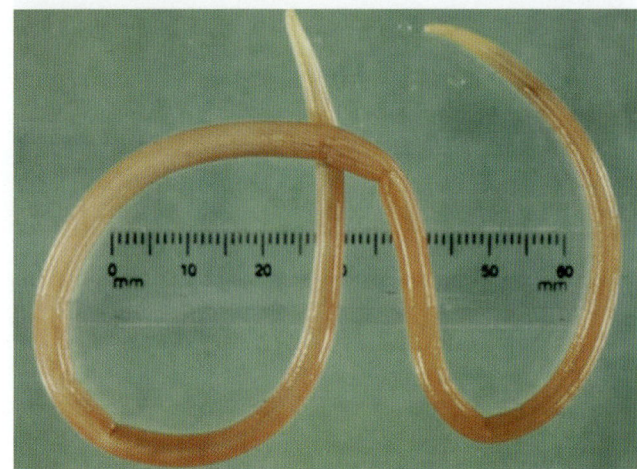

Fig. 28.17 *Ascaris* as seen on VCE

28.10.2 Development

Adult nematodes live in the human intestine, and therefore humans are the definitive host. The infection may be acquired through the oral ingestion of eggs or by larvae penetrating the skin. With strongyloidiasis or *E. vermicularis* infection, autoinfection can occur.

28.10.3 Endoscopy

Motile worms of varying size may be observed in the bowel lumen [56]. Ascarids can easily be identified by their large size (Figs. 28.17 and 28.18). On the other hand, the tiny *Strongyloides* is hardly visible at all (Fig. 28.19). Flexible endoscopy with the possibility of biopsy sampling may be desirable [57–59]. *Enterobius* usually occurs in the cecum, where multiple small worms may be seen (Fig. 28.20). *Trichuris* is a long worm (smaller than *Ascaris*) with a thin proximal end (Fig. 28.21), which is not seen in hookworms (Figs. 28.22 and 28.23). The largest helminths are tapeworms, consisting of multiple proglottides and reaching a length of several meters (Figs. 28.24 and 28.25) [60]. Visualization of adult worms at endoscopy or in stool, some-

Fig. 28.18 Adult *Ascaris*

times combined with microscopic detection of worm eggs, enables a correct classification of the parasites. Serology is rather insensitive because of frequent cross-reactions.

The outer cuticle of the parasites remains intact even after the worms have been killed. Wormlike structures with irregular outlines in the small bowel are usually food residues.

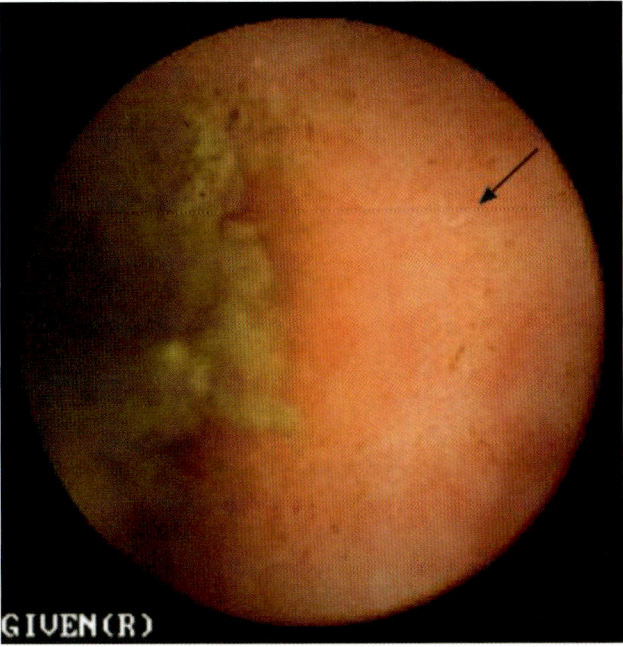

Fig. 28.19 *Strongyloides* (*arrow*). This small worm is hardly visible on the still image. (Courtesy of Annette Stelzer, MD)

Fig. 28.20 (**a**) Colonoscopy shows pinworms (*Enterobius vermicularis*) in the cecum of a man with chronic anal fissures. (**b**) Incidental finding of pinworms in the cecum by PillCam COLON 2, which was used to complement an incomplete colonoscopy. Additionally, a polyp in the right colon was detected. (Courtesy of Michael Philipper, MD)

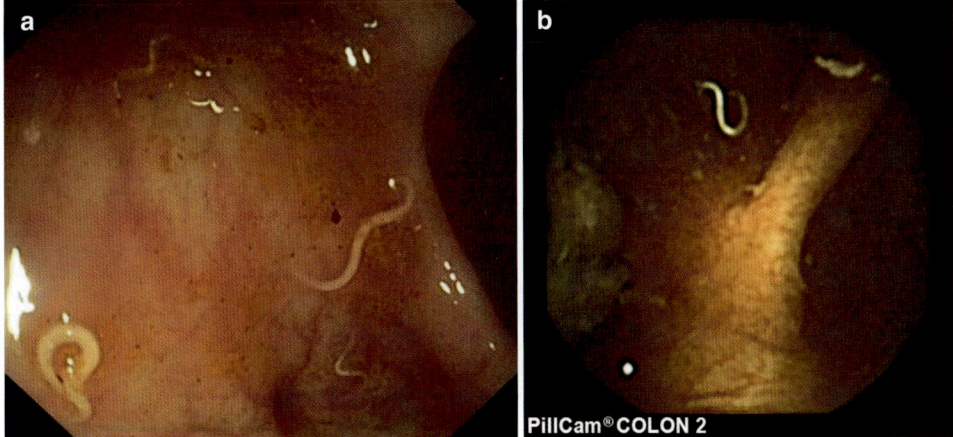

Fig. 28.21 Whipworm. (**a**) Image from VCE in the small intestine (Courtesy of Bruno Neu, MD.) (**b**) Adult whipworm

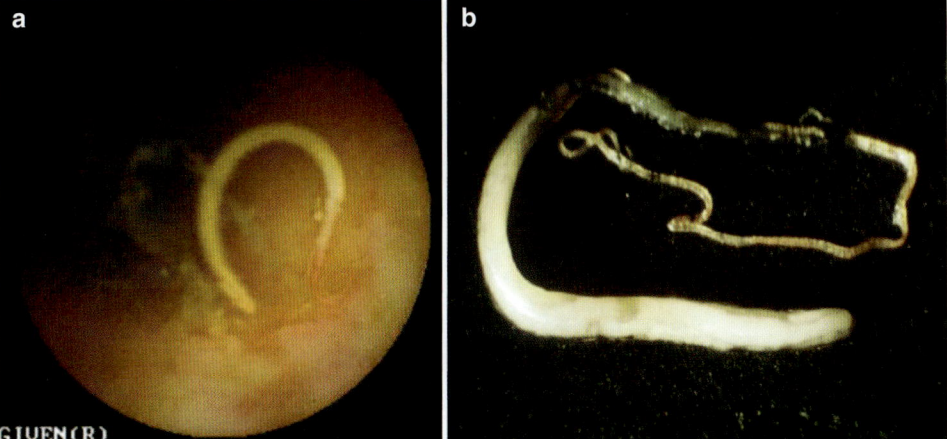

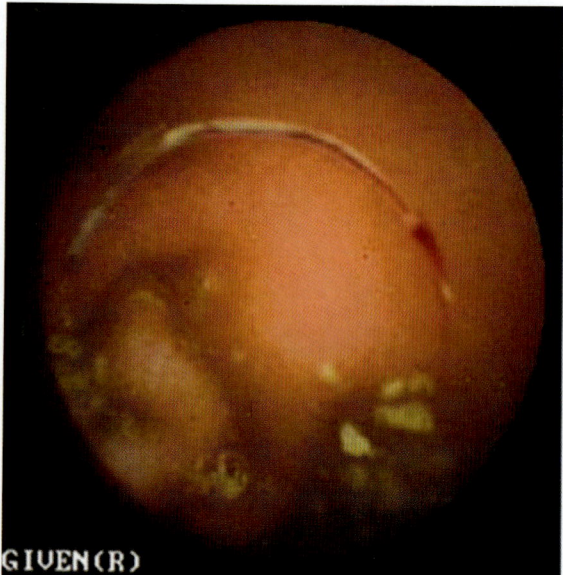

Fig. 28.22 Worm in the small intestine, most likely hookworm

Fig. 28.23 (**a**, **b**) Hookworms penetrating the small bowel mucosa with visible blood loss in a patient with anemia (Courtesy of Selva Mony, BSC, RN, and Tariq Iqbal, MD)

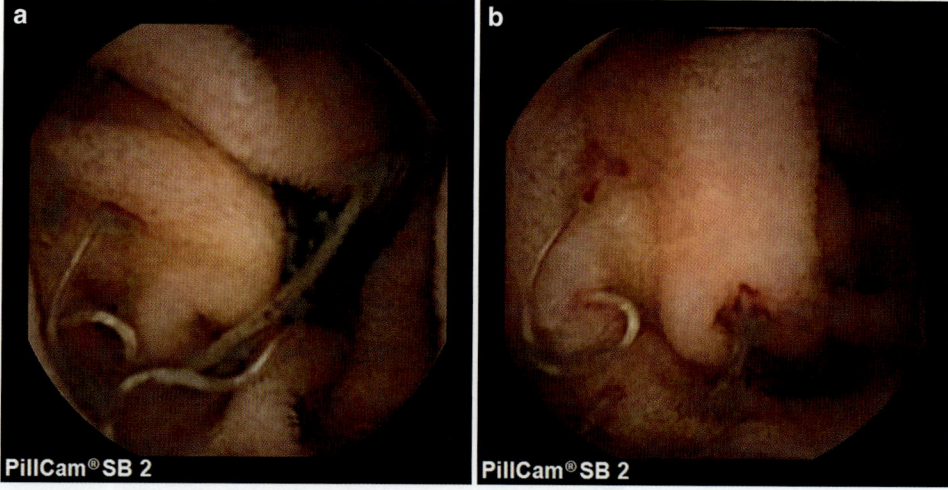

Fig. 28.24 *Taenia*. (**a**) The proglottides are clearly visible. (**b**) The head is visible (*arrow*) (Courtesy of Ingo Steinbrück, MD)

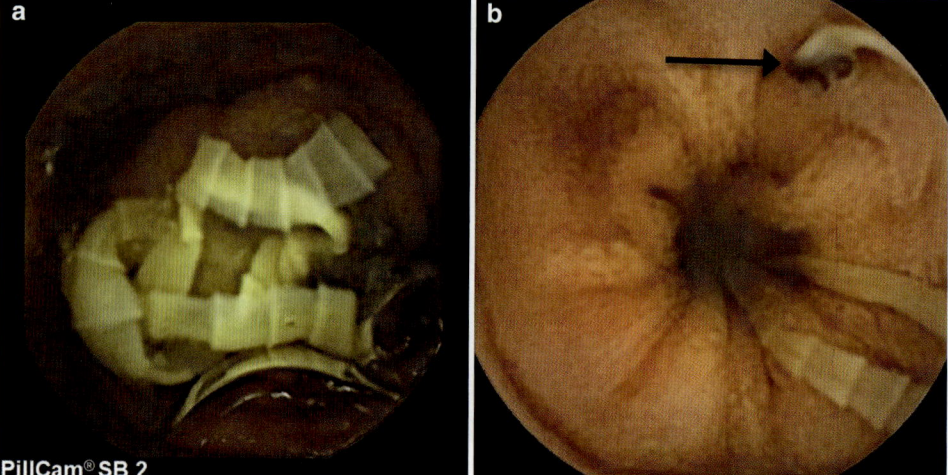

Fig. 28.25 (**a**, **b**) *Taenia*. Lumen-filling proglottides (Courtesy of Wolfgang Fortelny, MD)

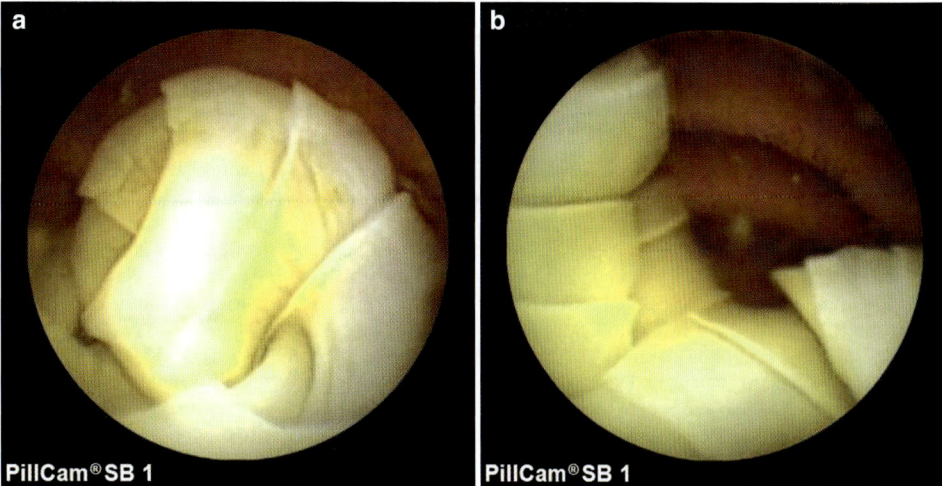

References

1. Bentley SD, Maiwald M, Murphy LD, et al. Sequencing and analysis of the genome of the Whipple's disease bacterium Tropheryma whipplei. Lancet. 2003;361:637–44.
2. Schneider T, Moos V, Loddenkemper C, et al. Whipple's disease: new aspects of pathogenesis and treatment. Lancet Infect Dis. 2008;8:179–90.
3. Kolfenbach S, Monkemuller K, Rocken C, Malfertheiner P. Whipple's disease: magnification endoscopy and histological characteristics. Endoscopy. 2008;40 Suppl 2:E112.
4. Fritscher-Ravens A, Swain CP, von Herbay A. Refractory Whipple's disease with anaemia: first lessons from capsule endoscopy. Endoscopy. 2004;36:659–62.
5. Gay G, Roche JF, Delvaux M. Capsule endoscopy, transit times, and Whipple's disease. Endoscopy. 2005;37:272–3.
6. Keane MG, Shariff M, Stocks J, et al. Imaging of the small bowel by capsule endoscopy in Whipple's disease. Endoscopy. 2009;41 Suppl 2:E139.
7. Mateescu BR, Bengus A, Marinescu M, et al. First Pillcam Colon 2 capsule images of Whipple's disease: case report and review of the literature. World J Gastrointest Endosc. 2012;4:575–8.
8. Bhat M, Laneuville P, Marliss EB, et al. Secondary intestinal lymphangiectasia due to multiple myeloma. Gastrointest Endosc. 2011;74:718–20.
9. Ratnaike RN. Whipple's disease. Postgrad Med J. 2000;76:760–6.
10. Dzirlo L, Blaha B, Muller C, et al. Capsule endoscopic appearance of the small-intestinal mucosa in Whipple's disease and the changes that occur during antibiotic therapy. Endoscopy. 2007;39 Suppl 1:E207–8.
11. Lagier JC, Fenollar F, Lepidi H, Raoult D. Failure and relapse after treatment with trimethoprim/sulfamethoxazole in classic Whipple's disease. J Antimicrob Chemother. 2010;65:2005–12.
12. Pantongrag-Brown L, Nelson AM, Brown AE, et al. Gastrointestinal manifestations of acquired immunodeficiency syndrome: radiologic-pathologic correlation. Radiographics. 1995;15:1155–78.
13. Aldeman NL, Guimaraes LM, Cabral MM. Atypical duodenal mycobacteriosis in a patient with AIDS. Braz J Infect Dis. 2012;16:209–10.
14. Escapa VM, Beltran VP, Viudez LA, et al. Intestinal involvement by Micobacterium genavense in an immunodepressed patient. Gastrointest Endosc. 2010;72:1108–10.
15. Collado C, Stirnemann J, Ganne N, et al. Gastrointestinal tuberculosis: 17 cases collected in 4 hospitals in the northeastern suburb of Paris. Gastroenterol Clin Biol. 2005;29:419–24.
16. Radzi M, Rihan N, Vijayalakshmi N, Pani SP. Diagnostic challenge of gastrointestinal tuberculosis: a report of 34 cases and an overview of the literature. Southeast Asian J Trop Med Public Health. 2009;40:505–10.
17. Cordova J, Shiloh R, Gilman RH, et al. Evaluation of molecular tools for detection and drug susceptibility testing of Mycobacterium tuberculosis in stool specimens from patients with pulmonary tuberculosis. J Clin Microbiol. 2010;48:1820–6.
18. Loureiro AI, Pinto CS, Oliveira AI, et al. Ulcerated lesion of the cecum as a form of presentation of gastrointestinal tuberculosis. [Article in Portuguese]. Acta Med Port. 2011;24:371–4.
19. Kim ES, Keum B, Jeen YT, Chun HJ. Isolated small bowel tuberculosis with stricture diagnosed by capsule endoscopy. Dig Liver Dis. 2012;44:84.
20. Lee CW, Chang WH, Shih SC, et al. Gastrointestinal tract pseudo-obstruction or obstruction due to Mycobacterium tuberculosis breakthrough. Int J Infect Dis. 2009;13:e185–7.
21. Pulimood AB, Amarapurkar DN, Ghoshal U, et al. Differentiation of Crohn's disease from intestinal tuberculosis in India in 2010. World J Gastroenterol. 2011;17:433–43.
22. Ramchandani M, Reddy DN, Gupta R, et al. Diagnostic yield and therapeutic impact of single-balloon enteroscopy: series of 106 cases. J Gastroenterol Hepatol. 2009;24:1631–8.
23. Reddy DN, Sriram PV, Rao GV, Reddy DB. Capsule endoscopy appearances of small-bowel tuberculosis. Endoscopy. 2003;35:99.
24. Chang DK, Kim JJ, Choi H, et al. Double balloon endoscopy in small intestinal Crohn's disease and other inflammatory diseases such as cryptogenic multifocal ulcerous stenosing enteritis (CMUSE). Gastrointest Endosc. 2007;66:S96–8.
25. Matsumoto T, Kudo T, Esaki M, et al. Prevalence of non-steroidal anti-inflammatory drug-induced enteropathy determined by double-balloon endoscopy: a Japanese multicenter study. Scand J Gastroenterol. 2008;43:490–6.
26. Park SH, Yang SK, Yang DH, et al. Prospective randomized trial of six-month versus nine-month therapy for intestinal tuberculosis. Antimicrob Agents Chemother. 2009;53:4167–71.
27. Tsinganou E, Gebbers JO. Human intestinal spirochetosis–a review. Ger Med Sci. 2010;8:Doc01. doi:10.3205/000090.
28. Lozano C, Arellano L, Yaquich P. Human intestinal spirochetosis: clinical series and literature review. [Article in Spanish]. Rev Chilena Infectol. 2012;29:449–52.
29. Koulaouzidis A, Campbell S, Ahmed S, et al. Colonic spirochetosis associated with dermatomyositis. Endoscopy. 2007;39 Suppl 1:E30–1.

30. Al-Saleem T, Al-Mondhiry H. Immunoproliferative small intestinal disease (IPSID): a model for mature B-cell neoplasms. Blood. 2005;105:2274–80.

31. Mesnard B, De VB, Maunoury V, Lecuit M. Immunoproliferative small intestinal disease associated with Campylobacter jejuni. Dig Liver Dis. 2012;44:799–800.

32. Mönkemüller K, Safatle-Ribeiro AV, Olano C, Fry LC. Unusual findings in the small bowel. VJGIEN. 2013;1:286–8. doi.10.1016/S2212-0971(13)70125-0.

33. Ersoy O, Akin E, Demirezer A, Atalay R, Buyukasik S. Capsule-endoscopic findings in immunoproliferative small-intestinal disease. Endoscopy. 2012;44(Suppl 2 UCTN):E61–2.

34. Safatle-Ribeiro AV, Iriya K, Couto DS, et al. Secondary lymphangiectasia of the small bowel: utility of double balloon enteroscopy for diagnosis and management. Dig Dis. 2008;26:383–6.

35. Cha JM, Lee JI, Choe JW, et al. Cytomegalovirus enteritis causing ileal perforation in an elderly immunocompetent individual. Yonsei Med J. 2010;51:279–83.

36. Kalaitzis J, Basioukas P, Karzi E, et al. Small-bowel necrosis complicating a cytomegalovirus-induced superior mesenteric vein thrombosis in an immunocompetent patient: a case report. J Med Case Rep. 2012;6:118.

37. Papadimitriou G, Koukoulaki M, Vardas K, et al. Small bowel obstruction caused by inflammatory cytomegalovirus tumor in a renal transplant recipient: report of a rare case and review of the literature. Transplant Infect Dis. 2012;14:E111–5.

38. Sakai E, Endo H, Tokoro C, et al. Cytomegalovirus-induced small-bowel bleeding detected by capsule endoscopy. Gastrointest Endosc. 2011;73:1058–60.

39. Kakugawa Y, Kim SW, Takizawa K, et al. Small intestinal CMV disease detected by capsule endoscopy after allogeneic hematopoietic SCT. Bone Marrow Transplant. 2008;42:283–4.

40. Jha AK, Uppal B, Chadha S, et al. Clinical and microbiological profile of HIV/AIDS cases with diarrhea in North India. J Pathog. 2012;2012:971958.

41. Nawabi DH, Ffolkes L, O'Bichere A. Cryptococcal small-bowel obstruction in an HIV-positive patient. J R Soc Med. 2005;98:513–4.

42. Tzimas D, Wan D. Small bowel perforation in a patient with AIDS. Diagnosis: small bowel infection with Cryptococcus neoformans. Gastroenterology. 2011;140:1882. 2150.

43. Marco-Lattur MD, Payeras A, Campins AA, et al. Intestinal lymphangiectasia: an undescribed cause of malabsorption and incomplete immunological recovery in HIV-infected patients. Enferm Infecc Microbiol Clin. 2011;29:117–20.

44. Cello JP, Day LW. Idiopathic AIDS enteropathy and treatment of gastrointestinal opportunistic pathogens. Gastroenterology. 2009;136:1952–65.

45. Venkataramani A, Behling CA, Lyche KD. Sclerosing mesenteritis: an unusual cause of abdominal pain in an HIV-positive patient. Am J Gastroenterol. 1997;92:1059–60.

46. Fonseca LC, Mignone C. Paracoccidioidomycosis of the small intestine. Radiologic and anatomo clinical aspects of 125 cases. Rev Hosp Clin Fac Med Sao Paulo. 1976;31:199–207.

47. Lemos LB, Baliga M, Guo M. Blastomycosis: the great pretender can also be an opportunist. Initial clinical diagnosis and underlying diseases in 123 patients. Ann Diagn Pathol. 2002;6:194–203.

48. Avritchir Y, Perroni AA. Radiological manifestations of small intestinal South American Blastomycosis. Radiology. 1978;127:607–9.

49. Sawatzki M, Peter S, Hess C. Therapy-resistant diarrhea due to Giardia lamblia in a patient with common variable immunodeficiency disease. Digestion. 2007;75:101–2.

50. Rossignol JF. Cryptosporidium and Giardia: treatment options and prospects for new drugs. Exp Parasitol. 2010;124:45–53.

51. Perez-Roldan F, Mate-Valdezate A, Villafanez-Garcia MC, et al. Nodular lymphoid hyperplasia by Giardia lamblia. Endoscopy. 2008;40 Suppl 2:E116–7.

52. Sriram PV, Rao GV, Reddy DN. Wireless capsule endoscopy: experience in a tropical country. J Gastroenterol Hepatol. 2004;19:63–7.

53. Croese J, Speare R. Intestinal allergy expels hookworms: seeing is believing. Trends Parasitol. 2006;22:547–50.

54. De Simone P, Feron P, Loi P, et al. Acute intestinal bleeding due to Taenia solium infection. Chir Ital. 2004;56:151–6.

55. Karanikas ID, Sakellaridis TE, Alexiou CP, et al. Taenia saginata: a rare cause of bowel obstruction. Trans R Soc Trop Med Hyg. 2007;101:527–8.

56. Floro L, Pak G, Sreter L, Tulassay Z. Wireless capsule endoscopy in the diagnosis of helminthiasis. Gastrointest Endosc. 2007;65:1078. discussion 9.

57. Mittal S, Sagi SV, Hawari R. Strongyloidiasis: endoscopic diagnosis. Clin Gastroenterol Hepatol. 2009;7:e8.

58. Somani SK, Goyal R, Awasthi G. Duodenal mucosal nodularity in Strongyloides stercoralis infection. Trop Gastroenterol. 2009;30:47–8.

59. Thompson BF, Fry LC, Wells CD, et al. The spectrum of GI strongyloidiasis: an endoscopic-pathologic study. Gastrointest Endosc. 2004;59:906–10.

60. Hosoe N, Imaeda H, Okamoto S, et al. A case of beef tapeworm (Taenia saginata) infection observed by using video capsule endoscopy and radiography (with videos). Gastrointest Endosc. 2011;74:690–1.

Involvement of the Small Intestine in Systemic Diseases

29

Adriana Safatle-Ribeiro, Gérard Gay, Eberhard Barth, and Martin Keuchel

Contents

Systemic diseases are rare and etiologically diverse. They can affect a variety of organs; involvement of the small bowel occurs with varying degrees of frequency [1]. The assignment of symptoms and findings (including endoscopic findings) to specific disease entities can be a formidable challenge. A diagnosis cannot be made from endoscopic findings alone.

29.1 Amyloidosis

29.1.1 Definition

Amyloidosis is a disorder characterized by the extracellular deposition of an abnormal fibrillar protein, which disrupts tissue structure and function.

29.1.2 Forms

Amyloidosis can be acquired or hereditary and can be systemic or localized to a single organ. Systemic amyloidosis can cause gastrointestinal (GI) complications,

The work was first published in 2006 by Springer Medizin Verlag Heidelberg with the following title: *Atlas of Video Capsule Endoscopy.*

A. Safatle-Ribeiro (✉)
Department of Gastroenterology,
University of Sao Paulo, Sao Paulo, Brazil
e-mail: adrisafatleribeiro@terra.com.br

G. Gay
Department of Gastroenterology and Hepatology,
University Hospital of Strasbourg, Nouvel Hôpital Civil,
Strasbourg, France
e-mail: gerard.gay@chru-strasbourg.fr

E. Barth
Gastroenterology and Rheumatology Practice, Hamburg, Germany
e-mail: e.barth-hamburg@t-online.de

M. Keuchel
Department of Internal Medicine,
Bethesda Krankenhaus Bergedorf,
Hamburg, Germany
e-mail: keuchel@bkb.info

M. Keuchel et al. (eds.), *Video Capsule Endoscopy: A Reference Guide and Atlas*,
DOI 10.1007/978-3-662-44062-9_29, © Springer-Verlag Berlin Heidelberg 2014

but primary diseases of the GI tract also may cause systemic amyloidosis [2]. The most common systemic form is lambda light chain amyloidosis (AL) associated with plasmacytoma. Less common are the kappa light chain form and primary amyloidosis not associated with plasmacytoma. Reactive amyloidosis (AA) caused by serum amyloid A may occur in patients with chronic inflammatory disorders such as Crohn's disease [3], rheumatoid arthritis, and Still's disease or in the setting of hereditary familial Mediterranean fever or chronic bacterial inflammations (e.g., osteomyelitis, tuberculosis, bronchiectasis). There is also a dialysis-associated amyloidosis (Aβ2M) caused by β2-microglobulin and numerous other hereditary forms involving different proteins [4, 5].

29.1.3 Diagnosis

Diagnosing GI amyloidosis requires high suspicion by the endoscopist because mucosal abnormalities are nonspecific. Pseudotumors may be seen [6] (Fig. 29.1). Submucosal hematomas, erosions, and ulcers can cause GI bleeding [7] (Fig. 29.2) or perforation [8]. Patients can have vascular fragility, and biopsies of the submucosal vessels may increase the diagnostic sensitivity by reason of the diffuse vascular involvement. Other manifestations include intestinal pseudo-obstruction [9] and malabsorption [10]. GI symptoms have a negative impact on quality of life and survival in amyloidotic patients. [2, 11–13]. The diagnosis is established by histologic examination (Fig. 29.3).

Fig. 29.1 Lambda light chain amyloidosis (AL), as seen with video capsule endoscopy (VCE) of the jejunum (**a**) and the ileum (**b**, **c**) and with enteroscopy (**d**) (Courtesy of Ingo Steinbrück, MD)

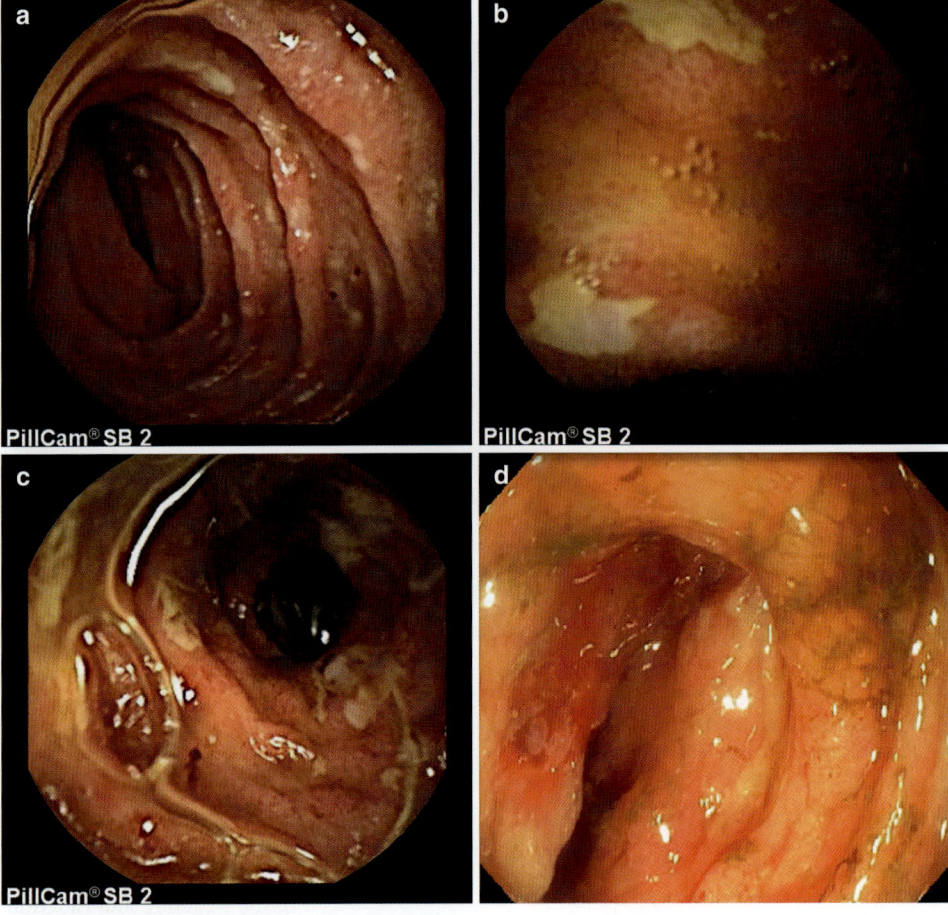

Fig. 29.2 Endoscopic appearance of colonic erosions, circular ulcers (**a**, **d**), and submucosal hematomas (**b**, **c**) in a patient with systemic amyloidosis who presented with hematochezia

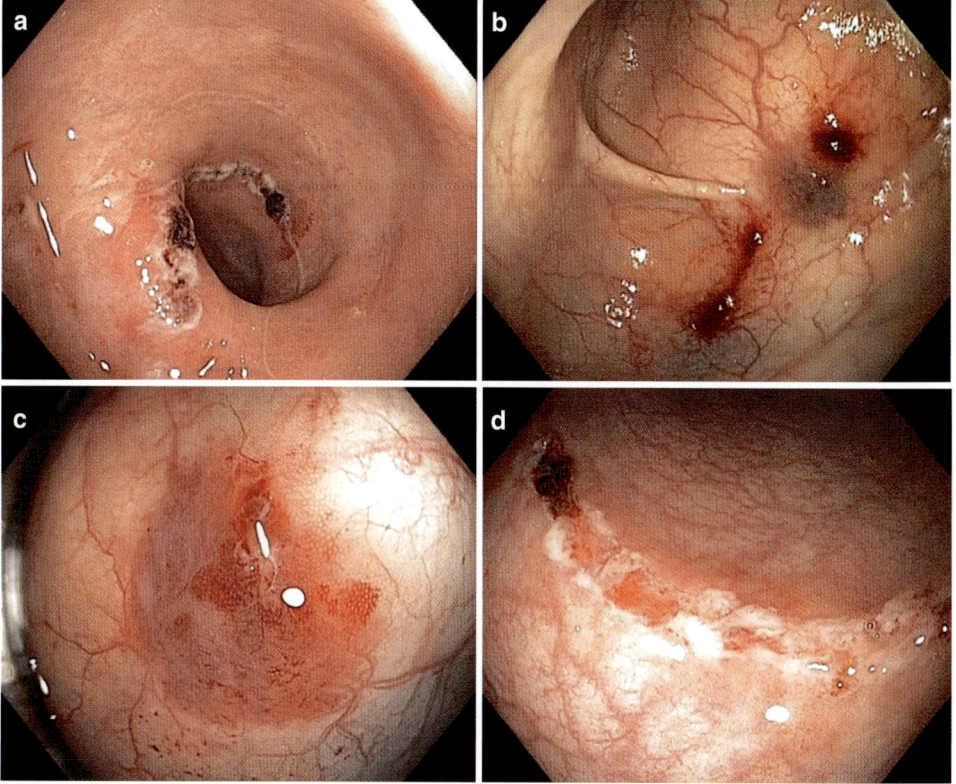

Fig. 29.3 Systemic amyloidosis. (**a**) Multiple bluish-purple masses. (**b**) Some of the masses are ulcerated. (**c**) Diffuse small bowel involvement seen at operation. (**d**) Histology shows massive amyloid infiltration of the small bowel (hematoxylin-eosin [H&E] stain) (Courtesy of Michael Amthor, MD). (**e**) Immunohistology: λ-amyloid (Courtesy of Wolfgang Saeger, MD). (**f**) The patient presented clinically with recurrent intestinal bleeding and involvement of the skin and tongue

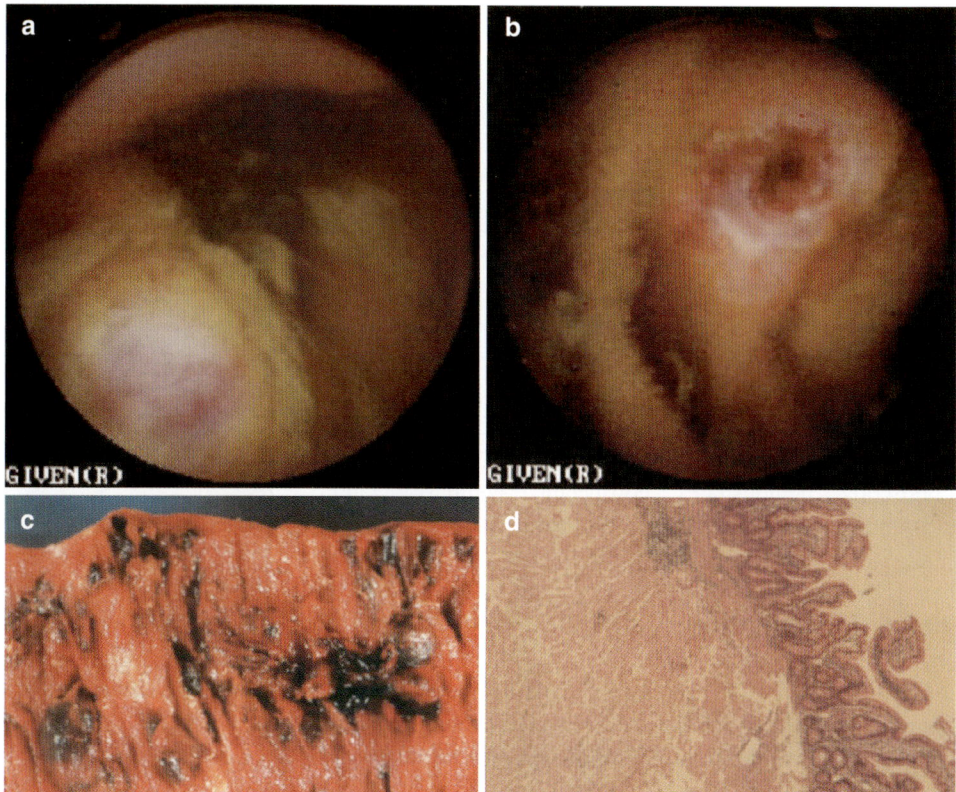

Fig. 29.3 (continued)

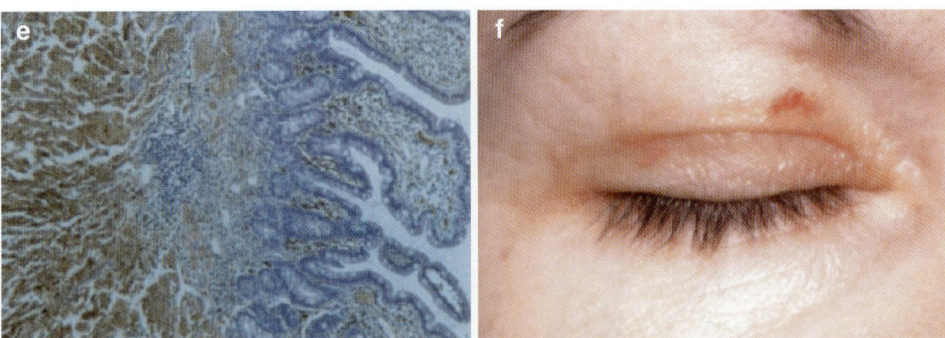

29.2 Sarcoidosis

29.2.1 Etiology

Sarcoidosis is a granulomatous systemic disease of unknown cause.

29.2.2 Clinical Features

The chronic form is frequently asymptomatic. Pulmonary involvement is usually predominant, but the disease may also involve the central nervous system, eyes, myocardium, skin, liver, and kidneys. Small bowel involvement is very rare [14, 15].

29.2.3 Diagnosis

The diagnosis is based on the histologic detection of noncaseating, epithelioid cell granulomas; radiologic evidence of bihilar lymphadenopathy; or bronchoalveolar lavage material with a CD4/CD8 ratio greater than 3.5 in the presence of typical clinical manifestations.

29.2.4 Endoscopy

Endoscopy demonstrates nonspecific nodularity and ulcerations of the bowel mucosa [16] (Fig. 29.4).

29.2.5 Treatment

Steroid therapy may be necessary, depending on the severity of pulmonary lesions and the involvement of extrapulmonary organs. Methotrexate or azathioprine can also be administered to reduce steroid use [17, 18].

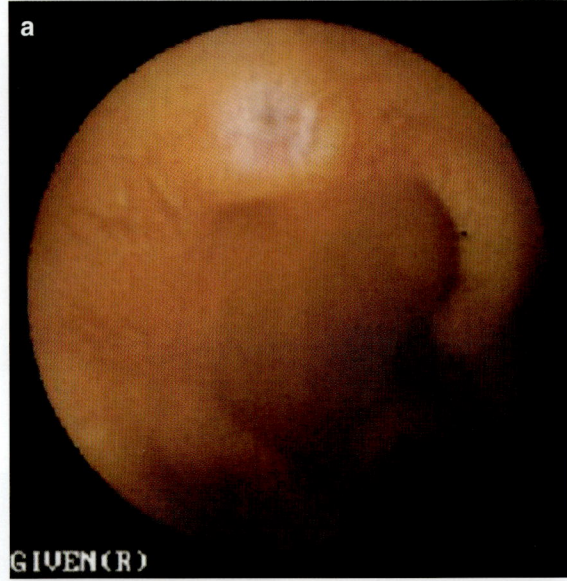

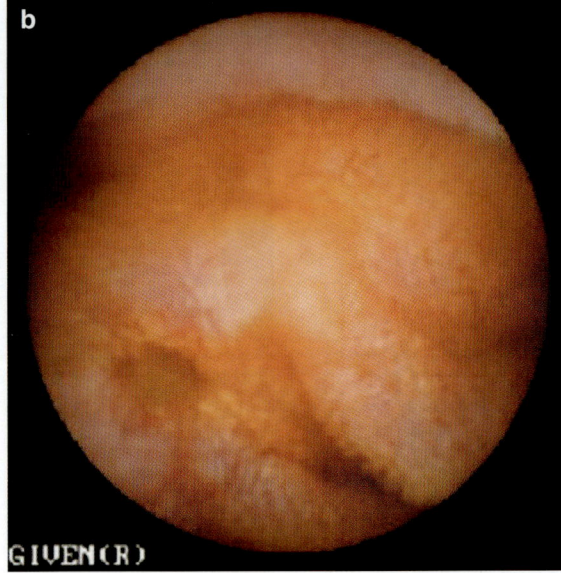

Fig. 29.4 Polypoid mucosal lesion (**a**) and a small ulcer (**b**) in the small bowel mucosa of a woman with confirmed pulmonary sarcoidosis (Courtesy of Ruprecht Botzler, MD)

29.3 Vasculitides

Vasculitides may occur as primary entities or may be secondary to other underlying diseases such as infections, tumors, and collagen diseases or drug side effects. The primary vasculitides were defined by the Chapel Hill Consensus Conference (1994) and were classified mainly according to the size of the affected blood vessels (large, medium-sized, or small vessels). Besides clinical and pathological criteria, immunologic findings are also taken into account, such as an association with antineutrophil cytoplasmic antibodies (ANCA) in "pauci-immune" vasculitides (no immune complex deposition by histology) or immune complex vasculitides with complement consumption [19].

In 2012, another International Chapel Hill Consensus Conference convened to develop nomenclature and definitions [20]. In simplified terms, the end-organ damage corresponds to the affected type of vessel and ranges from stenosis with hypoxemia and edema to organ infarction or vessel wall destruction with hemorrhage. Radiologic findings have a great overlap between the different types of affected vessels [21]. Vasculitic diseases in which intestinal involvement is relatively common include the following disease entities [22].

29.3.1 IgA Vasculitis (IgAV, Henoch-Schönlein)

IgA vasculitis (Henoch-Schönlein purpura) is an immune complex vasculitis with IgA1-dominant immune deposits and involvement of the skin, kidneys, GI tract, joints, and rarely the lung. It is characterized by a palpable purpura, abdominal pain, and the biopsy detection of leukocytoclastic vasculitis by granulocytic infiltrates in the walls of small blood vessels (arterioles and venules). Intestinal involvement occurs in a high percentage of patients [23, 24]. Endoscopic findings include edema, erythema, ulceration, and bleeding (Figs. 29.5, 29.6, and 29.7) [25, 26]. Abdominal pain and bloody diarrhea are occasionally the dominant complaints in oligosymptomatic forms and precede renal involvement and purpura. According to the EULAR (European League Against Rheumatism) criteria [27], diagnosis of Henoch-Schönlein purpura can be made from the presence of petechiae with lower limb predominance (Figs. 29.5a and 29.7c) along with three of the following four criteria: abdominal pain, histopathology (IgA, Fig. 29.5b, c), arthritis or arthralgia, and renal involvement (Fig. 29.6e, f).

IgAV occurs predominantly in children. Oligosymptomatic forms are more common in adults and can cause problems of differential diagnosis.

29.3.2 Eosinophilic Granulomatosis with Polyangiitis (EGPA, Churg-Strauss)

EGPA is a necrotizing vasculitis of small- and medium-sized blood vessels characterized by an eosinophilic granulomatous inflammation often involving the respiratory tract [28]. It is associated clinically with eosinophilia and with a bronchial asthma that often precedes the vasculitis. Particularly serious vasculitic manifestations are myocardial involvement, neuropathies, renal involvement, and alveolitis. Sporadic cases of small bowel ulcers and perforations have been described [29–32].

29.3.3 Behçet's Syndrome

Behçet's syndrome is a recurrent, systemic inflammatory disease predominated by vasculitis of small, medium, and large vessels (arteries and veins). Behçet's disease is associated with the presence of HLA-B51. The clinical picture is characterized by oral and genital mucous ulcers, uveitis, and skin lesions [33]. Thrombotic events and involvement of the central nervous system and GI tract are less frequent but can be life-threatening. About 10–25 % of patients present with involvement of the GI tract, particularly in the distal ileum and cecum, with ulcerations [34] (Figs. 29.8 and 29.9) that may lead to perforation. Inflammatory pseudotumor of the ileum has been described [35]. Behçet's disease is more prevalent in populations along the ancient Silk Road from Eastern Asia to the Mediterranean Basin, and it most commonly affects young adults between the second and fourth decades of life [36–38].

29.3.4 Polyarteritis Nodosa (PAN)

By definition, polyarteritis nodosa (also known as *panarteritis nodosa*) is a necrotizing inflammation of small- and medium-sized arteries. It is classified immunopathologically as an immune complex vasculitis. Researchers have found a serologic association with HBsAg carriers and, increasingly, with antibodies to the hepatitis C virus [39–41]. Conventional angiography demonstrates microaneurysms or vascular occlusions, occurring mainly in the mesenteric territory. Additional features are livedo reticularis, myalgias, painful skin nodules, testicular pain, and renal involvement in the form of a vascular nephropathy. Glomerulonephritis is not part of the clinical picture. The symptoms of intestinal involvement are abdominal pain, nausea, and vomiting. Small bowel involvement is a result of mesenteric ischemia, with lesions ranging from ulceration (Fig. 29.10) to mesenteric infarction and subsequent necrosis [42].

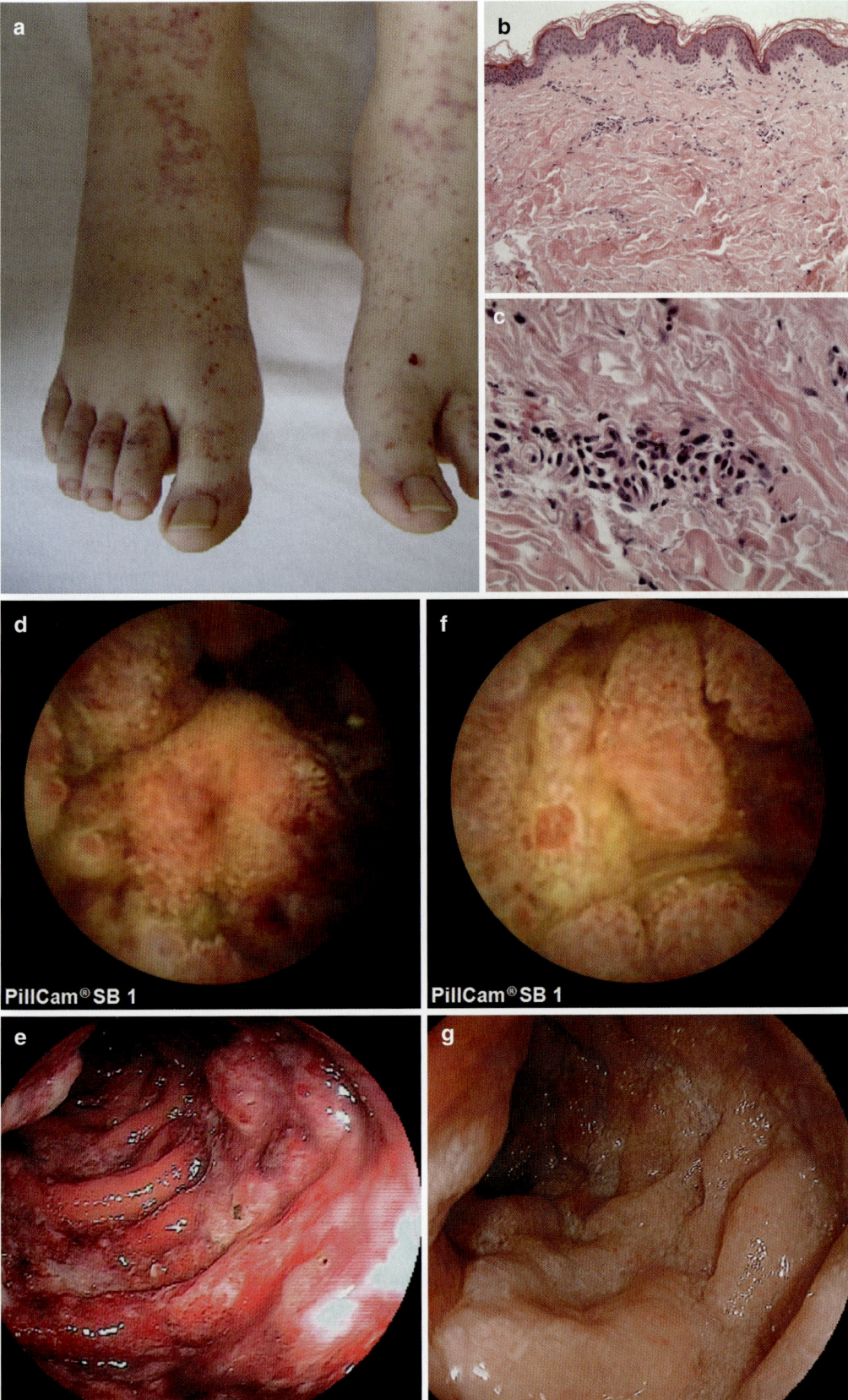

Fig. 29.5 IgA vasculitis (Henoch-Schönlein purpura) in young women with abdominal pain, petechiae, and later proteinuria and renal insufficiency. (**a**) Petechiae, typically with predominance on the lower extremities, are mandatory for diagnosis. (**b, c**) Skin biopsy shows leukocytoclastic vasculitis (Courtesy of Konstanze Holl-Ulrich, MD). (**d**, **e**) Capsule endoscopy reveals large segments of ulcerated, hemorrhagic small bowel. (**f**) Push enteroscopy initially showed severe, diffuse hemorrhagic ulcerations. (**g**) After 1 month, enteroscopy showed partially recovered mucosa with nonspecific edema and partial villous atrophy

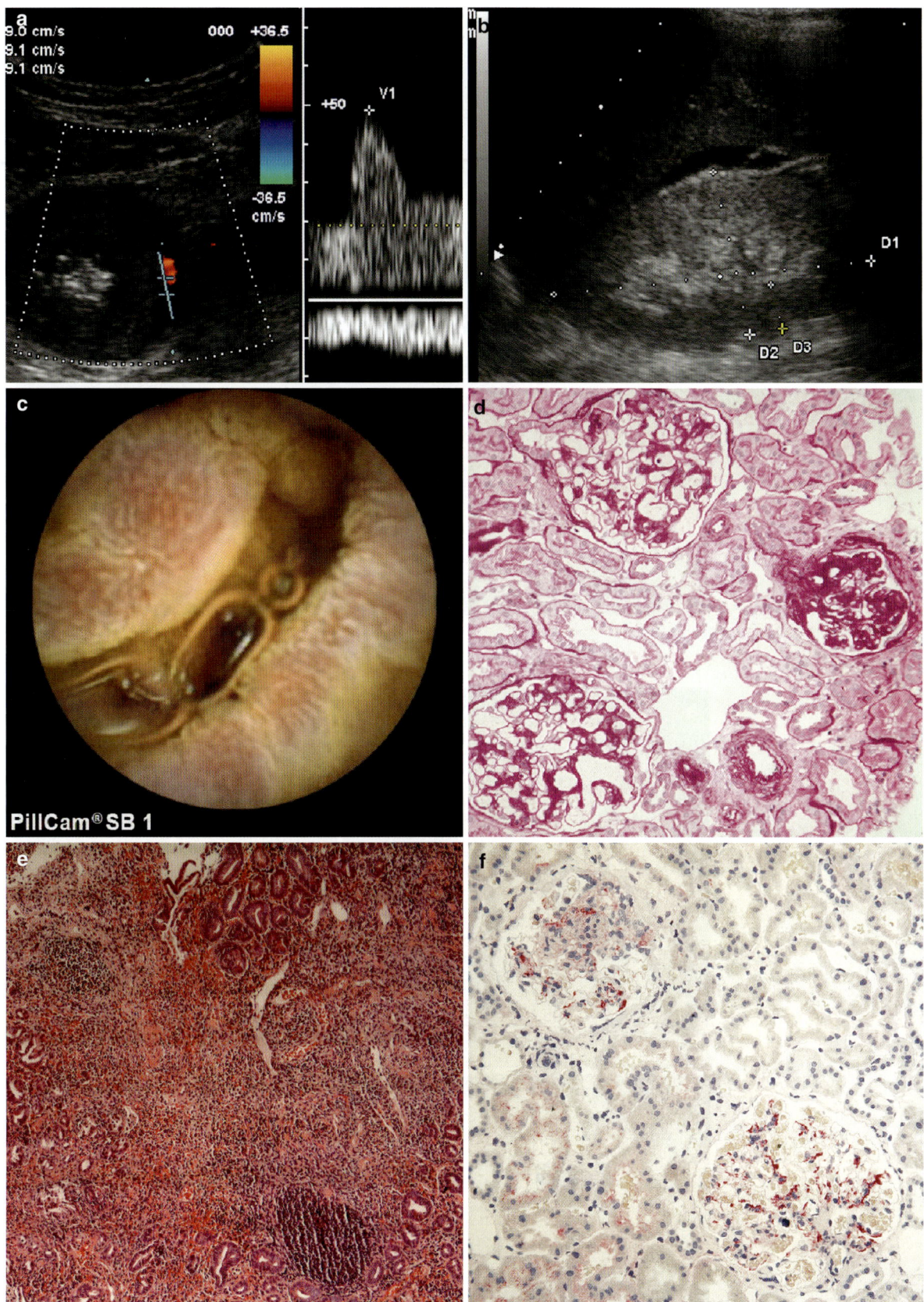

Fig. 29.6 IgA vasculitis in a young man with petechiae, abdominal pain, proteinuria, and prolonged renal insufficiency. (*Left*: **a**) Ultrasound shows thickened, well-perfused jejunum. (**c**) VCE findings in the phase of beginning recovery include edema and erythema. (**e**) Biopsy shows inflammatory infiltration of the small bowel (H&E stain, courtesy of Jörg Caselitz, MD). (*Right*: **b**) Sonographic signs of nephritis (bright kidney parenchyma, ascites). (**d, f**) Kidney biopsy demonstrated mesangioproliferative nephritis with IgA deposits (immunostain) (Courtesy of Udo Helmchen, MD)

Fig. 29.7 IgA vasculitis (Henoch-Schönlein) in an adult. Moderate ulcerative jejunitis, as seen using VCE (**a**) and push enteroscopy (**b**), rapidly improved with steroids. Later, systemic vasculitis developed, with relapse of petechiae (**c**) and renal and cerebral involvement

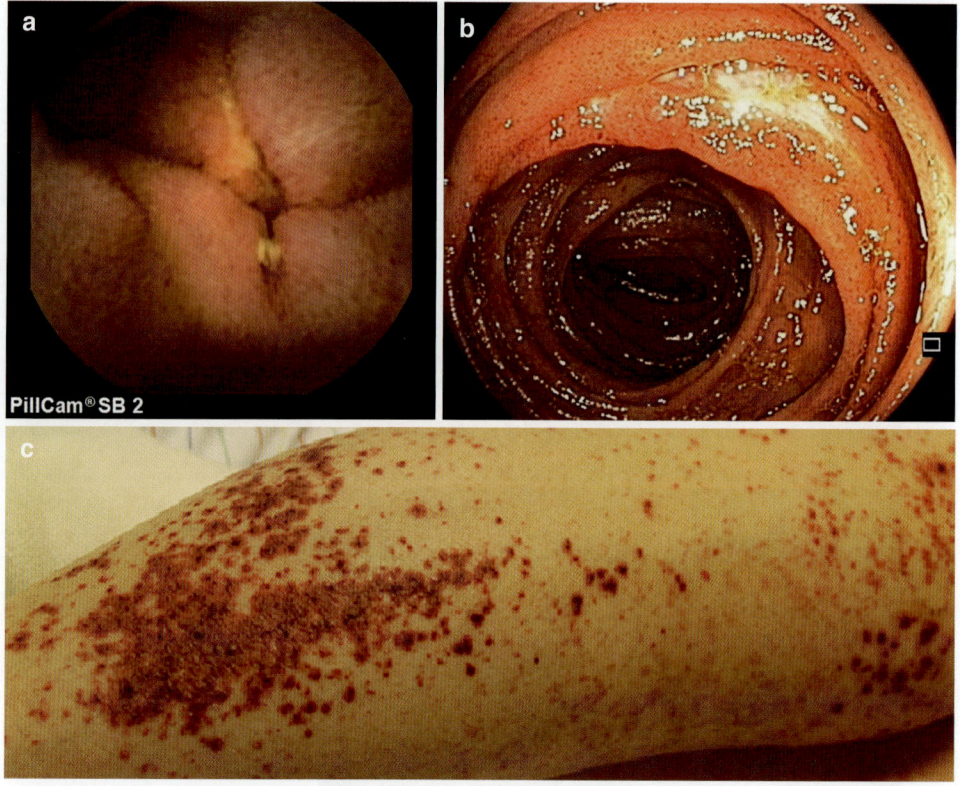

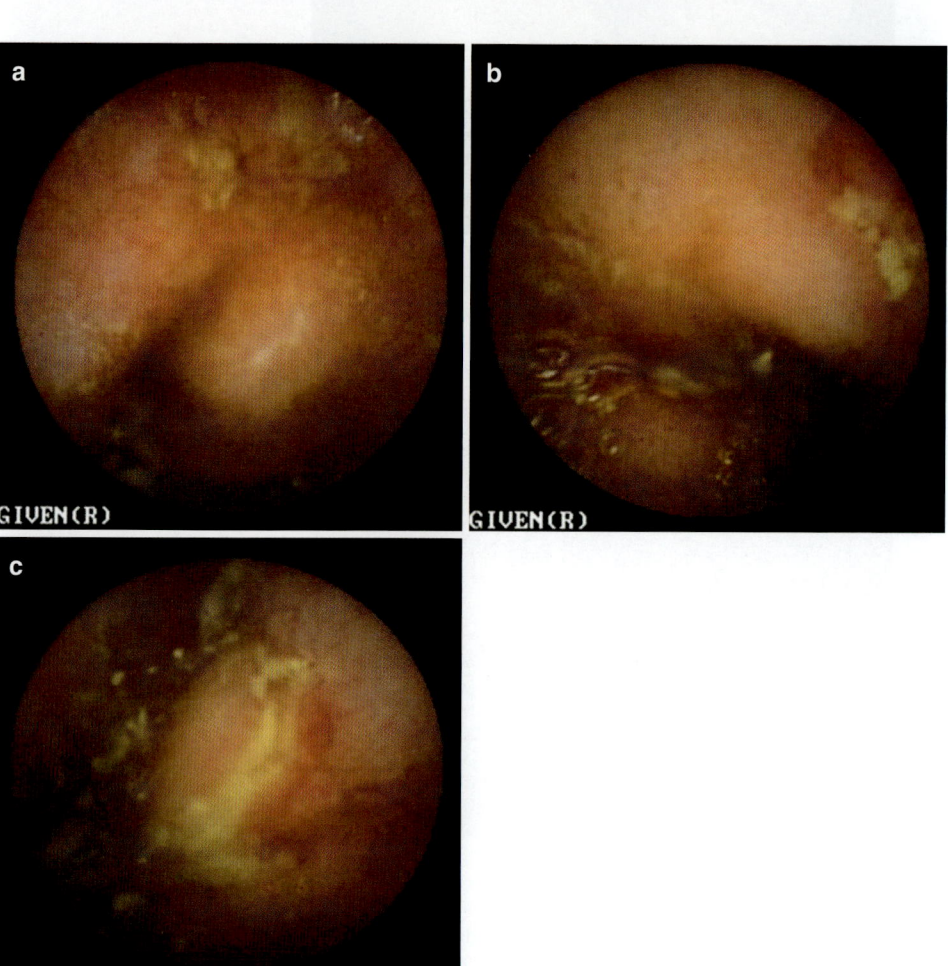

Fig. 29.8 (**a–c**) Capsule endoscopy images demonstrating aphthous ulcers at the ileum in a patient with Behçet's syndrome

Fig. 29.9 (**a–c**) Double-balloon endoscopy images showing ileum ulcers in a patient with Behçet's syndrome

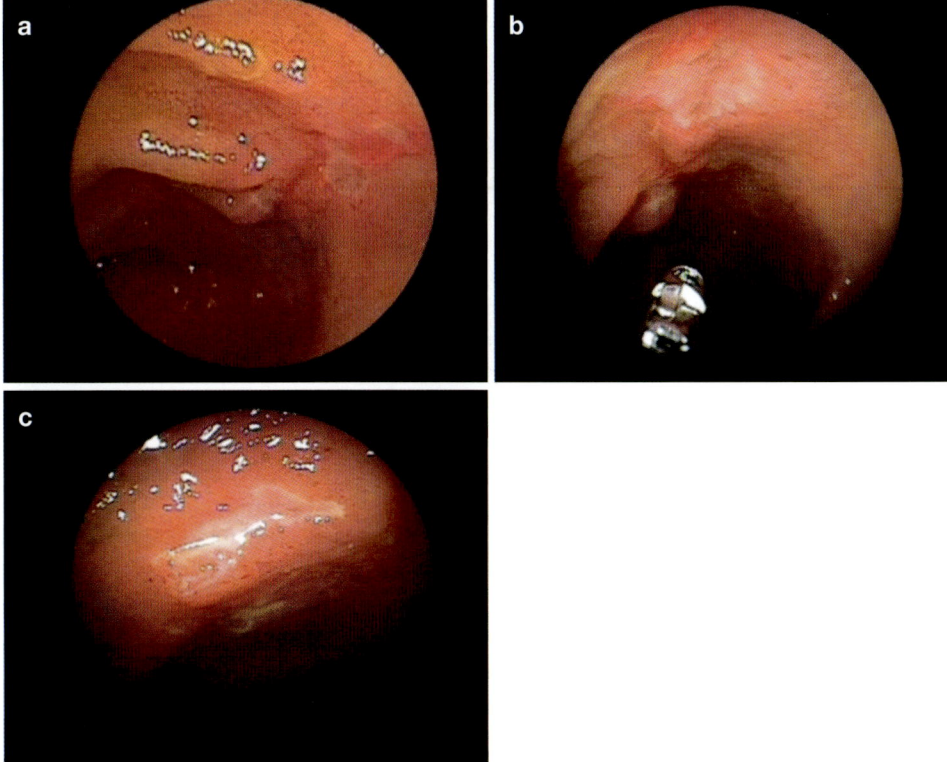

Fig. 29.10 Systemic vasculitis. (**a, b**) Single-balloon enteroscopy shows multiple serpiginous ulcers throughout the small bowel

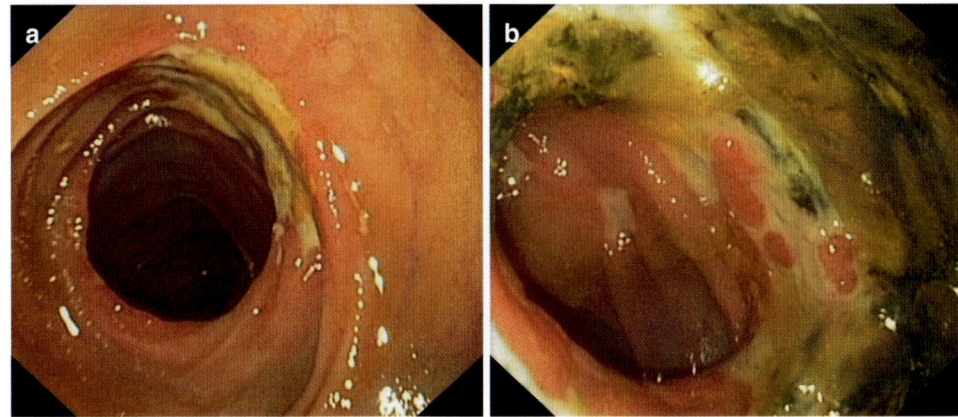

For historical reasons, PAN requires differentiation from microscopic polyangiitis (MPA), a microvascular vasculitis that chiefly affects the lungs and kidneys, causing an alveolitis or glomerulonephritis. MPA is a pauci-immune vasculitis and is associated with the detection of antineutrophil cytoplasmic antibodies (ANCAs) directed against myeloperoxidase. Intestinal involvement is rare, but sporadic cases with associated intestinal bleeding have been reported (Fig. 29.10) [43–45].

29.3.5 Granulomatosis with Polyangiitis (GPA, Wegener's)

GPA is a granulomatous inflammation of the upper respiratory tract that is associated with a necrotizing vasculitis of small blood vessels. All organ systems may be affected during the generalized vasculitic phase, particularly the lung (alveolitis), kidneys, peripheral nervous system, and central nervous system. GPA is another pauci-immune vasculitis and is associated with the serologic presence of an ANCA directed against proteinase 3. Small bowel involvement is rare; it is manifested by bloody stools, mucoid diarrhea, and abdominal pain resulting from ulcers, active vasculitis, and mucosal inflammation [46, 47].

29.3.6 Takayasu's Arteritis

Takayasu's arteritis is a rare systemic disease, presenting as a mostly granulomatous large vessel vasculitis that predominantly affects the aorta and its large branches, leading to stenosis and aneurysms. General symptoms include fatigue, muscle pain, subfebrile temperatures, and weight loss. The perfusion disorder can cause muscle pain, dizziness, and claudication. Abdominal pain, nausea, vomiting, and GI bleeding can also occur (Fig. 29.11). It generally occurs in female patients (80–90 % of the cases) younger than 50 years [48].

29.4 Collagen Diseases

Collagen diseases is a collective term for inflammatory systemic diseases that manifest common features such as the presence of antinuclear antibodies, elevated serum inflammatory markers, and systemic symptoms such as fever, debilitation, and joint pain. These diseases show considerable variation, however, in their dominant symptoms and prognosis. The named collagen diseases are systemic lupus erythematosus (SLE), Sjögren's syndrome, systemic sclerosis, CREST (calcinosis, Raynaud's phenomenon, esophageal dysfunction, sclerodactyly, telangiectasia) syndrome, myositis, and dermatomyositis. Additionally, mixed collagen diseases, undifferentiated collagen diseases, and overlap syndromes are also recognized.

SLE is characterized by aphthous lesions of the mucous membranes in the ENT (ear, nose, and throat) region. Small bowel involvement is generally rare but occurs in the setting of secondary vasculitis, for example. Small bowel involvement may be manifested by aphthae (Figs. 29.12 and 29.13), lymphangiectasia (Fig. 22.5), ulcers [49], perforations [50], or intestinal pseudo-obstruction [51].

Systemic sclerosis leads to intestinal motility disturbances, usually beginning in the esophagus, as a result of progressive sclerosis. Involvement of the arteries of the hands may lead to Raynaud's phenomenon. Small bowel involvement with hypomotility may be manifested by pseudo-obstruction or malabsorption caused by abnormal bacterial colonization [52–55]. Abnormal capillaries with distortion and parallel bundles may be observed in the small intestine. Capillary nail fold microscopy can be used to visualize capillary morphology noninvasively (Fig. 29.14).

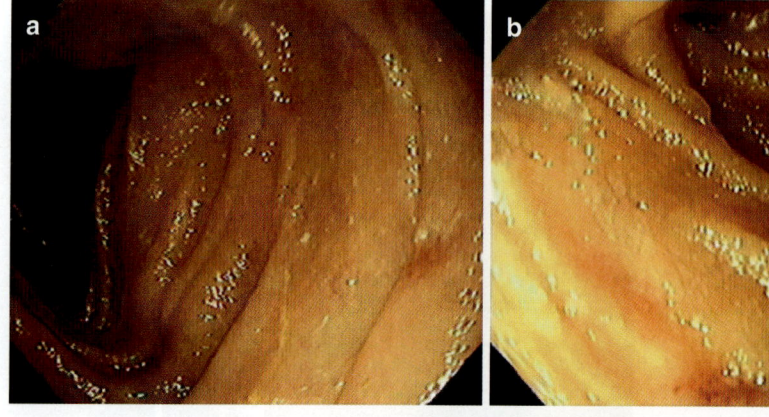

Fig. 29.11 (**a**, **b**) Endoscopic images of small bowel erosions seen in a female patient with Takayasu's arteritis who presented with aortic insufficiency, pulmonary hypertension, and symptoms of dyspnea, claudication of the lower limb, abdominal pain, and obscure gastrointestinal bleeding

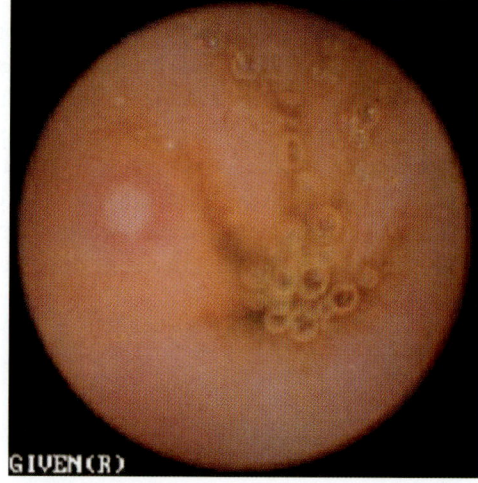

Fig. 29.12 Patient with systemic lupus erythematosus: multiple aphthae in the middle third of the small bowel, not clearly distinguishable from Crohn's disease by endoscopy. The patient presented with iron deficiency anemia, albuminuria, arthritis, and positive antinuclear antibodies

Fig. 29.13 Systemic lupus erythematosus. (**a**) Edematous and erythematous enteropathy seen with VCE. (**b**) Thickened small bowel loops and ascites on a CT scan (Courtesy of Ernst Malzfeldt, MD)

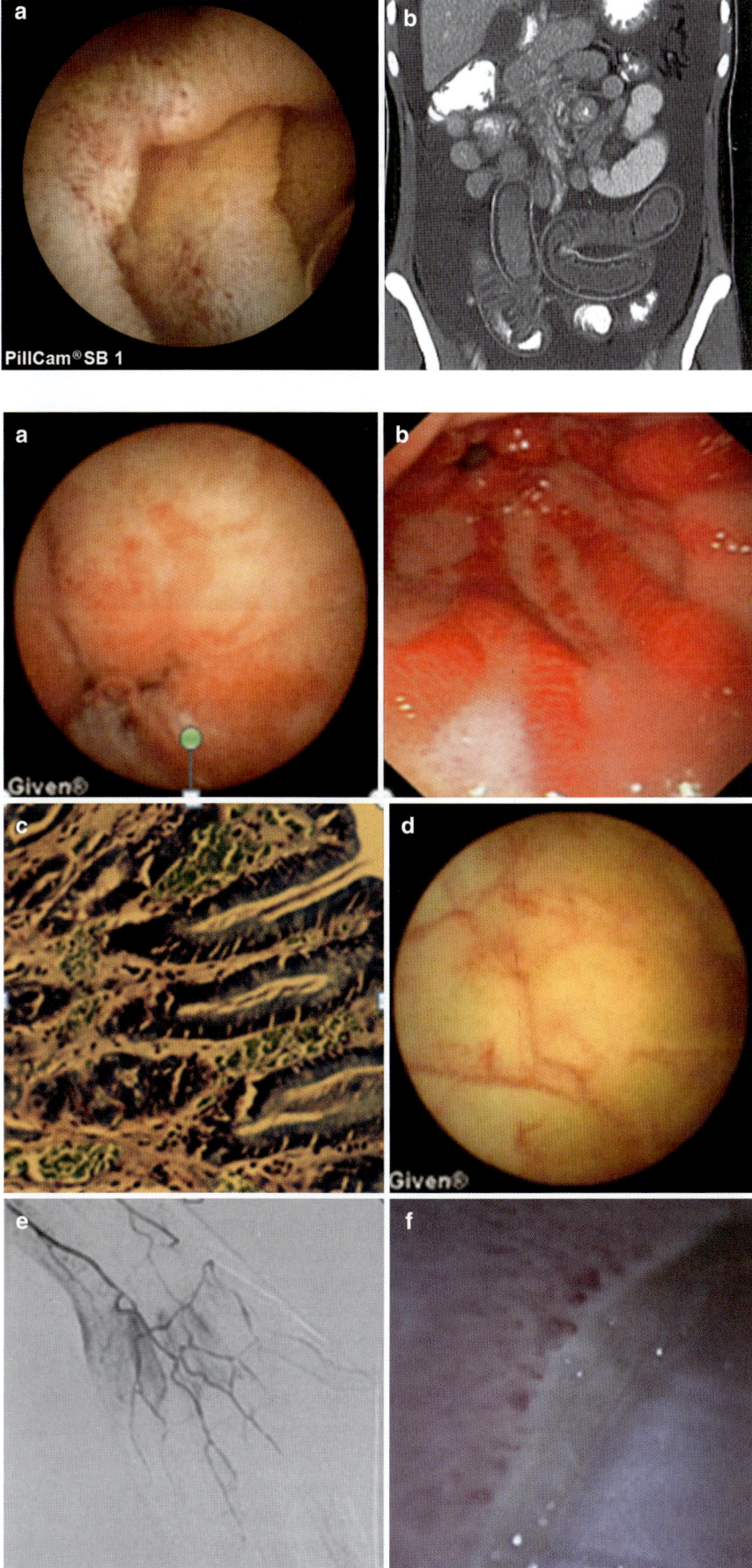

Fig. 29.14 Multiple blood vessels are affected in a patient with systemic sclerosis. (**a**) Digital subtraction angiography of the hand shows severe rarefaction of digital arteries (Courtesy of Doris Welger, MD). (**b–d**) Gastric antral vascular ectasia without portal hypertension is seen on VCE, gastroscopy, and histology (Giemsa stain showing dilated vessel, Courtesy of Renate Höhne, MD), respectively. (**e**) Irregular vessels of the small intestine seen with VCE. (**f**) Nail capillary microscopy

29.5 Common Variable Immunodeficiency Syndrome (CVID)

This heterogeneous group of congenital or acquired immunodeficiencies is characterized by the inability of B lymphocytes to differentiate to plasma cells, resulting in a pan-hypogammaglobulinemia. Clinical features include chronic pulmonary infections, lymphadenopathy, fever, diarrhea, and malabsorption [56, 57]. Endoscopy typically reveals diffuse intestinal lymphoid hyperplasia (Figs. 29.15 and 29.16) [58]. Histology shows a wide spectrum of findings such as nodular lymphoid hyperplasia, villous atrophy [59], granulomas, and lymphocytic infiltration [60].

Fig. 29.15 Common variable immunodeficiency syndrome (CVID). (**a**, **b**) Multiple lymph follicles throughout the small intestine (Courtesy of Emese Mihaly, MD)

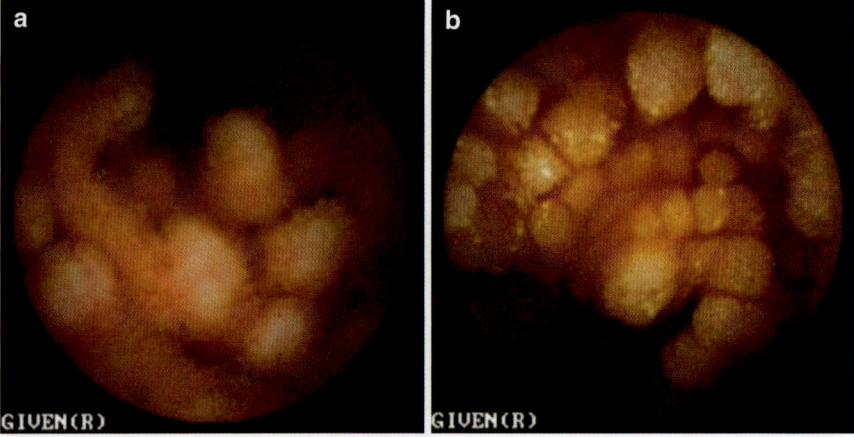

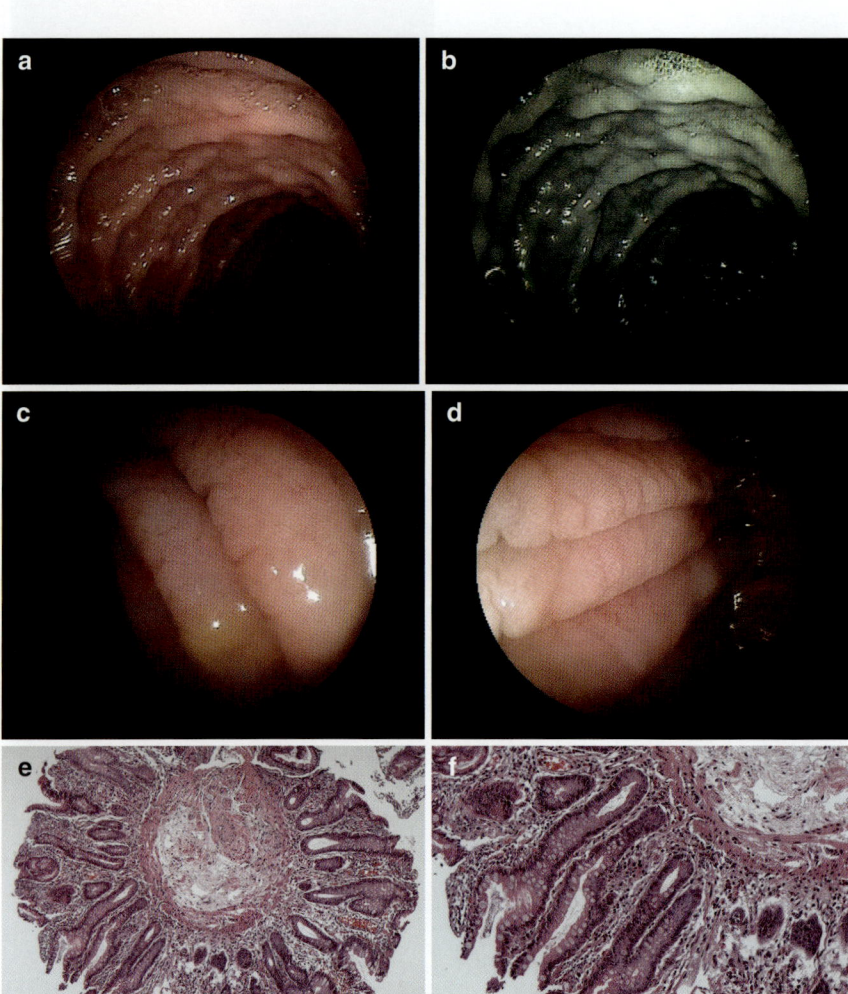

Fig. 29.16 (**a–d**) Endoscopic images of a patient with CVID and anemia, demonstrating mucosal changes suggestive of villous atrophy with duodenal nodularity and jejunal scalloping. (**e**, **f**) Histologic images of a jejunal biopsy specimen show villous atrophy with intraepithelial lymphocytes and decreased villous-crypt ratio (**e**, 100×; **f**, 200×)

29.6 Hemosiderosis

Hemosiderosis is a rare condition caused by iron overload, e.g., due to multiple blood transfusions in inherited anemia, but also in liver cirrhosis and kidney disease. Intestinal involvement is very rare. Diffuse punctate dark spots in the small intestine can be observed (Fig. 29.17) [61].

29.7 Inherited Diseases Involving the Small Intestine

29.7.1 Abetalipoproteinemia, Hypobetalipoproteinemia (Bassen-Kornzweig Syndrome)

This condition is a very rare, hereditary, autosomal recessive deficiency of β-lipoproteins (very-low-density lipoproteins [VLDL] and low-density lipoproteins [LDL]) with no measurable apolipoprotein B and associated malabsorption, with its sequelae. Abetalipoproteinemia is caused by mutations of the gene that encodes larger subunits of the microsomal triglyceride transfer protein (MTP). The deficiency of apolipoprotein B is a secondary phenomenon caused by increased breakdown in the endoplasmic reticulum [62].

Symptoms are malabsorption with steatorrhea, a deficiency of fat-soluble vitamins with its sequelae, retinitis pigmentosa, progressive neurologic symptoms (e.g., ataxia), mental retardation, and massive fatty infiltration of the liver [63].

Pathognomonic signs are hypocholesterolemia (<40 mg/dL), hypotriglyceridemia (<10 mg/dL), no detectable VLDL, and the deformation of erythrocytes (acanthocytosis) in blood smears due to membrane lipid abnormalities. Endoscopy shows a grayish-white discoloration of the entire small bowel mucosa caused by an accumulation of fat vacuoles (Fig. 29.18) [64].

Treatment consists of triglyceride replacement with medium-chain fatty acids, plus the strict avoidance of other fats. High doses of fat-soluble vitamins are also administered.

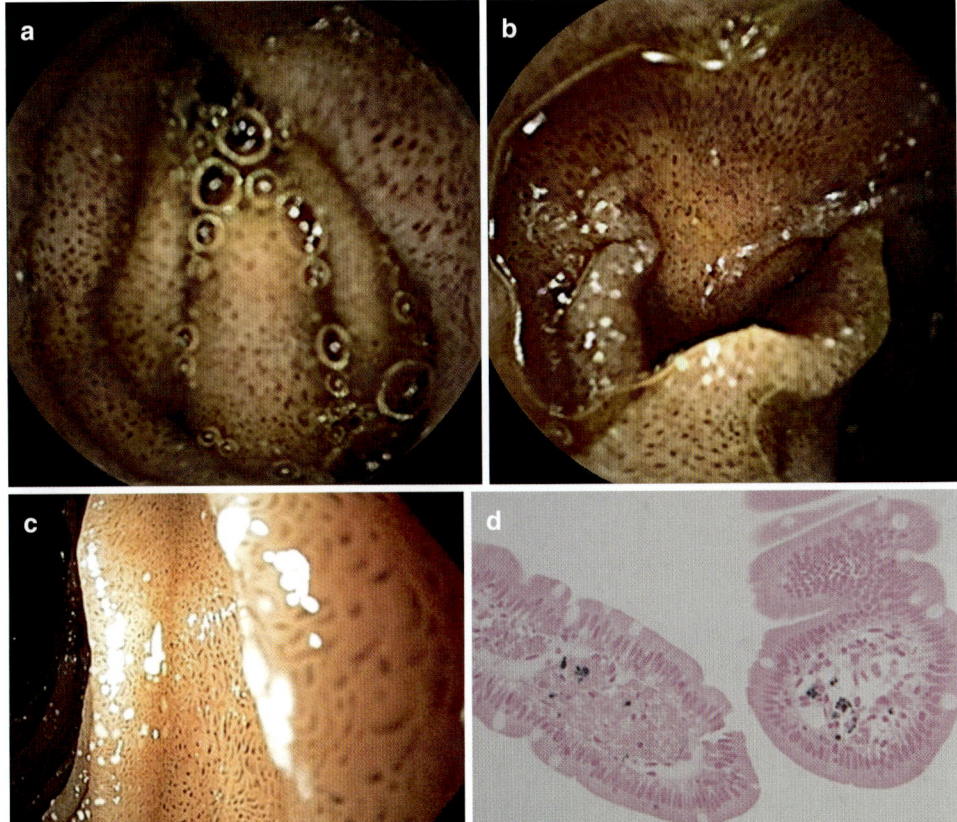

Fig. 29.17 Intestinal hemosiderosis in a patient with portal hypertension due to hepatitis C, end-stage renal disease, multiple transfusions, and iron supplementation. (**a, b**) VCE of jejunum and duodenoscopy (**c**) showing multiple diffusely distributed dark spots of the mucosa. (**d**) Biopsy of the small intestine with positive iron staining (Courtesy of Wilson Kwong, MD and Denise Kalmaz, MD)

Fig. 29.18 Hypobetalipoprotein-emia (single case report by G. Gay and M. Delvaux). (**a**) Diffuse white discoloration of the mucosa seen with VCE (Reprinted from Gay et al. [63], with permission from Given Imaging). (**b**) Discoloration of the mucosa seen with push enteroscopy. (**c**) Histology shows multiple small lipid vacuoles in the small bowel mucosa. (**d**) Immunohistochemistry: polar accumulation of truncated apolipoprotein B

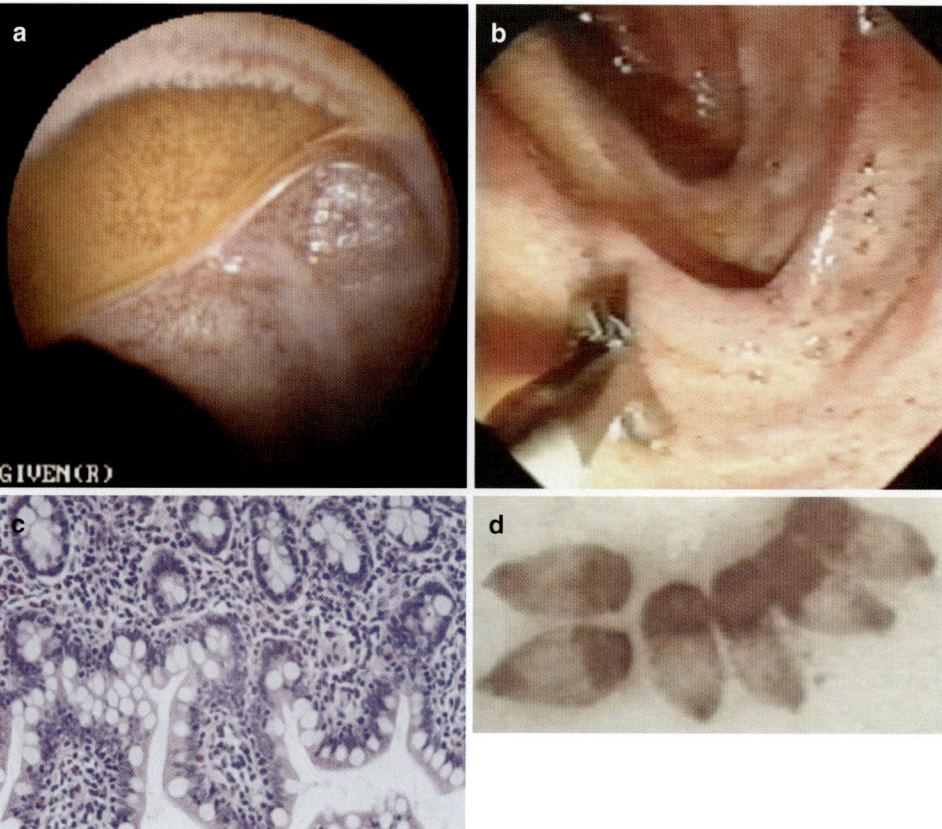

29.7.2 Sea-Blue Histiocytosis

Sea-blue histiocytosis is a disorder associated with both acquired conditions of increased cellular turnover and inborn errors of lipid metabolism. The common feature is the accumulation in various organs of lipid-laden histiocytes because of increased production or a failure of catabolism (Figs. 29.19, 29.20, and 29.21). Blood disorders such as chronic myeloid leukemia, idiopathic thrombocytopenic purpura, and myelodysplastic syndromes, in which cells are produced at an increased rate by the reticuloendothelial system, represent the acquired conditions. The inherited metabolic defects include sphingomyelinase deficiency (e.g., Niemann-Pick disease, Gaucher disease) and abnormalities of lipoprotein metabolism [65, 66].

Other conditions associated with sea-blue histiocytosis include infectious diseases such as lepromatous leprosy, mononucleosis, and visceral leishmaniasis; a pathological storage condition in patients receiving long-term parenteral nutrition with fat-emulsion sources; and thalassemia [67].

Clinically, sea-blue histiocytosis manifests with impaired liver and lung function, hepatosplenomegaly, and lymphadenopathy. It can be diagnosed in patients from the first year of life to their 80s, but it is usually diagnosed by the fourth decade. The incidence is similar in both men and women.

29.7.3 Noonan Syndrome

Noonan syndrome (NS) is a relatively common autosomal dominant, congenital disorder considered to be a type of dwarfism affecting both males and females equally. Heterozygous mutations in nine genes (*PTPN11*, *SOS1*, *KRAS*, *NRAS*, *RAF1*, *BRAF*, *SHOC2*, *MEK1*, and *CBL*) have been evolved to the disease, and the diagnosis can be confirmed molecularly in about 75 % of affected individuals [68]. The principal features include congenital heart defect (typically pulmonary valve stenosis), hypertrophic cardiomyopathy, short stature, learning problems, pectus excavatum, impaired blood clotting, and a characteristic configuration of facial features that includes a webbed neck and a flat nose bridge. Bleeding sometimes occurs in patients with NS. The small intestine may be affected (Fig. 29.22). Angioectasia at the small intestine has been described as the cause of obscure GI bleeding in a man with NS and aortic regurgitation [69]. Postbiopsy intramural hematoma of the duodenum in an adult with NS has also been reported [70].

Fig. 29.19 (**a**) Double-balloon endoscopy by the oral route revealed multiple, sessile, elevated, and confluent lesions at the duodenum in a female patient with sea-blue histiocytosis, who presented with abdominal pain and anemia. (**b**) At the jejunum, numerous sessile lesions can be observed, as well as pedunculated and multilobulated lesions of the small intestine

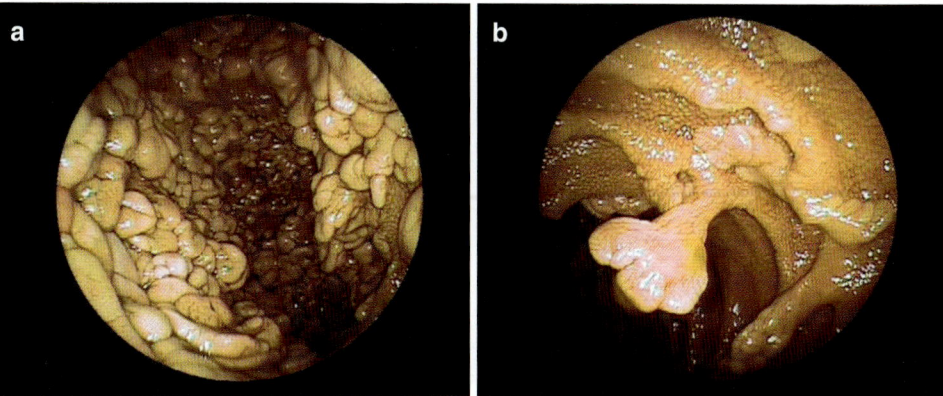

Fig. 29.20 Double-balloon endoscopy by the anal route demonstrated normal colonic mucosa (**a**). At the ileocecal valve (**b**) and ileum (**c**, **d**), several small sessile lesions are seen and enhanced with indigo carmine chromoscopy (**b**, **d**)

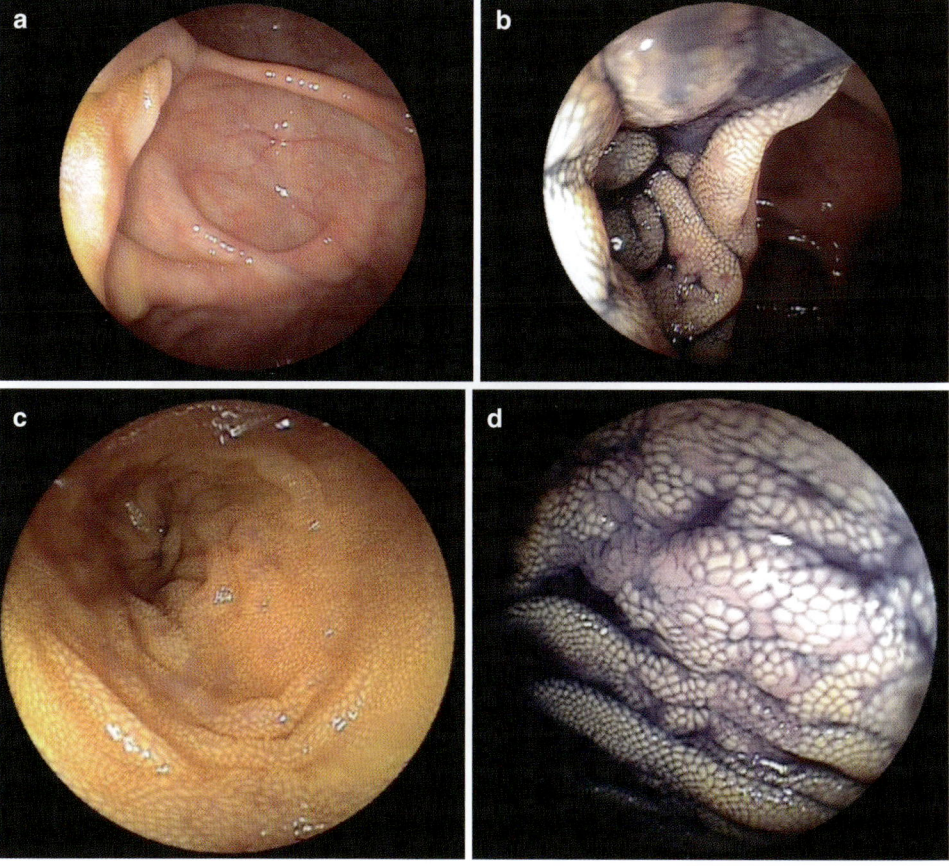

Fig. 29.21 (**a**) Biopsy samples of the lesions with H&E staining identified subepithelial macrophages, with the accumulation of lipofuscin, glycophospholipid, and sphingomyelin. (**b**) May-Giemsa staining revealed sea-blue macrophages, the reason for the name of sea-blue histiocytosis

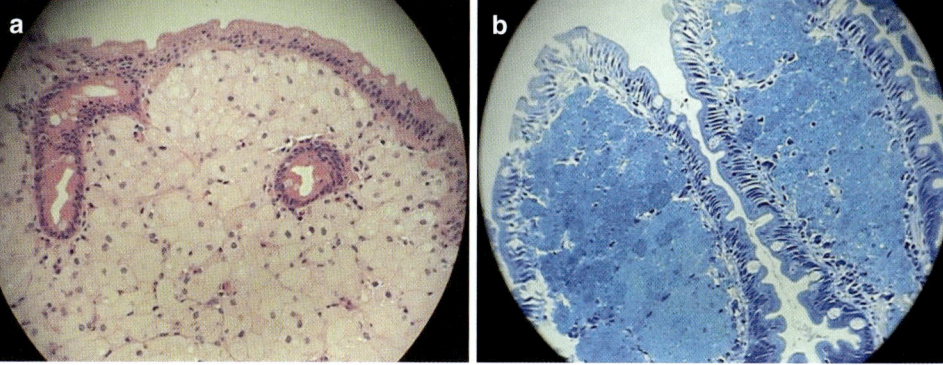

Fig. 29.22 Endoscopic pictures showing nodularity and friability of the small bowel mucosa in a patient with Noonan syndrome and anemia (**a**, **b**). Biopsies revealed inflammation and previous signs of hemorrhage

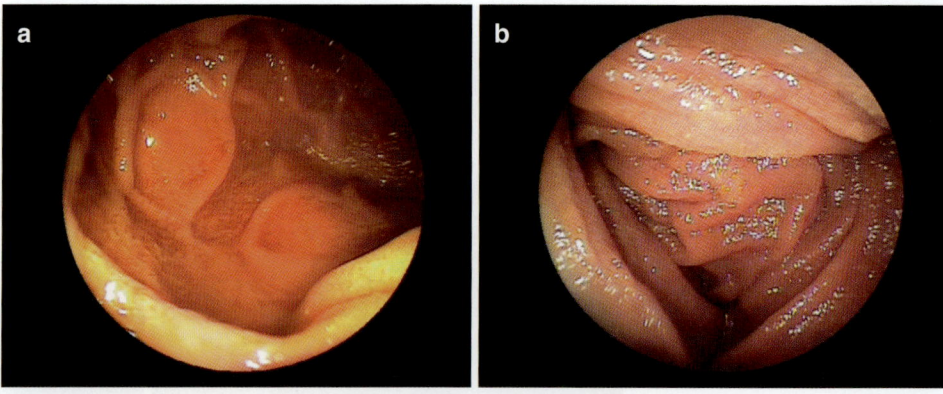

Fig. 29.23 (**a–c**) Endoscopic diagnosis of jejunal lymphangiectasia and multiple oozing angioectasias in a patient with Goldenhar syndrome, who presented with obscure gastrointestinal bleeding

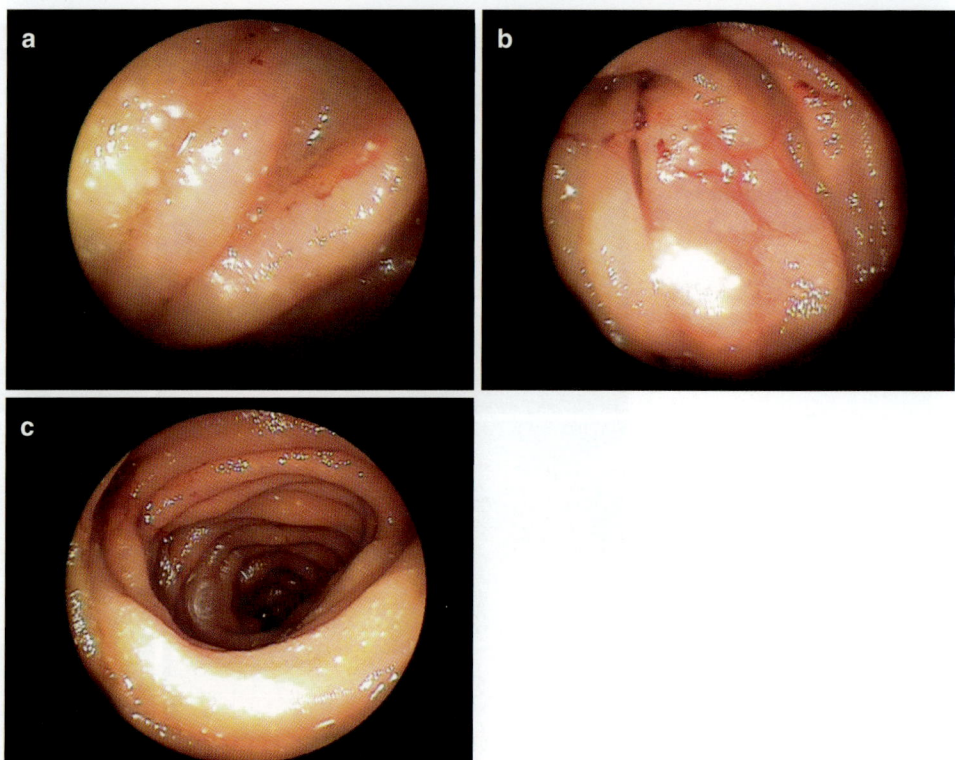

29.7.4 Goldenhar Syndrome

Goldenhar syndrome (oculoauriculovertebral dysplasia) is characterized by preauricular skin tags, microtia, facial asymmetry, ocular abnormalities, and vertebral anomalies of different size and shape. Chromosomal alterations are responsible for malformations of the central nervous system and heart and for many other abnormalities of the kidney, lung, and GI tract (Fig. 29.23) [71, 72].

References

1. Hagenmüller F. Funktionelle und morphologische Veränderungen des Dünndarms bei systemischen und extraintestinalen Erkrankungen. In: Caspary W, editor. Handbuch der Inneren Medizin. Bd III/3B: Dünndarm. Berlin: Springer; 1983. p. 611–30.

2. Sattianayagam PT, Hawkins PN, Gillmore JD. Systemic amyloidosis and the gastrointestinal tract. Nat Rev Gastroenterol Hepatol. 2009;10:608–17.

3. Ebert EC, Nagar M. Gastrointestinal manifestations of amyloidosis. Am J Gastroenterol. 2008;103:776–87.

4. Linke R, Altland K, Ernst J, et al. Praktische Hinweise zur Diagnose und Therapie generalisierter Amyloidosen. Dtsch Ärzteblatt. 1998;95:A2626–36.

5. Saeger W, Röcken C. Amyloid: microscopic demonstration, classification and clinical correlation. [Article in German]. Pathologe. 1998;19:345–54.

6. Peny MO, Debongnie JC, Haot J, van Gossum A. Localized amyloid tumor in small bowel. Dig Dis Sci. 2000;45:1850–3.

7. Barzola S, Lespi P, Fuentes R. Intestinal bleeding associated with systemic amyloidosis. [Article in Spanish]. Acta Gastroenterol Latinoam. 1998;28:257–9.

8. Stelzner M, Krug B. Gastrointestinal amyloidosis: differential diagnosis and indications for surgical therapy. Chirurg. 1991;62:493–9.

9. Koppelman RN, Stollman NH, Baigorri F, Rogers AI. Acute small bowel pseudoobstruction due to AL amyloidosis: a case report and literature review. Am J Gastroenterol. 2000;95:294–6.

10. Hayman SR, Lacy MQ, Kyle RA, Gertz MA. Primary systemic amyloidosis: a cause of malabsorption syndrome. Am J Med. 2001;111:535–40.

11. Hokama A, Kishimoto K, Nakamoto M, et al. Endoscopic and histopathological features of gastrointestinal amyloidosis. World J Gastrointest Endosc. 2011;3:157–61.

12. Yoshii S, Mabe K, Nosho K, et al. Submucosal hematoma is a highly suggestive finding for amyloid light-chain amyloidosis: two case reports. World J Gastrointest Endosc. 2012;4:434–7.

13. Cowan AJ, Skinner M, Seldin DC, et al. Amyloidosis of the gastrointestinal tract: a 13-year, single-center, referral experience. Haematologica. 2013;98:141–6.

14. Vahid B, Spodik M, Braun KN, et al. Sarcoidosis of gastrointestinal tract: a rare disease. Dig Dis Sci. 2007;52:3316–20.

15. Marie I, Sauvetre G, Levesque H. Small intestinal involvement revealing sarcoidosis. QJM. 2010;103:60–2.

16. Tsibouris P, Kalantzis C, Alexandrakis G, et al. Capsule endoscopy findings in a case of intestinal sarcoidosis. Endoscopy. 2009;41 Suppl 2:E191.

17. Culver DA. Sarcoidosis. Immunol Allergy Clin North Am. 2012;32:487–511.

18. Costabel U. Sarkoidose. In: Paumgartner G, Steinbeck G, editors. Therapie innerer Krankheiten, 10. Berlin: Springer; 2003. p. 414–9.

19. Jennette JC, Falk RJ, Andrassy K, et al. Nomenclature of systemic vasculitides. Proposal of an international consensus conference. Arthritis Rheum. 1994;37:187–92.

20. Jennette JC, Falk RJ, Bacon PA, et al. 2012 revised International Chapel Hill Consensus Conference Nomenclature of Vasculitides. Arthritis Rheum. 2013;65:1–11.

21. Ha HK, Lee SH, Rha SE, et al. Radiologic features of vasculitis involving the gastrointestinal tract. Radiographics. 2000;3:779–94.

22. Ahn E, Luk A, Chetty R, Butany J. Vasculitides of the gastrointestinal tract. Semin Diagn Pathol. 2009;2:77–88.

23. Esaki M, Matsumoto T, Nakamura S, et al. GI involvement in Henoch-Schönlein purpura. Gastrointest Endosc. 2002;56:920–3.

24. Szer IS. Gastrointestinal and renal involvement in vasculitis: management strategies in Henoch-Schönlein purpura. Cleve Clin J Med. 1999;66:312–7.

25. Skogestad E. Capsule endoscopy in Henoch-Schonlein purpura. Endoscopy. 2005;37:189.

26. Keuchel M, Baltes P, Stövesand-Ruge B, et al. Henoch Schönlein Purpura. VJGIEN. 2013;1:235–6.

27. Ozen S, Pistorio A, Iusan SM, et al. EULAR/PRINTO/PRES criteria for Henoch-Schonlein purpura, childhood polyarteritis nodosa, childhood Wegener granulomatosis and childhood Takayasu arteritis: Ankara 2008. Part II: final classification criteria. Ann Rheum Dis. 2010;69:798–806.

28. Churg J, Strauss L. Allergic granulomatosis, allergic angiitis, and periarteritis nodosa. Am J Pathol. 1951;27:277–301.

29. Nakamura Y, Sakurai Y, Matsubara T, et al. Multiple perforated ulcers of the small intestine associated with allergic granulomatous angiitis: report of a case. Surg Today. 2002;32:541–6.

30. Suzuki T, Matsushima M, Arase Y, et al. Double-balloon endoscopy-diagnosed multiple small intestinal ulcers in a Churg-Strauss syndrome patient. World J Gastrointest Endosc. 2012;4:194–6.

31. Ushiki A, Koizumi T, Kubo K, et al. Colonic sarcoidosis presenting multiple submucosal tumor-like lesions. Intern Med. 2009;48:1813–6.

32. Murakami S, Misumi M, Sakata H, et al. Churg-Strauss syndrome manifesting as perforation of the small intestine: report of a case. Surg Today. 2004;34:788–92.

33. Barnes CG. Behcet's syndrome – classification criteria. Ann Med Interne (Paris). 1999;150:477–82.

34. Korman U, Cantasdemir M, Kurugoglu S, et al. Enteroclysis findings of intestinal Behçet disease: a comparative study with Crohn's disease. Abdom Imaging. 2003;28:308–12.

35. Pretorius ES, Hruban RH, Fishman EK. Inflammatory pseudotumor of the terminal ileum mimicking malignancy in a patient with Behçet's disease. CT and pathological findings. Clin Imaging. 1996;20:191–3.

36. Neves FS, Fylyk SN, Lage LV, et al. Behçet's disease: clinical value of the video capsule endoscopy for small intestine examination. Rheumatol Int. 2009;5:601–3.

37. Wu QJ, Zhang FC, Zhang X. Adamantiades-Behcet's disease-complicated gastroenteropathy. World J Gastroenterol. 2012;18:609–15.

38. Hokama A, Kishimoto K, Ihama Y, et al. Endoscopic and radiographic features of gastrointestinal involvement in vasculitis. World J Gastrointest Endosc. 2012;4:50–6.

39. Carson CW, Conn DL, Czaja AJ, et al. Frequency and significance of antibodies to hepatitis C virus in polyarteritis nodosa. J Rheumatol. 1993;20:304–9.

40. Lidar M, Lipschitz N, Langevitz P, Shoenfeld Y. The infectious etiology of vasculitis. Autoimmunity. 2009;42:432–8.

41. Guillevin L. Infections in vasculitis. Best practice & research. Clin Rheumatol. 2013;27:19–31.

42. Becker A, Mader R, Elias M, et al. Duodenal necrosis as the presenting manifestation of polyarteritis nodosa. Clin Rheumatol. 2002;21:314–6.

43. Ueda C, Hirohata Y, Kihara Y, et al. Pancreatic cancer complicated by disseminated intravascular coagulation associated with production of tissue factor. J Gastroenterol. 2001;36:848–50.

44. Villiger PM, Guillevin L. Microscopic polyangiitis: clinical presentation. Autoimmun Rev. 2010;9:812–9.

45. Chung SA, Seo P. Microscopic polyangiitis. Rheum Dis Clin North Am. 2010;36:545–58.

46. Storesund B, Gran JT, Koldingsnes W. Severe intestinal involvement in Wegener's granulomatosis: report of two cases and review of the literature. Br J Rheumatol. 1998;37:387–90.

47. Deniz K, Ozşeker HS, Balas S, et al. Intestinal involvement in Wegener's granulomatosis. J Gastrointestin Liver Dis. 2007;16:329–31.

48. Simon S, Schittko G, Bösenberg H, et al. Fulminant course of a Takayasu's arteritis and rare mesenteric arterial manifestation. [Article in German]. Z Rheumatol. 2006;65(520):522–6.
49. Sasamura H, Nakamoto H, Ryuzaki M, et al. Repeated intestinal ulcerations in a patient with systemic lupus erythematosus and high serum antiphospholipid antibody levels. South Med J. 1991;84:515–7.
50. Moriuchi J, Ichikawa Y, Takaya M, et al. Lupus cystitis and perforation of the small bowel in a patient with systemic lupus erythematosus and overlapping syndrome. Clin Exp Rheumatol. 1989;7: 533–6.
51. Nguyen H, Khanna N. Intestinal pseudo-obstruction as a presenting manifestation of systemic lupus erythematosus: case report and review of the literature. South Med J. 2004;97:186–9.
52. Marie I, Levesque H, Ducrotte P, Courtois H. Involvement of the small intestine in systemic scleroderma. Rev Med Interne. 1999;20: 504–13.
53. Ebert EC, Ruggiero FM, Seibold JR. Intestinal perforation. A common complication of scleroderma. Dig Dis Sci. 1997;42:549–53.
54. Harrison E, Herrick AL, McLaughlin JT, Lal S. Malnutrition in systemic sclerosis. Rheumatology (Oxford). 2012;51:1747–56.
55. Savarino E, Mei F, Parodi A, et al. Gastrointestinal motility disorder assessment in systemic sclerosis. Rheumatology (Oxford). 2013;52:1095–100.
56. Díez R, García MJ, Vivas S, et al. Gastrointestinal manifestations in patients with primary immunodeficiencies causing antibody deficiency. Gastroenterol Hepatol. 2010;5:347–51.
57. Malamut G, Verkarre V, Suarez F, et al. The enteropathy associated with common variable immunodeficiency: the delineated frontiers with celiac disease. Am J Gastroenterol. 2010;10:2262–75.
58. Mihaly E, Nemeth A, Zagoni T, et al. Gastrointestinal manifestations of common variable immunodeficiency diagnosed by video- and capsule endoscopy. Endoscopy. 2005;37:603–4.
59. Biagi F, Bianchi PI, Zilli A, et al. The significance of duodenal mucosal atrophy in patients with common variable immunodeficiency: a clinical and histopathologic study. Am J Clin Pathol. 2012;2:185–9.
60. Washington K, Stenzel TT, Buckley RH, Gottfried MR. Gastrointestinal pathology in patients with common variable immunodeficiency and X-linked agammaglobulinemia. Am J Surg Pathol. 1996;20:1240–52.
61. Kwong W, Kalmaz D. Jejunal hemosiderosis detected with small bowel capsule endoscopy. VHJOE. 2013;12(1). http://www.vhjoe.org/index.php/vhjoe/article/viewFile/86/139

62. Sharp D, Blinderman L, Combs KA, et al. Cloning and gene defects in microsomal triglyceride transfer protein associated with abetalipoproteinaemia. Nature. 1993;365:65–9.
63. Gay G, Fassler I, Florent C, Delvaux M. Malabsorption. In: Halpern M, Jacob H, editors. Atlas of capsule endoscopy. Norcross: Given Imaging; 2002. p. 83–101.
64. Gay G, Delmotte JS. Abeta and hypobetalipoproteinemias. In: Rossini F, Gay G, editors. Atlas of enteroscopy. Berlin: Springer; 1998. p. 119–20.
65. Candoni A, Grimaz S, Doretto P, et al. Sea-blue histiocytosis secondary to Niemann-Pick disease type B: a case report. Ann Hematol. 2001;10:620–2.
66. Suzuki O, Abe M. Secondary sea-blue histiocytosis derived from Niemann-Pick disease. J Clin Exp Hematop. 2007;47:19–21.
67. Safatle-Ribeiro AV, Baba ER, Iriya K. Double-balloon endoscopy reveals sea-blue histiocytosis affecting the small bowel (with video). Gastrointest Endosc. 2010;6:1266; discussion 1266–7.
68. Tartaglia M, Gelb BD, Zenker M. Noonan syndrome and clinically related disorders. Best Pract Res Clin Endocrinol Metab. 2011;25:161–79.
69. Yoshino H, Okumachi Y, Akisaki T, et al. Bleeding from the small intestine and aortic regurgitation in Noonan syndrome. Intern Med. 2011;50:2611–3.
70. Sgouros SN, Karamanolis G, Papadopoulou E, et al. Postbiopsy intramural hematoma of the duodenum in an adult with Noonan's syndrome. J Gastroenterol Hepatol. 2004;10:1217–9.
71. Touliatou V, Fryssira H, Mavrou A, et al. Clinical manifestations in 17 Greek patients with Goldenhar syndrome. Genet Couns. 2006;17:359–70.
72. Engiz O, Balci S, Unsal M, et al. 31 cases with oculoauriculovertebral dysplasia (Goldenhar syndrome): clinical, neuroradiologic, audiologic and cytogenetic findings. Genet Couns. 2007;3:277–88.

Internet

www.amyloidosis.org: Amyloidosis Foundation
www.eular.org: The European League Against Rheumatism
www.lupus.org: Lupus Foundation of America
www.rheumatology.org: American College of Rheumatology

Physical–Chemical Small Intestinal Injury

30

Ingvar Bjarnason, Samuel N. Adler, and Choitsu Sakamoto

Contents

The small bowel has been the least accessible part of the gastrointestinal tract for diagnostic imaging, but with the introduction of push enteroscopy and wireless capsule enteroscopy, the diagnosis of small bowel disease has become routine. Furthermore, as capsule enteroscopy is so much more sensitive than radiologic procedures, Pandora's box has been opened. A number of small bowel diseases are now evident where none were thought to exist, and many more remain to be discovered. This chapter summarises the appearance of small bowel damage induced by drugs and radiation.

30.1 NSAID-Induced Enteropathy

30.1.1 Aetiology

The precise pathogenesis of enteropathy induced by nonsteroidal anti-inflammatory drugs (NSAIDs) is slowly coming to light. It seems likely that it is initiated through a local topical effect that involves an NSAID–membrane phospholipid interaction and/or uncoupling of mitochondrial oxidative phosphorylation that compromises intestinal integrity [1, 2]. The consequence of concomitant COX-1 inhibition prevents an increase in microvascular blood flow, while COX-2 inhibition may alter inflammatory (immunologic) responses to this injury. Together these factors lead to inflammation, erosions, ulcers and strictures.

The work was first published in 2006 by Springer Medizin Verlag Heidelberg with the following title: *Atlas of Video Capsule Endoscopy*.

I. Bjarnason (✉)
Department of Gastroenterology, King's College Hospital, London, UK
e-mail: Ingvar.Bjarnason@nhs.net

S.N. Adler
Department of Gastroenterology, Shaare Zedek Medical Center, Jerusalem, Israel
e-mail: nasnadler@gmail.com

C. Sakamoto
Department of Gastroenterology, Nippon Medical School
Graduate School of Medicine, Tokyo, Japan
e-mail: choitsu@nms.ac.jp

30.1.2 Frequency

NSAID-induced enteropathy occurs in up to 60 % of patients who take conventional NSAIDs, whether the use is short term [3–5] or long term [6, 7]. It is not evident in patients treated short term with COX-2 inhibitors [5], but may occur with long-term use [7]. The frequency of serious outcomes (discussed below) is comparable to that seen in the stomach [8], with 1–2 % of patients having problems with anaemia [9].

M. Keuchel et al. (eds.), *Video Capsule Endoscopy: A Reference Guide and Atlas*,
DOI 10.1007/978-3-662-44062-9_30, © Springer-Verlag Berlin Heidelberg 2014

30.1.3 Clinical Features

Many cases of NSAID-induced enteropathy are asymptomatic and are evident only if specifically looked for. Potential complications can be mild, with occult bleeding that may lead to iron deficiency anaemia or protein loss leading to hypoalbuminaemia, or they can be serious, with overt bleeding, perforation and strictures. This bleeding is often considered only after endoscopy and colonoscopy have not disclosed a bleeding site, and the strictures are particularly difficult to diagnose. Some patients with strictures present with weight loss, postprandial abdominal pain and a history of recurrent iron deficiency anaemia and hypoalbuminaemia. The unique "diaphragmatic" strictures are pathognomonic for NSAIDs [10], at least when assessed histologically, but macroscopically, the smooth, concentric strictures are on rare occasions found in other intestinal diseases.

30.1.4 Treatment

There are no rigorously tested and proven methods for reducing damage to the small bowel from NSAIDs. A COX-2-selective agent is certainly much safer when given short term or indeed long term [9]. Sulphasalazine, misoprostol and metronidazole have all been shown to be effective in reducing the inflammatory activity and bleeding. The serious complications of the enteropathy demand surgery, but some of these complications may come to attention only at a post-mortem [11].

30.1.5 Endoscopy

After short-term ingestion of NSAIDs, a range of abnormalities may be seen, none of which by themselves are pathognomonic for NSAID-induced damage; similar pathology may be seen in a number of diseases [12]. It has been suggested [4] that NSAIDs denude the mucosa via a topical effect (Fig. 30.1) with loss of villi and that this effect then progresses to erosions (Fig. 30.2) and ulcers (because of COX-1 and/or COX-2 inhibition). The damage may be very subtle, however, and interest in the short-term damage is largely confined to research.

The long-term damage seen with endoscopy is associated not with the high prevalence of denuded areas, but rather with erosions (Fig. 30.3) and ulcers (Fig. 30.4). The weblike diaphragmatic strictures are the most spectacular manifestations of the damage, however. These begin as subtle, linear ulcers (Fig. 30.5), progressing to characteristic circular ulcers (Fig. 30.6) with subsequent narrowing of the small bowel lumen (Fig. 30.7). Eventually they progress to fibrosing, stenotic

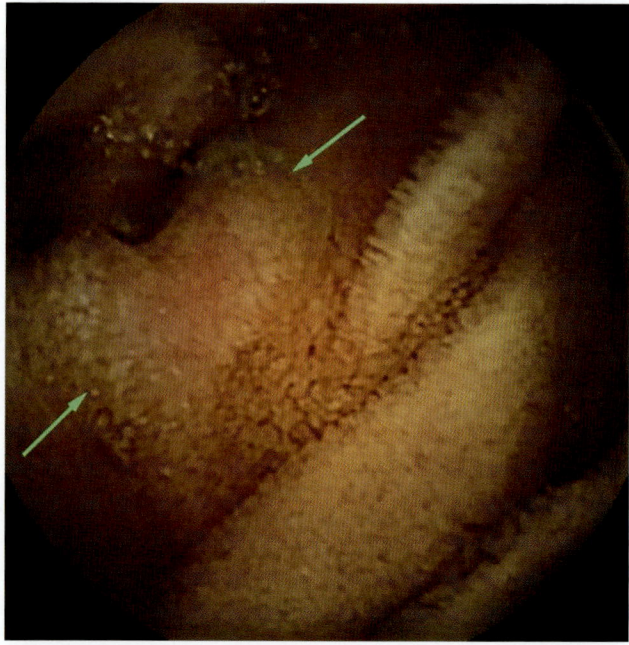

Fig. 30.1 Denuded area with villous blunting (*arrows*)

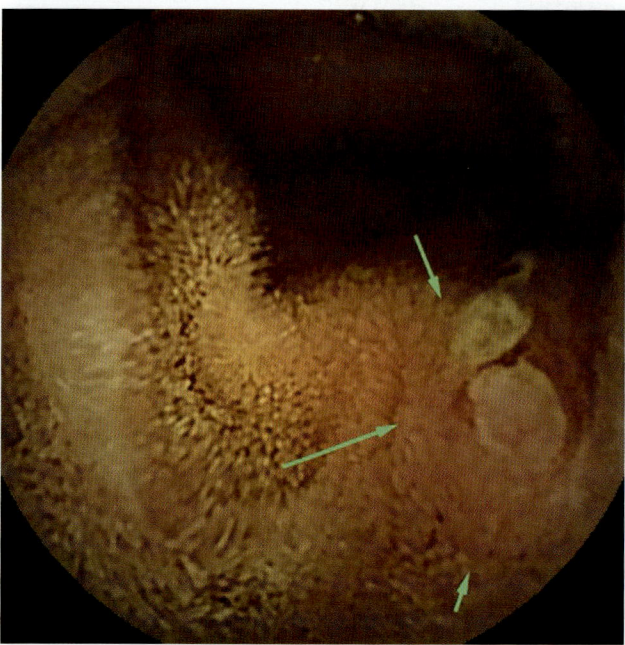

Fig. 30.2 Denuded area with loss of villi (*arrows*) and a central erosion/ulcer after short-term intake of nonsteroidal anti-inflammatory drugs (NSAIDs)

lesions (Fig. 30.8) that are highly suggestive of NSAID-induced damage [10, 13, 14]. Figure 30.9 shows how the critical strictures can be treated, but some may require open surgery.

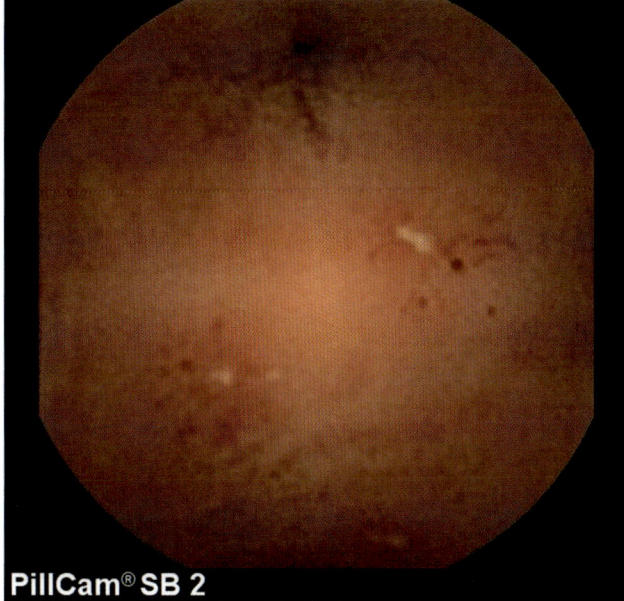

Fig. 30.3 Mucosal break resembling an erosion with central pallor and surrounding erythema

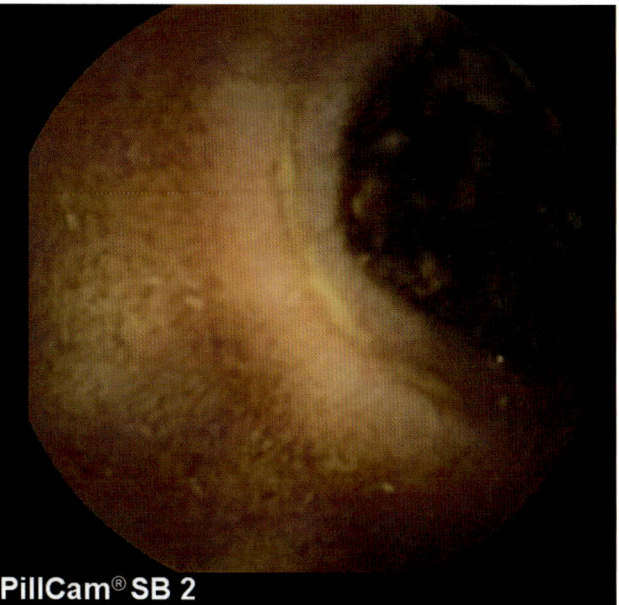

Fig. 30.5 Linear, circular NSAID-induced ulcer sitting on a fold

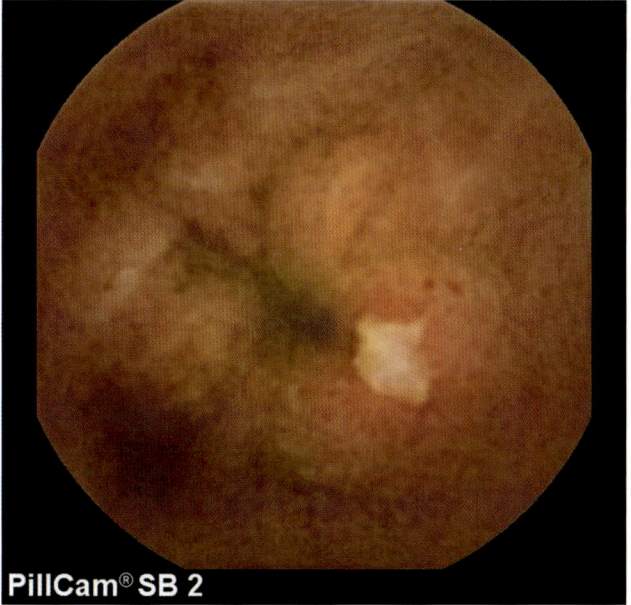

Fig. 30.4 Mucosal break resembling an ulcer. As neither this image nor Fig. 30.3 clearly demonstrates depth; however, these two lesions are lumped together. Of note is that without a history of NSAID intake, capsule endoscopy cannot positively distinguish these lesions from Crohn's disease

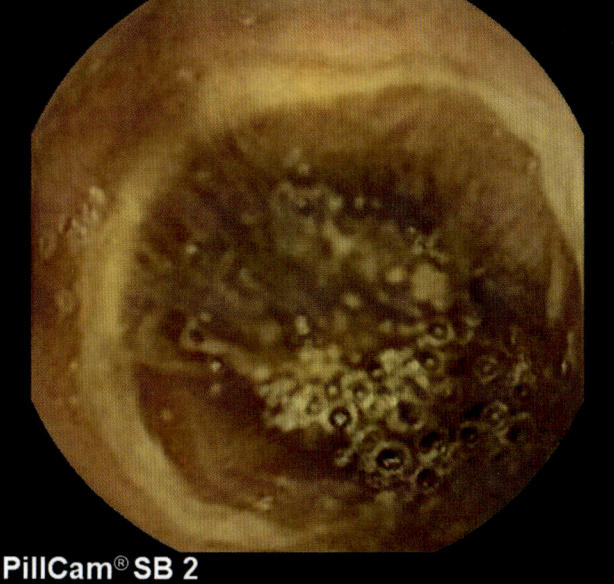

Fig. 30.6 Circular NSAID-induced ulcer causing some narrowing of the small bowel lumen

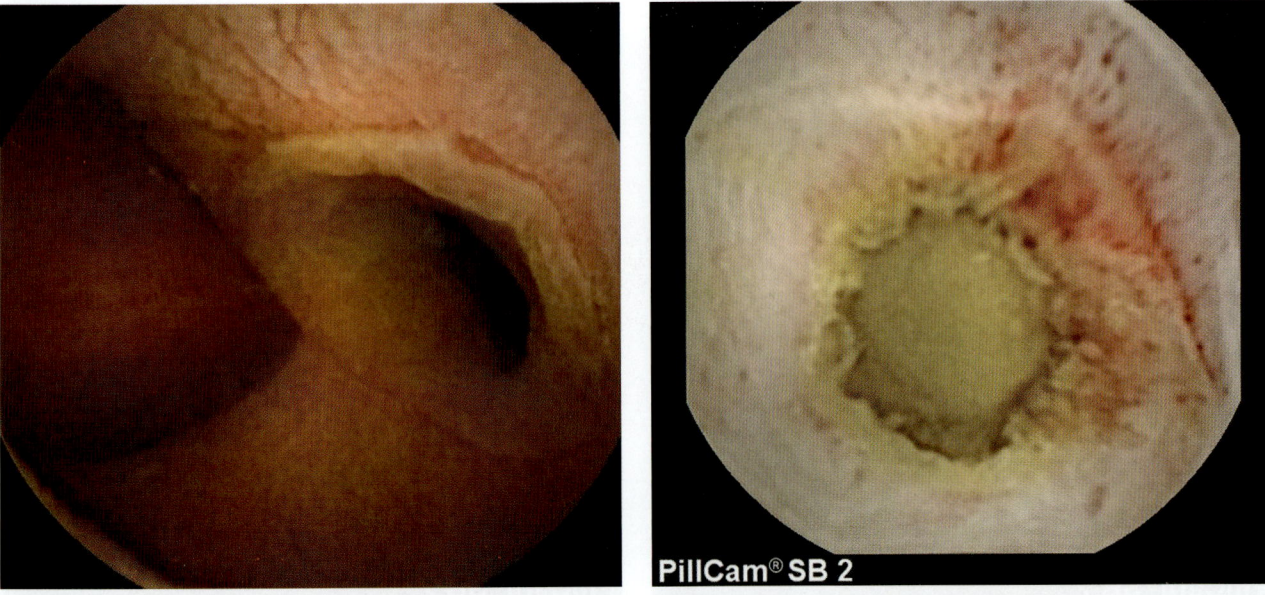

Fig. 30.7 Circular NSAID-induced ulcer causing stenosis in a patient with long-term NSAID use

Fig. 30.8 Circular NSAID-induced fibrous stricture

Fig. 30.9 NSAID-induced enteropathy. (**a**) Ulcerated stenosis in a patient with abdominal pain and anaemia. There is a fibrotic stricture, which is passed by the enteroscopy capsule. (**b, c**) Retrograde double-balloon enteroscopy allows dilation of the ulcerated stricture with wide prestenotic lumen. (**d**) Histology shows fibrosis and a chronic inflammatory cell infiltrate (H&E stain; *Courtesy of* Jörg Caselitz, MD)

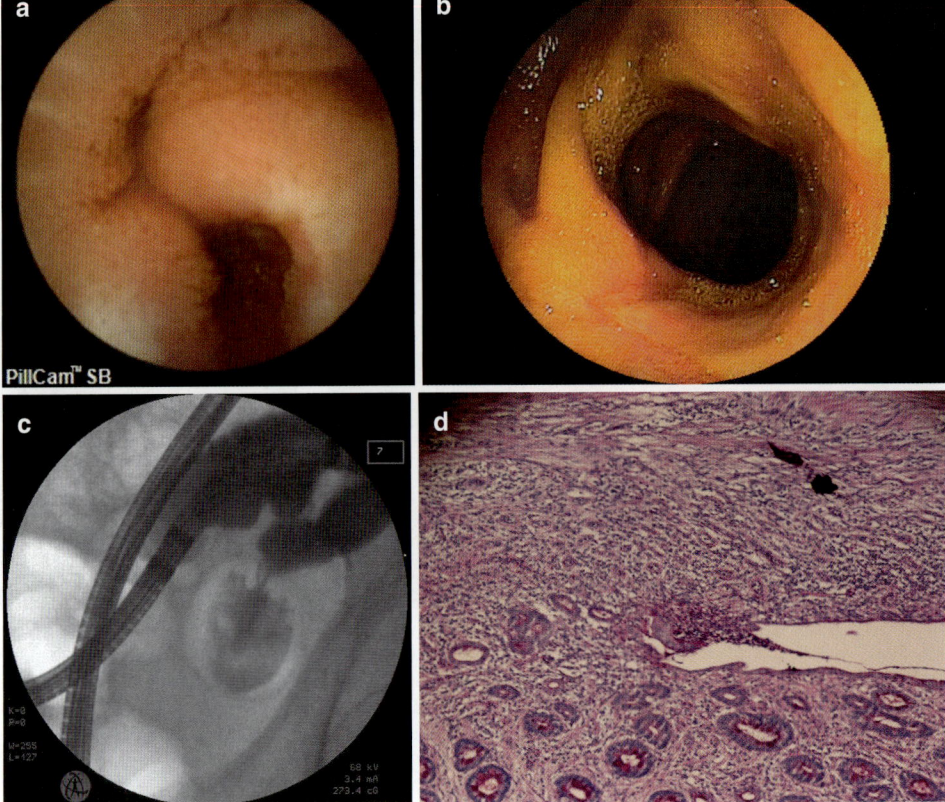

30.2 Chronic Radiation Enteritis

30.2.1 Occurrence

Chronic radiation enteritis can occur within 1 year after radiotherapy to the small bowel, or it may appear many years later, especially if the bowel is fixed due to adhesions or other lesions. The disease is caused by a progressive endarteritis, which leads to a state of chronic ischaemia.

30.2.2 Clinical Features

Symptoms include diarrhoea, maldigestion–malabsorption [15], vomiting and especially abdominal pain [16]. Perforation, bleeding and stenosis are potential complications, but these are very rare indeed.

30.2.3 Diagnosis

The diagnosis of chronic radiation enteritis is often difficult. Currently it relies on ileoscopy, enteroclysis and CT scans [17], which will identify only very advanced cases. The present experience with capsule endoscopy supports the notion that radiation-induced enteritis will be diagnosed earlier, with greater ease and certainty.

30.2.4 Treatment

Treatment is often targeted towards effects such as possible small bowel overgrowth and bile acid malabsorption. Symptomatic treatment (dietary management with obstipants and antispasmodics) is the norm. Surgical treatment for adhesions and strictures is associated with a high complication rate [18, 19].

30.2.5 Endoscopy

It is advisable to exclude significant stenosis by the ingestion of a patency capsule prior to carrying out a capsule study in patients who have been subjected to abdominal radiation, especially those with postprandial pain, nausea and vomiting.

By the nature of the problem, many patients undergoing chemotherapy and abdominal radiation have significant abdominal symptoms during active treatment, but many find their way to the gastroenterologist 5 years or more later. The early events in radiation enteritis damage to the small bowel are at present not known, but it is suggested that the damage may be similar to that seen following the use of conventional NSAIDs [12].

Long-term damage can include a range of lesions. A very common feature of radiation enteritis is the clubbing of villi with lymphangiectasia. These can be subtle or can be immediately obvious in severe cases lasting many years (Fig. 30.10a) [12]. These lesions can sometimes be distinguished from NSAID-induced strictures because the inflammatory activity is not on the leading edge of the diaphragm. Sometimes the strictures are evident because of capsule retention (Fig. 30.10b–d).

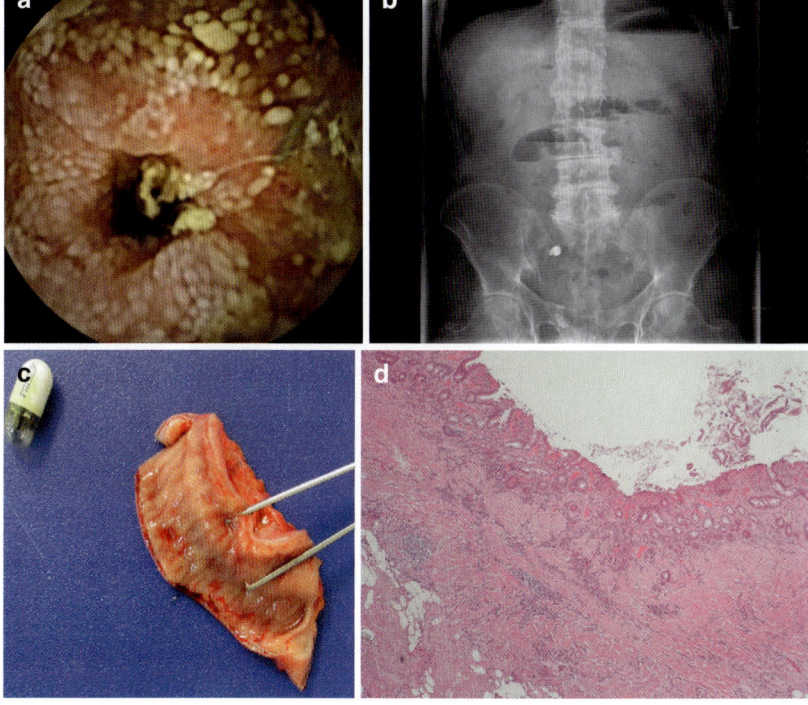

Fig. 30.10 Chronic radiation enteritis. (**a**) Lymphangiectasia, thickening of the small bowel wall and stenosis (*Courtesy of* Felix Wiedbrauck, MD). (**b**) Radiography demonstrates a retained capsule and partial obstruction. (**c**) At resection, a short stenotic segment is seen. (**d**) Histology reveals submucosal fibrosis (H&E stain; *Courtesy of* Peer Flemming, MD, and Axel Wellmann, MD)

30.3 Emerging Research

The small bowel is the main site of absorption of drugs. The suggestion that ingestion of a variety of drugs may lead to small bowel disease is therefore reasonable but has not been studied in a systematic way [20]. Most cases are therefore in the form of single case reports, but the field is open for much research and new discoveries. Nowhere is this more apparent than in patients undergoing chemotherapy, in whom diarrhoea may be the limiting factor for drug treatment. Figure 30.11 shows superficial damage shortly after induction of chemotherapy, and Fig. 30.12 shows more severe damage in a severely symptomatic patient receiving chemotherapy for breast cancer.

Mucositis is a common side effect during treatment of lymphoma and leukaemia. The upper gastrointestinal symptoms dominate the clinical picture, but small bowel damage can be documented, as shown in Fig. 30.13 (although this patient was also taking NSAIDs.)

Patients misusing cocaine may present with intestinal perforation, presumably due to excessive doses and the vasoconstrictive effect of this drug. Figure 30.14 demonstrates punched-out lesions in a man admitted to hospital following excessive use of the drug.

Proton pump inhibitors are one of the most widely prescribed medicines worldwide. It has always been suspected that ingestion of this class of drugs could damage the small bowel, perhaps via alterations in the microbial flora. Figure 30.15 demonstrates mucosal breaks following 2 weeks of ingestion of a proton pump inhibitor in a healthy volunteer participating in Prof. Sakamoto's ongoing research trial.

These illustrations are only intended to demonstrate areas of emerging research. More data are required before we can assign clinical importance to these findings.

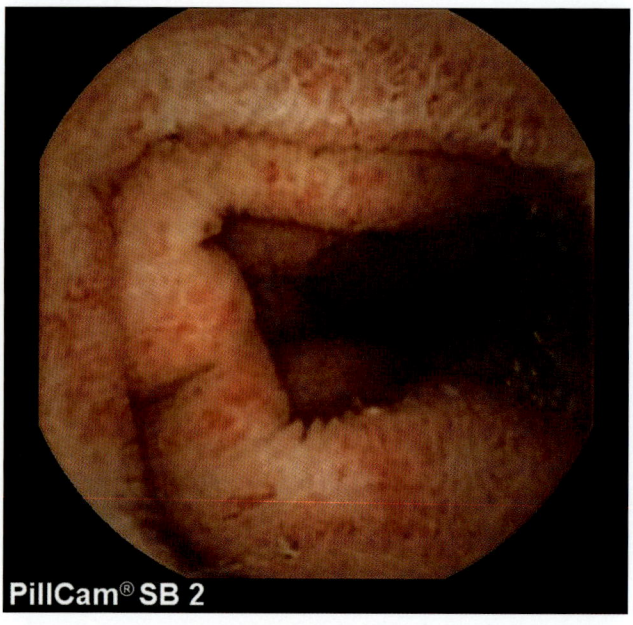

Fig. 30.12 Villous clubbing and inflammatory changes in a breast cancer patient with severe diarrhoea following long-term chemotherapy

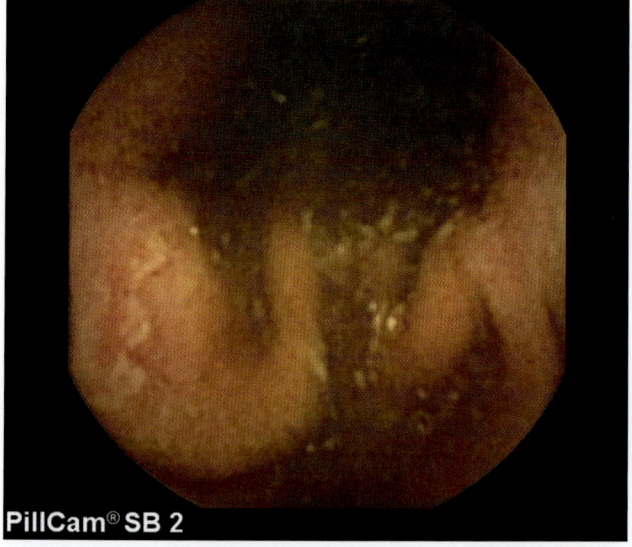

Fig. 30.11 A superficial erosion in a patient experiencing diarrhoea after a single session of chemotherapy

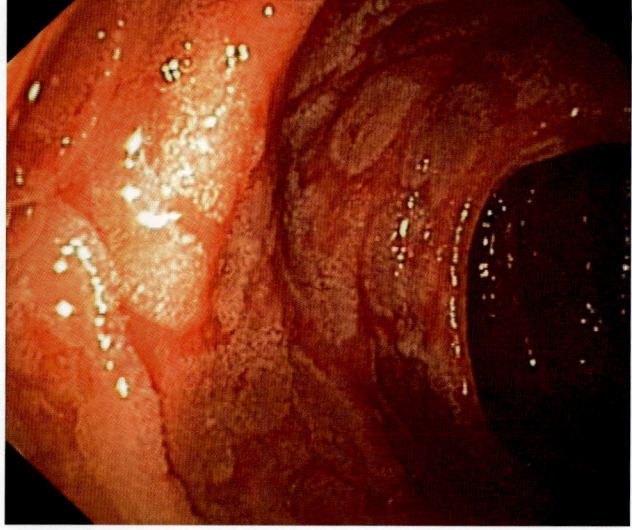

Fig. 30.13 Superficial lesions representing mucositis following chemotherapy in a patient additionally taking NSAIDs

Fig. 30.14 (**a, b**) Nonspecific mucosal breaks in a patient who was admitted to hospital with abdominal pain following long-term misuse of cocaine

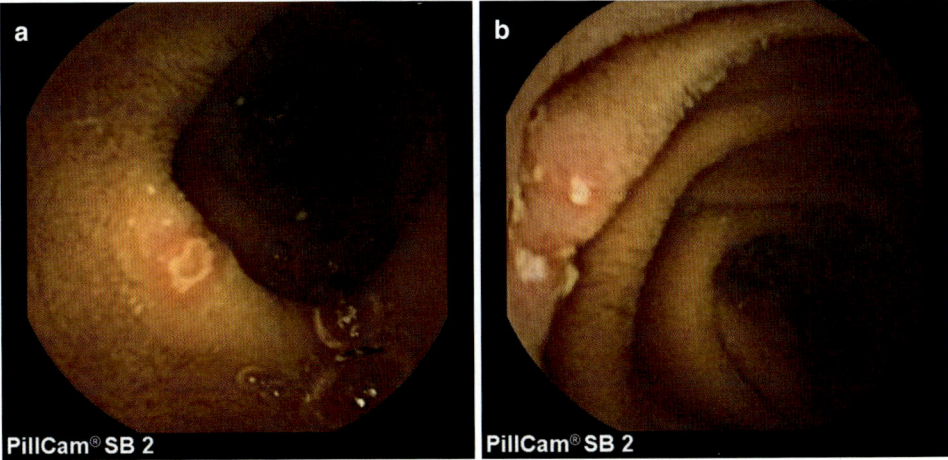

Fig. 30.15 (**a, b**) A healthy volunteer developed these punched-out small bowel lesions after 2 weeks of treatment with a proton pump inhibitor

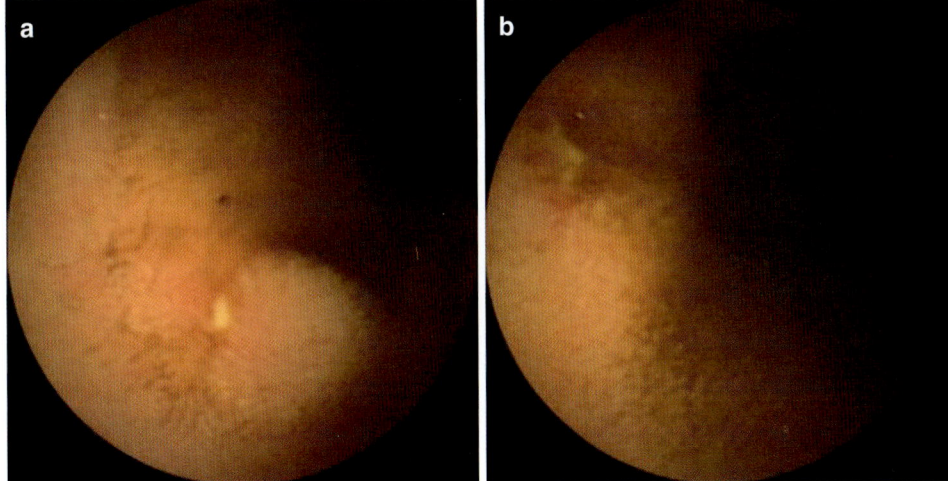

References

1. Smale S, Tibble J, Sigthorsson G, Bjarnason I. Epidemiology and differential diagnosis of NSAID-induced injury to the mucosa of the small intestine. Best Pract Res Clin Gastroenterol. 2001;15:723–38.
2. Bjarnason I, Hayllar J, Macpherson AJ, Russell AS. Side effects of nonsteroidal anti-inflammatory drugs on the small and large intestine in humans. Gastroenterology. 1993;104:1832–47.
3. Tibble JA, Foster R, Sigthorsson G, et al. Faecal calprotectin: a simple method for the diagnosis of NSAID-induced enteropathy. Gut. 1999;45:362–6.
4. Maiden L, Thjodleifsson B, Theodors A, et al. A quantitative analysis of NSAID-induced small bowel pathology by capsule enteroscopy. Gastroenterology. 2005;128:1172–8.
5. Goldstein JL, Eisen GM, Lewis B, et al. Video capsule endoscopy to prospectively assess small bowel injury with celecoxib, naproxen plus omeprazole, and placebo. Clin Gastroenterol Hepatol. 2005;3:133–41.
6. Graham DY, Opekun AR, Willingham FF, Qureshi WA. Visible small-intestinal mucosal injury in chronic NSAID users. Clin Gastroenterol Hepatol. 2005;3:55–9.
7. Maiden L, Thjodleifsson B, Seigal A, et al. Long-term effects of nonsteroidal anti-inflammatory drugs and cyclooxygenase-2 selective agents on the small bowel: a cross-sectional capsule enteroscopy study. Clin Gastroenterol Hepatol. 2007;5:1040–5.
8. Laine L, Connors LG, Reicin A, et al. Serious lower gastrointestinal clinical events with nonselective NSAID or coxib use. Gastroenterology. 2003;124:288–92.
9. Chan FK, Lanas A, Scheiman J, et al. Celecoxib versus omeprazole and diclofenac in patients with osteoarthritis and rheumatoid arthritis (CONDOR): a randomised trial. Lancet. 2010;376:173–9.
10. Bjarnason I, Price AB, Zanelli G, et al. Clinicopathological features of nonsteroidal antiinflammatory drug-induced small intestinal strictures. Gastroenterology. 1988;94:1070–4.
11. Allison MC, Howatson AG, Torrance CJ, et al. Gastrointestinal damage associated with the use of nonsteroidal anti-inflammatory drugs. N Engl J Med. 1992;327:749–54.
12. Bjarnason I, Takeuchi K, Bjarnason A, et al. The G.U.T. of gut. Scand J Gastroenterol. 2004;39:807–15.
13. Chutkan R, Toubia N. Effect of nonsteroidal anti-inflammatory drugs on the gastrointestinal tract: diagnosis by wireless capsule endoscopy. Gastrointest Endosc Clin N Am. 2004;14:67–85.
14. Morris AJ. Nonsteroidal anti-inflammatory drug enteropathy. Gastrointest Endosc Clin N Am. 1999;9:125–33.
15. Cosnes J, Laurent-Puig P, Baumer P, et al. Malnutrition in chronic radiation enteritis. Study of 100 patients. Ann Gastroenterol Hepatol (Paris). 1988;24:7–12.

16. Cosnes J, Gendre JP, Le Quintrec Y. Chronic radiation enteritis. II. General consequences and prognostic factors. Gastroenterol Clin Biol. 1983;7:671–6.

17. Chen S, Harisinghani MG, Wittenberg J. Small bowel CT fat density target sign in chronic radiation enteritis. Australas Radiol. 2003;47:450–2.

18. Frede KE, Bories-Azeau A. Strahlenfolgen am Darm. In: Siewert J, Harder F, Allgöwer M, et al., editors. Chirurgische Gastroenterololgie. Heidelberg: Springer; 1990. p. S1008–15.

19. Wobbes T, Verschueren RC, Lubbers EJ, et al. Surgical aspects of radiation enteritis of the small bowel. Dis Colon Rectum. 1984;27: 89–92.

20. Zeino Z, Sisson G, Bjarnason I. Adverse effects of drugs on small intestine and colon. Best Pract Res Clin Gastroenterol. 2010;24: 133–41.

Acute Gastrointestinal Graft-Versus-Host Disease After Bone Marrow Transplantation

31

Samuel N. Adler, Vincent Maunoury, Yasuo Kakugawa, and Yutaka Saito

Contents

31.1 Definition

Acute graft-versus-host disease (GVHD) is a major complication following allogeneic stem cell transplantation (allo-SCT) and carries a high morbidity and mortality rate [1]. This disease may affect the skin, liver, and gastrointestinal tract (acute GI GVHD). Mismatched histocompatibility antigens cause graft T cells to attack the host's tissues in acute GI GVHD. Histologic findings in the intestine include crypt epithelial cell apoptosis, crypt destruction, and variable lymphocytic infiltration of the epithelium and lamina propria. Severe GVHD (Table 31.1) affects the small bowel, causing extensive damage with a large spectrum of endoscopic findings [2]. Patients with acute GI GVHD have a higher mortality than patients without acute GI GVHD [3]. Treatment of acute GI GVHD requires aggressive immunosuppressive therapy, which is associated with infectious complications.

Chronic GVHD occurs months later after stem cell transplantation and primarily involves the skin. It may involve the GI tract, affecting the esophagus or leading to intestinal strictures.

The work was first published in 2006 by Springer Medizin Verlag Heidelberg with the following title: *Atlas of Video Capsule Endoscopy*.

S.N. Adler (✉)
Department of Gastroenterology, Shaare Zedek Medical Center, Jerusalem, Israel
e-mail: nasnadler@gmail.com

V. Maunoury
Department of Gastroenterology, Hôpital Huriez, Lille Cedex, France
e-mail: vmaunoury@chru-lille.fr

Y. Kakugawa • Y. Saito
Endoscopy Division, National Cancer Center Hospital, Tokyo, Japan
e-mail: yakakuga@gmail.com; ytsaito@ncc.go.jp

Table 31.1 Stages of acute gastrointestinal GVHD affecting the digestive tract

Stage	Endoscopic classification	Diarrhea
Stage 1	Focal mild erythema and edematous mucosa	>30 mL/kg or >500 mL/24 h
Stage 2	Rough, reddish, and atrophic mucosa	>60 mL/kg or >1,000 mL/24 h
Stage 3	Erosive changing and oozing	>90 mL/kg or >1,500 mL/24 h
Stage 4	Ulceration with extensive exudates	>90 mL/kg or >2,000 mL/24 h or severe abdominal pain with or without ileus

GVHD graft-versus-host disease

31.2   Diagnosis

The diagnosis of acute GI GVHD may be challenging. Whereas diarrhea is the most common symptom in acute GI GVHD, it is certainly not specific. Diarrhea may be treatment related or may be caused by GI infections such as cytomegalovirus (CMV), other viruses, *Clostridium difficile* toxin, toxoplasmosis, fungi, and other pathogens [4]. Diagnosis of acute GI GVHD usually requires upper or lower GI endoscopy with biopsies. Patients with Stage 3 and 4 GVHD are very ill, and can only with difficulty tolerate and upper GI endoscopy, which examines just the most proximal part of the small bowel. The diagnostic accuracy of endoscopy, when compared with histologic findings, is high [3]. The precise diagnosis of acute GI GVHD is important because treatment for GVHD-associated diarrhea requires increased immunosuppressive therapy, whereas diarrhea associated with infectious pathogens requires specific antiviral or antibacterial agents. Added immunosuppression will have grave consequences for patients with infection, who are already severely compromised.

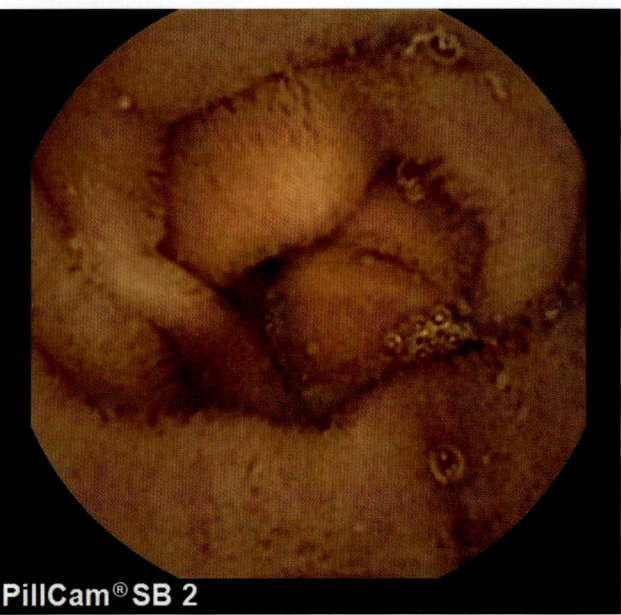

Fig. 31.1 Normal mucosa in a patient with suspected acute gastrointestinal (GI) graft-versus-host disease (GVHD)

31.3   Video Capsule Endoscopy in Acute GI GVHD

The authors used video capsule endoscopy (VCE) in patients with acute GI GVHD to evaluate the feasibility and diagnostic yield of this method. A total of 28 patients who had received allo-SCT were examined: 25 patients with acute GI GVHD and 3 patients with chronic GVHD. All patients had undergone intensive investigations in the evaluation of diarrhea, which included stool cultures; testing for *C. difficile* toxin; serum polymerase chain reaction (PCR) and serology for Epstein-Barr virus (EBV) and adenovirus; viral cultures of throat, stool, and urine; and an assay for CMV pp65 antigen in blood.

VCE was performed in all patients. One patient had difficulty swallowing the capsule, and in one patient the video capsule remained lodged in the esophagus for the entire study. No untoward adverse effects were noted in any of the 28 patients. VCE was performed safely even in the patients with the most severe acute GI GVHD, and it was far better tolerated than invasive endoscopic procedures.

A normal video capsule study (Fig. 31.1) essentially rules out acute GI GVHD. The normal findings at capsule endoscopy in some patients led to the reduction of immunosuppression [5]. In patients with chronic GVHD, the capsule endoscopy findings in the small bowel are normal even if they suffer from diarrhea [2]. However, all patients with Stage 2 to 4 acute GI GVHD have abnormal findings on capsule endoscopy of the small bowel. The extent and severity of the lesions parallel the stage of the disease. VCE was at least as sensitive as upper GI endoscopy and histology in diagnosing acute GI GVHD [5]. In two cases, despite invasive tests, only VCE made the diagnosis of acute GI GVHD [6]. Finally, VCE findings have a direct impact on clinical management in these critically ill patients.

31.4   Findings at Capsule Endoscopy in Acute GI GVHD

VCE findings characteristic of the mucosal damage include the following:
- Erythema (Fig. 31.2)
- Destruction of the mucosa (Fig. 31.3)
- Diffuse superficial mucosal disease, mucosal breaks
- Loss of villous formation, scalloped folds
- Ulcerations, aphthous lesions
- Mucosal erosive changes and inflammatory exudates (Fig. 31.4)
- Vascular malformation
- Mucosal hemorrhages, fresh bleeding (Fig. 31.5)
- Strictures (Fig. 31.6)

Video capsule endoscopy revealed new findings previously not described in patients with acute GI GVHD, such as strictures (Fig. 31.6). The anemia of some patients is worsened by spontaneous bleeding of friable mucosa (Fig. 31.5). Typical diffuse ulcerations of the small bowel in grade 4 GVHD are depicted in Figs. 31.7 and 31.8. The diffuse granular appearance of the small bowel mucosa with loss of villi is also typical for grade 4 GVHD (Fig. 31.9).

31.5   Transit Times in Acute GI GVHD

Gastric emptying of the video capsule was delayed, especially in grade 3 and 4 acute GI GVHD. This fact must be taken into account when VCE is performed in patients with severe acute GI GVHD. These patients may require prokinetic agents and should be kept in the right lateral position for an extended period to facilitate passage into the small bowel [7].

Small bowel transit time characteristically is prolonged, either because some segments of the small bowel have no propagated contractions or because of the presence of inflammatory strictures (Fig. 31.6).

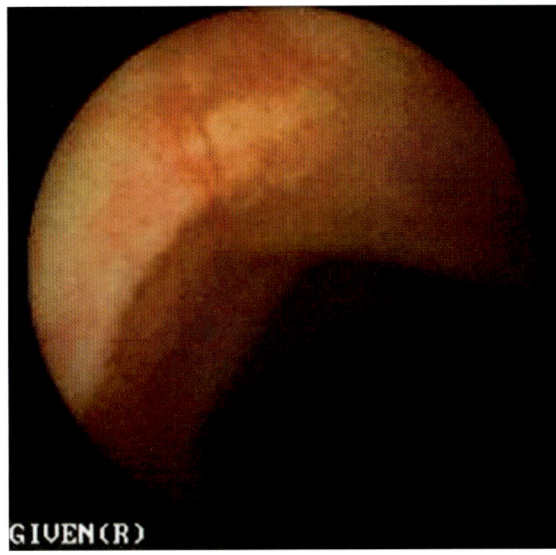

Fig. 31.2   Grade 1 acute GI GVHD with focal, mild erythema

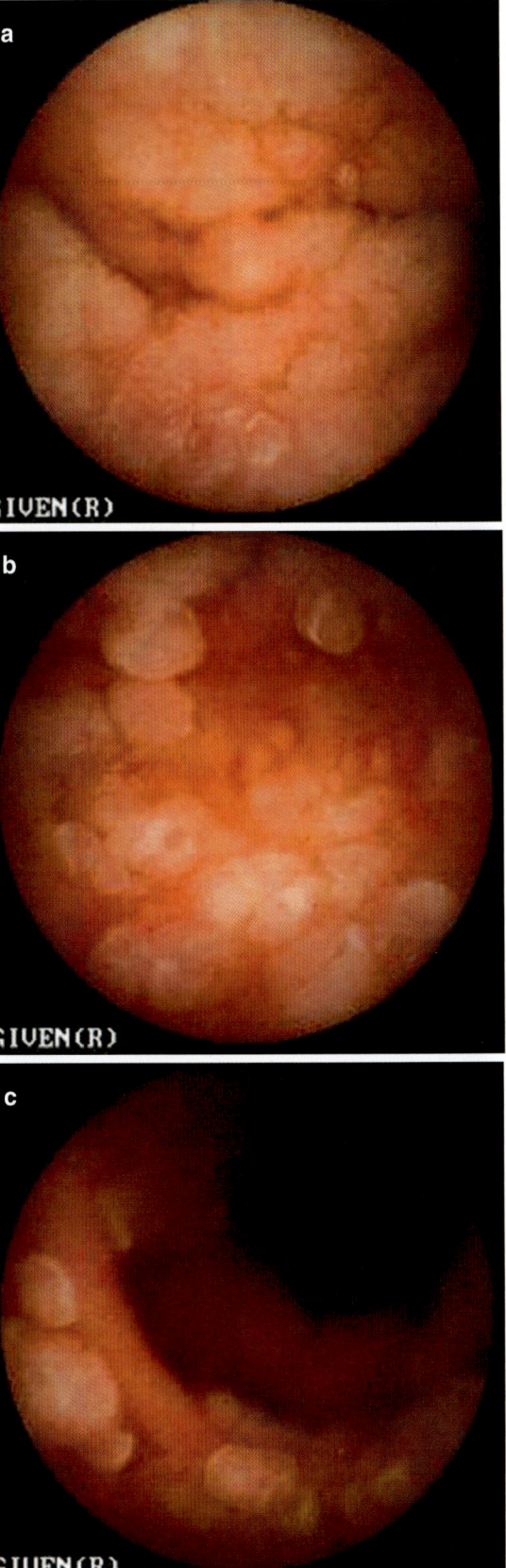

Fig. 31.3   (**a–c**) Grade 2 acute GI GVHD with rough, reddish, atrophic mucosa and erosive changes

Fig. 31.4 (**a, b**) Grade 3 acute
GI GVHD: erosive changes and
inflammatory exudates

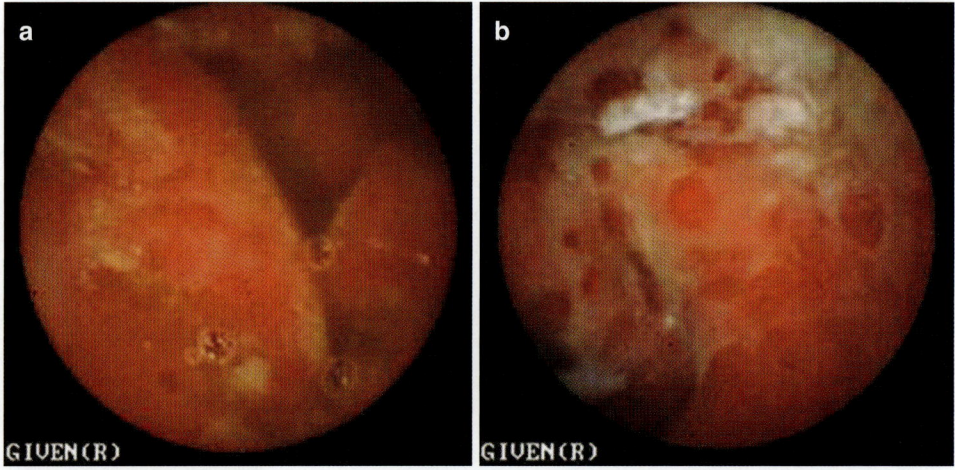

Fig. 31.5 Grade 3 acute GI GVHD. Spontaneous mucosal bleeding
(*arrow*) in a patient with acute GVHD

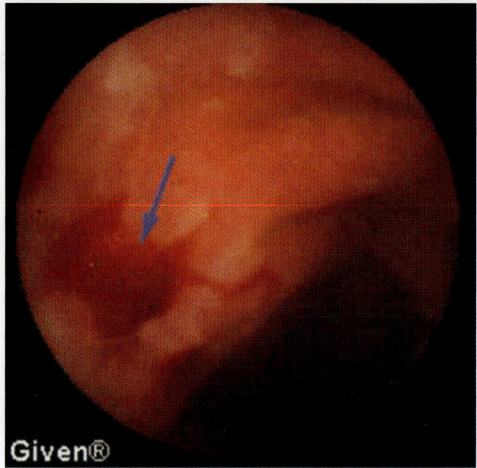

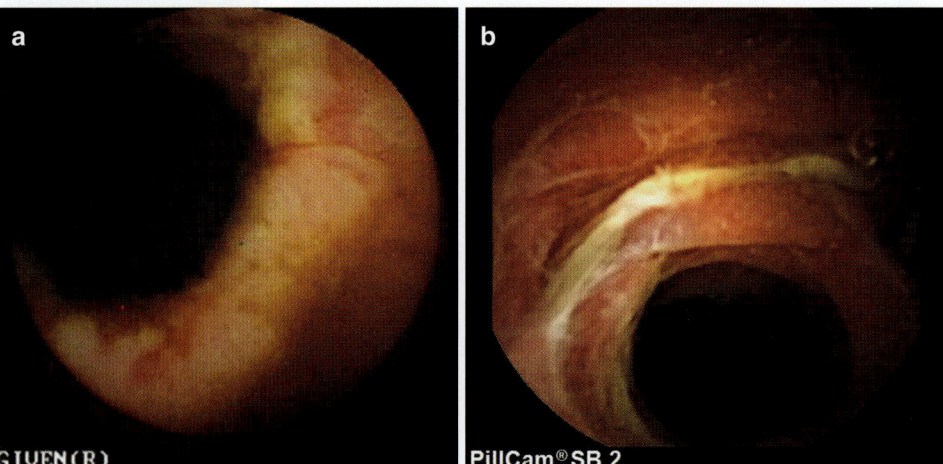

Fig. 31.6 (**a, b**) Inflammatory
strictures in a patient with
acute GVHD

Fig. 31.7 (**a, b**) Red spots, edema, erosions, and ulcerations of the small bowel in a patient with grade 4 GVHD

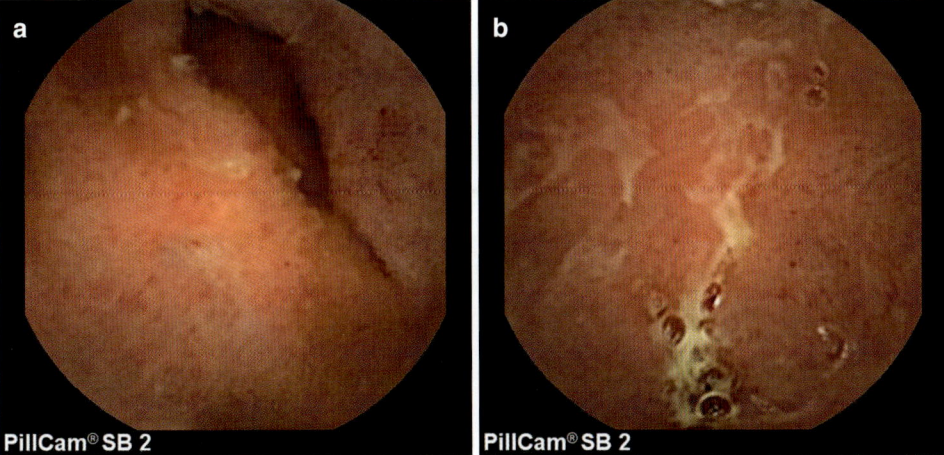

Fig. 31.8 (**a, b**) Extensive ulcerations of the small bowel in different patients with grade 4 GVHD

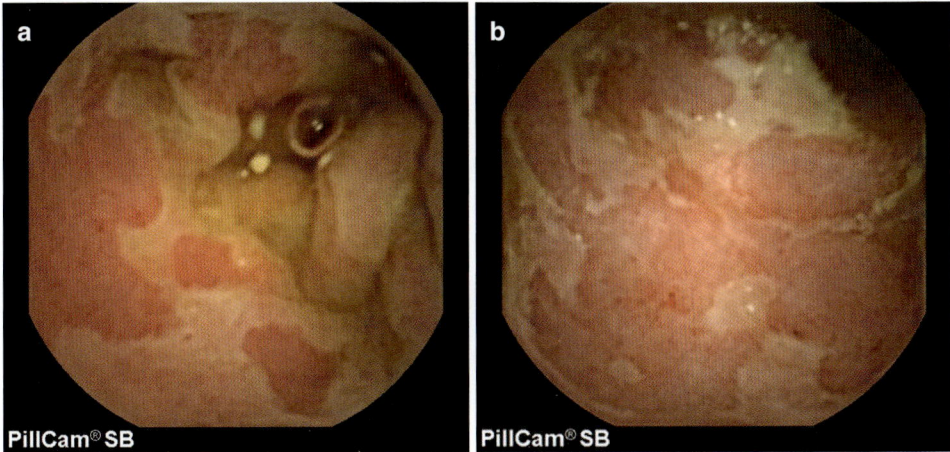

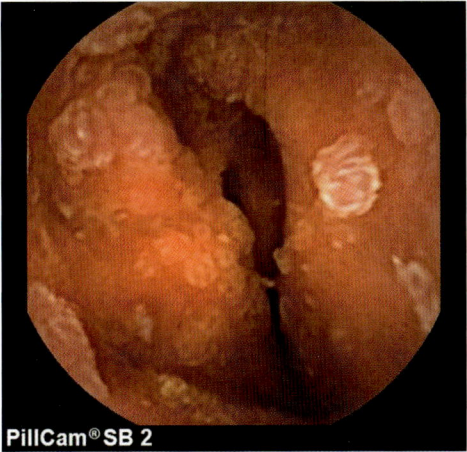

Fig. 31.9 Diffuse granular appearance of the mucosa in a patient with grade 4 GVHD

31.6   Differential Diagnosis

Yakoub-Agha et al. [5] and Adler et al. [2] describe two patients with deep ulcers with sharply demarcated borders (Figs. 31.10

and 31.11). Both patients were demonstrated to have CMV infections and were successfully treated with ganciclovir.

Fig. 31.10 (**a, b**) Sharply demarcated deep ulcer (*arrows*) in a patient with acute GVHD and CMV infection

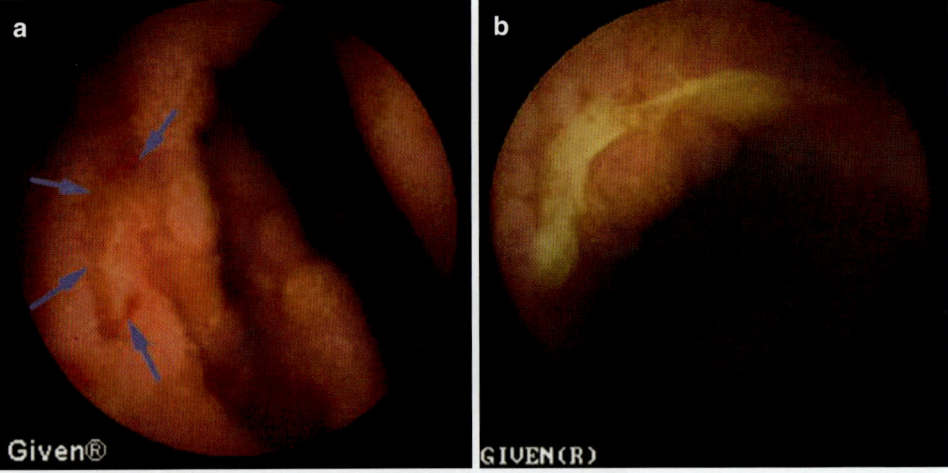

Fig. 31.11 (**a, b**) Necrotic ulcerations related to CMV in a patient with acute GVHD

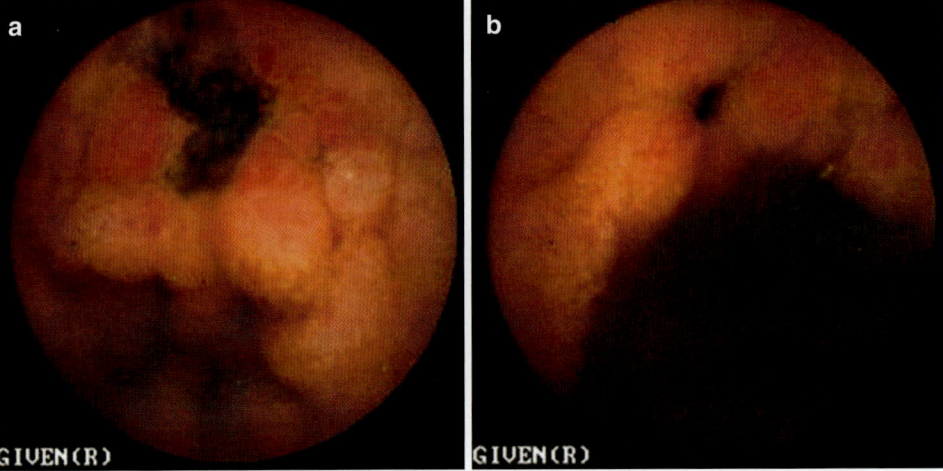

References

1. Ferrara JL, Deeg HJ. Graft-versus-host disease. N Engl J Med. 1991;324:667–74.
2. Adler SN, Jacob H, Shapira MY, et al. Capsule endoscopy of the small intestine in graft versus host disease. Gastrointest Endosc. 2004;59:AB174.
3. Cruz-Correa M, Poonawala A, Abraham SC, et al. Endoscopic findings predict the histologic diagnosis in gastrointestinal graft-versus-host disease. Endoscopy. 2002;34:808–13.
4. Einsele H, Ehninger G, Hebart H, et al. Incidence of local CMV infection and acute intestinal GVHD in marrow transplants recipients with severe diarrhoea. Bone Marrow Transplant. 1994; 14:955–63.
5. Yakoub-Agha I, Maunoury V, Wacrenier S, et al. Impact of small bowel exploration using video-capsule endoscopy in the management of acute gastrointestinal graft-versus-host disease. Transplantation. 2004;78:1697–701.
6. Shapira MY, Adler SN, Jacob H, et al. New insights into the pathophysiology of gastrointestinal graft-versus-host disease using capsule endoscopy. Haematologica. 2005;90:1003–4.
7. Sachdev R, Hibberd P, Mammen A, Cave DR. Reduction of gastric transit time of video capsule endoscopy by right lateral positioning. Gastrointest Endosc. 2004;59:AB176.

Internet

http://bethematch.org/Physicians: US National Marrow Donor

Chronic Nonspecific Multiple Ulcer of the Small Intestine

32

Kenji Watanabe

Contents

Chronic nonspecific multiple ulcer of the small intestine (CNSU) is an enteropathy characterized by persistent anemia and hypoproteinemia occurring in childhood or adolescence [1]. CNSU was advocated as an established disease entity in the 1960s. At one time, it was called "nonspecific ulcers in the small intestine," but this ragtag disease name was not suitable for an established disease entity.

32.1   Etiology

The etiology and pathogenesis of CNSU have not yet been clarified. Intermarriage has been reported in the family background of some patients, so a genetic factor may be involved.

32.2   Clinical Features

The lesions of CNSU are most common in the middle or lower ileum [2]; in some patients they appear in the jejunum or colon. Typical macroscopic findings are multiple, sharply marginated, circular, or oblique ulcers in the middle or lower ileum, except the terminal ileum [3] (Fig. 32.1). The ulcer is shallow, and the wall thickening of the small intestine is mild. Therefore, even though some strictures can be formed, endoscopic balloon dilation therapy is usually easier and safer than in Crohn's disease [4]. Recurrence after surgical resection often occurs.

CNSU occurs more often in women than in men [5]. Persistent anemia and hypoproteinemia result in easy fatigability, edema, growth impairment, or amenorrhea. Abdominal obstructive symptoms can occur because of stricture, but diarrhea or bloody stool is rare.

In spite of severe anemia or hypoproteinemia, the level of C-reactive protein (CRP) is normal or only mildly elevated. Fecal occult blood test is positive.

The work was first published in 2006 by Springer Medizin Verlag Heidelberg with the following title: *Atlas of Video Capsule Endoscopy*.

K. Watanabe
Department of Gastroenterology, Graduate School of Medicine, Osaka City University, Osaka, Japan
e-mail: kenjiw@med.osaka-cu.ac.jp

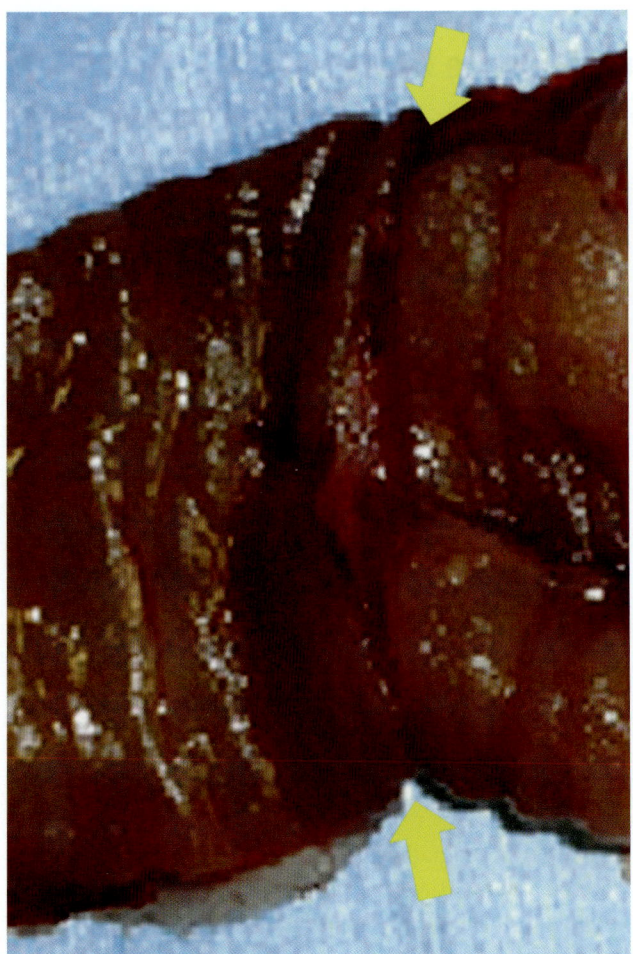

Fig. 32.1 This surgical specimen from a patient with chronic nonspecific multiple ulcer of the small intestine (CNSU) shows a sharply marginated, circular ulcer in the ileum. The *yellow arrows* point to sharply marginated circular ulcer

32.3 Histology

The ulcers are localized in the mucosal or submucosal layer (Fig. 32.2). Typical microscopic findings are mild inflammatory cell infiltrate with plasma cells, lymphocytes, and eosinophils.

32.4 Differential Diagnosis

The differential diagnosis of CNSU includes Crohn's disease, intestinal tuberculosis, radiation enteropathy, and nonsteroidal anti-inflammatory drug (NSAID) enteropathy. The typical findings for ulcer description, location, history,

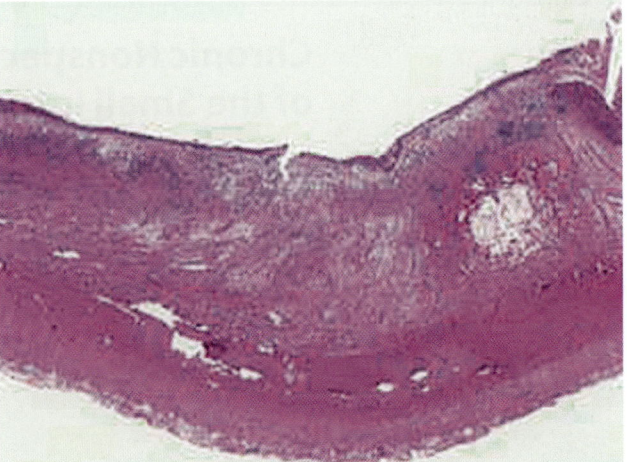

Fig. 32.2 Microscopic histological view of the surgical specimen shows that the ulcers are localized in the submucosal layer

response to treatment, and supportive laboratory data are useful in making the diagnosis.

32.5 Treatment

Anti-inflammatory treatments including steroids, 5-aminosalicylate, immunomodulators, and anti-TNFα agents have not been effective. At present, the only effective method to induce and maintain remission of CNSU is nutrition therapy with total parenteral nutrition or elemental diet.

32.6 Endoscopy

Circular or oblique, sharply marginated, shallow ulcers are observed mainly in the ileum [6] (Figs. 32.3 and 32.4). Scars, strictures, and pseudodiverticulosis also can be observed (Figs. 32.5 and 32.6). Double-balloon or single-balloon enteroscopy is useful for observation.

32.6.1 The Role of Capsule Endoscopy

Capsule endoscopy is useful for differential diagnosis or confirming treatment efficacy in some cases (Figs. 32.7 and 32.8). Confirming functional patency of the small intestine by using patency capsule is usually required prior to capsule endoscopy (Figs. 32.9 and 32.10) [7].

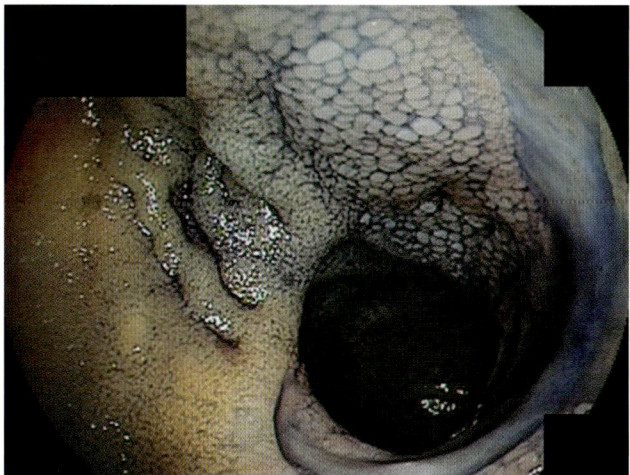

Fig. 32.3 Double-balloon enteroscopy (with chromoendoscopy using indigo carmine) shows a typical endoscopic finding in CNSU: an oblique, sharply marginated, shallow ulcer

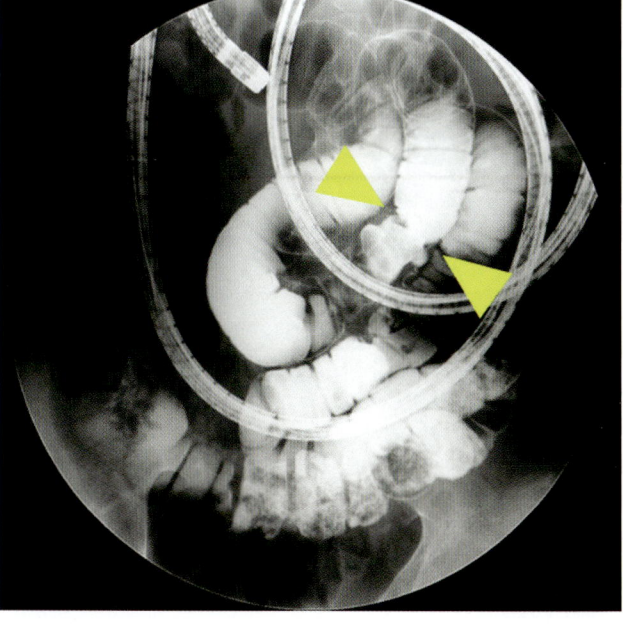

Fig. 32.5 Selective small bowel series with double-balloon enteroscopy shows mild stricture and pseudodiverticulosis. The *yellow arrows* point to mild stricture. And pseudodiverticulosis are shown at its oral side

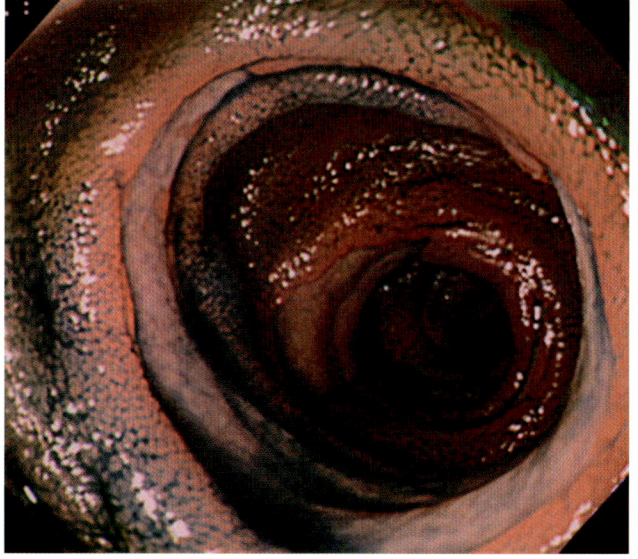

Fig. 32.4 Single-balloon enteroscopy (with chromoendoscopy using indigo carmine) shows a typical endoscopic finding in CNSU: a circular, sharply marginated, shallow ulcer

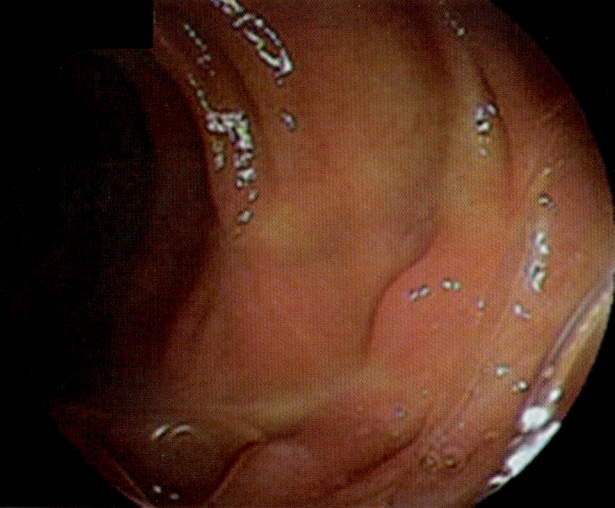

Fig. 32.6 Double-balloon enteroscopy shows mucosal healing with scars, achieved by treatment using total parenteral nutrition

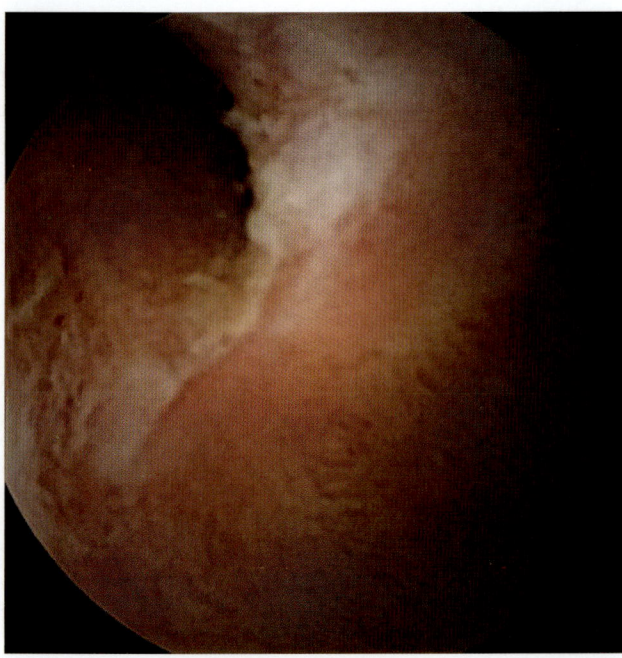

Fig. 32.7 Capsule endoscopy revealed part of an active, circular ileal ulcer in a patient with CNSU

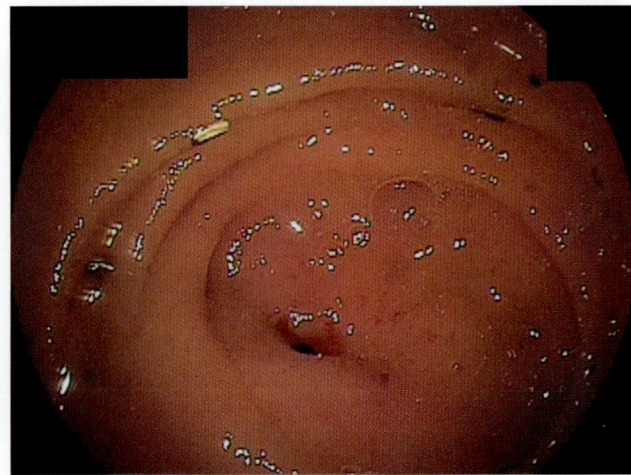

Fig. 32.9 Double-balloon enteroscopy shows severe stricture in the middle ileum

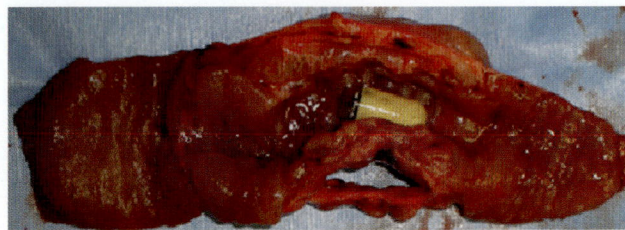

Fig. 32.10 Macroscopic findings of ileum resected because of severe stricture with capsule retention

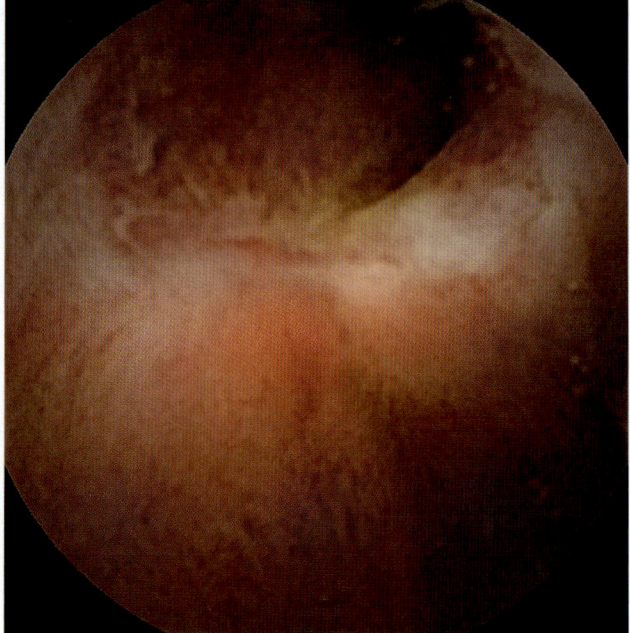

Fig. 32.8 Capsule endoscopy also revealed part of an active, circular ileal ulcer or scar in a patient with CNSU

References

1. Matsumoto T, Kubokura N, Matsui T, et al. Chronic nonspecific multiple ulcer of the small intestine segregates in offspring from consanguinity. J Crohns Colitis. 2011;5:559–65.
2. Matsumoto T, Iida M, Matsui T, et al. Non-specific multiple ulcers of the small intestine unrelated to non-steroidal anti-inflammatory drugs. J Clin Pathol. 2004;57:1145–50.
3. Matsumoto T, Nakamura S, Esaki M, et al. Endoscopic features of chronic nonspecific multiple ulcers of the small intestine: comparison with nonsteroidal anti-inflammatory drug-induced enteropathy. Dig Dis Sci. 2006;51:1357–63.
4. Ohmiya N, Arakawa D, Nakamura M, et al. Small-bowel obstruction. Diagnostic comparison between double-balloon endoscopy and fluoroscopic enteroclysis, and the outcome of enteroscopic treatment. Gastrointest Endosc. 2009;69:84–93.
5. Chen Y, Ma WQ, Chen JM, et al. Multiple chronic non-specific ulcer of small intestine characterized by anemia and hypoalbuminemia. World J Gastroenterol. 2010;16:782–4.
6. Matsumoto T, Iida M, Matsui T, Yao T. Chronic nonspecific multiple ulcers of the small intestine: a proposal of the entity from Japanese gastroenterologists to Western enteroscopists. Gastrointest Endosc. 2007;66 Suppl 3:S99–107.
7. Tokuhara D, Watanabe K, Okano Y, et al. Wireless capsule endoscopy in pediatric patients: the first series from Japan. J Gastroenterol. 2010;45:683–91.

Benign Tumors

33

Felix Wiedbrauck, Warwick S. Selby, and Ervin Tóth

Contents

The work was first published in 2006 by Springer Medizin Verlag Heidelberg with the following title: *Atlas of Video Capsule Endoscopy.*

F. Wiedbrauck (✉)
Department of Gastroenterology,
Allgemeines Krankenhaus Celle,
Celle, Germany
e-mail: felix.wiedbrauck@akh-celle.de

W.S. Selby
AW Morrow Gastroenterology and Liver Centre,
Royal Prince Alfred Hospital, Camperdown University of Sydney,
Sydney, Australia

Faculty of Medicine, University of Sydney,
Sydney, Australia
e-mail: warwicks@sydney.edu.au

E. Tóth
Department of Gastroenterology,
Skåne University Hospital,
Malmö, Sweden
e-mail: ervin.toth@med.lu.se

33.1 Introduction

Neoplasms of the small bowel are rare, accounting for only 2 % of all primary gastrointestinal tumors. The incidence is less than 1.0 per 100,000 in the world [1]. Men have a slightly higher incidence than women, and the median age of diagnosis is in the mid-60s [2]. About 20 % are localized in the duodenum. Approximately 40 different histologic types have been identified; only one third of those are benign [3].

33.1.1 Definition

Benign tumors of the small intestine consist of various rare entities such as tumorlike inflammatory or hyperplastic lesions, hamartomas (organoid malformations), ectopic tissues, and true neoplasms of epithelial or mesenchymal origin (Table 33.1).

33.1.2 Clinical Features

Benign tumors of the small intestine often stay asymptomatic for years, with small lesions frequently remaining undiscovered. They may be manifested clinically by bleeding, iron deficiency anemia, or abdominal pain. Possible complications are obstruction, intussusception, and perforation. These symptoms depend on the tumor's size, location, and histopathology. Adenomas may progress to carcinoma.

Table 33.1 Benign small bowel tumors

Inflammatory lesions
Inflammatory polyps
Inflammatory fibroid polyps
Hyperplasias
Hyperplastic polyps
Brunneromas
Nodular lymphoid hyperplasia
Hamartomas
Juvenile polyps
Peutz–Jeghers polyps
Ectopic tissues
Pancreatic heterotopia
Gastric heterotopia
Endometriosis
Epithelial neoplasms
Adenomas
Mesenchymal tumors
Hemangiomas
Lymphangiomas
Leiomyomas
Lipomas
Neurofibromas

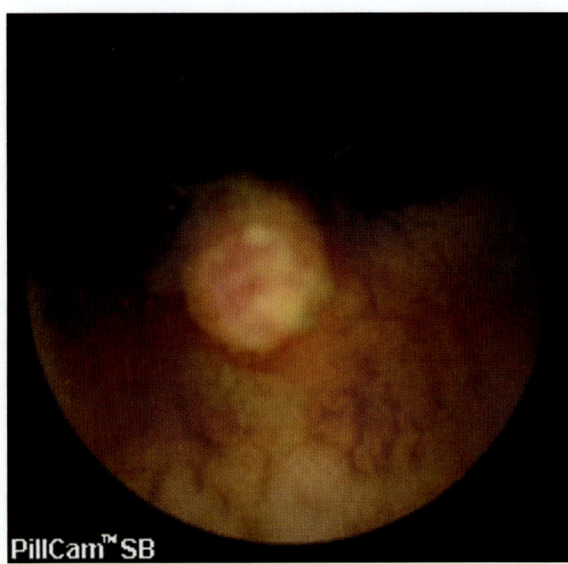

Fig. 33.1 Inflammatory ileal polyp of unknown etiology

33.1.3 Endoscopy

Hyperplasias, hamartomas, ectopic gastric mucosa, and adenomas may appear as flat or raised lesions on the mucosal surface. Ectopic pancreatic tissue and mesenchymal tumors usually are located beneath normal mucosa, have smooth margins, and are raised. The surface may show a generally circumscribed ulceration, which can cause bleeding. Vascular tumors often have a reddish or bluish appearance.

Endoscopic examination cannot reliably differentiate between benign and malignant tumors of the small intestine.

33.2 Inflammatory Lesions

33.2.1 Inflammatory Polyps

Various nonneoplastic inflammatory lesions may present as a polyp anywhere in the small intestine. The etiology of erosive pseudopolyps (Fig. 33.1) often remains unclear, but they have been described in association with ileoileal invagination [4]. Inflammatory suture granulomas may be seen at anastomoses, sometimes together with ulcers (Fig. 33.2).

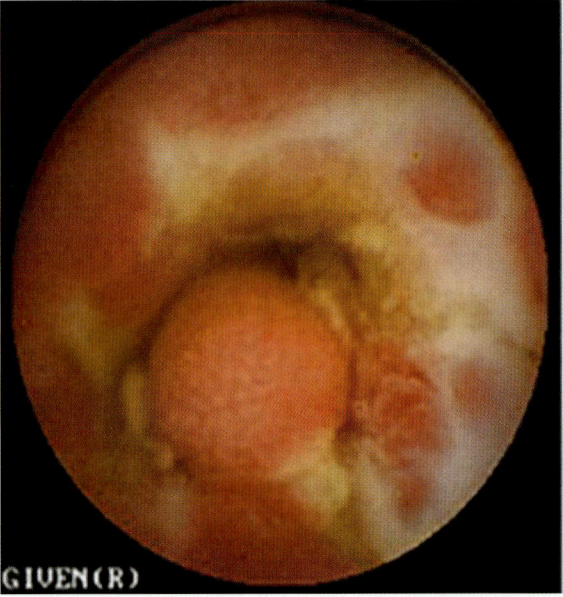

Fig. 33.2 Tumorlike suture granuloma and ulcerated stricture in the ileum in a patient with previously resected small bowel Crohn's disease

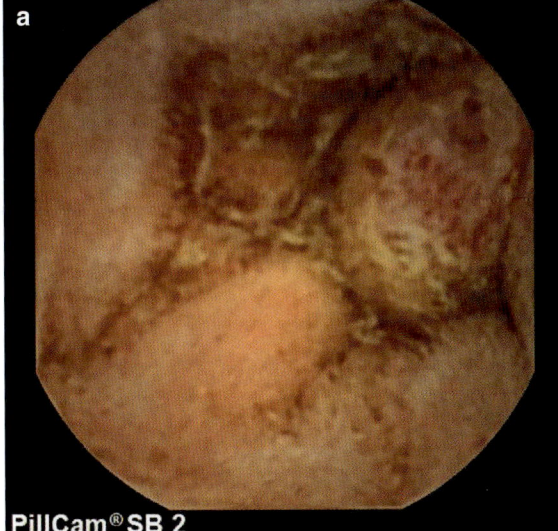

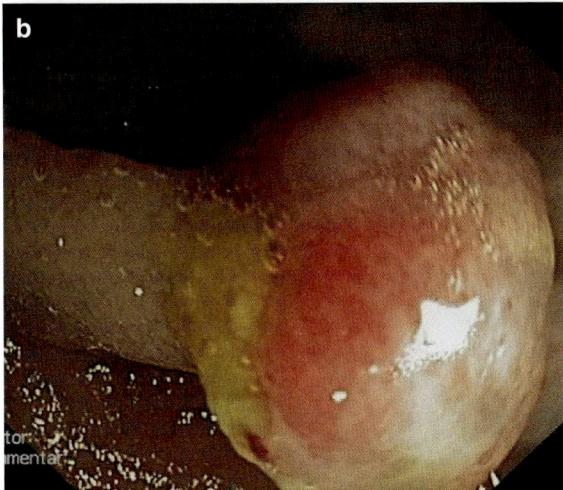

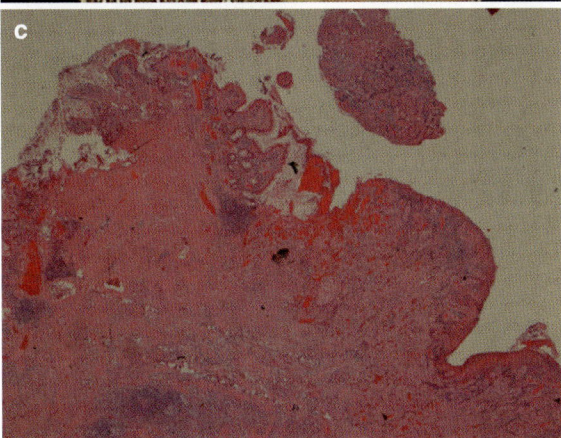

Fig. 33.3 Pedunculated inflammatory pseudopolyp in the ileum. (**a**) The polyp as seen with video capsule endoscopy (VCE). (**b**) The stalk is only visible with ileoscopy. (**c**) Histology (*Courtesy of Peer Fleming, MD, and Axel Wellmann, MD*)

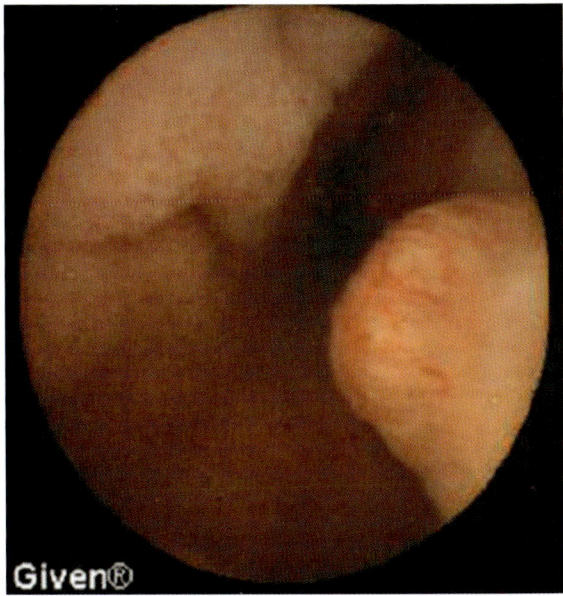

Fig. 33.4 Pyloric inflammatory fibroid polyp seen at VCE

33.2.2 Inflammatory Fibroid Polyp (IFP, Vanek's Tumor)

The etiology of these submucosal benign polyps is unknown. They may occur throughout the entire gastrointestinal tract, but about 70 % are localized in the stomach. Histologically, they show a fibroblast proliferation and eosinophilia [5]. Immunohistology and endoscopic ultrasound (EUS) in the stomach and duodenum may be helpful to distinguish them from other submucosal lesions [6].

On endoscopy, sessile or pedunculated polyps (Figs. 33.3, 33.4, and 33.5) may be seen, sometimes with ulceration, hemorrhage, or hematoma.

These polyps can cause intussusception or bleeding [7]. Treatment is resection, depending on the size and location.

33.3 Hyperplasias

33.3.1 Hyperplastic Polyps

Hyperplastic polyps are rare in the small intestine. They are found mostly in the duodenum [8] and are usually small, but bleeding has been reported [9].

On endoscopy, these small sessile or pedunculated polyps look soft, sometimes with a lobulated surface. Usually there is no evident discoloration or ulceration (Fig. 33.6).

Fig. 33.5 Inflammatory fibroid polyp. (**a**) Endoscopic view. (**b**) Resected specimen. (**c**) Histology (*Courtesy of Peer Fleming, MD, and Axel Wellmann, MD*)

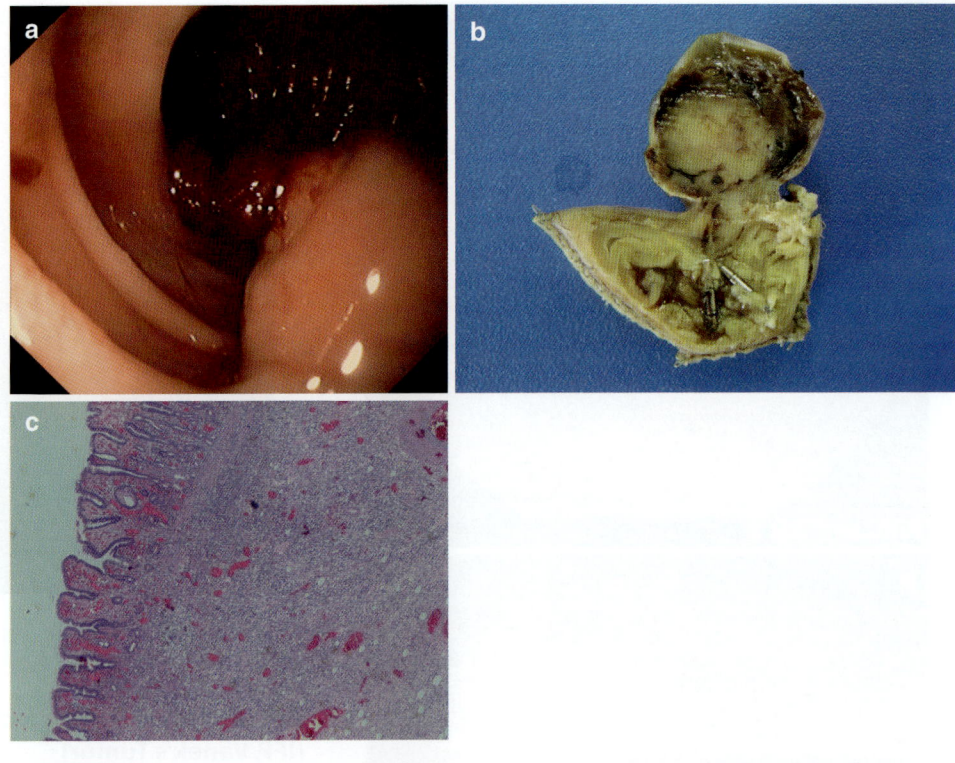

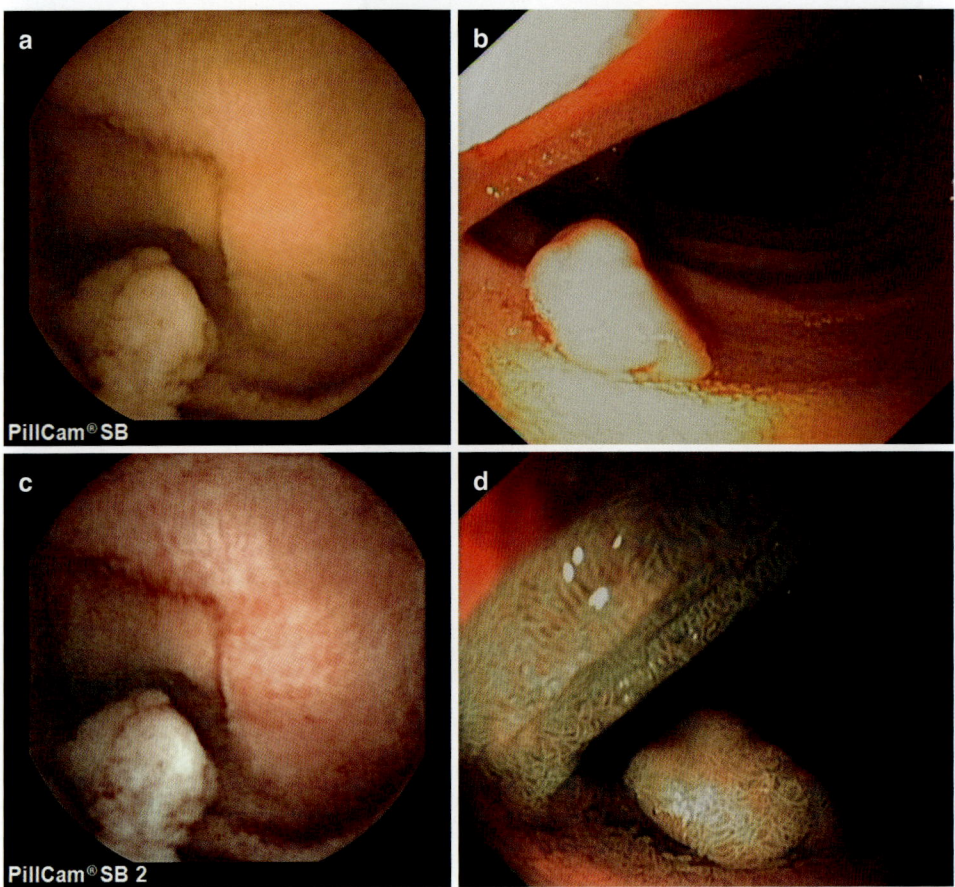

Fig. 33.6 Hyperplastic polyp of the jejunum. (**a**) VCE (visible on one single frame only). (**b**) Single-balloon enteroscopy. (**c**) VCE with flexible spectral imaging color enhancement (FICE1) mode. (**d**) Single-balloon enteroscopy with narrow band imaging (NBI) mode

33.3.2 Brunneromas

It is postulated that Brunner's gland hyperplasia in the duodenal bulb is induced by increased acid secretion or inflammation with causes such as *Helicobacter pylori* [6]. Rarely, hyperplasia can develop into a large pedunculated polyp, known as Brunner's gland adenoma (Figs. 33.7 and 33.8).

Brunneromas account for 7 % of all tumorlike lesions in the duodenum [10]. They are asymptomatic and need no therapy. Only the large pedunculated Brunner's gland adenomas, which can result in bleeding or obstruction, should be managed endoscopically or surgically (Fig. 33.9).

Endoscopy often reveals multiple, polypoid elevations isocolor to the surrounding mucosa (Figs. 33.7 and 33.8).

Fig. 33.7 Biopsy-confirmed hyperplasia of Brunner's glands in the duodenal bulb and retrograde view of the pylorus

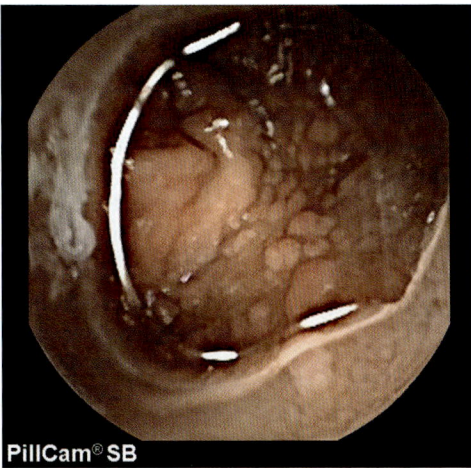

Fig. 33.8 Biopsy-confirmed hyperplasia of Brunner's glands in the duodenal bulb with superficial villi. (**a**) VCE. (**b**) Side-viewing duodenoscopy

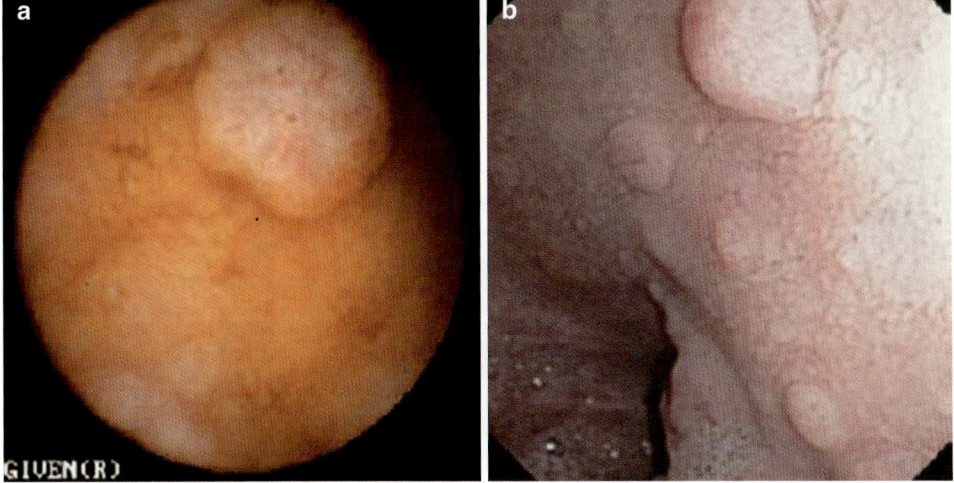

Fig. 33.9 Brunner's gland adenoma. (**a**) Duodenoscopic view. (**b**) Histology (*Courtesy of* Peer Fleming, MD, and Axel Wellmann, MD)

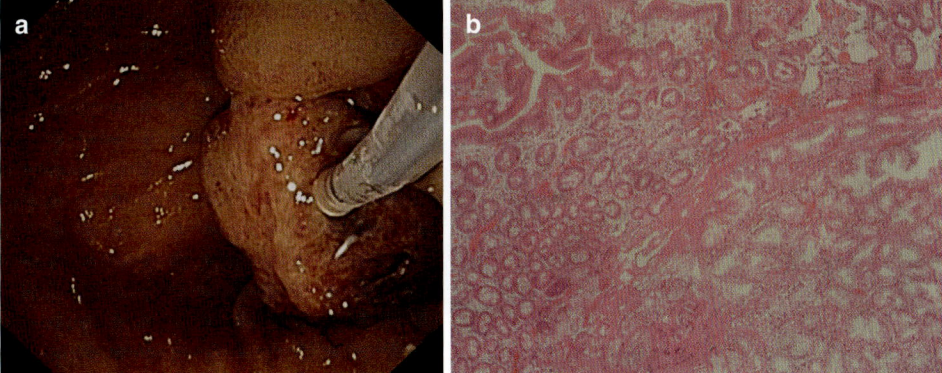

33.3.3 Lymphoid Hyperplasia

Some degree of hyperplasia of lymphoid tissue in the terminal ileum is not uncommon, especially in children (Chap. 38) but also in healthy adults or patients undergoing video capsule endoscopy (VCE) for mid-gastrointestinal bleeding originating from unrelated sources (Fig. 33.10a). If infections (e.g., *Yersinia*, *Salmonella*, *Mycobacteria*) are found in adults (Fig. 33.10b), they should be taken into account. Diffuse duodenal nodular lymphoid hyperplasia due to *H. pylori* infection has also been described [11]. In localized tumorous and asymmetric manifestations, lymphoma should also be considered.

On endoscopy, nodular or polypoid lesions, typically diffuse and symmetrically distributed, sometimes aggregated, are typically found in the terminal ileum (Fig. 33.10a).

33.4 Hamartomas

Hamartomas are tumorlike developmental anomalies in which different tissue components are abnormally combined. They may occur sporadically, but most of them are part of one of the polyposis syndromes, as Peutz–Jeghers polyposis (Chap. 36) or juvenile polyposis (Chap. 37) (Figs. 33.11, 33.12, and 33.13).

Large hamartomatous polyps may cause intestinal obstruction or intussusception, or they may bleed. They are often pedunculated.

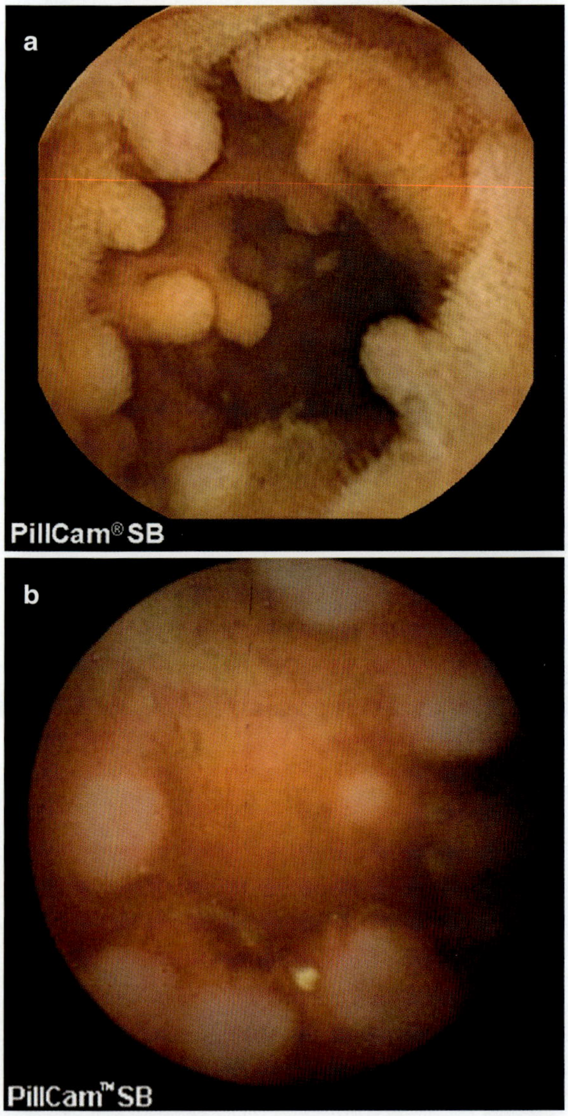

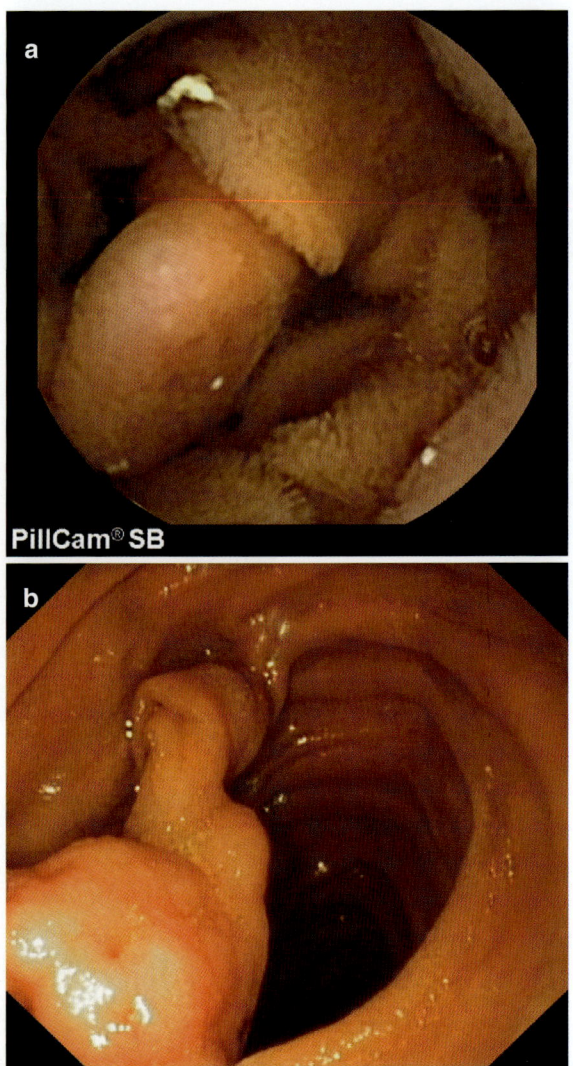

Fig. 33.11 Hamartomatous (Peutz–Jeghers) polyp in a young man with anemia without history of polyposis syndrome. (**a**) VCE. (**b**) Single-balloon enteroscopy

Fig. 33.10 Lymphoid hyperplasia in the terminal ileum. (**a**) A variant of normal in a patient with mid-gastrointestinal bleeding. (**b**) Lymphoid hyperplasia in a patient in whom mycobacteriosis was diagnosed months later

Fig. 33.12 Hamartomatous polyp (15×15 mm in size) in the proximal jejunum. The patient had a 1-year history of persistent iron deficiency anemia (the lowest hemoglobin level 60 g/L). Preoperative enteroclysis was normal. After 2 years of follow-up, the patient is symptom-free, with normal laboratory tests. (**a**) VCE finding. (**b**) Intraoperative view. (**c**) Resected surgical specimen. (**d**) Histology of benign hamartomatous polyp (*Courtesy of* Otto Ljungberg, MD)

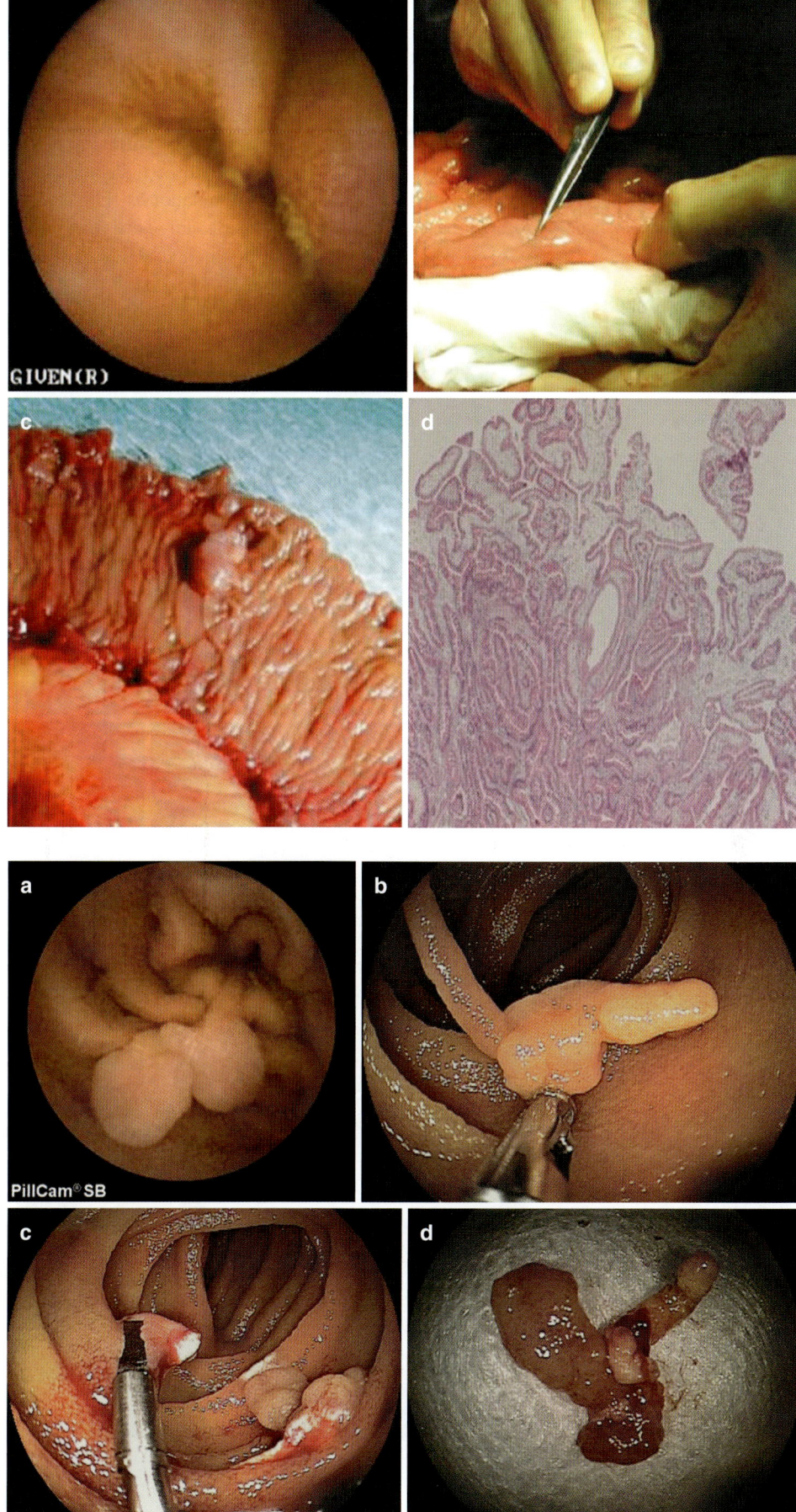

Fig. 33.13 Juvenile polyp. (**a**) VCE shows a pedunculated polyp in the distal part of the jejunum. (**b**) With double-balloon enteroscopy, a long-stalked polyp was identified about 2 m from the pylorus in the distal jejunum and was removed by snare polypectomy. (**c**) A clip was placed on the base of the stalk and the polyp retrieved (**d**). Histology showed a juvenile polyp (*Courtesy of* Jörgen Nielsen, MD; Gabrielle Wurm Johansson, MD, PhD; and Artur Nemeth, MD)

33.5   Ectopic Tissues

Ectopic tissues are structurally normal but occur at an abnormal location in the body.

33.5.1 Pancreatic Heterotopia

Heterotopic rests of pancreatic tissue represent a congenital abnormality and are usually located beneath the normal mucosa. The most frequent location is the stomach, followed by the small bowel [12].

Pancreatic heterotopia usually is asymptomatic, but it may become relevant if growth or inflammation occurs [13]. Bleeding has been reported [12]. Larger heterotopias can be a leading point for invagination (Figs. 33.14 and 33.15), potentially causing obstructive symptoms.

Endoscopy demonstrates a submucosal mass. Histologic examination establishes the diagnosis. If invagination occurs, the leading head may be hardly visible, and only the alteration in mucosal folds may be seen.

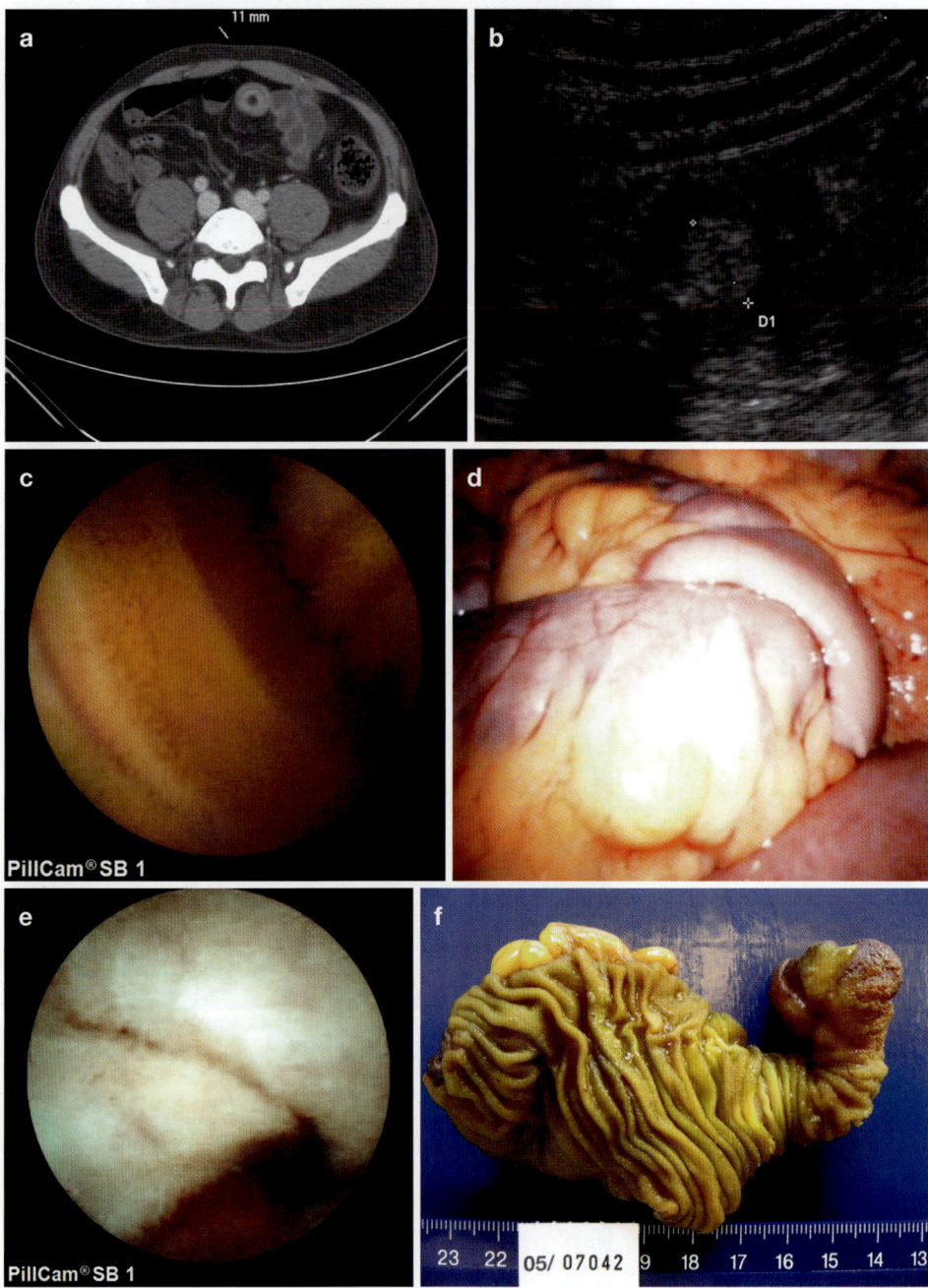

Fig. 33.14 Ectopic pancreas in a patient with anemia and mild abdominal pain. (**a**) Intussusception is seen on a CT scan (*Courtesy of* Ernst Malzfeldt, MD). (**b**) Consecutive ultrasound also shows intussusception. (**c**) Invagination is seen by VCE. (**d**) Laparoscopy also shows invagination (*Courtesy of* Christopher Pohland, MD). (**e**) Leading point is hardly visible in VCE with FICE1-enhanced contrast. (**f**) Resected specimen with ectopic, ulcerated pancreas (*Courtesy of* Jörg Caselitz, MD)

Fig. 33.15 (**a**) Lilac polypoid mass and atypical folds (*arrows*) at VCE. (**b**) Rectal double-balloon-enteroscopy does not reach the process; lilac tumor can be seen 100 cm from the ileocecal valve. (**c**) Atypical folds can be seen in ectopic pancreas between 9 and 12 o'clock and in **a** between 11 and 4 o'clock. (**d**, **e**) Resection of ileum segment with ectopic pancreatic tissue (*Courtesy of* Peer Fleming, MD, and Axel Wellmann, MD)

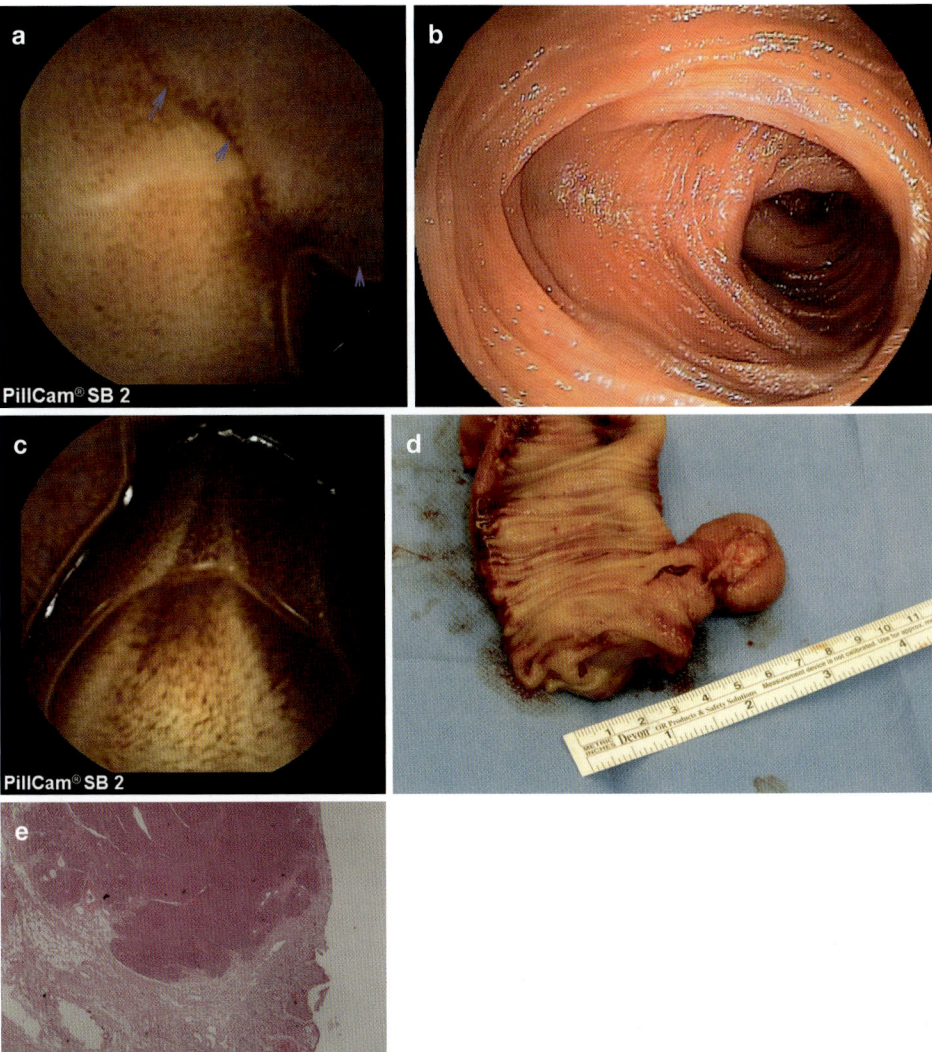

33.5.2 Gastric Heterotopia

Congenital ectopic rests of the gastric mucosa may be seen in the duodenum (Fig. 44.22), jejunum, ileum, and Meckel's diverticula (Fig. 20.11). Heterotopias are benign, but they may cause ulceration and even bleeding.

On endoscopy, a typical raised, brightly colored mosaic pattern of the gastric mucosa with no villi is seen. The surface of the affected area is more reddish than the surrounding normal mucosa (Fig. 33.16).

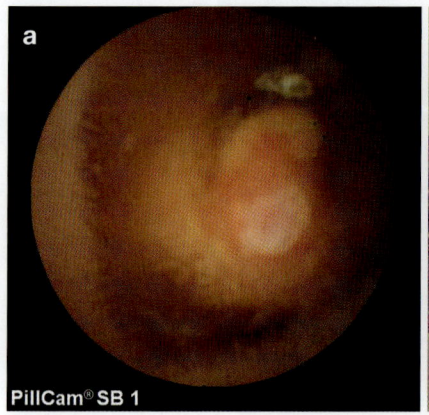 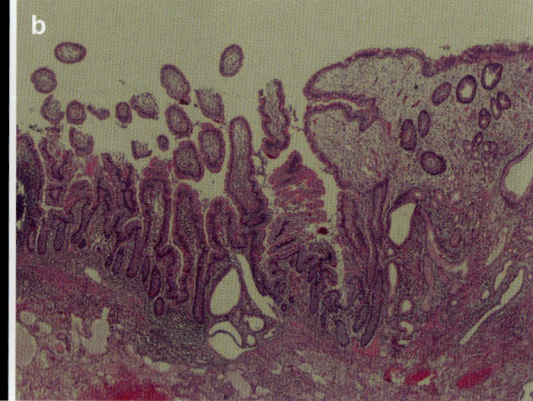

Fig. 33.16 Lymphangioma with gastric heterotopia. (**a**) VCE. (**b**) Histology (*Courtesy of* Peer Fleming, MD, and Axel Wellmann, MD)

33.5.3 Endometriosis

Ectopic endometrial tissue has been found in the gastrointestinal tract in 3–37 % of menstruating women. These benign lesions may cause obstructive symptoms predominantly in the ileal area [14]. Endoluminal endometriosis in the small bowel seems to be very rare, as no reports of diagnosis by VCE are available. For appendiceal endometriosis, see Fig. 46.19.

33.6 Epithelial Neoplasms

33.6.1 Adenomas

An adenoma is a benign neoplasm that arises from the crypt epithelium. Adenomas in the small intestine occur predominantly in the duodenum, often in the peripapillary region, where they present a greater risk of malignant transformation [6]. They occur sporadically (Figs. 33.17 and 33.18), and their incidence is increased in patients with polyposis syndromes (Chap. 35). The frequency of adenoma detection by capsule endoscopy was increased in patients with sporadic duodenal adenomas without familial adenomatous polyposis (FAP) [15]. More data are needed for recommendations about whether small bowel screening should be recommended for all patients with sporadic duodenal adenomas.

Pyloric gland adenomas are very rare (Fig. 33.17). They can arise in gastric metaplasia or heterotopia in the whole gastrointestinal tract [16].

For larger adenomas, endoscopic therapy or surgical intervention is recommended. A colonoscopy also should be considered. Currently, there are no surveillance guidelines.

On endoscopy, adenomas in the duodenum often appear as flat lesions with a typical whitish surface (Figs. 33.18 and 33.19). Adenomatous polyps of the small intestine can be of any size and may be sessile, broad based, or pedunculated (Fig. 33.20).

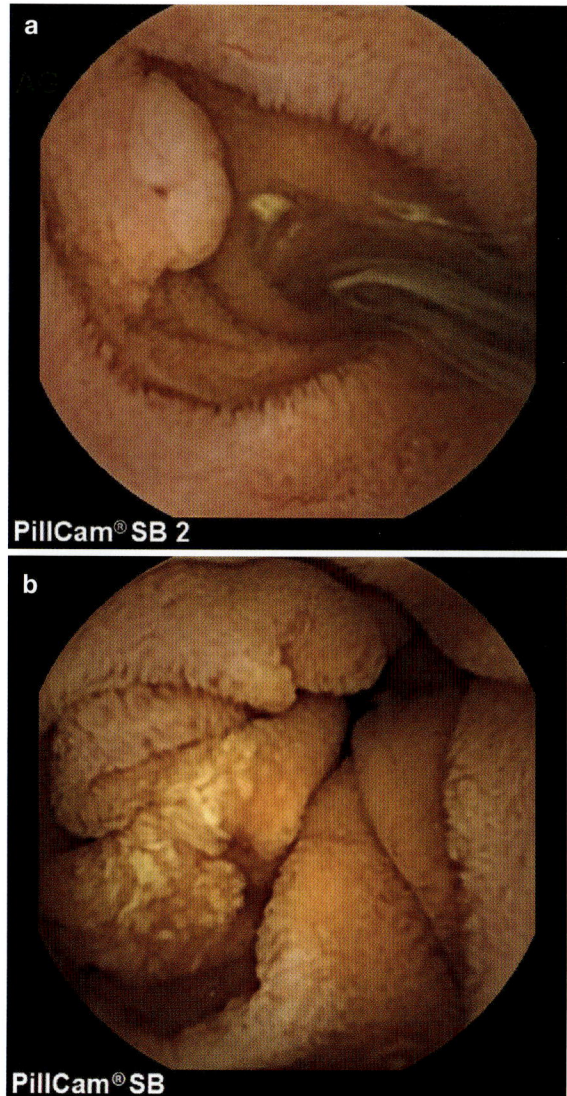

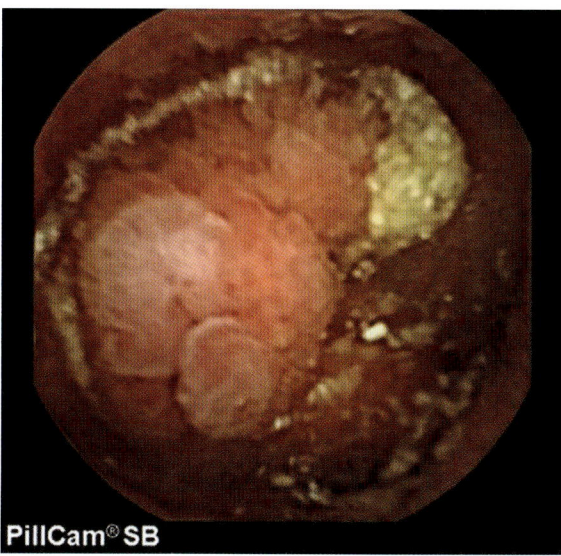

Fig. 33.17 Pyloric gland adenoma in the duodenum

Fig. 33.18 (**a**, **b**) Sporadic duodenal adenomas in two patients

Fig. 33.19 Circular sporadic adenomas of the distal duodenum. (**a**) VCE. (**b**) Duodenoscopy. These lesions were confirmed histologically after duodenal resection

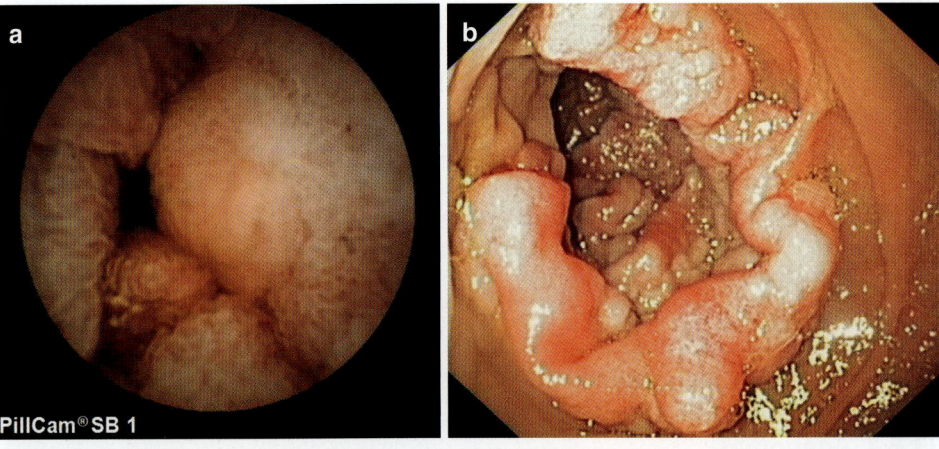

Fig. 33.20 (**a**) Jejunal pedunculated tubular adenoma. (**b**) Touch by the capsule caused bleeding

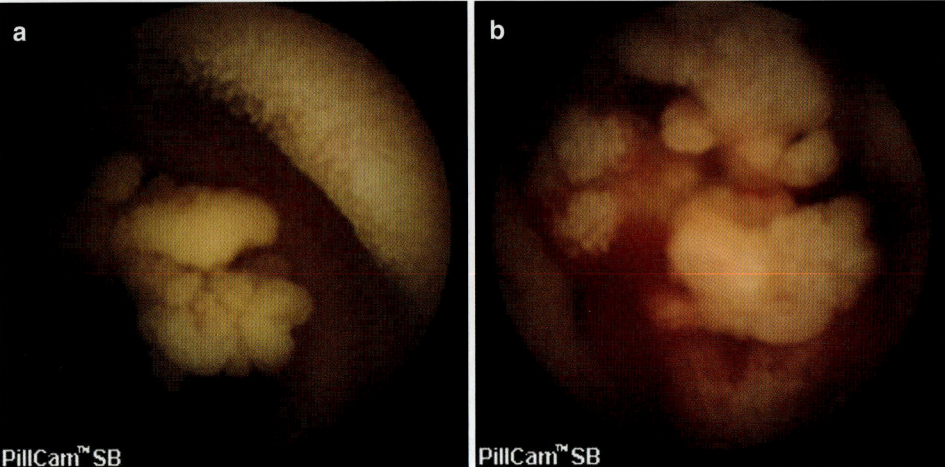

33.7 Mesenchymal Tumors

Mesenchymal tumors are benign neoplasms that arise from various mesodermal cells. They are classified according to the underlying cell type, which often can be characterized only with the help of additional immunohistochemical methods. Mesenchymal tumors can lead to problems such as intestinal obstruction, erosion, or bleeding.

33.7.1 Hemangiomas

Hemangiomas of the small intestine are rare. Types include capillary (Fig. 33.21) [17], cavernous [18], and mixed. Hemangiomas may occur as single lesions or may be multiple, such as in blue rubber bleb nevus syndrome [19, 20], which also includes cutaneous lesions (Figs. 21.7 and 21.8). The main symptom is episodes of bleeding.

On endoscopy, hemangiomas appear as soft, bluish, vascular tumors, and sometimes reaching giant dimensions (Fig. 33.22). Occasionally, active bleeding is observed during VCE.

33.7.2 Lymphangiomas and Cystic Lymphangiectasia

Cystic lymphangiectasia is a frequent incidental finding in VCE of the small intestine. It was found in up to 20 % of cases in an older autopsy series [21] and in 13 % of patients undergoing double-balloon enteroscopy, with a range from one to five lesions [22]. Peristaltic waves can change the appearance of the lesions (Fig. 33.23).

The lesion itself apparently has no clinical significance. Smaller lesions can occasionally cause bleeding (Figs. 33.24 and 33.25), and an extremely large lesion (Fig. 33.26) can lead to intestinal obstruction and erosion [23].

On endoscopy, a submucosal, yellowish–whitish mass is observed (Fig. 33.24). Occasionally, the villi over the cyst are white and thickened (Fig. 33.25). The submucosal vessels are often clearly visible in lesions with the normal mucosa and normal villi. Sometimes they look flat, and sometimes like a protruding polyp (Fig. 33.23).

Fig. 33.21 Bleeding capillary hemangioma occurring in an 82-year-old woman with a 6-week history of obscure gastrointestinal bleeding requiring transfusion. (**a**) VCE shows ongoing bleeding and a narrow lumen in the proximal jejunum. (**b**) Large (1 cm), polypoid bleeding tumor (push enteroscopy). (**c**) Histology of the surgically resected tumor, showing a benign capillary hemangioma with dilated submucosal blood vessels (*Courtesy of* Otto Ljungberg, MD). After 2 years of follow-up, the patient is symptom-free, with no further bleeding

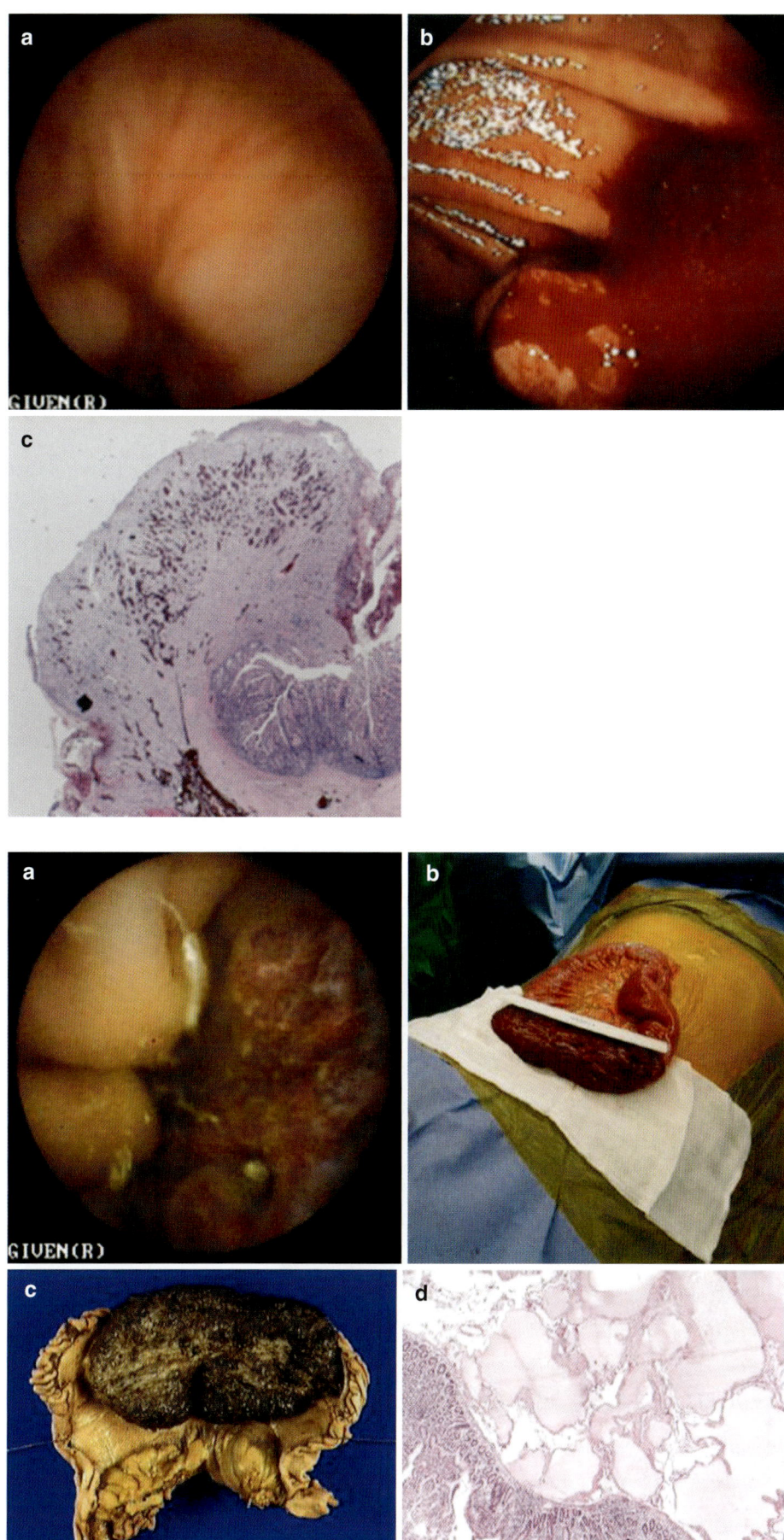

Fig. 33.22 Giant hemangioma. (**a**) VCE shows a vascular polypoid lesion. (**b**) Laparotomy reveals the presence of a giant intestinal hemangioma. (**c**) Surgical specimen. (**d**) Histology showing dilated vessels (*Case courtesy of* Andre Van Gossum, MD)

Fig. 33.23 (**a**) Cystic lymphangiectasia with blood vessels. (**b**) 1 s later, the same lesion looks polypoid because of the peristaltic wave

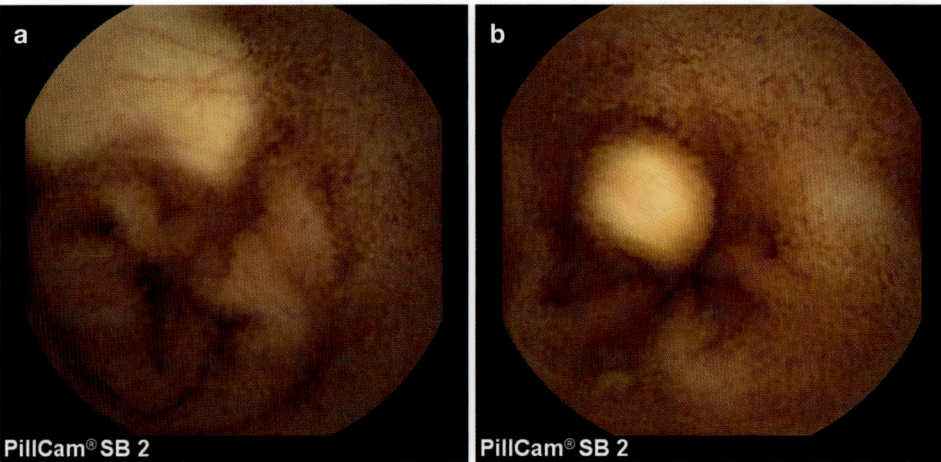

Fig. 33.24 Cystic lymphangiectasias. (**a**) Double-balloon enteroscopy shows white lymph exudate. (**b**) Histology with bleeding (*Courtesy of* Peer Fleming, MD, and Axel Wellmann, MD)

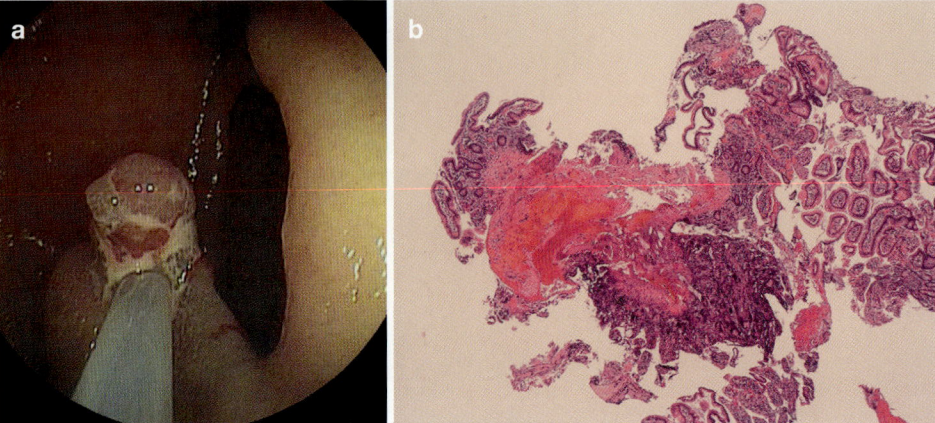

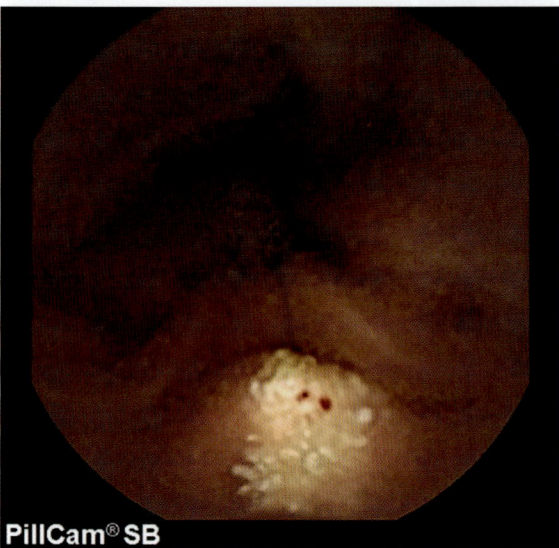

Fig. 33.25 Microcystic lymphangiectasia: white, thickened villi with two small bleeding points

Fig. 33.26 (**a**, **b**) Large, segmental lymphangiectasia completely filling the intestinal lumen. Motion from the swift passage of the capsule through the stenotic segment of the small intestine reduced the sharpness of the images. (**c**) Resected specimen. (**d**) Histology showed marked cystic dilation of the lymph vessels (*Case courtesy of Siegbert Faiss, MD*)

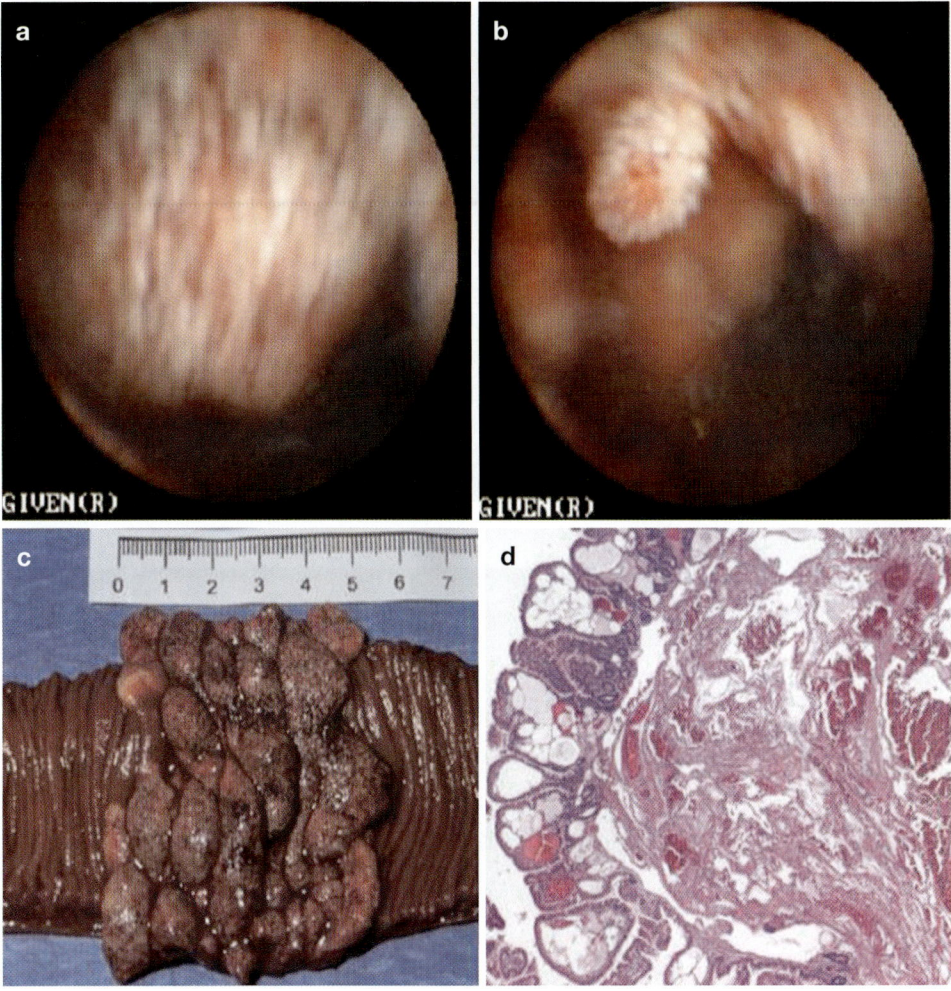

33.7.3 Leiomyomas

Leiomyoma is a benign mesenchymal tumor of smooth muscle cells. It can be distinguished immunohistologically from a gastrointestinal stromal tumor (GIST) [24]. Leiomyomas are frequently asymptomatic.

Endoscopy demonstrates a submucosal tumor [25] (Fig. 33.27) of highly variable size, occasionally with ulceration of the otherwise normal-appearing mucosa. Endoscopic biopsies are often unrewarding because of the submucosal tumor location, as only the normal mucosa overlying the submucosal tumor is evaluated.

33.7.4 Lipomas

Lipomas are benign mesenchymal tumors derived from adipocytes. Although small intestinal lipomas are mainly asymptomatic, they can cause intestinal bleeding or obstruction, requiring surgery [26].

Endoscopy reveals a soft, yellowish–whitish, mobile, sometimes pedunculated tumor (Fig. 33.28), sometimes with ulcers and inflammation (Fig. 33.29). VCE often underestimates these tumors. The capsule may stay for a long time near the obstructing tumor.

Rarely, multiple lipomas present as intestinal lipomatosis (Fig. 33.30), potentially causing intussusception [27]. Fibrolipomas are characterized by additional fibrosis of the stroma, changing the endoscopic appearance to a more consistent, reddish tumor with a somewhat irregular surface (Fig. 33.31).

33.7.5 Neurofibromas

Neurofibromas are benign tumors with neural and connective tissue differentiation. They occur rarely in the setting of neurofibromatosis type I (Recklinghausen's disease) due to a mutation of the NF-1 gene on chromosome 17. Other small intestinal tumors, including malignant lesions, may also occur [28]. Sporadic neurofibroma of the small intestine is a rarity [29].

The endoscopic features of neurofibromas are nonspecific. They appear as firm, submucosal tumors on the mesenteric side of the intestine. They are occasionally ulcerated (Fig. 33.32).

Fig. 33.27 Small leiomyoma of the ileum. (**a**) VCE shows the submucosal tumor. (**b**) Histologically, the tumor is composed of smooth muscle cells. Note the normal mucosa over the tumor (Periodic acid–Schiff [PAS]) (*Courtesy of* Renate Höhne, MD)

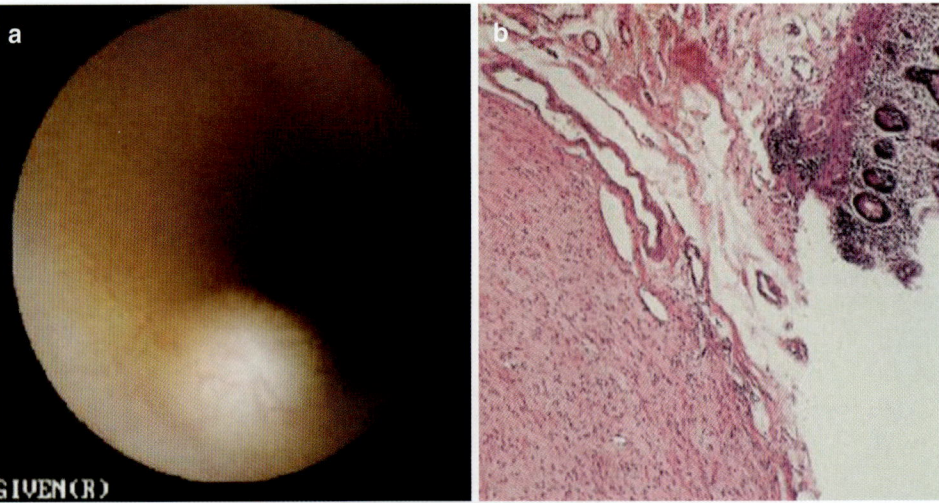

Fig. 33.28 Duodenal lipoma. (**a**) VCE. (**b**) Side-viewing duodenoscopy

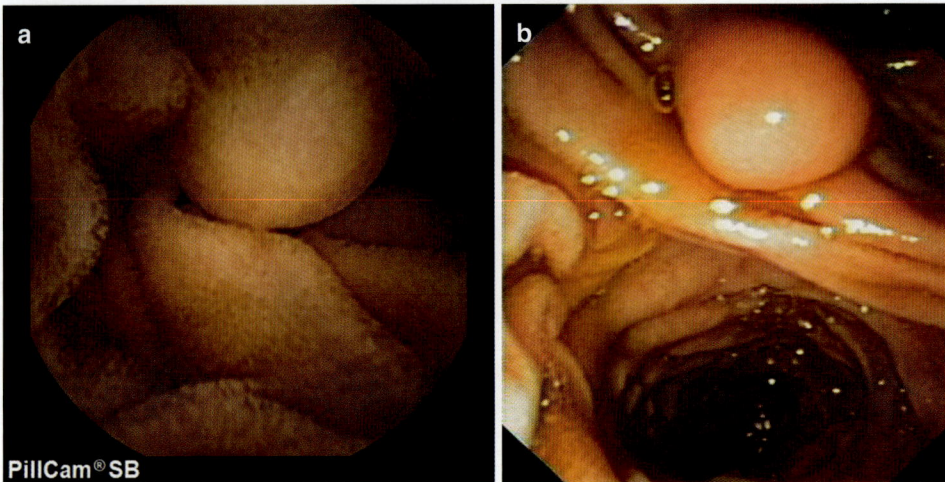

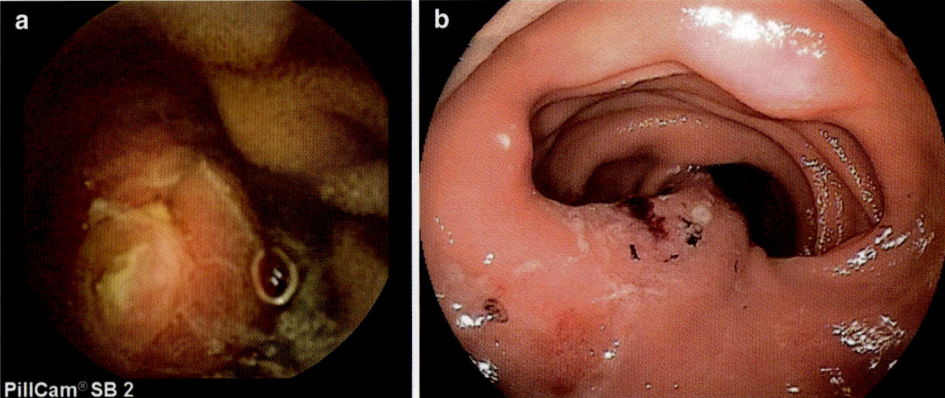

Fig. 33.29 Lipoma. (**a**, **c**) VCE shows a large, possibly pedunculated tumor with an ulcer. (**b**, **d**) Double-balloon enteroscopy shows a large, pedunculated tumor with ulceration. (**e**) Intussusception. (**f**) Resected specimen (*Courtesy of* Peer Fleming, MD, and Axel Wellmann, MD)

Fig. 33.29   (continued)

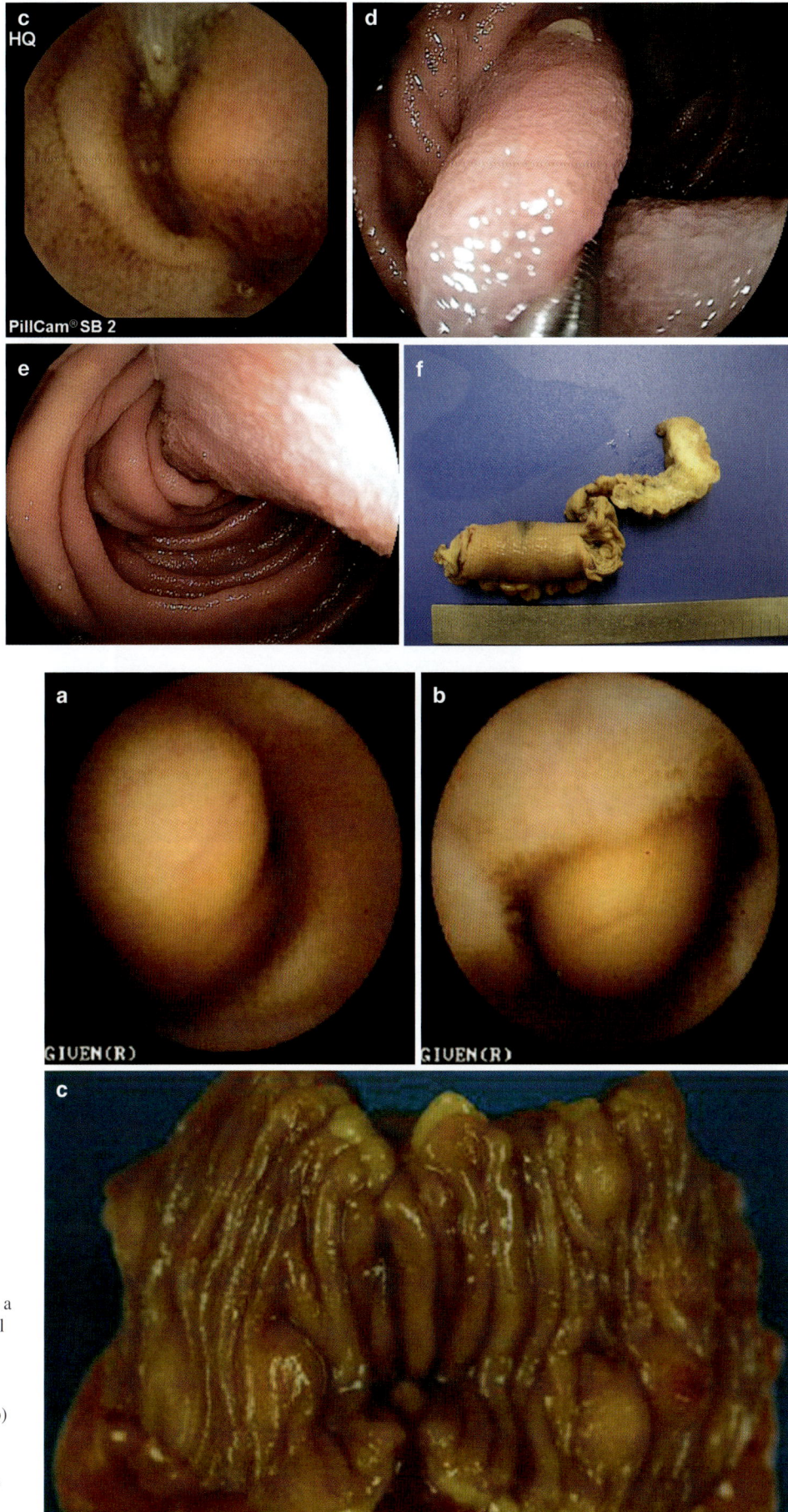

Fig. 33.30   Intestinal lipomatosis in a 48-year-old patient with postprandial abdominal pain and weight loss of 20 kg. After resection of 110 cm of the small intestine, complete resolution of the pain occurred. (**a**, **b**) Multiple, bulging, yellowish, submucosal tumors of the jejunum. (**c**) Resected specimen with multiple lipomas (*Courtesy of* Frank Stenschke, MD, and Henryk Dancygier, MD)

Fig. 33.31 Fibrolipoma of the jejunum in a patient referred because of relapsing, severe intestinal hemorrhage. (**a**) VCE demonstrates a submucosal tumor. (**b**) Push enteroscopy. (**c**) Sonography in power Doppler mode shows a tumor with hyperechogenic, inhomogeneous pattern and hypervascularization. (**d**) A CT scan reveals an intraluminal, inhomogeneous tumor of low density, typical of fat (*arrow*) (*Courtesy of* Ernst Malzfeldt, MD)

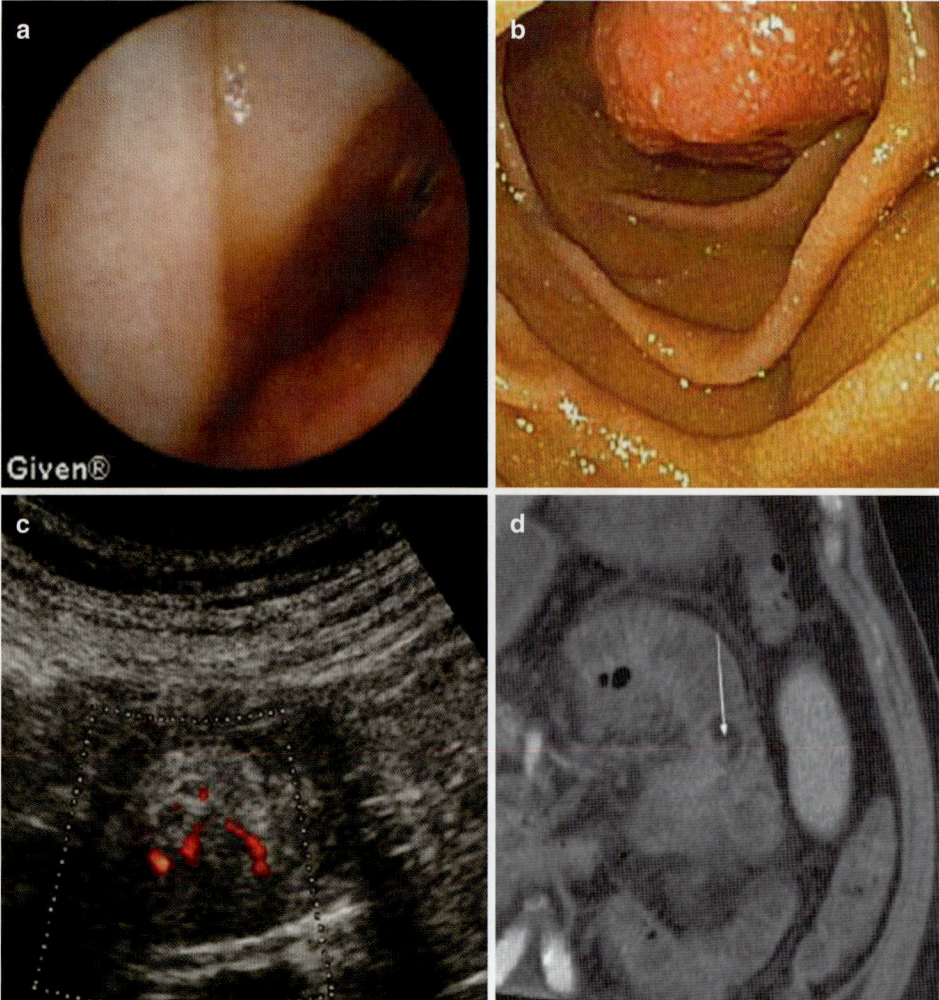

Fig. 33.32 Neurofibromas.
(**a**) Cutaneous lesions. (**b**) VCE
shows firm, white submucosal
tumors that are partly ulcerated.
(**c**) Resected fibrotic tumor.
(**d**) Histology shows a
neurofibroma covered by the
normal small bowel mucosa
(H&E) (*Courtesy of* Jörg
Caselitz, MD)

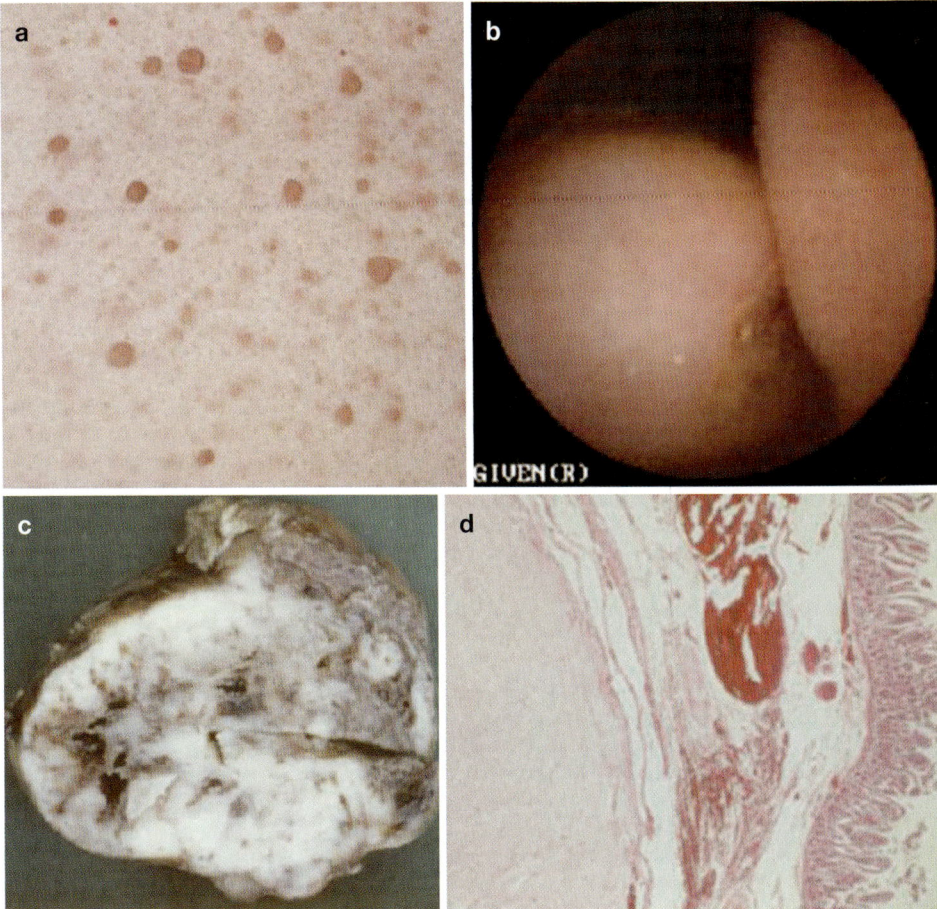

References

1. Schottenfeld D, Beebe-Dimmer JL, Vigneau FD. The epidemiology and pathogenesis of neoplasia in the small intestine. Ann Epidemiol. 2009;19:58–69.
2. Paski CC, Semrad CE. Small bowel tumors. Gastrointest Endosc Clin N Am. 2009;19:461–79.
3. Cheung DY, Lee I-S, Chang DK, et al. Capsule endoscopy in small bowel tumors: a multicenter Korean study. J Gastroenterol Hepatol. 2010;25:1079–86.
4. May A, Schoen M, Nachbar L, et al. Ileo-ileal invagination – a cause of recurrent mid-gastrointestinal bleeding: diagnostic and endoscopic therapy by means push-and-pull enteroscopy. Dig Liver Dis. 2008;40:477–80.
5. Santos G, Alves AF, Wakamatsu A, Zucoloto S. Inflammatory fibroid polyp. An immunohistochemical study. Arq Gastroenterol. 2004;41:104–7.
6. Culver EL, McIntyre AS. Sporadic duodenal polyps: classification, investigation, and management. Endoscopy. 2011;43:144–55.
7. Morales-Fuentes GA, de Arino-Suarez M, Zarate-Osorno A, et al. Vanek's polyp or inflammatory fibroid polyp. Case report and review of the literature. Cir Cir. 2011;79:242–5.
8. Matsuura H, Kuwano H, Kanematsu T, et al. Clinicopathological features of elevated lesions of the duodenal bulb. J Surg Oncol. 1990;45:79–84.
9. Kawaratani H, Tsujimoto T, Nishimura N, et al. A case of lobulated and pedunculated duodenal hyperplastic polyp treated with snare polypectomy. Case Rep Gastroenterol. 2011;5:404–10.
10. Stolte M, Lux G. Duodenum und Papilla Vateri: Tumoren und tumorähnliche Läsionen – ein klinisch pathologisches Gespräch. Leber Magen Darm. 1983;13:227–41.
11. Khuroo MS, Khuroo NS, Khuroo MS. Diffuse duodenal nodular lymphoid hyperplasia: a large cohort of patients etiologically related to Helicobacter pylori infection. BMC Gastroenterol. 2011;11:36.
12. Lee MJ, Chang JH, Maeng IH, et al. Ectopic pancreas bleeding in the jejunum revealed by capsule endoscopy. Clin Endosc. 2012;45:194–7.
13. Eisenberger CF, Gocht A, Knoefel WT, et al. Heterotopic pancreas–clinical presentation and pathology with review of the literature. Hepatogastroenterology. 2004;51:854–8.
14. De Ceglie A, Bilardi C, Blanchi S, et al. Acute small bowel obstruction caused by endometriosis: a case report and review of the literature. World J Gastroenterol. 2008;14:3430–4.
15. Riemann JF, Hartmann D, Schilling D, et al. Frequency of small bowel polyps in patients with duodenal adenoma but without familial adenomatous polyposis. Z Gastroenterol. 2006;44:235–8.
16. Vieth M, Vogel C, Kushima R, et al. Pyloric gland adenoma–how to diagnose? Cesk Patol. 2006;42:4–7.
17. Kim YS, Chun HJ, Jeen YT, et al. Small bowel capillary hemangioma. Gastrointest Endosc. 2004;60:599.
18. Khurana V, Dala R, Barkin JS. Small bowel cavernous hemangioma. Gastrointest Endosc. 2004;60:96.
19. Fish L, Fireman Z, Kopelman Y, Sternberg A. Blue rubber bleb nevus syndrome: small-bowel lesions diagnosed by capsule endoscopy. Endoscopy. 2004;36:836.
20. Maunoury V, Turck D, Brunetaud JM, et al. Blue rubber bleb nevus syndrome. 3 cases treated with a Nd:YAG laser and bipolar electrocoagulation. [In French]. Gastroenterol Clin Biol. 1990;14:593–5.
21. Shilkin KB, Zerman JB, Blackwell JB. Lymphangiectatic cysts of the small bowel. J Pathol Bacteriol. 1968;96:353–8.
22. Bellutti M, Mönkemüller K, Fry LC, et al. Characterization of yellow plaques found in the small bowel during double-balloon enteroscopy. Endoscopy. 2007;39:1059–63.
23. Kida A, Matsuda K, Hirai S, et al. A pedunculated polyp-shaped small-bowel lymphangioma causing gastrointestinal bleeding and treated by double-balloon enteroscopy. World J Gastroenterol. 2012;18:4798–800.
24. Miettinen M, Sobin LH, Sarlomo-Rikala M. Immunohistochemical spectrum of GISTs at different sites and their differential diagnosis with reference to CD 117 (KIT). Mod Pathol. 2000;13:1134–42.
25. Maeda M, Kanke K, Sasai T, et al. (1)(8)F-fluorodeoxyglucose PET/CT and small bowel endoscopy in a patient with small bowel leiomyoma. Nihon Shokakibyo Gakkai Zasshi. 2012;109:1561–6.
26. Zissin R. Enteroenteric intussusception secondary to a lipoma: CT diagnosis. Emerg Radiol. 2004;11:107–9.
27. Lee BJ, Park JJ, Joo MK, et al. A case of small-bowel intussusception caused by intestinal lipomatosis: preoperative diagnosis and reduction of intussusception with double-balloon enteroscopy. Gastrointest Endosc. 2010;71:1329–32.
28. Behranwala KA, Spalding DR, Wotherspoon A, et al. Small bowel gastrointestinal stromal tumours and ampullary cancer in type 1 neurofibromatosis. World J Surg Oncol. 2004;2:1–4.
29. Watanuki F, Ohwada S, Hosomura Y, et al. Small ileal neurofibroma causing intussusception in a non-neurofibromatosis patient. J Gastroenterol. 1995;30:113–6.

Internet

http://ghr.nlm.nih.gov: *Genetics Home Reference (US National Library of Medicine)*
http://www.nfnetwork.org: *Neurofibromatosis Network*
http://www.rarediseases.org: National Organization for Rare Disorders

Malignant Tumors

34

Blair S. Lewis, Martin Keuchel, Felix Wiedbrauck,
Jörg Caselitz, Yasuo Kakugawa, and Yutaka Saito

Contents

The work was first published in 2006 by Springer Medizin Verlag Heidelberg with the following title: *Atlas of Video Capsule Endoscopy*.

B.S. Lewis (✉)
Mount Sinai Hospital, New York, NY, USA
e-mail: blairslewismdpc@me.com

M. Keuchel
Department of Internal Medicine,
Bethesda Krankenhaus Bergedorf,
Hamburg, Germany
e-mail: keuchel@bkb.info

F. Wiedbrauck
Department of Gastroenterology,
Allgemeines Krankenhaus Celle, Celle, Germany
e-mail: felix.wiedbrauck@akh-celle.de

J. Caselitz
Department for Pathology, Asklepios Klinik Altona,
Hamburg, Germany
e-mail: j.caselitz@asklepios.com

Y. Kakugawa • Y. Saito
Endoscopy Division, National Cancer Center Hospital,
Tokyo, Japan
e-mail: yakakuga@gmail.com; ytsaito@ncc.go.jp

34.1 Introduction

34.1.1 Prevalence

Tumors of the small bowel account for 5 % of all gastrointestinal tract tumors and 2 % of the cancers (Table 34.1). Before the advent of capsule endoscopy, however, the methods for examining the small bowel were inadequate, so the accuracy of these figures may be questioned. The diagnosis of small-bowel tumors is often delayed, contributing to the poor prognosis in patients with malignant tumors. In 1995, 4,600 new cases of cancer in the small intestine were reported, with 1,120 deaths [1]. Tumors are typically missed by most radiographic tests, and thus tumors of the small bowel generally carried a dismal prognosis before small intestinal endoscopy. In 1980, Herbsman et al. [2] reported that survival of more than 6 months for adenocarcinoma of the small bowel was rare. More recently, with earlier detection due to small-bowel endoscopic techniques, the overall 5-year survival is reported to be 57 %, and the median survival is 52 months [3]. The prognosis for adenocarcinoma generally is less favorable than for other small-bowel malignancies [4], depending on tumor stage [5]. In a review of 1,260 cases, 305 were located in the ileum, 25 % in the duodenum, and 15 % in the jejunum [6].

M. Keuchel et al. (eds.), *Video Capsule Endoscopy: A Reference Guide and Atlas*,
DOI 10.1007/978-3-662-44062-9_34, © Springer-Verlag Berlin Heidelberg 2014

Table 34.1 Types of malignant small-bowel tumors

Primary small-bowel malignancies
Adenocarcinomas (47 %)
Neuroendocrine tumors (28 %)
Sarcomas (12 %)
Lymphomas (12 %)
Metastases
Small-bowel infiltration by extraintestinal malignancies

34.1.2 Clinical Features

Malignant tumors of the small bowel are asymptomatic in their early stages. Later, the complaints are often uncharacteristic, causing a delay in diagnosis. An important warning sign is gastrointestinal bleeding or iron deficiency anemia of unknown cause. Abdominal pain, weight loss, (partial) bowel obstruction, or perforation is seen with advanced tumors [7].

34.1.3 Endoscopy

The endoscopic appearance of a small-bowel mass can be deceiving. The variety of pathologies seen within the small bowel cannot be matched by the colon or the stomach. Even a well-trained endoscopist may be able to say only that a tumor is present and may not know the true pathology. Many small-bowel tumors are submucosal, adding to the difficulty of visual diagnosis or even diagnosis by endoscopic biopsy. Submucosal tumors include leiomyomas, neuroendocrine tumors (NET)/carcinoids, lipomas, and metastatic disease. With the small space of the small bowel and the large nature of a tumor, the typical changes suggestive of a submucosal process may be missed. Typically the endoscopist looks for visible mucosa and a vascular pattern across the tumor to confirm its submucosal nature. Bridging folds may also help in this regard. In the small bowel, the mucosa may be pulled so tightly over the mass that it becomes transparent, masking the standard changes.

Leiomyomas can vary in size, and the endoscopic appearance does not disclose the size of the extramucosal component. Occasionally, central ulceration or umbilication may be seen. Lymphomas can have several different appear-ances. A classification of these appearances has been created and includes a nodular pattern, an infiltrative pattern, and an ulcerating pattern [8]. Halphen et al. [9], in a review of 120 patients with primary small-bowel lymphoma, found the infiltrative pattern, in which the mucosa is firm and motionless, to be most indicative of lymphoma. The other patterns may be mimicked by celiac disease, radiation enteritis, and other disorders. Adenocarcinoma is circumferential and often quite exophytic, resembling the endoscopic appearance of colon cancer. Metastatic melanoma can often be suspected by its pigmented nature. Neuroendocrine tumors often appear as multiple submucosal nodules.

Most small-bowel tumors diagnosed by video capsule endoscopy (VCE) have been detected in patients evaluated for intestinal bleeding [10–14]. VCE is more sensitive than imaging procedures in detecting these lesions. False-negative VCE findings have been described in cases where the viewing axis of the capsule was deflected by a tumor-related stricture [15], or vision was obscured due to tumor bleeding [16, 17] or inadequate preparation [18].

34.1.4 Treatment

Complete surgical or in early stages endoscopical removal of the tumor is the treatment of choice [19]. Other adjuvant or alternative treatment modalities may be considered, depending on the tumor entity and stage.

34.2 Adenocarcinoma

From 41 % to 76 % of adenocarcinomas are located in the duodenum, and approximately 38 % can be reached by esophagogastroduodenoscopy (Fig. 34.1) [20].

Risk factors for small-bowel adenocarcinoma include several polyposis syndromes, sprue, Crohn's disease, and previous radiotherapy.

Endoscopy may reveal an infiltrating lesion or exophytic tumor (Figs. 34.2, 34.3, and 34.4), which may show ulceration, stricturing, and/or bleeding. As in other tumors, infiltration of the mesentery may additionally lead to mucosal alterations like erythema in the proximity of the tumor (Fig. 34.3c).

Fig 34.1 (**a**) 25-mm 0–IIa lesion located in the duodenum. (**b**) After indigo-carmine was sprayed, the margin became apparent. (**c**) Crystal-violet staining demonstrated an irregular pit pattern corresponding to Type V pit on the nodular change. Endoscopic diagnosis was 0–IIa, intramucosal carcinoma in the duodenum. (**d**) Endoscopic en bloc resection was achieved using hybrid endoscopic mucosal resection (EMR) technique on this lesion. (**e–g**) Histopathological diagnosis was an intramucosal, well-differentiated adenocarcinoma. Curative resection was achieved

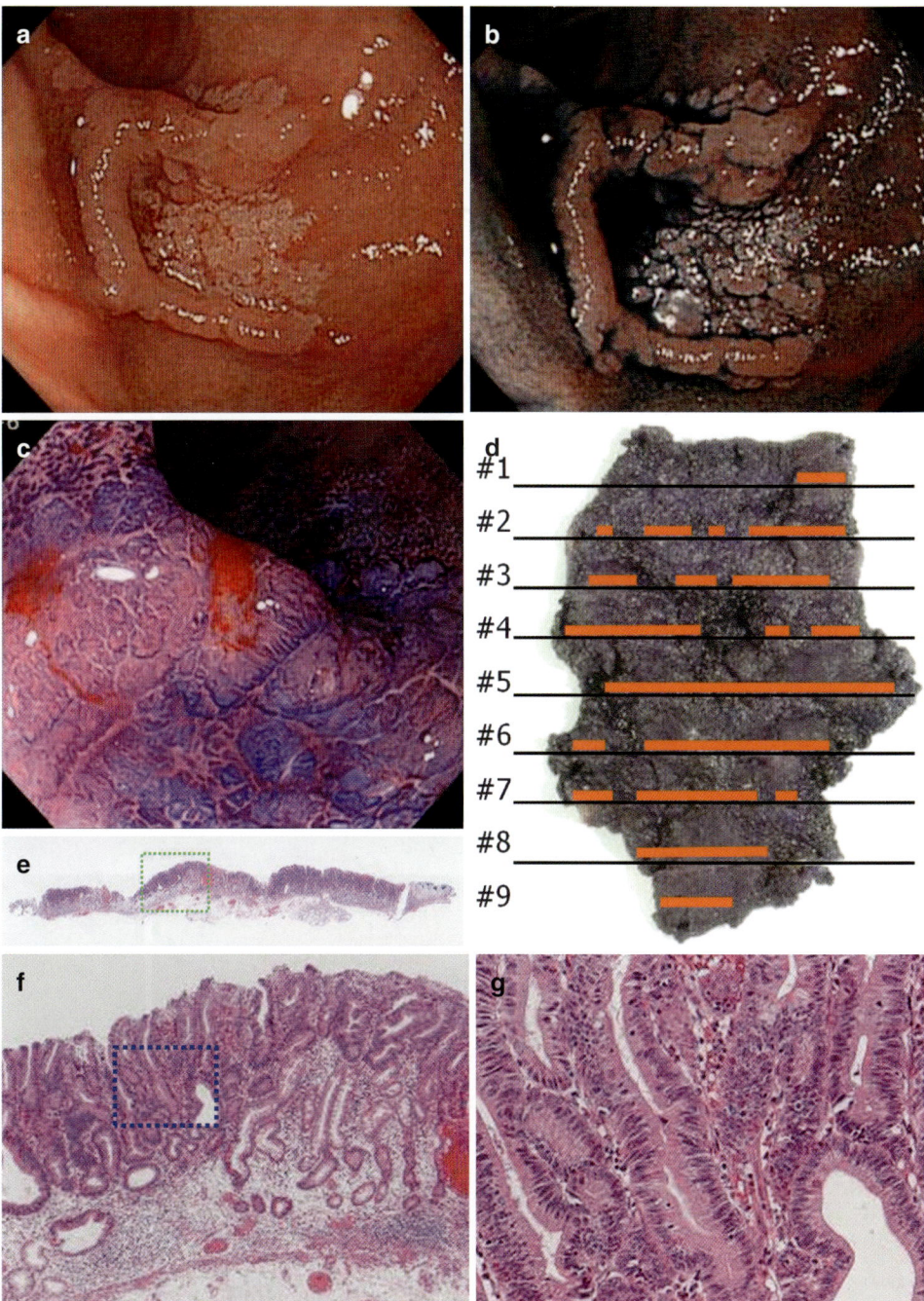

Fig. 34.2 A 58-year-old man with iron deficiency anemia, tarry stool, weight loss, anorexia, and general fatigue, but no symptoms of stenosis. CT scan showed wall thickening of the small intestine, para-aortic lymph node swelling, and multiple metastatic liver tumors. (**a**) Capsule endoscopy revealed a protruding lesion with central ulceration in the jejunum. (**b**) Double-balloon endoscopy also revealed a protruding lesion with sharply demarcated ulceration in the jejunum. The lesion size was estimated as 2.5 cm in diameter. (**c**) Biopsy of the tumor revealed moderately differentiated adenocarcinoma by hematoxylin-eosin (H&E) staining (×200). Genetic analysis for hereditary polyposis syndromes did not reveal mutations in *APC*, *MYH*, *MLH1*, *MSH2*, or *MSH6*

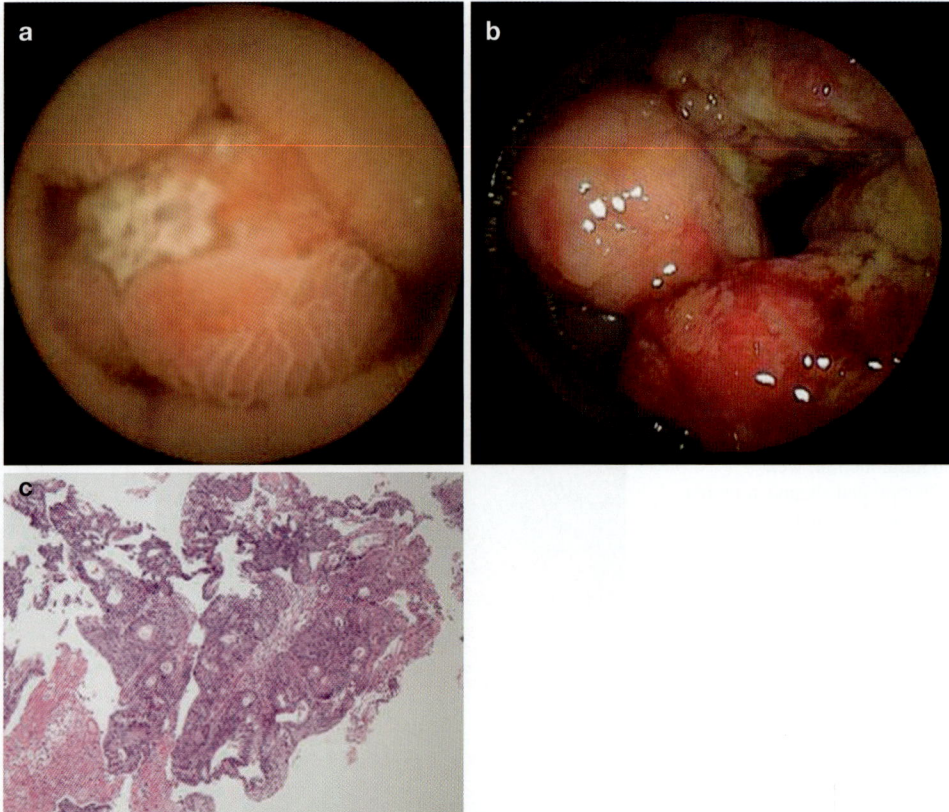

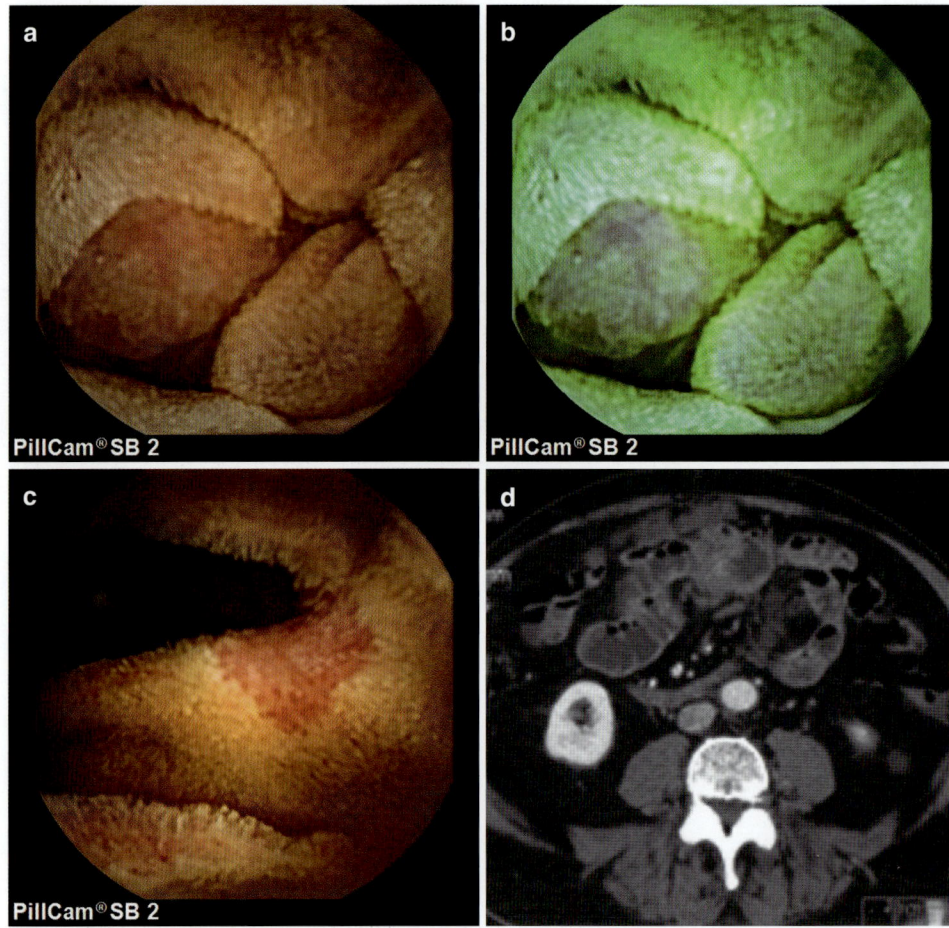

Fig. 34.3 Adenocarcinoma of the jejunum. (**a**) Video capsule endoscopy (VCE). (**b**) VCE with flexible spectral imaging color enhancement (FICE2). (**c**) Patchy erythema caused by infiltration of the mesentery. (**d**) CT scan (*Courtesy of* Roman Fischbach, MD)

Fig. 34.4 Adenocarcinoma of the jejunum from a patient who had anemia and abdominal pain. (**a**) VCE shows a large mass. (**b**) VCE in FICE 3 mode. (**c**) Resected specimen with a short, stenotic segment and prestenotic dilatation. (**d**) Circumferential tumor. The VCE capsule was retained and was retrieved at surgery (*Courtesy of* Christopher Pohland, MD)

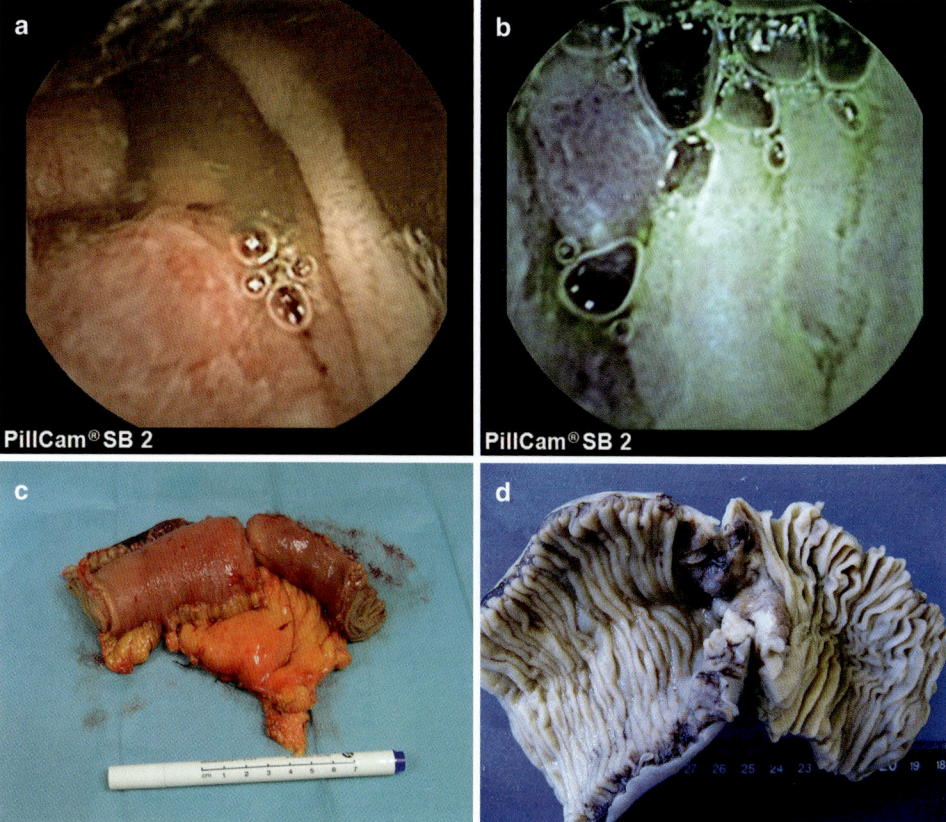

34.3 Neuroendocrine Tumors (Carcinoids)

Neuroendocrine tumors originate from neuroendocrine cells, are often hormone-producing, and are of varying biologic behavior. Neuroendocrine tumors of the gastroenteropancreatic system are subdivided into well-differentiated neuroendocrine tumors with a benign pattern of behavior (e.g., carcinoid) and well-differentiated or poorly differentiated neuroendocrine carcinomas (e.g., malignant carcinoid) [21, 22].

Most neuroendocrine tumors (NET) occur in the small intestine [23]. They are considered one of the most common malignant tumors of the small bowel and are most frequently found in the ileum [6].

Localized NET of the small bowel are frequently asymptomatic [24]. Pain, bleeding, and bowel obstruction may occur, and symptoms of carcinoid syndrome can occur with hepatic metastases. Increased consumption of saturated fats seems to be a risk factor for small-bowel NET [25].

Diagnostic tests include the serum determination of chromogranin A, specific hormone determinations (e.g.,

gastrin, insulin, glucagon, vasoactive intestinal peptide [VIP]), the determination of breakdown products (urinary 5-hydroxyinsolacetic acid with NET), and somatostatin receptor scintigraphy as a localizing study [26]. Scintigraphy and CT scans may complement endoscopy, especially for tumors infiltrating to the mesentery [27, 28].

Endoscopy usually shows submucosal, infiltrating, or exophytic tumors (Figs. 34.5 and 34.6) of varying size. They can be classified only by histologic examination. NET are often located in the terminal ileum and can be found incidentally at routine ileocolonoscopy. VCE can be considered to exclude additional intestinal tumors, as multiple tumors may occur.

Surgery is the first choice for treatment. Hormone-related symptoms in advanced cases may respond to treatment with somatostatin [29]. Other options are interferon, chemotherapy if necessary, and experimental radiation therapy [30].

Fig. 34.5 Multiple neuroendocrine tumors. (**a–c**) Several submucosal tumors with umbilication, discoloration, and bridging folds seen with VCE. (**d**) Double balloon enteroscopy. (**e**) Resected jejunal segment with multiple tumors

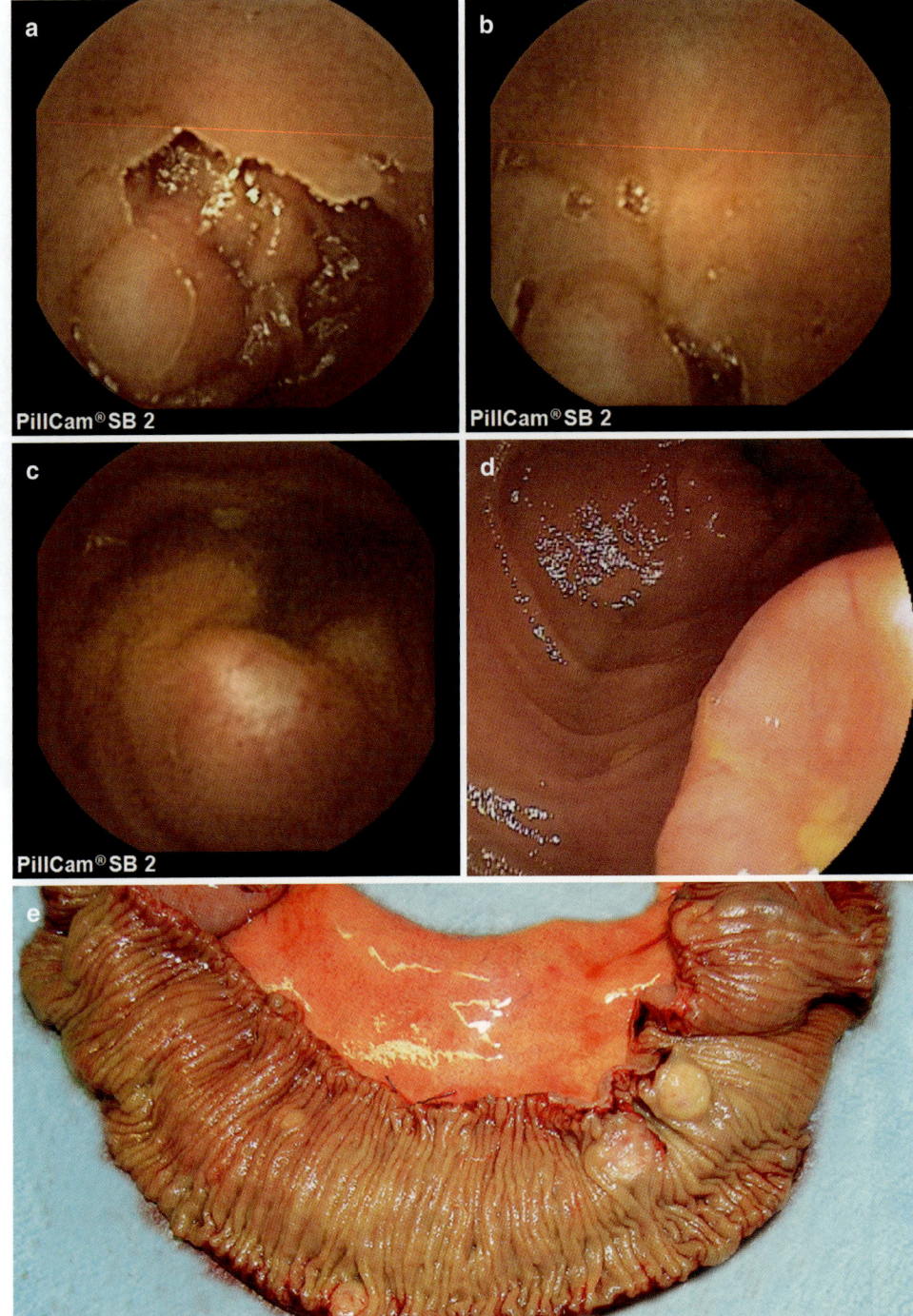

Fig. 34.6 Neuroendocrine carcinoma. (**a** and **b**) Circular infiltrating tumor of the jejunum with stenosis, erythema, and lymphangiectasia. (**c**) Resected specimen. (**d**) Histology showing small tumor cells and desmoplastic reaction. H&E stain

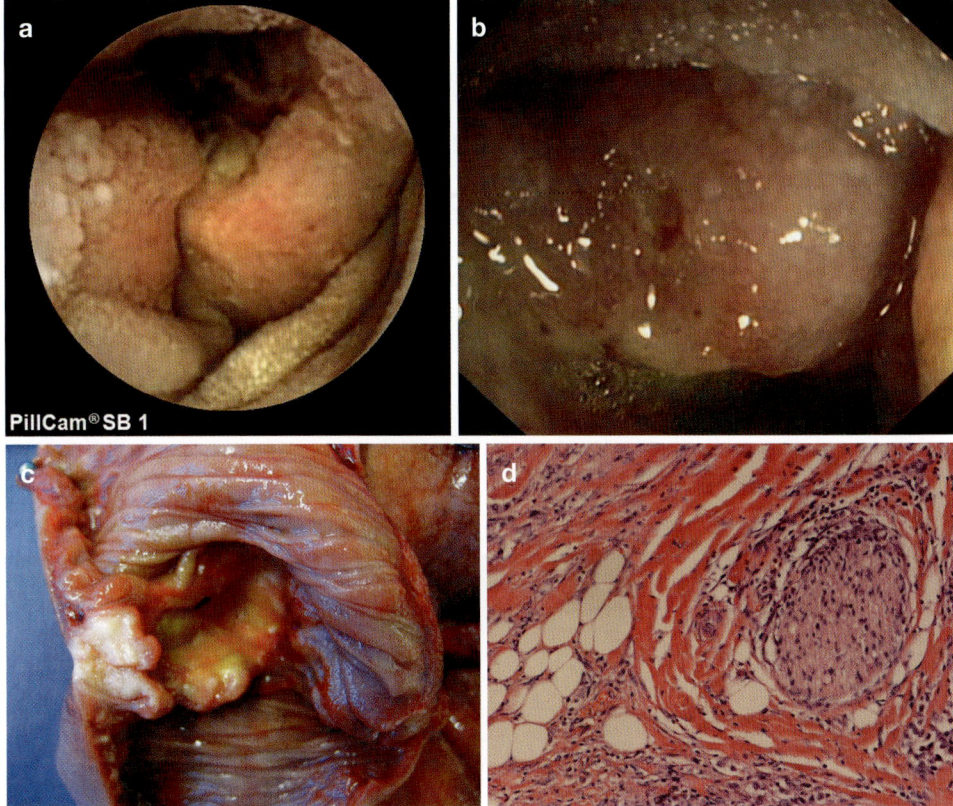

34.4 Sarcomas

34.4.1 Gastrointestinal Stromal Tumors

Gastrointestinal stromal tumors (malignant GISTs) are mesenchymal tumors that express the CD117 marker. In a large series they were the second most common malignant tumor of the small bowel [6]. They presumably have a similar origin to intestinal pacemaker cells [31]. Their biologic behavior is variable. In the absence of metastasis and local invasion, their prognosis (ranging from favorable to unfavorable) can be assessed on the basis of criteria such as tumor size, histologic type, and rate of mitosis.

GISTs are rare, with an incidence of 1 or 2 cases per 100,000 population per year, but they are the most common mesenchymal tumor of the small bowel. They are generally more common in the stomach than in the small bowel, but the malignant form tends to be located in the small bowel [32]. The malignant potential of the tumor correlates with its size and intestinal location [33].

Endoscopy often shows a firm, submucosal tumor, which may be smooth (Fig. 34.7) or cauliflower-like. An extraintestinal tumor site may produce a visible mucosal impression of another bowel loop (Fig. 34.7b), but this is a nonspecific sign. Large size and extramural growth have been suggested as risk factors for missing a GIST on VCE [34].

Besides surgery, an option for treatment of GISTs at advanced tumor stages is treatment with the specific tyrosine kinase inhibitor imatinib or sunitinib in case of resistance.

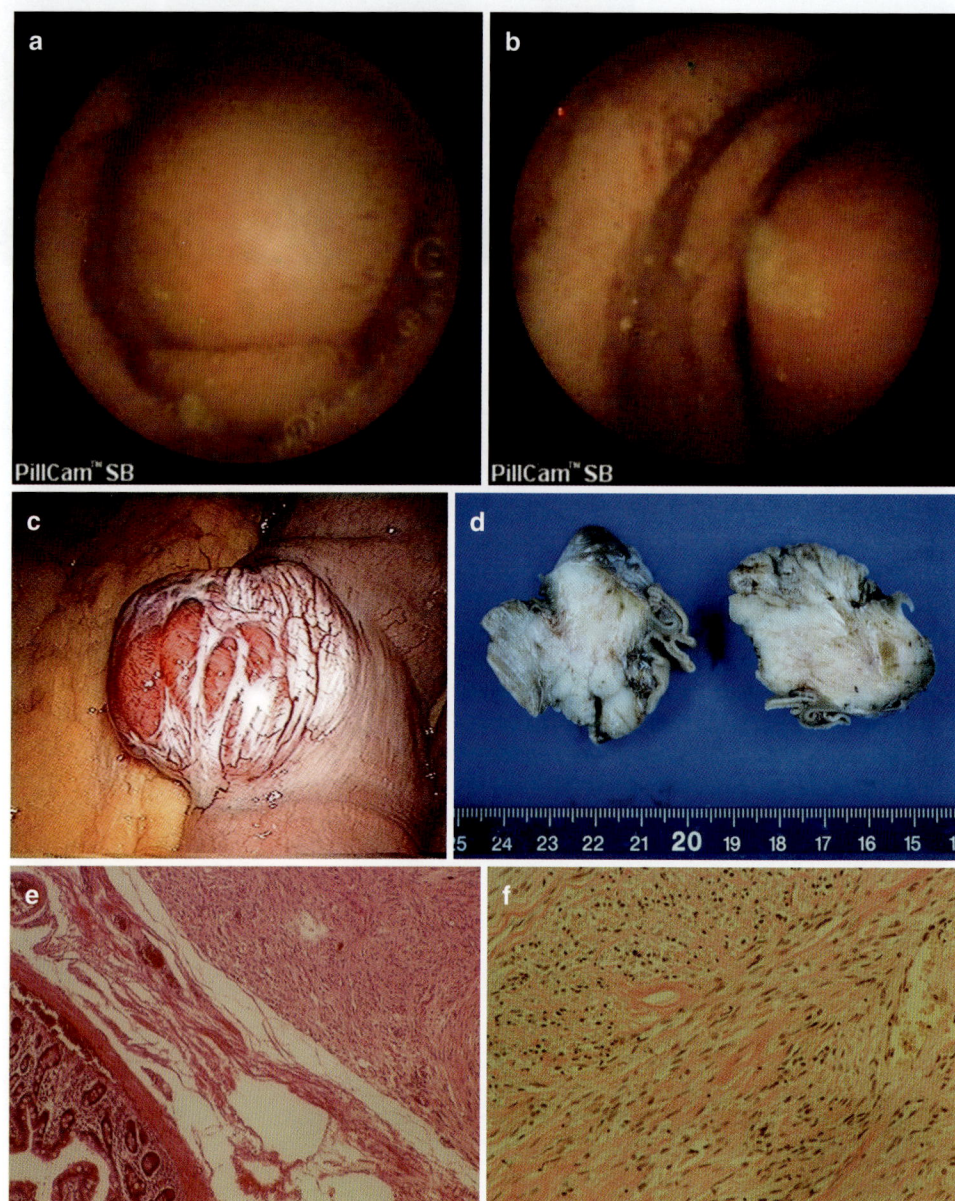

Fig. 34.7 Gastrointestinal stromal tumor (GIST). (**a**) VCE shows a protruding lesion in the duodenum. (**b**) VCE shows a slightly reddish, submucosal mass in the jejunum. (**c**) Laparoscopy with large extraluminal mass (probably causing impression of the duodenum). (**d**) Resected specimen. (**e**) Histology shows spindle cell tumor. (**f**) CD 117 (c-kit) positive staining

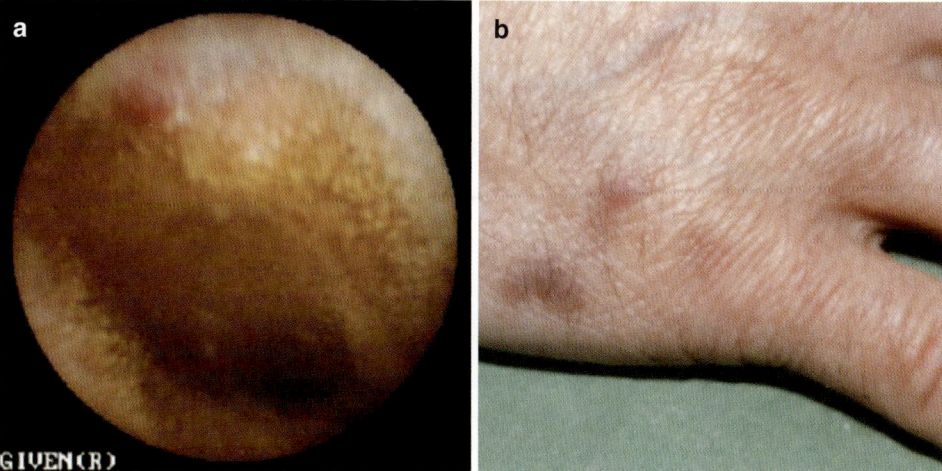

Fig. 34.8 Kaposi's sarcoma. (**a**) Bluish-red polypoid lesions in the jejunum. (**b**) AIDS patient with recurrent intestinal bleeding and cutaneous Kaposi's sarcoma

34.4.2 Kaposi's Sarcoma

Kaposi's sarcoma is a malignant angiosarcoma that is associated with human herpesvirus 8. The epidemic form is associated with HIV infection, in contrast to the classic or endemic form.

The most common lesion is the cutaneous Kaposi's sarcoma observed in patients with AIDS, but internal organs, including the small bowel, can be involved. Small-bowel involvement is usually asymptomatic, but some patients present with bleeding [35], intussusception, or exudative enteropathy.

Endoscopic findings typically consist of bluish-red nodules or tumors (Figs. 34.8 and 34.9) [36].

Treatment for the AIDS-associated form consists of antiretroviral therapy. Other options are chemotherapy and radiation. Resection is advised only in emergencies because of the high risk of recurrence.

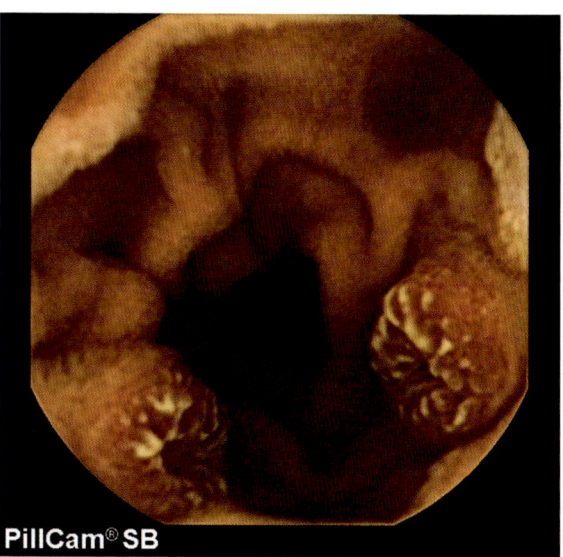

Fig. 34.9 Classic Kaposi's sarcoma (*Courtesy of* Nikolaos Viazis, MD) (Reprinted from Viazis et al. [36] with permission from Thieme Verlag)

34.4.3 Other Types of Sarcoma

Hemangiosarcoma, a very rare malignant tumor deriving from endothelial cells, can cause intestinal perforation or bleeding [16]. Pleomorphic sarcoma, an undifferentiated variant, cannot be related to a distinct originating tissue.

Endoscopy may show reddish or black polypoid or submucosal tumors (Figs. 34.10 and 34.11). Rarely, multiple nodules may be distributed throughout the small intestine (Fig. 34.12).

Fig. 34.10 (**a** and **b**) Angiosarcoma

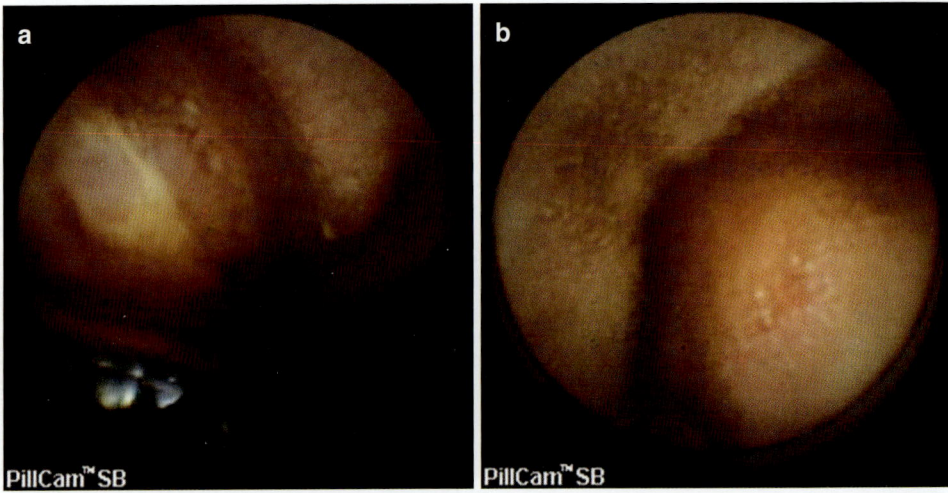

Fig. 34.11 Epithelioid angiosarcoma in a transplanted patient under immunosuppression. (**a**) VCE. (**b**) Enteroscopy (*Courtesy of Virender Sharma, MD*)

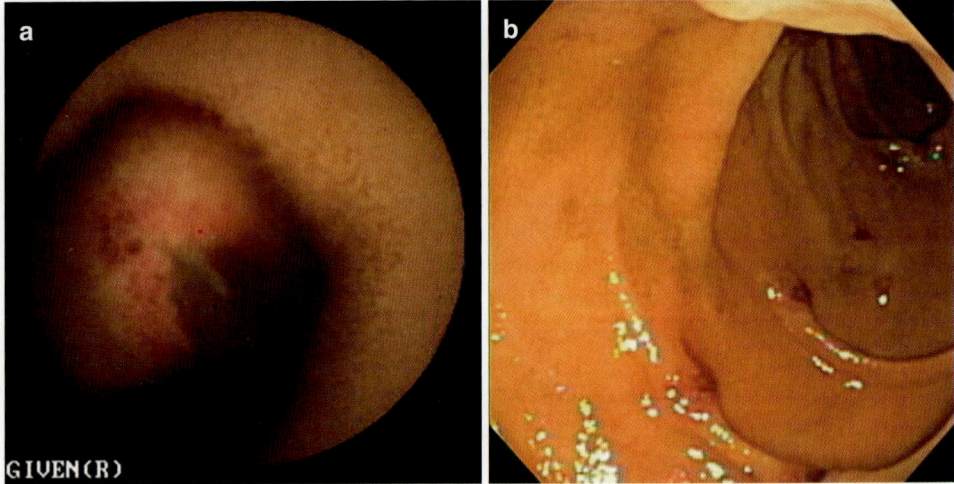

Fig. 34.12 Multilocular pleomorphic cellular sarcoma. (**a**) VCE, (**b**) endoscopy

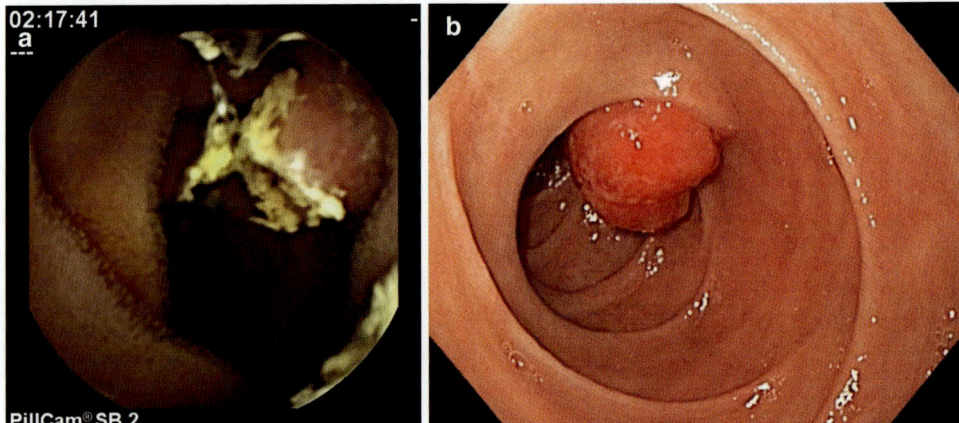

34.5 Intestinal Lymphomas

Gastrointestinal lymphomas are the most common extranodal manifestation of non-Hodgkin's lymphoma [37], with 90 % originating from B lymphocytes and 10 % from T lymphocytes (Table 34.2). Most are highly malignant. The most common site of occurrence is the stomach, followed by the small bowel and the colon. Celiac disease and immunoproliferative small intestinal disease (IPSID) are considered predisposing factors.

These tumors can be classified by clinical characteristics (primary small-bowel lymphomas tend to be localized, whereas immunoproliferative lymphomas are diffuse) [38]. Follicular lymphomas frequently involve the duodenum [39]. Endoscopy shows a variegated pattern of nodular polypoid tumors, ulcerations, infiltrative growth, thickened folds, and focal atrophy (Figs. 34.13, 34.14, 34.15, 34.16, 34.17, 34.18,

Table 34.2 Intestinal lymphomas

B-cell lymphomas

High-grade malignancies

Diffuse large-cell B-cell lymphomas: centroblastic (Fig. 34.17), immunoblastic

Burkitt's lymphoma (mainly in the terminal ileum, more prevalent in developing countries)

Low-grade malignancies

Extranodal marginal zone lymphoma of the MALT type (Western-type lymphoma; Fig. 34.18)

Mantle cell lymphoma (Fig. 34.13)

Alpha heavy-chain disease: Mediterranean-type lymphoma; follicular lymphoma (rare as primary intestinal tumor) (Figs. 34.14, 34.15, and 34.16)

T-cell lymphomas

Enteropathy-associated T-cell lymphoma (EATL) (Figs. 34.19 and 34.20)

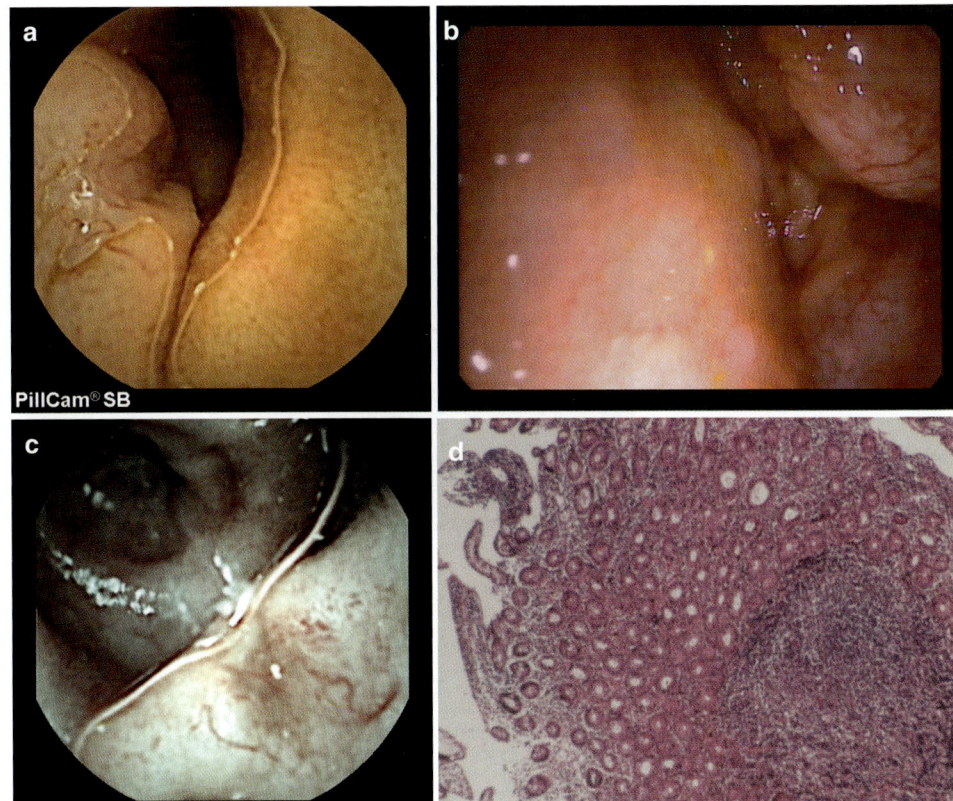

Fig. 34.13 Mantle cell lymphoma of the ileum. (**a**) VCE shows tumor with central depression. (**b**) Enteroscopy. (**c**) VCE in FICE1 mode shows enhanced visualization of pathologic vessels. (**d**) Histology (H&E stain)

Fig. 34.14 Follicular lymphoma of the terminal ileum. (**a**) Incidental finding during screening colonoscopy showing atypical, asymmetric aggregation of unusually large nodules. (**b**) Same aspect in VCE, which was performed to rule out additional small-bowel manifestations before resection

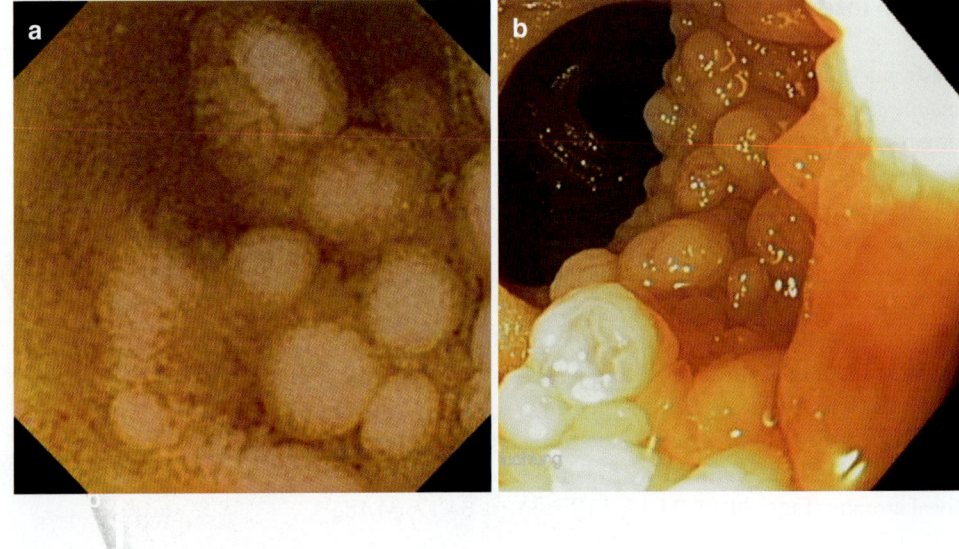

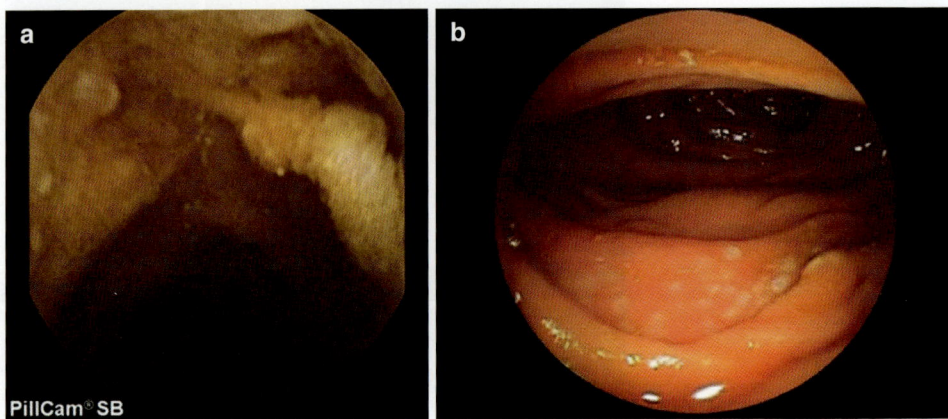

Fig. 34.15 Follicular lymphoma. (**a**) VCE. (**b**) Double-balloon enteroscopy

Fig. 34.16 Intestinal follicular lymphoma grade 1. (**a** and **b**) Ulcerated weblike stricture seen with small-bowel capsule endoscopy, mimicking a lesion from the use of nonsteroidal anti-inflammatory drugs (NSAIDs). (**c** and **d**) With double-balloon enteroscopy, the retained capsule was retrieved. (**e** and **f**) Bioptic diagnosis of lymphoma (**e**, CD10 positive staining) was confirmed at segmental resection (**e** and **f** *courtesy of* Axel Wellmann, MD)

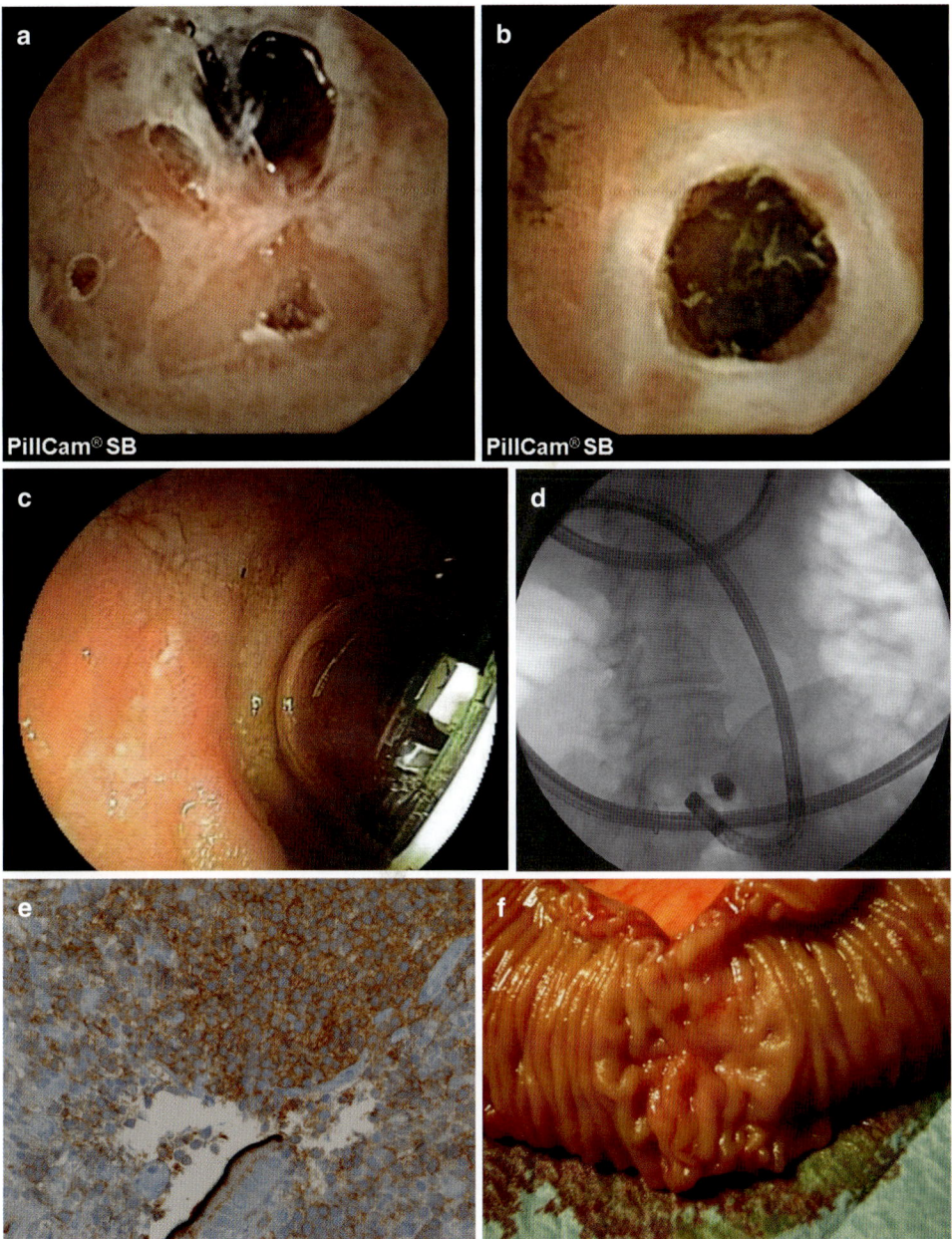

34.19, and 34.20) [40, 41]. Immunoproliferative small intestinal disease (IPSID) is characterized by a cobblestone appearance and multiple sessile polyps (Fig. 28.7) [42].

Whenever possible, treatment should be provided within the framework of studies based on the histology and stage of the tumor, with consideration of all modalities, including chemotherapy (CHOP regimen/high dose), radiotherapy, and surgical resection [43].

Fig. 34.17 Localized jejunal, highly malignant, diffuse B-cell lymphoma of the centroblastic type in a 70-year-old patient with melena, anemia, and weight loss. (**a** and **b**) VCE shows infiltration, concentric stenosis, and ulceration. The capsule is retained. (**c**) CT scan reveals circumscript thickening of jejunal wall (*Courtesy of* Roman Fischbach, MD). (**d**) Double-balloon enteroscopy for capsule retrieval, biopsy, and ink marking confirms short stenotic small-bowel segment

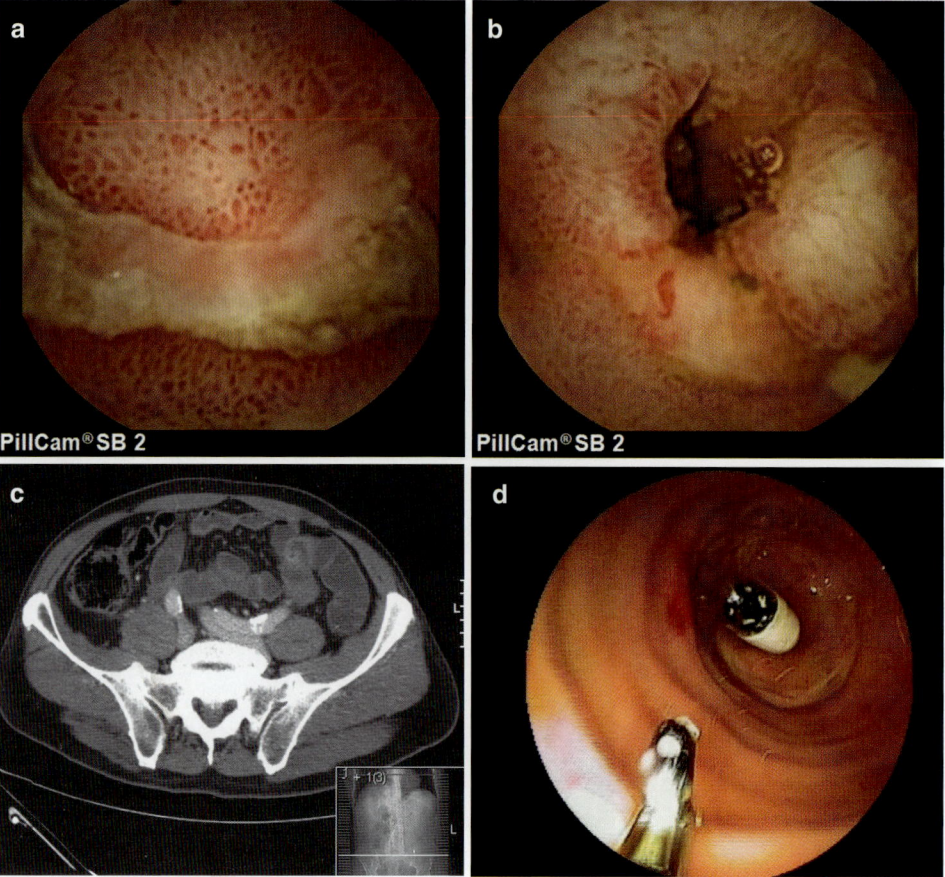

Fig. 34.18 (**a** and **b**) MALT lymphoma. Infiltrating, polypoid tumor (*Courtesy of* Markus Oeyen, MD)

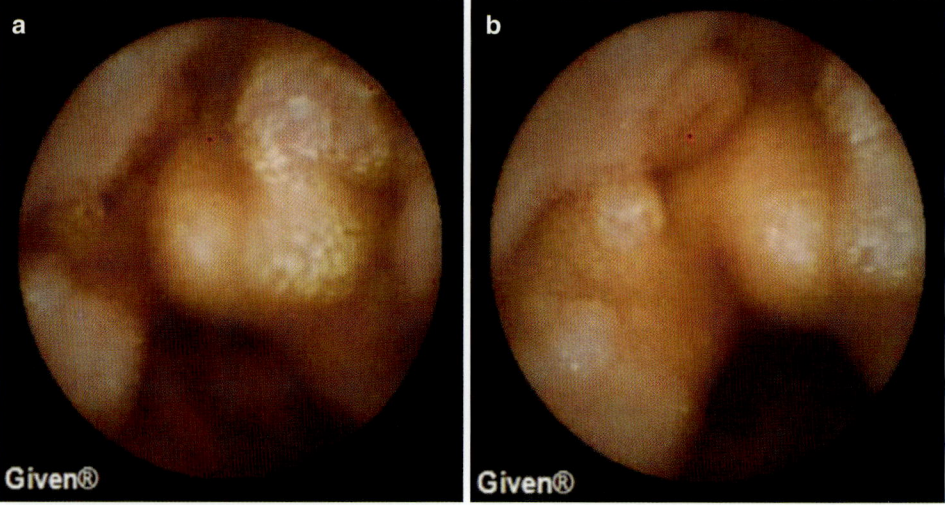

Fig. 34.19 Refractory villous atrophy in a patient with T-cell lymphoma. (**a**) VCE. (**b**) Push enteroscopy. (**c**) Ulcerative jejunoileitis is also present. (**d**) Lymphocytic T-cell infiltrate. Molecular biology: monoclonal T-cell receptor (*Case courtesy of* Michel Delvaux, MD, and Gerard Gay, MD)

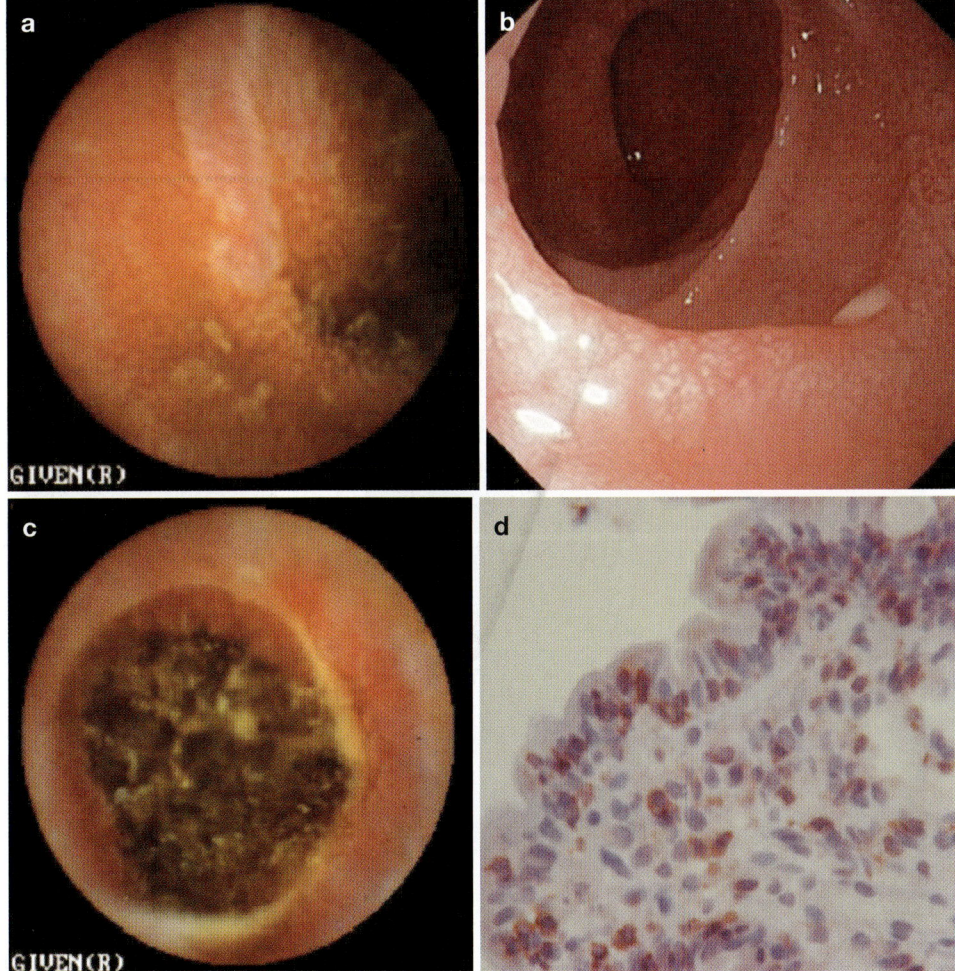

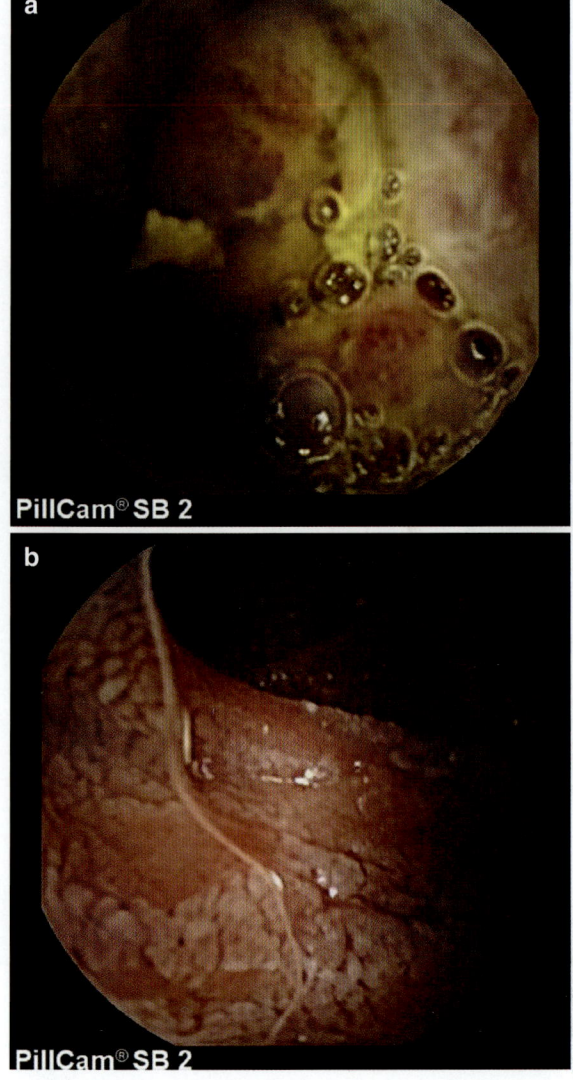

Fig. 34.20 Enteropathy-associated T-cell lymphoma (EATL). (**a**) Obstructing mass. (**b**) Villous atrophy

34.6   Melanoma of the Small Intestine

Melanoma is the most common metastatic tumor to the small bowel. Small-bowel capsule endoscopy has a high diagnostic yield in detecting melanoma metastasis [44], especially in advanced stages (Clarke level IV) and in patients with additional anemia [45]. Primary small-bowel melanoma (Fig. 34.21) is a rarity [46].

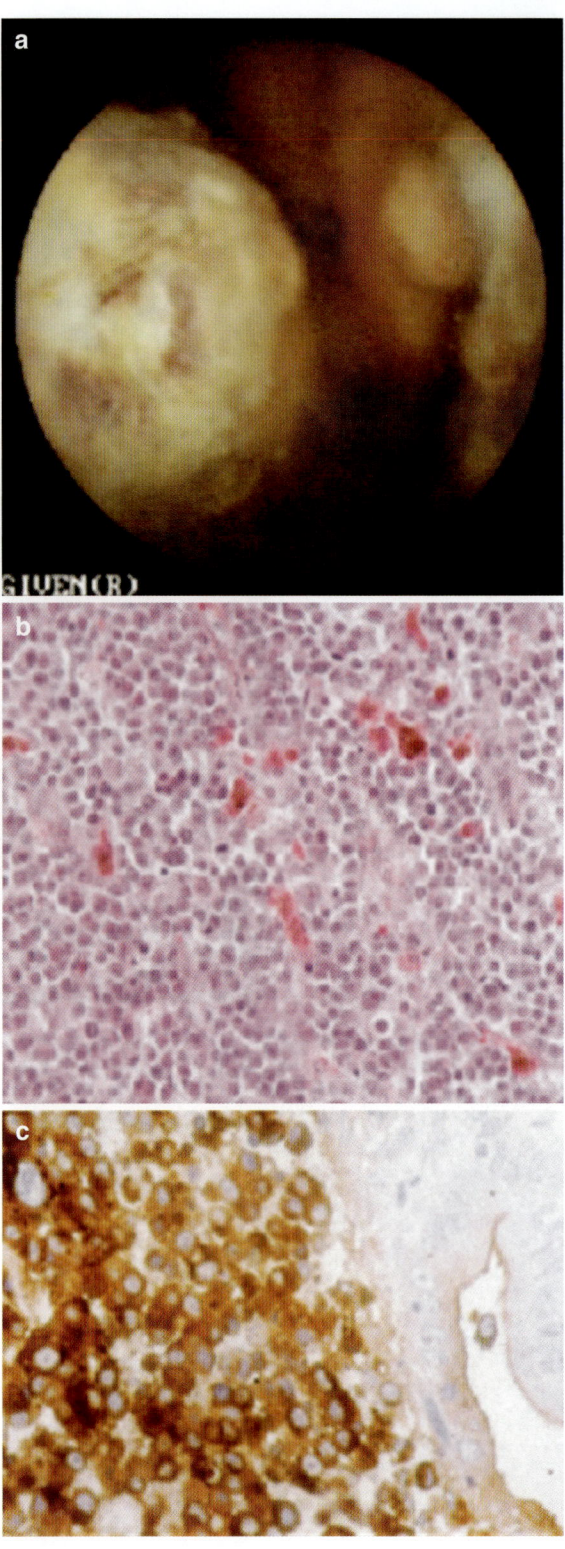

Fig. 34.21 Primary melanoma of the small bowel. The patient presented with intestinal bleeding and normal enteroclysis with no additional foci of melanoma. (**a**) Exophytic ulcerated tumor of the ileum causing partial stenosis, with active bleeding. (**b**) Histology: small-cell tumor with melanin pigment (H&E). (**c**) Strongly positive expression of the melanoma marker HMB 45 (**b** and **c** *courtesy of* Stefan Krüger, MD)

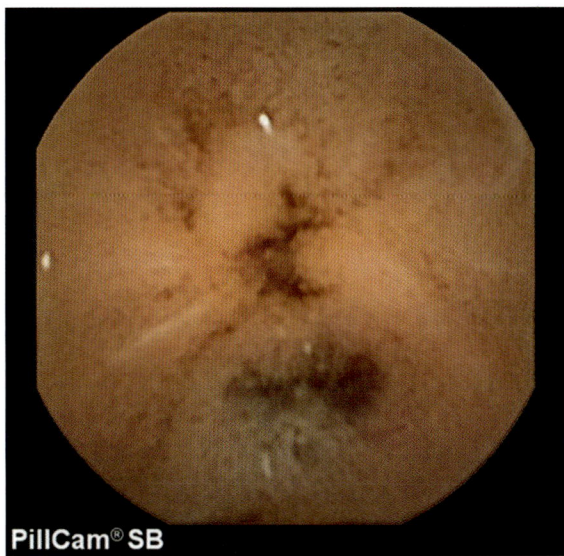

Fig. 34.22 Small metastasis of malignant melanoma

On endoscopy, the typical aspect of small-bowel melanoma is a black tumor, reaching in size from small black spots (Fig. 34.22) to an obstructing mass (Fig. 34.23). However, it should be noted that amelanotic melanoma (Fig. 34.24) is not uncommon [44]. These cases cannot be differentiated endoscopically from other malignant tumors.

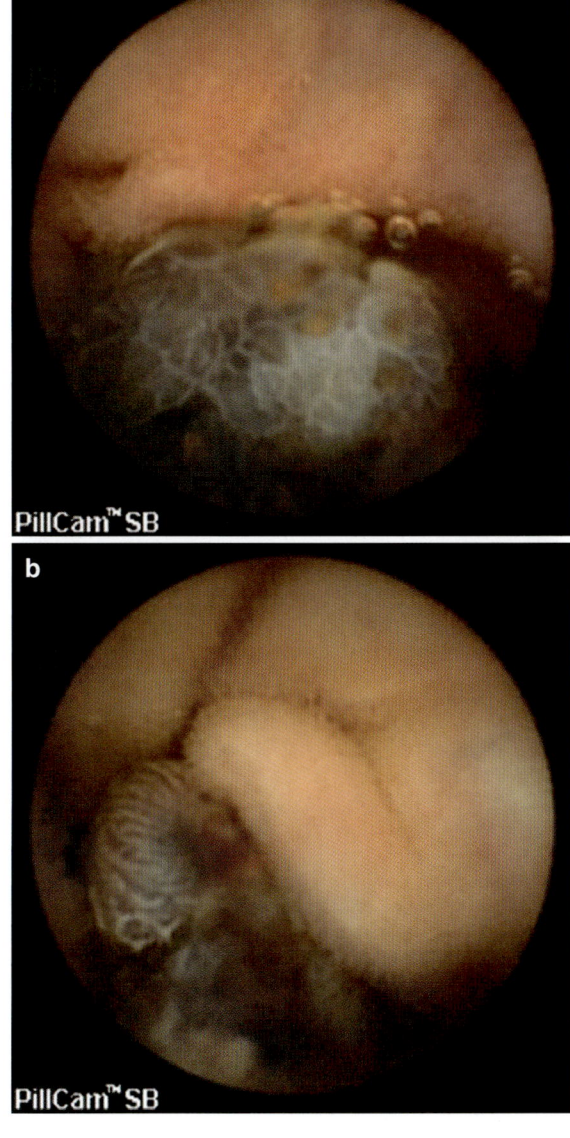

Fig. 34.23 (**a** and **b**) Larger metastasis of black melanoma

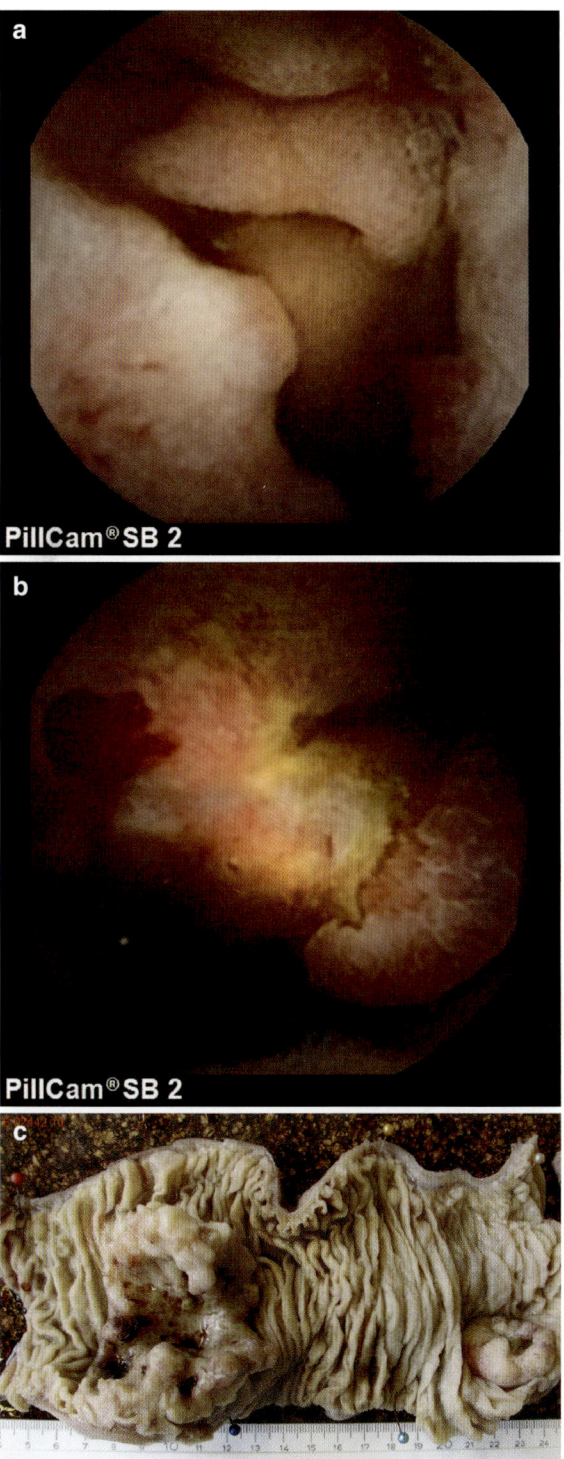

Fig. 34.24 Multilocular amelanotic melanoma. (**a** and **b**) VCE. (**c**) Resected specimen

34.7 Metastases

Metastases in the small bowel are very rare. They originate most often from melanomas (Figs. 34.22, 34.23, and 34.24) and less commonly from carcinomas of the colon, stomach, uterus, ovaries, bladder, breast, bronchi, kidney, pancreas, and others (Figs. 34.25, 34.26, 34.27, 34.28, and 34.29) [47].

Endoscopy reveals polypoid, exophytic, or submucosal, ulcerated tumors that cannot be differentiated by VCE from other malignant small-bowel tumors without knowledge of the primary.

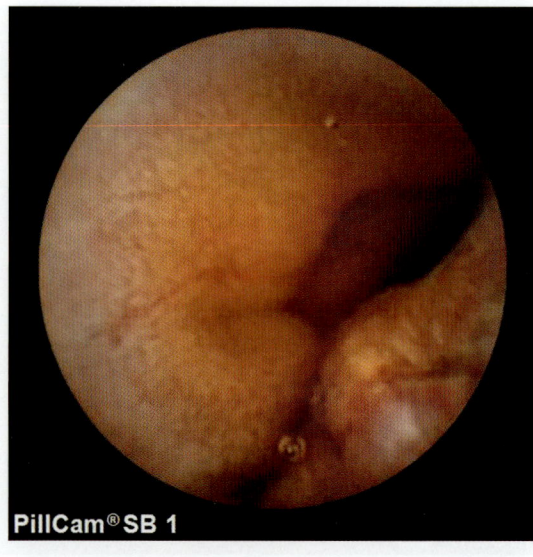

Fig. 34.26 Metastatic ovarian cancer

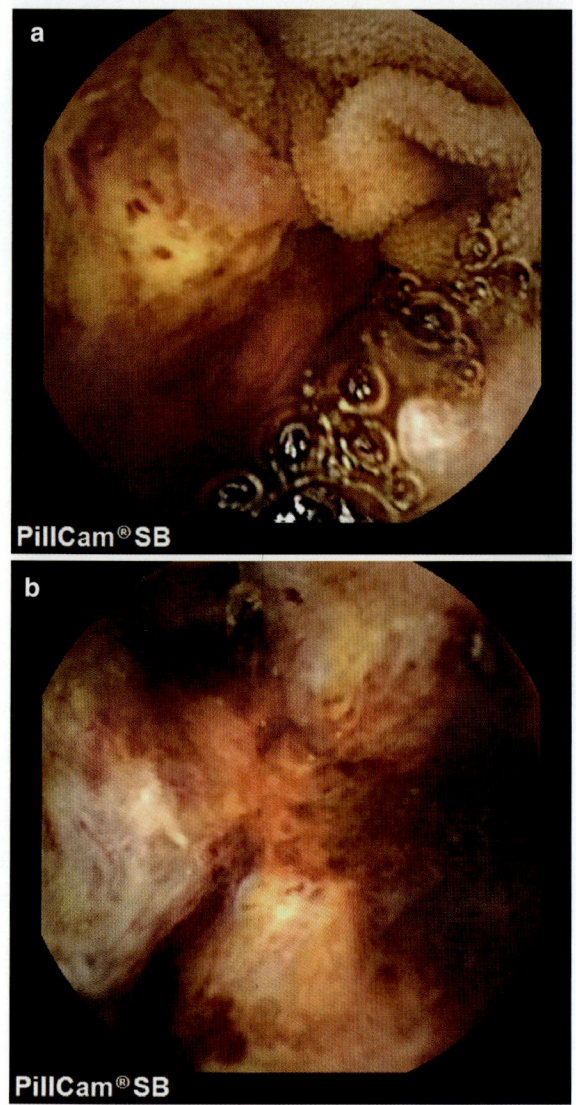

Fig. 34.25 (**a** and **b**) Metastasis of endometrial adenocarcinoma

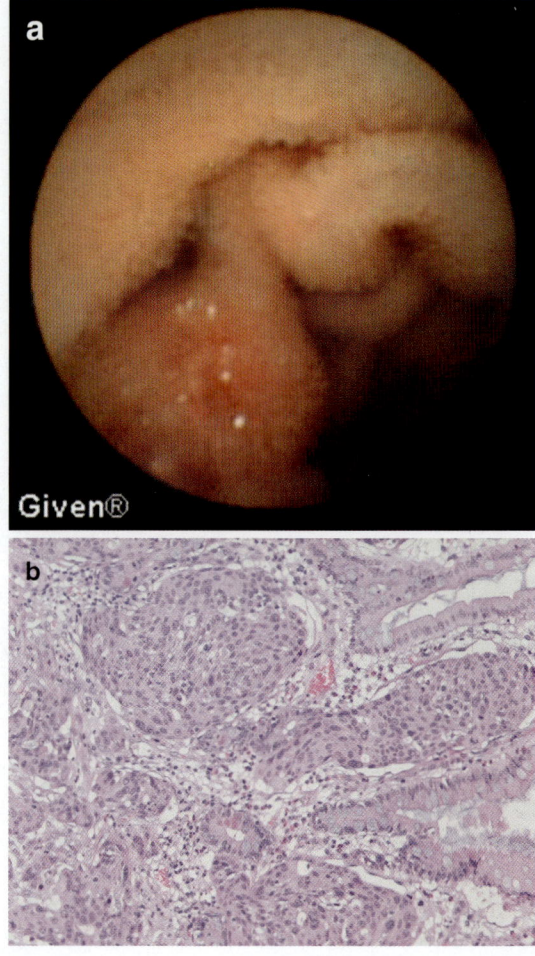

Fig. 34.27 Metastasis of large-cell lung cancer. (**a**) VCE (*Courtesy of* Felix Wiedbrauck, MD). (**b**) Histology (*Courtesy of* Peer Flemming, MD, and Axel Wellmann, MD)

Fig. 34.28 Small-bowel metastasis of gastric cancer. (**a**) VCE shows submucosal infiltration with central loss of villi owing to infiltration and surrounding lymphangiectasia. (**b**) Histology (*Courtesy of* Peer Flemming, MD, and Axel Wellmann, MD)

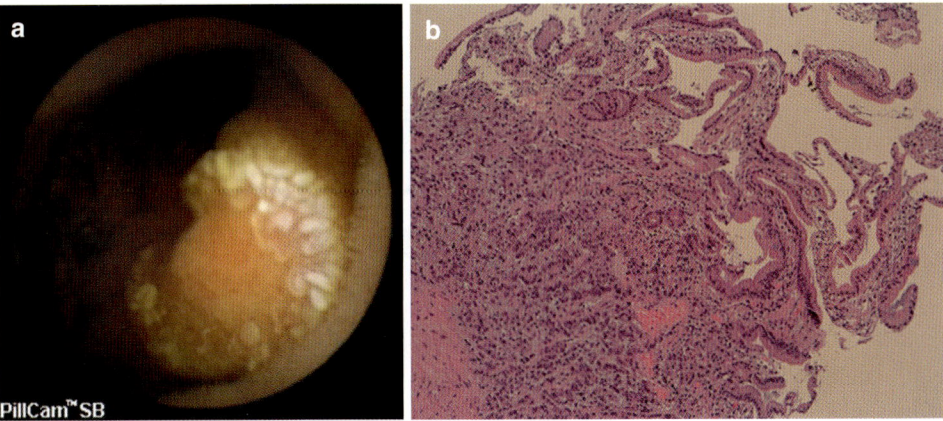

Fig. 34.29 Metastasis of kidney carcinoma to the small bowel. (**a**) VCE. (**b**) Double-balloon enteroscopy. (**c**) CT scan. (**d**) Resected specimen (*Courtesy of* Peer Flemming, MD, and Axel Wellmann, MD)

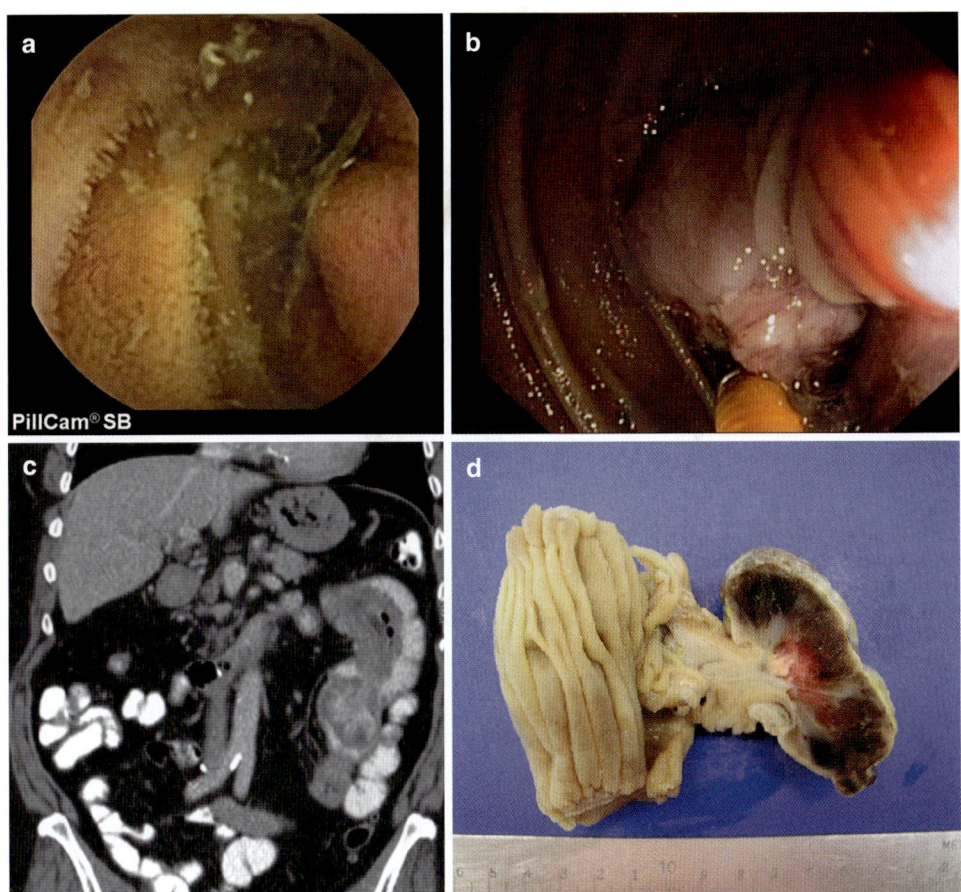

34.8 Contiguous Invasion of the Small Intestine

When VCE findings in the small bowel are equivocal, the examiner should also consider the rare possibility of small-bowel invasion by the contiguous spread of malignant tumors from neighboring organs. Ultrasound, endosonography, CT scans, MRI, and laparoscopy can accomplish the diagnosis in these patients (Fig. 34.30).

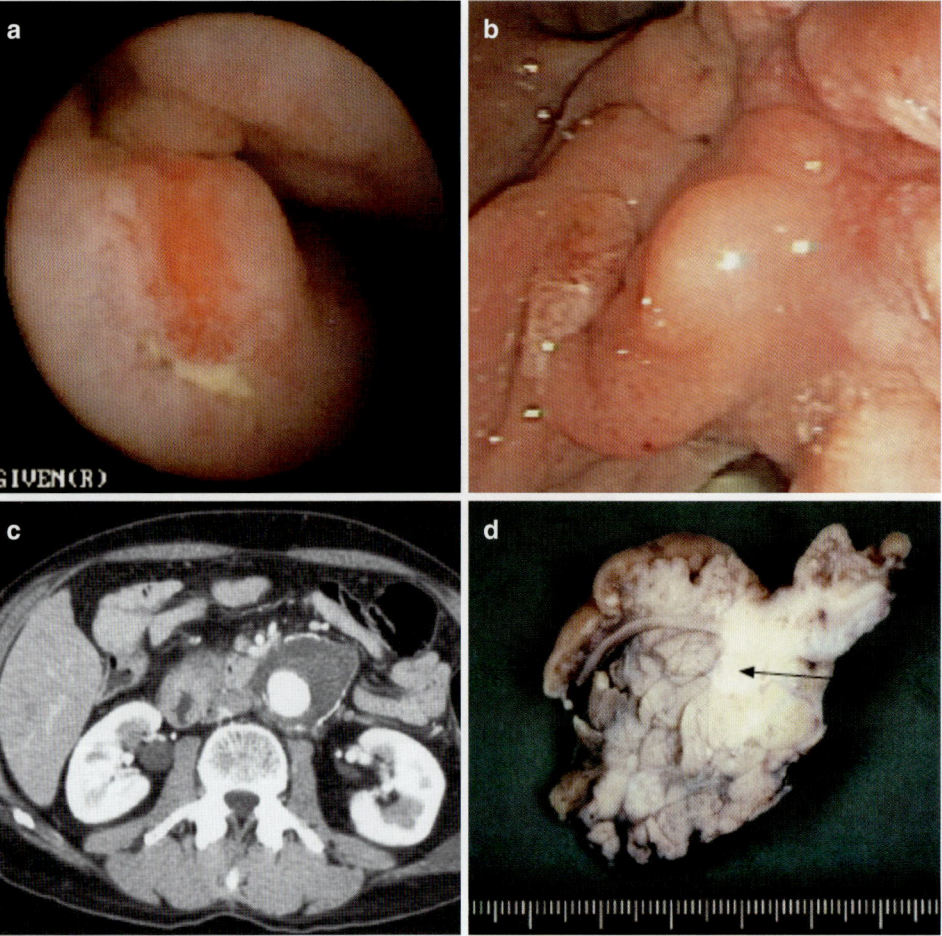

Fig. 34.30 Duodenal infiltration. VCE was performed to investigate chronic diarrhea and a 15-kg weight loss. Several prior esophagogastroduodenoscopic examinations showed nonspecific duodenitis. MR cholangiopancreatography was normal. (**a**) Duodenal infiltration seen on VCE. (**b**) A side-viewing duodenoscope confirmed the finding. (**c**) CT scan demonstrates a pancreatic head tumor (with an aortic aneurysm as an incidental finding) (*Courtesy of* Ernst Malzfeldt, MD). (**d**) Tumor resected by a pancreaticoduodenectomy (Whipple's operation): pancreatic head carcinoma (*arrow*)

References

1. Conn M. Tumors of the small intestine. In: DiMarino A, Benjamin S, editors. Gastrointestinal disease: an endoscopic approach. Malden: Blackwell Science; 1997. p. 551–66.
2. Herbsman H, Wetstein L, Rosen Y, et al. Tumors of the small intestine. Curr Probl Surg. 1980;17:121.
3. North JH, Pack MS. Malignant tumors of the small intestine: a review of 144 cases. Am Surg. 2000;66:46–51.
4. Qubaiah O, Devesa SS, Platz CE, et al. Small intestinal cancer: a population-based study of incidence and survival patterns in the United States, 1992 to 2006. Cancer Epidemiol Biomarkers Prev. 2010;19:1908–18.
5. Wu TJ, Yeh CN, Chao TC, et al. Prognostic factors of primary small bowel adenocarcinoma: univariate and multivariate analysis. World J Surg. 2006;30:391–8.
6. Hatzaras I, Palesty A, Abir F, et al. Small bowel tumors, epidemiologic and clinical characteristics of 1260 cases from the Connecticut Tumor Registry. Arch Surg. 2007;142:229–35.
7. Rossini FP, Risio M, Pennazio M. Small bowel tumors and polyposis syndromes. Gastrointest Endosc Clin N Am. 1999;9:93–114.
8. Barakat M. Endoscopic features of primary small bowel lymphoma: a proposed endoscopic classification. Gut. 1982;23:36–41.
9. Halphen M, Najjar T, Jaafoura H, et al. Diagnostic value of upper intestinal fiber endoscopy in primary small intestinal lymphoma. Cancer. 1986;58:2140–5.
10. Mascarenhas-Saraiva MN, da Silva Araujo Lopes LM. Small-bowel tumors diagnosed by wireless capsule endoscopy: report of five cases. Endoscopy. 2003;35:865–8.
11. Cobrin GM, Pittman RH, Lewis BS. Diagnosing small bowel tumors with capsule endoscopy. Gastroenterology. 2004;126 Suppl 2:A194–5.
12. Bailey AA, Debinski HS, Appleyard MN, et al. Diagnosis and outcome of small bowel tumors found by capsule endoscopy: a three-center Australian experience. Am J Gastroenterol. 2006;101: 2237–43.
13. Rondonotti E, Pennazio M, Toth E, et al. Small-bowel neoplasms in patients undergoing video capsule endoscopy: a multicenter European study. Endoscopy. 2008;40:488–95.
14. Achour J, Serraj I, Amrani L, Amrani N. Small bowel tumors: what is the contribution of video capsule endoscopy? Clin Res Hepatol Gastroenterol. 2012;36:222–6.
15. Madisch A, Schimming W, Kinzel F, et al. Locally advanced small-bowel adenocarcinoma missed primarily by capsule endoscopy but diagnosed by push enteroscopy. Endoscopy. 2003;35:861–4.
16. Knop FK, Hansen MB, Meisner S. Small-bowel hemangiosarcoma and capsule endoscopy. Endoscopy. 2003;35:637.
17. Ross A, Mehdizadeh S, Tokar J, et al. Double balloon enteroscopy detects small bowel mass lesions missed by capsule endoscopy. Dig Dis Sci. 2008;53:2140–3.
18. Hara AK, Leighton JA, Sharma VK, Fleischer DE. Small bowel: preliminary comparison of capsule endoscopy with barium study and CT. Radiology. 2004;230:260–5.
19. Brucher BL, Roder JD, Fink U, et al. Prognostic factors in resected primary small bowel tumors. Dig Surg. 1998;15:42–51.
20. Abrahams NA, Halverson A, Fazio VW, et al. Adenocarcinoma of the small bowel: a study of 37 cases with emphasis on histologic prognostic factors. Dis Colon Rectum. 2002;45:1496–502.
21. Klöppel G, Perren A, Heitz PU. The gastroenteropancreatic neuroendocrine cell system and its tumors: the WHO classification. Ann N Y Acad Sci. 2004;1014:13–27.
22. Klimstra DS, Modlin IR, Adsay NV, et al. Pathology reporting of neuroendocrine tumors: application of the Delphic consensus process to the development of a minimum pathology data set. Am J Surg Pathol. 2010;34:300–13.
23. Modlin IM, Lye KD, Kidd M. A 5-decade analysis of 13,715 carcinoid tumors. Cancer. 2003;97:934–59.
24. Hemminki K, Li X. Incidence trends and risk factors of carcinoid tumors: a nationwide epidemiologic study from Sweden. Cancer. 2001;92:2204–10.
25. Cross AJ, Leitzmann MF, Subar AF, et al. A prospective study of meat and fat intake in relation to small intestinal cancer. Cancer Res. 2008;68:9274–9.
26. Horton KM, Kamel I, Hofmann L, Fishman EK. Carcinoid tumors of the small bowel: a multitechnique imaging approach. AJR Am J Roentgenol. 2004;182:559–67.
27. Johanssen S, Boivin M, Lochs H, Voderholzer W. The yield of wireless capsule endoscopy in the detection of neuroendocrine tumors in comparison with CT enteroclysis. Gastrointest Endosc. 2006;63:660–5.
28. van Tuyl SA, van Noorden JT, Timmer R, et al. Detection of small-bowel neuroendocrine tumors by video capsule endoscopy. Gastrointest Endosc. 2006;64:66–72.
29. Oberg K, Kvols L, Caplin M, et al. Consensus report on the use of somatostatin analogs for the management of neuroendocrine tumors of the gastroenteropancreatic system. Ann Oncol. 2004; 15:966–73.
30. Buscombe JR, Caplin ME, Hilson AJ. Long-term efficacy of high-activity 111 in-pentetreotide therapy in patients with disseminated neuroendocrine tumors. J Nucl Med. 2003;44:1–6.
31. Logrono R, Jones DV, Faruqi S, Bhutani MS. Recent advances in cell biology, diagnosis, and therapy of gastrointestinal stromal tumor (GIST). Cancer Biol Ther. 2004;3:251–8.
32. Burkill GJ, Badran M, Al Muderis O, et al. Malignant gastrointestinal stromal tumor: distribution, imaging features, and pattern of metastatic spread. Radiology. 2003;226:527–32.
33. Tazawa K, Tsukada K, Makuuchi H, Tsutsumi Y. An immunohistochemical and clinicopathological study of gastrointestinal stromal tumors. Pathol Int. 1999;49:786–98.
34. Nakatani M, Fujiwara Y, Nagami Y, et al. The usefulness of double-balloon enteroscopy in gastrointestinal stromal tumors of the small bowel with obscure gastrointestinal bleeding. Intern Med. 2012;51:2675–82.
35. Neville CR, Peddada AV, Smith D, et al. Massive gastrointestinal hemorrhage from AIDS-related Kaposi's sarcoma confined to the small bowel managed with radiation. Med Pediatr Oncol. 1996;26:135–8.
36. Viazis N, Vlachogiannakos J, Georgiadis D, et al. Classic Kaposi's sarcoma and involvement of the small intestine as shown by capsule endoscopy. Endoscopy. 2008;40 Suppl 2:E209.
37. Feller AC, Diebold J. Histopathology of nodal and extranodal non-Hodgkin's lymphomas. 3rd ed. Berlin/Heidelberg/New York: Springer; 2004.
38. Chaaya A, Heller SJ. Introduction to small bowel tumors. Tech Gastrointest Endosc. 2012;14:88–93.
39. Nakamura M, Ohmiya N, Hirooka Y, et al. Endoscopic diagnosis of follicular lymphoma with small-bowel involvement using video capsule endoscopy and double-balloon endoscopy: a case series. Endoscopy. 2013;45:67–70.
40. Flieger D, Keller R, May A, et al. Capsule endoscopy in gastrointestinal lymphomas. Endoscopy. 2005;37:1174–80.

41. Hartmann D, Schilling D, Rebel M, et al. Diagnosis of a high-grade B-cell lymphoma of the small bowel by means of wireless capsule endoscopy. Z Gastroenterol. 2003;41:171–4.

42. Ersoy O, Akin E, Demirezer A, et al. Capsule endoscopic findings in immunoproliferative small intestinal disease. Endoscopy. 2012;44:E61–2.

43. Fischbach W. Gastrointestinal lymphomas. [Article in German]. Z Gastroenterol. 2004;42:1067–72.

44. Prakoso E, Selby WS. Polypoid and non-pigmented small-bowel melanoma in capsule endoscopy is common. Endoscopy. 2010;42:979.

45. Albert JG, Fechner M, Fiedler E, et al. Algorithm for detection of small-bowel metastasis in malignant melanoma of the skin. Endoscopy. 2011;43:490–8.

46. Khosrowshahi E, Horvath W. Primary malignant melanoma of the small intestine – a case report. Rontgenpraxis. 2002;54:220–3.

47. Washington K, McDonagh D. Secondary tumors of the gastrointestinal tract: surgical pathologic findings and comparison with autopsy survey. Mod Pathol. 1995;8:427–33.

Internet

www.cancer.org: American Cancer Society

www.carcinoid.org: The Carcinoid Cancer Foundation

www.eortc.be: European Organisation for Research and Treatment of Cancer (EORTC)

www.liferaftgroup.org: The Life Raft Group (support organization for patients with GIST)

www.lymphoma.org: Lymphoma Research Foundation

Familial Adenomatous Polyposis

35

Carol Burke, Christian P. Pox, Wolff Schmiegel, and Martin Keuchel

Contents

The work was first published in 2006 by Springer Medizin Verlag Heidelberg with the following title: *Atlas of Video Capsule Endoscopy*.

C. Burke (✉)
Department of Medicine,
Cleveland Clinic Foundation, Cleveland, OH, USA
e-mail: burkec1@ccf.org

C.P. Pox • W. Schmiegel
Department of Medicine, Ruhr-University Bochum,
Knappschaftskrankenhaus, Bochum, Germany
e-mail: christian.p.pox@rub.de; wolff.schmiegel@rub.de

M. Keuchel
Department of Internal Medicine,
Bethesda Krankenhaus Bergedorf, Hamburg, Germany
e-mail: keuchel@bkb.info

35.1   Genetics and Clinical Manifestation

The incidence of small-bowel polyps is very low in the general population, but it is significantly increased in hereditary polyposis syndromes such as familial adenomatous polyposis (FAP). FAP is caused by an autosomal dominant inherited defect in the *APC* gene, a classical tumor suppressor gene (Figs. 35.1 and 35.2). Colon polyposis is the most striking clinical manifestation, with more than 100 polyps (Fig. 35.3), leading in almost all patients to colorectal carcinoma. Prophylactic colectomy is recommended after adolescence.

Other manifestations such as retinopathy, osteomas, and connective tissue involvement occur less often. The combination of FAP with osteomas and other abnormalities is called Gardner's syndrome. Desmoid tumors, often located in the mesentery, may be especially challenging in these patients [1].

Attenuated forms of FAP have fewer colonic polyps, which will probably progress to cancer later in life. These patients have different gene mutations, only a part of which can be tested today. *MUTYH* mutation polyposis clinically resembles an attenuated form of AFP.

In patients with hereditary colon cancer syndromes, polyps occur not only in the colon and rectum but also in the stomach and small bowel with varying frequency. The risk for intestinal and extraintestinal malignancies is significantly increased in these patients [2]. Additional screening for thyroid cancer also is recommended for female patients [3].

Fundic gland polyps (Fig. 35.4) are very frequent in FAP. Larger sizes and advanced duodenal adenomas were associated with dysplasia [4], but they generally do not advance to cancer.

M. Keuchel et al. (eds.), *Video Capsule Endoscopy: A Reference Guide and Atlas*,
DOI 10.1007/978-3-662-44062-9_35, © Springer-Verlag Berlin Heidelberg 2014

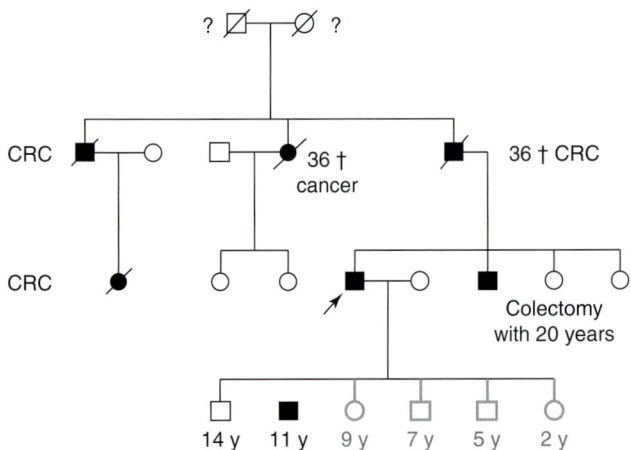

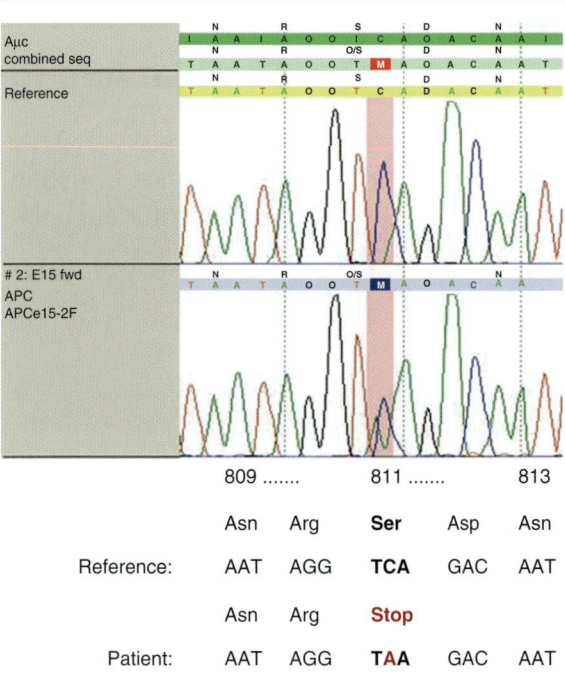

Fig. 35.1 Family pedigree in familial adenomatous polyposis (FAP). Index person (*black square with arrow*) with FAP and confirmed heterozygous *APC* gene mutation (Fig. 35.10). The two oldest children were tested for *APC* mutation; one was positive. Patients with FAP (*black symbols*); females (*circles*); males (*squares*); deceased individuals (*slashes*). (*Courtesy of* Britta Fiebig, MD)

	Asn	Arg	**Ser**	Asp	Asn
Reference:	AAT	AGG	**TCA**	GAC	AAT
	Asn	Arg	**Stop**		
Patient:	AAT	AGG	**TAA**	GAC	AAT

Fig. 35.2 Genetic testing with gene sequencing detected heterogenic *APC* gene mutation leading to a new stop codon at amino acid position 811, leading to a truncated *APC* protein. (*Courtesy of* Britta Fiebig, MD)

Fig. 35.3 Multiple polyps (tubular adenomas) of the colon in FAP. (**a**) Colonoscopy. (**b**) Video capsule endoscopy (VCE)

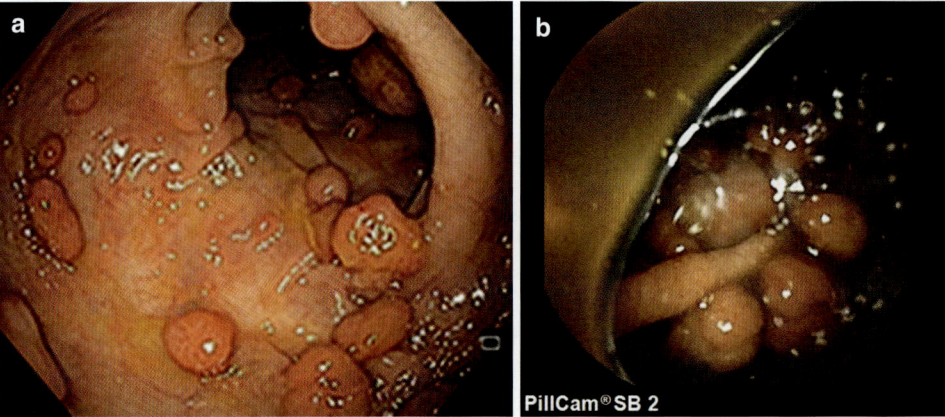

Fig. 35.4 Multiple small fundic gland polyps clearly seen at gastroscopy with insufflation (**a**), but hardly detectable at VCE (blue mode) (**b**)

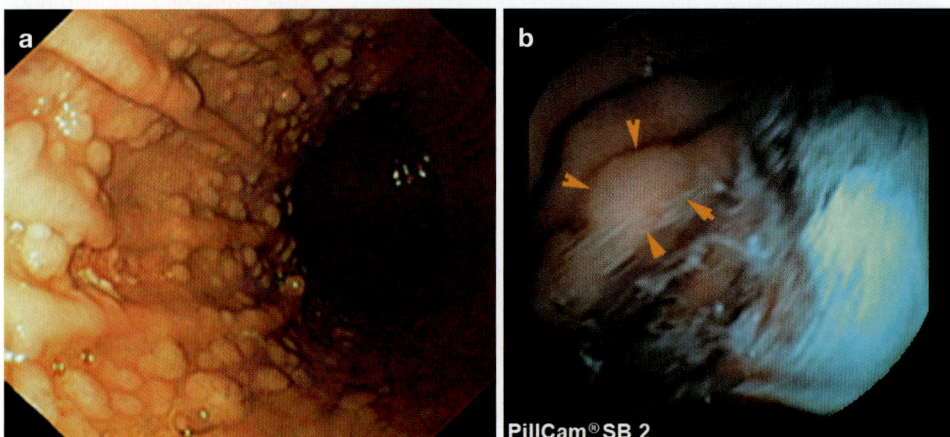

35.1.1 Duodenal Adenomas

Duodenal adenomas develop in a high percentage of FAP patients, so regular forward-viewing and side-viewing endoscopy with careful inspection of the papilla is recommended in FAP [5, 6]. The Spigelman score for staging duodenal adenomas is shown on Table 35.1 [7].

Duodenal carcinoma after colectomy is the leading cause of cancer death in patients with FAP [8]. Small intestinal adenomas are predominantly diagnosed in the duodenum [9] (Fig. 35.5). Adenomas can be treated endoscopically, depending on their size. Some polyps have turned out to be malignant at surgery in spite of previous benign biopsy, however. Furthermore, local treatment had a higher rate of recurrence than segmental or radical duodenectomy [10].

Table 35.1 Spigelman score for staging duodenal adenomas

Points	1	2	3
Number of adenomas	1–4	5–20	>20
Size	1–4 mm	5–10 mm	>10 mm
Histology	Tubular	Tubulovillous	Villous
Dysplasia	Mild	Moderate	Severe

From Spigelman et al. [7]
Zero points = stage 0; 1–4 points = stage I; 5–6 points = stage II; 7–8 points = stage III; 9–12 points = stage IV

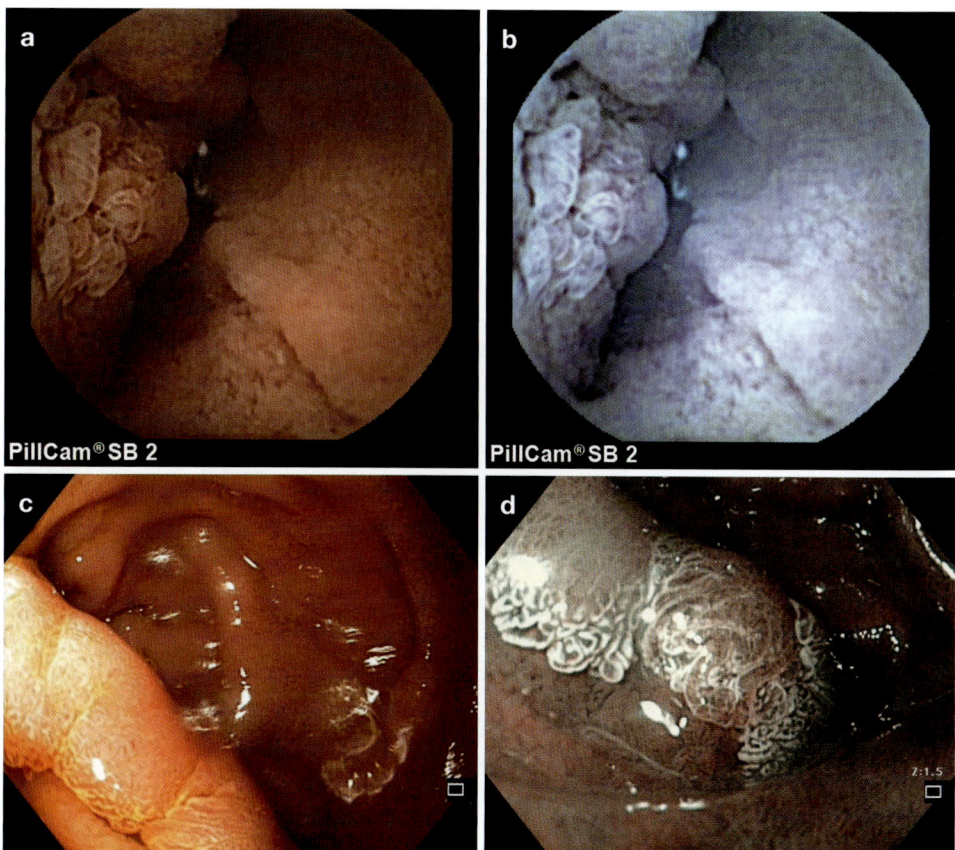

Fig. 35.5 Large duodenal adenoma (tubular adenoma with low-grade intraepithelial neoplasia) distal to the papilla. (**a** and **b**) VCE (**b** in flexible spectral imaging color enhancement [FICE] 3 mode). (**c** and **d**) Duodenoscopy (**d** in narrow-band imaging [NBI] mode)

35.1.2 Intestinal Adenomas

Additional small intestinal polyps are detectable in FAP patients, depending on the severity of duodenal polyposis [11–13] (Figs. 35.6, 35.7, 35.8, 35.9, and 35.10). However, there is not yet enough evidence on their relevance for recommendations on surveillance and follow-up [14].

35.2 Impact of VCE in FAP

Among 11 FAP patients with duodenal adenomas, 7 had jejunal or ileal polyps detected at VCE; none were found in FAP patients without duodenal adenomas [15]. The Spigelman stage of duodenal polyposis (Table 35.1) correlated with the presence of jejunal and ileal polyps [16].

Fig. 35.6 Small- to medium-sized jejunal polyps, seen at VCE (**a**) and double-balloon enteroscopy (**b**)

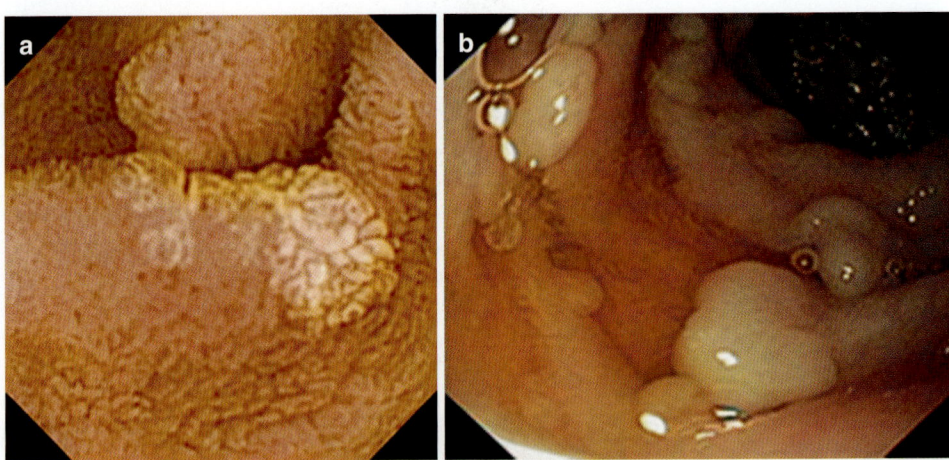

Fig. 35.7 Large jejunal polyp, seen at VCE (**a**) and single-balloon enteroscopy (NBI) (**b**)

Fig. 35.8 Medium-sized jejunal polyp, seen at VCE (**a**) and in FICE3 mode (**b**)

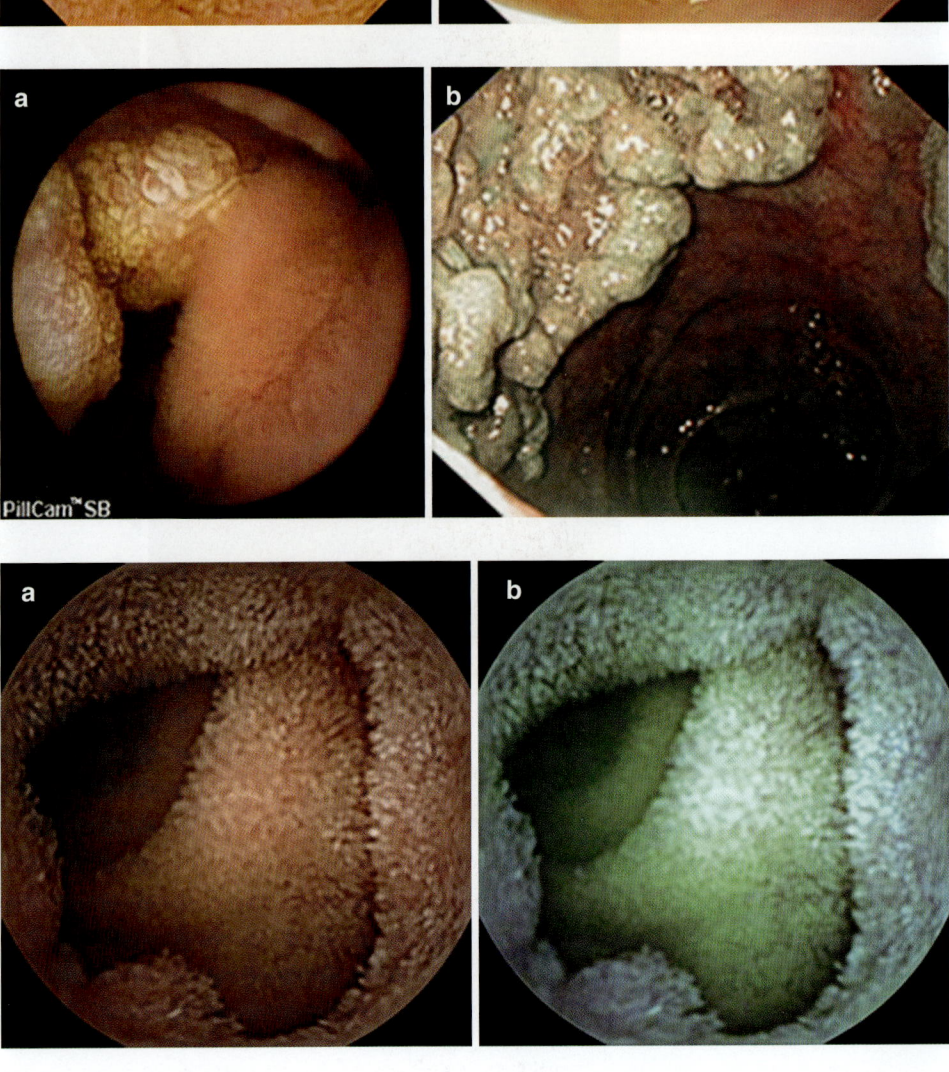

Fig. 35.9 Ileal polyp in a patient with FAP and duodenal adenoma, seen at VCE (**a**) and in blue mode (**b**). Tubular adenoma was confirmed at retrograde enteroscopy

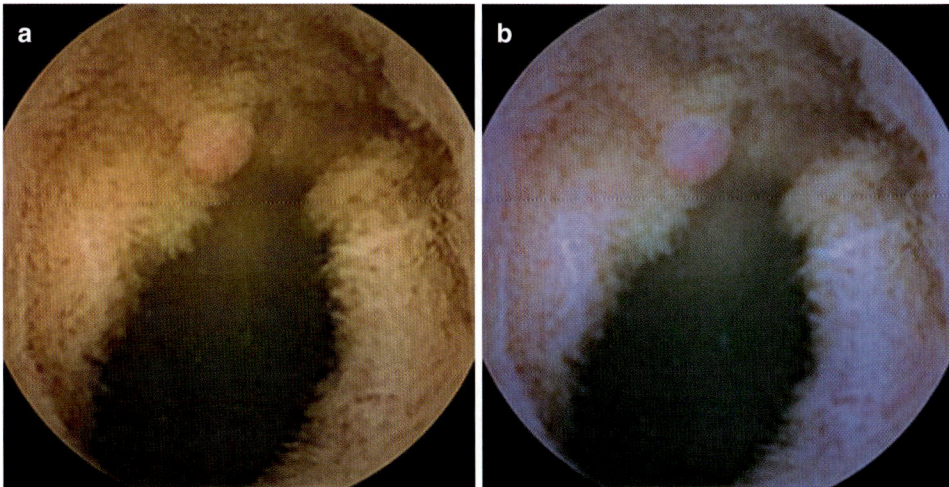

Fig. 35.10 Ileal polyps in an FAP patient. (**a**) VCE. (**b**) VCE localization trace (*blue*, stomach; *orange*, small intestine). (**c**) Retrograde single-balloon enteroscopy. (**d**) Bioptic removal with biopsy forceps (NBI mode). Histology showed tubular adenoma

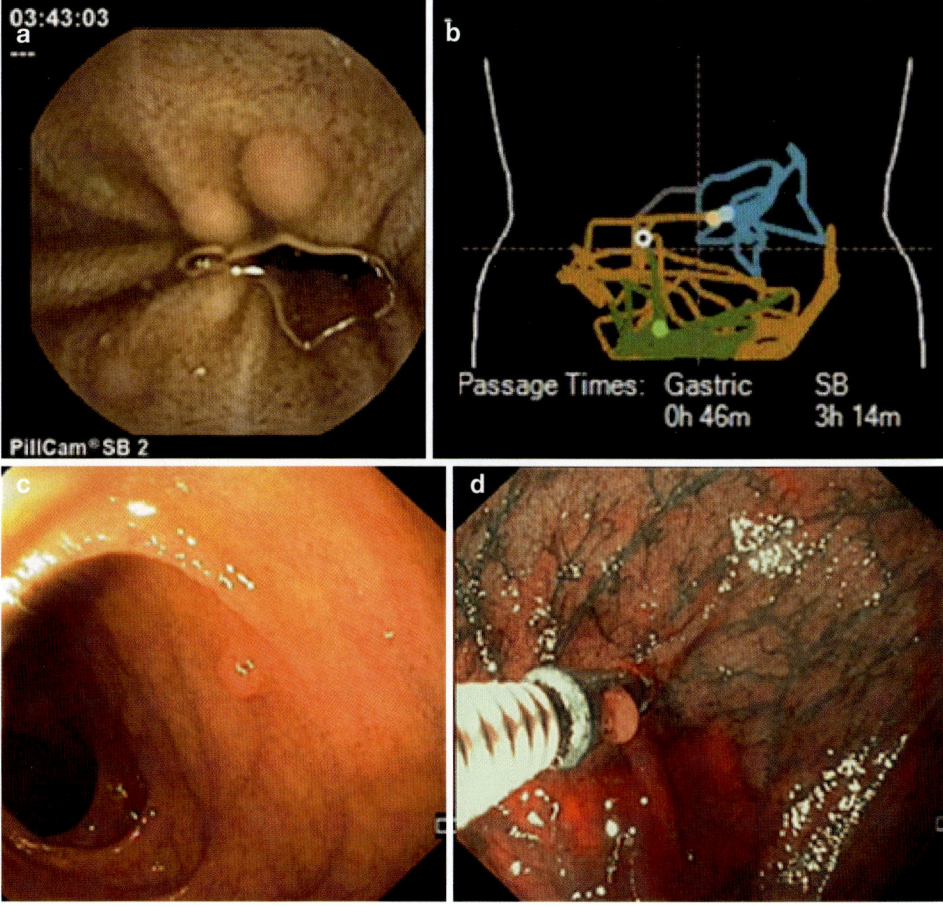

Polyps of medium or large size were located in the proximal jejunum (Figs. 35.6 and 35.7), not in the distal jejunum or ileum [17].

APC mutations between codons 499 and 805 were associated with the absence of small-bowel polyps in a small series [15]. Compare Fig. 35.2, showing a codon 811 mutation in an FAP patient with small intestinal polyps.

In one study of 20 patients, VCE was superior to small-bowel follow-through in detecting small-bowel polyps [18].

In a comparison with MRI, VCE detected small polyps, but MRI was more accurate in localization and size estima-

tion [19]. In another small series, VCE tended to find more small intestinal polyps than did MRI; the MRI showed additional extraintestinal pathology, such as desmoid tumors [20].

VCE identified fewer polyps in the stomach (Fig. 35.4) and duodenum than upper-GI endoscopy, but VCE was superior in the detection of jejunal and ileal polyps when compared with small-bowel follow-through and MRI (*n* = 20) [21]. Overall, VCE was the only modality to find polyps in all segments.

Wong et al. [22] found no additional benefit of VCE versus standard ileoscopy and push enteroscopy in the detection of small intestinal polyps in 32 FAP patients after colectomy.

Plum et al. [23], however, detected intestinal polyps that were beyond the reach of push enteroscopy and ileoscopy in 12 of 23 patients. Enteroclysis had false negative results in 19 of 23 patients, and eight of these polyps were larger than 10 mm.

35.3   Findings at VCE

Duodenal adenomas in general have a typical flat, white appearance, which should not be confused with focal lymphangiectasia. In the lymphangiectasia, the white color is clearly restricted to each single villus, whereas adenomas often are somewhat irregular, are slightly elevated, and do not respect villous morphology (see Fig. 5.24). Larger adenomas are seen as protruding lesions. Jejunal and ileal polyps may appear rather nodular, without a white surface. Occasionally, pedunculated polyps are seen.

Spectral color selection can be helpful in enhancing the contrast of polyps detected in VCE standard mode (Figs. 35.5c, 35.8b, and 35.9b). However, all three settings for flexible spectral imaging color enhancement (FICE) [24] and contrast image capsule endoscopy [25] were not helpful in the detection of polyps.

35.4   Limitations of VCE

Polyp detection in the duodenum with capsule endoscopy is limited. Duodenal polyps detected endoscopically were seen by VCE in only 4 of 11 patients [15], and four papillary adenomas were missed by VCE [16]. Hence, VCE cannot replace duodenoscopy. Nevertheless, special attention should be paid to the duodenal images in VCE as well, because esophagogastroduodenoscopy (EGD) may miss duodenal adenomas seen in VCE [26]. VCE seems to underestimate the number of polyps when compared with the combination of push enteroscopy and ileoscopy [22] or duodenoscopy [15].

In the published series, VCE was performed without complication. However, single cases of capsule retention in FAP patients and prior colectomy have been observed (Fig. 35.11) [27]. Probably severe adhesions and desmoid tumors are risk factors (Fig. 35.12). In doubtful cases, a prior patency capsule test (Chap. 9) may be considered.

In summary, small-bowel VCE seems to be safe and effective in diagnosing jejunal and ileal polyps in FAP patients, but the clinical relevance of detecting these polyps is yet unclear [28]. VCE cannot replace duodenoscopy. In FAP patients without duodenal adenomas, VCE is not helpful, as the incidence of jejunal and ileal polyps is very low.

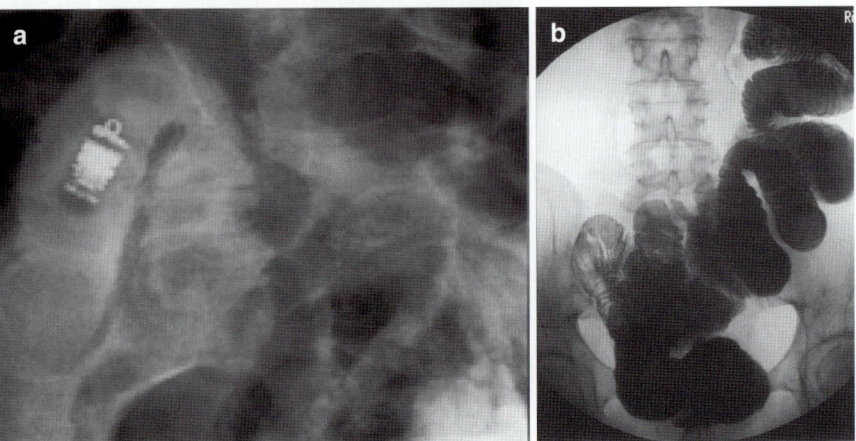

Fig. 35.11 (**a**) Retained capsule in a patient with FAP. (The patency capsule was not yet available.) After colectomy and small-bowel resection, there were adhesions and intra-abdominal desmoid tumors. (**b**) Short small intestine seen at enteroclysis

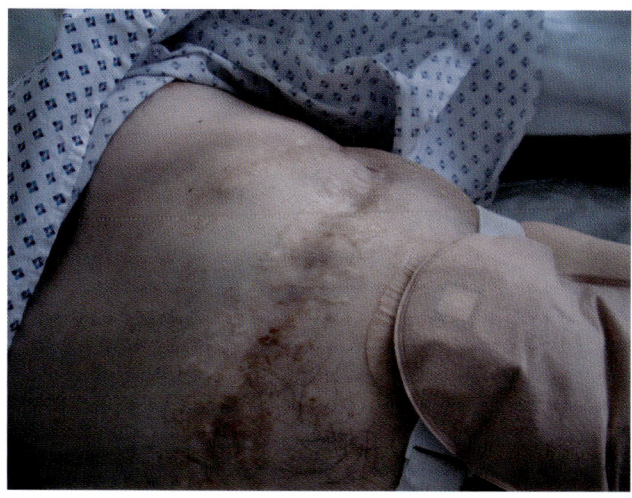

Fig. 35.12 Abdominal wall of an FAP patient with desmoid tumors after colectomy, small intestinal resection for obstruction, and ileostoma. A patency capsule was not excreted intact but dissolved within the GI tract, thus clearly indicating that VCE was contraindicated

References

1. Turina M, Pavlik CM, Heinimann K, et al. Recurrent desmoids determine outcome in patients with Gardner syndrome: a cohort study of three generations of an APC mutation-positive family across 30 years. Int J Colorectal Dis. 2013;28:865–72.
2. Giardiello FM, Brensinger JD, Petersen GM. AGA technical review on hereditary colorectal cancer and genetic testing. Gastroenterology. 2001;121:198–213.
3. Jarrar AM, Milas M, Mitchell J, et al. Screening for thyroid cancer in patients with familial adenomatous polyposis. Ann Surg. 2011;253:515–21.
4. Bianchi LK, Burke CA, Bennett AE, et al. Fundic gland polyp dysplasia is common in familial adenomatous polyposis. Clin Gastroenterol Hepatol. 2008;6:180–5.
5. Burke CA, Beck GJ, Church JM, van Stolk RU. The natural history of untreated duodenal and ampullary adenomas in patients with familial adenomatous polyposis followed in an endoscopic surveillance program. Gastrointest Endosc. 1999;49:358–64.
6. Pox C, Aretz S, Bischoff SC, et al. S3-guideline colorectal cancer version 1.0. Z Gastroenterol. 2013;51:753–854.
7. Spigelman AD, Williams CB, Talbot IC, et al. Upper gastrointestinal cancer in patients with familial adenomatous polyposis. Lancet. 1989;2(8666):783–5.
8. Galle TS, Juel K, Bulow S. Causes of death in familial adenomatous polyposis. Scand J Gastroenterol. 1999;34:808–12.
9. Saurin JC, Chayvialle JA, Ponchon T. Management of duodenal adenomas in familial adenomatous polyposis. Endoscopy. 1999;31:472–8.
10. Johnson MD, Mackey R, Brown N, et al. Outcome based on management for duodenal adenomas: sporadic versus familial disease. J Gastrointest Surg. 2010;14:229–35.
11. Schulmann K, Schmiegel W. Capsule endoscopy for small bowel surveillance in hereditary intestinal polyposis and non-polyposis syndromes. Gastrointest Endosc Clin N Am. 2004;14:149–58.
12. Schulmann K, Hollerbach S, Kraus K, et al. Feasibility and diagnostic utility of video capsule endoscopy for the detection of small bowel polyps in patients with hereditary polyposis syndromes. Am J Gastroenterol. 2005;100:27–37.
13. Burke CA, Santisi J, Church J, Levinthal G. The utility of capsule endoscopy small bowel surveillance in patients with polyposis. Am J Gastroenterol. 2005;100:1498–502.
14. Dunlop MG. Guidance on gastrointestinal surveillance for hereditary non-polyposis colorectal cancer, familial adenomatous polyposis, juvenile polyposis and Peutz-Jeghers syndrome. Gut. 2002;51:21–7.
15. Iaquinto G, Fornasarig M, Quaia M, et al. Capsule endoscopy is useful and safe for small-bowel surveillance in familial adenomatous polyposis. Gastrointest Endosc. 2008;67:61–7.
16. Katsinelos P, Kountouras J, Chatzimavroudis G, et al. Wireless capsule endoscopy in detecting small-intestinal polyps in familial adenomatous polyposis. World J Gastroenterol. 2009;15:6075–9.
17. Gunther U, Bojarski C, Buhr HJ, et al. Capsule endoscopy in small-bowel surveillance of patients with hereditary polyposis syndromes. Int J Colorectal Dis. 2010;25:1377–82.
18. Mata A, Llach J, Castells A, et al. A prospective trial comparing wireless capsule endoscopy and barium contrast series for small-bowel surveillance in hereditary GI polyposis syndromes. Gastrointest Endosc. 2005;61:721–5.
19. Caspari R, von Falkenhausen M, Krautmacher C, et al. Comparison of capsule endoscopy and magnetic resonance imaging for the detection of polyps of the small intestine in patients with familial adenomatous polyposis or with Peutz-Jeghers' syndrome. Endoscopy. 2004;36:1054–9.
20. Akin E, Demirezer BA, Buyukasik S, et al. Comparison between capsule endoscopy and magnetic resonance enterography for the detection of polyps of the small intestine in patients with familial adenomatous polyposis. Gastroenterol Res Pract. 2012:215028.
21. Tescher P, Macrae FA, Speer T, et al. Surveillance of FAP: a prospective blinded comparison of capsule endoscopy and other GI imaging to detect small bowel polyps. Hered Cancer Clin Pract. 2010;8:3.
22. Wong RF, Tuteja AK, Haslem DS, et al. Video capsule endoscopy compared with standard endoscopy for the evaluation of small-bowel polyps in persons with familial adenomatous polyposis (with video). Gastrointest Endosc. 2006;64:530–7.
23. Plum N, May A, Manner H, Ell C. Small-bowel diagnosis in patients with familial adenomatous polyposis: comparison of push enteroscopy, capsule endoscopy, ileoscopy, and enteroclysis. Z Gastroenterol. 2009;47:339–46.
24. Kobayashi Y, Watabe H, Yamada A, et al. Efficacy of flexible spectral imaging color enhancement on the detection of small intestinal diseases by capsule endoscopy. J Dig Dis. 2012;13:614–20.
25. Hatogai K, Hosoe N, Imaeda H, et al. Role of enhanced visibility in evaluating polyposis syndromes using a newly developed contrast image capsule endoscope. Gut Liver. 2012;6:218–22.
26. Yamada A, Watabe H, Iwama T, et al. The prevalence of small intestinal polyps in patients with familial adenomatous polyposis: a prospective capsule endoscopy study. Fam Cancer. 2013 Jun 7 (Epub ahead of print).
27. Perez-Segura P, Siso I, Luque R, et al. Iatrogenic intestinal obstruction: a rare complication of capsule endoscopy in a patient with familial adenomatous polyposis. Endoscopy. 2007;39 Suppl 1:E298–9.
28. Koornstra JJ. Small bowel endoscopy in familial adenomatous polyposis and Lynch syndrome. Best Pract Res Clin Gastroenterol. 2012;26:359–68.

Peutz-Jeghers Syndrome

36

Christopher Fraser and Edward J. Despott

Content

Peutz-Jeghers syndrome (PJS) is an autosomal dominant polyposis syndrome with high penetrance. It is associated with a germline mutation in the *STK11/LKB1* gene (19p13.3) in 80–94 % of patients [1] and has an incidence of about 1 in 8,500 to 1 in 200,000 live births [2–5]. The characteristics of the PJS phenotype include mucocutaneous melanin pigmentation (Fig. 36.1), gastrointestinal (GI) polyposis [6] and a predisposition to GI and extra-GI malignancies [2, 4–10].

GI polyps in PJS have distinct hamartomatous histopathological features, with "frond-like" epithelial lengthening and "arborisation" of a smooth muscle core (Fig. 36.2), and are thought to arise as a result of GI mucosal prolapse [3, 8]. Although PJS polyps may occur anywhere within the GI tract, they predominantly occur within the small bowel, particularly the jejunum [6, 10, 11]. Large ($\geq$1.5 cm) PJS polyps in the small bowel frequently result in intussusception (Fig. 36.3) and small-bowel obstruction or bleeding with iron deficiency anaemia [3–5, 10, 12, 13] and contribute to a major part of the disease burden in patients with this condition. Complications arising from small-bowel polyps often manifest themselves early in life [3, 14–16]. The cumulative risk of intussusception may be as high as 50 % by the age of 20 years [10], and many patients require multiple laparotomies throughout their life [17].

To facilitate early detection of these large PJS polyps and to examine for possible occult small-bowel malignancies, current guidelines recommend that patients should undergo small-bowel surveillance on a biennial to triennial basis starting at 8–10 years of age [3, 12, 13]. This surveillance may be undertaken by minimally invasive technologies such as small-bowel capsule endoscopy (SBCE) and/or radiologic diagnostic imaging.

SBCE has the advantage of being very well tolerated by patients and is a less invasive test for surveillance [12]. The potential to miss significant lesions has been reported, however, particularly if the lesions are located within the proximal small bowel [12, 13, 18–20]. Further limitations associated with the use of SBCE for this indication include challenges relating to the estimation of polyp size (Fig. 36.4), estimation of polyp location and possible "double counting" of visualised polyps [12, 13].

The work was first published in 2006 by Springer Medizin Verlag Heidelberg with the following title: *Atlas of Video Capsule Endoscopy*.

C. Fraser (✉)
Wolfson Unit for Endoscopy, St. Mark's Hospital and Academic Institute, Imperial College London, London, UK
e-mail: chris.fraser@imperial.ac.uk

E.J. Despott
Centre for Gastroenterology,
The Royal Free Hospital and UCL School of Medicine, London, UK
e-mail: edespott@doctors.org.uk

M. Keuchel et al. (eds.), *Video Capsule Endoscopy: A Reference Guide and Atlas*,
DOI 10.1007/978-3-662-44062-9_36, © Springer-Verlag Berlin Heidelberg 2014

Owing to its low sensitivity, two-dimensional quality (with poor differentiation of overlapping small-bowel loops), and risks associated with ionising radiation [12, 21–23], small-bowel follow-through has been superseded by magnetic resonance enterography (or enteroclysis) (MRE) for radiologic surveillance of the small bowel in patients with PJS [12, 13]. A recent prospective comparative study of SBCE and MRE for this indication [12] showed that although MRE was less well tolerated and less preferred by patients than SBCE, MRE is likely comparable to SBCE for the detection of large PJS polyps (≥1.5 cm). Currently, MRE may also allow for more accurate estimation of PJS polyp size and location (Fig. 36.5), while reducing "miss rates" [12, 13, 24]. MRE therefore appears to be a useful alternative modality to SBCE for the surveillance of PJS small-bowel polyps, if it is available [12, 13].

Detection of these large PJS polyps within the small bowel by minimally invasive surveillance allows for their pre-emptive removal before an episode of intussusception occurs, avoiding the need for emergency surgery and small-bowel resection [3, 17]. Until recently, laparotomy with intraoperative enteroscopy (IOE) was the sole option available for removal of PJS polyps deep within the small bowel [25, 26]. Laparotomy with IOE exposes patients to the hazards inherent in major abdominal surgery, however, and the potential postoperative complications such as intra-abdominal adhesions and short-bowel syndrome [27–29]. The introduction of device-assisted enteroscopy (DAE) permits endoscopic removal of PJS polyps located deep within the small bowel [30–40] without the need for operative surgery (Fig. 36.6). Published data on DAE for this indication (mainly relating to double-balloon enteroscopy) are

promising, and a strategy incorporating the use of DAE may offer a lower-morbidity alternative for selected patients with PJS by potentially avoiding the need for a laparotomy [11, 12, 33–35, 37]. Because the success of DAE may be hindered by the presence of postsurgical intra-abdominal adhesions [41, 42], however, the application of DAE earlier in life may enhance the effectiveness of endoscopic removal of small-bowel polyps. The combination of DAE and laparoscopic assistance (lap-DAE) should also be considered in patients with PJS who have established postsurgical adhesive disease, as lap-DAE may provide a less invasive alternative to laparotomy with IOE [43]. Nevertheless, laparotomy with IOE will continue to play a major role in managing small-bowel polyps in certain patients with PJS. The overall management strategy should be tailored to each patient on an individual basis. Figure 36.7 presents a proposed algorithm (based on current recommendations) for the surveillance and management of small-bowel polyps in patients with PJS.

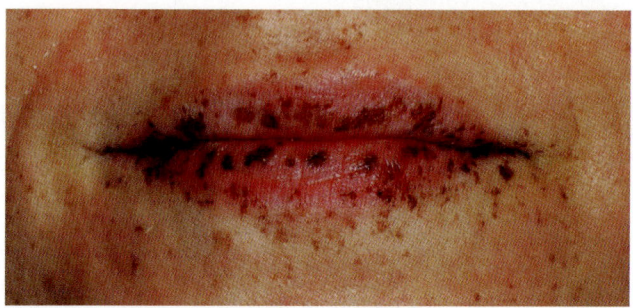

Fig. 36.1 Macular melanin pigmentation of the lips and perioral region affecting a patient with Peutz-Jeghers syndrome (PJS)

Fig. 36.2 Photomicrograph of a PJS small-bowel polyp. A low-power, sagittal section through the polyp head shows "arborisation" of the smooth muscle core. Haematoxylin and eosin (H&E) stain (**a**); smooth muscle actin stain (**b**). (*Courtesy of* Morgan Moorghen, MD)

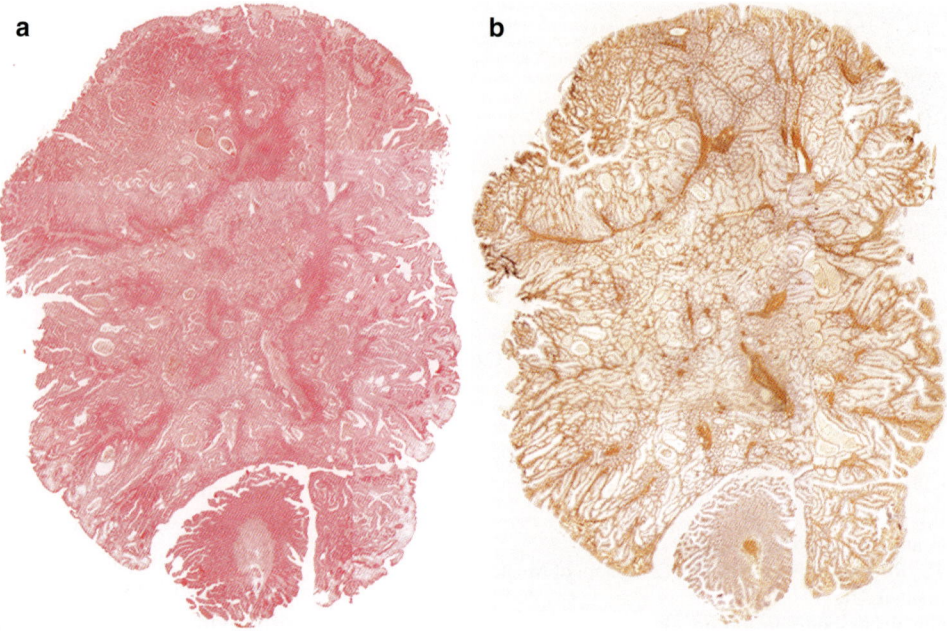

Fig. 36.3 CT scan of the abdomen and pelvis showing a large ileocolonic intussusception caused by a small-bowel PJS polyp "lead point". (**a**) An axial section demonstrates the typical "target" sign (*white arrow*). (**b**) A coronal section shows the ileal intussusceptum (*red arrow*) within the colonic intussuscipiens (*blue arrow*). (*Courtesy of Niall Power, MD*)

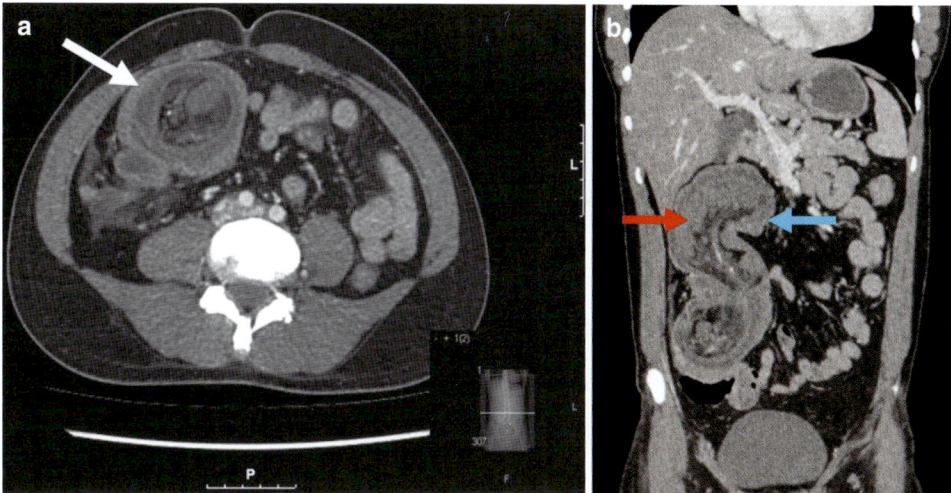

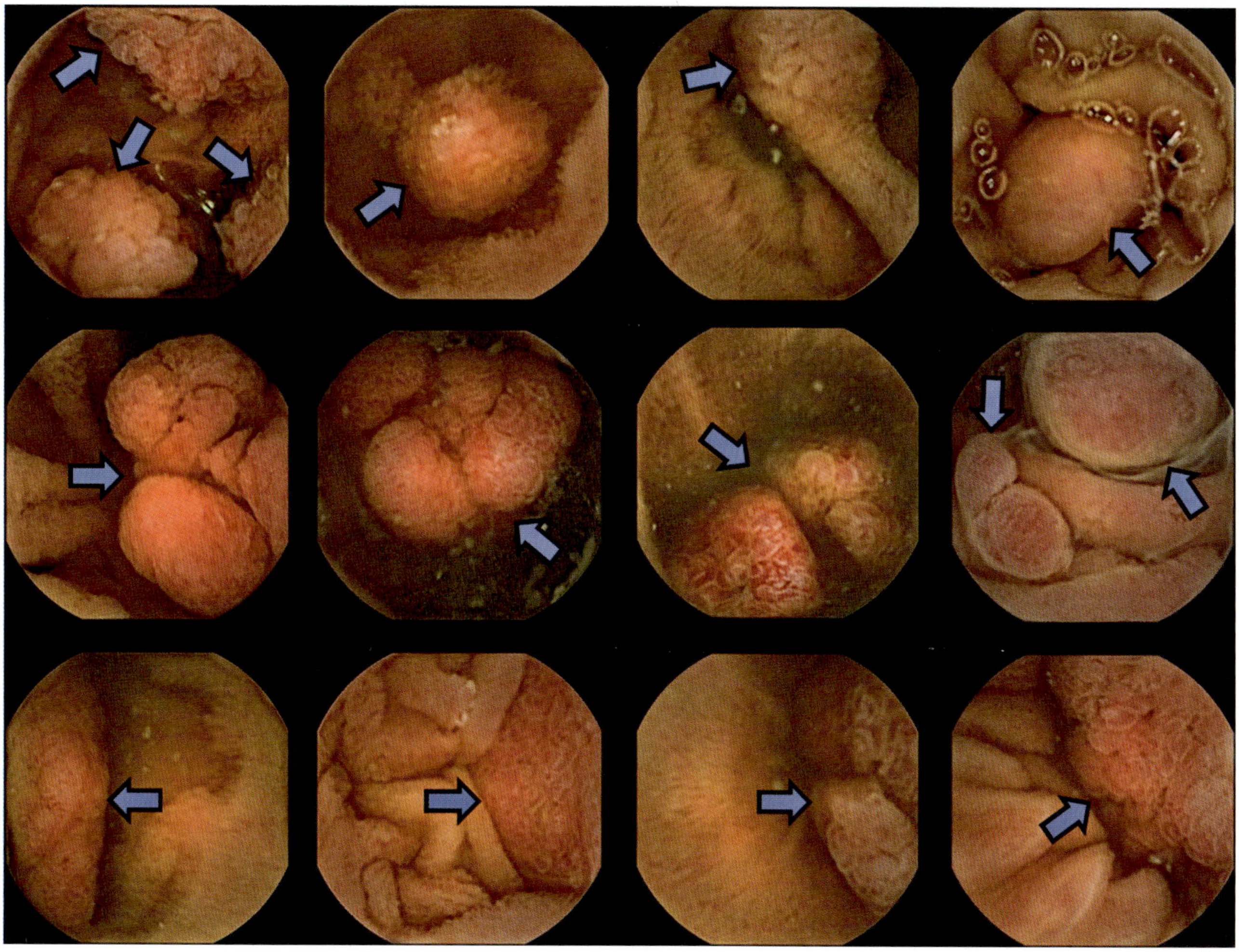

Fig. 36.4 A variety of PJS small-bowel polyps as seen at small-bowel capsule endoscopy (SBCE). Polyp tissue is usually darker than the surrounding small-bowel mucosa (*blue arrows*). Estimation of polyp size and number can be challenging, and often only a small portion of larger polyps can be identified (*row C*) (*Courtesy of* Aine O'Rourke and Chris Fraser, MD)

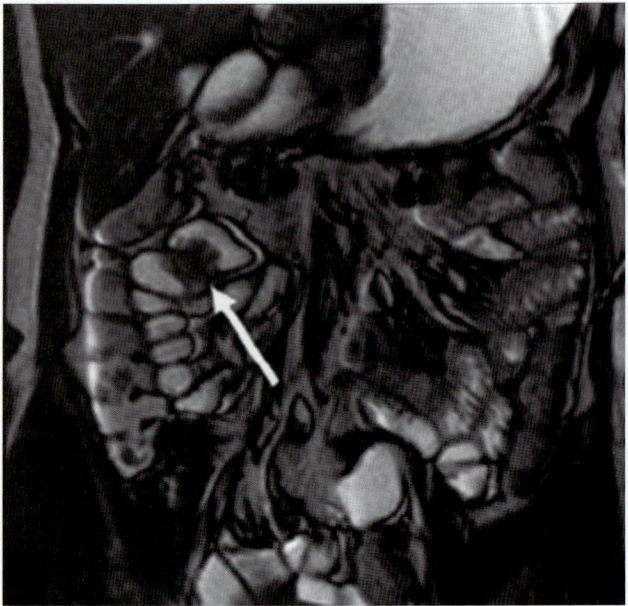

Fig. 36.5 A large (2.5 cm) PJS ileal polyp (*white arrow*) as seen at magnetic resonance enterography (MRE) (*Courtesy of* Arun Gupta, MD)

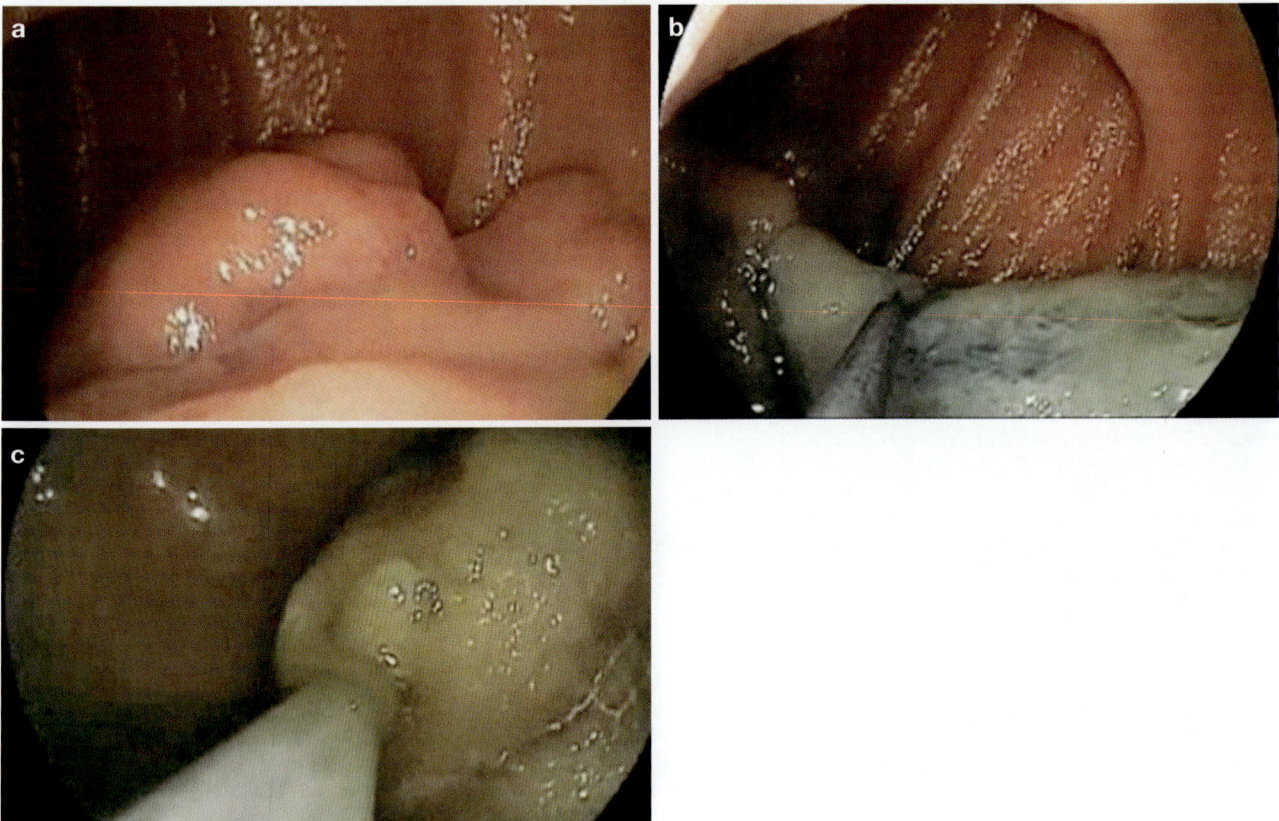

Fig. 36.6 (**a**) Large (2 cm) semi-pedunculated PJS jejunal polyp as seen at double-balloon enteroscopy (DBE). (**b**) Prior to polypectomy, the submucosa of the polyp base/stalk is injected with a dilute solution of adrenaline (1 in 100,000) in normal saline and 2 drops of 0.005 % methylene blue, to reduce the risk of perforation and bleeding at polypectomy. (**c**) After polypectomy, the polyp is retrieved using a Roth net

Fig. 36.7 A proposed algorithm (based on current recommendations [3]) for the surveillance and management of small-bowel (SB) polyps in patients with Peutz-Jeghers syndrome (PJS)

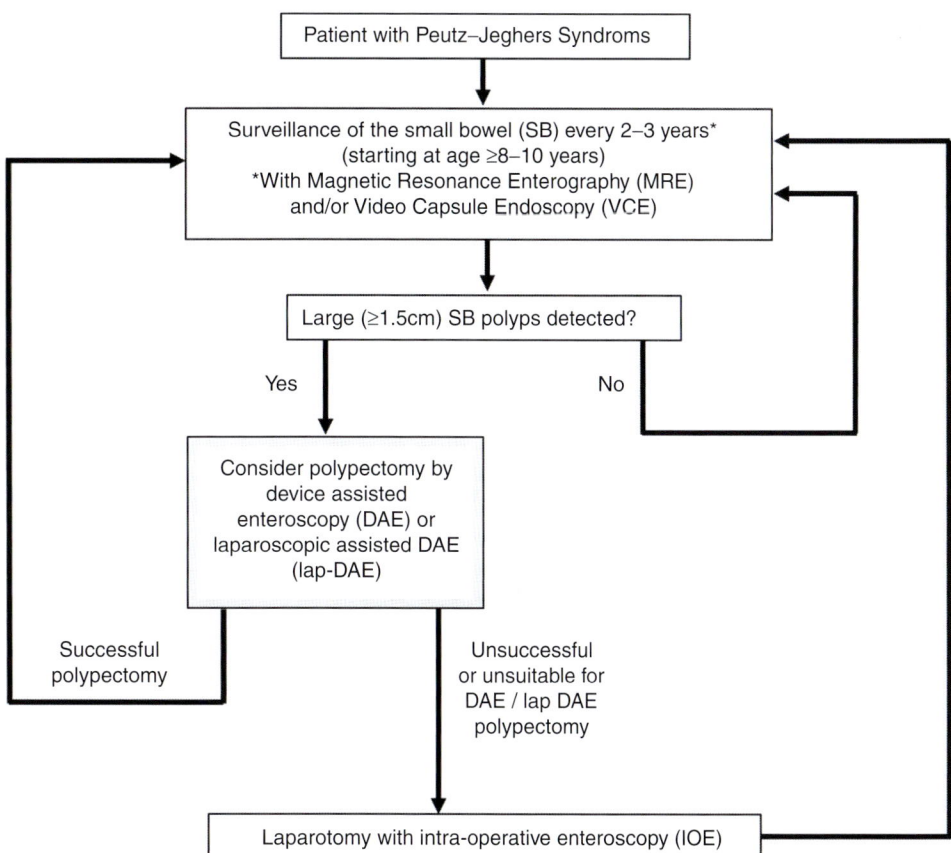

References

1. Aretz S, Stienen D, Uhlhaas S, et al. High proportion of large genomic STK11 deletions in Peutz-Jeghers syndrome. Hum Mutat. 2005;26:513–9.
2. Riegert-Johnson D, Gleeson FC, Westra W, et al. Peutz-Jeghers syndrome. In: Riegert-Johnson DL, Boardman LA, Hefferon T, et al., editors. Cancer syndromes [Internet]. Bethesda: National Center for Biotechnology Information; 2009.
3. Beggs AD, Latchford AR, Vasen HF, et al. Peutz-Jeghers syndrome: a systematic review and recommendations for management. Gut. 2010;59:975–86.
4. Giardiello FM, Welsh SB, Hamilton SR, et al. Increased risk of cancer in the Peutz-Jeghers syndrome. N Engl J Med. 1987;316:1511–4.
5. Giardiello FM, Trimbath JD. Peutz-Jeghers syndrome and management recommendations. Clin Gastroenterol Hepatol. 2006;4: 408–15.
6. Utsunomiya J, Gocho H, Miyanaga T, et al. Peutz-Jeghers syndrome: its natural course and management. Johns Hopkins Med J. 1975;136:71–82.
7. Latchford AR, Phillips RK. Gastrointestinal polyps and cancer in Peutz-Jeghers syndrome: clinical aspects. Fam Cancer. 2011;10:455–61.
8. Latchford AR, Neale K, Phillips RK, Clark SK. Peutz-Jeghers syndrome: intriguing suggestion of gastrointestinal cancer prevention from surveillance. Dis Colon Rectum. 2011;54:1547–51.
9. van Lier MG, Westerman AM, Wagner A, et al. High cancer risk and increased mortality in patients with Peutz-Jeghers syndrome. Gut. 2011;60:141–7.
10. van Lier MG, Mathus-Vliegen EM, Wagner A, et al. High cumulative risk of intussusception in patients with Peutz-Jeghers syndrome: time to update surveillance guidelines? Am J Gastroenterol. 2011;106:940–5.
11. Gao H, van Lier MG, Poley JW, et al. Endoscopic therapy of small-bowel polyps by double-balloon enteroscopy in patients with Peutz-Jeghers syndrome. Gastrointest Endosc. 2010;71:768–73.
12. Gupta A, Postgate AJ, Burling D, et al. A prospective study of MR enterography versus capsule endoscopy for the surveillance of adult patients with Peutz-Jeghers syndrome. AJR Am J Roentgenol. 2010;195:108–16.
13. Korsse SE, Dewint P, Kuipers EJ, van Leerdam ME. Small bowel endoscopy and Peutz-Jeghers syndrome. Best Pract Res Clin Gastroenterol. 2012;26:263–78.
14. Hyer W. Polyposis syndromes: pediatric implications. Gastrointest Endosc Clin N Am. 2001;11:659–82.
15. Hyer W. Implications of Peutz-Jeghers syndrome in children and adolescents. In: Riegert-Johnson DL, Boardman LA, Hefferon T, et al., editors. Cancer syndromes [Internet]. Bethesda: National Center for Biotechnology Information; 2009.
16. Will OC, Phillips RK, Hyer W, Clark SK. Symptomatic polyposis in a 4-year-old: the exception proves the rule. J Paediatr Child Health. 2009;45:320–1.
17. Hinds R, Philp C, Hyer W, Fell JM. Complications of childhood Peutz-Jeghers syndrome: implications for pediatric screening. J Pediatr Gastroenterol Nutr. 2004;39:219–20.
18. Postgate A, Despott E, Burling D, et al. Significant small-bowel lesions detected by alternative diagnostic modalities after negative capsule endoscopy. Gastrointest Endosc. 2008;68:1209–14.

19. Ross A, Mehdizadeh S, Tokar J, et al. Double balloon enteroscopy detects small bowel mass lesions missed by capsule endoscopy. Dig Dis Sci. 2008;53:2140–3.
20. Soares J, Lopes L, Vilas BG, Pinho C. Wireless capsule endoscopy for evaluation of phenotypic expression of small-bowel polyps in patients with Peutz-Jeghers syndrome and in symptomatic first-degree relatives. Endoscopy. 2004;36:1060–6.
21. Berrington de Gonzalez A, Darby S. Risk of cancer from diagnostic X-rays: estimates for the UK and 14 other countries. Lancet 2004;363:345–51.
22. Bessette JR, Maglinte DD, Kelvin FM, Chernish SM. Primary malignant tumors in the small bowel: a comparison of the small-bowel enema and conventional follow-through examination. AJR Am J Roentgenol. 1989;153:741–4.
23. Maglinte DD, Kelvin FM, O'Connor K, et al. Current status of small bowel radiography. Abdom Imaging. 1996;21:247–57.
24. Maccioni F, Al Ansari N, Mazzamurro F, et al. Surveillance of patients affected by Peutz-Jeghers syndrome: diagnostic value of MR enterography in prone and supine position. Abdom Imaging. 2012;37:279–87.
25. Oncel M, Remzi FH, Church JM, et al. Benefits of 'clean sweep' in Peutz-Jeghers patients. Colorectal Dis. 2004;6:332–5.
26. Spigelman AD, Thomson JP, Phillips RK. Towards decreasing the relaparotomy rate in the Peutz-Jeghers syndrome: the role of preoperative small bowel endoscopy. Br J Surg. 1990;77:301–2.
27. Parker MC, Ellis H, Moran BJ, et al. Postoperative adhesions: ten-year follow-up of 12,584 patients undergoing lower abdominal surgery. Dis Colon Rectum. 2001;44:822–9.
28. Parker MC, Wilson MS, Menzies D, et al. The SCAR-3 study: 5-year adhesion-related readmission risk following lower abdominal surgical procedures. Colorectal Dis. 2005;7:551–8.
29. You YN, Wolff BG, Boardman LA, et al. Peutz-Jeghers syndrome: a study of long-term surgical morbidity and causes of mortality. Fam Cancer. 2010;9:609–16.
30. Akarsu M, Ugur KF, Akpinar H. Double-balloon endoscopy in patients with Peutz-Jeghers syndrome. Turk J Gastroenterol. 2012;23:496–502.
31. Akerman PA, Agrawal D, Cantero D, Pangtay J. Spiral enteroscopy with the new DSB overtube: a novel technique for deep peroral small-bowel intubation. Endoscopy. 2008;40:974–8.
32. Akerman PA, Cantero D. Spiral enteroscopy and push enteroscopy. Gastrointest Endosc Clin N Am. 2009;19:357–69.
33. Kopacova M, Tacheci I, Rejchrt S, Bures J. Peutz-Jeghers syndrome: diagnostic and therapeutic approach. World J Gastroenterol. 2009;15:5397–408.
34. Ohmiya N, Taguchi A, Shirai K, et al. Endoscopic resection of Peutz-Jeghers polyps throughout the small intestine at double-balloon enteroscopy without laparotomy. Gastrointest Endosc. 2005;61:140–7.
35. Ohmiya N, Nakamura M, Takenaka H, et al. Management of small-bowel polyps in Peutz-Jeghers syndrome by using enteroclysis, double-balloon enteroscopy, and videocapsule endoscopy. Gastrointest Endosc. 2010;72:1209–16.
36. Riccioni ME, Urgesi R, Cianci R, et al. Single-balloon push-and-pull enteroscopy system: does it work? A single-center, 3-year experience. Surg Endosc. 2011;25:3050–6.
37. Sakamoto H, Yamamoto H, Hayashi Y, et al. Nonsurgical management of small-bowel polyps in Peutz-Jeghers syndrome with extensive polypectomy by using double-balloon endoscopy. Gastrointest Endosc. 2011;74:328–33.
38. Thomson M, Venkatesh K, Elmalik K, et al. Double balloon enteroscopy in children: diagnosis, treatment, and safety. World J Gastroenterol. 2010;16:56–62.
39. Yamamoto H, Sekine Y, Sato Y, et al. Total enteroscopy with a nonsurgical steerable double-balloon method. Gastrointest Endosc. 2001;53:216–20.
40. Yamamoto H, Yano T, Kita H, et al. New system of double-balloon enteroscopy for diagnosis and treatment of small intestinal disorders. Gastroenterology. 2003;125:1556–7.
41. Despott EJ, Murino A, Fraser C. Management of deep looping when failing to progress at double-balloon enteroscopy. Endoscopy. 2011;43(Suppl 2 UCTN):E275–6.
42. Gerson LB, Flodin JT, Miyabayashi K. Balloon-assisted enteroscopy: technology and troubleshooting. Gastrointest Endosc. 2008;68:1158–67.
43. Ross AS, Dye C, Prachand VN. Laparoscopic-assisted double-balloon enteroscopy for small-bowel polyp surveillance and treatment in patients with Peutz-Jeghers syndrome. Gastrointest Endosc. 2006;64:984–8.

HNPCC and Rare Syndromes

37

Jean-Christophe Saurin, Robert Benamouzig, and Uwe Seitz

Contents

37.1   Lynch Syndrome (HNPCC)

Lynch syndrome, previously called hereditary nonpolyposis colorectal cancer (HNPCC), is one of the most common digestive genetic diseases, occurring in 1 person out of 2,000. Involvement of the small bowel is much less frequent (about 4 % cumulative risk of cancer) than colorectal involvement (50–60 % cumulative risk). However, prospective studies have shown an 8.5 % detection rate of neoplasia (adenoma, cancer) at capsule endoscopy in asymptomatic patients [1] (Figs. 37.1 and 37.2), including advanced cancer without anemia. It is likely that capsule endoscopy has lower sensitivity for adenocarcinoma detection [2, 3]. Systematic screening using capsule endoscopy is not recommended for these patients and is probably not cost-effective, but capsule endoscopy should be performed if unexplained anemia is present. Some specialized centers do routinely perform capsule endoscopy in these patients as screening for small-bowel cancer. Whenever upper digestive endoscopy is performed, careful attention should be paid to flat, distal duodenal adenomas, best detected by classic, forward-viewing gastroscopy.

The work was first published in 2006 by Springer Medizin Verlag Heidelberg with the following title: *Atlas of Video Capsule Endoscopy*.

J.-C. Saurin (✉)
Department of Gastroenterology, Hôpital Edouard Herriot,
Lyon, France
e-mail: jean-christophe.saurin@chu-lyon.fr

R. Benamouzig
Department of Gastroenterology, Avicenne Hospital,
Bobigny, France
e-mail: robert.benamouzig@avc.aphp.fr

U. Seitz
Internal Medicine/Gastroenterology,
Kreiskrankenhaus Bergstrasse, Heppenheim, Germany
e-mail: u.seitz@kkh-bergstrasse.de

M. Keuchel et al. (eds.), *Video Capsule Endoscopy: A Reference Guide and Atlas*,
DOI 10.1007/978-3-662-44062-9_37, © Springer-Verlag Berlin Heidelberg 2014

Fig. 37.1 (**a** and **b**) Adenomas detected in asymptomatic patients with Lynch syndrome (*From* Saurin et al. [1], reprinted with permission from Thieme Verlag)

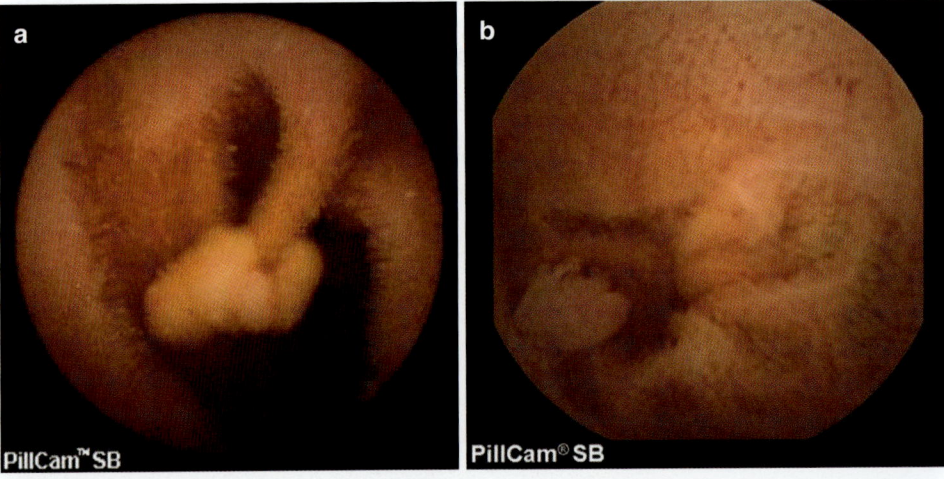

Fig. 37.2 (**a** and **b**) Jejunal adenocarcinoma detected in an asymptomatic patient with Lynch syndrome (*From* Saurin et al. [1], reprinted with permission from Thieme Verlag)

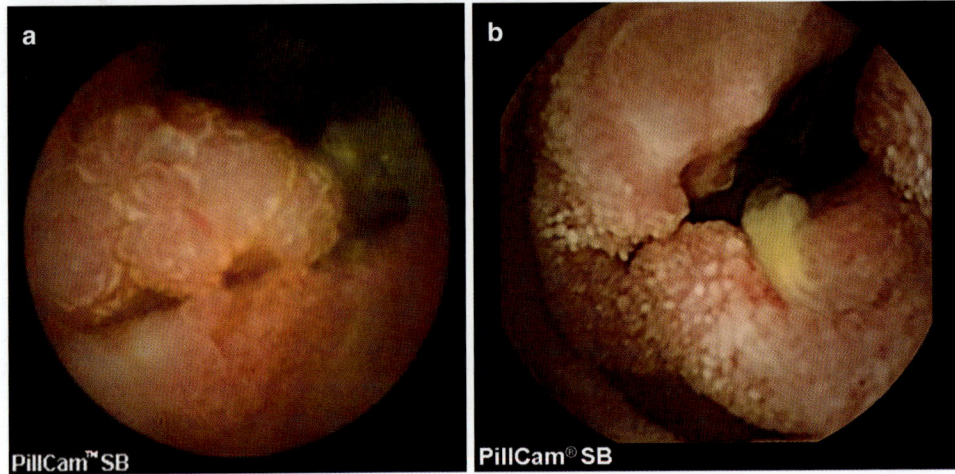

37.2 Rare Syndromes

Rare syndromes involving the intestines are heterogeneous. Some (juvenile polyposis, Cowden disease) have genetic origins. Others, such as Cronkhite-Canada syndrome, are unexplained inflammatory diseases.

37.2.1 Juvenile Polyposis

No screening for small-bowel neoplasia is recommended for patients with juvenile polyposis, as the main epidemiologic study by Giardiello et al. [4] did not reveal any increased risk of cancer at this level. Tiny duodenal polyps can be observed at usual upper endoscopy, but most lesions are located in the stomach (especially in the subgroup of juvenile polyposis patients with an *SMAD4* mutation) or in the colon (especially in the *BMPR1A* mutation subgroup). Video capsule endoscopy (VCE) may demonstrate small-bowel polyps (Fig. 37.3). Inflammatory alterations in histology define juvenile polyps [5], which are not restricted to young patients.

37.2.2 Cowden Disease

Cowden disease (PTEN hamartoma tumor syndrome) is autosomal dominant inherited [6]. SBCE may show hamartomatous small-bowel polyps [7] (Figs. 37.4 and 37.5). However, digestive surveillance is seldom recommended for patients with Cowden disease, as their risk of gastric, small bowel, or colorectal cancer may be comparable to that of the general population. In contrast, these patients have a high cumulative risk of breast and thyroid cancer [8].

Fig. 37.3 Juvenile polyposis. (**a** and **b**) Pedunculated and partially ulcerated jejunal polyp. (**c**) Enteroscopic image. (**d**) Histology with typical inflammatory infiltration (*Courtesy of* Jörg Caselitz, MD). (**e** and **f**) Inflammatory appearance of juvenile polyps in the colon of the same patient

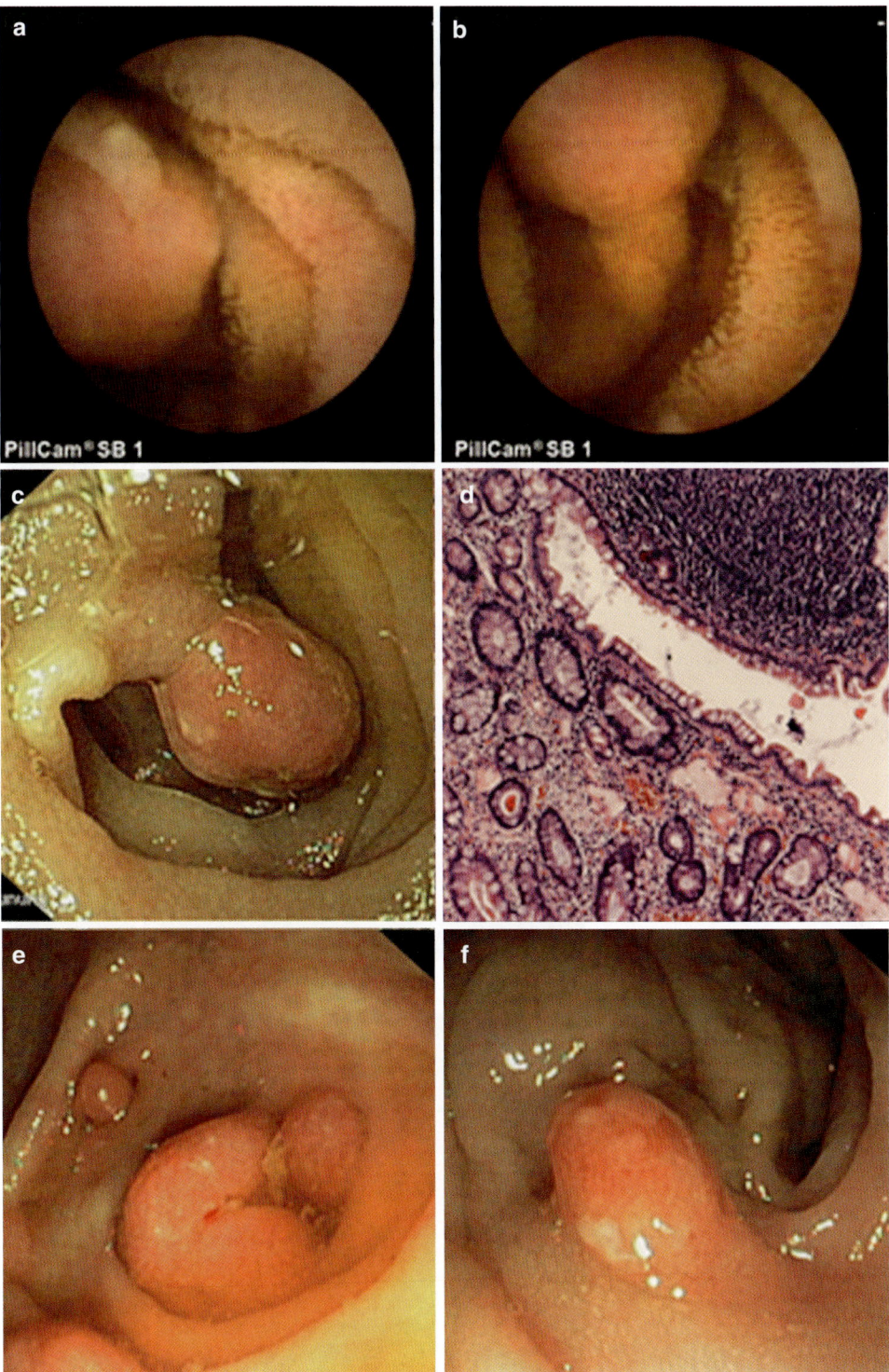

Fig. 37.4 Cowden disease. (**a**) Gingival papillomatosis. (**b** and **c**) Jejunal hamartomas as seen by small-bowel capsule endoscopy (SBCE). (**d**) Acrokeratosis (*Courtesy of* Christian Florent, MD) (*From* Bencheqroun et al. [7]; *with permission*)

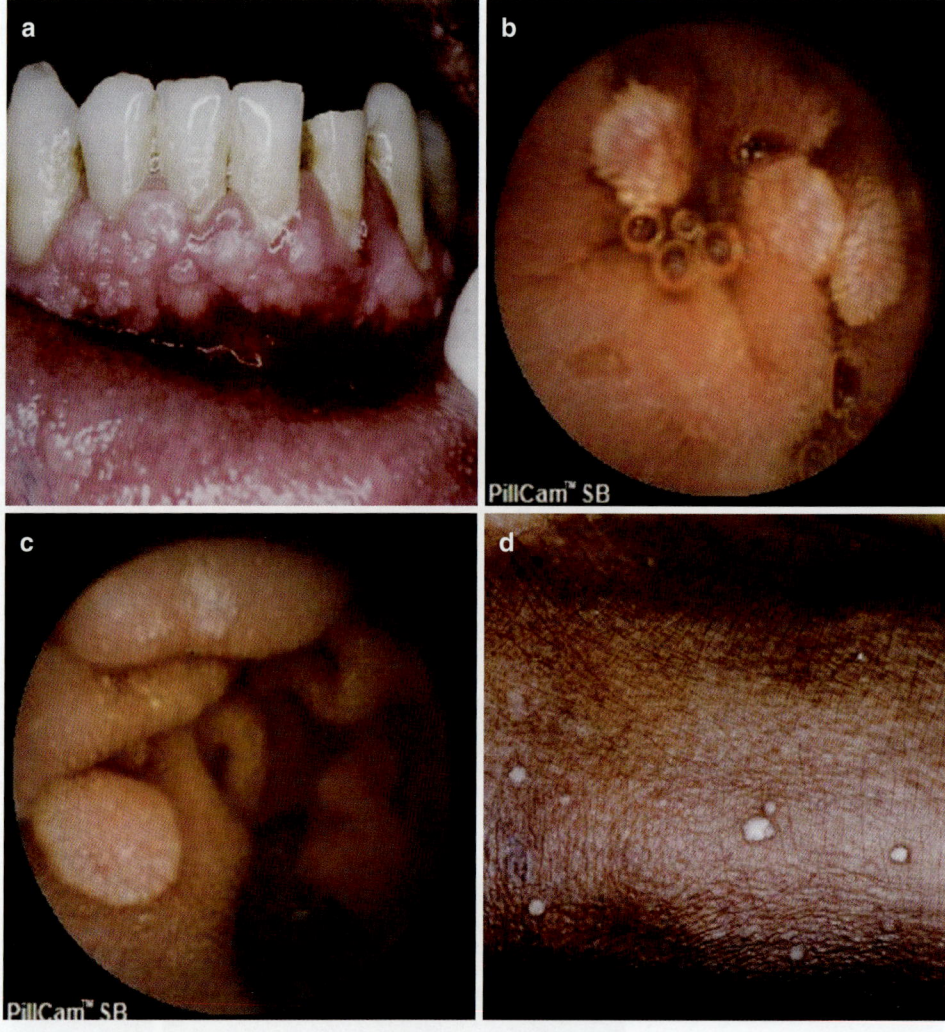

Fig. 37.5 Cowden disease. (**a**, **b**) Small-bowel hamartomas (small polyps) and lymphangiectasia (white villi) (Courtesy of Bakhtiar Bejou, MD)

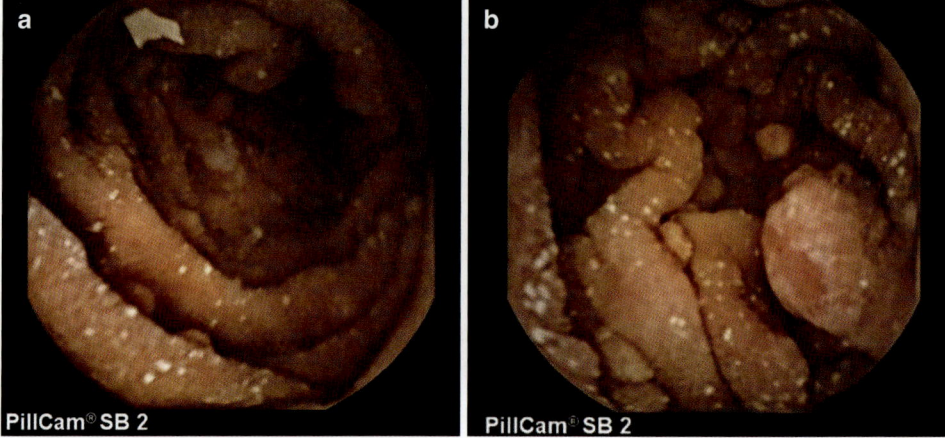

37.2.3 Cronkhite-Canada Syndrome

Cronkhite-Canada syndrome corresponds to a diffuse digestive, pseudopolypoid, inflammatory process; an autoimmune genesis has been suggested (Sweetser et al. 2011). Presentation may include diarrhea, weight loss, alopecia, onychodystrophy, and skin hyperpigmentation. Treatment with anti-inflammatory agents such as corticosteroids and azathioprine is very difficult and prolonged. Only a few uses of VCE in these patients have been reported [9–11] (Figs. 37.6 and 37.7).

Fig. 37.6 Cronkhite-Canada syndrome.
(**a**) Polypoid lesions in the stomach.
(**b**) Corresponding endoscopic image.
(**c**) Polypoid lesion in the jejunum with
lymphangiectasia (white villi).
(**d**) Enteroscopy. (**e** and **f**) VCE pictures
of colonic polyps. (**g**) Alopecia.
(**h**) Dystrophic nails

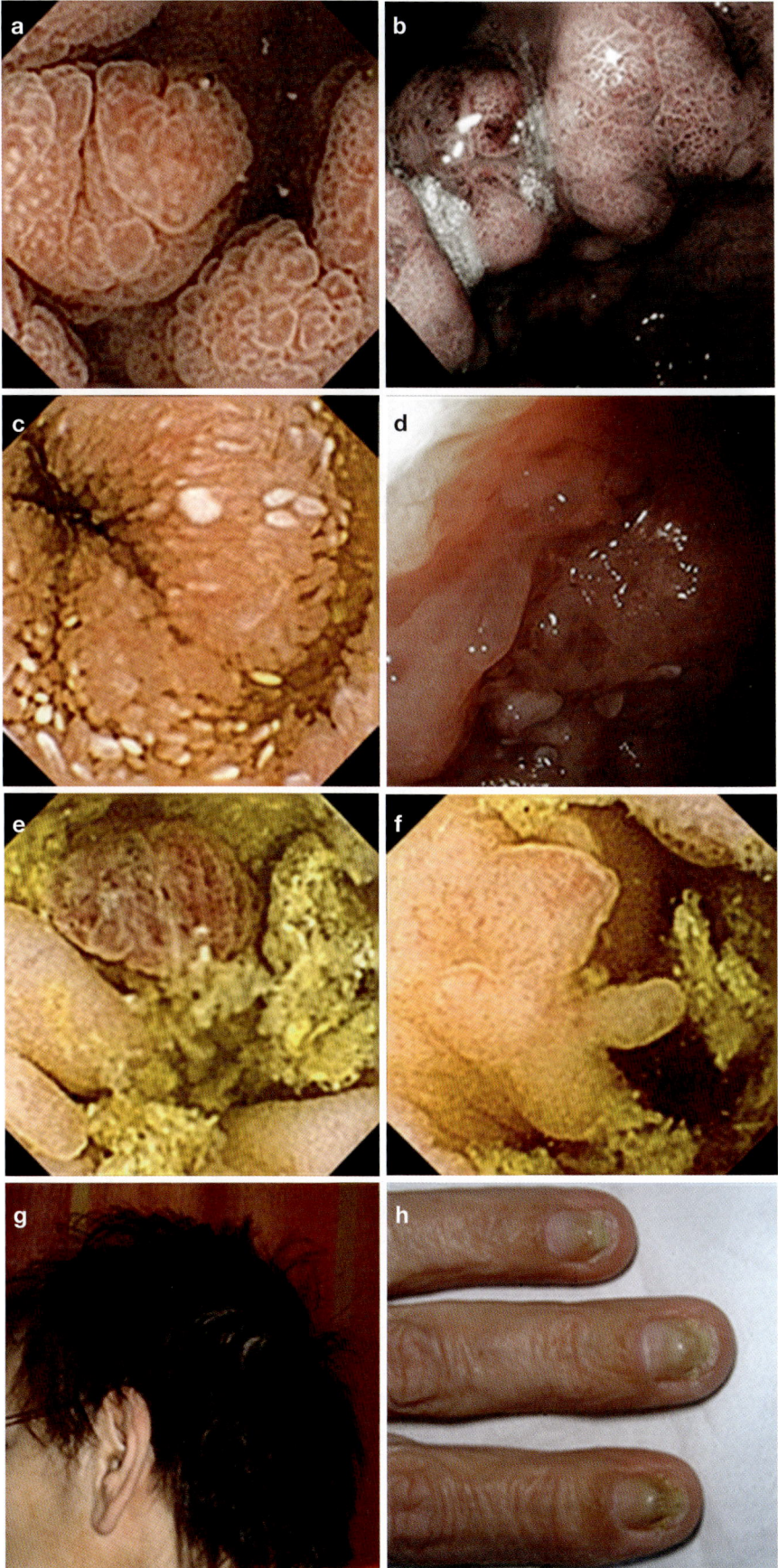

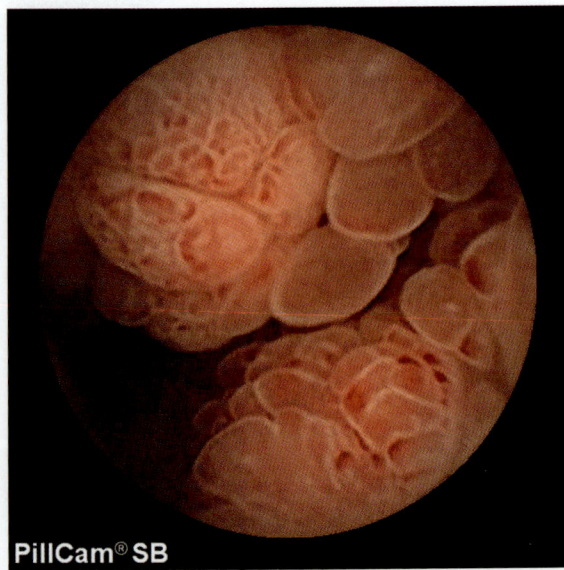

Fig. 37.7 Diffuse polypoid infiltration of the stomach in a patient with Cronkhite-Canada syndrome

37.2.4 Intestinal Ganglioneuromatosis

Intestinal ganglioneuromatosis is a rare condition with polypoid small-bowel ganglioneuromas (Fig. 37.8). The condition can be idiopathic or may occur in association with other inherited diseases such as multiple endocrine neoplasia type 2B (MEN 2B) (medullary thyroid cancer, pheochromocytoma, marfanoid habitus) [12, 13] or in Cowden disease [14].

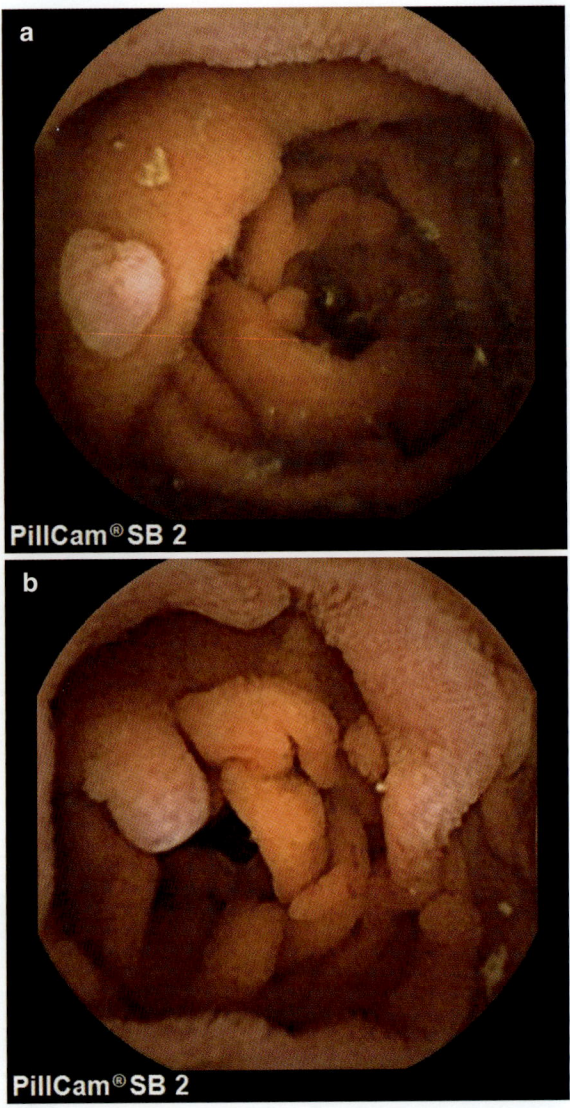

Fig. 37.8 (**a** and **b**) Sporadic ganglioneuromatosis of the proximal small bowel with multiple small polyps seen on VCE (*Courtesy of* Jörg Albert, MD)

References

1. Saurin JC, Pilleul F, Soussan EB, et al. Small-bowel capsule endoscopy diagnoses early and advanced neoplasms in asymptomatic patients with Lynch syndrome. Endoscopy. 2010;42:1057–62.

2. Baichi MM, Arifuddin RM, Mantry PS. Small-bowel masses found and missed on capsule endoscopy for obscure bleeding. Scand J Gastroenterol. 2007;42:1127–32.

3. Ross A, Mehdizadeh S, Tokar J, et al. Double balloon enteroscopy detects small bowel mass lesions missed by capsule endoscopy. Dig Dis Sci. 2008;53:2140–3.

4. Brosens LA, van Hattem A, Hylind LM, et al. Risk of colorectal cancer in juvenile polyposis. Gut. 2007;56:965–7.

5. Postgate AJ, Will OC, Fraser CH, et al. Capsule endoscopy for the small bowel in juvenile polyposis syndrome: a case series. Endoscopy. 2009;41:1001–4.

6. Pilarski R, Eng C. Will the real Cowden syndrome please stand up (again)? Expanding mutational and clinical spectra of the PTEN hamartoma tumour syndrome. J Med Genet. 2004;41:323–6.

7. Bencheqroun R, Meary N, Laroche L, et al. Cowden syndrome, first case investigated using electronic video capsule. Acta Endosc. 2005;35:227–32.

8. Tan MH, Mester JL, Ngeow J, et al. Lifetime cancer risks in individuals with germline PTEN mutations. Clin Cancer Res. 2012;18:400–7.

9. Sweetser S, Ahlquist DA, Osborn NK, et al. Clinicopathologic features and treatment outcomes in Cronkhite-Canada syndrome: support for autoimmunity. Dig Dis Sci. 2011;57:496–502.

10. Sweetser S, Boardman LA. Cronkhite-Canada syndrome: an acquired condition of gastrointestinal polyposis and dermatologic abnormalities. Gastroenterol Hepatol (NY). 2012;8:201–3.

11. Cao XC, Wang BM, Han ZC. Wireless capsule endoscopic finding in Cronkhite-Canada syndrome. Gut. 2006;55:899–900.

12. Camacho CP, Hoff AO, Lindsey SC, et al. Early diagnosis of multiple endocrine neoplasia type 2B: a challenge for physicians. Arq Bras Endocrinol Metabol. 2008;52:1393–8.

13. Carney JA, Go VL, Sizemore GW, Hayles AB. Alimentary-tract ganglioneuromatosis. A major component of the syndrome of multiple endocrine neoplasia, type 2b. N Engl J Med. 1976;295:1287–91.

14. Coriat R, Mozer M, Caux F, et al. Endoscopic findings in Cowden syndrome. Endoscopy. 2012;43:723–6.

Video Capsule Endoscopy in Children

38

Ernest G. Seidman, Gian Luigi de' Angelis,
Anna Sant'Anna, Martha H. Dirks, and Michael Thomson

Contents

The work was first published in 2006 by Springer Medizin Verlag Heidelberg with the following title: *Atlas of Video Capsule Endoscopy*.

E.G. Seidman (✉)
McGill IBD Research Group, Digestive Lab, Research Institute of McGill University Health Center, Montreal, QC, Canada
e-mail: ernest.seidman@mcgill.ca

G.L. de' Angelis
Gastroenterology and Endoscopy Unit,
University of Parma, Parma, Italy
e-mail: gianluigi.deangelis@unipr.it

A. Sant'Anna
McMaster University, Hamilton, ON, Canada
e-mail: santann@mcmaster.ca

M.H. Dirks
Division of Gastroenterology, Hepatology and Nutrition,
Hôpital Sainte-Justine, University of Montreal,
Montreal, QC, Canada
e-mail: Martha.dirks.hsj@ssss.gouv.qc.ca

M. Thomson
Centre for Pediatric Gastroenterology,
The Children's Hospital, Sheffield, UK
e-mail: m.thomson@hspg.org.uk

Almost all but the most proximal and distal segments of the small bowel are essentially out of range of standard endoscopes. Push enteroscopy generally allows visualization only of the proximal areas of the jejunum, up to about 150 cm distal to the pylorus. Moreover, the need for an overtube (15 mm) limits the applicability of this relatively invasive technique in children [1]. Intraoperative enteroscopy necessitates more invasive abdominal laparotomy or laparoscopy, with potential complications such as prolonged postoperative ileus, obstruction, perforation, and fistula formation [2]. Balloon-assisted enteroscopy is a novel method that has shown promising initial results for achieving complete enteroscopy and providing therapy without requiring laparotomy [3]. This technique generally entails a long period of manipulation, however, so general anesthesia is often needed. Moreover, its availability is limited, with little experience in pediatric patients reported to date [4]. Thus, the small bowel has been deemed the last unexplored frontier in terms of pediatric endoscopy [5].

The invention of wireless video capsule endoscopy has, for the first time, enabled the visualization of the entire small bowel in a truly noninvasive manner. This ingenious technological discovery was achieved by scientists in Israel who miniaturized the components necessary to transmit video signals to an external data recorder [6]. The ultrashort focal length of the lens (1 mm) permits highly detailed imaging of the intestinal mucosa as the capsule travels through the lumen in a forward or backward orientation, without requiring insufflation of air. "Redouts" (as may occur in standard endoscopic procedures when the lens is too close to the mucosa) are thus not a problem. The remarkable resolution of the lens (0.1 mm) yields extraordinarily detailed, high-quality images of the mucosa, including the ability to visualize the normal villi (Fig. 38.1a). Consequently, the clear identification of areas of even mild villous atrophy is made possible as never before seen by any endoscopic device (Fig. 38.1b and c). The goals of this review are to provide representative images that illustrate the key indications and findings of capsule endoscopy in the pediatric age group.

Fig. 38.1 (a) The extraordinary resolution of the capsule endoscope is capable of revealing the minute features of normal small bowel mucosa, such as the feathery, hairlike microvilli. (b) Capsule study in a child with atopic dermatitis and food allergies, showing discrete changes in the small bowel mucosa that were not detected by other endoscopic or imaging studies: edematous proximal jejunal folds, atrophy of the microvilli, and focal erythema. (c) Capsule study reveals focal inflammatory changes in the small bowel mucosa in an adolescent with indeterminate colitis. The microvilli are broad and "white tipped" and focally atrophied, with a small linear mucosal break. The numerous small bowel lesions observed by the capsule were suggestive of the ultimate diagnosis of Crohn's disease

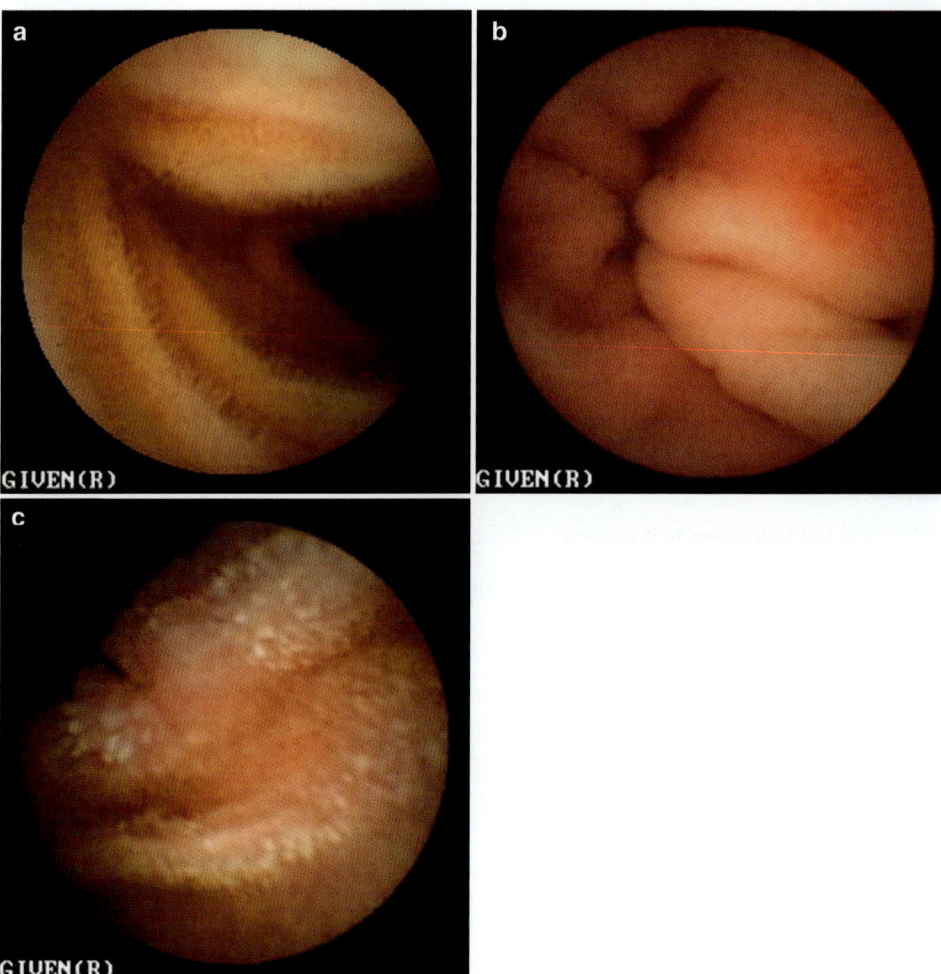

38.1 Clinical Indications in Pediatrics

Several studies in adult populations have demonstrated that capsule endoscopy is a highly effective and safe method to explore the small bowel for obscure causes of bleeding inflammatory mucosal disorders such as Crohn's and celiac disease, as well as tumors [7–12]. On the basis of our pioneering trial in Montreal [13], the Given M2A capsule (Given Imaging; Yoqneam, Israel) was first approved for the investigation of disorders of the small bowel in children and adolescents above age 10 by both the US Food and Drug Administration and the Health Protection Branch of Health and Welfare Canada. Potential indications of capsule endoscopy in the pediatric age group are summarized in Table 38.1.

In a review of the use of video capsule endoscopy performed in pediatric patients in Belgium [14], relevant findings having an impact on the diagnosis were found in 60 % of cases investigated for obscure gastrointestinal (GI) bleeding or iron deficiency anemia. In the group with chronic abdominal pain, capsule endoscopy revealed relevant findings in 43 %. The capsule findings had an impact on therapy in 44 % of the patients overall. In an Italian series [15], the

Table 38.1 Potential indications for capsule endoscopy in pediatric patients

Small bowel inflammatory disorders
Crohn's disease, celiac disease, allergic or eosinophilic enteropathies, intestinal vasculitis, Henoch-Schönlein purpura, drug-induced mucosal injury (*e.g.*, nonsteroidal anti-inflammatory drugs or chemotherapy), radiation enteropathy, graft-versus-host disease, intestinal transplantation
Small bowel polyps and tumors
Peutz-Jeghers syndrome, other familial and nonfamilial polyposes; lymphoma, leiomyoma, carcinoid, and other tumors; Kaposi's sarcoma in AIDS
Occult or obscure intestinal bleeding
Angiectasia, arteriovenous malformations, tumors, portal hypertension, and small bowel varices
Unexplained abnormal findings on small bowel imaging
Unexplained malabsorption and protein-losing enteropathies
Intestinal lymphangiectasia, allergic or congestive enteropathies, etc.
Chronic abdominal pain with high suspicion of small bowel pathology
Motility disorders
Esophageal disorders[a]
Esophagitis, Barrett's esophagus, esophageal varices

[a]Requires use of the two-sided PillCam ESO capsule. (Given Imaging, Yoqneam, Israel) with placement of chest leads

video capsule exam revealed pathological findings in 71 % of patients.

In the largest retrospective study to date, Cohen et al. [16] reported on 284 consecutive studies performed in 277 patients with a mean age of 15 (±3.7) years over a 5-year period. The youngest to swallow the capsule was 4.6 years old, but 7 % of the capsules had to be placed. Overall, 86 % of the studies were done for suspected (65 %) or known (21 %) Crohn's disease. Among the others, 9.5 % were carried out for anemia or GI bleeding, 2 % for polyposis, and 1.4 % for celiac disease. Positive findings were observed in 72 % of the studies (54 % with small bowel findings); of these, 47 % were diagnostic. Gastric (33 %) and colonic (11 %) abnormalities were also identified. Five capsules (1.8 %) were retained. A patency capsule was used first in 23 cases, 19 of which proceeded with the video capsule; only 1 of these capsules was retained. In 21 % of cases, the video capsule did not reach the colon. Nevertheless, 65 % of these had significant findings, including 49 % documenting small bowel Crohn's disease [16].

Finally, a recent meta-analysis of over 700 capsule exams was reported [17]. Once again, suspicion or evaluation of inflammatory bowel disease (IBD) was the most common indication (54 %) for capsule endoscopy (34 % for patients suspected to have Crohn's disease, 16 % for patients known to have Crohn's disease, 1 % for patients with ulcerative colitis, and 3 % for patients with indeterminate colitis). The completion rate was 86 % and the retention rate was 2.6 %. Retention rates for children were similar to those of adults, by indication. The authors reported that 65.4 % (95 % CI, 54.8–75.2) of procedures resulted in positive findings. Where reported, 69.4 % (95 % CI, 46.9–87.9) of the examinations resulted in a new diagnosis, and 68.3 % (95 % CI, 43.6–88.5) led to a change in therapy [17].

38.1.1 Inflammatory Disorders

Whereas in adults obscure bleeding is the most common indication for capsule endoscopy, suspected Crohn's disease accounted for the majority of the studies in the pediatric age group [16, 18]. In our prospective study [13], capsule endoscopy was found to be highly useful for the investigation of "obscure" small bowel Crohn's disease, defined as Crohn's disease that is clinically suspected but not proven by conventional methods such as complete ileocolonoscopy with biopsies and barium imaging of the upper GI tract and small bowel [13]. The diagnostic yield was high in this inflammatory category, with Crohn's disease or eosinophilic gastroenteritis diagnosed only by capsule in 60 % of the cases, compared with 0 % using conventional imaging [13]. Another study in adolescents yielded similar results (58.3 % vs. 0 %) for Crohn's disease missed by conventional imaging [19]. In some cases, identification of lesions

compatible with Crohn's disease by capsule endoscopy (Fig. 38.2a and b) precluded laparoscopic assessment to rule out a possible intestinal lymphoma. Moreover, in the approximately 40 % of cases with negative upper endoscopy, colonoscopy, and small bowel capsule exams, Crohn's disease could be definitively excluded. Other imaging techniques have been shown to have higher false-positive results. Capsule endoscopy is also potentially useful for the reassessment of small bowel Crohn's disease after therapy, to objectively demonstrate the degree of mucosal healing of the small bowel or to diagnose a relapse (Fig. 38.2c) in a noninvasive manner.

Findings of obscure small bowel Crohn's disease uncovered by capsule endoscopy may also include the detection of unsuspected inflammatory strictures in addition to typical mucosal ulcerations (Fig. 38.2d), and other inflammatory changes such as pseudopolyps (Fig. 38.2e), or the presence of edematous mucosa with white-tipped villi (Fig. 38.1c). A normal barium small bowel study or CT or MR enterography does not completely exclude the risk that one or more small bowel strictures may result in capsule retention [5, 13]. The use of a patency capsule is thus advocated for all cases of known Crohn's disease or for suspected cases in which obstructive-type symptoms are reported [20].

Capsule endoscopy may also be helpful in identifying (as well as excluding) small bowel lesions in patients with "indeterminate" colitis [21], allowing for a change in diagnosis and precluding colectomy with an ileal pouch for the wrong indication (Figs. 38.1c and 38.2f). In a pediatric series of known or suspected IBD, capsule endoscopy altered medical or surgical decisions in 13 cases (72 %), leading to a change in management in 79 % [22].

The small bowel endoscopic findings found to be most characteristic of eosinophilic gastroenteropathy (reviewed in Chap. 27) include marked focal villous atrophy, with clearly delineated areas of erythematous, glossy, denuded mucosa adjacent to the normal villi (Fig. 27.2). Strictures and inflammatory polyps may also be found in this disorder (Figs. 27.7 and 27.8). The children with eosinophilic gastroenteritis diagnosed by capsule endoscopy often presented with a protein-losing enteropathy. Capsule endoscopy in this clinical setting in pediatric patients has also been reported to yield a diagnosis of obscure Crohn's disease [23].

Although nonsteroidal anti-inflammatory drugs are less commonly used by children, they certainly may cause significant mucosal injury, including ulcerations that mimic Crohn's disease [24, 25]. The drug-induced lesions may include mucosal breaks and focal ulcerations (Fig. 38.3a–d), as well as circumferential, ulcerated strictures (Fig. 38.3e). Histologic confirmation of specific diagnoses suggested by capsule endoscopy should thus always be considered, where feasible.

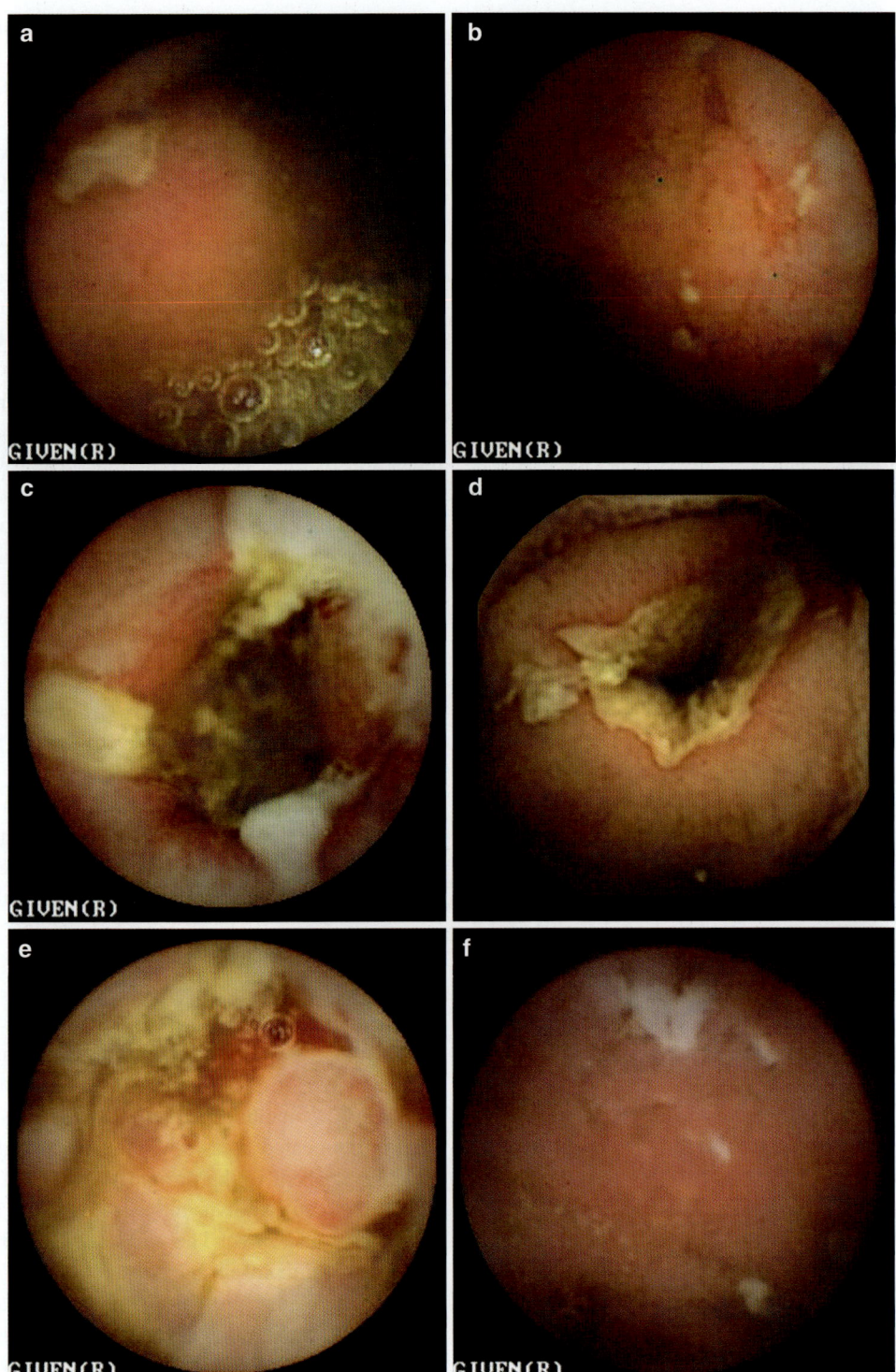

Fig. 38.2 (**a**) Capsule image of one of numerous small bowel ulcerations in an 11-year-old boy with "obscure" Crohn's disease. Despite suggestive characteristic symptoms and signs, as well as biological markers (anemia, high C-reactive protein [CRP], serology positive for antibodies against *Saccharomyces cerevisiae* [ASCA]), all other imaging, endoscopic findings, and even histopathological evidence of Crohn's disease had been lacking. The focal ulceration is characteristically covered with an exudate and surrounded by erythema. (**b**) Focal ulcerations and mucosal fissuring in an adolescent female whose initial presentation of Crohn's disease was massive obscure gastrointestinal (GI) bleeding. The capsule exam was able to establish the diagnosis of Crohn's disease, avoiding a laparotomy. A prior colonoscopy had only revealed active bleeding coming from the small bowel. The barium small bowel follow through was normal. (**c**) Relapse of Crohn's disease diagnosed at the ileocolonic anastomosis in an 18-year-old male patient with abdominal pain. The capsule was evacuated spontaneously. (**d**) Ileal stenosis in patients with Crohn's disease. (**e**) A follow-up capsule study in a 16-year-old boy treated for Crohn's disease shows inflammatory pseudopolyps in the ileum. (**f**) Capsule endoscopy in an 8-year-old girl with steroid-resistant indeterminate colitis revealed numerous lesions of the small bowel suggestive of Crohn's disease. In view of these findings, a colectomy was averted in favor of further medical therapy with infliximab

Fig. 38.3 Small bowel lesions associated with the use of nonsteroidal anti-inflammatory drugs (NSAIDs), uncovered by capsule endoscopy in pediatric patients. (**a**) Ileal bleeding detected by capsule endoscopy in adolescent patients treated with NSAIDs. (**b**) Focal erosion on an ileal fold in a 15-year-old boy with spina bifida and use of NSAIDs for back pain. (**c**) Small aphthous-like ulcers in the proximal jejunum of an 11-year-old girl with NSAID use for juvenile rheumatoid arthritis. (**d**) Ulcerated, circumferential stricture in an adolescent patient with chronic use of NSAIDs and methotrexate for polyarticular arthritis. The ulcerated, stenotic lesion cannot be distinguished endoscopically from a lesion caused by Crohn's disease

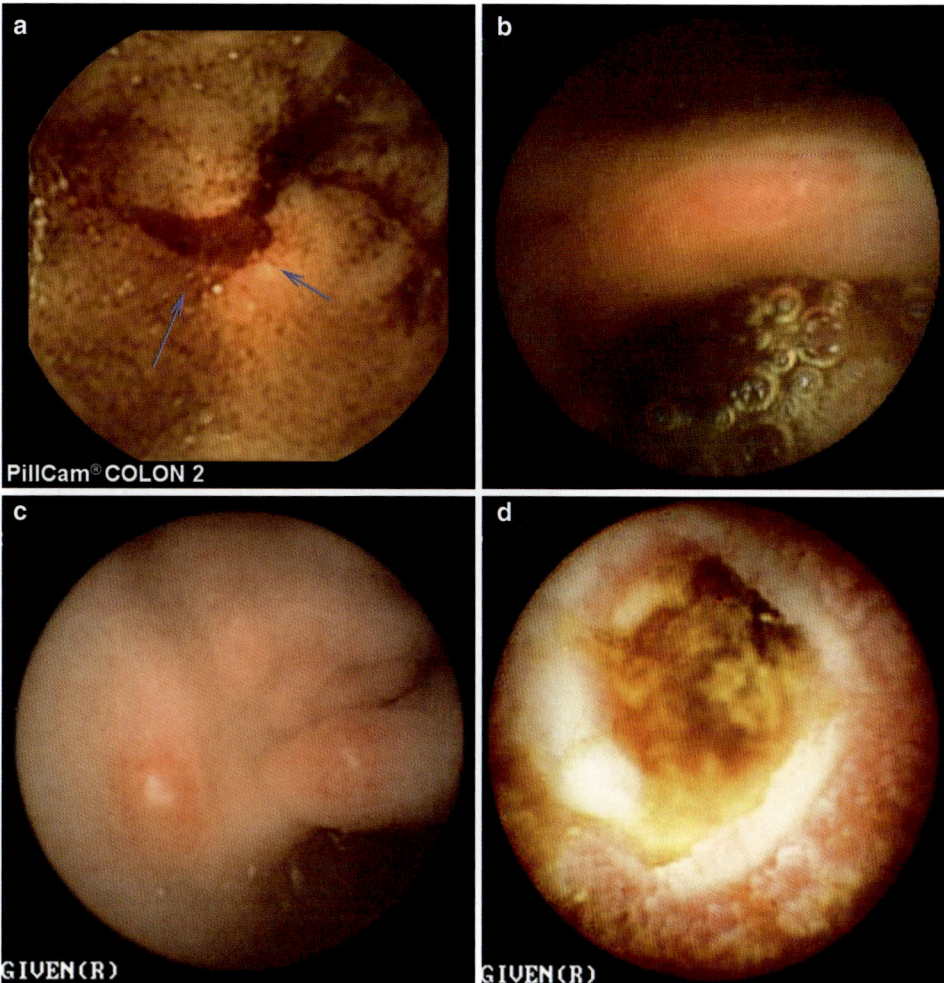

38.1.2 Polyposis Syndromes and Other Intestinal Tumors

Among adult patients, capsule endoscopy has been shown to be highly efficient in detecting small bowel tumors that were missed by conventional endoscopic and imaging methods, including push enteroscopy [12, 26]. Although small bowel malignancies are rare in children, inherited gastrointestinal polyposis disorders such as Peutz-Jeghers syndrome are not uncommonly seen by pediatric gastroenterologists and surgeons. Complications of these tumors include small bowel intussusception, bleeding, anemia, and infrequent malignancy. Surveillance of the small bowel for polyps in these disorders is difficult, and current recommendations for management of these syndromes are ambiguous. In our pediatric capsule study [13], intestinal polyposes such as Peutz-Jeghers syndrome constituted the second most common indication for capsule endoscopy. We observed 100 % concordance of capsule identification between the presence and absence of small bowel polyps compared with previous imaging modalities (endoscopic and radiologic) [13]. Capsule endoscopy was able to identify a far greater number

of polyps per patient than the other imaging and endoscopic procedures in a noninvasive manner and without exposure to radiation [13]. Others have reported similar results in familial adenomatous polyposis and Peutz-Jeghers syndrome [27–29]. Polyps less than 15 mm are better detected with capsule endoscopy than with MRI or other imaging studies [28]. Furthermore, 24 % of patients with hereditary polyposis had jejunal or ileal polyps that were detected only by capsule endoscopy [29]. Iaquinto et al. [30] found that capsule endoscopy was highly accurate in identifying jejunal and ileal polyps in patients with familial adenomatous polyposis (FAP). However, most cancers in FAP are in the duodenum or periampullary area. Identification of the ampulla of Vater was not achieved accurately with capsule endoscopy, and duodenal polyps were identified endoscopically in only 4 of 11 patients, with an underestimation of polyp numbers [30]. The authors concluded that capsule endoscopy is useful and safe for the surveillance of jejunal and ileal polyps in selected patients with FAP, but not for surveillance of the duodenum, where most small bowel cancers occur. The latter may require forward-viewing and side-viewing endoscopy. Postgate et al. [31] carried out a blinded comparison study of

Fig. 38.4 Peutz-Jeghers syndrome (PJS) in a 13-year-old boy with perioral pigmentation (**a**), hyperplastic gastric polyps (**b**), pedunculated hamartomatous polyps in the jejunum and ileum (**c**) as well as in the colon (**d**)

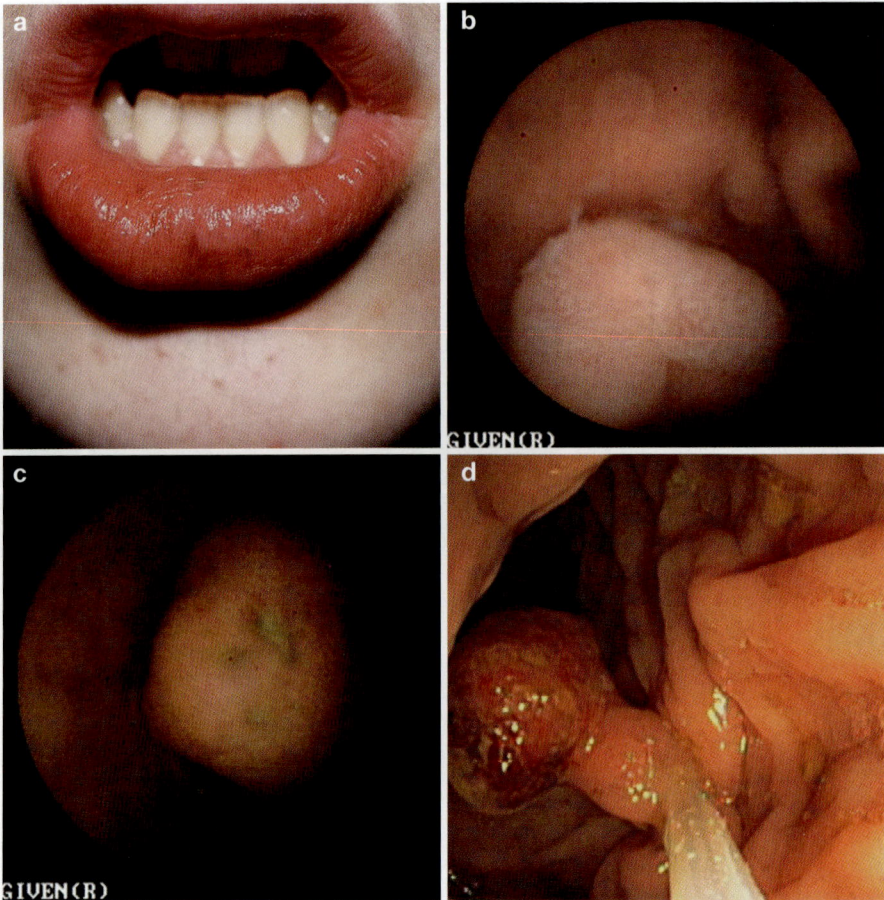

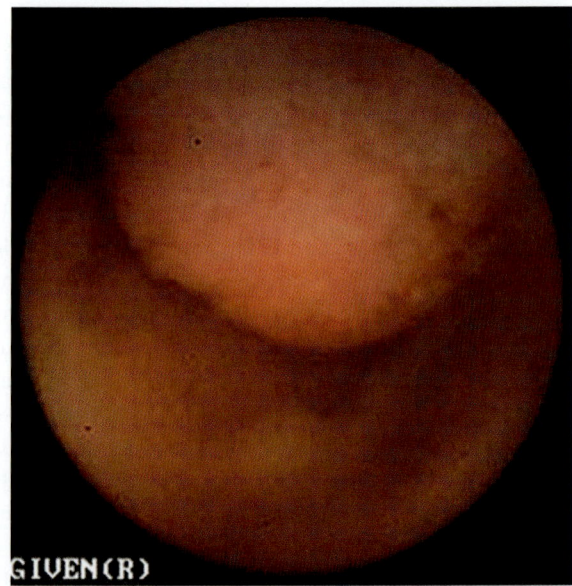

Fig. 38.5 Large PJS polyp in the ileum of a 17-year-old male, as revealed by capsule endoscopy

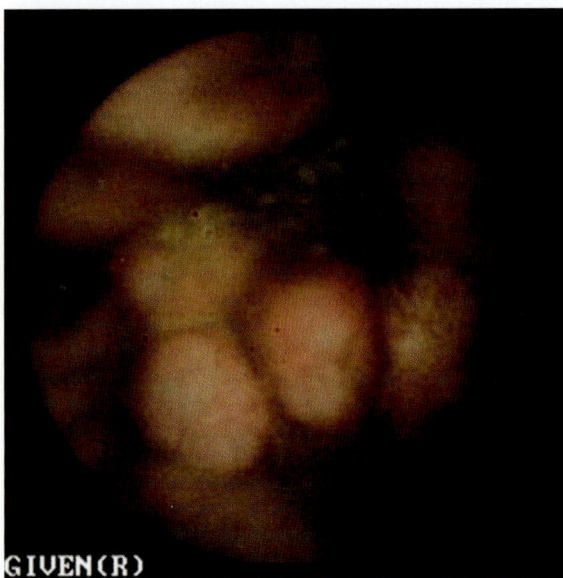

Fig. 38.6 Several small colonic PJS polyps seen at capsule endoscopy in an 11-year-old girl

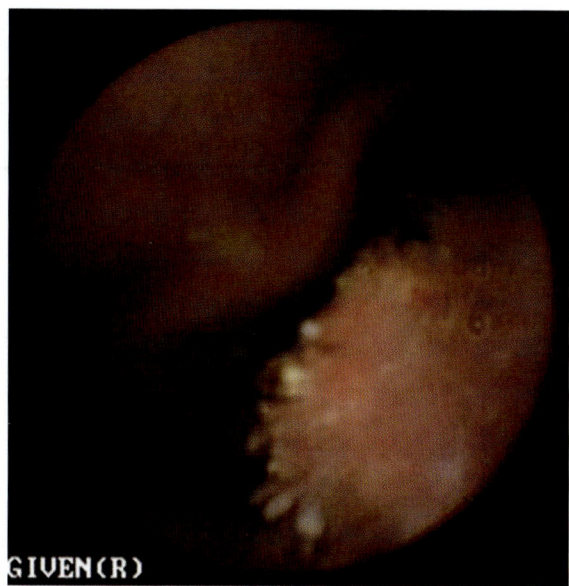

Fig. 38.7 Distal duodenal polyp discovered by capsule endoscopy in a 12-year-old patient with a familial polyposis syndrome. The polyp was missed in upper GI endoscopy and barium series. The capsule study directed the endoscopic removal and retrieval of the polyp

barium enterography with capsule endoscopy in Peutz-Jeghers syndrome. Among the 11 children, equal numbers of polyps >10 mm were detected, but 61 polyps <10 mm were found by capsule versus only 6 by barium studies ($p=0.02$). Capsule endoscopy was preferred over barium study by 90 % of the patients. The available data thus suggest that capsule endoscopy should replace barium X-rays, MRI, and push enteroscopy for the identification of small bowel polyps in the pediatric age group. The localization software can also guide the clinician to the possibility of reaching a polyp for removal endoscopically. Representative images are shown in Figs. 38.4, 38.5, 38.6, and 38.7.

38.1.3 Occult or Obscure Intestinal Bleeding

The most common indication for capsule endoscopy in adult studies remains the identification of a source of GI bleeding of obscure origin [32]. Obscure bleeding is defined as bleeding of unknown origin that persists or recurs (recurrent or persistent visible bleeding or iron-deficiency anemia with positive fecal occult blood testing) after negative initial endoscopies (upper and lower) [32, 33]. The source of bleeding is frequently located in the small bowel. The bleeding may result from a number of conditions, including vascular lesions, inflammatory lesions, or tumors. Imaging techniques for evaluation of the small bowel are relatively insensitive for intestinal bleeding lesions that are flat, small, infiltrative, or inflammatory. Angiography and radioisotope bleeding scans are insensitive in the absence of brisk, active

bleeding. Intraoperative enteroscopy, although potentially the most thorough means to visualize the entire small bowel, is also the most invasive. Although push enteroscopy is an effective diagnostic procedure, it is time-consuming and allows exploration only of the proximal jejunum. Double-balloon enteroscopy is the newest method that offers the possibility of achieving complete small bowel enteroscopy and providing therapy without the need for laparotomy, but access to this method is not widespread and pediatric experience is limited.

The key advantages of capsule endoscopy for patients with obscure intestinal bleeding have recently been reviewed [32]. They include the ability to image the entire small bowel noninvasively and without radiation exposure; the superior clarity of the images compared with other endoscopic devices; the ability to review and share images, patient preference; the safety profile; and the ability to conduct the testing in a variety of settings.

In adult patients, a lesion is generally detected in about two thirds of cases. A study with a median follow-up of 19 months [34] reported that among patients with a negative capsule exam, the cumulative rebleeding rate was significantly lower (5.6 %) than in patients with a positive capsule study (48.4 %, $p=0.03$ log-rank test). The sensitivity and negative predictive value of capsule endoscopy in predicting rebleeding were 93.8 % and 94.4 %, respectively. In a cohort of 55 adults with severe obscure bleeding, a recent study [35] showed that emergency capsule endoscopy within 48 h of negative bidirectional endoscopy was able to identify the approximate location of bleeding in 49 (89 %) of the 55 patients. The lesion-specific diagnostic yield was 67 %, with culprit lesions identified in 37 patients. Subsequent therapeutic interventions as guided by capsule findings were carried out in 42 (76 %) of 55 patients, including endotherapy in 30 patients (54 %) and surgery in 12 patients (22 %).

Data regarding experience with capsule endoscopy in the clinical setting of pediatric patients with obscure GI bleeding are much less extensive. In our study [13], a diagnosis of arteriovenous malformations or angiodysplasia as the source of obscure bleeding in the small bowel was confirmed using the capsule in three fourths of children and adolescents. Other imaging techniques (upper and lower endoscopies, as well as selective mesenteric angiography) had failed to identify the source of bleeding in any of these patients. Capsule endoscopy has been found to be a useful tool for diagnosing and monitoring the effects of therapy in patients with blue rubber bleb nevus syndrome [36]. We have also diagnosed cases of bleeding from small bowel varices in pediatric patients with portal hypertension (Fig. 38.8) and from ulcers due to Crohn's disease or NSAIDs (Figs. 38.2b and 38.3). Other bleeding lesions can include erosions, angiodysplastic lesions, tumors, and Meckel's diverticulum (Figs. 38.9, 38.10, and 38.11).

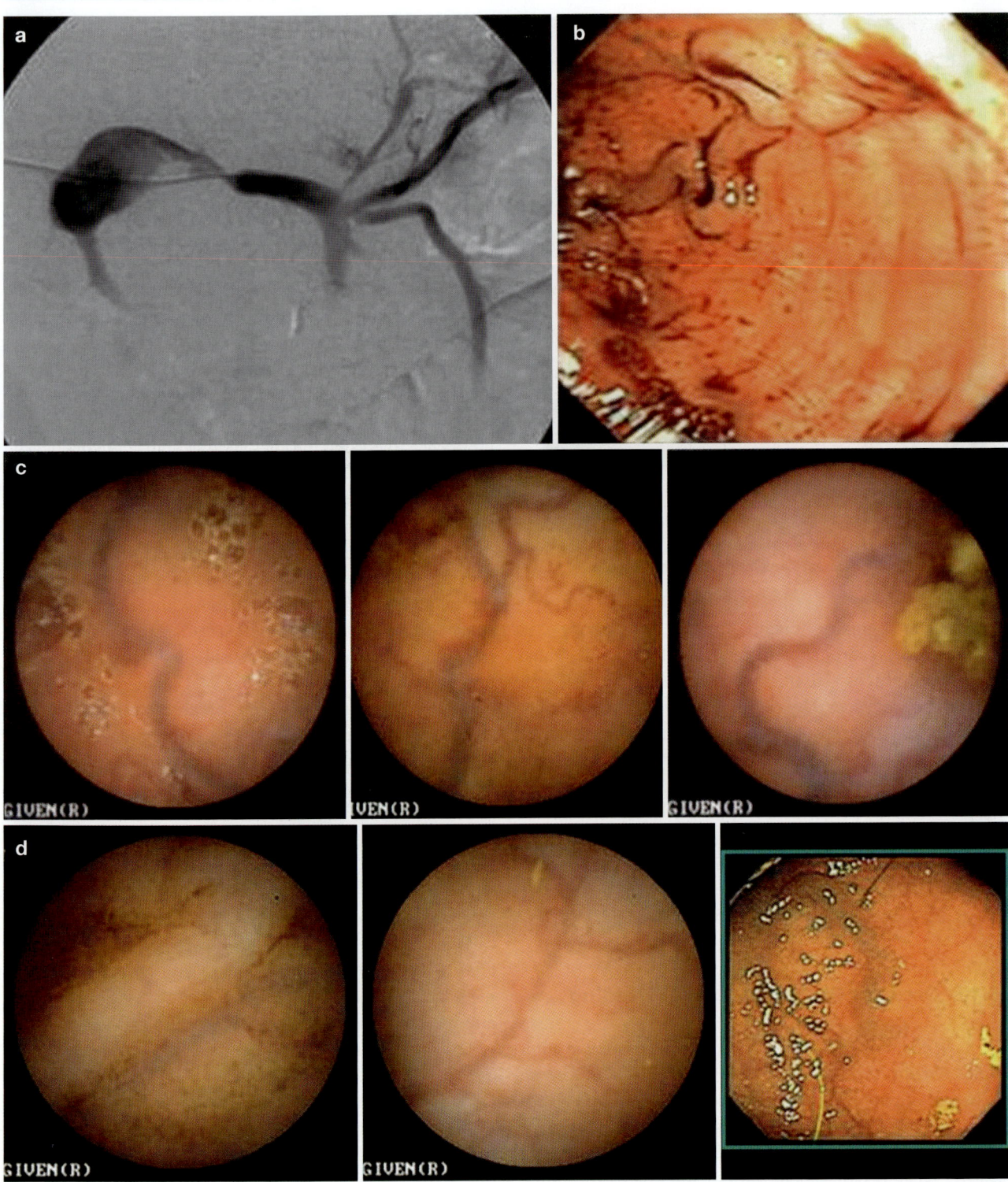

Fig. 38.8 Capsule endoscopy reveals small bowel varices undetected by other endoscopic and imaging tests. The patient is a 15-year-old girl with Alagille syndrome, presenting with obscure GI bleeding 12 years after a liver transplant. (**a**) Transhepatic portography revealing portal vein stenosis with poststenotic dilatation. Contrast demonstrates perigastric and perisplenic varices (portal and mesenteric pressures were 18 mmHg). (**b**) Colonoscopy revealed nonbleeding rectosigmoid varices. Active bleeding was seen to be coming from proximal to the ileocecal valve. (**c**) Capsule endoscopy revealed several varices in the distal small bowel. The portal vein stenosis was dilated angiographically and a stent was placed. Small bowel bleeding subsequently stopped. (**d**) Repeat capsule endoscopy revealed only one slightly prominent small bowel vein (*left image*), and colonoscopy confirmed the disappearance of the rectosigmoid varices (*right*)

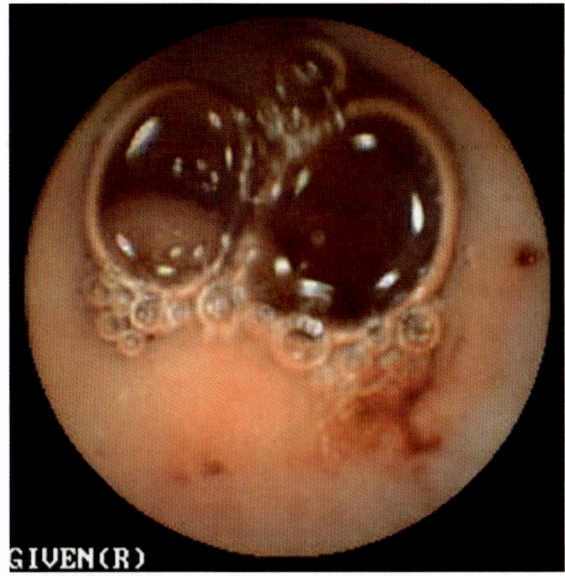

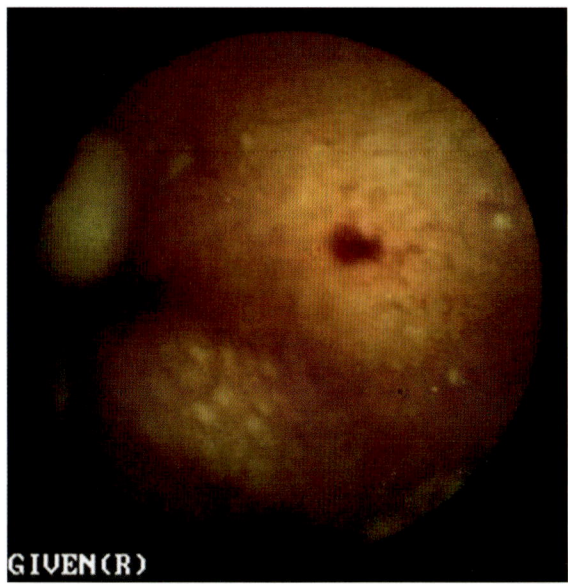

Fig. 38.9 Bleeding erosion in the ileum of an 8-year-old boy with anemia and positive fecal occult blood tests

Fig. 38.10 Angiodysplastic lesion in the ileum of a 3-year-old child with anemia and occult GI bleeding. Previous investigations had failed to reveal a source of bleeding

Fig. 38.11 (**a**) and (**b**) Meckel's diverticulum in a 14-year-old boy with iron deficiency anemia (hemoglobin 6.4 g/dL) and positive fecal occult blood tests. The patient was referred to surgery without prior scintigraphy, and the diagnosis was confirmed

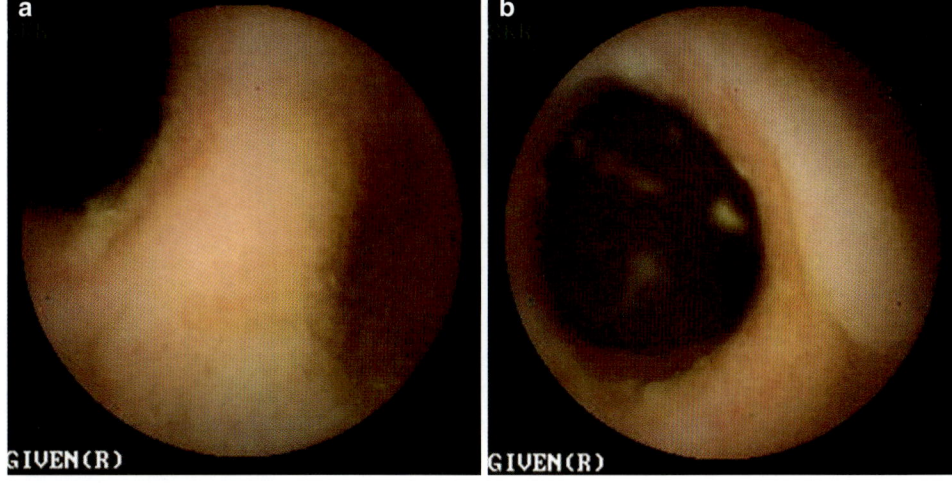

38.1.4 Celiac Disease

A pilot study [11] showed that capsule endoscopy, as interpreted by an experienced observer, was highly sensitive and specific for the diagnosis of untreated celiac disease in adult patients with moderate to severe villous atrophy. However, little prospective data have been reported. Murray et al. [37] reported on 38 adult patients ultimately shown to have celiac disease, in whom about 90 % had changes suggestive of atrophy on capsule study. This was substantially higher than the rate of atrophic changes on prior upper endoscopy. There is adequate evidence to support the use of capsule endoscopy in patients with previously confirmed, treated celiac disease who have developed alarm symptoms [38]. However, such cases of "refractory sprue" or lymphoma complicating celiac disease are exceedingly rare in pediatrics. A consensus panel [39] did feel that capsule

Table 38.2 Capsule endoscopy findings of the small bowel mucosa suggestive of celiac disease[a]

Fissuring
Scalloping
Mosaic pattern
Nodularity
Late appearance of the villi (absence of villi detected in the duodenum and proximal jejunum)
Loss of circular folds

[a]The identification of at least two of these findings, confirmed by experienced observers, is considered suggestive of celiac disease

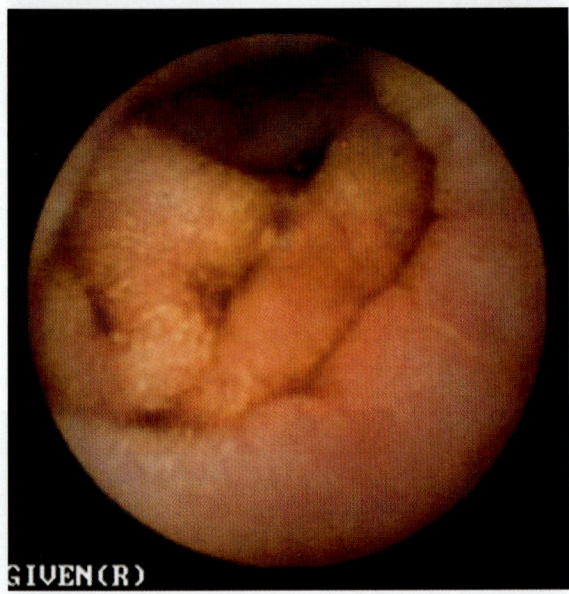

Fig. 38.12 Capsule endoscopy in an adolescent with an uncertain diagnosis of celiac disease, undergoing a gluten challenge (3 months). Capsule endoscopy reveals a scalloped fold in the distal duodenum (D3–4) with focal villous atrophy

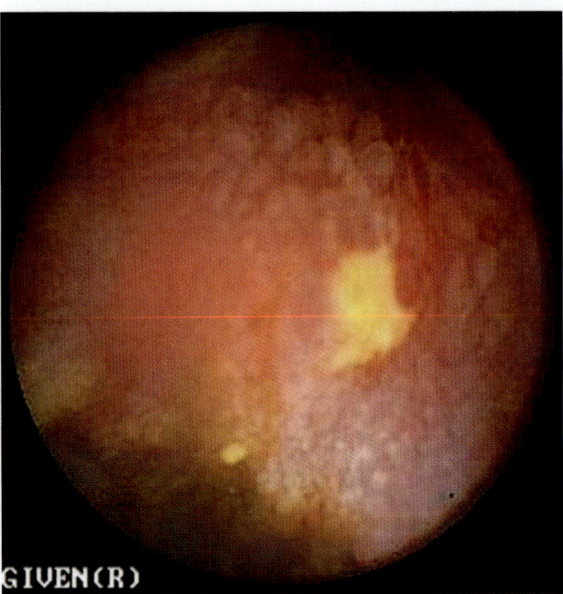

Fig. 38.13 This adolescent male with a history of a previously treated lymphoma presented with abdominal pain of uncertain etiology. Capsule endoscopy revealed an ulcerated "bulge" in the distal ileum. Surgical resection confirmed a recurrence of the lymphoma

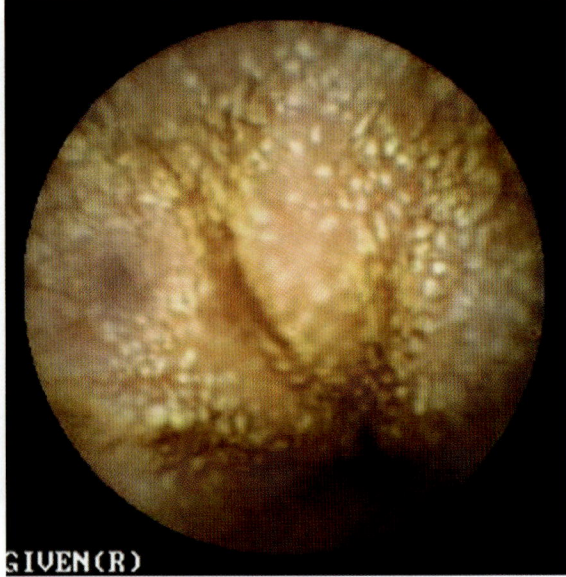

Fig. 38.14 Intestinal lymphangiectasia diagnosed by capsule in a 30-month-old child referred for a protein-losing enteropathy and anasarca. An incidental phlebectasia is noted

endoscopy may have a future role as an initial diagnostic test for confirming atrophy in patients who are seropositive. Capsule endoscopy was recommended as an alternative to biopsy in selected patients who are unwilling or unable to undergo upper endoscopy for confirmation of villous atrophy [39]. The findings that are characteristic of celiac disease are summarized in Table 38.2, and a representative case is illustrated in Fig. 38.12.

38.1.5 Other Indications

In addition to the more common indications discussed above, capsule endoscopy is clinically useful for a variety of other potential disorders of the small bowel in the pediatric age group (see Table 38.1). The identification of abnormal but undiagnosed findings on small bowel imaging is a worthwhile

indication for capsule study. Pathologies that have been uncovered include small bowel lymphomas (Fig. 38.13). In our experience [40], capsule endoscopy represents the diagnostic imaging method of choice to detect intestinal lymphangiectasia (Fig. 38.14). We have also used capsule endoscopy to diagnose chronic intussusception and ischemic bowel disease as causes of recurrent abdominal pain in adolescent patients

Fig. 38.15 (**a**) Jejunal intussusception, with a small mucosal erosion on the lead point. (**b**) Persistence of the same intussusception for well over an hour, as recorded by capsule endoscopy. The patient is an adolescent male who presented with abdominal pain of uncertain relation to the intussusception. The small bowel was otherwise normal

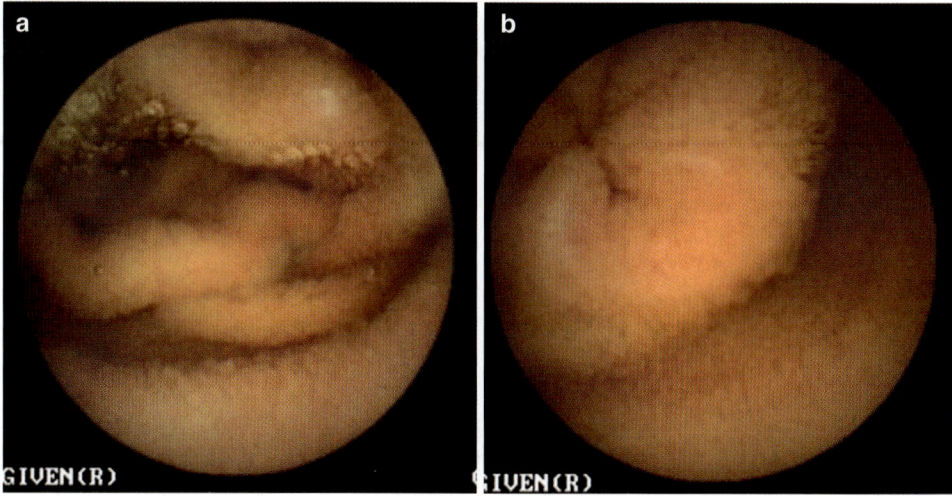

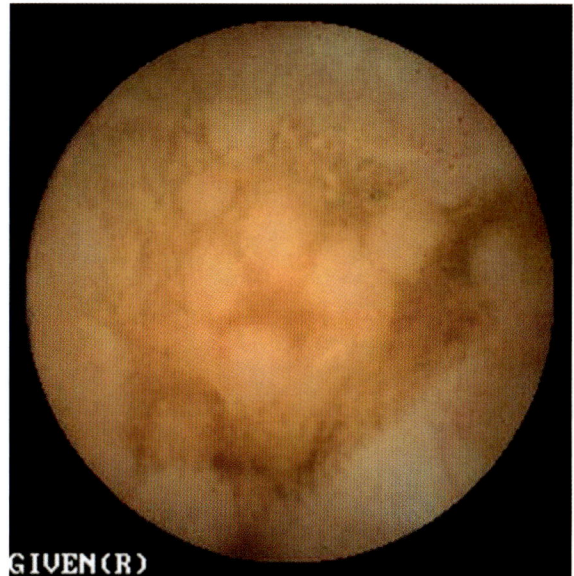

Fig. 38.16 Benign nodular lymphoid hyperplasia in a 9-year-old boy observed at capsule endoscopy

(Fig. 38.15). Capsule endoscopy can also be useful to ascertain the intestinal manifestations of immunodeficiency disorders [41]. In suspected graft-versus-host disease [42], capsule endoscopy revealed GI lesions even where upper endoscopy was negative. It is not uncommon to observe lymphoid hyperplasia of the distal ileum in normal children and adolescents (Figs. 38.16 and 38.17). However, an immunodeficiency was evoked by a capsule study that showed extensive multifocal lymphoid hyperplasia of the duodenum and ileum (Fig. 38.18). The ultimate diagnosis was IgA deficiency. A pilot study [43] in 10 pediatric patients suggested that capsule endoscopy has a higher yield than upper endoscopy in patients referred for functional abdominal pain. The timed

movement of the capsule through various segments of the GI tract (gastric emptying time, small bowel transit time) can also serve as a useful tool in the assessment of children with motility disorders.

38.2 Practical Issues

Capsule endoscopy is very well tolerated in children able to swallow the capsule. Several studies have reported that young patients prefer it to other imaging techniques. Patients can return to school or go about their usual daily activities during the exam. In our experience, capsule endoscopy in children does not routinely require bowel preparation or the use of a prokinetic drug. However, the clinician should ascertain if there is any history suggestive of gastroparesis or if medications (e.g., narcotics) are being used that may interfere with gastric emptying. Patients should be fasting for at least 8 h prior to the test. We generally permit patients to drink clear fluids 1–2 h after the study has begun and to eat a light meal about 2 h after ingesting the capsule. The use of a real-time viewer can provide reassurance that the video capsule has exited the stomach and is viewing the small bowel mucosa.

One of the key considerations before undertaking capsule endoscopy is to ascertain whether the child is able to swallow the capsule. Inability to swallow the capsule is a common problem in children under the age of 8, but it may even be encountered in older children and adolescents. For individuals judged unable to swallow the capsule, or for patients with gastroparesis, severe dysphagia, or swallowing disorders, the study can be safely undertaken by introducing the capsule into the proximal duodenum endoscopically under direct vision, as discussed in Chap. 7. Currently, our preferred method is to "front load" the

Fig. 38.17 (**a**) Lymphoid follicular hyperplasia in an 18-year-old male with rectal bleeding. (**b**) Small, prominent vessels are seen in the same patient

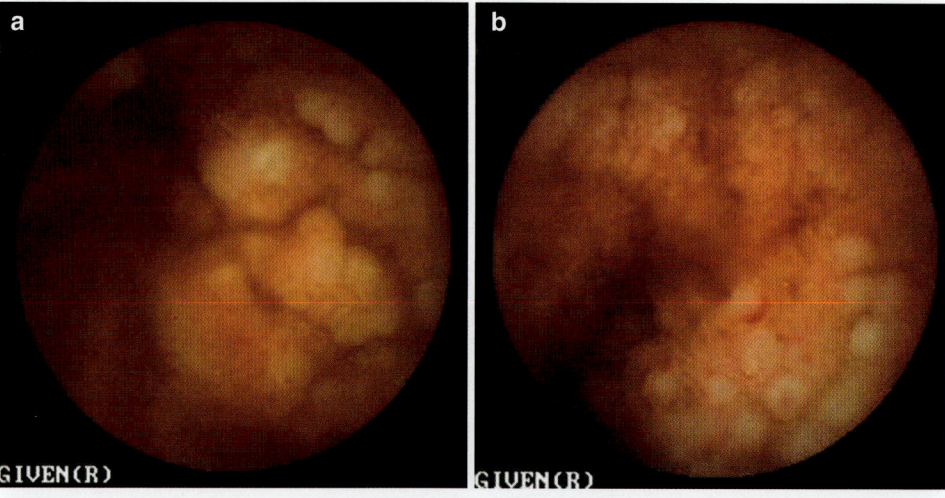

Fig. 38.18 Lymphoid hyperplasia in atypical locations – the duodenum (A) and mid-small bowel (**b**) revealed by a capsule study suggested that this 9-year-old patient had an immunodeficiency. Selective IgA deficiency was subsequently confirmed

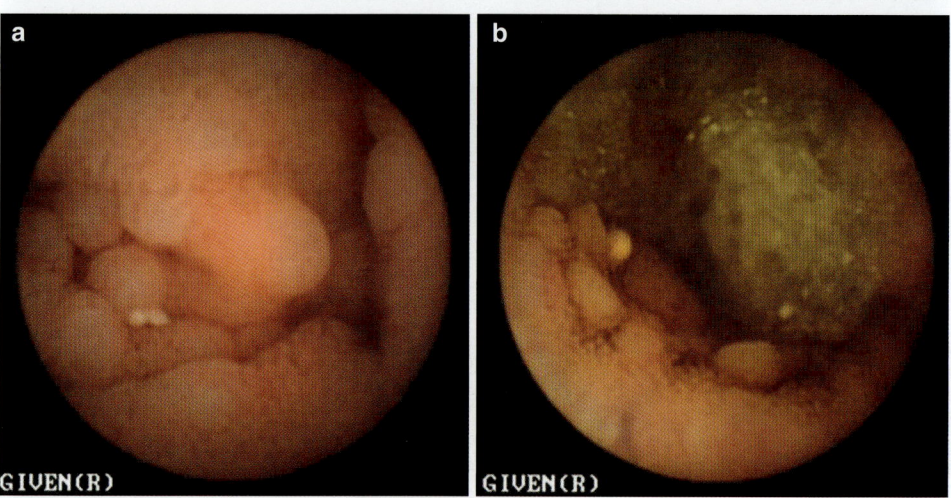

Fig. 38.19 Methods of "front loading" the small bowel capsule onto a gastroscope: (**a**) using a Roth net, (**b**) using an AdvanCE delivery device (US Endoscopy, Mentor, OH, USA)

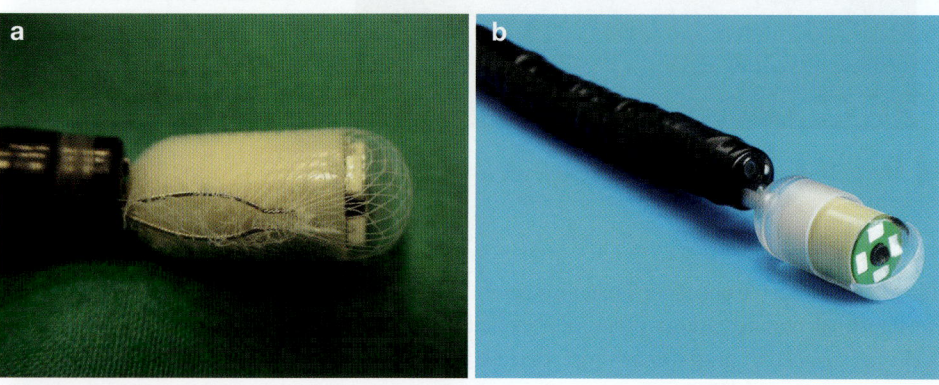

Fig. 38.20 Endoscopic insertion of a video capsule using the capsule delivery device in a 17-year-old girl who was unable to swallow the capsule. (**a**) Endoscopic view of the larynx. (**b**) The front-loaded capsule is advanced into the esophagus under direct visualization

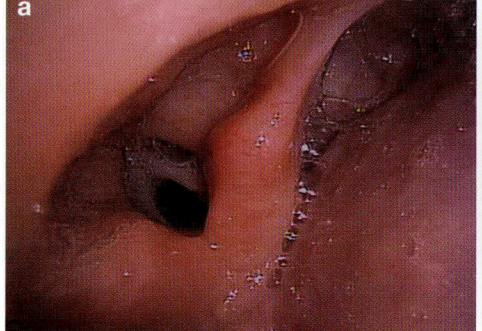
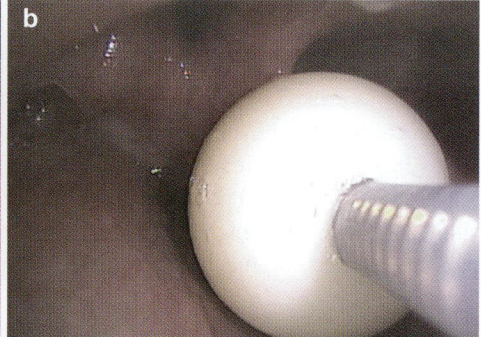

capsule on a gastroscope [5, 44], holding it in place using either a Dormia basket, the Roth net, or the "AdvanCE" delivery device designed for the PillCam video capsule (US Endoscopy, Mentor, OH, USA) (Figs. 38.19 and 38.20). The real-time viewer should be used to confirm that the capsule is in the small bowel before removing the gastroscope and extubating the patient [45].

Another important consideration is whether the patient's age or size will permit the capsule to traverse the pylorus and ileocecal valve. Guidelines are not yet available, but we have successfully used the capsule in children as young as 16 months of age. The critical limiting factor appears to be the size, rather than the age, of the child. In our experience, the lower weight limit is approximately 16 kg. A study recently established the safety and utility of capsule endoscopy in 83 children under age 8 [46], the youngest being 1.5 years of age. Twenty children over the age of 4 swallowed the capsule.

Finally, intestinal strictures or other obstructing lesions (tumors, adhesions) are a contraindication, as they may preclude the capsule's passage, and bowel obstruction may theoretically ensue. It is advisable to demonstrate luminal patency in patients with Crohn's disease or in those with obstructive symptoms prior to a capsule study. However, stenoses are not always excluded despite negative cross-sectional imaging studies. In one report [47], capsule retention occurred in 3 (5.2 %) of 58 pediatric patients with known Crohn's disease, similar to the result in adult series. The risk of capsule retention for patients with suspected IBD and all other indications was 0 %. We recommend the routine use of a dissolvable patency capsule for all patients with known Crohn's disease.

References

1. MacKenzie JF. Push enteroscopy. Gastrointest Endosc Clin N Am. 1999;9:29–36.
2. Waye JD. Small-bowel endoscopy. Endoscopy. 2003;35:15–21.
3. Yamamoto H, Kita H, Sunada K, et al. Clinical outcomes of double-balloon endoscopy for the diagnosis and treatment of small-intestinal diseases. Clin Gastroenterol Hepatol. 2004;2:1010–6.
4. Thomson M, Venkatesh K, Elmalik K, et al. Double balloon enteroscopy in children: diagnosis, treatment, and safety. World J Gastroenterol. 2010;16:56–62.
5. Seidman EG, Sant'Anna AMGA, Dirks MH. Potential applications of wireless capsule endoscopy in the pediatric age group. Gastrointest Endosc Clin N Am. 2004;14:207–18.
6. Iddan G, Meron G, Glukhovsky A, Swain P. Wireless capsule endoscopy. Nature. 2000;405:417.
7. Costamagna G, Shah SK, Riccioni ME, et al. A prospective trial comparing small bowel radiographs and video capsule endoscopy for suspected small bowel disease. Gastroenterology. 2002;123:999–1005.
8. Ell C, Remke S, May A, et al. The first prospective controlled trial comparing wireless capsule endoscopy in chronic gastrointestinal bleeding. Endoscopy. 2002;34:685–9.
9. Pennazio M, Santucci R, Rondonotti E, et al. Outcome of patients with obscure gastrointestinal bleeding after capsule endoscopy: report of 100 consecutive cases. Gastroenterology. 2004;126:643–53.
10. Triester SL, Leighton JA, Gurudu SR, et al. A meta-analysis of capsule endoscopy (CE) compared to other modalities in patients with non-stricturing small bowel Crohn disease (NSCD). Am J Gastroenterol. 2004;99:S271–2.
11. Petroniene R, Dubenco E, Baker JP, et al. Given capsule endoscopy in celiac disease: evaluation of diagnostic accuracy and interobserver variation. Am J Gastroenterol. 2005;100:685–94.
12. de Mascarenhas-Saraiva MN, da Silva Araujo Lopes LM. Small-bowel tumors diagnosed by wireless capsule endoscopy: report of five cases. Endoscopy. 2003;35:865–8.
13. Sant'Anna AMGA, Dubois J, Miron MJ, Seidman EG. Wireless capsule endoscopy for obscure small bowel disorders: final results of the first pediatric controlled trial. Clin Gastroenterol Hepatol. 2005;3:264–70.
14. Urbain D, Tresinie M, De Looz D, et al. Capsule endoscopy in paediatrics: multicentric Belgian study. Acta Gastroenterol Belg. 2007;70:11–4.
15. de Angelis GL, Fornaroli F, de Angelis N, et al. Wireless capsule endoscopy for pediatric small-bowel diseases. Am J Gastroenterol. 2007;102:1749–57.
16. Cohen SA, Ephrath H, Lewis JD, et al. Pediatric capsule endoscopy: review of the small bowel and patency capsules. J Pediatr Gastroenterol Nutr. 2012;54:409–13.
17. Cohen SA, Klevens AI. Use of capsule endoscopy in diagnosis and management of pediatric patients, based on meta-analysis. Clin Gastroenterol Hepatol. 2011;9:490–6.
18. Sant'Anna AMGA, Seidman EG. Wireless capsule endoscopy: comparison study in pediatric and adult patients. J Pediatr Gastroenterol Nutr. 2003;37:332.
19. Arguelles-Arias F, Caunedo A, Romero J, et al. The value of capsule endoscopy in pediatric patients with a suspicion of Crohn's disease. Endoscopy. 2004;36:869–73.
20. Cohen SA, Gralnek IM, Ephrath H, et al. The use of patency capsule in pediatric Crohn's disease: a prospective evaluation. Dig Dis Sci. 2011;56:860–5.
21. Cohen SA, Gralnek IM, Ephrath H, et al. Capsule endoscopy may reclassify pediatric inflammatory bowel disease: a historical analysis. J Pediatr Gastroenterol Nutr. 2008;47:31–6.
22. Gralnek IM, Cohen SA, Ephrath H, et al. Small bowel capsule endoscopy impacts diagnosis and management of pediatric inflammatory bowel disease: a prospective study. Dig Dis Sci. 2012;57:465–71.
23. Barkay O, Moshkowitz M, Reif S. Crohn's disease diagnosed by wireless capsule endoscopy in adolescents with abdominal pain, protein-losing enteropathy, anemia and negative endoscopic and radiologic findings. Isr Med Assoc J. 2005;7:262–3.
24. Maiden L, Thjodleifsson B, Theodors A, et al. A quantitative analysis of NSAID-induced small bowel pathology by capsule enteroscopy. Gastroenterology. 2005;128:1172–8.
25. Goldstein JL, Eisen GM, Lewis B, et al. Video capsule endoscopy to prospectively assess small bowel injury with celecoxib, naproxen plus omeprazole, and placebo. Clin Gastroenterol Hepatol. 2005;3:133–41.
26. Mata A, Bordas JM, Feu F, et al. Wireless capsule endoscopy in patients with obscure gastrointestinal bleeding: a comparative study with push enteroscopy. Aliment Pharmacol Ther. 2004;20:189–94.
27. Soares J, Lopes L, Vilas Boas G, Pinho C. Wireless capsule endoscopy for evaluation of phenotypic expression of small-bowel polyps in patients with Peutz-Jeghers syndrome and in symptomatic first-degree relatives. Endoscopy. 2004;36:1060–6.
28. Caspari R, von Falkenhausen M, Krautmacher C, et al. Comparison of capsule endoscopy and magnetic resonance imaging for the detection of polyps of the small intestine in patients with familial adenomatous polyposis or with Peutz-Jeghers' syndrome. Endoscopy. 2004;36:1054–9.
29. Schulmann K, Hollerbach S, Kraus K, et al. Feasibility and diagnostic utility of video capsule endoscopy for the detection of small

bowel polyps in patients with hereditary polyposis syndromes. Am J Gastroenterol. 2005;100:27–37.

30. Iaquinto G, Fornasarig M, Quaia M, et al. Capsule endoscopy is useful and safe for small-bowel surveillance in familial adenomatous polyposis. Gastrointest Endosc. 2008;67:61–7.

31. Postgate A, Hyer W, Phillips R, et al. Feasibility of video capsule endoscopy in the management of children with Peutz-Jeghers syndrome: a blinded comparison with barium enterography for the detection of small bowel polyps. J Pediatr Gastroenterol Nutr. 2009;49:417–23.

32. Pennazio M. Enteroscopy in the diagnosis and management of obscure gastrointestinal bleeding. Gastrointest Endosc Clin N Am. 2009;19:409–26.

33. Rondonotti E, Marmo R, Petracchini M, et al. The American Society for Gastrointestinal Endoscopy (ASGE) diagnostic algorithm for obscure gastrointestinal bleeding: eight burning questions from everyday clinical practice. Dig Liver Dis. 2013;45:179–85.

34. Lai LH, Wong GLH, Chow DKL, et al. Long-term follow-up of patients with obscure gastrointestinal bleeding after negative capsule endoscopy. Am J Gastroenterol. 2006;101: 1224–8.

35. Lecleire S, Iwanicki-Caron I, Di-Fiore A, et al. Yield and impact of emergency capsule enteroscopy in severe obscure-overt gastrointestinal bleeding. Endoscopy. 2012;44:337–42.

36. De Bona M, Bellumat A, De Boni M. Capsule endoscopy for the diagnosis and follow-up of blue rubber bleb nevus syndrome. Dig Liver Dis. 2005;37:451–3.

37. Murray JA, Brogan D, Van dyke C, et al. Mapping the extent of untreated celiac disease with capsule enteroscopy. Gastrointest Endosc. 2004;59:AB101.

38. Collin P, Rondonotti E, Lundin K, et al. Video capsule endoscopy in celiac disease: current clinical practice. J Dig Dis. 2012;13: 94–9.

39. Cellier C, Green PH, Collin P, Murray J. ICCE consensus for celiac disease. Endoscopy. 2005;37:1055–9.

40. Peretti N, Sant'Anna AMGA, Dirks MH, Seidman EG. Capsule endoscopy detects lymphangiectasia missed by other means. 4th International conference on capsule endoscopy, Miami, 2005 Mar 7–8, p. 189.

41. Mihaly F, Nemeth A, Zagoni T, et al. Gastrointestinal manifestations of common variable immunodeficiency diagnosed by video- and capsule endoscopy. Endoscopy. 2005;37:603–4.

42. Yakoub-Agha I, Maunoury V, Wacrenier A, et al. Impact of small bowel exploration using video-capsule endoscopy in the management of acute gastrointestinal graft-versus-host disease. Transplantation. 2004;78:1697–701.

43. Shamir R, Hino B, Hartman C, et al. Wireless video capsule in pediatric patients with functional abdominal pain. J Pediatr Gastroenterol Nutr. 2007;44:45–50.

44. Barth BA, Donovan K, Fox VL. Endoscopic placement of the capsule endoscope in children. Gastrointest Endosc. 2004;60:818–21.

45. Bass LM, Misiewicz L. Use of a real-time viewer for endoscopic deployment of capsule endoscope in the pediatric population. J Pediatr Gastroenterol Nutr. 2012;55:552–5.

46. Fritscher-Ravens A, Scherbakov P, Bufler P, et al. The feasibility of wireless capsule endoscopy in detecting small intestinal pathology in children under the age of 8 years: a multicentre European study. Gut. 2009;58:1467–72.

47. Atay O, Mahajan L, Kay M, et al. Risk of capsule endoscope retention in pediatric patients: a large single-center experience and review of the literature. J Pediatr Gastroenterol Nutr. 2009;49:196–201.

Postoperative and Postinterventional Changes

39

Lisa Rundt, Martin Keuchel, Roberto de Franchis, and Wolfgang Teichmann

Contents

The work was first published in 2006 by Springer Medizin Verlag Heidelberg with the following title: *Atlas of Video Capsule Endoscopy*.

L. Rundt (✉) • M. Keuchel
Department of Internal Medicine, Bethesda Krankenhaus Bergedorf, Hamburg, Germany
e-mail: rundt@bkb.info; keuchel@bkb.info

R. de Franchis
Gastroenterology Unit, Luigi Sacco University Hospital, University of Milan, Milan, Italy
e-mail: roberto.defranchis@unimi.it

W. Teichmann
Hamburg, Germany
e-mail: w.teichmann1@web.de

As postoperative changes can cause difficulties in the interpretation of video capsule endoscopy (VCE), knowledge of these differences is as important as in radiology [1]. It is not uncommon to examine patients who have had a previous fundoplication, some type of gastrectomy, a partial small bowel resection, or an ileocecal resection [2]. The findings obtained with VCE, especially at anastomotic sites, are often less than spectacular, at most demonstrating portions of the anastomosis.

39.1 Esophagus

39.1.1 Fundoplication

Today, fundoplication is usually performed laparoscopically in selected patients with a hiatal hernia and significant reflux. This procedure can lead to relative stenosis of the gastroesophageal junction, causing a delay in capsule passage (Fig. 39.1).

39.1.2 Esophagojejunostomy

An esophagojejunostomy is performed after a total gastrectomy (Fig. 39.2), usually constructing an end-to-side anastomosis with a terminolateral pouch and an efferent loop. A Roux-en-Y anastomosis is also necessary for the bile-carrying limb of the small bowel.

39.2 Stomach

39.2.1 Partial Gastrectomy

Passage through the stomach after a partial gastrectomy is hard to predict, as a capsule may pass within seconds without visualization of the anastomosis (Fig. 39.3). In other cases, passage of the capsule may be delayed for a long time at the anastomosis.

Fig. 39.1 Fundoplicated stomach. (**a**) Video capsule endoscopy (VCE) shows a relative stenosis of the gastroesophageal junction within the hiatal hernia, evidenced by the gastric folds; some secretion is also present. (**b**) Retroflexed gastroscopic view of the tight plication cuff

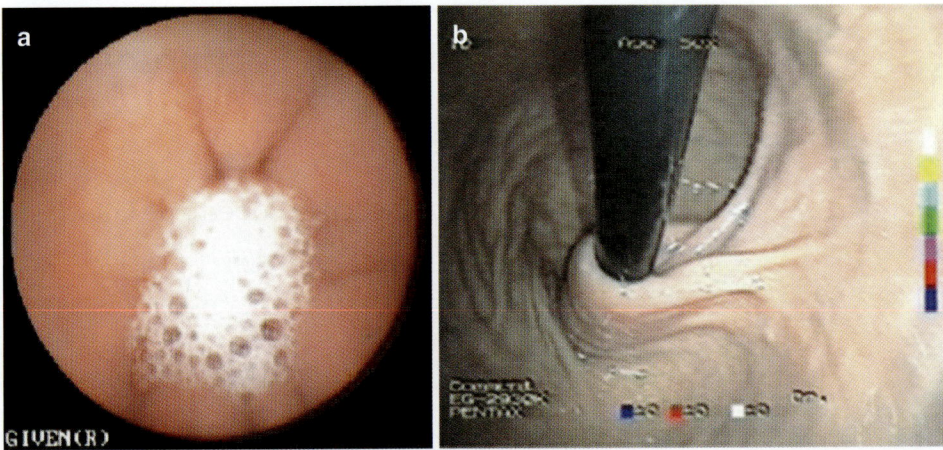

Fig. 39.2 Esophagojejunostomy with an end-to-side anastomosis. (**a**) Anastomotic septum viewed from the esophagus. (**b**) Reverse view of the anastomosis and esophagus from the small bowel. (**c**) Endoscopic view

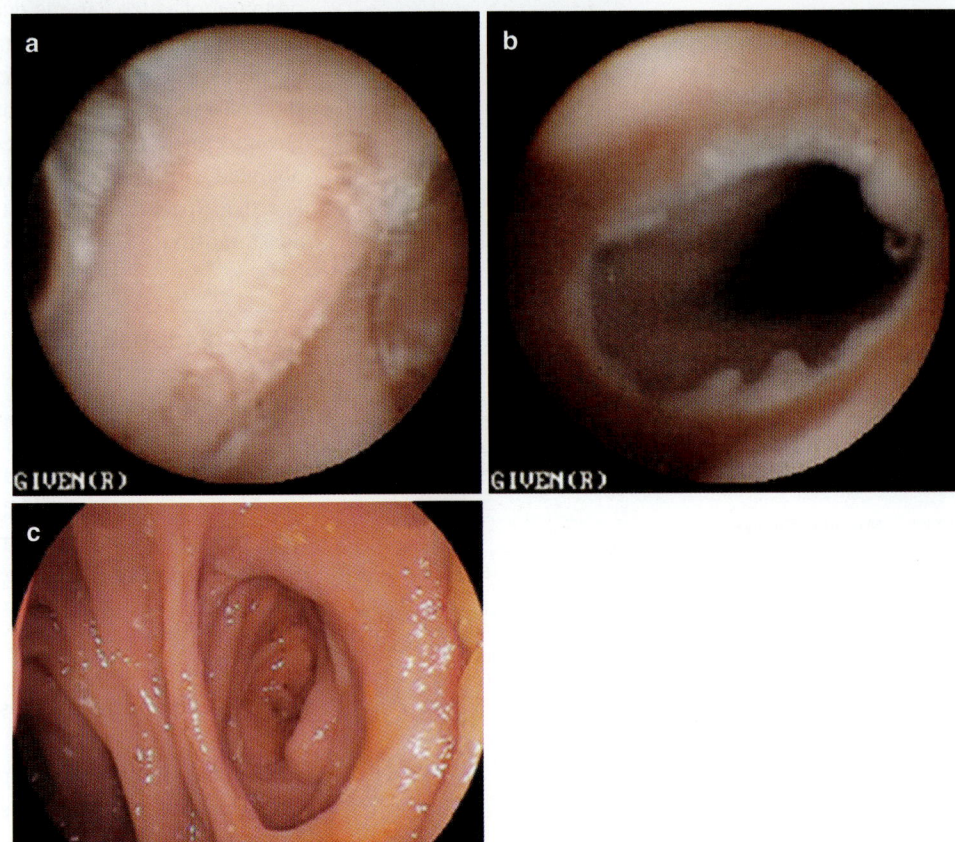

39.2.1.1 Billroth I

In this reconstruction technique, the end of the distally resected stomach is anastomosed to the end of the duodenum (Fig. 39.4), leaving passage through the stomach and duodenum essentially intact. Biliary reflux into the stomach may occur. A narrow stenosis may hold up the capsule in the stomach for some time, and the use of a real-time viewer to document passage is advisable.

39.2.1.2 Billroth II

The Billroth II (BII) operation is an end-to-side gastrojejunostomy with afferent and efferent loops of the jejunum (Fig. 39.5). Because the anastomosis is usually wide, the first images of the small bowel are often visible after a few minutes, but as the capsule can stay in the anastomotic region for hours, the starting point of small bowel transit time ("first duodenal image") should be marked at the point where the

Fig. 39.3 Four-fifths distal gastrectomy with gastrojejunostomy. The capsule passes within seconds through the esophagus (**a**) and stomach (**b**) to the jejunum (**c**) with a Roux-en-Y anastomosis (**d**)

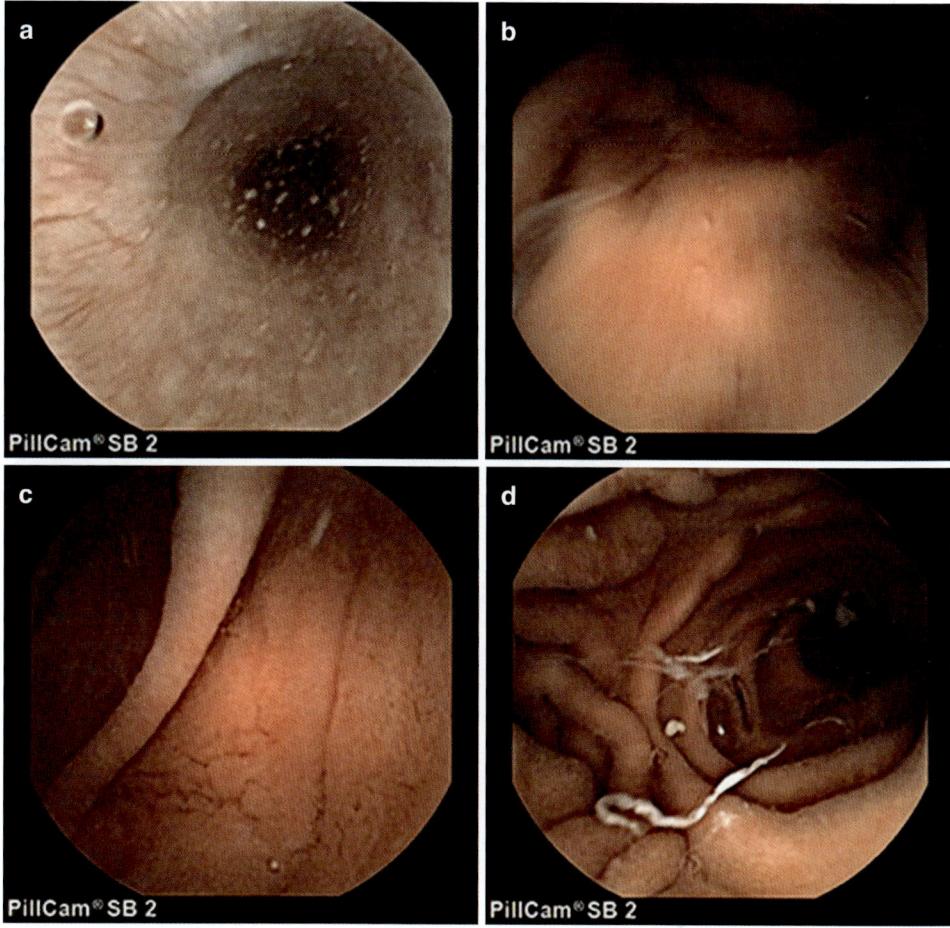

Fig. 39.4 Billroth I anastomosis. (**a**) Partially displayed by VCE. (**b**) Corresponding endoscopic view

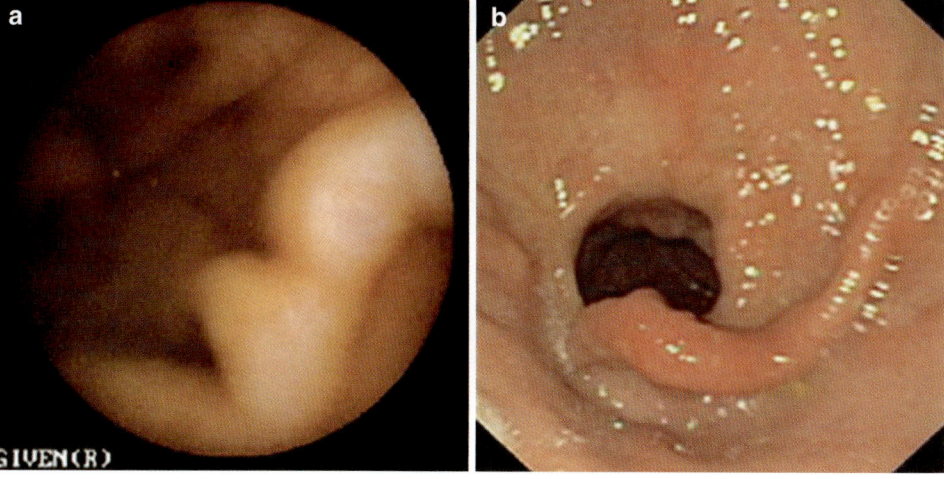

localization trace shows progressive movement of the capsule and no more gastric mucosa is seen. Endoscopic placement of the capsule in BII anatomy may avoid this problem [3], but it is generally not necessary. However, complete endoscopic inspection of the afferent loop is required, as this area is usually not seen with VCE. The bridge between the two limbs may be seen with VCE (Fig. 39.5). A limited experience with

VCE in BII shows no increased risk of retention [4, 5] but a higher percentage of incomplete small bowel visualization. Probably this limitation is less relevant with the longer battery life of current capsules. A Braun side-to-side anastomosis (see below) can be added distally between the afferent and efferent loops to prevent biliary reflux into the stomach, which can cause irritation seen as marked gastric reddening (Fig. 39.6b).

Fig. 39.5 Small ulcer at the bridge of a Billroth II anastomosis. (**a**) The ulcer was not described in unsedated transnasal endoscopy (used because of severe respiratory insufficiency). (**b**) VCE clearly shows the small ulcer

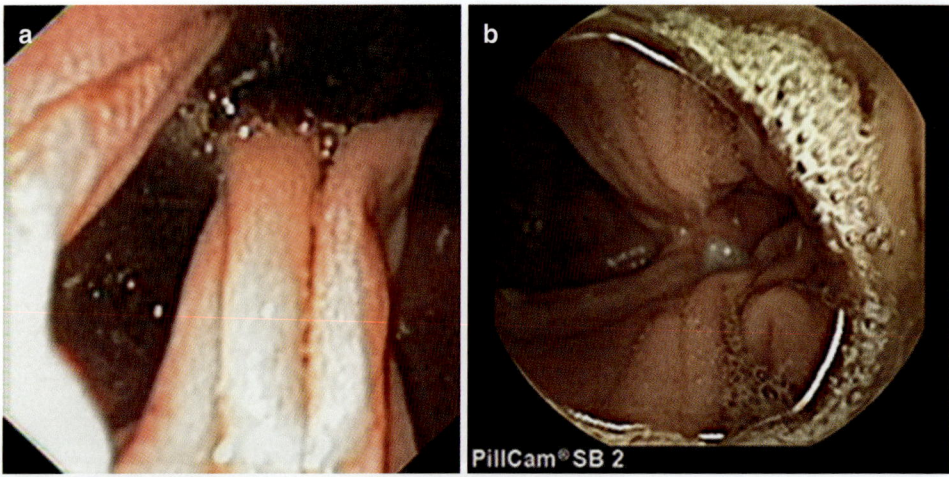

Fig. 39.6 Billroth II anastomosis. (**a** and **c**) VCE. (**b**) Endoscopic appearance: showing reddish gastric and paler small bowel mucosa. Although the anastomosis is seen shortly after entrance into the stomach, capsule stays for about 2 h in the anastomotic region. The first "duodenal" image is marked once the capsule progresses through the efferent jejunal loop. Note the extraordinarily long esophageal transit in this case. (**d**) Localization trace. (**e**) Time and color bar

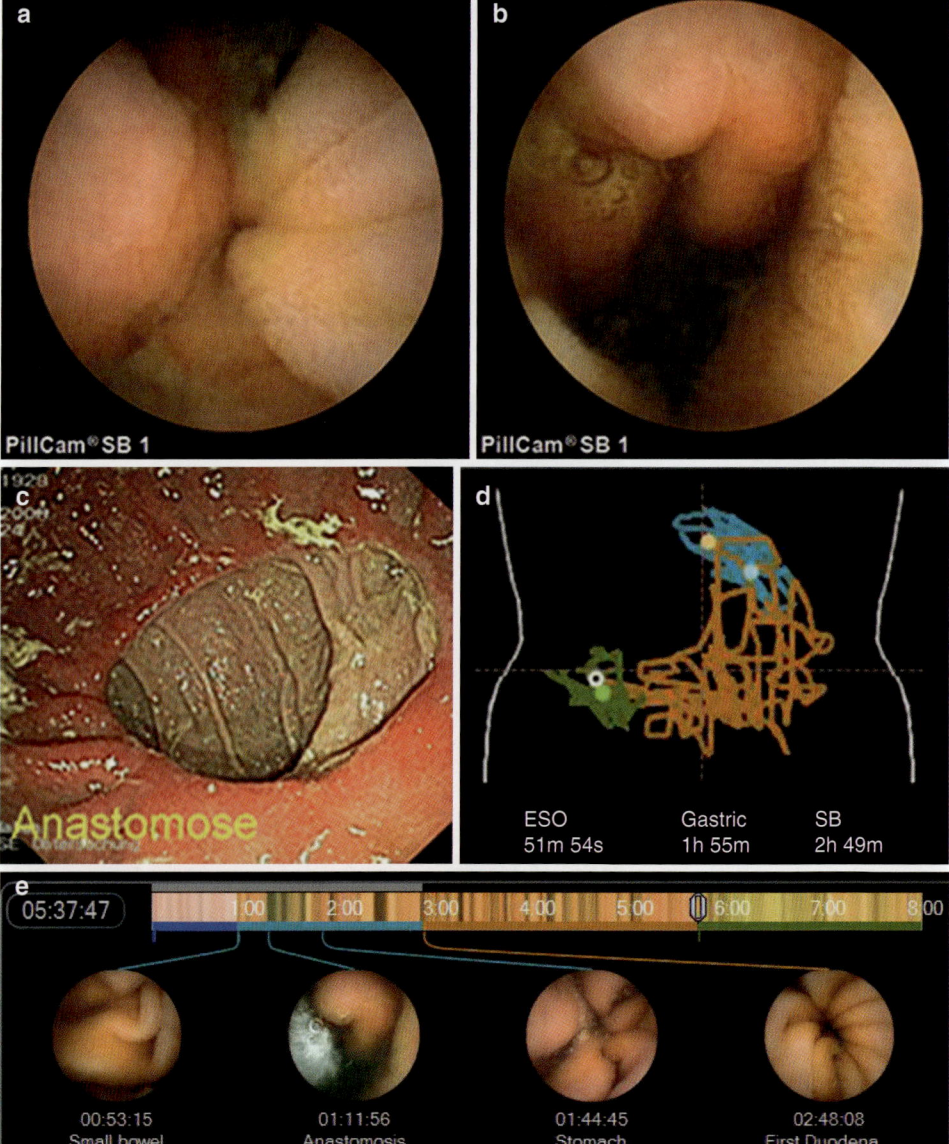

39.3 Small Intestine

Besides a Braun side-to-side or a Roux-en-Y anastomosis after gastrectomy, small intestinal anastomoses are most commonly found after partial resections of the intestine, ileocecal resections, or colectomy. Rare postoperative situations include previous diverticulectomy and mesenteric plication.

39.3.1 Braun Side-To-Side Anastomosis

The endoscopic appearance of a distal side-to-side anastomosis consists of two lumina separated by a narrow septum (Fig. 39.7). The afferent loop must be inspected using upper gastrointestinal (GI) endoscopy (Fig. 39.8)

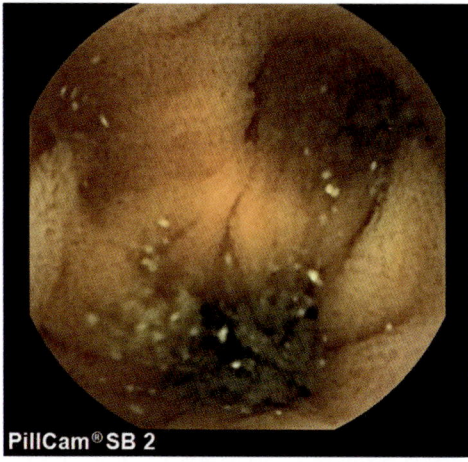

Fig. 39.7 Braun side-to-side anastomosis in VCE

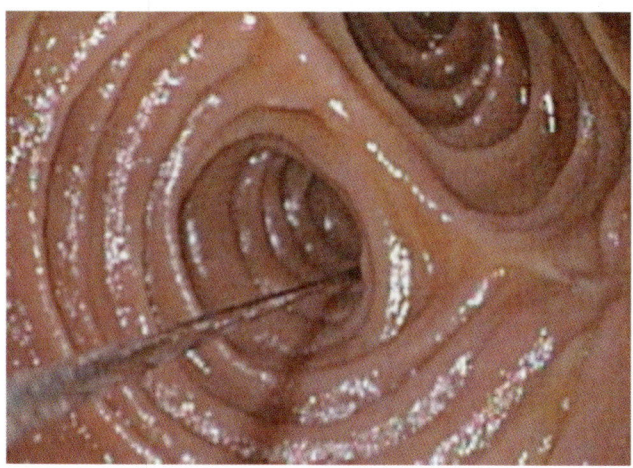

Fig. 39.8 Braun side-to-side anastomosis with two lumina and intervening septum at push enteroscopy

39.3.2 Roux-en-Y

This technique involves an end-to-end gastrojejunostomy with a Y-shaped distal anastomosis of the bile-carrying loop of the jejunum (Figs. 39.9 and 39.10). The risk of capsule retention does not seem to be higher in these patients. However, additional enteroscopy of the afferent limb is necessary, as VCE cannot show this region.

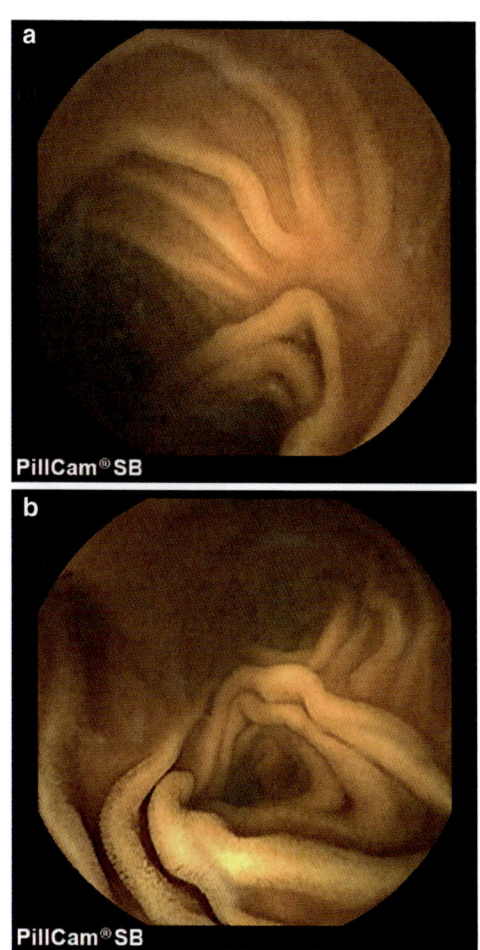

Fig. 39.9 (**a** and **b**) Roux-en-Y anastomosis at VCE

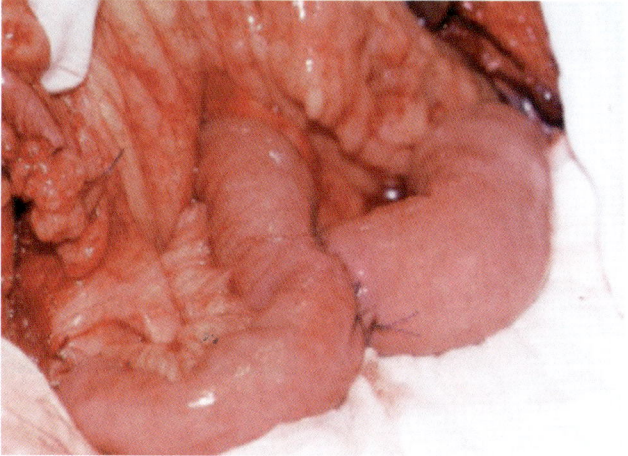

Fig. 39.10 Roux-en-Y anastomosis: appearance at operation

39.3.3 Enteroenteral Anastomoses

In patients with previous partial small bowel resection, often VCE does not show the anastomoses or only partially shows them. End-to-end anastomoses are predominant. In side-to-end or side-to-side anastomoses, luminal alterations as narrowing, dilatation, septum, blind pouches, and small diverticula may be observed (Fig. 39.11). Ulceration at an anastomosis may be detected by VCE as a source of mid-GI bleeding (Fig. 39.12).

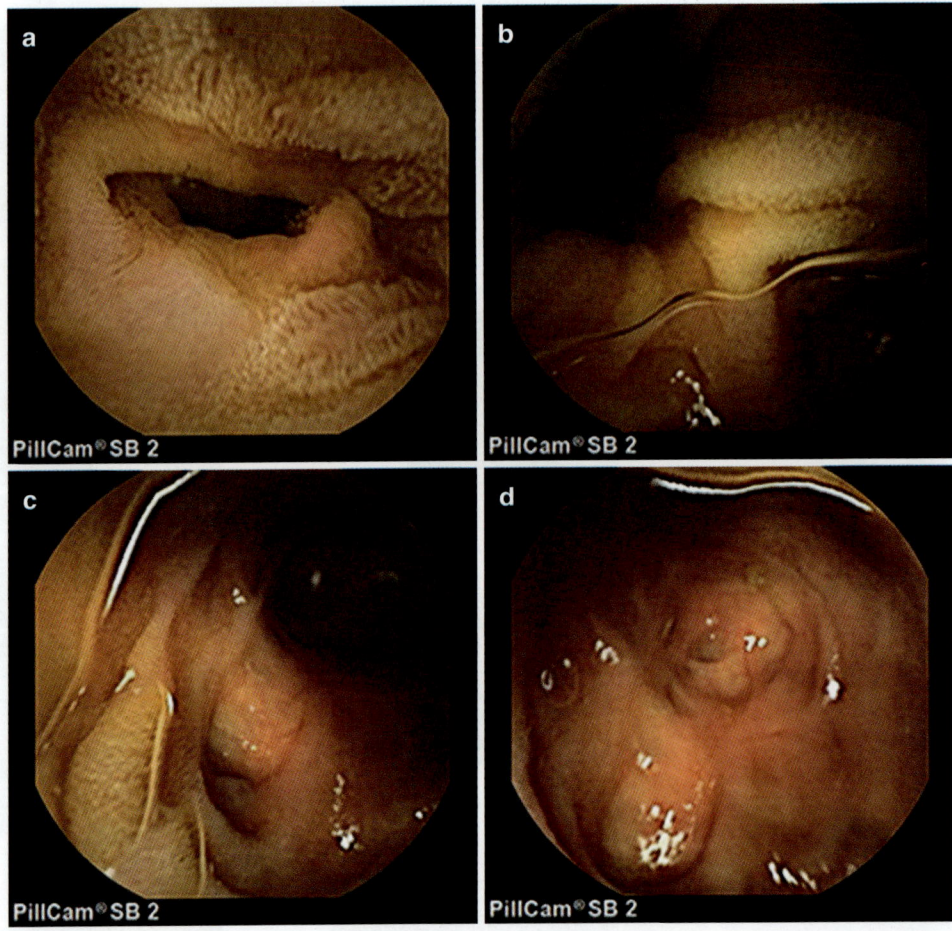

Fig. 39.11 Luminal alterations after small bowel resection: narrowing (**a**), two lumina (**b**), blind pouch (**c**), small diverticula (**d**)

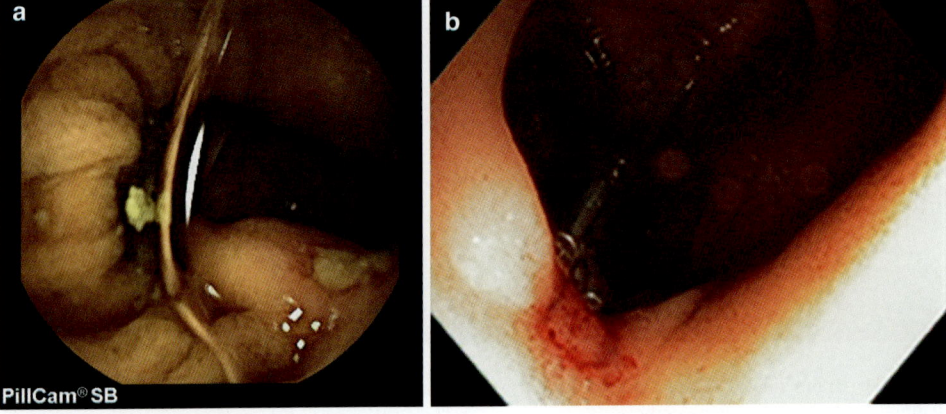

Fig. 39.12 Anastomotic ulcer after small bowel resection. (**a**) VCE. (**b**) Single-balloon enteroscopy with clipping for recurrent bleeding

39.3.4 Anastomotic Strictures

Rarely, stricturing anastomotic ulcers may be seen (Figs. 39.13 and 39.14). Stenotic anastomoses can lead to capsule impaction [6]. Additional radiotherapy may increase this risk [7]. It may be prudent, therefore, to include imaging procedures in the initial workup. After exclusion of stenoses by small bowel X-ray series, VCE was performed safely in a group of 10 patients with prior small bowel resec-tion [8]. However, normal radiologic findings do not guarantee uncomplicated passage of the capsule. In doubtful cases, the use of a patency capsule (Chap. 9) prior to VCE may be prudent to exclude relevant stenoses. Though the risk of capsule retention is low, the number of incomplete small bowel investigations is elevated after abdominal surgery [9].

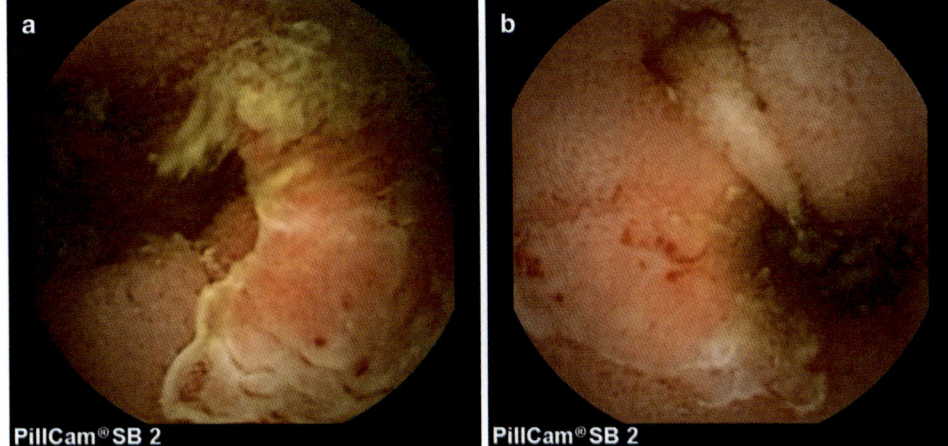

Fig. 39.13 (**a** and **b**) Stenotic and ulcerated small intestinal anastomoses

Fig. 39.14 Complex anatomy
after small bowel resection with
several anastomoses and circular
loops. Side-to-side anastomosis
with two lumina and ulcerated
weblike strictures. (**a** and **b**) VCE.
(**c–e**) Single-balloon enteroscopy;
panel (**d**) demonstrates a small
bowel circuit by panel (**e**)
demonstrates a small bowel
circuit by reaching the endoscope
again. (**f**) MRI shows thickened,
partially parallel small bowel
loops (*Courtesy of* Roman
Fischbach, MD)

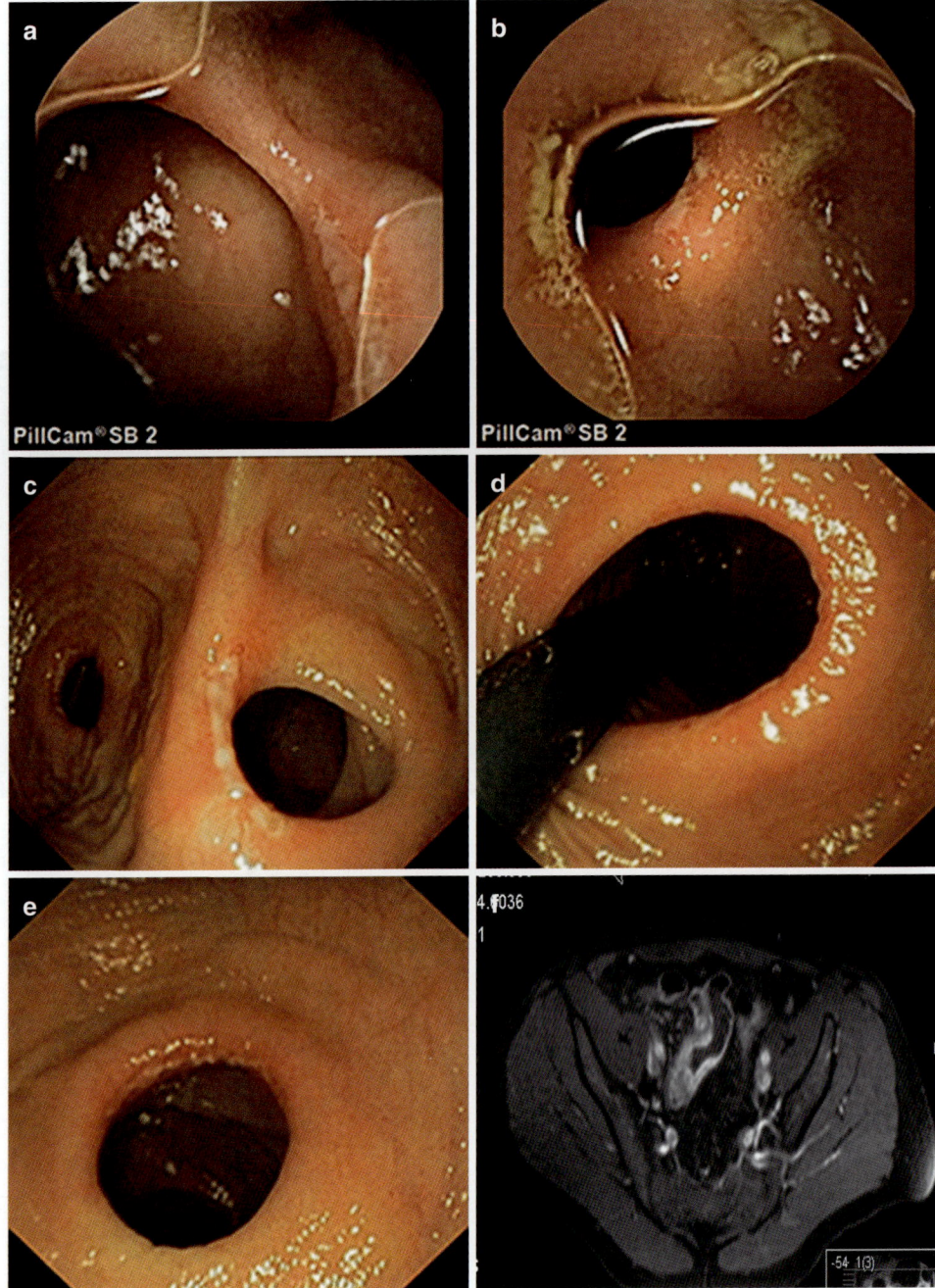

39.3.5 Previous Diverticulectomy

Especially after resection of a Meckel's diverticulum (Fig. 39.15a) rather than segmental small intestinal resection, persisting ulcers (Fig. 39.15b and c) rarely may cause relapsing bleeding. Retention of two consecutive capsules proximal to the anastomosis many years after repeated operations for Meckel's diverticulum and complications has been reported [10].

39.4 Mesenteric Plication

Mesenteric plication itself or the underlying disease may hamper the passage of the capsule. Endoscopy can show sharply bent small bowel loops (Fig. 39.16).

Fig. 39.15 Diverticulectomy. (**a**) Initial laparoscopic removal with a GIA stapler (Covidien, Mansfield, MA). (**b**) A second capsule endoscopy was done 1 year later for recurrence of intestinal blood loss showing shallow ulcers approximately 2 cm from the diverticulectomy site. (**c**) Surgical specimen after segmental resection with two ulcers (*Courtesy of* Jörg Caselitz, MD)

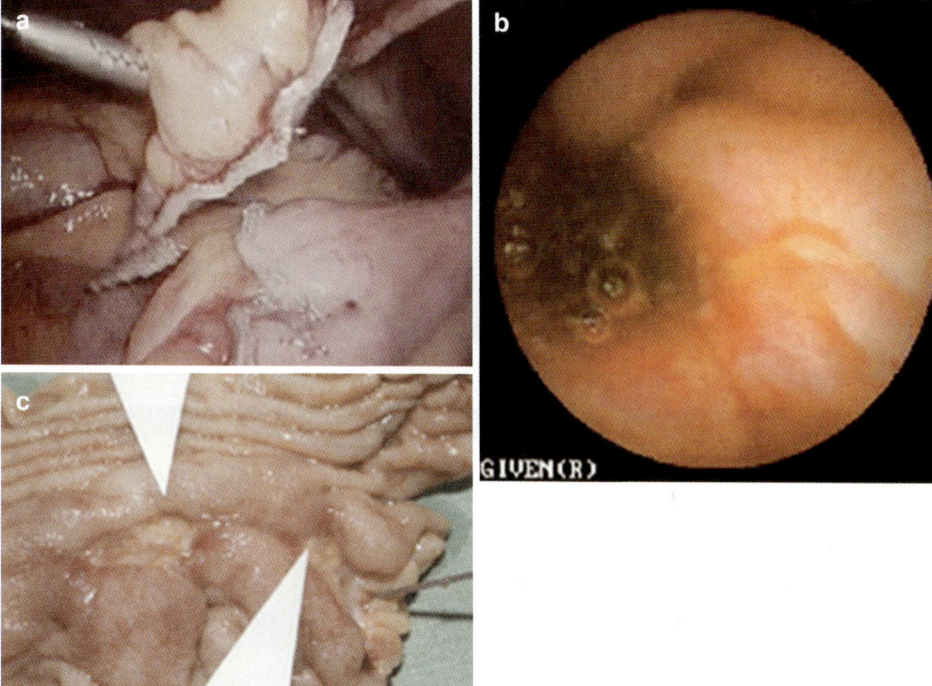

Fig. 39.16 Mesenteric plication. The patient had a previous Noble operation with a meandering arrangement of the small bowel loops followed by a Childs-Phillips mesenteric plication. (**a**) Closely spaced valvulae conniventes. (**b**) Sharp bend of the small bowel lumen with a 360° loop

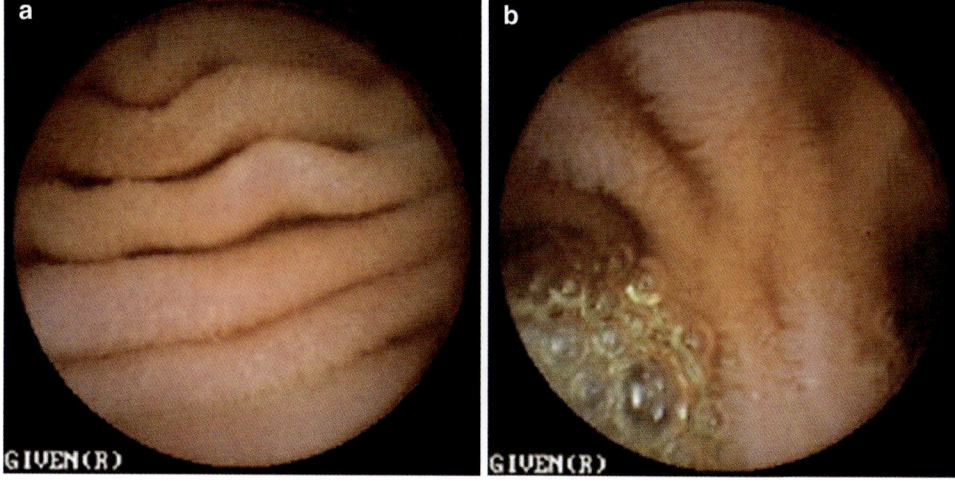

39.5   Ileocolostomy

Anastomoses after right-sided colectomy or ileocecal resection (Figs. 39.17 and 39.18) are sometimes difficult to visualize by VCE if the capsule passes quickly through a wide anastomosis or if reflux of feces from the colon reduces the quality of images. Frequently, switching of the capsule from the small bowel to colon and back can be observed (Fig. 39.18). Although these anastomoses are inspected routinely at preceding colonoscopy, VCE can detect ulcers in more proximal parts, especially in a side-to-end anastomosis (Fig. 39.19).

Fig. 39.17 Ileocolostomy. (**a**) VCE: smooth, relatively pale colonic mucosa is visible on the left side of the image, separated by a scar (*arrows*) from the darker ileal mucosa with villi on the right side. (**b**) Colonoscopy

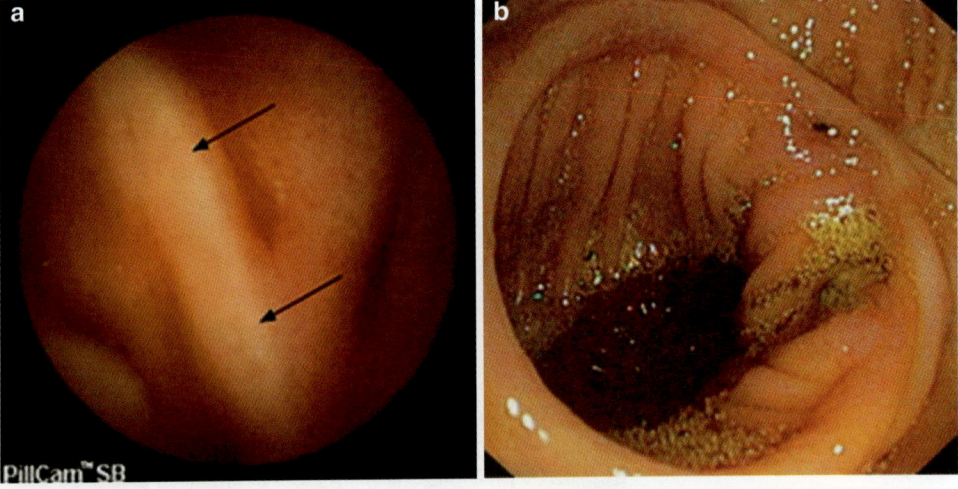

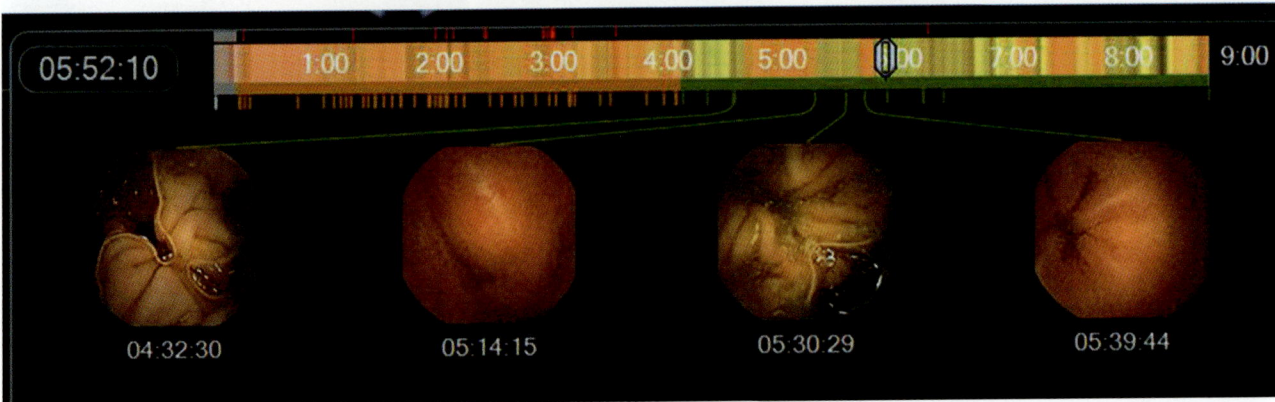

Fig. 39.18 Ileocecal anastomosis: time bar and thumbnails show capsule switching between the ileum and colon

Fig. 39.19 VCE shows an ileocolostomy (**a**) with a flat ulcer (**b**) in the ileal region of the anastomosis

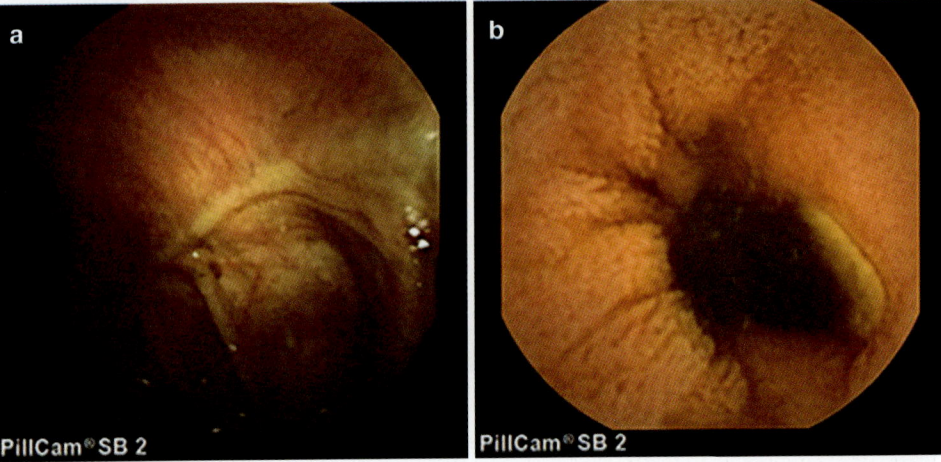

39.6 Surgical Fixation Material

VCE can show scars, sewing material, or staples (Figs. 39.20 and 39.21). Suture granulomas may have a tumorlike appearance (Fig. 33.2).

Fig. 39.20 Surgical fixation materials. (**a** and **b**) Metal. (**c** and **d**) Suture

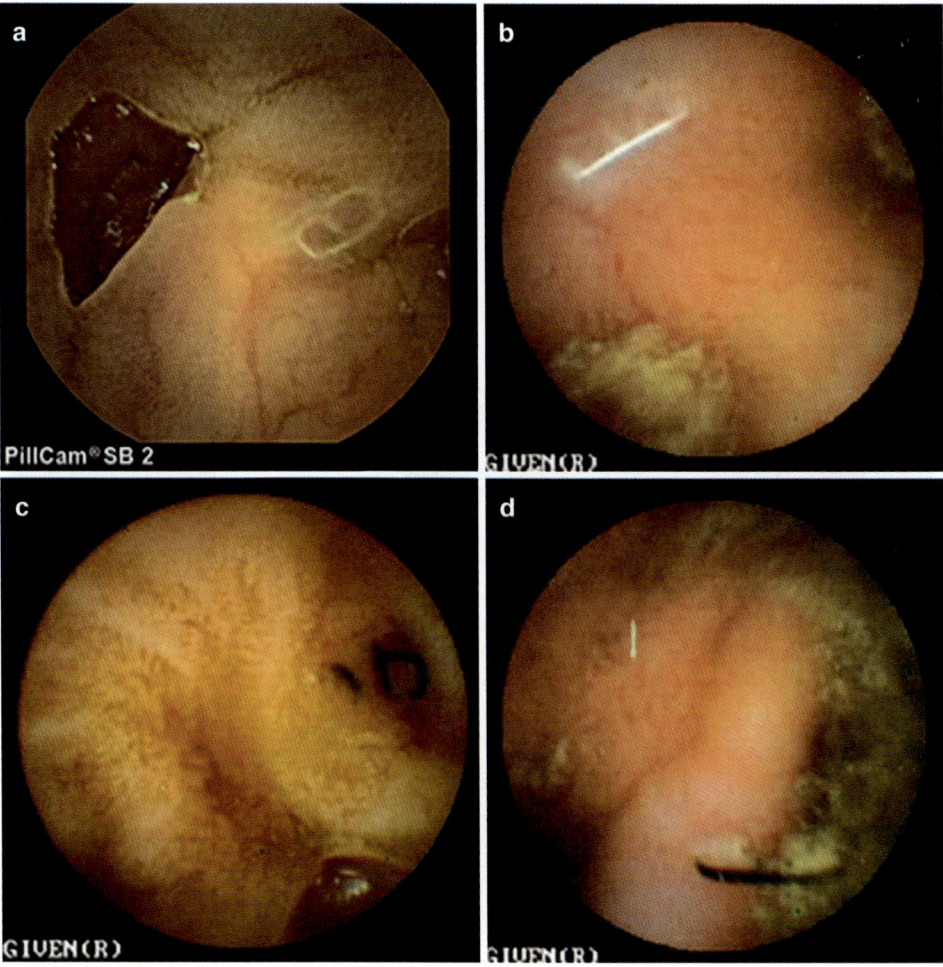

Fig. 39.21 Serosal suture. (**a**) Surgical aspect (*Courtesy of* Carsten Möllmann, MD.) (**b**) VCE with intraluminal aspect

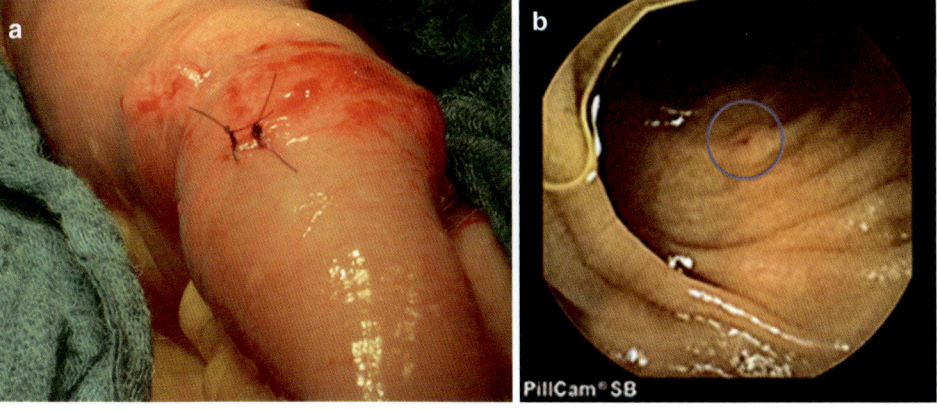

39.7 Adhesions

VCE currently does not appear to be a reliable tool for the diagnosis of adhesions. Suspicious indirect signs include strangulation (Fig. 39.22), sharp angulation, segmental dilatation of small intestinal loops, and the arrest of capsule progression. Minor changes seen at capsule endoscopy (Fig. 39.22a) may be associated with severe adhesions (Fig. 39.22b). Moreover, dilatation of the small bowel in some cases may be due entirely to bowel cleansing with lavage. In other patients, adhesions can lead to capsule retention.

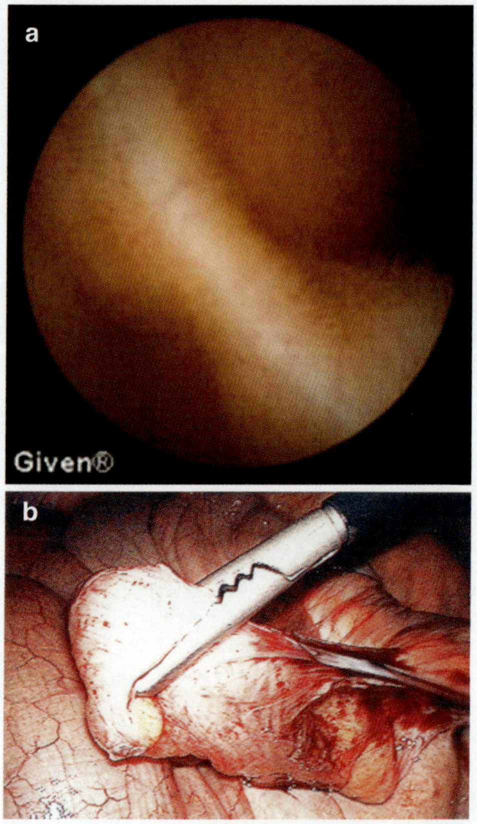

39.8 Vascular Surgery

In our personal experience, we have had no problems with passage of a video capsule after graft implantation for abdominal aortic aneurysm or after aortofemoral bypass, but aortoduodenal fistula is a rare but hazardous complication after aortic graft surgery. A case of such a fistula demonstrated by VCE has already been described [11] (Fig. 39.23). The standard diagnostic procedure is urgent deep duodenoscopy and angio-CT (Fig. 39.24).

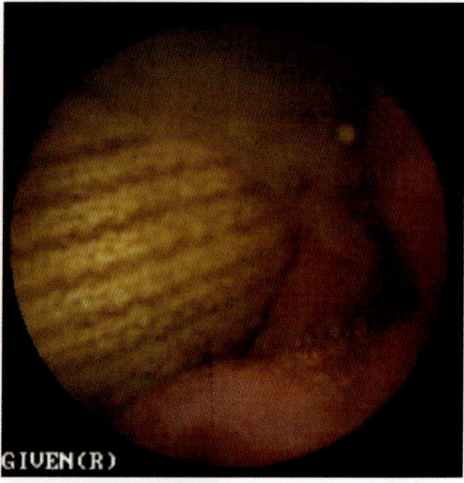

Fig. 39.23 Aortoduodenal fistula after aortic graft for aneurysm repair. VCE shows vascular prosthesis from the duodenum (*Courtesy of* Begoña González-Suárez, MD., *reprinted from* González-Suárez et al. [11] with permission from Georg Thieme Verlag, Stuttgart)

Fig. 39.22 Adhesion after prior resection of a Meckel's diverticulum in a 24-year-old woman with crampy abdominal pain. (**a**) Strangulation of an ileal loop. (**b**) Laparoscopic view of adhesion (*arrow*)

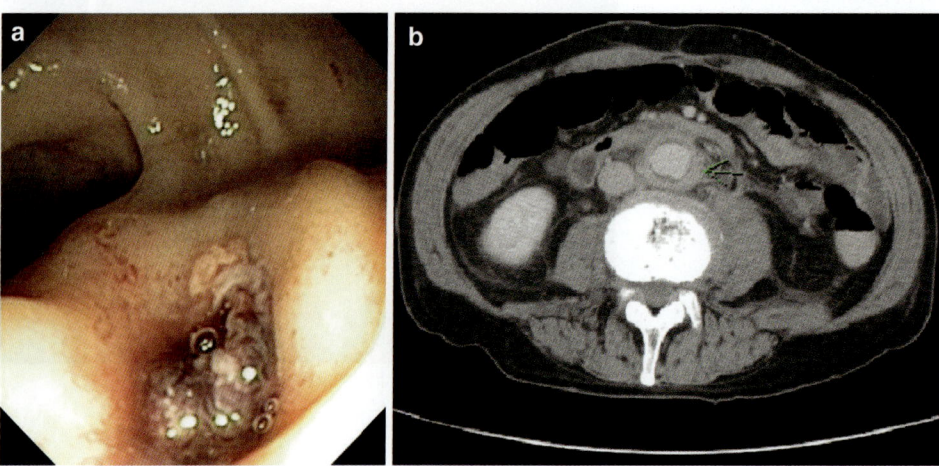

Fig. 39.24 Aortoduodenal fistula in the deep duodenum after implantation of an aortic prosthesis, seen at emergency endoscopy (**a**) (*Courtesy of* Harald Grosse, MD.) and at contrast CT scan (**b**) (*Courtesy of* Jörg Sievers, MD)

39.9   Ileostomy, Ileoanal Pouch, and Ileorectostomy

If the ileum must perform a reservoir function after removal or exclusion of the colon, the mucosa is sometimes affected by cdematous changes (Fig. 39.25a).

Small residual polyps are occasionally found in patients with polyposis (Fig. 39.25b). Special attention should be paid to polyps in patients with familial adenomatous polyposis and remaining rectum after colectomy. Passage of the capsule through an ileostomy (Fig. 39.26) may be delayed.

Fig. 39.25 (**a**) Ileostomy; slight edema. (**b**) Ileoanal pouch after colectomy for familial adenomatous polyposis (FAP), with multiple small polyps (confirmed by biopsy)

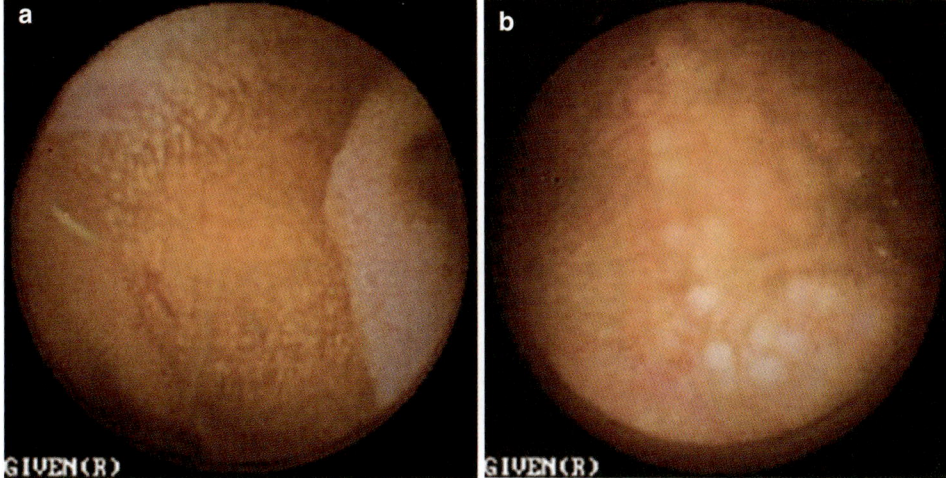

Fig. 39.26 Ileostomy. (**a**) Capsule dropping from small bowel into bag. (**b**) Capsule within the bag

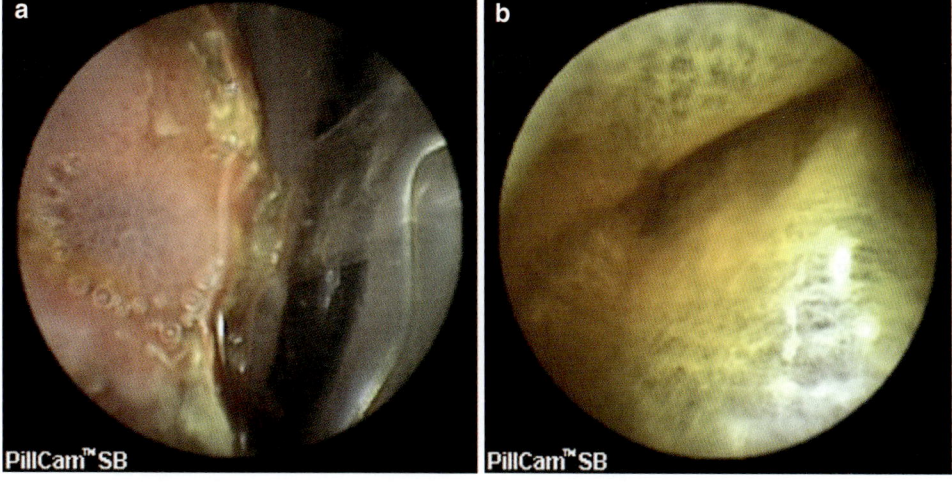

39.10 Previous Small Intestinal Transplantation

Small bowel transplantation may be indicated in patients with a short-bowel syndrome that necessitates parenteral nutrition for the patient's lifetime. With modified operating techniques and recent advances in immunosuppressant drugs, survival rates for the transplant and the patient have improved markedly [12]. Regular endoscopic examinations should be performed initially through an ileostomy placed temporarily for easy access, so that complications such as rejection or infection can be detected at an early stage. VCE can be used in selected patients with normal ileoscopy to detect abnormalities in inaccessible portions of the small bowel (Fig. 39.27) [13, 14] or for exclusion [15].

39.11 Findings Following Endoscopic Intervention

As VCE is used as a diagnostic tool in concert with upper and lower GI endoscopy, VCE may show changes following endoscopic intervention. Most frequently, small focal lesions are seen after endoscopic biopsy of the duodenum (Fig. 39.28a) or terminal ileum (Fig. 39.28b). These small reddish or ulcerated lesions may persist. If VCE is performed directly following upper GI endoscopy, blood clots on the biopsy site may be seen, and sometimes small traces of blood may be mistaken for small bowel bleeding. Knowledge of previous biopsy also helps to avoid confusion with ulcers caused by inflammatory bowel disease.

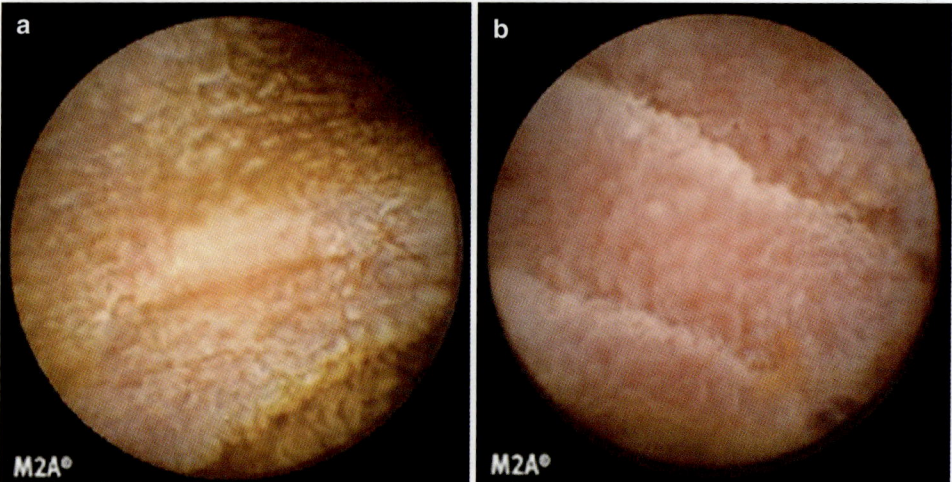

Fig. 39.27 VCE after small bowel transplantation. (**a**) Swollen, whitish villi and circumscribed hyperemia 20 days after transplantation. (**b**) Diffuse edema with thickened villi 64 days postoperatively (*Reprinted from* de Franchis et al. [14] with permission from Given Imaging)

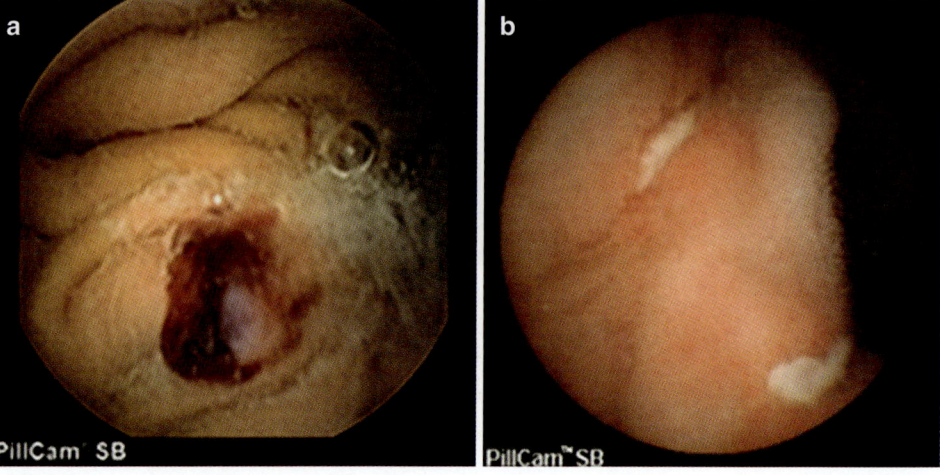

Fig. 39.28 VCE findings after endoscopic biopsy. (**a**) Small duodenal defect with minimal mucosal hemorrhage. (**b**) Ulcers in the terminal ileum

Other findings may include ulcer following coagulation (Fig. 39.29) or mucosectomy (Fig. 39.30). Also visible may be ink marks that are sometimes injected during balloon enteroscopy to document the extent of investigation (Fig. 39.31). Endoscopic interventions also may leave behind clips that are seen on later VCE (Figs. 39.32 and 39.33).

Fig. 39.29 Findings after prior argon plasma coagulation in a patient with hereditary hemorrhagic telangiectasia. (**a**) Superficial lesions after coagulation of multiple angiectasias. (**b**) Small ulcer. (**c**) Ulceration, edema, lymphangiectasia, and erythema. (**d**) Large, deep defect after coagulation of multiple confluent angiectasias

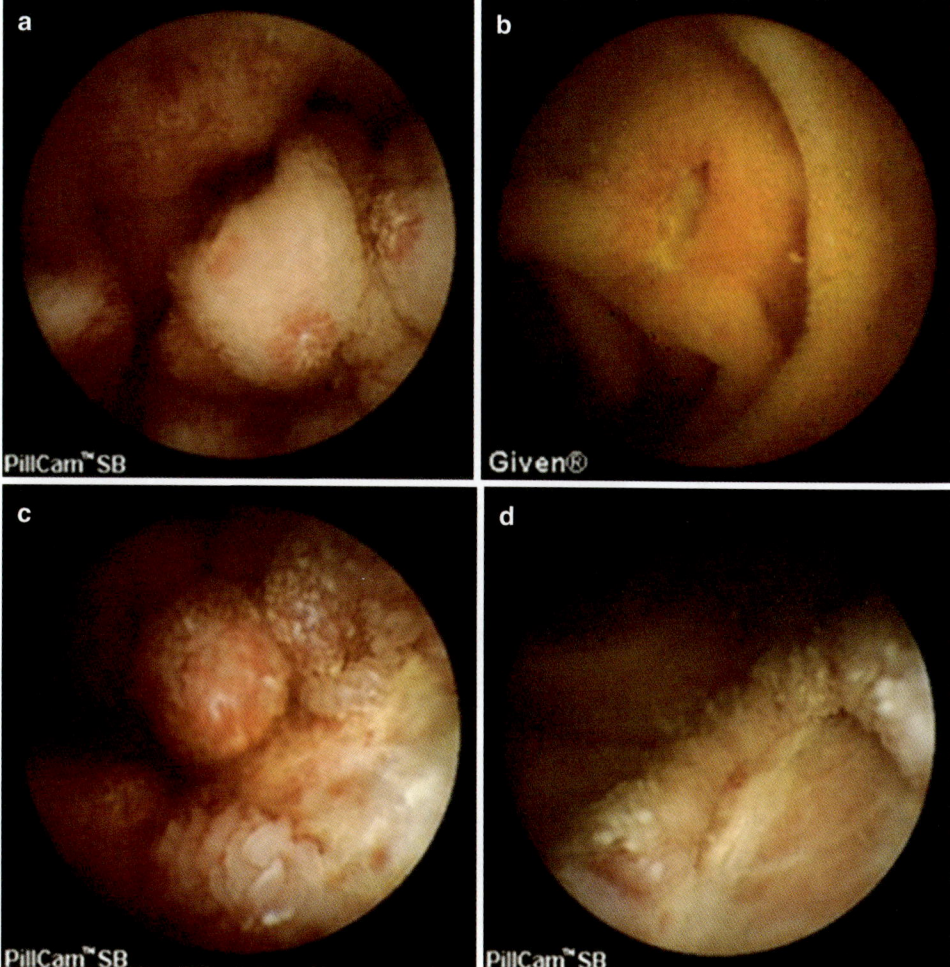

Fig. 39.30 (**a**) Large sporadic duodenal adenoma. (**b**) After mucosectomy. (**c** and **d**) VCE (performed to exclude additional adenomas of the small bowel) shows ulcerated mucosa. The capsule stayed in the duodenum for a long time. Follow-up duodenoscopies did not show residual adenoma

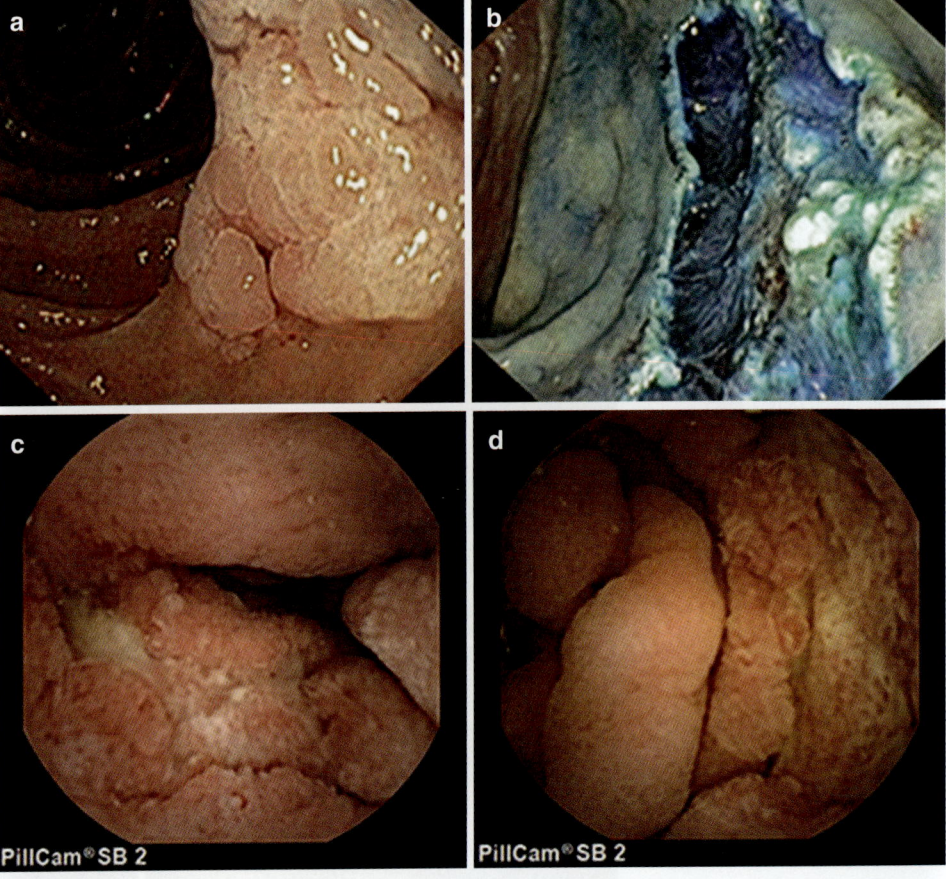

Fig. 39.31 Ink mark. (**a**) Injection during single-balloon enteroscopy. (**b**) Image of the tattoo at VCE

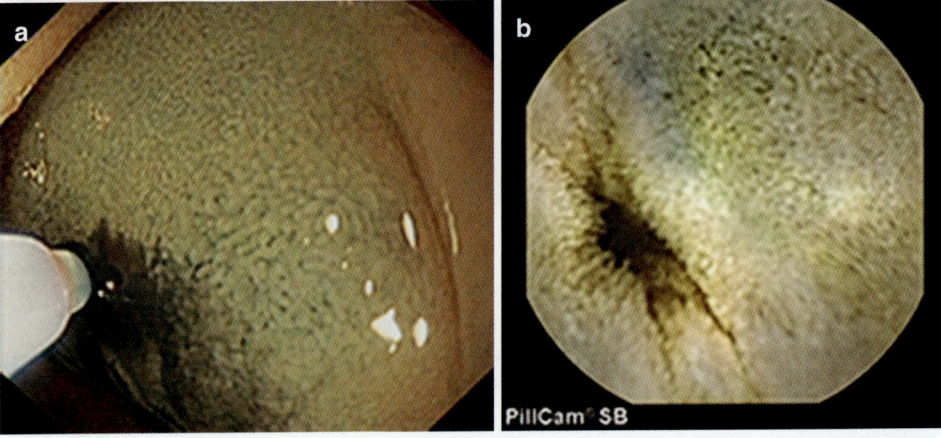

Fig. 39.32 Jejunal carcinoid. (**a**) Clip marking at double-balloon enteroscopy. (**b**) Clip seen at subsequent VCE in the search for additional tumors. (*See also* Fig. 34.5)

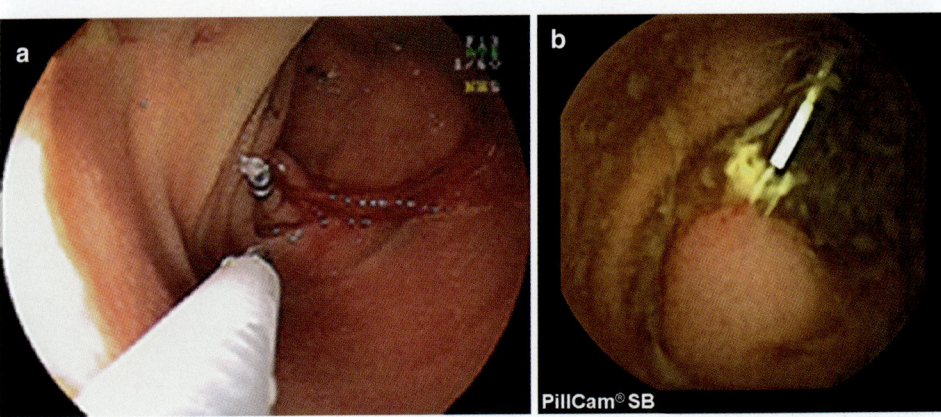

Fig. 39.33 Bleeding cecal angiectasia after argon plasma coagulation (**a**) and after hemostasis with clip (**b**). At VCE (**c**), the clip is visible with small remnants of old blood. At follow-up colonoscopy (**d**), one remaining clip without signs of bleeding is visible

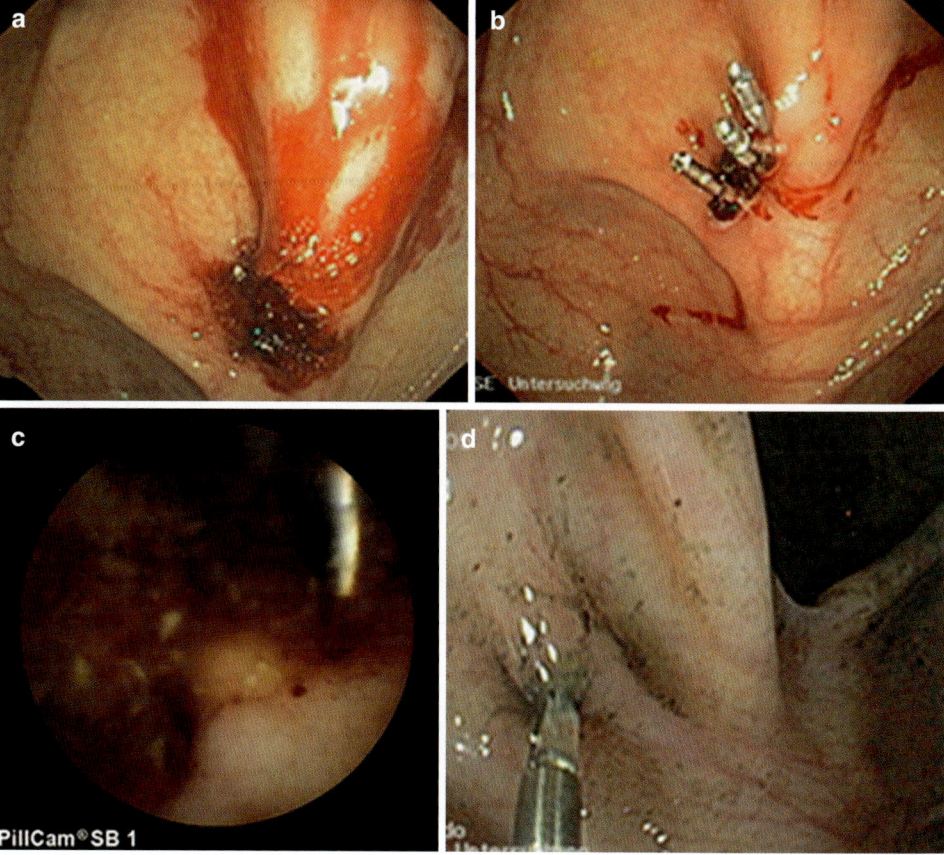

References

1. Lappas JC. Imaging of the postsurgical small bowel. Radiol Clin N Am. 2004;41:305–26.
2. Wu GY, Aziz K, Whalen GF. An internist's illustrated guide to gastrointestinal surgery. Totowa: Humana Press; 2003.
3. Spera G, Spada C, Riccioni ME, et al. Video capsule endoscopy in a patient with a Billroth II gastrectomy and obscure bleeding. Endoscopy. 2004;36:931.
4. Wei W, Ge ZZ, Gao YJ, et al. An analysis of failure and safety profiles of capsule endoscopy. Zhonghua Nei Ke Za Zhi. 2008;47:19–22.
5. Keuchel M, Störring U, Bruhn JP, et al. Influence of major gastrointestinal surgery on video capsule endoscopy. Endoscopy. 2005;37 Suppl 1:A529.
6. de Franchis R, Avesani EM, Abbiati C, et al. Unsuspected ileal stenosis causing obscure GI bleeding in patients with previous abdominal surgery–diagnosis by capsule endoscopy: a report of two cases. Dig Liver Dis. 2003;35:577–84.
7. Majeski J. Endoscopic capsule retention in an intestinal anastomosis. Int Surg. 2009;94:254–7.
8. De Palma GD, Rega M, Puzziello A, et al. Capsule endoscopy is safe and effective after small-bowel resection. Gastrointest Endosc. 2004;60:135–8.
9. Lee MM, Jacques A, Lam E, et al. Factors associated with incomplete small bowel capsule endoscopy studies. World J Gastroenterol. 2010;16:5329–33.
10. Miehlke S, Tausche AK, Bruckner S, et al. Retrieval of two retained endoscopy capsules with retrograde double-balloon enteroscopy in a patient with a history of complicated small-bowel disease. Endoscopy. 2007;39 Suppl 1:E157.
11. González-Suárez B, Guarner C, Escudero JR, et al. Wireless capsule video endoscopy: a new diagnostic method for aortoduodenal fissure. Endoscopy. 2002;34:938.
12. Fishbein TM, Gondolesi GE, Kaufman SS. Intestinal transplantation for gut failure. Gastroenterology. 2003;124:1615–28.
13. de Franchis R, Rondonotti E, Abbiati C, et al. Capsule enteroscopy in small bowel transplantation. Dig Liver Dis. 2003;35:728–31.
14. de Franchis R, Rondonotti E, Abbiati C, et al. Transplantation. In: Halpern M, Jacob H, editors. Atlas of capsule endoscopy. Norcross: Given Imaging; 2002.
15. Beckurts KT, Stippel D, Schleimer K, et al. First case of isolated small bowel transplantation at the University of Cologne: rejection-free course under quadruple immunosuppression and endoluminal monitoring with video-capsule. Transplant Proc. 2004;36:340–2.

Internet

Intestinal Transplant Registry (international). www.intestinaltransplant.org

Complications: Prevention and Management

40

Emanuele Rondonotti, Fernando J. Martinez,
Jamie Barkin, Gérard Gay, and Michael W. Cheng

Contents

Video capsule endoscopy (VCE) is a noninvasive procedure with few contra-indications (which are listed in Table 40.1) and complications. Among them the most frequent, and clinically relevant, are capsule retention and aspiration. Both of them should be explained to the patient during procedure counseling to obtain a fully informed consent.

40.1   Aspiration

A recently published review [2] reported the incidence of VCE aspiration to be 1 case out of 800 to 1,000 procedures. This figure has been confirmed by prospective data coming from a multicenter complication registry [3]. This complication typically occurs in elderly men with comorbidities such as neurologic diseases, swallowing disorders, or both. In the most cases, the capsule aspiration resolved quickly because patients expectorated the capsule [4], and the patients experienced no effects [5] or only minor symptoms such as mild respiratory distress or foreign-body sensation [6–8] (Fig. 40.1). In a few cases, however, emergent rigid or flexible bronchoscopy was necessary for extraction of these capsules [9]. If any patient experiences coughing, dyspnea, or a foreign-body sensation after ingestion of the capsule, an x-ray of the chest should be considered.

The work was first published in 2006 by Springer Medizin Verlag Heidelberg with the following title: *Atlas of Video Capsule Endoscopy.*

E. Rondonotti (✉)
Gastrointestinal Endoscopy Unit, Valduce Hospital, Como, Italy
e-mail: ema.rondo@gmail.com

F.J. Martinez • J. Barkin
Division of Gastroenterology, Mount Sinai Medical Center,
University of Miami, Miami, FL, USA
e-mail: fmartinez@med.miami.edu; jsbarkin@miami.edu

G. Gay
Department of Gastroenterology and Hepatology, Nouvel Hôpital Civil, University Hospital of Strasbourg, Strasbourg, France
e-mail: gerard.gay@chru-strasbourg.fr

M.W. Cheng
Southern Gastroenterology Specialists, Locust Grove, GA, USA

Table 40.1 Contraindications to video capsule endoscopy

Contraindications
Known or suspected gastrointestinal obstruction, strictures, or fistulae—unless surgery is warranted or patency is proven
Pseudo-obstruction
Relative contraindications
Pregnancy
Cardiac pacemaker or defibrillator
Extensive Crohn's disease
Prior pelvic or abdominal surgery—if signs of chronic obstruction
Prior pelvic or abdominal radiotherapy—unless patency is proven
Severe adhesions—unless patency is proven

M. Keuchel et al. (eds.), *Video Capsule Endoscopy: A Reference Guide and Atlas*,
DOI 10.1007/978-3-662-44062-9_40, © Springer-Verlag Berlin Heidelberg 2014

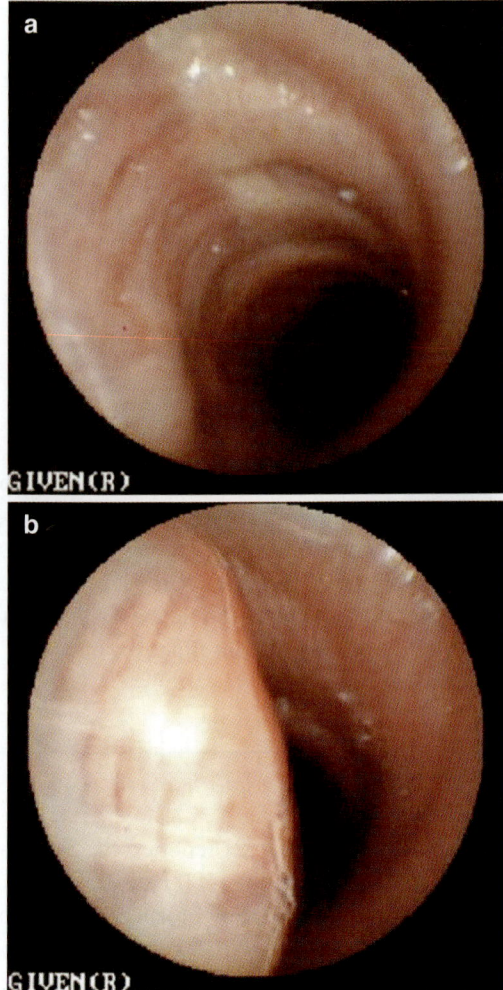

Fig. 40.1 Aspiration. View into the trachea (**a**); prolapse of the membranous trachea on coughing (**b**)

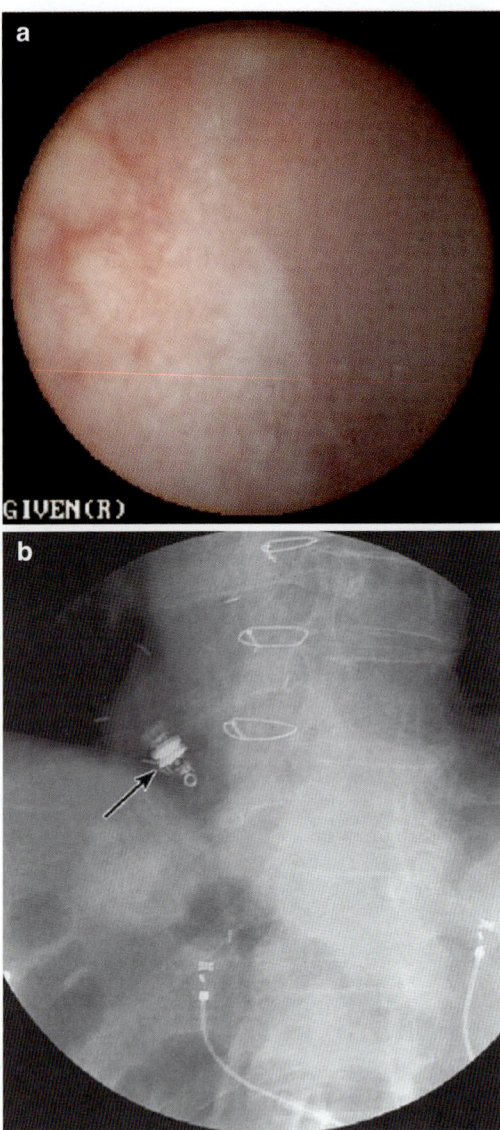

Fig. 40.2 Capsule retention in an epiphrenic diverticulum. (**a**) VCE. (**b**) Fluoroscopy. Capsule in air-filled diverticulum (*arrow*), also electrodes for VCE and cerclage wires after sternotomy

40.2 Capsule Retention in the Upper GI Tract

Although capsule retention in the upper gastrointestinal (GI) tract (esophagus and stomach) is uncommon, some conditions may lead to impaction of the capsule or slow passage through the upper GI tract. Some cases of capsule retention in Zenker's or epiphrenic diverticula (Fig. 40.2), requiring endoscopic removal and placement into the stomach, have been reported [10, 11]. Leung and Sung [12] reported a case of esophageal retention of the capsule in an elderly diabetic woman, presumably due to impaired esophageal motility and cardiomegaly compressing the esophagus. Another risk factor for impaired esophageal transit abnormalities is previous esophageal surgery such as resection or fundoplication (Fig. 40.3). To minimize the risk of esophageal retention, it is recommended to exclude swallowing problems by collect-

ing a detailed history of swallowing disorders. Patients with dysphagia should undergo further evaluation with video esophagograms and possibly endoscopy prior to VCE to rule out any potential lesions that may cause retention of the capsule. Nevertheless, these conditions are not contraindications for VCE; they can be overcome by endoscopic placement of the capsule into the stomach or duodenum (Fig. 40.4).

Gastric retention of the endoscopy capsule may occur in patients with gastroparesis (Fig. 40.5), with upside-down stomach, after vagotomy, or with anatomic narrowing of the pylorus or duodenum. In one patient, the capsule had to be extracted endoscopically from the stomach after 2 weeks, although the endoscope could be easily passed to the duodenum [13]. Complete capsule examination of the small bowel occurs in

70 % to 85 % of wireless capsule endoscopy procedures. The most common cause of incomplete examinations is decreased motility, including delayed gastric emptying and delayed small bowel transit [14]. The gastric transit time can be delayed in inpatients [15] and in patients with reduced physical activity during the procedure [16]. Therefore, capsule endoscopy can be postponed in these inpatients, especially if they are bedridden. The administration of prokinetics can decrease the gastric transit time in such patients, although it does not seem to affect the completeness of the small bowel evaluation [17].

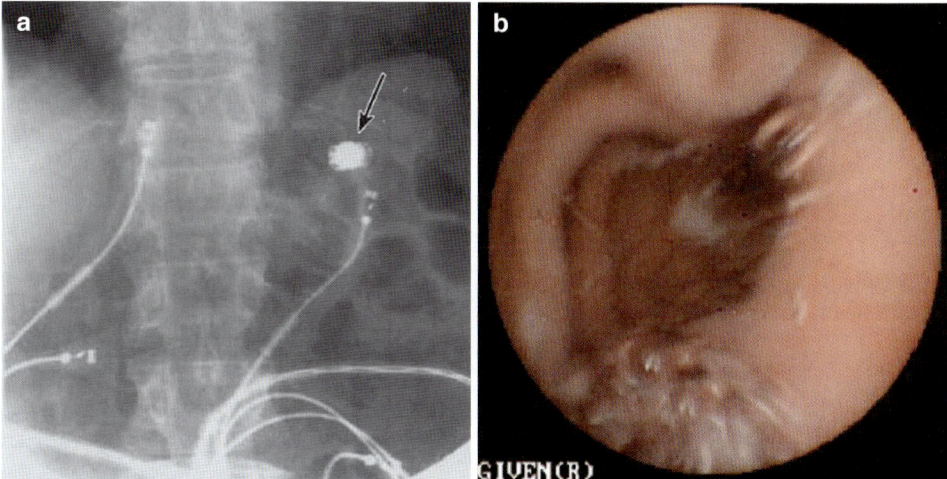

Fig. 40.3 (**a, b**) Capsule (*arrow*) temporarily retained in the curved limb of an esophagojejunostomy, later passed spontaneously. (**a**) Radiology; (**b**) VCE

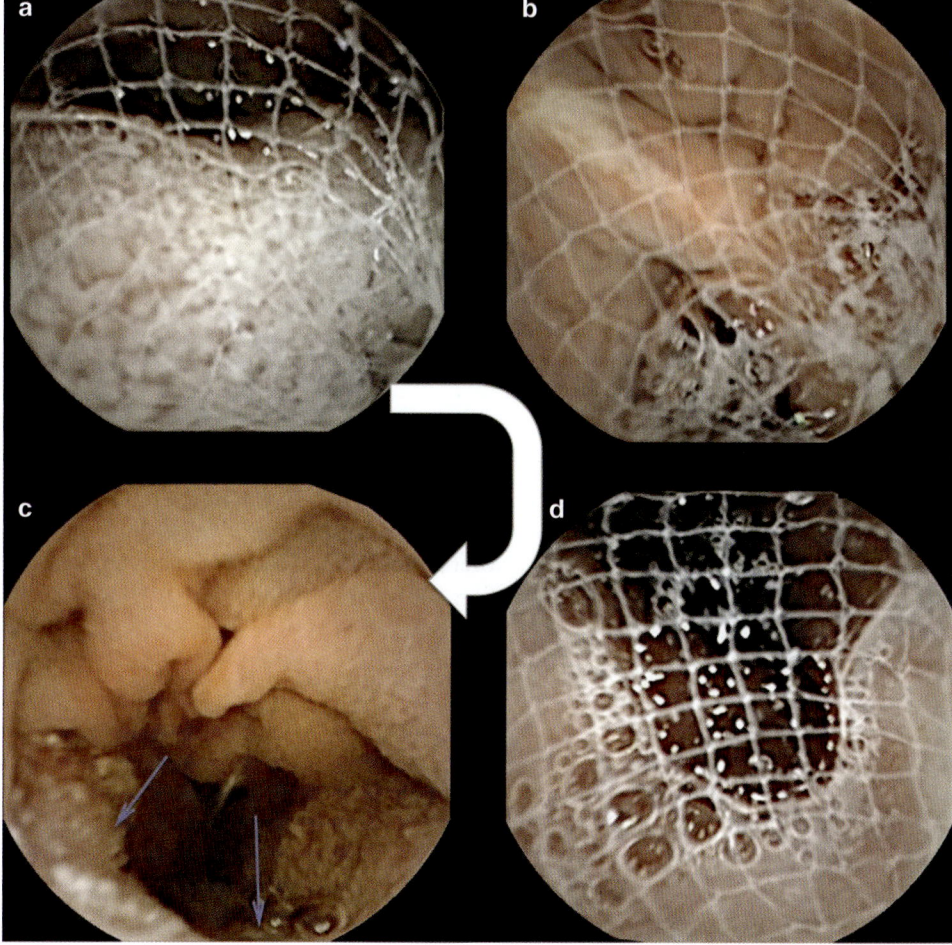

Fig. 40.4 Patient (with history of obscure gastrointestinal bleeding, frontal ischemia, and swallowing disorders) in which capsule has been placed in the stomach by means of a basket. The capsule showed (through the basket meshes) pictures of the oral cavity (**a**), pharynx (**b**), and stomach (**c**). After being released in the duodenum, the capsule continued its navigation through the small bowel and showed an adenocarcinoma (**d**, *blue arrows*) in the distal jejunum

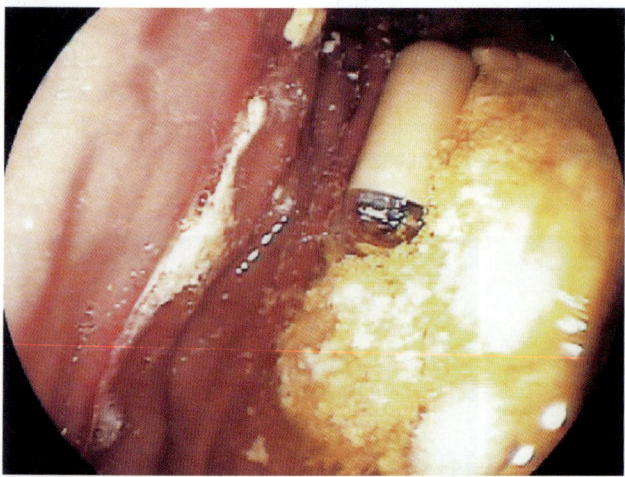

Fig. 40.5 Diabetic gastroparesis. Video capsule, food, and tablet residues retained in the stomach

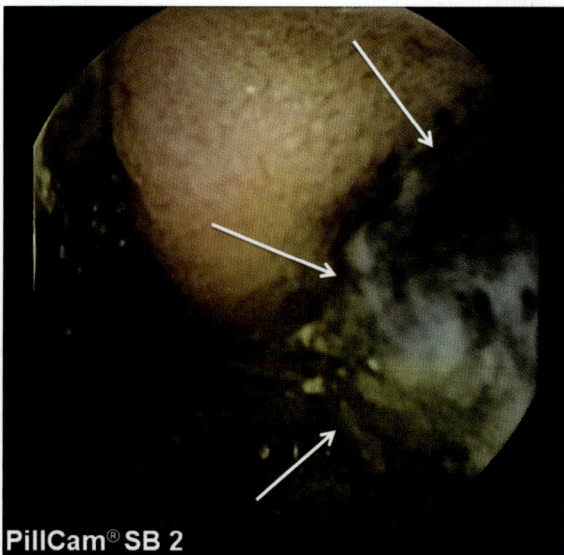

PillCam® SB 2

Fig. 40.6 Jejunal melanoma causing capsule retention

Table 40.2 Risk of capsule retention according to indication

Indication	Retention risk, %
Healthy volunteers	0
Obscure gastrointestinal bleeding	1–2
Suspected Crohn's disease	1–2
Known Crohn's disease	5–15
Small bowel tumours	10–25
Obstruction	20

Various techniques of "endoscopically assisted VCE" have been described in patients with proven or suspected slow esophageal/gastric capsule transit. The capsule may be inserted endoscopically, or, after the patient has swallowed the capsule, it can be grasped with an endoscopic device and then placed into the duodenum. Another technique incorporates the use of a real-time viewing system, which enables the physician to check the position of the capsule in real time to identify patients with slow transit. The physician then can administer prokinetics or can plan gastroscopy to ensure a complete small bowel examination [14]. In the near future (preliminary studies are ongoing), the development of maneuverable capsules or of biologically inspired steering mechanisms could help to control capsule movements through the stomach [18].

40.3 Capsule Retention in the Small Intestine

Small bowel retention is the most feared complication of capsule endoscopy, and the risk of capsule retention with the possible requirement of surgical or endoscopic retrieval is the major issue of the informed consent. Nevertheless, the impaction of a capsule is a complication only if neither the clinical features nor the diagnosis justifies an operation or endoscopic intervention.

40.3.1 Incidence

Anatomic narrowings in the small bowel (e.g., angulations, small bowel stricturing diseases, surgical anastomoses) or diverticula [19] can cause retention or nonnatural passage of the capsule (Fig. 40.6). Recently published studies [20–22]

in a large number of patients undergoing capsule endoscopy worldwide showed that the overall retention rate ranges from 1.0 to 2.1 %. These studies have also confirmed that there is a strict correlation between the retention rate and the clinical indication for capsule endoscopy. In the subset of patients undergoing capsule endoscopy for obscure GI bleeding or unexplained anemia, which account for about 70 % of all capsule endoscopy patients, the retention rate was about 1.2 %, whereas in patients with known Crohn's disease, the rate of retention ranges from 5 to 15 % [23] (Table 40.2).

40.3.2 Discovery of Retention

Patients who retain the capsule in the small bowel usually display no clinical signs or symptoms of obstruction. Transient pain may occur as the capsule passes into the narrowing or through a stenosis. Discovery of nonpassage of the capsule is elicited by findings of an obstructing lesion on review of the VCE study or by the patient's history showing that the capsule has not been excreted. Nonvisualization of the cecum may be the only evidence of stenosis during review of the video, if the capsule approaches the stenosis with the blind back [24]. The pre-

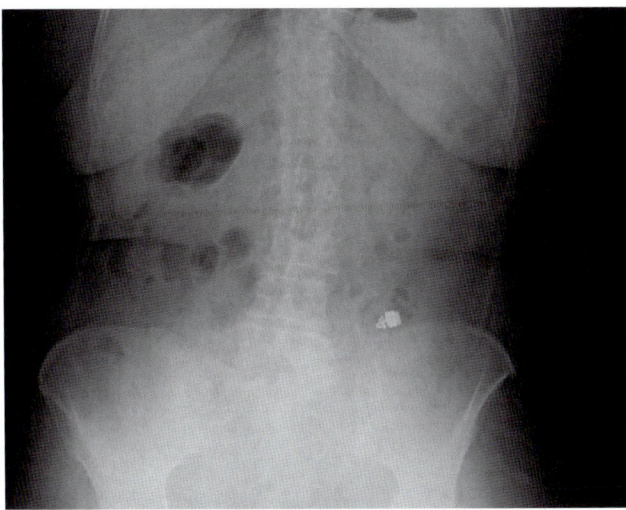

Fig. 40.7 Retained capsule (radiographic detection)

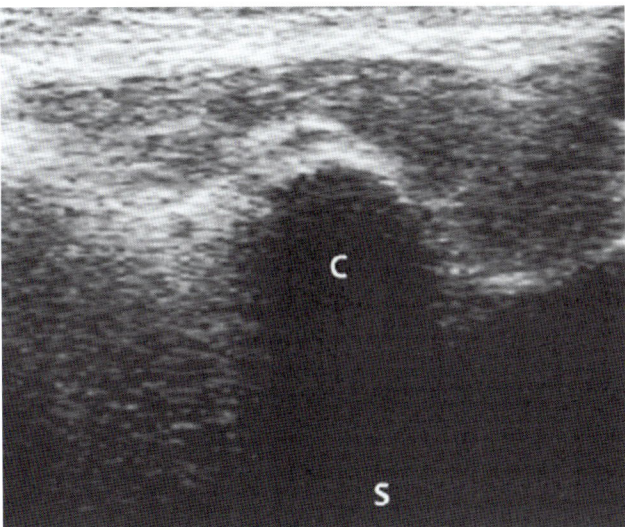

Fig. 40.8 Capsule retained for 4 weeks: sonographic detection of a video capsule (*C*) with acoustic shadow (*S*)

sumed degree of stenosis does not furnish definite information on whether the lumen is still passable. In normal individuals, the capsule is expelled naturally after an average time of 72 h (range, 24–222 h) [25]. If retention is suspected, an abdominal flat-plate radiograph can be done to verify retention and to follow the capsule's progression (Fig. 40.7). Ultrasound can also demonstrate the capsule, with an associated acoustic shadow [26] (Fig. 40.8). A CT scan can provide additional information on extraluminal changes. The timing of the test aimed at verifying the presence of the capsule within the patient's body has been suggested, by consensus, to be 2 weeks after its ingestion in asymptomatic patients [27]. If the endoscopy capsule is still present at least 2 weeks after ingestion, then the patient is deemed to have a retained capsule. Nevertheless,

about 50 % of asymptomatically retained capsules are eventually excreted [21].

Although capsule retention occurs without obstructive symptoms in most patients (even in cases of tight stenoses or large obstructing masses), some cases of acute obstruction [28, 29] with capsule fracture [30] and small bowel perforations [31] have been described. Clinically, these patients overwhelmingly manifest appropriate symptoms of these exacerbations.

40.3.3 Management of Retention

The most reasonable approach to a retained capsule in an asymptomatic patient depends on the findings shown by the VCE images. If review of the capsule images shows a lesion, it is reasonable to initiate therapy. This can include a medical course of steroids, an endoscopic attempt at removal of the capsule, or a surgical approach. The medical approach with a course of corticosteroids is to decrease inflammation, thus allowing capsule passage. This approach has been used in patients with Crohn's disease and ulcerative jejunitis complicating celiac disease.

Whether the capsule is entrapped in the proximal or distal small bowel, it can be easily retrieved by means of a gastroscope, colonoscope, or push enteroscope (Fig. 40.9). In these cases, previous endoscopic dilation of a stricture may be necessary to facilitate retrieval [32, 33] (Fig. 40.10). In the past 10 years, new device-assisted endoscopes, specifically designed to evaluate the small bowel, have become available. These newer devices assist in the exploration of the entire small bowel through the combination of the oral and anal approach, making endoscopic retrieval possible even when the capsule is located in the deep small bowel [34, 35] (Fig. 40.11). In addition, device-assisted enteroscopy is not only a reliable method for removing retained capsules (and preventing unnecessary surgery), but it also is the method of choice for obtaining an accurate diagnosis (Fig. 40.12), for adequate staging, and for optimal surgical planning if surgery is required.

Surgery may be needed when endoscopic retrieval fails or when the capsule findings, combined with results of other diagnostic techniques (e.g., CT enterography) suggest the presence of a disease requiring resection, such as small bowel neoplasms. Laparotomy is used to treat the underlying disease leading to capsule retention as well as retrieving the capsule [30] (Fig. 40.13). A recent systematic review showed that of 164 retained capsules reported in 122 articles, 58 % required surgical removal [20].

Asymptomatic patients with a retained capsule proximal to a partially obstructing lesion have been observed for over 2 years without sequelae [36]. Nevertheless, when the capsule remains entrapped in the small bowel for a long time, capsule fragmentation and eventually small bowel perforation can

Fig. 40.9 (**a**, **b**) A capsule that had been retained in the cecum for more than 20 days was easily retrieved by means of a basket

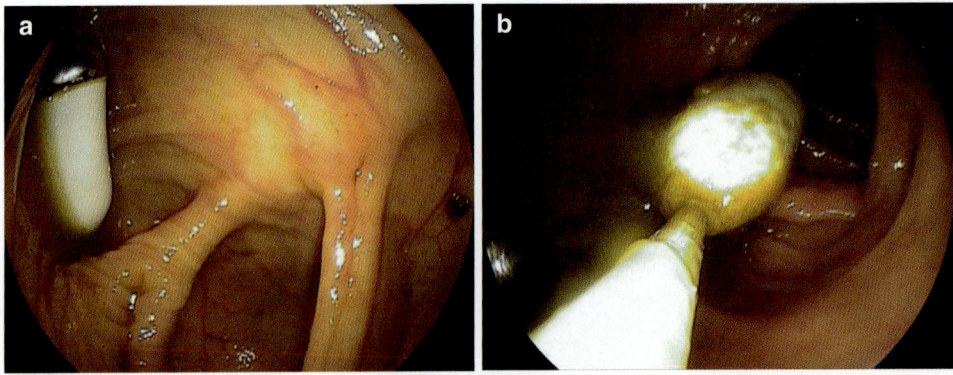

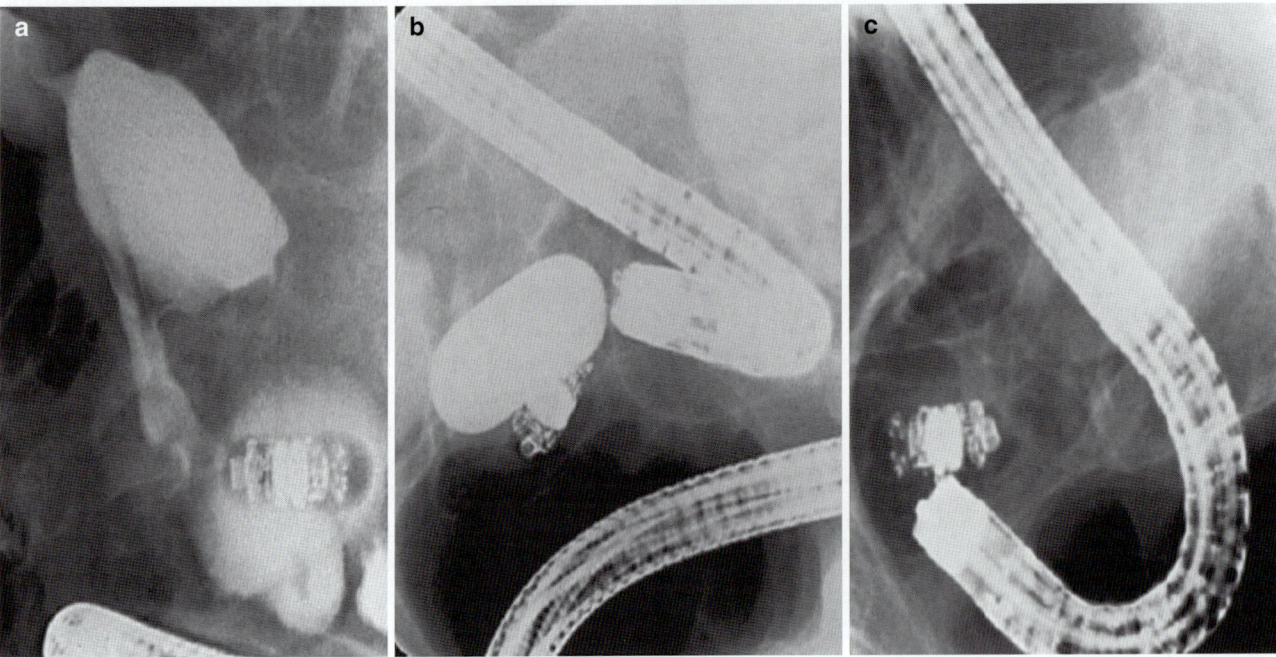

Fig. 40.10 Endoscopic retrieval of retained capsules. Balloon dilation. (**a**) Endoscopic contrast visualization of the terminal ileum shows multiple stenoses and an impacted capsule. (**b**) Balloon dilation. (**c**) Now the capsule can be reached with the endoscope. The patient presented with obscure gastrointestinal bleeding and known, asymptomatic Crohn's disease (Reprinted from Keuchel and Hagenmüller [33] with permission from Deutsches Ärzteblatt)

occur. Therefore, although asymptomatic capsule retention does not warrant urgent measures, a watchful approach, together with a plan for capsule retrieval, is generally recommended.

40.3.4 Prevention of Retention

The first step for minimizing the risk of capsule retention is to obtain a detailed medical history and look for symptoms suggestive of obstruction or for conditions that predispose patients to obstruction. These include ongoing symptoms at the time of capsule endoscopy (e.g., vomiting, nausea, abdominal distension), previous small bowel resection, previous episodes of small bowel obstruction, previous radiation therapy, or the chronic use of potentially harmful agents such as nonsteroidal anti-inflammatory drugs (NSAIDs). This history helps to identify patients at risk for capsule retention and to select those who need further studies before undergoing VCE. At the beginning of the capsule endoscopy era, radiologic examination with a small bowel series was recommended prior to VCE to exclude anatomic narrowing in patients at risk. Nevertheless, a normal x-ray examination of the small bowel does not guarantee uneventful passage of the capsule; several patients with negative small bowel series and

Fig. 40.11 Patient with weight loss, anemia, and abdominal pain experiencing capsule retention. CT enterography (**a**), performed 15 days after capsule endoscopy, showed the retained capsule (*red arrow*) and a bowel mass (*white arrows*), which was confirmed by device-assisted enteroscopy (**b**). During this procedure, a tattoo was placed close to the lesion (**c**), and the capsule was retrieved by means of a basket (**d**)

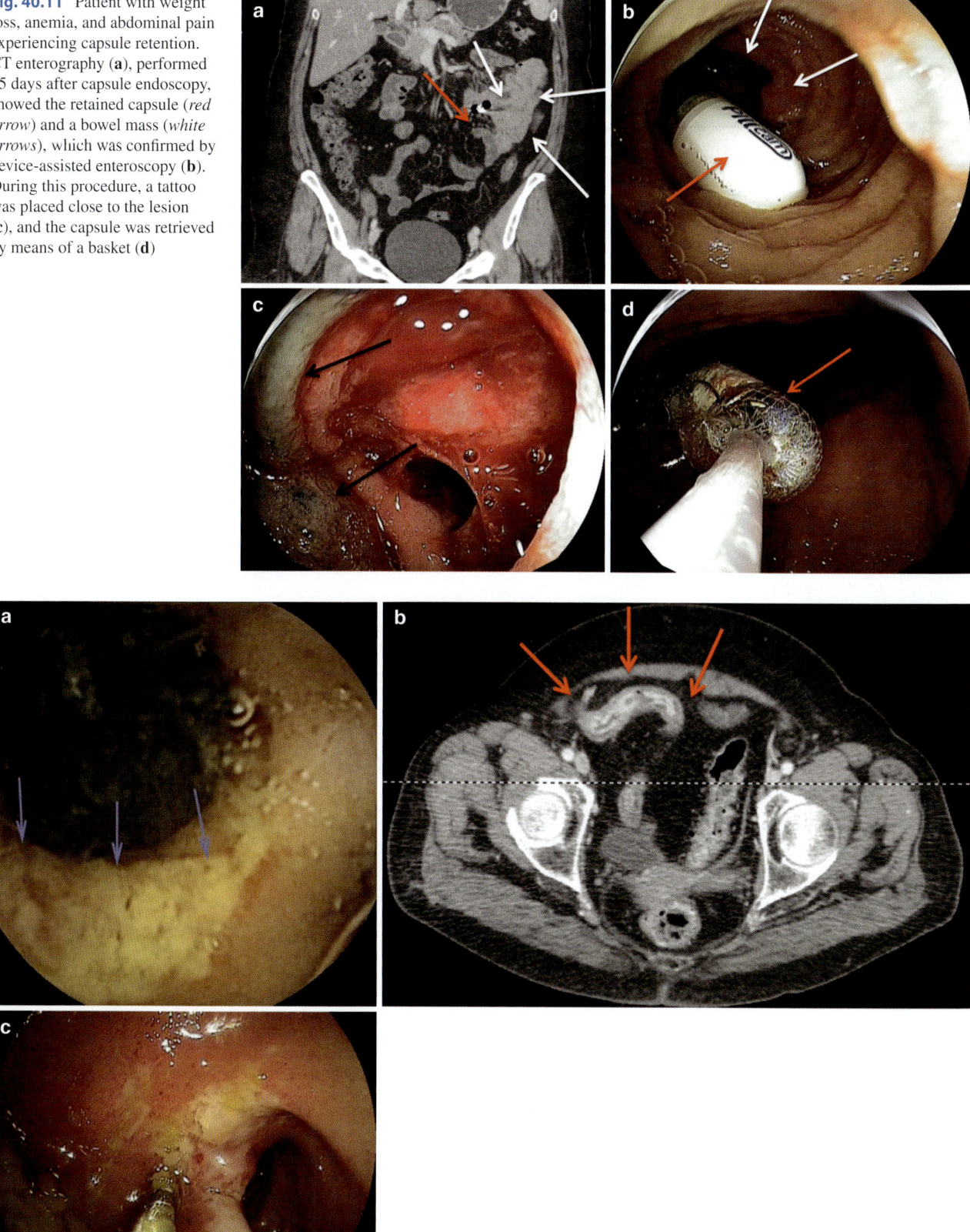

Fig. 40.12 Patient with suspected Crohn's disease (increased fecal calprotectin, history of abdominal pain, chronic diarrhea, and persistent anemia), in whom gastroscopy and colonoscopy were both unremarkable. Capsule endoscopy showed small bowel ulcerations (**a**). Although the capsule did not reach the ileocecal valve during the examination time, it was naturally excreted 25 h after ingestion. The CT enterography confirmed an ileal stricture with small bowel wall thickening (**b**, *red arrows*). Anal double-balloon enteroscopy was eventually performed, and both macroscopic findings (**c**) and histology confirmed the diagnosis of Crohn's disease

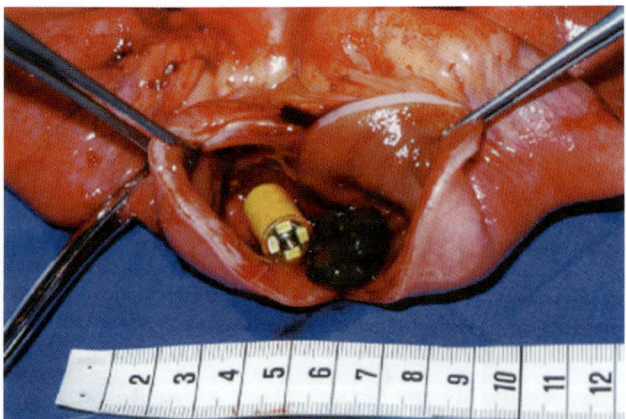

Fig. 40.13 Ileal stricture due to Crohn's disease seen at operation. The capsule was surgically retrieved proximal to the stricture. Capsule endoscopy was done to exclude additional proximal stenoses with a known stenosis requiring surgical treatment (Courtesy of Dirk Hartmann, MD, and Jürgen F. Riemann, MD)

capsule retention have been described [37, 38]. Conversely, studies have shown that a radiologically confirmed stenosis sometimes can be naturally passed by the capsule without retention [39]. To screen patients at risk for capsule retention and for those patients with documented small bowel stenosis, Given Imaging (Yokneam Israel) developed the blind, time-dependent dissolvable patency capsule (PC). The PC consists of a small identification tag detectable by radiofrequency (RFID), which is surrounded by an absorbable material with a small amount of barium. The PC has the same dimensions (11.4×26.4 mm) and shape as the usual capsules available in the market (PillCam SB, Given Imaging Inc. [Yokneam Israel] and EndoCapsule, Olympus [Tokyo, Japan]). It is designed to remain intact in the gastrointestinal tract for about 80 h. After this period, if it is still within the body, enzymes enter the capsule through a permeable cap and disintegrate the capsule body. The presence of the PC

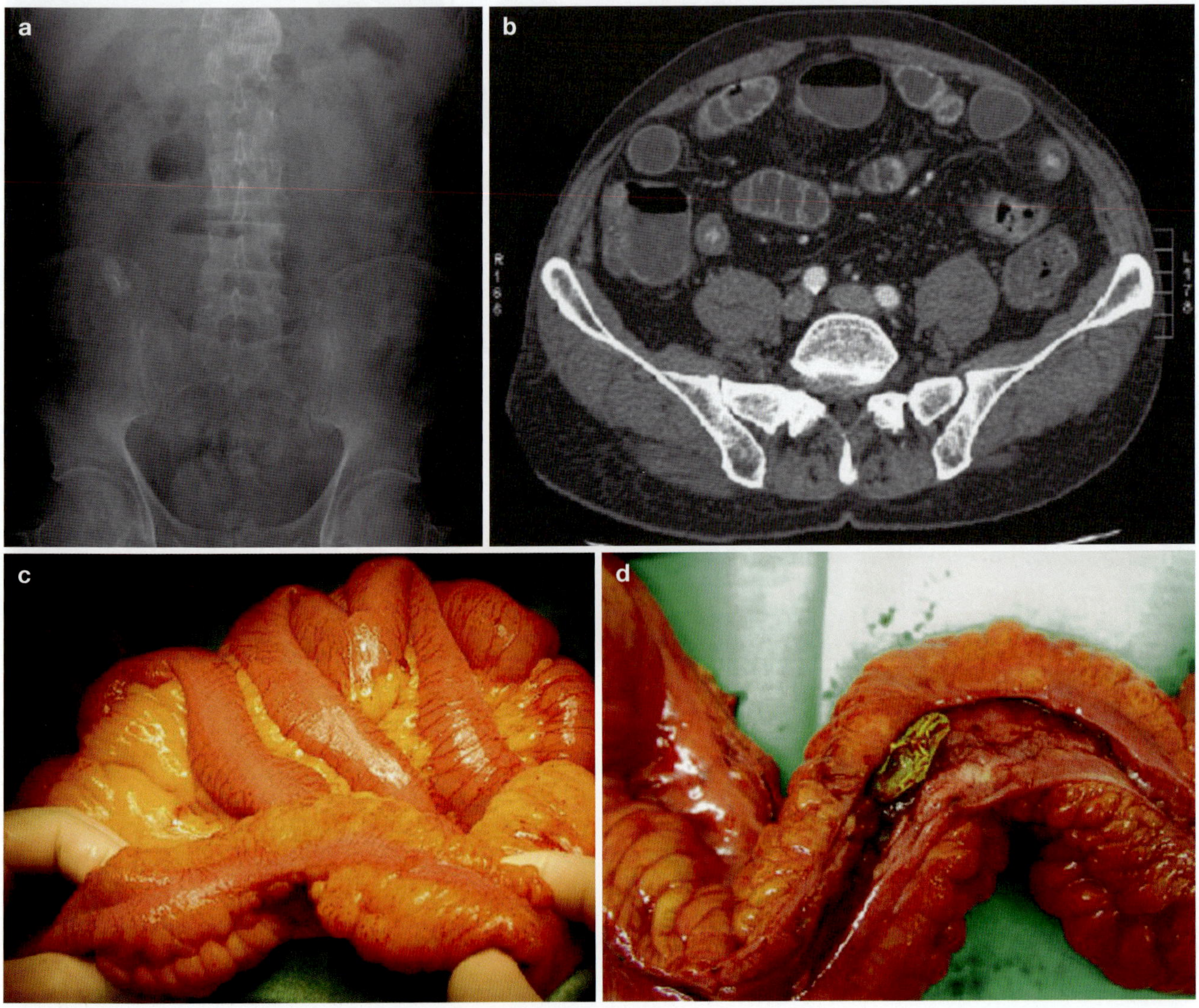

Fig. 40.14 Long stricture of the ileum with remnants of the patency capsule within the stenosis. (**a**) Plain abdominal radiograph with intact patency capsule. (**b**) CT scan with partially dissolved patency capsule proximal to an ileal stenosis. (**c**) Surgical situs with ileal stenosis. (**d**) Remnants of the dissolved patency capsule within the stenosis

inside the gastrointestinal lumen can be verified by means of radiology or by a radiofrequency-emitting external detector device locating the identification tag. Several studies [39–42] have demonstrated that if the PC is excreted intact and its passage does not induce abdominal pain, or if the RFID is no longer detectable inside the patient before the start of capsule dissolution, a regular capsule study can be performed safely. It should be noted, however, that in patients with long and tight stenoses of the small intestine, such as those with established Crohn's disease, the biodegradable PC can cause symptomatic obstruction [38, 40] (Fig. 40.14). Some authors have reported a possible "diagnostic" role for the PC: In the study by Boivin et al. [40], five of six patients experiencing abdominal pain during a PC test required a surgical intervention during the follow-up period.

Recently, a new PC (Agile patency capsule®), with two permeable windows, which begins to dissolve at approximately 30–40 h after ingestion, has been released by Given Imaging. A large multicenter study [43] confirmed a good safety profile and an excellent negative predictive value. Unfortunately, there are no data comparing the performances of patency capsules and new radiologic techniques such as CT enterography in the evaluation of small bowel patency. A recent study [44] reported that the negative predictive value for the PC and for radiologic tests were not significantly different. Therefore, this study suggests that if findings on either test are negative before capsule endoscopy, the patient will most likely pass the capsule without any incident. Taking into account the risk related to radiation exposure, the PC may be the method of choice to test small bowel patency, whereas radiologic tests can be used to minimize false-positive results of PC studies by confirming or excluding the presence of a significant stricture suspected by the PC and to localize the PC if its passage is delayed.

40.4 Pacemakers: Interactions with VCE

The use of a cardiac pacemaker has been considered a contraindication to the use of wireless capsule endoscopy. Unfortunately, pacemakers are being used in an increasing percentage of the population, and these individuals subsequently will be excluded from the benefits of VCE. Although a possible negative effect of the pacemaker on VCE (loss of images) has been described, the reason for excluding these patients from a wireless capsule endoscopy study is mostly related to the possible interference of the endoscopy study's magnetic field with the activity of the pacemaker or implantable cardioverter defibrillator (ICD). To minimize and/or monitor possible cardiovascular events during capsule endoscopy in patients with a pacemaker or ICD, it has been suggested that the capsule endoscopy could be performed under continuous ECG monitoring (telemetry). In all the studies investigating the safety of capsule endos-

copy in patients with different types of pacemakers and ICDs in vivo, interactions between the pacemaker and capsule were reported, but none of them resulted in clinically significant events [45–47]. A recently published paper by Cuschieri et al. [48] conducted a chart review of patients with a cardiac pacemaker who underwent continuous ECG monitoring (telemetry) during capsule endoscopy examinations and confirmed these results. Therefore, the authors concluded that it appears safe to perform capsule endoscopy in these individuals without the use of telemetry monitoring.

References

1. Barkin JS, O'Loughlin C. Capsule endoscopy contraindications: complications and how to avoid their occurrence. Gastrointest Endosc Clin N Am. 2004;14:61–5.
2. Lucendo AJ, Gonzalez-Castillo S, Fernandez-Fuente M, et al. Tracheal aspiration of a capsule endoscope: a new case report and literature compilation of an increasingly reported complication. Dig Dis Sci. 2011;56:2758–62.
3. Soncini M, et al. Diagnostic yield and safety of small bowel capsule endoscopy in clinical practice: prospective data from a regional registry. Gut. 2012;61(S3):A147.
4. Schneider AR, Hoepffner N, Rösch W, Caspary WF. Aspiration of an M2A capsule. Endoscopy. 2003;35:713.
5. Morandi E, Passoni GR, Stillittano D, et al. An unusual complication: capsule endoscopy in the bronchial tree. 2nd international conference on Capsule Endoscopy; Berlin; 23–25 Mar 2003.
6. Buchkremer F, Herrmann T, Stremmel W. Mild respiratory distress after wireless capsule endoscopy. Gut. 2004;53:472.
7. Sinn I, Neef B, Andus T. Aspiration of a capsule endoscope. Gastrointest Endosc. 2004;59:926–7.
8. Tabib S, Fuller C, Daniels J, Lo SK. Asymptomatic aspiration of a capsule endoscope. Gastrointest Endosc. 2004;60:845–8.
9. Girdhar A, Usman F, Bajwa A. Aspiration of capsule endoscope and successful bronchoscopic extraction. J Bronchology Interv Pulmonol. 2012;19:328–31.
10. Knapp AB, Ladetsky L. Endoscopic retrieval of a small bowel enteroscopy capsule lodged in a Zenker's diverticulum. Clin Gastroenterol Hepatol. 2005;3:xxxiv.
11. Ziachehabi A, Maieron A, Hoheisel U, et al. Capsule retention in a Zenker's diverticulum. Endoscopy. 2011;43(Suppl 2 UCTN):E387.
12. Leung WK, Sung JJY. Endoscopically assisted video capsule endoscopy. Endoscopy. 2004;36:562–4.
13. Mow WS, Lo SK, Targan SR, et al. Initial experience with wireless capsule enteroscopy in the diagnosis and management of inflammatory bowel disease. Clin Gastroenterol Hepatol. 2004;2:31–40.
14. Shiotani A, Honda K, Kawakami M, et al. Use of an external real-time image viewer coupled with prespecified actions enhanced the complete examinations for capsule endoscopy. J Gastroenterol Hepatol. 2011;26:1270–4.
15. Yazici C, Losurdo J, Brown MD. Inpatient capsule endoscopy leads to frequent incomplete small bowel examinations. World J Gastroenterol. 2012;18:5051–7.
16. Shibuya T, Mori H, Takeda T, et al. The relationship between physical activity level and completion rate of small bowel examination in patients undergoing capsule endoscopy. Intern Med. 2012;51:997–1001.
17. Zhang JS, Ye LP, Zhang JL, et al. Intramuscular injection of metoclopramide decreases the gastric transit time and does not increase the complete examination rate of capsule endoscopy: a prospective randomized controlled trial. Hepatogastroenterology. 2011;58:110–1.

18. Keller J, Fibbe C, Rosien U, et al. Recent advances in capsule endoscopy: development of maneuverable capsules. Expert Rev Gastroenterol Hepatol. 2012;6:561–6.

19. Gortzak Y, Lantsberg L, Odes HS. Video capsule entrapped in a Meckel's diverticulum. J Clin Gastroenterol. 2003;37:270–1.

20. Liao Z, Gao R, Xu C, et al. Indications and detection, completion, and retention rates of small-bowel capsule endoscopy: a systematic review. Gastrointest Endosc. 2010;71:280–6.

21. Rondonotti E, Soncini M, Girelli C, et al. Small bowel capsule endoscopy in clinical practice: a multicenter 7-year survey. Eur J Gastroenterol Hepatol. 2010;22:1380–6.

22. Höög CM, Bark LA, Arkani J, et al. Capsule retentions and incomplete capsule endoscopy examinations: an analysis of 2300 examinations. Gastroenterol Res Pract. 2012;2012:518718.

23. Ge ZZ, Hu YB, Xiao SD. Capsule endoscopy in diagnosis of small bowel Crohn's disease. World J Gastroenterol. 2004;10:1349–52.

24. Madisch A, Schimming W, Kinzel F, et al. Locally advanced small-bowel adenocarcinoma missed primarily by capsule endoscopy but diagnosed by push enteroscopy. Endoscopy. 2003;35:861–4.

25. De Luca L, Di George P, Rivellini G, et al. Capsule endoscopy: experience in southern Italy. 2nd international conference on Capsule Endoscopy; Berlin; 23–25 Mar 2003.

26. Girelli CM, Amato A, Rocca F. Easy ultrasound detection of retained video endoscopy capsule. J Gastroenterol Hepatol. 2004; 19:241.

27. Lewis BS. How to prevent endoscopic capsule retention. Endoscopy. 2005;37:852–3.

28. Levsky JM, Milikow DL, Rozenblit AM, et al. Small bowel obstruction due to an impacted endoscopy capsule. Abdom Imaging. 2008;33:579–81.

29. Guillèn-Paredes MP, Gòmez-Espìn R, Soria-Aledo V, et al. Intestinal obstruction secondary to endoscopic capsule retention. Rev Esp Enferm Dig. 2012;104:286–7.

30. Fry LC, De Petris G, Swain JM, Fleischer DE. Impaction and fracture of a video capsule in the small bowel requiring laparotomy for removal of the capsule fragments. Endoscopy. 2005;37:674–6.

31. Strosberg JR, Shibata D, Kvols LK. Intermittent bowel obstruction due to a retained wireless capsule endoscope in a patient with a small bowel carcinoid tumour. Can J Gastroenterol. 2007;21:113–5.

32. Arifuddin RM, Baichi MM, Mantry PS. Small bowel capsule impaction and successful endoscopic retrieval. Clin Gastroenterol Hepatol. 2005;3:A34.

33. Keuchel M, Hagenmüller F. Small bowel endoscopy with the wireless video capsule. Dtsch Arztebl. 2002;99:A2702–10.

34. Van Weyenberg SJ, Van Turenhout ST, Bouma G, et al. Double-balloon endoscopy as the primary method for small-bowel video capsule endoscope retrieval. Gastrointest Endosc. 2010;71:535–41.

35. May A, Nachbar L, Ell C. Extraction of entrapped capsules from the small bowel by means of push-and-pull enteroscopy with the double-balloon technique. Endoscopy. 2005;37:591–3.

36. Sears DM, Avots-Avotins A, Culp K, Gavin MW. Frequency and clinical outcome of capsule retention during capsule endoscopy for GI bleeding of obscure origin. Gastrointest Endosc. 2004;60: 822–7.

37. Barkin JS, Friedman S. Wireless capsule endoscopy requiring surgical intervention: the world's experience. Am J Gastroenterol. 2002;97(Suppl):S298.

38. Gay G, Delvaux M, Laurent V, et al. Temporary intestinal occlusion induced by a "patency capsule" in a patient with Crohn's disease. Endoscopy. 2005;37:174–7.

39. Spada C, Spera G, Riccioni M, et al. A novel diagnostic tool for detecting functional patency of the small bowel: the Given patency capsule. Endoscopy. 2005;37:793–800.

40. Boivin ML, Voderholzer W, Lochs H. Does passage of a Patency Capsule indicate small bowel patency? A prospective trial. Endoscopy. 2005;37:808–15.

41. Signorelli C, Rondonotti E, Villa F, et al. Use of the given Patency System for the screening of patients at high risk for capsule retention. Dig Liver Dis. 2006;38:326–30.

42. Caunedo A, Rodriguez-Tellez M, Romero J, et al. Evaluation of the M2A Patency capsule in the gastrointestinal tract: one centre preliminary data from a multicentre prospective trial. Endoscopy. 2003;35:A182.

43. Herrerias JM, Leighton JA, Costamagna G, et al. Agile patency system eliminates risk of capsule retention in patients with known intestinal strictures who undergo capsule endoscopy. Gastrointest Endosc. 2008;67:902–9.

44. Yadav A, Heigh RI, Hara AK, et al. Performance of the patency capsule compared with nonenteroclysis radiologic examinations in patients with known or suspected intestinal strictures. Gastrointest Endosc. 2011;74:834–9.

45. Bandorski D, Jakobs R, Bruck M, et al. Capsule endoscopy in patients with cardiac pacemakers and implantable cardioverter defibrillators: (re)evaluation of the current state in Germany, Austria, and Switzerland 2010. Gastroenterol Res Pract. 2012;2012:717408.

46. Payeras G, Piqueras J, Moreno VJ, et al. Effects of capsule endoscopy on cardiac pacemakers. Endoscopy. 2005;37:1181–5.

47. Dubner S, Dubner Y, Gallino S, et al. Electromagnetic interference with implantable cardiac pacemakers by video capsule. Gastrointest Endosc. 2005;61:250–4.

48. Cuschieri JR, Osman MN, Wong RC, et al. Small bowel capsule endoscopy in patients with cardiac pacemakers and implantable cardioverter defibrillators: Outcome analysis using telemetry review. World J Gastrointest Endosc. 2012;4:87–93.

Influence of Small Bowel Capsule Endoscopy on Clinical Outcome

41

Lucia C. Fry, Friedrich Hagenmüller, Jörg G. Albert, and David E. Fleischer

Contents

The work was first published in 2006 by Springer Medizin Verlag Heidelberg with the following title: *Atlas of Video Capsule Endoscopy*.

L.C. Fry (✉)
Department of Internal Medicine, Gastroenterology, and Infectious Diseases, Marien Hospital, Bottrop, Germany
e-mail: luciafry@yahoo.com

F. Hagenmüller
1st Medical Department, Asklepios Klinik Altona, Hamburg, Germany
e-mail: f.hagenmueller@asklepios.com

J.G. Albert
Medical Clinic I, University Hospital Frankfurt, Frankfurt, Germany
e-mail: j.albert@med.uni-frankfurt.de

D.E. Fleischer
Division of Gastroenterology, Mayo Clinic Arizona, Scottsdale, AZ, USA
e-mail: fleischer.david@mayo.edu

Video capsule endoscopy (SBCE) has become the first choice in the evaluation of suspected small bowel bleeding [1–4]. The positive impact of SBCE on clinical outcomes in patients with obscure gastrointestinal bleeding (OGIB) has been demonstrated in several studies [5–7]. SBCE showed a better diagnostic yield in detecting mucosal lesions in patients with OGIB when compared with radiologic investigations such as small bowel follow-through (SBFT), small bowel enteroclysis (SBE), or cross-sectional imaging such as CT scans or MRI [2, 4, 8–10]. Device-assisted enteroscopy (DAE), which comprises single-balloon, double-balloon, and spiral enteroscopy, also enables inspection of the whole small bowel mucosa and permits the performance of therapeutic interventions [1]. DAE is time-consuming, however; so SBCE and DAE should be considered complementary procedures. The effect of SBCE on diagnosis and outcome in patients with established Crohn's disease (CD) and clinically suspected CD has been also demonstrated in several studies [11–15]. Recent studies have also shown that SBCE is useful for screening and surveillance of patients with polyposis syndromes [16, 17]. Furthermore, the usefulness of SBCE for patients with celiac disease or for patients with symptoms such as chronic diarrhea and chronic abdominal pain (when accompanied by inflammatory markers), and for less frequent small bowel diseases, has been increasingly demonstrated in recent publications [18–22].

One measure of clinical outcome is the impact of this diagnostic technique on subsequent patient management and the patient's health. The findings of SBCE may lead to a therapeutic consequence or intervention, which can be active (invasive or medical therapy) or inactive (no therapy). Negative as well as positive findings on SBCE could minimize further examinations, resulting in improved quality of life for the patient, reduced economic costs, and prompt treatment [23]. The evaluation of clinical outcome must also include the evaluation of adverse effects and complications, which could have a negative impact on patient health and quality of life [24, 25]. There are very few data on clinical outcomes in most diagnostic areas of gastroenterology. Nevertheless, many of the large studies using SBCE have enough variables to analyze patients' clinical outcomes [5, 6, 26–28].

M. Keuchel et al. (eds.), *Video Capsule Endoscopy: A Reference Guide and Atlas*,
DOI 10.1007/978-3-662-44062-9_41, © Springer-Verlag Berlin Heidelberg 2014

This chapter reviews the evidence as to whether the use of SBCE in the daily praxis improves health outcomes. The focus is on small bowel bleeding and CD, but we also delineate the use of SBCE for conditions such as abdominal pain or diarrhea, polyposis syndromes, celiac disease, and less frequent clinical settings.

41.1　Outcome in Obscure Gastrointestinal Bleeding

Small bowel bleeding represents about 5–10 % of gastrointestinal (GI) bleeding events [29]. Obscure GI bleeding (OGIB) is defined as bleeding from the GI tract that persists or recurs without an obvious etiology after esophagogastroduodenoscopy (EGD), colonoscopy, and radiologic evaluation of the small bowel such as SBFT [1]. OGIB is categorized into obscure overt and obscure occult bleeding, based on the presence or absence of visible blood loss [1]. Since the availability of SBCE and DAE, the localization of GI bleeding has been reclassified into three categories: upper, mid-, and lower GI bleeding. Bleeding above the ampulla of Vater, within the reach of an EGD, is defined as upper GI bleeding; bleeding from the ampulla of Vater to the terminal ileum, best investigated by SBCE and DAE, is defined as mid-GI bleeding; and colonic bleeding is defined as lower GI bleeding, which can be evaluated by colonoscopy.

SBCE represents the first noninvasive method for the examination of the small bowel that visualizes the complete small bowel mucosa in about 80–90 % of patients and has a better detection rate in most studies when compared with other techniques such as push enteroscopy (PE), intraoperative enteroscopy (IOE), small bowel radiography (SBFT and small bowel enteroclysis), and cross-sectional imaging (CT, MRI) (Table 41.1) [2, 9, 10, 27, 30–34]. The most often used cross-sectional imaging methods, which have been compared to SBCE in patients with OGIB, are CT or CT enterography (CTE), followed by magnetic resonance (MR) enterography [2, 9, 10, 12, 14, 27, 28, 31–37]. SBCE has consistently been reported to be superior for detecting flat or mucosal lesions, such as angiectasias, whereas CT or CTE have been shown to be superior in detecting small bowel wall tumors [9, 35]. It might therefore be recommended to include CT/CTE if SBCE is negative. Some authors recommend performing CT scans first in patients with OGIB, using SBCE if the CT findings are negative [9, 38].

SBCE has now become the method of choice for the evaluation of OGIB, reaching a diagnostic yield of about 60 % in patients with OGIB (Table 41.2) [1–6, 39–41]. The most common lesions reported in patients with OGIB are angiectasia, ulcers (including those induced by nonsteroidal anti-inflammatory drugs (NSAIDs)), erosions, and tumors (Figs. 41.1, 41.2, and 41.3) [1, 3–7, 28]. Nevertheless, it may be necessary to repeat endoscopies in patients referred for SBCE because up to 30 % of lesions found with SBCE (i.e., Cameron lesions, gastric ulcers, gastric or colonic angiectasias) may be located within the reach of conventional endoscopy (EGD, colonoscopy) [1, 26, 42, 43]. One more important issue to consider is the timing of the examination. It has been demonstrated that the earlier SBCE is performed, the higher the diagnostic yield achieved for patients with overt OGIB, thus resulting in a higher intervention rate [44]. The same study demonstrated that the duration between bleeding and SBCE was shorter for patients with angiectasia than for those with other abnormalities [44].

SBCE and DAE are complementary methods with similar detection rates reported in several studies; combining them in the same patient increases detection rates [45–48]. One of the advantages of the DAE is the possibility of directly visualizing the small bowel mucosa and performing biopsies and therapy. The implementation of therapy during DAE after the detection of lesions with SBCE represents an immense improvement in

Table 41.1　Yield of SBCE compared with small bowel imaging in suspected small bowel bleeding

Study	Type	N	Comparator	Yield of SBCE (%)	Yield of comparator (%)	Incremental yield of SBCE
Lewis and Swain [30]	Prospective	20	PE	55	30	p=n.s.
Ell et al. [31]	Prospective	32	PE	66	28	$p<0.001$
Saurin et al. [27]	Prospective	58	PE	69	38	$p<0.04$
Mata et al. [32]	Prospective	42	PE	74	19	$p=0.05$
Triester et al. [2]	Meta-analysis	396	PE	63	28	35 % ($p<0.00001$; 95 % CI=26–43 %)
Triester et al. [2]	Meta-analysis	88	Small bowel radiography	67	8	59 % ($p<0.00001$; 95 % CI=48–70 %)
Hartmann et al. [33]	Prospective	47	Intraoperative enteroscopy	74	72	p=n.s.
Zhang et al. [34]	Prospective	123	CT	57	30	27 %, $p=0.01$
Huprich et al. [9]	Prospective	58	CTE	38	88	$p=0.008$ (CTE better yield than SBCE)
Wiarda et al. [10]	Prospective	34	MRI	61	21	40 %, $p=0.0015$

CTE computed tomography enterography, *PE* push enteroscopy, *SBCE* video capsule endoscopy

Table 41.2 Role of SBCE in detection of small bowel lesions in patients with unexplained iron deficiency anemia

Study	Year	Analysis of data	N	Diagnostic yield (%)
Apostolopoulos et al. [39]	2006	Retrospective	51	57
Riccioni et al. [40]	2010	Retrospective	138	65.9
Milano et al. [4]	2011	Prospective	45	77.8
Holleran et al. [41]	2012	Retrospective	65	53
Koulaouzidis et al. [3]	2012	Retrospective	221	30.7

After negative endoscopic workup with esophagogastroduodenoscopy and colonoscopy

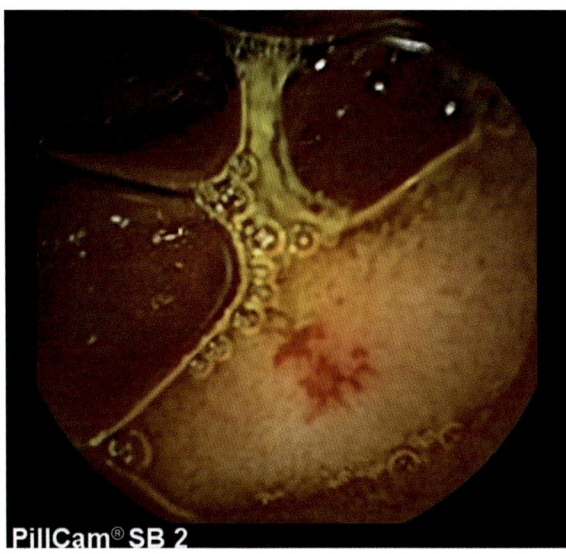

Fig. 41.1 Small angiectasia of the proximal jejunum

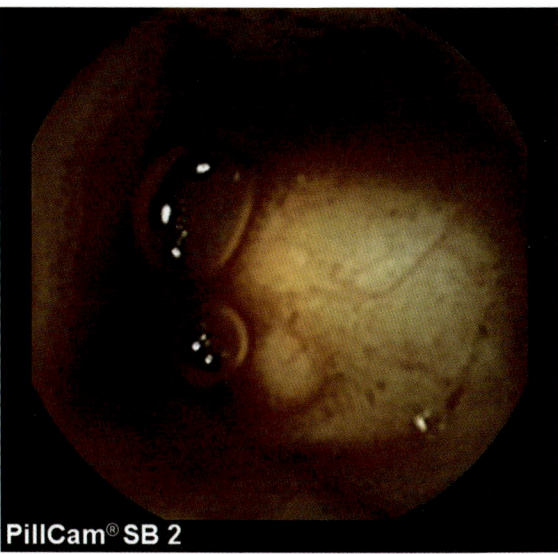

Fig. 41.3 Gastrointestinal stromal tumor (GIST) in a patient with iron deficiency anemia. This patient has a submucosal lesion covered by normal mucosa; the final diagnosis was made after surgery

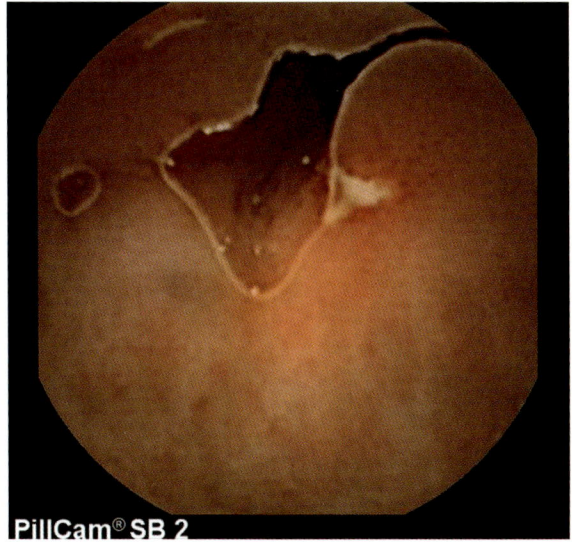

Fig. 41.2 Superficial fibrin-coated ulcers in a patient with intake of nonsteroidal anti-inflammatory drugs (NSAIDs)

the outcomes of SBCE. Given the fact that SBCE is able to assess the complete small bowel mucosa, it is easier to perform and often improve the results of DAE if SBCE is performed initially and then followed by DAE. However, in patients with severe, ongoing bleeding of the small intestine,

in whom intervention by DAE may be expected, DAE should be the first method of choice [45–47, 49]. In these patients, SBCE often only demonstrates fresh intraluminal blood without identifying the bleeding lesion (Fig. 41.4) [45].

Some published studies have included long-term follow-up data and evaluation of clinical outcome (Table 41.3) [5–7, 26–28, 37, 50–54]. Penazzio et al. reported that the subsequent therapeutic approach after the findings on SBCE led to a resolution of the clinical problem in 87 % of patients with ongoing overt OGIB, in 41 % of patients with previously overt OGIB, and in 69 % of patients with occult OGIB [5]. Others point out a high negative predictive value in patients without significant SBCE findings, and negative SBCE is followed by a low rebleeding rate of 0–12 % [6, 33, 50, 51, 53–55]. Also, they reported an important reduction of further endoscopies after a therapy was implemented, such as argon plasma coagulation (APC) for the treatment of angiectasias (Fig. 41.5).

The pathology revealed during SBCE has influenced further therapy (i.e., therapy was stopped or initiated) in 58–66 % of patients. Improvement of the clinical outcome was reported in 16–66 % of cases [26, 28, 33, 52]. One study reported 100 % resolution of OGIB observed after a long-term follow-up in

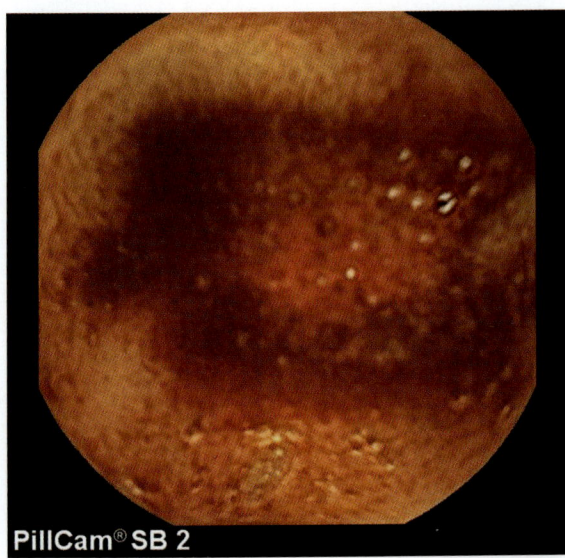

Fig. 41.4 Video capsule endoscopy (SBCE) shows active bleeding, but the underlying lesion cannot be seen

young patients and concluded that angiectasias were a predictor of less favorable clinical outcome [52].

A major deficiency in these studies is the failure to compare the outcomes of SBCE to outcomes with other methods. Neu et al. [28] compared the impact of SBCE versus PE, angiography, and SBE in 56 patients with OGIB. As the diagnostic yield was 68 % for SBCE and 38 % for all other tests, the authors concluded that SBCE may be able to replace the other tests in the clinical decision-making process.

Long-term follow-up of 47 patients with OGIB who underwent SBCE followed by IOE with APC or resection showed a rebleeding rate of 26 %, mainly due to angiectasias. None of the six patients with negative SBCE examination had signs of rebleeding [33]. Several studies reported that angiectasias discovered during SBCE were treated with APC during DAE, which significantly reduced the rebleeding rate and blood transfusion requirements; nevertheless, rebleeding occurred in more than 40 % of patients despite adequate treatment (Table 41.3) [55, 56].

Table 41.3 Long-term follow-up after SBCE for obscure gastrointestinal bleeding

Study	Follow-up N	Months	Diagnostic yield (%)	Diagnostic SBCE Angiectasias (%)	Therapy (%)	Rebleed (%)	Negative SBCE Rebleed (%)	Comments
Delvaux et al. [6]	44	12	61	50	100	12	0	1 death after surgery
Pennazio et al. [5]	91	18	47	46	88	22	54	5 retentions
			92		100	14	0	Overt ongoing
			13		50	50	62	Overt previous
			44		74	20	50	Occult
Rastogi et al. [26]	41	6.7	42	72	67	38	–	
Neu et al. [28]	56	13	68	71	45	56	22	SBCE *vs* PE, SBCE *vs* radiology; 2 deaths after surgery
Saurin et al. [27]	58	12	72	71	40	19	23	
					61			High bleeding potential
					28			Intermediate bleeding potential
Estevez et al. [7]	95	11.4	68	34	76	22	34	
Hartmann et al. [33]	47	11.5	72	47	100	26	0	SBCE *vs* IOE
Fujimori et al. [50]	45	18.8	49	5	89	5	12	SBCE *vs* DBE
Albert et al. [51]	285	20.7	76	51	52	31	11	
Hindryckx et al. [52]	92	21	60	40	76	40	24	
Apostolopoulos et al. [53]	37	12	92	78	57	16	0	
Iwamoto et al. [54]	78	6	45	46	53	26	4	

DAE device-assisted enteroscopy, *IOE* intraoperative enteroscopy, *PE* push enteroscopy
Criteria for definition of therapy and rebleeding may vary amongst the studies.

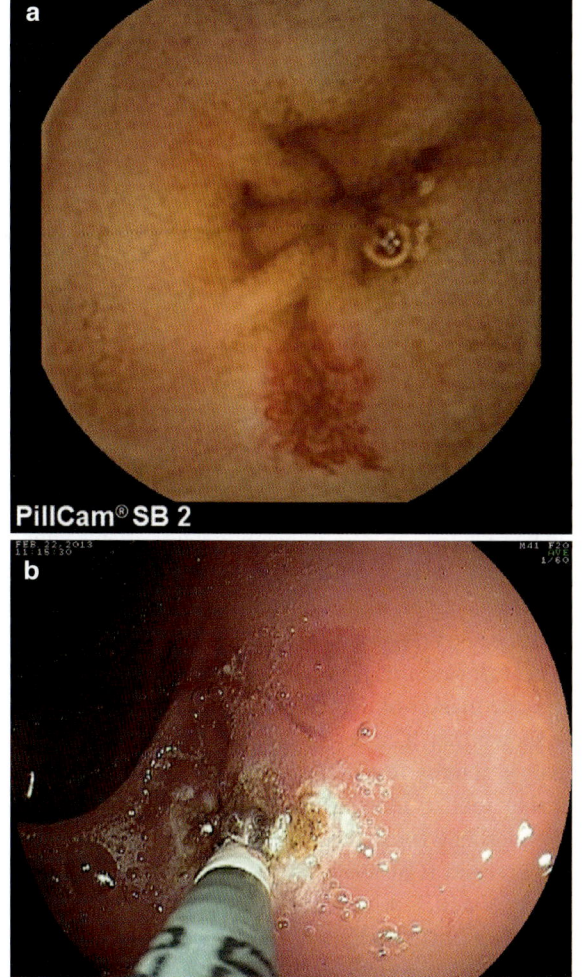

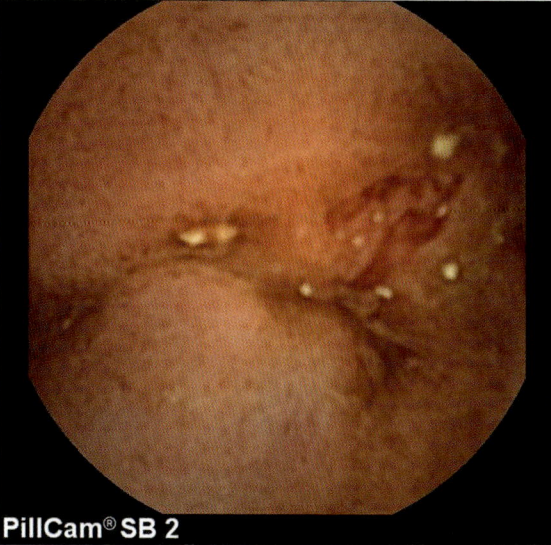

Fig. 41.6 Fissures and spontaneous bleeding at the time of diagnosis of Crohn's disease

Fig. 41.5 (**a**, **b**) Angiectasia of the jejunum was identified during SBCE and was treated with argon plasma coagulation during device-assisted enteroscopy

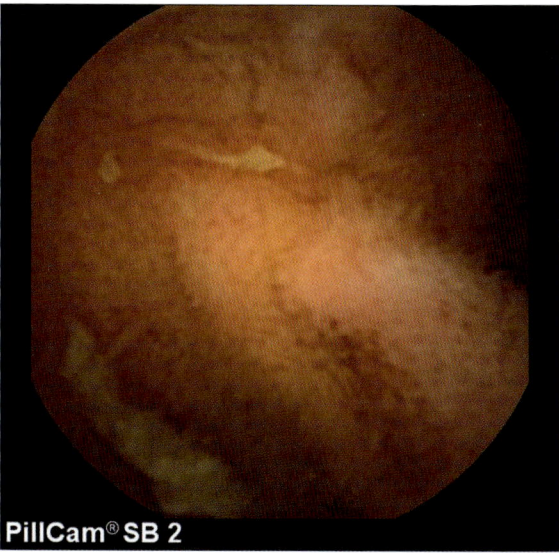

41.2   Outcome in Crohn's Disease

Fig. 41.7 Linear fibrin-coated ulcerations in a patient with Crohn's disease

Another important indication for SBCE is the diagnosis of suspected inflammatory bowel disease (IBD) or the evaluation of patients with known IBD (response to therapy, extent of the disease) (Figs. 41.6 and 41.7). SBCE has proven to be an effective diagnostic procedure for patients with suspected IBD when previous conventional studies (SBFT, CT enterography, MR enterography) have shown negative results. Clinical trials report a diagnostic yield of SBCE of 43–71 % for lesions suggestive of CD [11]. Furthermore, SBCE has shown an incremental yield (compared with PE, CTE, and small bowel radiography) of 22–47 % in patients who were suspected of having CD and from 32 % to 57 % in patients with established CD (Table 41.4) [57–67]. In patients with perianal disease and a negative conventional workup to exclude CD, the incremental diagnostic yield of SBCE is 24 % [68].

Eliakim et al. [12] compared the yield of SBCE versus SBFT and CTE in patients with suspected CD. SBCE detected lesions in addition to those found on other modalities in 47 % of patients. Patients newly diagnosed with CD were medically treated with significant clinical improvement. In the comparative study of Voderholzer et al. [37], a therapeutic impact of SBCE was reported in 24 % of all patients: 17 % of patients with an established diagnosis of CD and 100 % in patients with suspected CD. Mow et al. [69] analyzed 50 patients with known or suspected IBD; symptoms improved after the implementation of specific therapy in 17 of 20 patients with diagnostic SBCE and in 7 of 10 patients with

Table 41.4 Comparing the diagnostic yield or sensitivity of cross-sectional imaging and SBCE in diagnosing small bowel Crohn's disease

Study	N	SBCE yield	Comparator (cross-sectional imaging)	Comparator yield	Statistical significance
Eliakim et al. [57]	35	77 %	CTE	20 %	p<0.05
Voderholzer et al. [58]	41	25/41 (61 %)	CTE	12/41 (29 %)	p=0.004
Albert et al. [59]	52	25/27 (93 %)	MRI	21/27 (78 %)	n.s.
Golder et al. [60]	18	12/18 (66 %)	MRI	1/18 (5 %)	p=0.016
Hara et al. [61]	17	12/17 (71 %)	CT	9/17 (53 %)	n.s.
Solem et al. [62]	28	83 %	CTE	83 %	n.s.
Tillack et al. [63]	19	18/19 (95 %)	MRI	18/19 (95 %)	n.s.
Böcker et al. [64]	21	9/21 (43 %)	MRI	6/21 (29 %)	Significant for proximal small bowel
Jensen et al. [65]	93	100 %	MRI and CTE	81 % (MRI)	p<0.05 (for proximal small bowel)
				76 % (CTE)	
Casciani et al. [66]	37	10/11 (91 %)	MRI	19/19	n.s.

CTE computed tomography enterography, *SBCE* video capsule endoscopy

Table 41.5 Therapeutic impact and clinical improvement with therapeutic measure in patients with suspected or established Crohn's disease

Study	N	Therapeutic impact	Clinical improvement
Voderholzer et al. [37]	56	17.8 %	100 %
Liangpunsakul et al. [14]	40	7.5 %	100 %
Herrerias et al. [15]	21	42.8 %	100 %
Chong et al. [70]	42	66 % (suspected CD)	57 % (suspected CD)
		72 % (established CD)	56 % (known CD)
Mow et al. [69]	50	60 %	80 %
Dussault et al. [71]	77	53 % (established CD)	–

CD Crohn's disease

suspicious findings during SBCE (Table 41.5) [14, 15, 41, 69–72]. Even if not all studies included a sufficiently long period of follow-up, in one study with 12 months of follow-up, Tukey et al. [73] found a sensitivity of 77 % and a specificity of 89 % to diagnose small bowel ulcers in 102 patients suspected of having CD [73]. One year later, CD had been diagnosed in 13 % of the patients. It is important to note that SBCE had a high negative predictive value (96 %) in excluding the presence of CD. SBCE also decreased the delay until a diagnosis of CD was reached, specifically in those patients with a negative previous workup [73].

In colitis with an unclassified type of inflammatory bowel disease (IBDU), the presence of inflammatory lesions in the small bowel may reveal CD in some patients. In one such study, the detection of small bowel ulcerations led to a diagnosis of CD in 18 (15 %) of 120 patients with IBDU [74].

One important consideration at the time of performing SBCE in patients with confirmed or suspected CD is the possibility of capsule retention [24, 25]. In two trials, 27 % of the patients were excluded because suspected strictures were seen at CT enteroclysis, causing concern that the capsule

could be retained [58, 59]. In symptomatic patients with suspicion of an intestinal stricture, the so-called patency capsule should be used before SBCE to detect strictures that might lead to capsule retention [75].

Fecal calprotectin (fCal) has recently been investigated as a surrogate marker of ileocolonic inflammation [76]. Studies have shown that fCal levels correlate with endoscopic and histologic activity in patients with IBD, also being a useful screening tool to identify patients who are most likely to need endoscopy for suspected IDB [76]. Koulaouzidis et al. [77] correlated fCal levels with SBCE findings in patients referred for SBCE with clinical suspicion of CD and negative bidirectional endoscopies. They demonstrated that all the patients with normal fCal levels (≤50 µg/g) had normal SBCE. An fCal level greater than 100 µg/g was a good predictor of positive SBCE findings, and fCal greater than 200 µg/g was associated with higher SBCE yield (65 %) and confirmed CD in 50 % of patients. Patients with fCal levels between 50 and 100 µg/g had normal SBCE despite symptoms suggestive of IBD [77]. However, these findings were not confirmed in a later study [78]. Sipponen et al. [78] found that fecal biomarkers such as fCal and S100A12 (also a fecal biomarker of inflammation) have moderate specificity but low sensitivity in predicting SBCE results in patients with suspected CD. Neither fCal nor S100A12 was useful for screening or excluding small bowel CD [78]. Larger prospective studies should help to clarify the significance of this test to select patients with nonspecific symptoms for SBCE.

41.3 Outcome in Abdominal Pain or Diarrhea/Irritable Bowel Syndrome

Patients with chronic abdominal pain or diarrhea usually undergo several diagnostic procedures until a final diagnosis is reached. The likelihood of positive findings from SBCE in those patients has been low (Table 41.6) [79]. In one published study involving 20 patients with chronic abdominal pain, none of the patients had significant findings on SBCE [80]. Another retrospective review of 64 patients who underwent CE because of chronic abdominal pain and/or diarrhea showed a yield of SBCE of 6 % in patients with abdominal pain, 14 % in patients with diarrhea, and 13 % in patients with both symptoms [81].

A multicenter study including 72 patients with chronic (>3 months) abdominal pain with or without diarrhea, in whom the diagnosis could not be reached by conventional modalities, found the highest diagnostic yield in patients with abdominal pain and positive inflammatory markers (66 %), when compared with patients with abdominal pain and negative inflammatory markers (21 %), but interestingly, SBCE was negative in the group of patients with both abdominal pain and diarrhea and negative inflammatory markers [18]. Thus, it is possible to conclude that this latter group of patients probably have irritable bowel syndrome [18]. The comparative findings of SBCE in patients with suspected CD and/or abdominal pain are outlined in Table 41.6 [18, 80–86]. The usefulness of SBCE in patients with abdominal pain increases in the presence of weight loss, anemia, or inflammatory markers.

In patients with irritable bowel syndrome, abnormal transit time in SBCE has been shown to be a possible positive finding that can cause abdominal pain or diarrhea in this group of patients [87]. Interestingly, in recent years, small bowel transit times, symptoms, and changes after the administration of prokinetic drugs in patients with irritable bowel syndrome have been evaluated using SBCE. After the administration of a prokinetic (mosapride citrate) to patients with constipation-predominant irritable bowel syndrome, symptomatic changes as well as alteration in the transit time were assessed using SBCE. After 4 weeks under prokinetics, symptoms improved, gastric transit time was not significantly changed, but small bowel transit time was significantly reduced, which also correlated with changes in the times of defecation [88].

SBCE also has been used to evaluate the prokinetic effect of lubiprostone in healthy subjects [89]. This drug was approved for treatment of chronic idiopathic constipation and constipation-predominant irritable bowel syndrome. Lubiprostone produced a significant increase in gastric transit time but did not result in a significant decrease in small bowel transit time compared with placebo. The administration of lubiprostone before capsule ingestion did not result in improved overall preparation of the small bowel for SBCE or increase the percentage of visualized small bowel [89].

41.4 Outcome in Polyposis Syndromes

When compared with SBFT, CT, and MRI, SBCE identified a considerably higher number of polyps with lesion sizes ranging between 1 and 30 mm (Fig. 41.8) [16, 17, 90]. MRI was more accurate in terms of localization, whereas SBCE was more arbitrary [16]. Soares et al. [90] found SBCE an effective method for evaluation of the small bowel in patients with Peutz-Jeghers syndrome (PJS). Given that PJS has a high prevalence of small intestinal polyps and risks of obstruction and malignant degeneration of those polyps, SBCE appears to be a useful test for initial staging and also for regular follow-up. The management of small bowel polyps in patients with PJS who underwent different diagnostic methods was evaluated by Ohmiya et al. [17]. When the authors compared SBCE, enteroscopy, and enteroclysis, SBCE had a better diagnostic yield to detect polyps. The resection of polyps during enteroscopy showed adenoma or adenocarcinoma in 30 % of polyps larger than 20 mm and only 1.3 % of polyps smaller than 20 mm [17]. The use of SBCE in patients with familial adenomatous polyposis (FAP) is less well substantiated, given the fact that polyps of the small bowel (except for the duodenum) are very rare.

41.5 Outcome in Small Bowel Tumors

The outcomes of small bowel tumors newly diagnosed using SBCE have been addressed in some studies (Figs. 41.3, 41.9, 41.10, and 41.11) [91, 92]. A single center reported 13 newly

Table 41.6 SBCE in patients with chronic abdominal pain or suspected Crohn's disease

Study	N	Indication	Findings (%)	Predictive factor
De Bona et al. [82]	38	Suspected CD	34	Inflammatory marker
Valle et al. [83]	18	Suspected CD	26	Inflammatory marker
Fidder et al. [84]	112	Suspected CD	6	Diarrhea
Bardan et al. [80]	20	Abdominal pain	0	None
Fry et al. [81]	64	Abdominal pain	9	Diarrhea
Shim et al. [85]	110	Abdominal pain	17.3	Weight loss, CRP, anemia
May et al. [86]	50	Abdominal pain	36	CRP, other symptoms
Katsinelos et al. [18]	72	Abdominal pain	44	Inflammatory markers

CD Crohn's disease, *CRP* C-reactive protein, *SBCE* video capsule endoscopy
Positive findings only when additional predictive factors were present

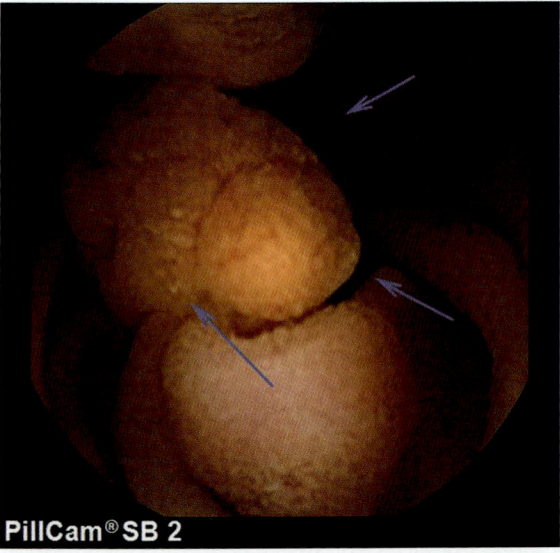

Fig. 41.8 Jejunal polyps in a patient with Peutz-Jeghers syndrome. (*courtesy of* Carolina Olano, MD)

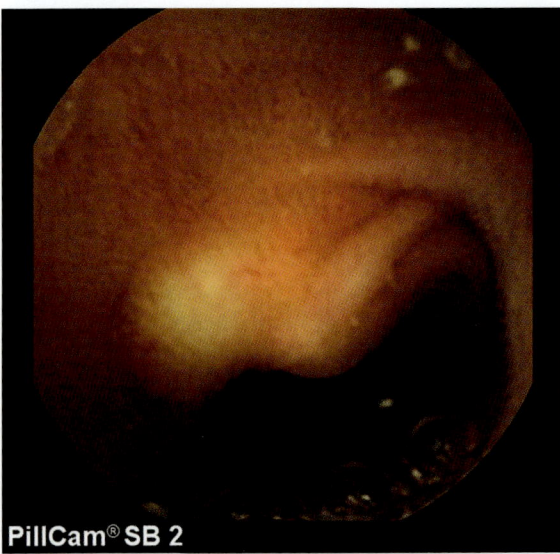

Fig. 41.10 Neuroendocrine tumor in a patient with liver metastases

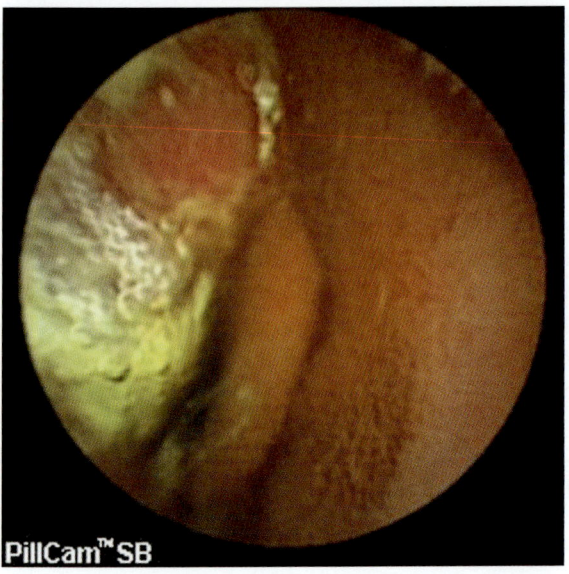

Fig. 41.9 Adenocarcinoma of the proximal jejunum: the lumen is partially occluded by a lobulated mass

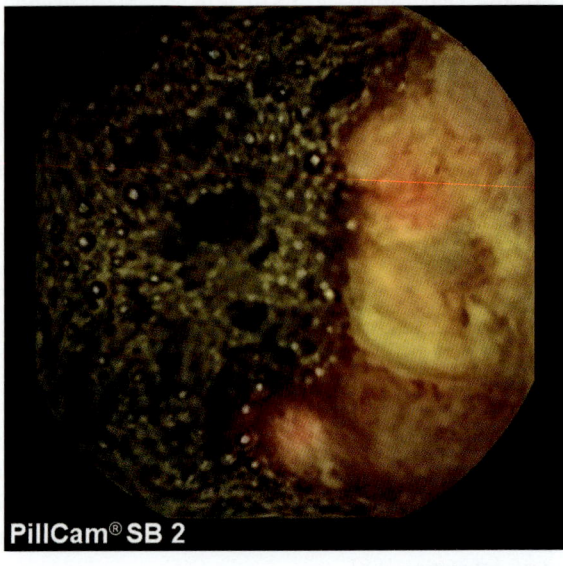

Fig. 41.11 B-cell lymphoma in a patient with warm antibody autoimmune hemolytic anemia seen as an ulcerated, stenosing mass. Capsule passage was delayed at this point

diagnosed malignant small bowel tumors in 380 consecutive patients who underwent SBCE [91]. The indication for SBCE in these 13 patients was mainly GI bleeding. Interestingly, these patients had undergone a total of 65 diagnostic procedures before SBCE. Six patients had a history of previous malignancies, including colonic adenocarcinoma, melanoma, chronic lymphocytic leukemia, and enteropathy-associated T-cell lymphoma. In 10 (77 %) of the 13 patients, SBCE was considered to have influenced the diagnosis and management. In the remaining patients, SBCE confirmed lesions already diagnosed by other imaging methods and

thus did not have an impact on the final diagnosis. Three patients with small bowel lymphoma were treated with chemotherapy, and two of them also had surgical resection of a stenosing segment. All other patients underwent radical tumor resection [91].

In a multicenter Korean study including a total of 1,332 SBCE procedures with all indications, small bowel tumors were diagnosed in 57 (4.3 %) [92]. The tumors were malignant in 33 cases and included adenocarcinomas, lymphomas, gastrointestinal stromal tumors (GISTs), and metastatic cancers. Of the 57 tumors, 30 were identified exclusively by SBCE (diagnostic impact=30/57); these tumors were smaller than the tumors detected using radiologic studies. Of the 33 malignant tumors, 9 were exclusively seen by SBCE and 7 patients underwent surgical resection (therapeutic impact=7/57). The 57 patients underwent a total of 182 diagnostic procedures prior to SBCE (average, 3.19 per patient). CT was performed in 36 patients (52.9 %). After SBCE, 28 sessions of additional gastrointestinal imaging were employed [92].

In a retrospective chart review of 500 patients who underwent SBCE for all indications, 20 small bowel tumors were detected (4 %) and 9 tumors turned out to be GISTs (45.0 %) (Fig. 41.3). In all these patients with newly diagnosed GIST, traditional endoscopic and radiologic imaging failed to detect the lesion. All patients underwent surgical treatment and showed normalized hemoglobin levels at follow-up [93].

The usefulness of CTE, small bowel enteroclysis, SBCE, and DAE for the diagnosis of small bowel tumors was evaluated in a large retrospective study [48]. CTE and small bowel enteroclysis had significantly lower diagnostic yields for the diagnosis of small bowel tumors (≤10 mm), but SBCE and DAE had high yields regardless of size. CTE had a significantly lower diagnostic yield of epithelial tumors than subepithelial tumors. The diagnostic yield of SBCE for small bowel tumors located only in the distal duodenum or the proximal jejunum (73 %) was significantly lower than for those located in other areas (90 %). SBCE and DAE had significantly higher diagnostic yields than CTE, and DAE had a significantly higher diagnostic yield than SBCE, but a combination of CTE and SBCE had a diagnostic yield similar to that of DAE. The histologic diagnostic yield of small bowel tumors by DAE was 92, and 25 % of the tumors were enteroscopically treated. Metastatic tumors had the poorest overall survival, followed by adenocarcinomas and malignant lymphomas [48].

A study including 390 patients with malignant melanoma was conducted in order to identify patients with small bowel metastasis (Fig. 41.12) [94]. All patients in stage I–III disease with a positive fecal occult blood test (FOBT) and/or anemia, as well as all patients in stage IV, were offered gastrointestinal panendoscopy. Small bowel metastases were detected in 28 % of patients in stage IV, 1.7 % in stage III, and 0 in stage I/II. In FOBT-positive patients, the detection rates of small bowel metastases were 72.7 % in stage IV,

14.3 % in stage III, and 0 % in stage I/II. In two patients (18 %), the diseased bowel segment was palliatively resected [94]. In these two patients, anemia was detected during follow-up, and small bowel endoscopy revealed recurrent small bowel metastases. In one case, the metastasis was again resected. Immunochemotherapy was initiated in all patients. Of 15 patients with stage IV disease, 6 (40 %) were found to have small bowel metastases, and palliative resection was done in 1 (7 %). Therefore, this study shows that in some patients, SBCE can lead to therapeutic consequences such as palliative resection of the metastasis or initiation of immunochemotherapy [94]. The authors concluded that small bowel metastases were more frequent in patients with advanced melanoma. The indication in patients with stage IV should be individually established, depending on the consequences. In patients with stage III disease, screening for intestinal blood loss by panendoscopy may help to identify small bowel metastases that can be treated, with improvement of quality of life and survival. More studies are needed to confirm these results.

41.6 Outcome in Celiac Disease

The main role of SBCE in celiac disease is for patients with known celiac disease who are symptomatic despite a gluten-free diet and in whom there is a suspected complication such as ulcerative jejunitis and associated T-cell lymphoma (Figs. 41.13, 41.14, and 41.15). In patients with refractory celiac disease, SBCE has led to the adjustment of immunosuppressive therapy and increased support for patients in achieving better dietary compliance [20]. Also, the improvement of the mucosal atrophy in response to therapy was confirmed for many authors [20, 94–96]. Furthermore, SBCE was proven to be helpful in the follow-up of patients after gluten-free diet in newly diagnosed celiac disease. Twelve months after starting a gluten-free diet, patients underwent symptom assessment, celiac serology, upper endoscopy, and SBCE. This SBCE demonstrated mucosal healing from distal to proximal, and the percentage of villous atrophy was significantly reduced, from 18 % to 3 %. This improvement of the villous

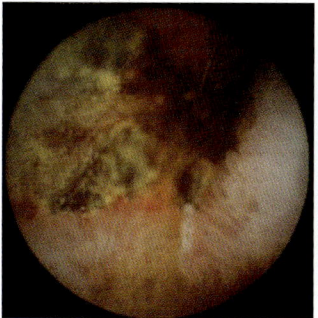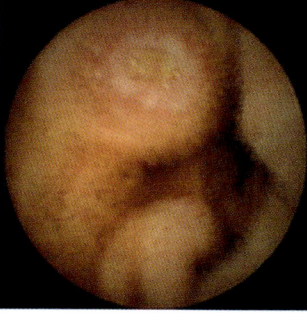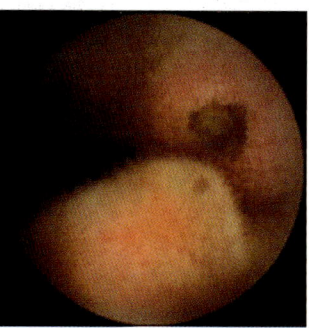

Fig. 41.12 Ulcerated pigmented lesions and ulcerated masses throughout the small bowel in a patient with metastatic melanoma

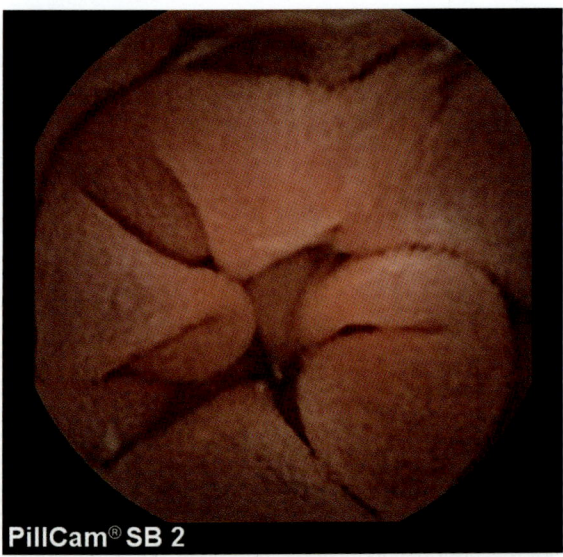

Fig. 41.13 Villous atrophy in a patient with celiac disease

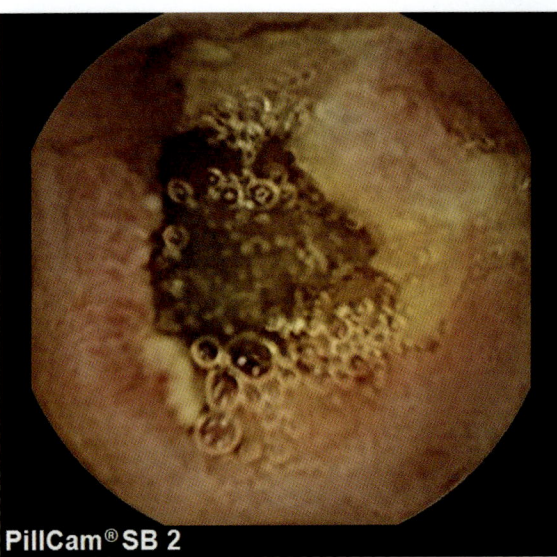

Fig. 41.15 T-cell lymphoma in a patient with refractory celiac disease (Courtesy of Carolina Olano, MD)

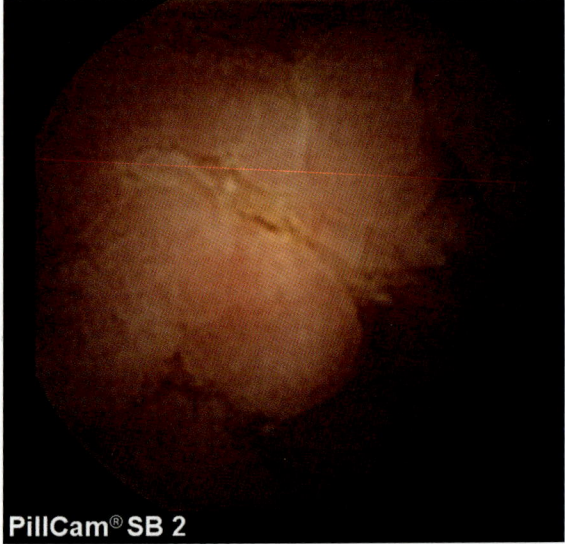

Fig. 41.14 Ulcerative jejunitis: Fissures and villous atrophy in a young patient with celiac disease despite a gluten-free diet

atrophy correlated with improvement of symptom score and reduction in immunoglobulin A-tTG levels. However, 42 % of patients had persistent villous abnormality as assessed by duodenal histology [21].

41.7 Outcomes in Less Frequent Clinical Settings

Several case reports have shown unsuspected lesions diagnosed by SBCE and missed by other techniques. The pathologies discovered by SBCE, resulting in an important change in the therapeutic approach, have included Whipple's disease, autoimmune enteropathy, Meckel's diverticulum, helminthiasis (*Ascaris lumbricoides*, *Enterobius vermicularis*, *Taenia saginata*), tuberculosis of the small bowel, graft-versus-host disease of the small bowel, Dieulafoy's lesion of the colon, radiation-induced enteritis, ileal ulcers in a long-distance runner, varices of the small bowel, and NSAID-induced diaphragms of the intestine (Figs. 41.16 and 41.17).

Soon SBCE will be able to analyze the small bowel effect of different drugs. As already mentioned, SBCE has been used to evaluate the effect of prokinetic drugs on small bowel transit time. Potential injury to the small bowel mucosa from the use of NSAIDs also has been investigated (Figs. 41.2 and 41.16). A study comparing two NSAIDs analyzed the effect on small bowel mucosa of celecoxib (a selective cyclooxygenase-2 inhibitor) versus loxoprofen (a nonselective NSAID), the most frequently used NSAIDs in Japan [97]. When given to healthy adults, 10 % of patients taking celecoxib experienced small bowel mucosal injury versus 70 % in the group taking loxoprofen [97]. Risk factors associated with NSAID-induced damage to the small intestine were also assessed using SBCE. A cross-sectional study was conducted in patients with rheumatoid arthritis. After taking NSAIDs for more than 3 months, SBCE showed severe small bowel mucosal damage in 28 % of patients, as well as significantly decreased hemoglobin levels. Independent risk factors for severe damage included age of 65 years or more and the use of a proton-pump inhibitor or a histamine H_2 receptor antagonist [98].

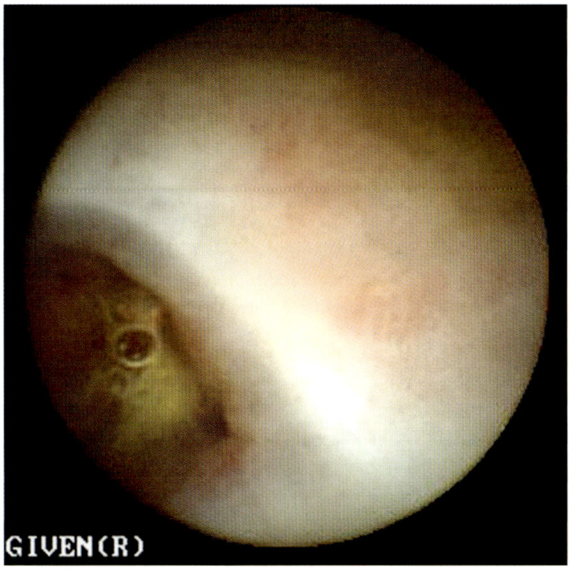

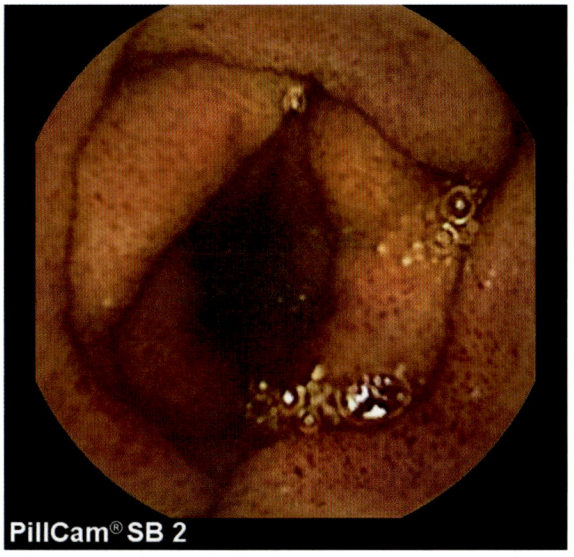

Fig. 41.16 Small bowel diaphragms seen in a patient with long-term NSAID use

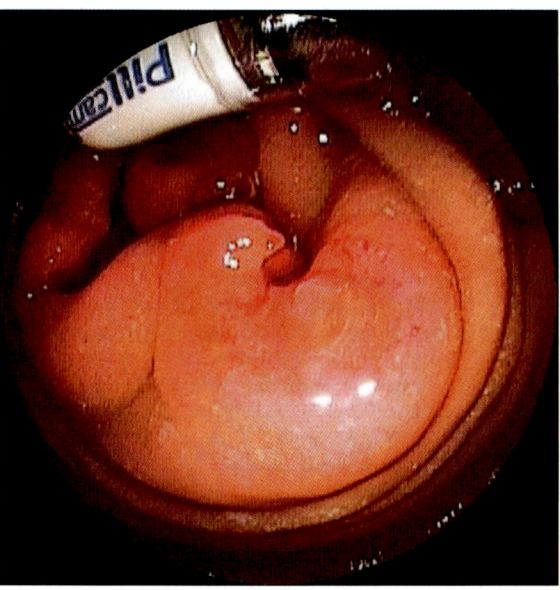

Fig. 41.17 Intramural hematomas in a patient with an overdose of the anticoagulant drug phenprocoumon and acute anemia

HIV-infected patients also may benefit from SBCE. The diagnostic yield of SBCE in HIV-infected patients was evaluated in a study that included 49 patients divided into three groups [22]: Group A included 19 HIV-positive patients with a CD4 cell count less than 200/μL and with GI symptoms, group B had 19 similar patients without GI symptoms, and a non-HIV control group comprised 11 healthy volunteers. In group A, there were a total of 30 pathologic findings, 15 of which had therapeutic implications. In group B, there were 22 pathologic findings, 5 of which were relevant for therapy. In group C, there were 13 pathologic findings, including 3 with therapeutic relevance. In 89 % (group A) versus 26 % (group B), pathologic

findings were detected distal to the ligament of Treitz, not within the reach of standard endoscopy. In this study, SBCE proved to be definitely helpful in providing additional information and influencing therapy in HIV-positive patients with a CD4 cell count less than 200/μL and GI symptoms [22].

The major complication of SBCE is capsule retention, occurring with an overall incidence of 1–2 % (Fig. 41.18) [23–25, 99]. In some circumstances, however, retention rates as high as 21 % have been reported, depending on the indication [99]. Even though retention is often asymptomatic, symptoms of small bowel obstruction may be present. The retained capsule can be retrieved using DAE [100], but sometimes surgery is necessary, with resection of the affected segment, called "therapeutic complication" [101]. A retrospective study that included data from 2,300 SBCE procedures showed capsule retention in 1.3 % (n=31) [25]. The risk factors for this capsule retention included known Crohn's disease and suspected tumor. Surgery was performed on 27 patients with retained capsule; acute obstructive symptoms and acute or subacute surgery occurred in six cases. Two patients died within days after surgery: One had widespread malignant disease and died of multiorgan failure. The second patient had an uneventful recovery until 6 days after surgery, when he suddenly died because of rupture of the anastomosis. One patient with CD and a stricture had the capsule retained for 2.5 years, and then spontaneous passage occurred. During this time, the patient was treated with TNF-alpha antibodies [25]. Capsule retention in patients with Crohn's disease can be clinically followed while the patient receives medical therapy, leading in many cases to excretion of the capsule [102].

Fig. 41.18 SBCE capsule retention in a patient with small bowel adenocarcinoma. The capsule was removed at the time of enteroscopy (Courtesy of Carolina Olano, MD)

41.8 Summary

SBCE has become an established method for the diagnosis of small bowel diseases. The diagnostic yield of SBCE ranges from 43 % to 92 %. In OGIB, SBCE is superior to other methods. The usefulness of SBCE for the diagnosis of suspected IBD has been also demonstrated. There is insufficient evidence to permit conclusions about the effect of SBCE on health outcomes for other clinical indications, but many studies have shown positive effects of SBCE on patient outcomes.

The practicing clinician should consider that even negative results can influence therapies and outcomes. A definite diagnosis has led to a change in management in up to 87 % of patients studied with SBCE, which in turn has an impact on patient outcomes. The issues of patient reassurance at having reached a diagnosis, patient preferences, and quality of life also need further evaluation in clinical outcomes. Thus, it is clear that patient outcomes are a very relevant standard for the assessment of the clinical utility of SBCE.

References

1. Raju GS, Gerson L, Das A, Lewis B. American Gastroenterological Association (AGA) Institute Technical Review on obscure gastrointestinal bleeding. Gastroenterology. 2007;133:1697–717.
2. Triester SL, Leighton JA, Leontiadis GI, et al. A meta-analysis of the yield of capsule endoscopy compared to other diagnostic modalities in patients with obscure gastrointestinal bleeding. Am J Gastroenterol. 2005;100:2407–18.
3. Koulaouzidis A, Rondonotti E, Giannakou A, Plevris JN. Diagnostic yield of small-bowel capsule endoscopy in patients with iron-deficiency anemia: a systematic review. Gastrointest Endosc. 2012; 76:983–92.
4. Milano A, Balatsinou C, Filippone A, et al. A prospective evaluation of iron deficiency anemia in the GI endoscopy setting: role of standard endoscopy, videocapsule endoscopy, and CT-enteroclysis. Gastrointest Endosc. 2011;73:1002–8.
5. Pennazio M, Santucci R, Rondonotti E, et al. Outcome of patients with obscure gastrointestinal bleeding after capsule endoscopy: report of 100 consecutive cases. Gastroenterology. 2004;126: 643–53.
6. Delvaux M, Fassler I, Gay G. Clinical usefulness of the endoscopic video capsule as the initial intestinal investigation in patients with obscure digestive bleeding: validation of a diagnostic strategy based on the patient outcome after 12 months. Endoscopy. 2004;36: 1067–73.
7. Estevez E, Gonzalez-Conde B, Vazquez-Iglesias JL, et al. Diagnostic yield and clinical outcomes after capsule endoscopy in 100 consecutive patients with obscure gastrointestinal bleeding. Eur J Gastroenterol Hepatol. 2006;18:881–8.
8. Costamagna G, Shah SK, Riccioni ME, et al. A prospective trial comparing small bowel radiographs and video capsule endoscopy for suspected small bowel disease. Gastroenterology. 2002;123: 999–1005.
9. Huprich JE, Fletcher JG, Fidler JL, et al. Prospective blinded comparison of wireless capsule endoscopy and multiphase CT enterography in obscure gastrointestinal bleeding. Radiology. 2011;260: 744–51.
10. Wiarda BM, Heine DGN, Mensink P, et al. Comparison of magnetic resonance enteroclysis and capsule endoscopy with balloon-assisted enteroscopy in patients with obscure gastrointestinal bleeding. Endoscopy. 2012;44:668–73.
11. Triester SL, Leighton JA, Leontiadis GI, et al. A meta-analysis of the yield of capsule endoscopy compared to other diagnostic modalities in patients with non-stricturing small bowel Crohn's disease. Am J Gastroenterol. 2006;101:954–64.
12. Eliakim R, Fischer D, Suissa A, et al. Wireless capsule video endoscopy is a superior diagnostic tool in comparison to barium follow-through and computerized tomography in patients with suspected Crohn's disease. Eur J Gastroenterol Hepatol. 2003;15: 363–7.
13. Fireman Z, Mahajna E, Broide E, et al. Diagnosing small bowel Crohn's disease with wireless capsule endoscopy. Gut. 2003;52: 390–2.
14. Liangpunsakul S, Chadalawada V, Rex DK, et al. Wireless capsule endoscopy detects small bowel ulcers in patients with normal results from state of the art enteroclysis. Am J Gastroenterol. 2003;98:1295–8.
15. Herrerias JM, Caunedo A, Rodriguez-Tellez M, et al. Capsule endoscopy in patients with suspected Crohn's disease and negative endoscopy. Endoscopy. 2003;35:564–8.
16. Caspari R, von Falkenhausen M, Krautmacher C, et al. Comparison of capsule endoscopy and magnetic resonance imaging for the detection of polyps of the small intestine in patients with familial adenomatous polyposis or with Peutz-Jeghers' syndrome. Endoscopy. 2004;36:1054–9.
17. Ohmiya N, Nakamura M, Takenaka H, et al. Management of small-bowel polyps in Peutz-Jeghers syndrome by using enteroclysis, double-balloon enteroscopy, and videocapsule endoscopy. Gastrointest Endosc. 2010;72:1209–16.
18. Katsinelos P, Fasoulas K, Beltsis A, et al. Diagnostic yield and clinical impact of wireless capsule endoscopy in patients with chronic abdominal pain with or without diarrhea: a Greek multicenter study. Eur J Intern Med. 2011;22:e63–6.
19. Kurien M, Evans KE, Aziz I, et al. Capsule endoscopy in adult celiac disease: a potential role in equivocal cases of celiac disease? Gastrointest Endosc. 2013;77:227–32.
20. Collin P, Rondonotti E, Lundin KE, et al. Video capsule endoscopy in celiac disease: current clinical practice. J Dig Dis. 2012;13:94–9.
21. Lidums I, Teo E, Field J, Cummins AG. Capsule endoscopy: a valuable tool in the follow-up of people with celiac disease on a gluten-free diet. Clin Transl Gastroenterol. 2011;2:e4.
22. Oette M, Stelzer A, Göbels K, et al. Wireless capsule endoscopy for the detection of small bowel diseases in HIV-1-infected patients. Eur J Med Res. 2009;14:191–4.
23. Chami G, Raza M, Bernstein CN. Usefulness and impact on management of positive and negative capsule endoscopy. Can J Gastroenterol. 2007;21:577–81.
24. Barkin JS, O'Loughlin C. Capsule endoscopy contraindications: complications and how to avoid their occurrence. Gastrointest Endosc Clin N Am. 2004;14:61–5.
25. Höög CM, Bark LÅ, Arkani J, et al. Capsule retentions and incomplete capsule endoscopy examinations: an analysis of 2300 examinations. Gastroenterol Res Pract. 2012;2012:518718.
26. Rastogi A, Schoen RE, Slivka A. Diagnostic yield and clinical outcomes of capsule endoscopy. Gastrointest Endosc. 2004;60: 959–64.
27. Saurin JC, Delvaux M, Gaudin JL, et al. Diagnostic value of endoscopic capsule in patients with obscure digestive bleeding: blinded comparison with video push-enteroscopy. Endoscopy. 2003;35: 576–84.
28. Neu B, Ell C, May A, et al. Capsule endoscopy versus standard tests in influencing management of obscure digestive bleeding:

results from a German multicenter trial. Am J Gastroenterol. 2005;100:1736–42.

29. Lewis BS. Small intestinal bleeding. Gastroenterol Clin North Am. 1994;23:67–91.

30. Lewis BS, Swain P. Capsule endoscopy in the evaluation of patients with suspected small intestinal bleeding: results of a pilot study. Gastrointest Endosc. 2002;56:349–53.

31. Ell C, Remke S, May A, et al. The first prospective controlled trial comparing wireless capsule endoscopy with push enteroscopy in chronic gastrointestinal bleeding. Endoscopy. 2002;34:685–9.

32. Mata A, Bordas JM, Feu F, et al. Wireless capsule endoscopy in patients with obscure gastrointestinal bleeding: a comparative study with push enteroscopy. Aliment Pharmacol Ther. 2004;20:189–94.

33. Hartmann D, Schmidt H, Schilling D, et al. Follow-up of patients with obscure gastrointestinal bleeding after capsule endoscopy and intraoperative enteroscopy. Hepatogastroenterology. 2007;54: 780–3.

34. Zhang B, Jiang L, Chen C, et al. Diagnosis of obscure gastrointestinal hemorrhage with capsule endoscopy in combination with multiple-detector computed tomography. J Gastroenterol Hepatol. 2010;25:75–9.

35. Khalife S, Soyer P, Alatawi A, et al. Obscure gastrointestinal bleeding: preliminary comparison of 64-section CT enteroclysis with video capsule endoscopy. Eur Radiol. 2011;21:79–86.

36. Saperas E, Dot J, Videla S, et al. Capsule endoscopy versus computed tomographic or standard angiography for the diagnosis of obscure gastrointestinal bleeding. Am J Gastroenterol. 2007;102:731–7.

37. Voderholzer WA, Ortner M, Rogalla P, et al. Diagnostic yield of wireless capsule enteroscopy in comparison with computed tomography enteroclysis. Endoscopy. 2003;35:1009–14.

38. Heo HM, Park CH, Lim JS, et al. The role of capsule endoscopy after negative CT enterography in patients with obscure gastrointestinal bleeding. Eur Radiol. 2012;22:1159–66.

39. Apostolopoulos P, Liatsos C, Gralnek IM, et al. The role of wireless capsule endoscopy in investigating unexplained iron deficiency anemia after negative endoscopic evaluation of the upper and lower gastrointestinal tract. Endoscopy. 2006;38:1127–32.

40. Riccioni ME, Urgesi R, Spada C, et al. Unexplained iron deficiency anaemia: is it worthwhile to perform capsule endoscopy? Dig Liver Dis. 2010;42:560–6.

41. Holleran GE, Barry SA, Thornton OJ, et al. The use of small bowel capsule endoscopy in iron deficiency anaemia: low impact on outcome in the medium term despite high diagnostic yield. Eur J Gastroenterol Hepatol. 2013;25:327–32.

42. Tang SJ, Christodoulou D, Zanati S, et al. Wireless capsule endoscopy for obscure gastrointestinal bleeding: a single-centre, one-year experience. Can J Gastroenterol. 2004;18:559–65.

43. Fry LC, Bellutti M, Neumann H, et al. Incidence of bleeding lesions within reach of conventional upper and lower endoscopes in patients undergoing double-balloon enteroscopy for obscure gastrointestinal bleeding. Aliment Pharmacol Ther. 2009;29:342–9.

44. Yamada A, Watabe H, Kobayashi Y, et al. Timing of capsule endoscopy influences the diagnosis and outcome in obscure-overt gastrointestinal bleeding. Hepatogastroenterology. 2012;59:676–9.

45. Marmo R, Rotondano G, Casetti T, et al. Degree of concordance between double-balloon enteroscopy and capsule endoscopy in obscure gastrointestinal bleeding: a multicenter study. Endoscopy. 2009;41:587–92.

46. Shishido T, Oka S, Tanaka S, et al. Diagnostic yield of capsule endoscopy vs double-balloon endoscopy for patients who have undergone total enteroscopy with obscure gastrointestinal bleeding. Hepatogastroenterology. 2012;59:955–9.

47. Teshima CW, Kuipers EJ, van Zanten SV, Mensink PBF. Double balloon enteroscopy and capsule endoscopy for obscure gastrointestinal bleeding: an updated meta-analysis. J Gastroenterol Hepatol. 2011;26:796–801.

48. Honda W, Ohmiya N, Hirooka Y, et al. Enteroscopic and radiologic diagnoses, treatment, and prognoses of small-bowel tumors. Gastrointest Endosc. 2012;76:344–54.

49. Mönkemüller K, Neumann H, Meyer F, et al. A retrospective analysis of emergency double-balloon enteroscopy for small-bowel bleeding. Endoscopy. 2009;41:715–7.

50. Fujimori S, Seo T, Gudis K, et al. Diagnosis and treatment of obscure gastrointestinal bleeding using combined capsule endoscopy and double balloon endoscopy: 1-year follow-up study. Endoscopy. 2007;39:1053–8.

51. Albert JG, Schulbe R, Hahn L, et al. Impact of capsule endoscopy on outcome in mid-intestinal bleeding: a multicentre cohort study in 285 patients. Eur J Gastroenterol Hepatol. 2008;20: 971–7.

52. Hindryckx P, Botelberge T, De Vos M, De Looze D. Clinical impact of capsule endoscopy on further strategy and long-term clinical outcome in patients with obscure bleeding. Gastrointest Endosc. 2008;68:98–104.

53. Apostolopoulos P, Liatsos C, Gralnek IM, et al. Evaluation of capsule endoscopy in active, mild-to-moderate, overt, obscure GI bleeding. Gastrointest Endosc. 2007;66:1174–81.

54. Iwamoto J, Mizokami Y, Shimokobe K, et al. The clinical outcome of capsule endoscopy in patients with obscure gastrointestinal bleeding. Hepatogastroenterology. 2011;58:301–5.

55. May A, Friesing-Sosnik T, Manner H, et al. Long-term outcome after argon plasma coagulation of small-bowel lesions using double-balloon enteroscopy in patients with mid-gastrointestinal bleeding. Endoscopy. 2011;43:759–65.

56. Samaha E, Rahmi G, Landi B, et al. Long-term outcome of patients treated with double balloon enteroscopy for small bowel vascular lesions. Am J Gastroenterol. 2012;107:240–6.

57. Eliakim R, Suissa A, Yassin K, et al. Wireless capsule video endoscopy compared to barium follow-through and computerised tomography in patients with suspected Crohn's disease–final report. Dig Liver Dis. 2004;36:519–22.

58. Voderholzer WA, Beinhoelzl J, Rogalla P, et al. Small bowel involvement in Crohn's disease: a prospective comparison of wireless capsule endoscopy and computed tomography enteroclysis. Gut. 2005;54:369–73.

59. Albert JG, Martiny F, Krummenerl A, et al. Diagnosis of small bowel Crohn's disease: a prospective comparison of capsule endoscopy with magnetic resonance imaging and fluoroscopic enteroclysis. Gut. 2005;54:1721–7.

60. Golder SK, Schreyer AG, Endlicher E, et al. Comparison of capsule endoscopy and magnetic resonance (MR) enteroclysis in suspected small bowel disease. Int J Colorectal Dis. 2006;21: 97–104.

61. Hara AK, Leighton JA, Heigh RI, et al. Crohn disease of the small bowel: preliminary comparison among CT enterography, capsule endoscopy, small-bowel follow-through, and ileoscopy. Radiology. 2006;238:128–34.

62. Solem CA, Loftus EVJ, Fletcher JG, et al. Small-bowel imaging in Crohn's disease: a prospective, blinded, 4-way comparison trial. Gastrointest Endosc. 2008;68:255–66.

63. Tillack C, Seiderer J, Brand S, et al. Correlation of magnetic resonance enteroclysis (MRE) and wireless capsule endoscopy (CE) in the diagnosis of small bowel lesions in Crohn's disease. Inflamm Bowel Dis. 2008;14:1219–28.

64. Böcker U, Dinter D, Litterer C, et al. Comparison of magnetic resonance imaging and video capsule enteroscopy in diagnosing small-bowel pathology: localization-dependent diagnostic yield. Scand J Gastroenterol. 2010;45:490–500.

65. Jensen MD, Nathan T, Rafaelsen SR, Kjeldsen J. Diagnostic accuracy of capsule endoscopy for small bowel Crohn's disease is superior to that of MR enterography or CT enterography. Clin Gastroenterol Hepatol. 2011;9:124–9.

66. Casciani E, Masselli G, Di Nardo G, et al. MR enterography versus capsule endoscopy in paediatric patients with suspected Crohn's disease. Eur Radiol. 2011;21:823–31.

67. Dionisio PM, Gurudu SR, Leighton JA, et al. Capsule endoscopy has a significantly higher diagnostic yield in patients with suspected and established small-bowel Crohn's disease: a meta-analysis. Am J Gastroenterol. 2010;105:1240–8.

68. Adler SN, Yoav M, Eitan S, et al. Does capsule endoscopy have an added value in patients with perianal disease and a negative work up for Crohn's disease? World J Gastrointest Endosc. 2012; 4:185–8.

69. Mow WS, Lo SK, Targan SR, et al. Initial experience with wireless capsule enteroscopy in the diagnosis and management of inflammatory bowel disease. Clin Gastroenterol Hepatol. 2004; 2:31–40.

70. Chong AK, Taylor A, Miller A, et al. Capsule endoscopy vs push enteroscopy and enteroclysis in suspected small-bowel Crohn's disease. Gastrointest Endosc. 2005;61:255–61.

71. Dussault C, Gower-Rousseau C, Salleron J, et al. Small bowel capsule endoscopy for management of Crohn's disease: a retrospective tertiary care centre experience. Dig Liver Dis. 2013;45:558–61.

72. Albert JG, Kotsch J, Köstler W, et al. Course of Crohn's disease prior to establishment of the diagnosis. Z Gastroenterol. 2008; 46:187–92.

73. Tukey M, Pleskow D, Legnani P, et al. The utility of capsule endoscopy in patients with suspected Crohn's disease. Am J Gastroenterol. 2009;104:2734–9.

74. Maunoury V, Savoye G, Bourreille A, et al. Value of wireless capsule endoscopy in patients with indeterminate colitis (inflammatory bowel disease type unclassified). Inflamm Bowel Dis. 2007;13: 152–5.

75. Liao Z, Gao R, Xu C, Li Z. Indications and detection, completion, and retention rates of small-bowel capsule endoscopy: a systematic review. Gastrointest Endosc. 2010;71:280–6.

76. Burri E, Beglinger C. Faecal calprotectin – a useful tool in the management of inflammatory bowel disease. Swiss Med Wkly. 2012;142:w13557.

77. Koulaouzidis A, Douglas S, Rogers MA, et al. Fecal calprotectin: a selection tool for small bowel capsule endoscopy in suspected IBD with prior negative bi-directional endoscopy. Scand J Gastroenterol. 2011;46:561–6.

78. Sipponen T, Haapamaki J, Savilahti E, et al. Fecal calprotectin and S100A12 have low utility in prediction of small bowel Crohn's disease detected by wireless capsule endoscopy. Scand J Gastroenterol. 2012;47:778–84.

79. Keuchel M, Hagenmüller F. Video capsule endoscopy in the workup of abdominal pain. Gastrointest Endosc Clin N Am. 2004;14:195–205.

80. Bardan E, Nadler M, Chowers Y, et al. Capsule endoscopy for the evaluation of patients with chronic abdominal pain. Endoscopy. 2003;35:688–9.

81. Fry LC, Carey EJ, Shiff AD, et al. The yield of capsule endoscopy in patients with abdominal pain or diarrhea. Endoscopy. 2006;38:498–502.

82. De Bona M, Bellumat A, Cian E, et al. Capsule endoscopy findings in patients with suspected Crohn's disease and biochemical markers of inflammation. Dig Liver Dis. 2006;38:331–5.

83. Valle J, Alcántara M, Pérez-Grueso MJ, et al. Clinical features of patients with negative results from traditional diagnostic work-up and Crohn's disease findings from capsule endoscopy. J Clin Gastroenterol. 2006;40:692–6.

84. Fidder HH, Nadler M, Lahat A, et al. The utility of capsule endoscopy in the diagnosis of Crohn's disease based on patient's symptoms. J Clin Gastroenterol. 2007;41:384–7.

85. Shim KN, Kim YS, Kim KJ, et al. Abdominal pain accompanied by weight loss may increase the diagnostic yield of capsule endoscopy: a Korean multicenter study. Scand J Gastroenterol. 2006;41:983–8.

86. May A, Manner H, Schneider M, et al. Prospective multicenter trial of capsule endoscopy in patients with chronic abdominal pain, diarrhea and other signs and symptoms (CEDAP-Plus Study). Endoscopy. 2007;39:606–12.

87. Mele C, Infantolino A, Conn M, et al. The diagnostic yield of wireless capsule endoscope in patients with unexplained abdominal pain. Am J Gastroenterol. 2003;98:S298.

88. Nakamura M, Ohmiya N, Miyahara R, et al. Are symptomatic changes in irritable bowel syndrome correlated with the capsule endoscopy transit time? A pilot study using the 5-HT4 receptor agonist mosapride. Hepatogastroenterology. 2011;58:453–8.

89. Hooks 3rd SB, Rutland TJ, Di Palma JA. Lubiprostone neither decreases gastric and small-bowel transit time nor improves visualization of small bowel for capsule endoscopy: a double-blind, placebo-controlled study. Gastrointest Endosc. 2009;70:942–6.

90. Soares J, Lopes L, Vilas Boas G, Pinho C. Wireless capsule endoscopy for evaluation of phenotypic expression of small-bowel polyps in patients with Peutz-Jeghers' syndrome and in symptomatic first-degree relatives. Endoscopy. 2004;36:1060–6.

91. Spada C, Riccioni ME, Familiari P, et al. Video capsule endoscopy in small-bowel tumours: a single centre experience. Scand J Gastroenterol. 2008;43:497–505.

92. Cheung DY, Lee IS, Chang DK, et al. Capsule endoscopy in small bowel tumors: a multicenter Korean study. J Gastroenterol Hepatol. 2010;25:1079–86.

93. Urgesi R, Riccioni ME, Bizzotto A, et al. Increased diagnostic yield of small bowel tumors with PillCam: the role of capsule endoscopy in the diagnosis and treatment of gastrointestinal stromal tumors (GISTs). Italian single-center experience. Tumori. 2012;98:357–63.

94. Albert JG, Fiedler E, Marsch WC, Helmbold P. Consequences of detecting small bowel metastasis of malignant melanoma by capsule endoscopy. Am J Gastroenterol. 2008;103:244–5.

95. Katsinelos P, Fasoylas K, Chatzimavroudis G, et al. Diagnostic yield and clinical management after capsule endoscopy in daily clinical practice: a single-center experience. Hippokratia. 2010;14: 271–6.

96. Murray JA, Rubio-Tapia A, Van Dyke CT, et al. Mucosal atrophy in celiac disease: extent of involvement, correlation with clinical presentation, and response to treatment. Clin Gastroenterol Hepatol. 2008;6:186–93.

97. Mizukami K, Murakami K, Yamauchi M, et al. Evaluation of selective cyclooxygenase-2 inhibitor-induced small bowel injury: randomized cross-over study compared with loxoprofen in healthy subjects. Dig Endosc. 2013;25:288–94.

98. Watanabe T, Tanigawa T, Nadatani Y, et al. Risk factors for severe nonsteroidal anti-inflammatory drug-induced small intestinal damage. Dig Liver Dis. 2013;45:390–5.

99. Karagiannis S, Faiss S, Mavrogiannis C. Capsule retention: a feared complication of wireless capsule endoscopy. Scand J Gastroenterol. 2009;44:1158–65.

100. Lee BI, Choi H, Choi KY, et al. Retrieval of a retained capsule endoscope by double-balloon enteroscopy. Gastrointest Endosc. 2005;62:463–5.

101. Cheifetz AS, Lewis BS. Capsule endoscopy retention: is it a complication? J Clin Gastroenterol. 2006;40:688–91.

102. Figueiredo P, Almeida N, Lopes S, et al. Small-bowel capsule endoscopy in patients with suspected Crohn's disease—diagnostic value and complications. Diagn Ther Endosc. 2010;2010:pii: 101284.

Esophageal Capsule Endoscopy

42

Rami Eliakim and Virender K. Sharma

Contents

42.1 Technique and Application

The esophageal video capsule (PillCam ESO; Given Imaging Ltd, Yoqneam, Israel) is a capsule developed for visualization of esophageal disorders, similar in design to the small bowel capsule developed by Given Imaging (Fig. 42.1). A feasibility study found it to have high sensitivity, specificity, positive predictive value (PPV), and negative predictive value (NPV); a subsequent prospective, international seven-center study confirmed the earlier results [1]. These studies led to US Food and Drug Administration clearance of the new capsule for clinical use in 2004. Later studies demonstrated similar sensitivity and specificity rates in detecting esophageal varices [2, 3]. Over the years, more studies were conducted on both Barrett's esophagus and the detection and grading of esophageal varices, with sensitivity rates around 80–85 % and specificities around 90 %, slightly lower than rates for optical endoscopy that were published earlier [4, 5]. A second generation of the capsule was developed, which captures more frames per second and has a broader angle of view (Fig. 42.2).

The work was first published in 2006 by Springer Medizin Verlag Heidelberg with the following title: *Atlas of Video Capsule Endoscopy*.

R. Eliakim (✉)
Department of Gastroenterology, Sheba Medical Center, Sackler School of Medicine, Tel-Aviv University, Tel-Hashomer, Israel
e-mail: abraham.eliakim@sheba.health.gov.il

V.K. Sharma
Arizona Digestive Health, Gilbert, AZ, USA
e-mail: vksharma@azcdh.com

M. Keuchel et al. (eds.), *Video Capsule Endoscopy: A Reference Guide and Atlas*,
DOI 10.1007/978-3-662-44062-9_42, © Springer-Verlag Berlin Heidelberg 2014

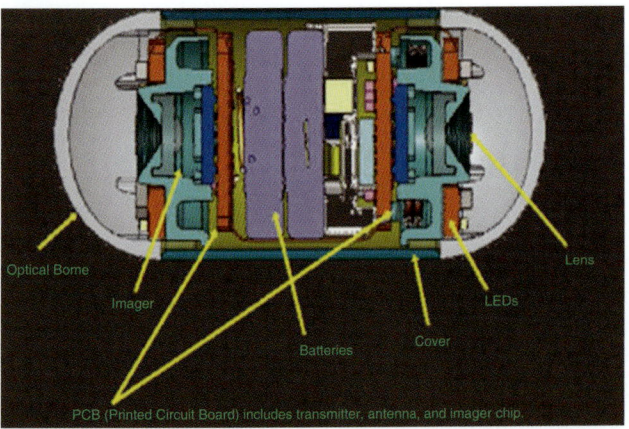

Fig. 42.1 A view of PillCam ESO. (Courtesy of Given Imaging Ltd, Yoqneam, Israel)

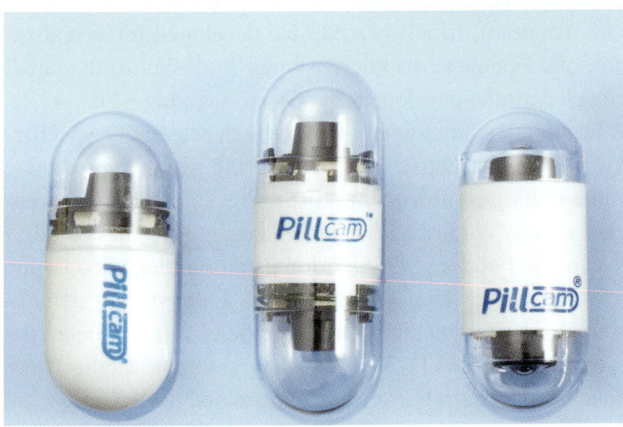

Fig. 42.2 A view of the new PillCam ESO2 capsule (*right*) as compared to PillCam SB2 (*left*) and PillCam Colon2 (*middle*)

Table 42.1 Technical specifications of PillCam ESO2

Height 11 mm, width 26 mm, weight 3.7 g
2 cameras, 3 lenses each
Field of view 169°, magnification 1:8 at both sides
Advanced illumination control
18 frames/s
Operating time 30 min

Given Imaging Ltd., Yoqneam, Israel

42.2 Technology

The new capsule differs from the conventional small bowel capsule in that it has two optical domes at either end of the capsule (Fig. 42.1, Table 42.1). When the capsule is activated, three light-emitting diodes (LEDs) emit a strobe light at the rate of 9 flashes per second from each end (18 total flashes per second) (Fig. 42.2). All the other elements and transmission techniques of this capsule are similar to the small bowel capsule. Normal esophageal capsule operating time is 30 min.

42.3 Procedure

The procedure for use of the esophageal capsule is markedly different from the procedure for the traditional small bowel capsule. There is no need for more than an hour of fasting. Three sensors are attached to the patient's chest, from the xyphoid upwards (Fig. 42.3). After first drinking water, the patient swallows the PillCam ESO in the left lateral decubitus position in order to prolong esophageal passage time (Fig. 42.4) [6]. The swallowing portion of the procedure lasts up to 7 min, and when the capsule is seen in the stomach (using the real-time viewer attached to the data recorder), the patient can stand; after a total of 30 min or when the battery wears out, the sensors and recorder are disconnected and the patient is discharged. The recorder is downloaded into a computer analysis program (Rapid 7 or Rapid 8 system), and the data are read, with the two separate camera images simultaneously displayed on the screen (Figs. 42.5 and 42.6). During the review process, the reviewer can mark specific image frames (thumbnails) and save them, as in the small bowel procedure. The same images can be saved to the final written report and provide a complete summary for the patient file. Additionally, the entire video image can be saved in an audio video interleave (AVI) format.

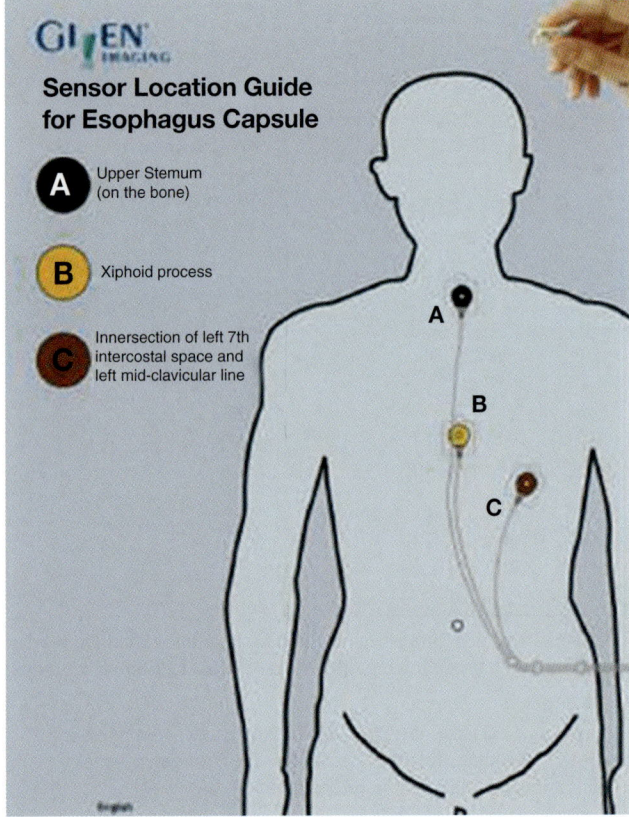

Fig. 42.3 Sensor location guide for PillCam ESO (Courtesy of Given Imaging)

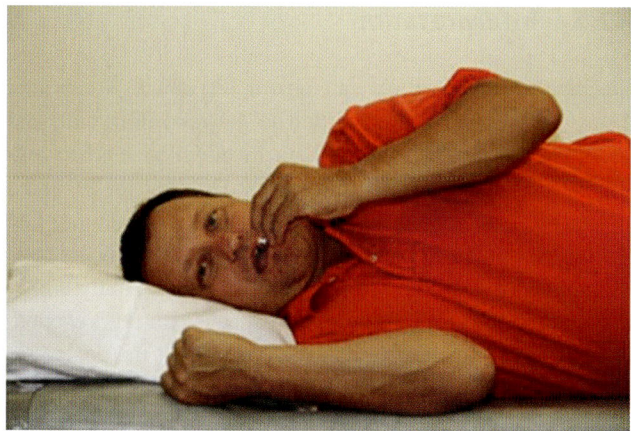

Patient ingests capsule while lying
on right side

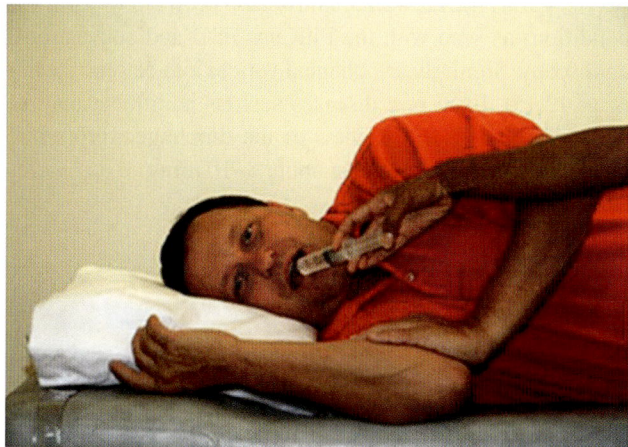

Capsule propelled by water
(15ml every 30 sec)

Fig. 42.4 The simplified swallowing procedure for PillCam ESO (Courtesy of Given Imaging)

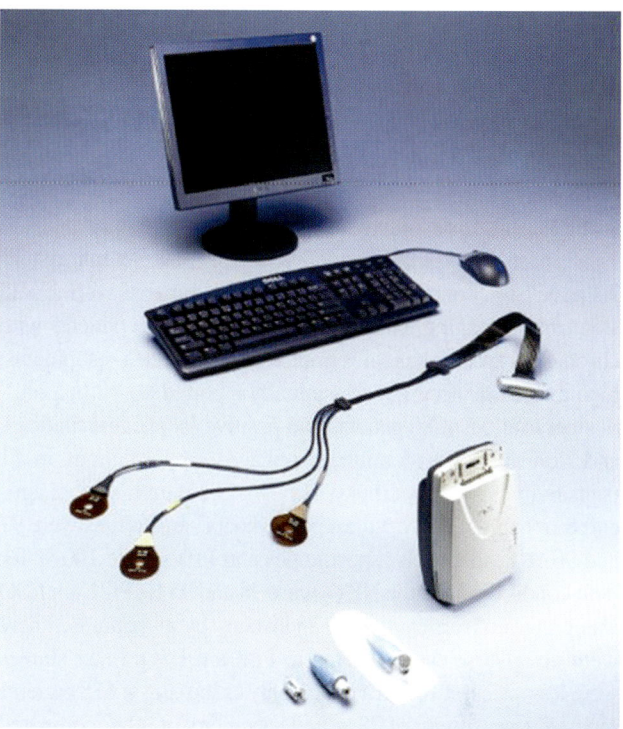

Fig. 42.5 Capsule endoscopy equipment. *Front left:* ESO capsule, capsule in holder, blister. *Front right:* DR 2C data recorder with integrated power supply. *Middle:* three sensor areas. *Rear:* workstation (Courtesy of Given Imaging)

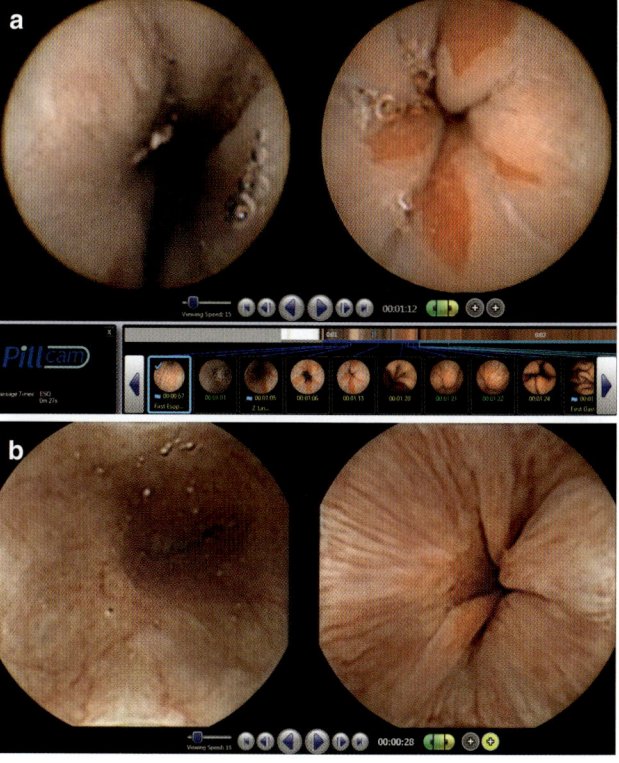

Fig. 42.6 (**a**) The RAPID 8.0 screen. (**b**) *Left* camera showing normal esophagus and *right* camera showing normal Z line

Impediments to visualization with PillCam ESO include bubbles, food residue, and rapid transit across the esophagogastric junction. The water swallowed just prior to the procedure and breathing through an open mouth after swallowing (to prevent swallowing more saliva) is meant to reduce the number of bubbles during the procedure. The use of the simplified ingestion procedure decreases the number of procedures in which the view is obscured by bubbles and allows better evaluation of the esophagogastric junction.

Space requirements for use of the PillCam ESO are similar to those for use of the small bowel capsule. The only additional equipment needed is a bed. The patient is discharged 20 min after swallowing the capsule and returns to the doctor's office only to consult with the physician about the results of the examination.

42.4   Application of PillCam ESO

There are three main indications for the use of the
PillCam ESO:

- Screening for esophagitis
- Screening for Barrett's esophagus
- Screening for esophageal varices

Because this type of capsule is relatively new, not many studies have been completed with it. When compared with a gold
standard of imaging with traditional endoscopy in patients with
chronic gastroesophageal symptoms or Barrett's esophagus,
high diagnostic accuracy was initially reported [1, 7]. In a multicenter trial, 55 of 80 patients had positive esophageal findings,
and PillCam ESO identified esophageal abnormalities in 51
(sensitivity, 93 %; specificity, 100 %). For Barrett's esophagus
and esophagitis, the capsule's per protocol sensitivities were 97
and 90 %, respectively; specificities and PPVs were 100 % for
both conditions; and the NPVs were 98 and 95 %. PillCam ESO
was preferred over traditional endoscopy by all patients. There
were no adverse events related to PillCam ESO. Later studies
were less successful, and a meta-analysis looking at 618 patients
reported a sensitivity of 78 % and specificity of 90 % compared
with traditional endoscopy for the diagnosis of Barrett's esophagus [5]. Pilot studies assessing the accuracy of the new capsule
in visualizing varices in patients with chronic liver disease
revealed very promising results [2]. These were followed by a
big, prospective multicenter trial of 288 patients, in which the
sensitivity of the capsule for detecting varices was 84 % and the
specificity was 88 %, with optical esophagoscopy serving as the
gold standard [3]. A meta-analysis looking at 446 patients found
a pooled sensitivity of 86 % and specificity of 81 % compared
with regular endoscopy [4].

The patient should be informed about the conduct of the
procedure and its associated risks and contraindications,
which are no different from those of the small bowel capsule:

- Dysphagia
- Zenker's diverticulum
- Strictures of the gastrointestinal tract
- Electronic implants
- Pregnancy
- Planned MRI within the near future

All limitations and possible complications mentioned in
Chaps. 4 and 40 are also relevant to the esophageal capsule.

A printed information sheet should be provided and a
written informed consent form signed prior to the beginning
of the procedure.

42.5   Interpretation

During the procedure, a mean of over 700 images is captured
from the esophagus, transmitted to the recording unit, and
recorded on its hard disk. The data are downloaded to a computer using a special software system (Rapid 7 or 8), and a
digital video is created. The video playback can be controlled
on the computer. Images from both camera heads are seen
simultaneously on the screen (Fig. 42.6), potentially allowing measurement of the length of suspected Barrett's esophagus or of a hiatus hernia, although the use of the device for
this purpose has yet to be established. Clear views of the
esophagus (Fig. 42.7), Z line (squamocolumnar junction,
Fig. 42.8), and pathologies such as esophagitis and suspected
Barrett's esophagus can often be obtained. Figures 42.9,
42.10, 42.11, 42.12, 42.13, and 42.14 show views of these
conditions as seen with the PillCam ESO and conventional
endoscopy. Similarly, esophageal varices can be seen clearly
(Fig. 42.15). Even rare diseases such as papilloma may be
detected (Fig. 42.16). Review of the esophageal procedure
generally takes the physician about 8–10 min.

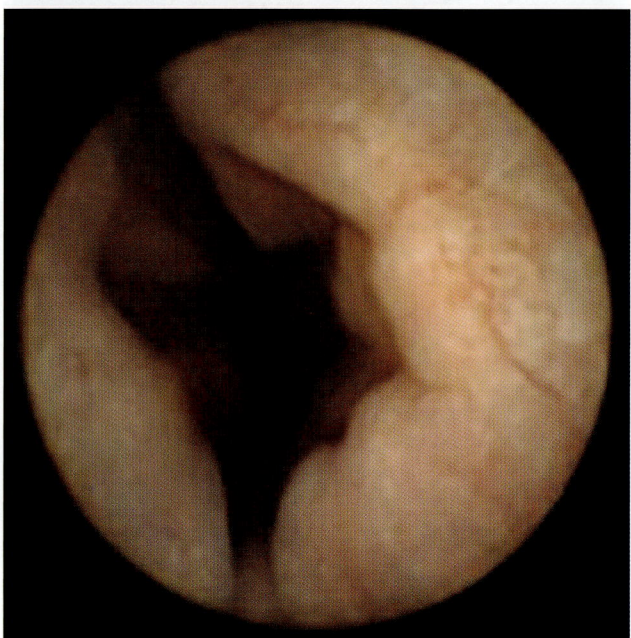

Fig. 42.7 A longitudinal view of a normal esophagus captured by
PillCam ESO

Fig. 42.8 Images of a normal Z line captured by PillCam ESO

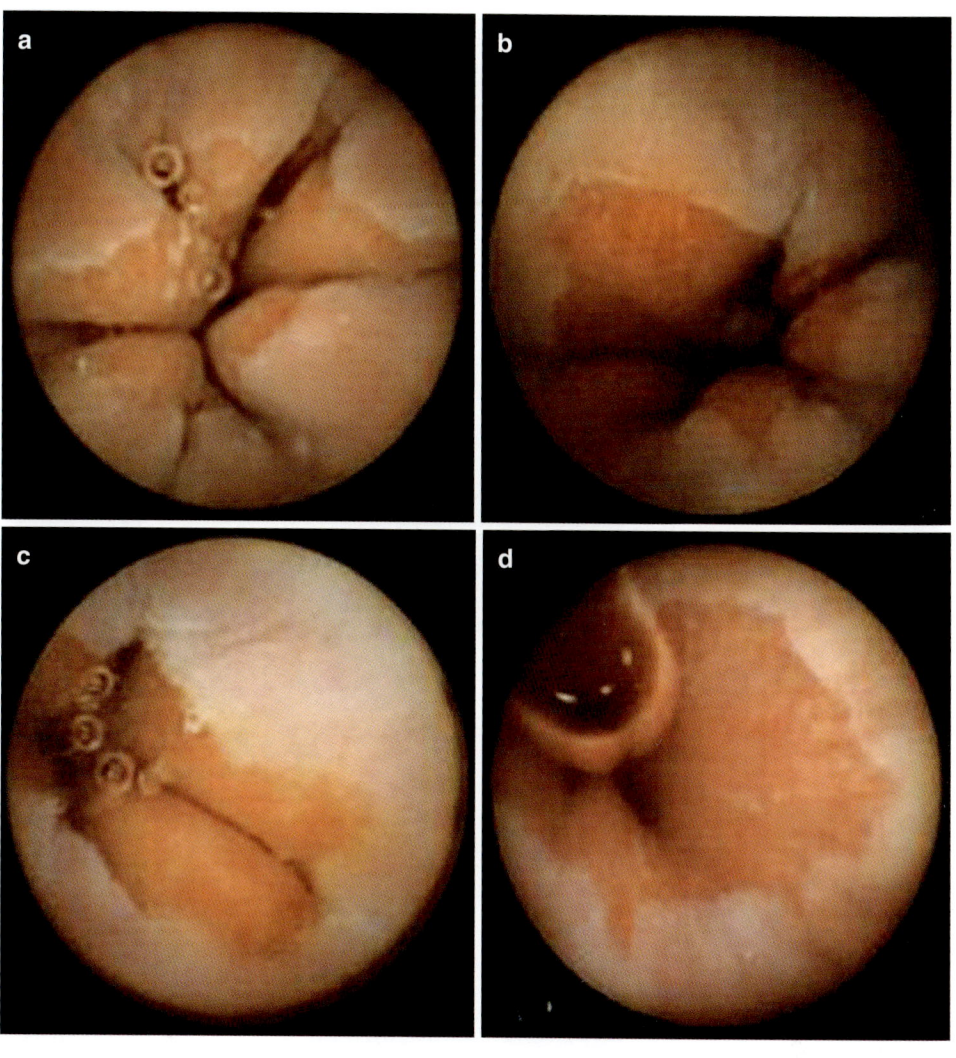

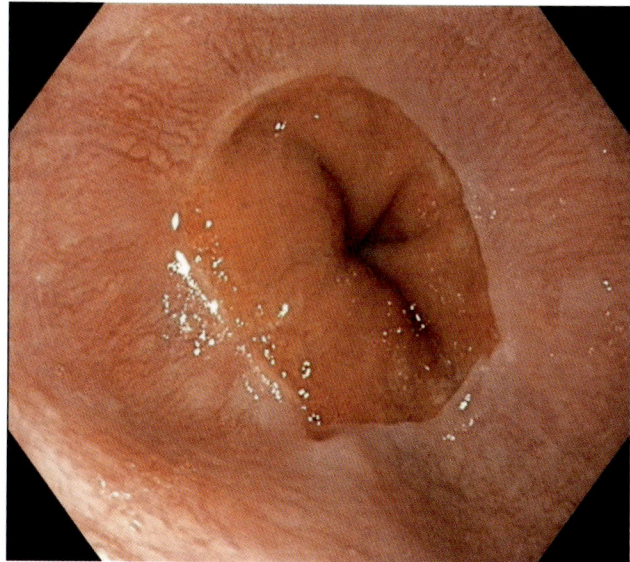

Fig. 42.9 A normal Z line as seen on traditional endoscopy

Fig. 42.10 (**a–d**) Images of esophagitis captured by PillCam ESO

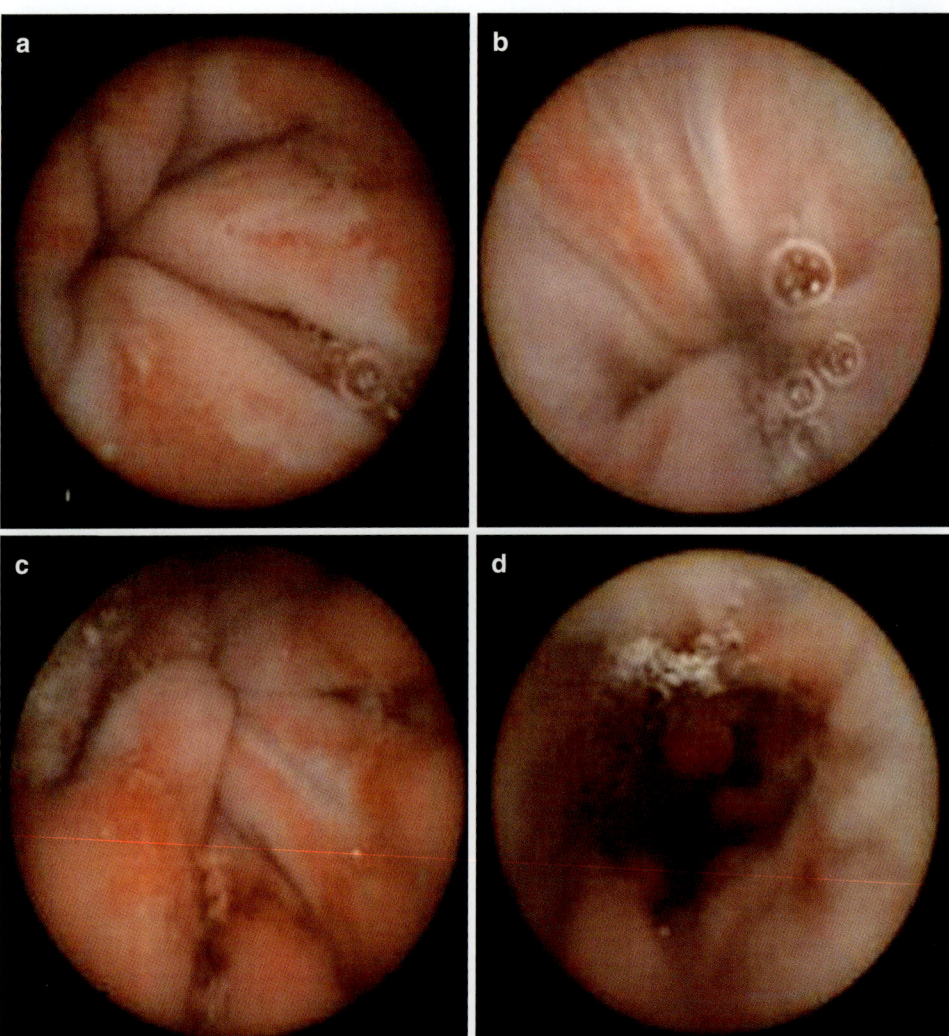

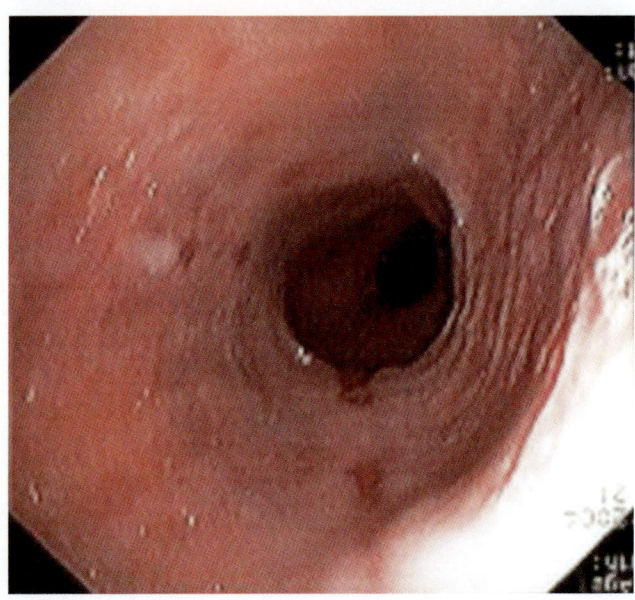

Fig. 42.11 Grade A esophagitis seen on traditional endoscopy

Fig. 42.12 (**a–d**) Images of suspected Barrett's metaplasia captured by PillCam ESO

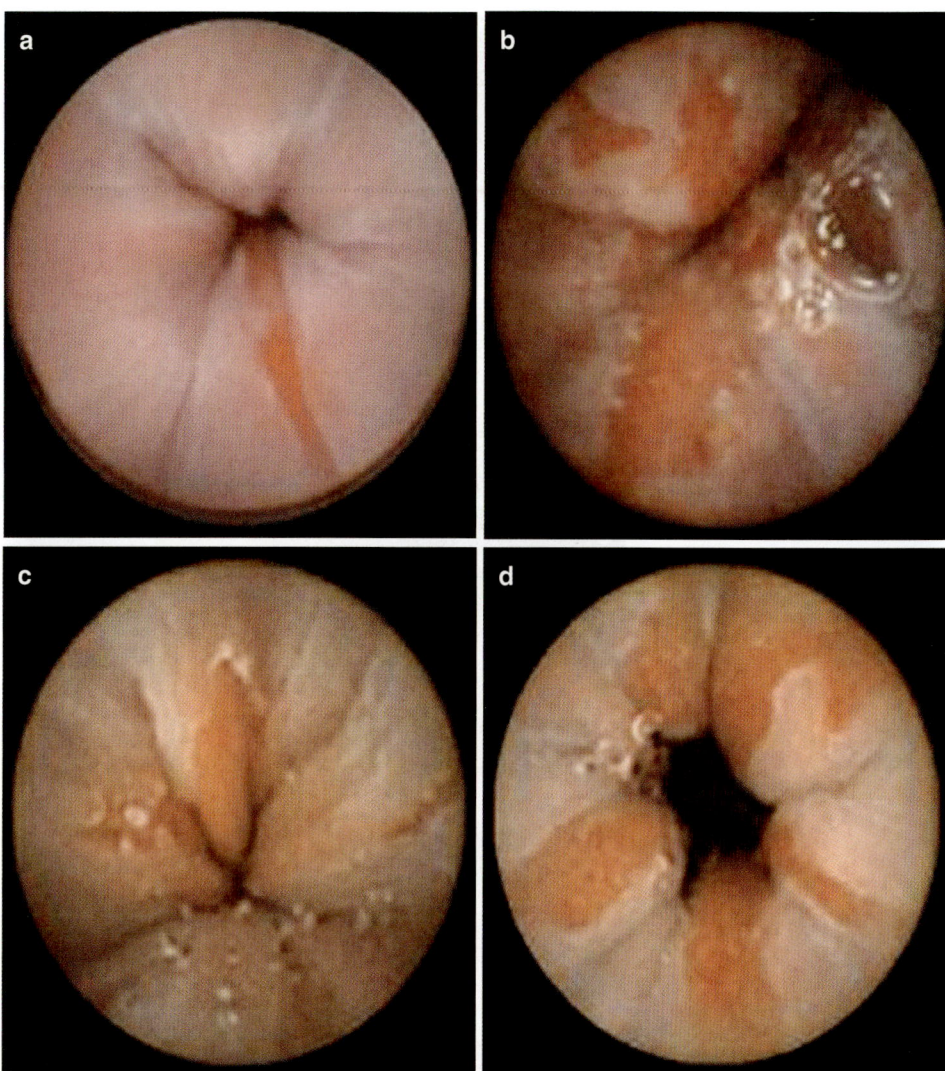

Fig. 42.13 (**a, b**) Barrett's metaplasia seen on traditional endoscopy

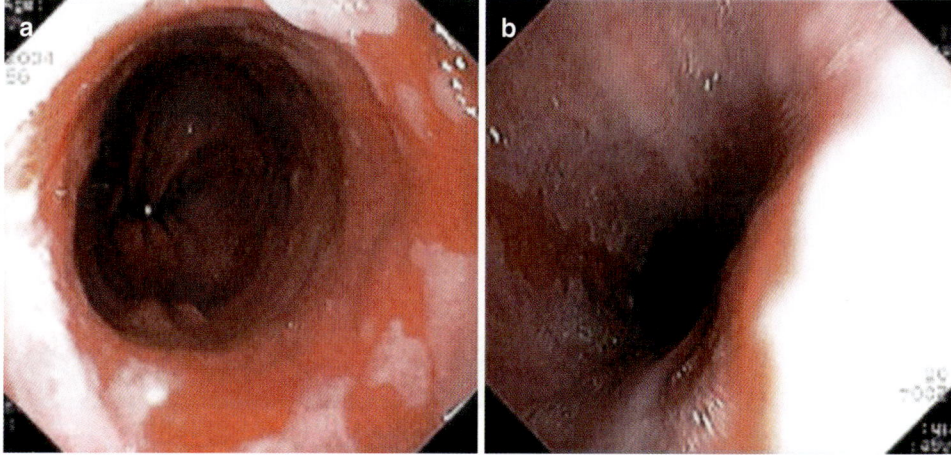

Fig. 42.14 Barrett's metaplasia and erosion. (**a**, **b**) Images captured by PillCam ESO. (**c**) Zoom endoscopy. (**d**) Histology showing Barrett's intestinal metaplasia (alcian blue stain) (Courtesy of Jörg Caselitz, MD)

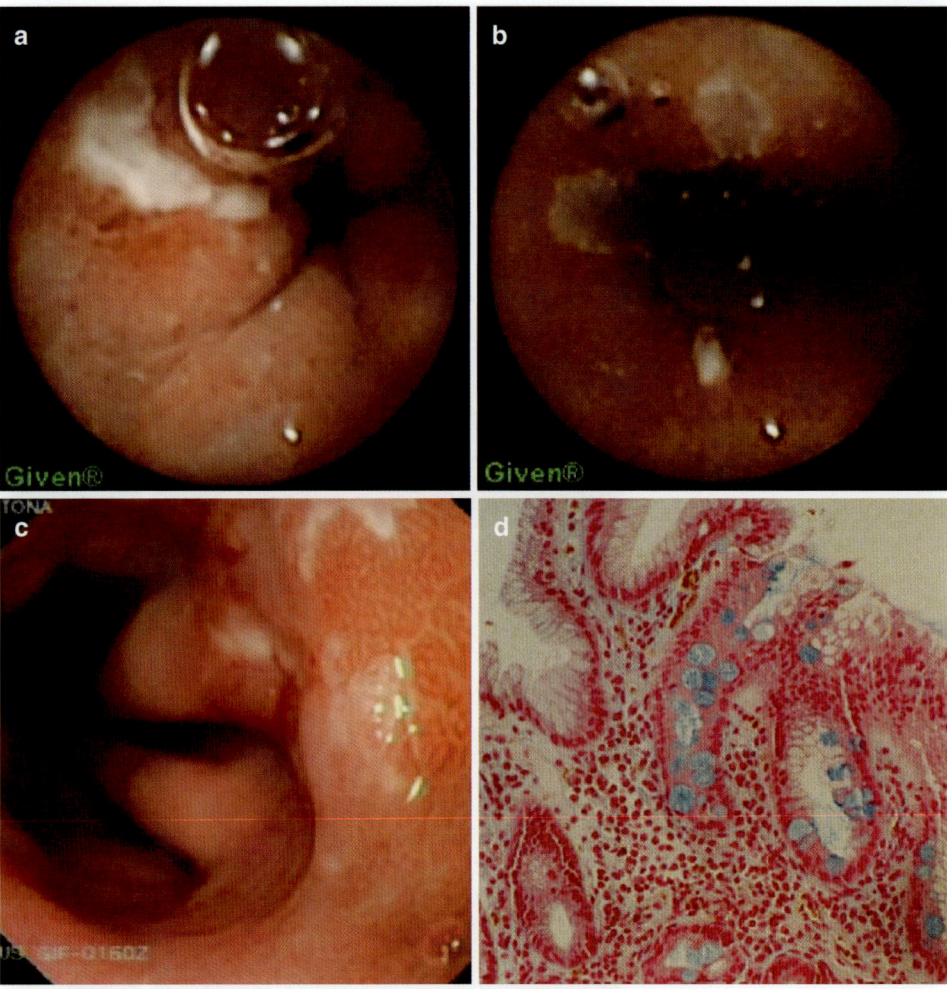

Fig. 42.15 (**a**, **b**) Esophageal varices captured by PillCam ESO

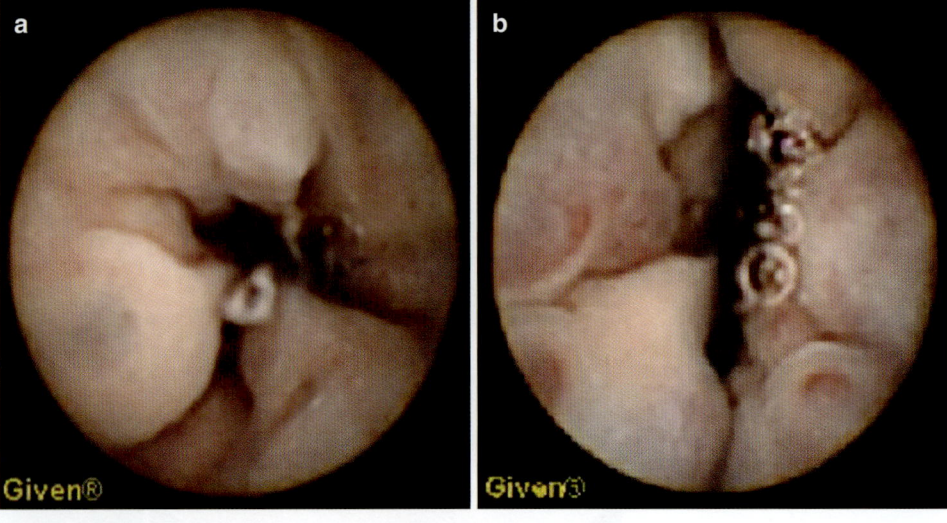

Fig. 42.16 Papilloma of the esophagus (proven by histology)

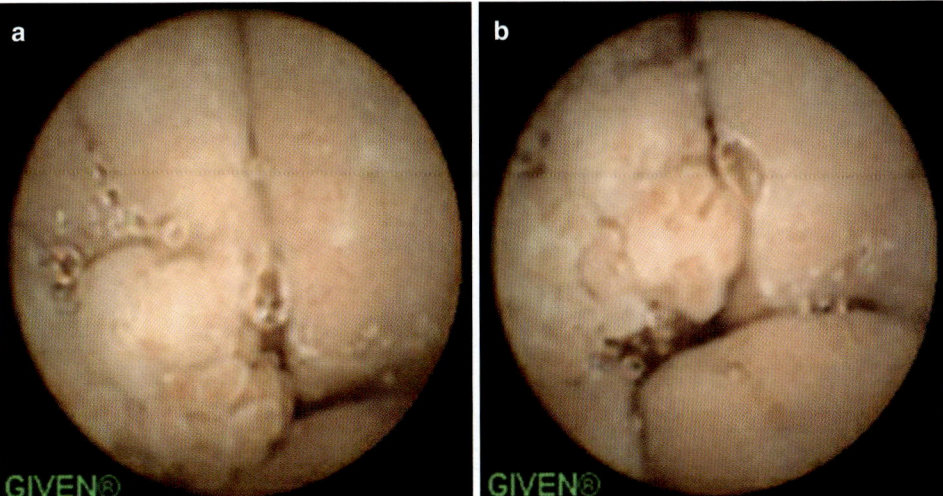

References

1. Eliakim R, Sharma VK, Yassin K, et al. A prospective study of the diagnostic accuracy of Given® esophageal capsule endoscopy versus conventional upper endoscopy in patients with chronic gastroesophageal reflux diseases. J Clin Gastroenterol. 2005;39:572–8.
2. Eisen GM, Eliakim R, Zaman A, et al. The accuracy of PillCam ESO capsule endoscopy versus conventional upper endoscopy for the diagnosis of esophageal varices: a prospective three-center pilot study. Endoscopy. 2006;38:31–5.
3. De Franchis R, Eisen GM, Laine L, et al. Esophageal capsule endoscopy for screening and surveillance of esophageal varices in patients with portal hypertension. Hepatology. 2008;47:1595–603.
4. Lu Y, Gao R, Liao Z, et al. Meta-analysis of capsule endoscopy in patients diagnosed or suspected with esophageal varices. World J Gastroenterol. 2009;15:1154–8.
5. Bhardwaj A, Hollenbeak CS, Pooran N, Mathew A. A meta-analysis of the diagnostic accuracy of esophageal capsule endoscopy for Barrett's esophagus in patients with gastroesophageal reflux disease. Am J Gastroenterol. 2009;104:1533–9.
6. Gralnek IM, Rabinovitz R, Afik D, Eliakim R. A simplified ingestion procedure for esophageal capsule endoscopy: initial evaluation in healthy volunteers. Endoscopy. 2006;38:913–8.
7. Eliakim R, Yassin K, Shlomi I, et al. A novel diagnostic tool for detecting oesophageal pathology: PillCam oesophageal video capsule. Aliment Pharmacol Ther. 2004;20:1083–9.

Incidental Findings in the Mouth, Pharynx, and Esophagus

43

Dani Dajani, Virender K. Sharma, and Martin Keuchel

Contents

43.1   Mouth and Pharynx

Some images of the oral cavity are frequently seen during video capsule endoscopy (VCE). Improved illumination allows better visualization of native or treated teeth (Figs. 43.1 and 43.2) or dentures (Fig. 43.3). Images of the oral cavity with tongue and palatine (Fig. 43.4) are often captured, whereas the uvula and epiglottis are less frequently seen (Fig. 43.5). Detailed visualization of the arytenoid cartilage or larynx is rare and suggestive for swallowing disorder (Figs. 43.6 and 43.7), especially in conjunction with a long stay of the capsule in the oropharyngeal region.

The work was first published in 2006 by Springer Medizin Verlag Heidelberg with the following title: *Atlas of Video Capsule Endoscopy*.

D. Dajani (✉) • M. Keuchel
Department of Internal Medicine,
Bethesda Krankenhaus Bergedorf, Hamburg, Germany
e-mail: dajani@bkb.info; keuchel@bkb.info

V.K. Sharma
Arizona Digestive Health, Gilbert, AZ, USA
e-mail: vksharma@azcdh.com

M. Keuchel et al. (eds.), *Video Capsule Endoscopy: A Reference Guide and Atlas*,
DOI 10.1007/978-3-662-44062-9_43, © Springer-Verlag Berlin Heidelberg 2014

Fig. 43.1 (**a**, **b**) Teeth

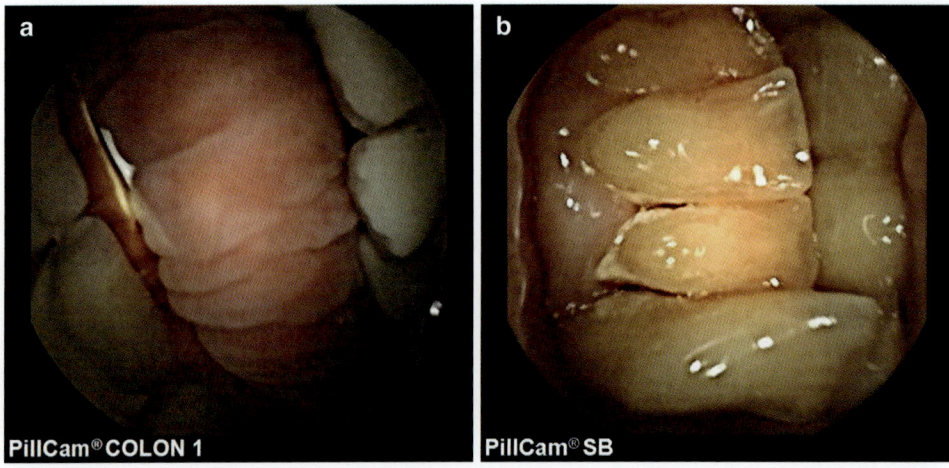

Fig. 43.2 (**a**) Dental caries. (**b**) Corona

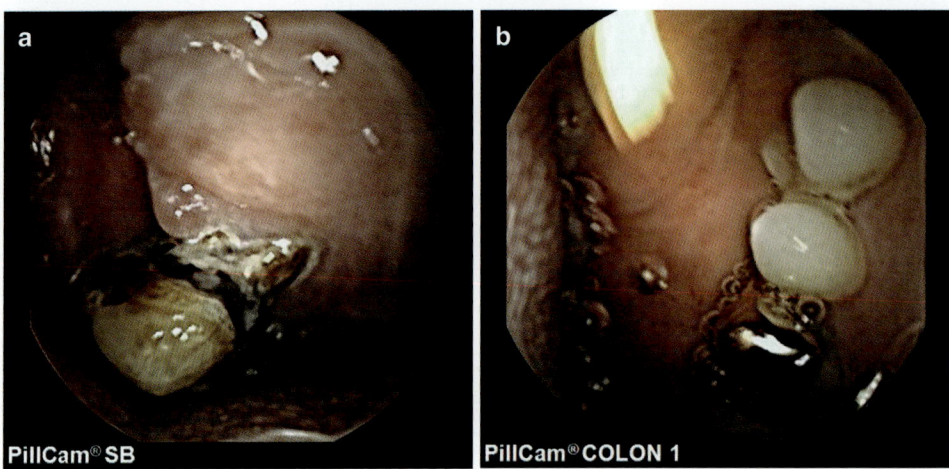

Fig. 43.3 (**a**, **b**) Denture

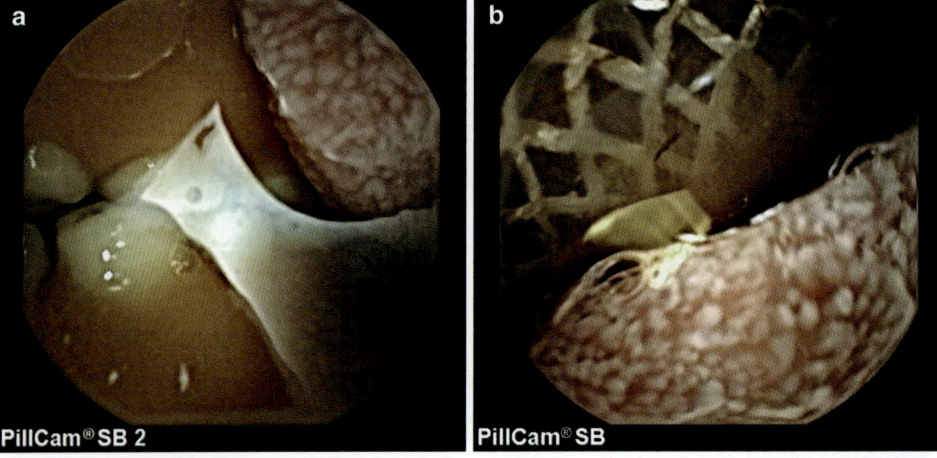

Fig. 43.4 (**a**, **b**) Tongue, palatine

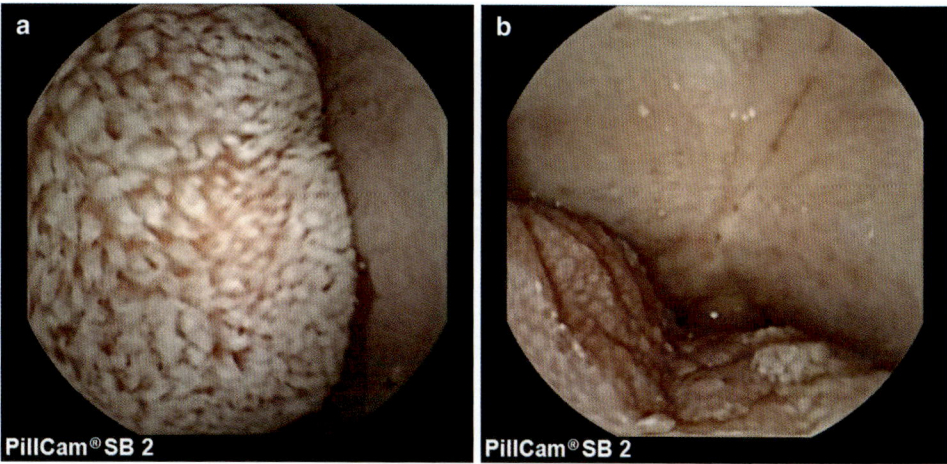

Fig. 43.5 (**a**, **b**) Uvula

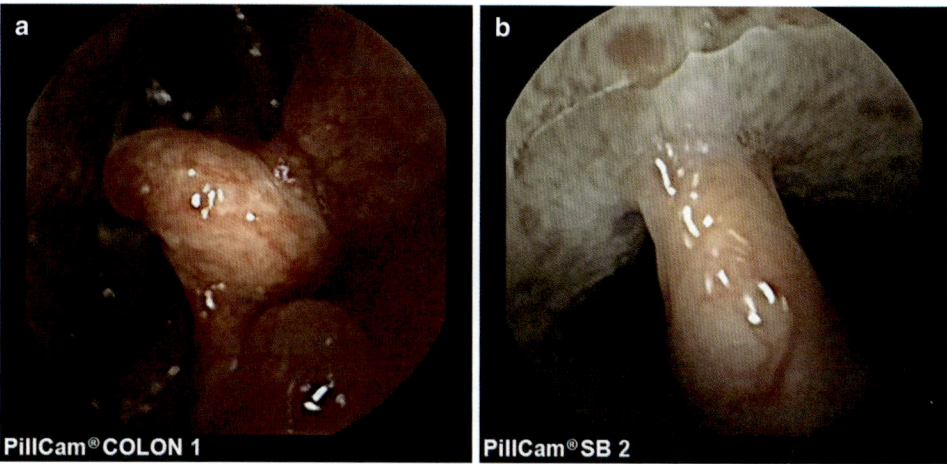

Fig. 43.6 (**a**) Piriform recessus. (**b**) Arytenoid

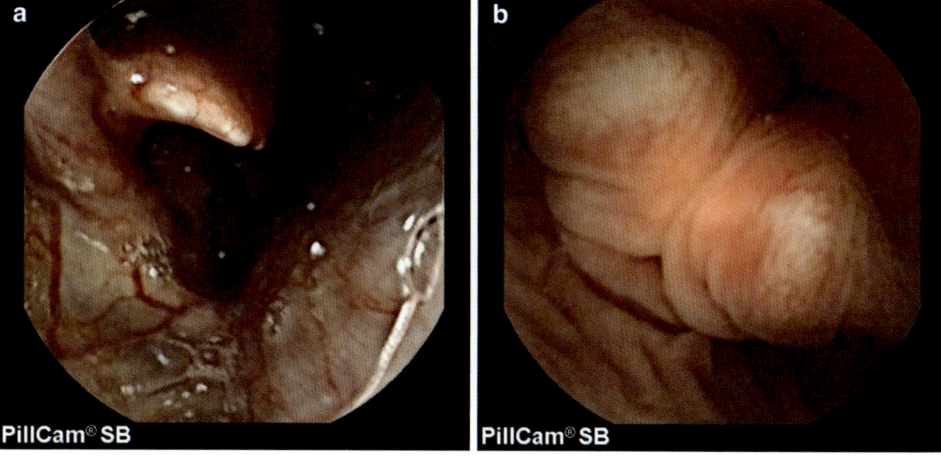

Fig. 43.7 Glottis and vocal cords open (**a**) and closed (**b**)

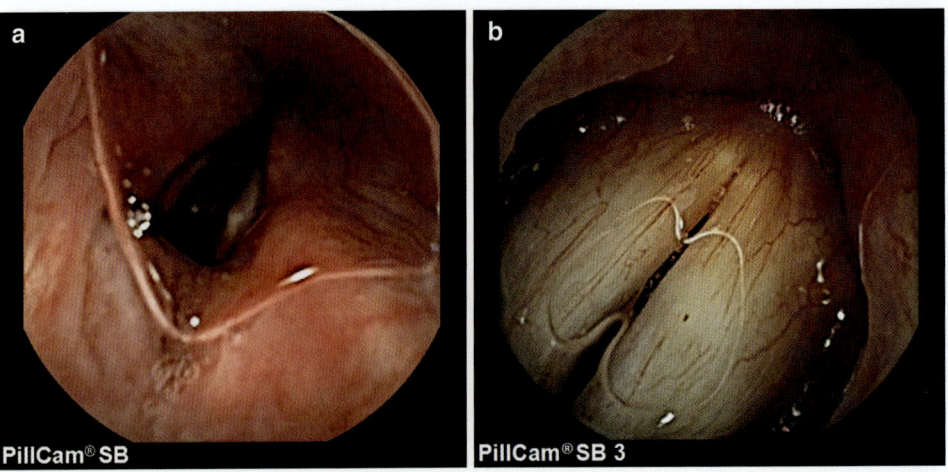

43.2   Esophagus

VCE for the small bowel or colon supplies only a few recognizable images of the esophagus. The upper esophageal sphincter is rarely identified, and the entire esophagus cannot be reliably evaluated because of the exceptionally swift passage of the capsule (Fig. 43.8) [1]. Pathologic findings are occasionally seen, most commonly at the cardioesophageal junction. Resolution in these cases is equal to that achieved with modern flexible video endoscopes. With the first generation of double-headed colon capsule, the Z-line (Fig. 43.9) can be visualized in 60 % of patients [2]. This capability may be an additional benefit in screening patients undergoing colon capsule endoscopy for suspected Barrett's esophagus as well. However, there

are no data yet beyond the percentage of patients in whom the Z-line can be visualized. Sensitivity and specificity compared with flexible endoscopy in this setting have not yet been determined. Z-line visualization can be accurately achieved in most cases when the small bowel capsule is swallowed in the right supine position [3]. Because of the usually swift passage of the capsule, however, variants of normal in the esophagus such as glycogen acanthosis are detected less frequently than with flexible esophagoscopy (Figs. 43.10 and 43.11).

Better results are achieved with the Pillcam ESO 2 (Given Imaging, Yoqneam, Israel), which is equipped with a camera on each end of the capsule, each of them flashing at a rate of 9 times per second. Findings with this special esophageal capsule are addressed in Chap. 42.

Fig. 43.8 Passage through the esophagus. (**a**) Upper esophageal sphincter. (**b**) Tubular esophagus with air. (**c**) Tubular esophagus with water. (**d**) Longitudinal vessels in the distal esophagus

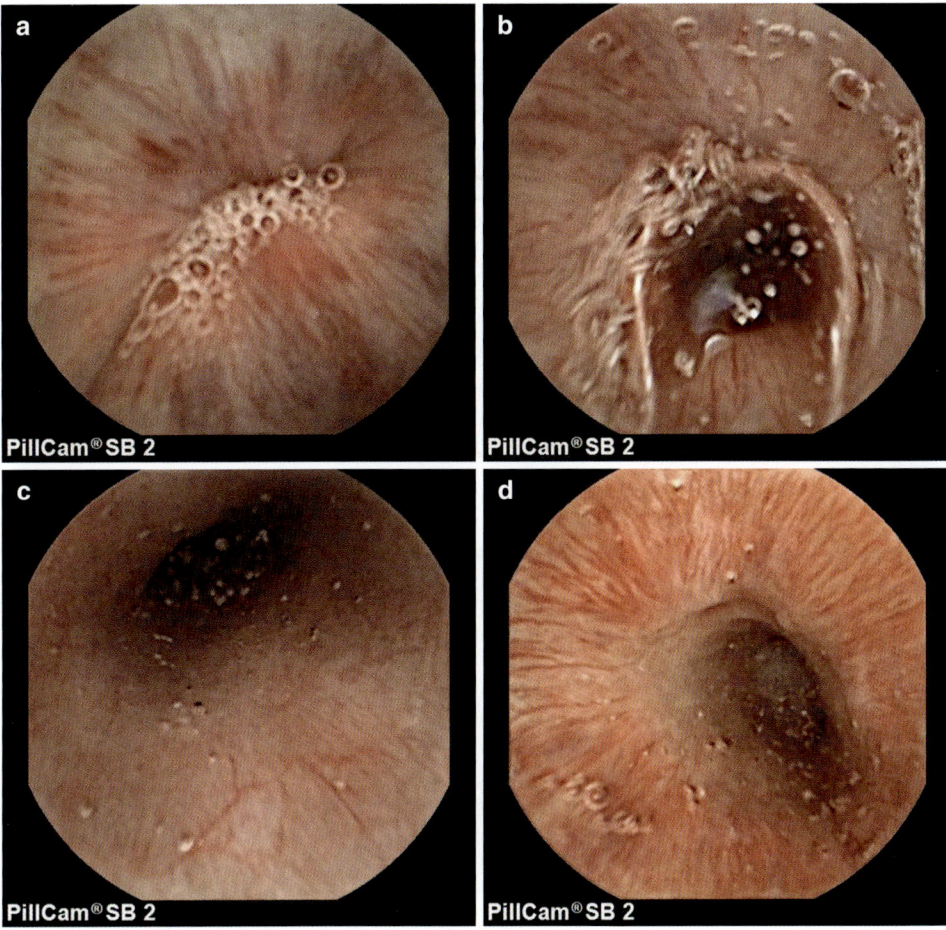

Fig. 43.9 (**a–c**) Normal Z-line opening up in a patient with prolonged esophageal passage of 18 min. (**d**) Enhanced contrast with FICE3 (flexible spectral imaging color enhancement)

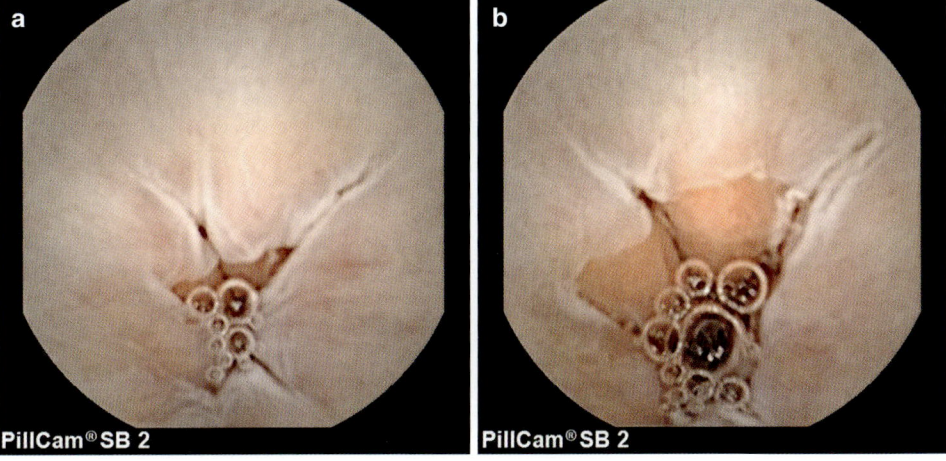

Fig. 43.9 (continued)

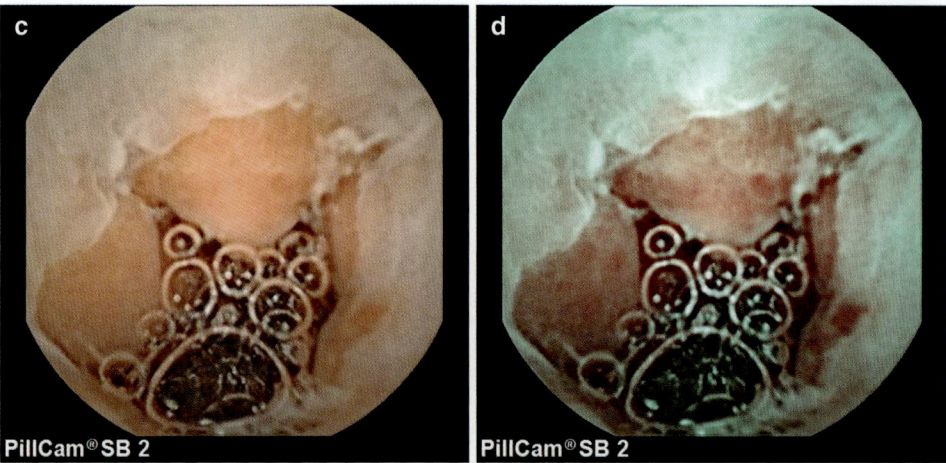

Fig. 43.10 Glycogen acanthosis.
(**a**) Native VCE image. (**b**) Image
in FICE2 mode

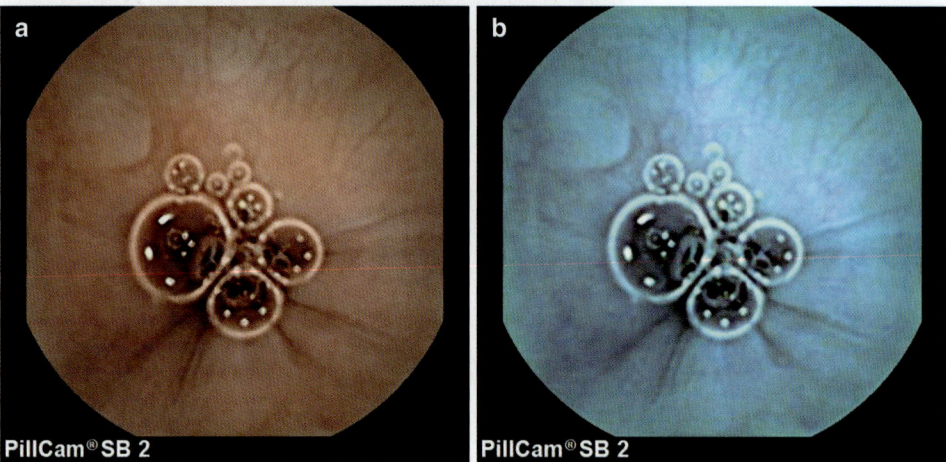

Fig. 43.11 Glycogen acanthosis.
(**a**) VCE image. (**b**) Flexible
esophagoscopy

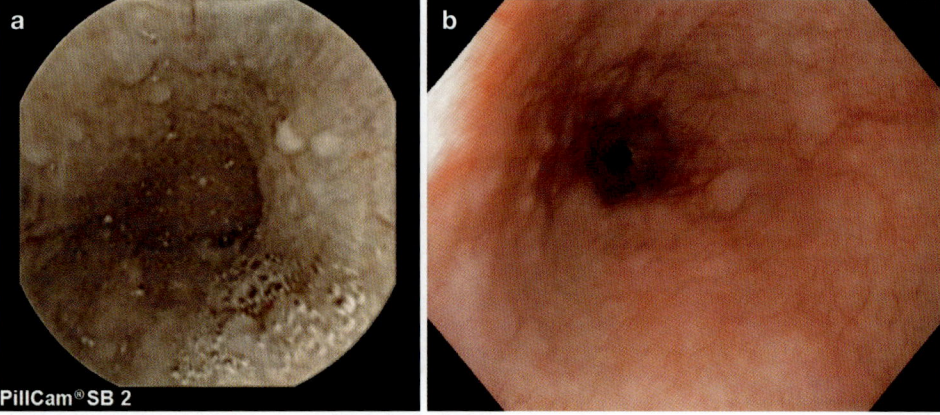

43.2.1 Sliding Hiatal Hernia

The Z-line is not visualized with the standard capsule in most cases [4, 5]. A Z-line that is clearly visible at VCE may signify a sliding hiatal hernia. A characteristic feature of a hiatal hernia is the presence of longitudinal gastric folds above the hiatal constriction. The hernia cannot be examined from within the stomach by capsule endoscopy (as it can with a retroflexed endoscope), but with a favorable position of the capsule, a retrograde view of the Z-line occasionally can be obtained (Fig. 43.12). The capsule may become trapped in a very large hernia for some time.

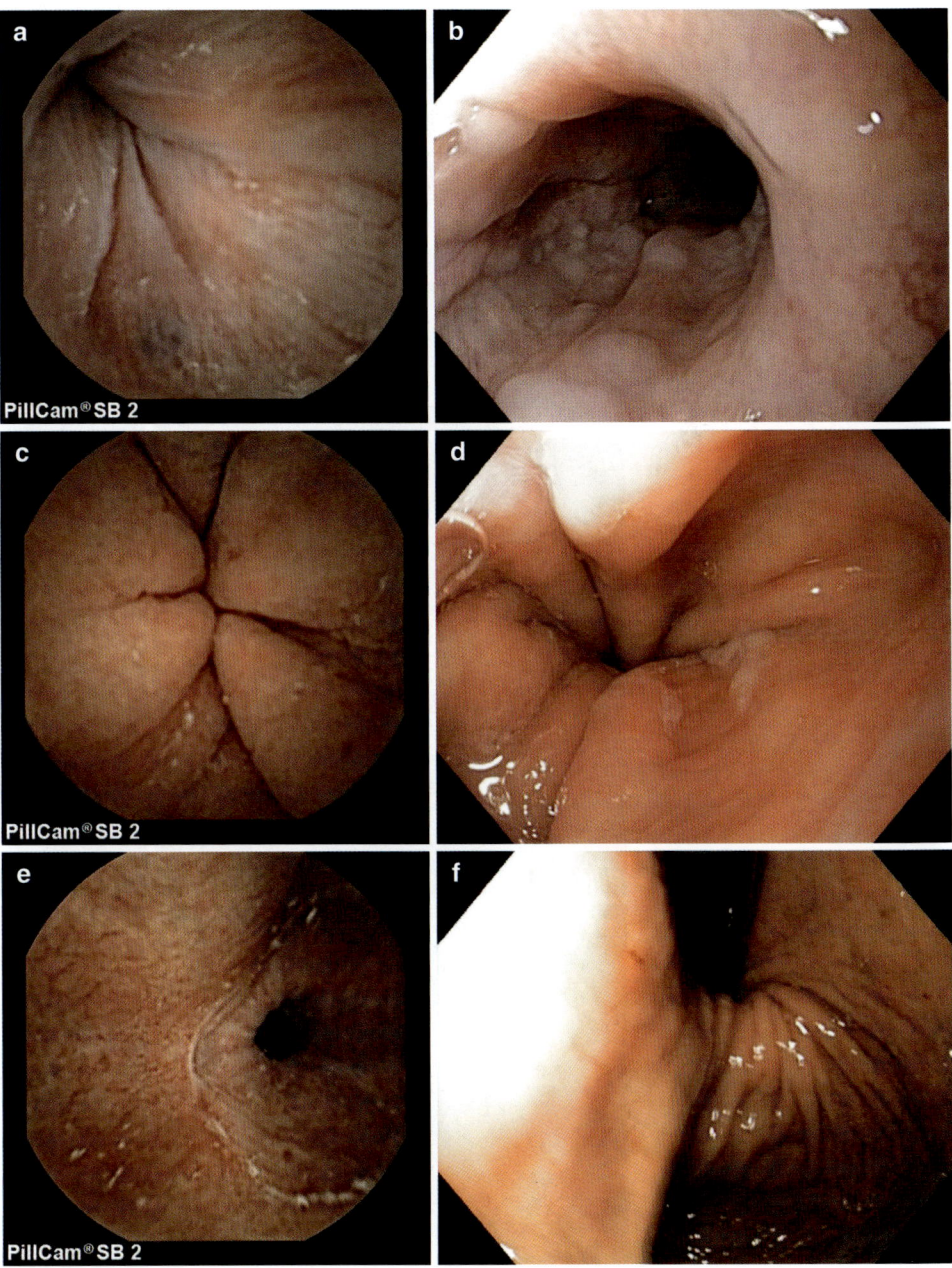

Fig. 43.12 Tubular esophagus with squamous cell epithelium as seen with VCE (**a**) and esophagoscopy (**b**). Hiatal hernia with columnar cell epithelium and gastric folds as seen with VCE (**c**) and esophagoscopy (**d**). In this case, a retrograde view in VCE (**e**) clearly delineates the Z-line, which is not documented in the image of retroflexion during routine gastroscopy in the same patient (**f**)

43.2.2 Barrett's Esophagus

Barrett's esophagus is discussed in detail in Chap. 42. During standard capsule endoscopy aimed at the small bowel (SBCE) or colon (CCE), the gastroesophageal junction cannot be investigated reliably without applying a special swallowing procedure. In many patients, however, relevant images can be obtained (Figs. 43.13, 43.14, and 43.15), making it worthwhile to include the esophagus in the evaluation of SBCE or CCE videos.

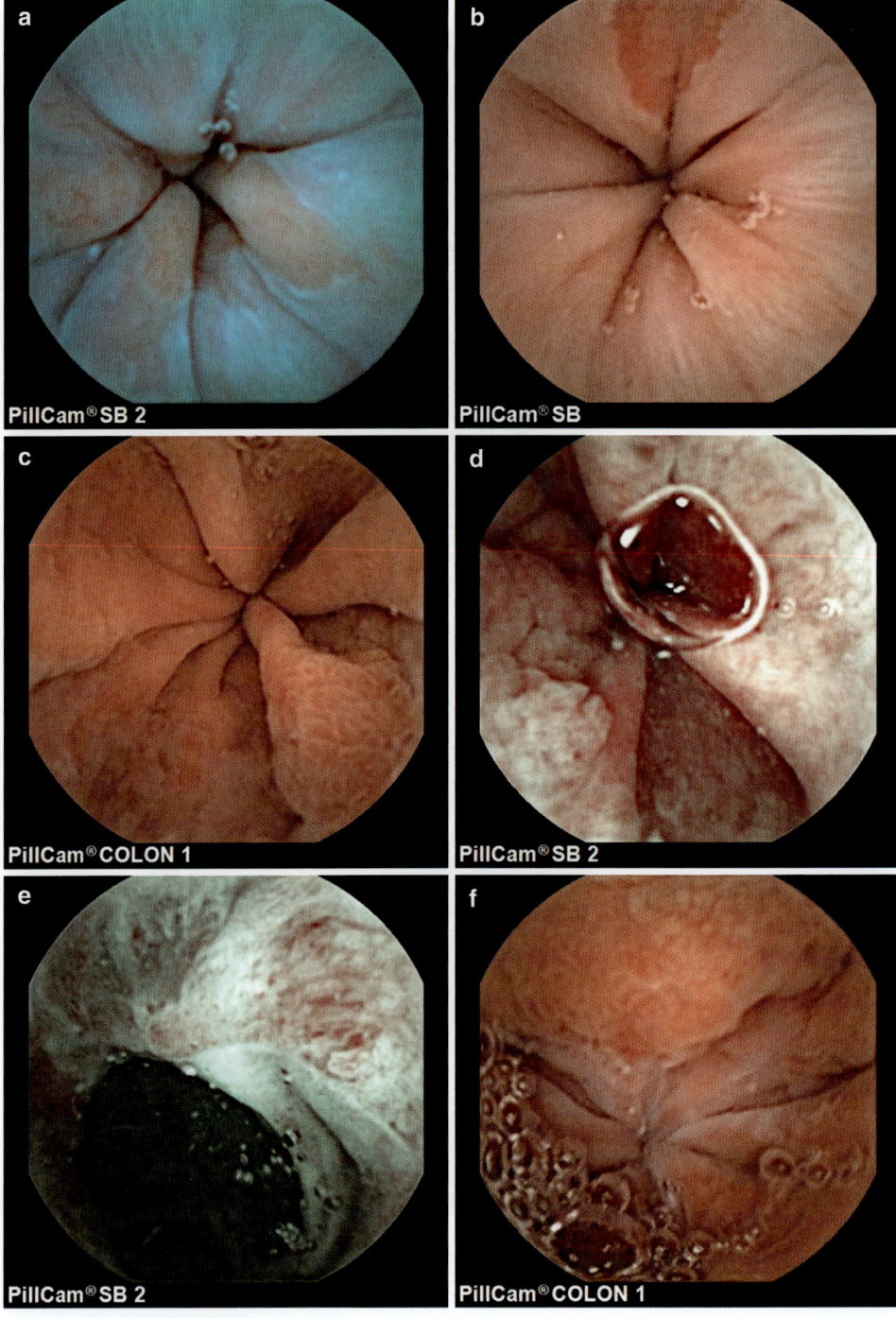

Fig. 43.13 VCE findings at the gastroesophageal junction include diminutive villous areas at the Z-line (*arrows*) (**a**) and Barrett's tongue (**b**). Slightly elevated villous area in a hernia, seen using PillCam Colon (**c**) and PillCam SB2 in FICE1 mode (**d**). Retrograde view of an irregular Z-line seen using PillCam SB2 in FICE1 mode (**e**) and PillCam Colon (**f**)

Fig. 43.14 Short-segment
Barrett's esophagus in a patient
undergoing small bowel capsule
endoscopy for Crohn's disease.
Previous
esophagogastroduodcnoscopy
(EGD) had reported reflux
esophagitis. VCE (**a**) and flexible
endoscopy (**b**) show tongues
suspicious for Barrett's esophagus
without reflux esophagitis. VCE
image in FICE mode (**c**) and EGD
with narrowband imaging (**d**).
Histology shows Barrett's
esophagus with intestinal
metaplasia (periodic acid-Schiff
[PAS] stain) (**e**) and strong alcian
blue staining of goblet cells (**f**). (**e,
f** Courtesy of Jörg Caselitz, MD)

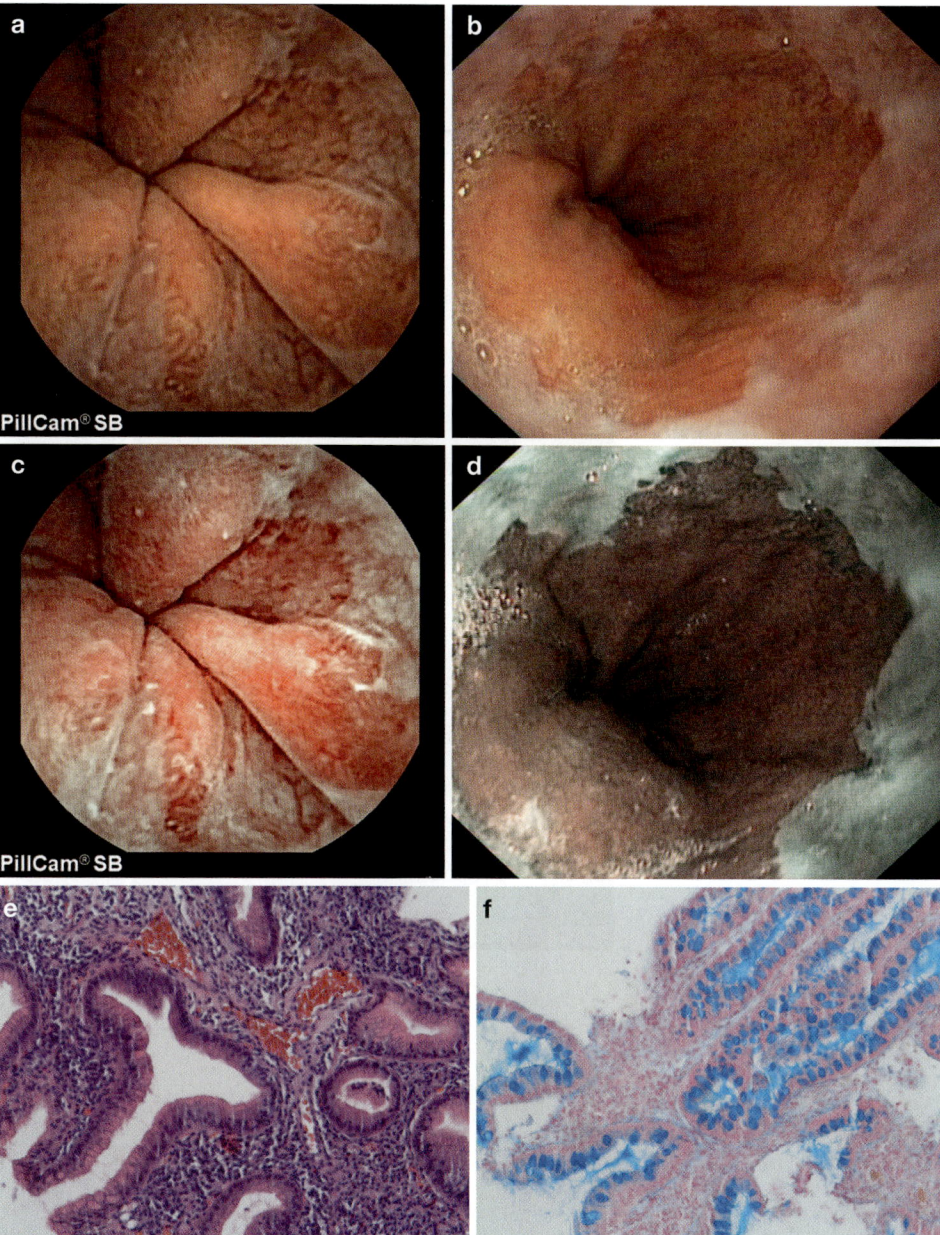

Fig. 43.15 Barrett's esophagus in VCE (**a**) and in endoscopic confocal laser microscopy (**b**). Barrett's mucosa with goblet cells: squamous cell mucosa in VCE (**c**) and confocal laser microscopy (**d**)

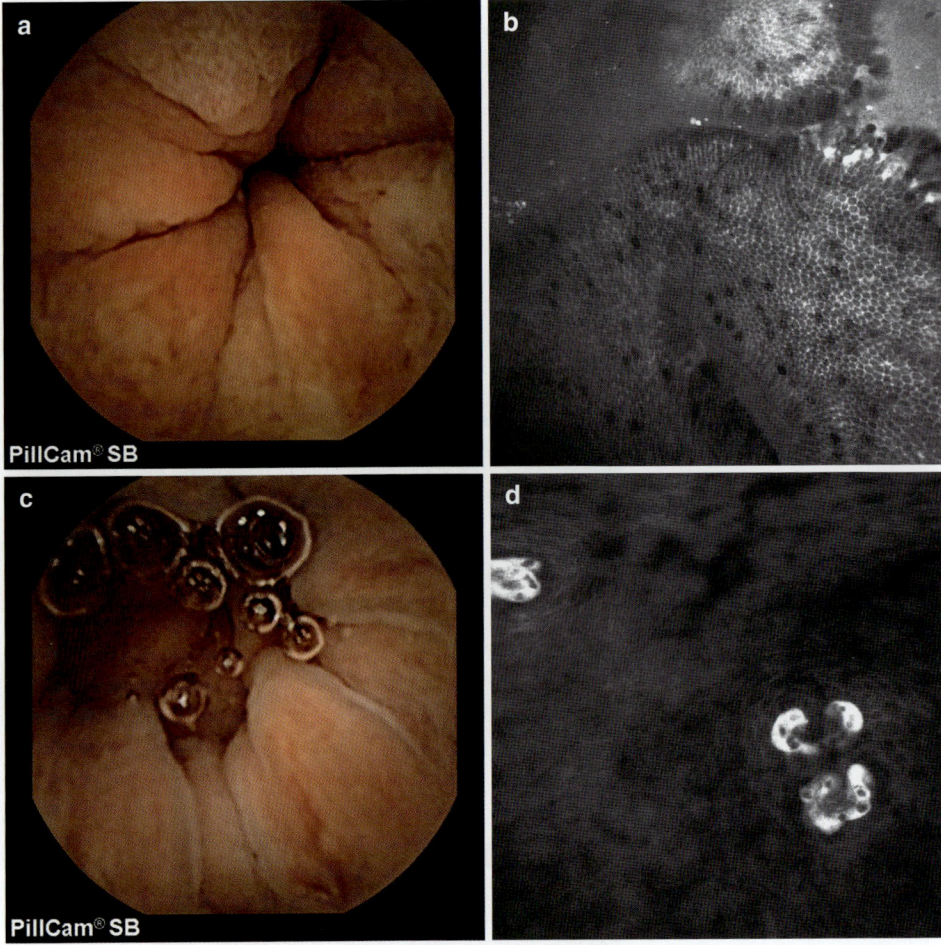

43.2.3 Esophageal Diverticula

Both Zenker's diverticula and epiphrenic diverticula (Fig. 43.16) can lead to capsule retention. Capsule endoscopy should be avoided in patients with large esophageal diverticula or dysphagia [6], or the capsule should be placed with endoscopic guidance in these patients [7].

43.2.4 Esophagitis

Reflux esophagitis with patchy or streaky erosions may be found incidentally (Fig. 43.17), even after inconclusive esophagogastroduodenoscopy (EGD) [8]. Previously unknown esophagitis may be diagnosed more often during CCE than during SBCE, because an EGD does not routinely precede CCE. Systematic studies are pending.

Fig. 43.16 Epiphrenic diverticulum on VCE (**a**) and esophagoscopy (**b**)

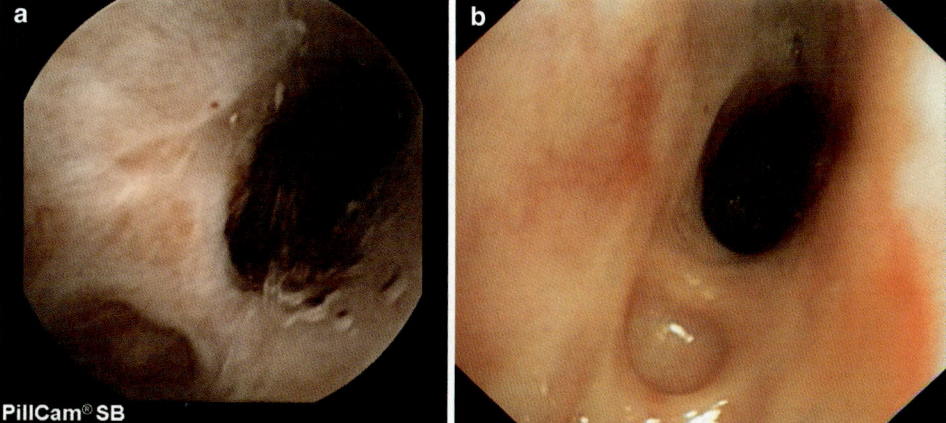

Fig. 43.17 (**a**) Reflux esophagitis. (**b**) Monilial esophagitis

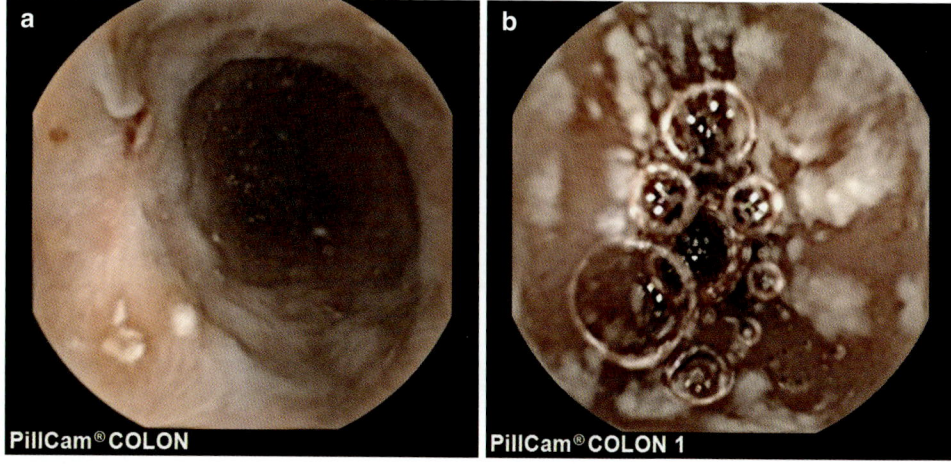

43.2.5 Motility Disorders

Ingesting the standard capsule while lying down can significantly delay passage of the capsule through the esophagus, but it does not guarantee a complete survey [1]. Even when the capsule is ingested in an upright position, motility disorders can greatly delay its passage through the esophagus (Figs. 43.18 and 43.19).

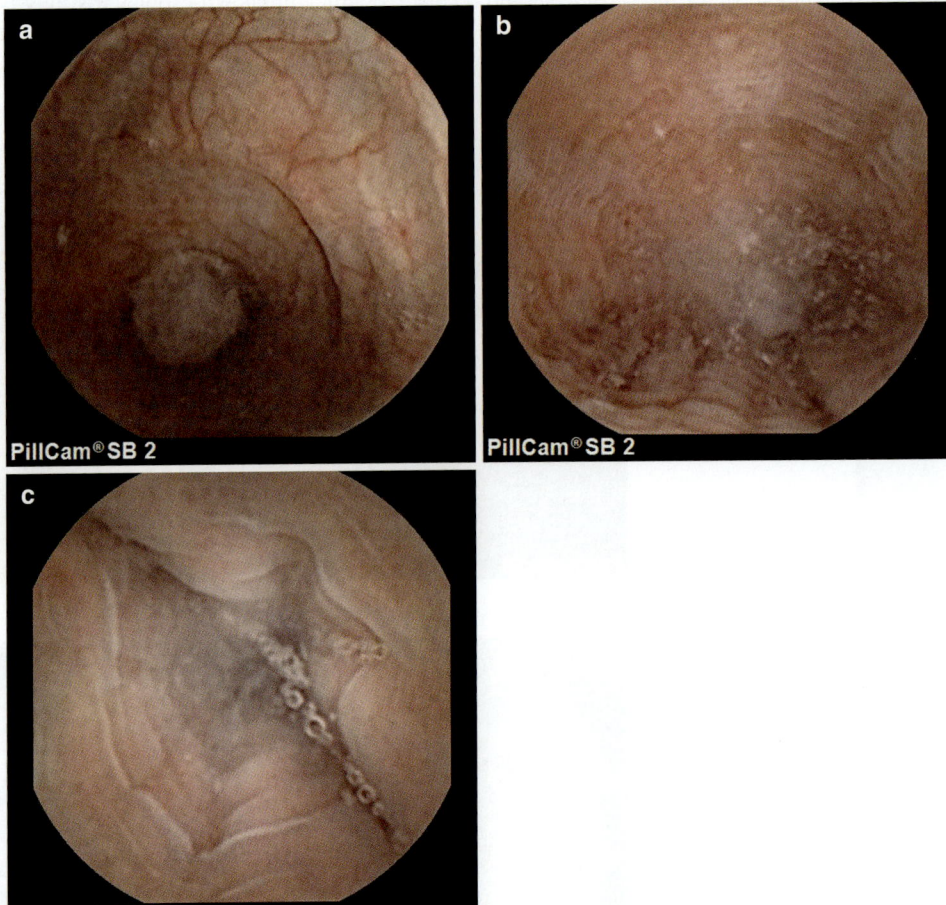

Fig. 43.18 Prolonged esophageal passage with simultaneous contractions (**a**, **b**) and dilated esophageal lumen (**c**)

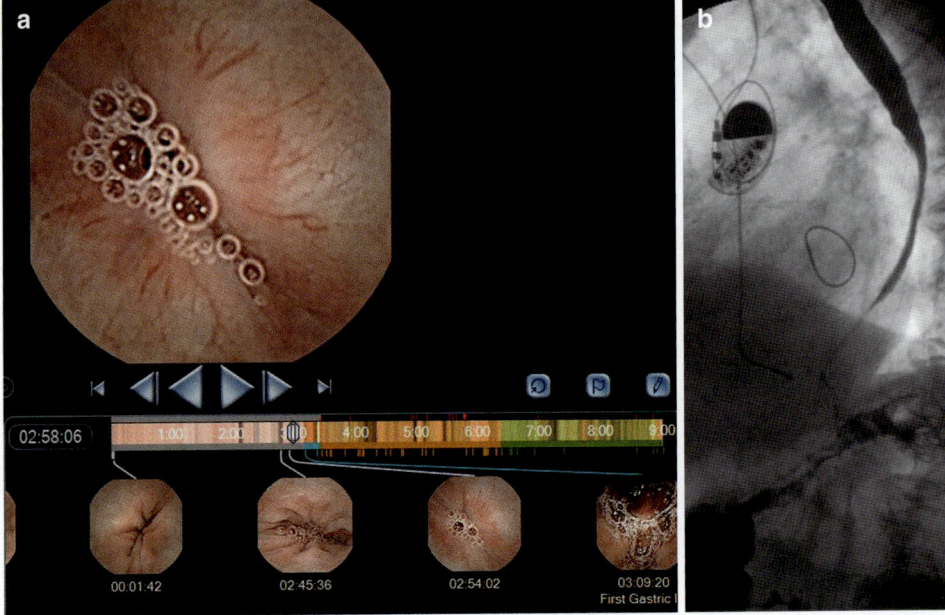

Fig. 43.19 (**a**, **b**) Prolonged esophageal transit time of the small bowel video capsule caused by compression due to cardiac disease. On VCE, a good visualization of localization was provided by the color bar. Note the esophageal transit time of 3 h

43.2.6 Stenosis

Esophageal stenoses are rarely discovered by SBCE (Fig. 43.20), as the procedure is usually preceded by upper gastrointestinal (GI) endoscopy. The risk of esophageal retention may increase with increasing use of CCE without prior upper GI endoscopy. Eosinophilic esophagitis has been reported as a cause of capsule retention [9].

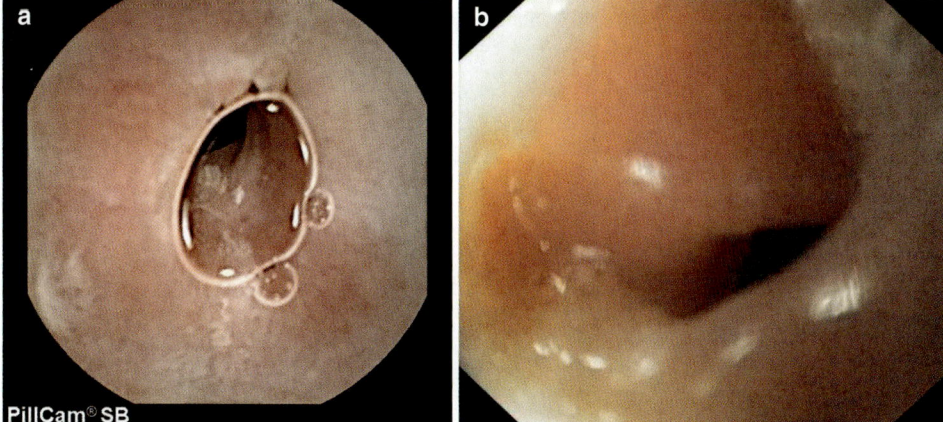

Fig. 43.20 Idiopathic stenosis of the proximal esophagus prohibiting passage of the capsule. (**a**) Capsule image. (**b**) Esophagoscopy. Capsule placement through an overtube was performed later

43.2.7 Esophageal Varices

Dedicated esophageal capsule endoscopy is applied in protocols to screen patients with portal hypertension for varices. Nevertheless, besides esophagitis, esophageal varices have been found in patients supposed to have obscure GI bleeding (i.e., after inconclusive EGD) [10] or in patients undergoing SBCE for suspected portal hypertensive enteropathy (Figs. 43.21, 43.22, and 43.23).

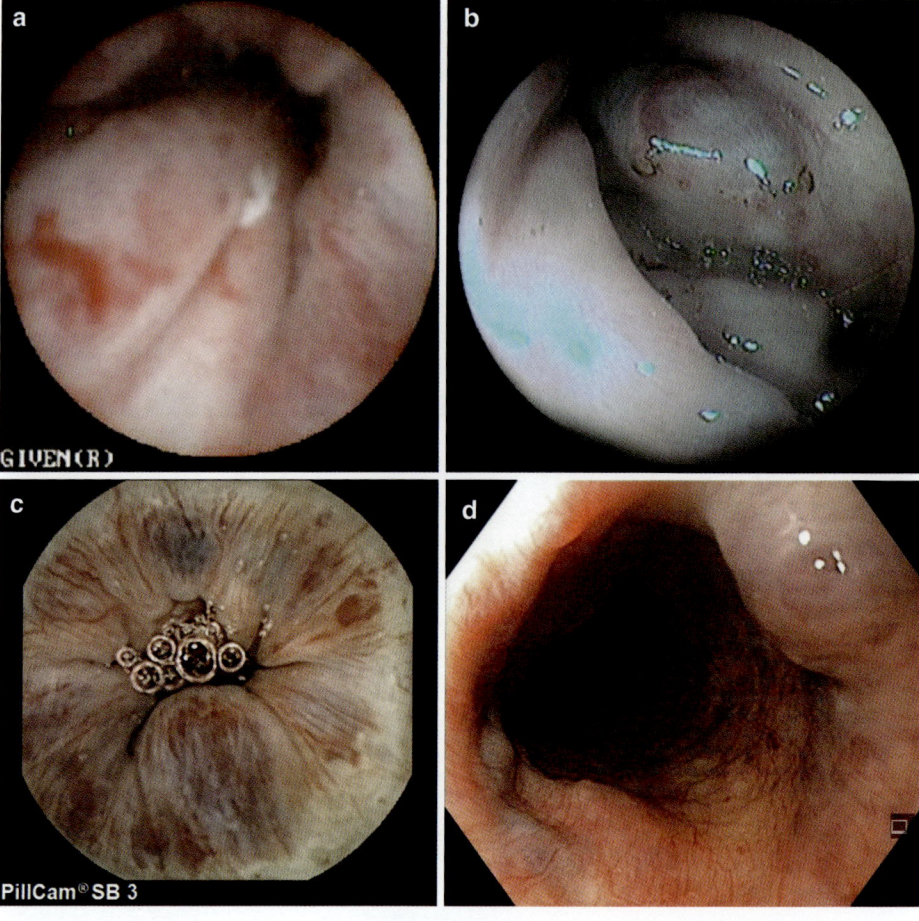

Fig. 43.21 Esophageal varices. Distal varices Grade II with vasa vasorum (**a**) VCE. (**b**) Esophagoscopy. Proximal downhill varices (**c**) VCE. (**d**) Esophagoscopy

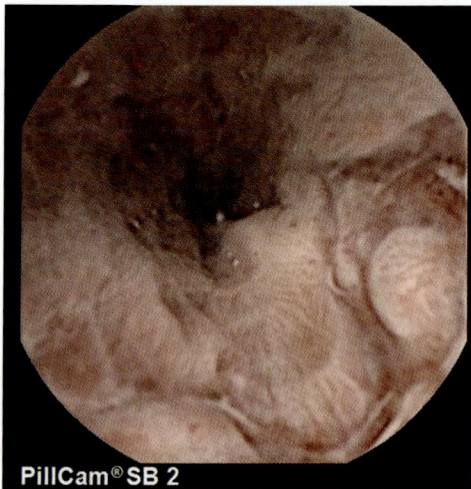
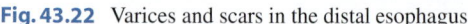

Fig. 43.22 Varices and scars in the distal esophagus

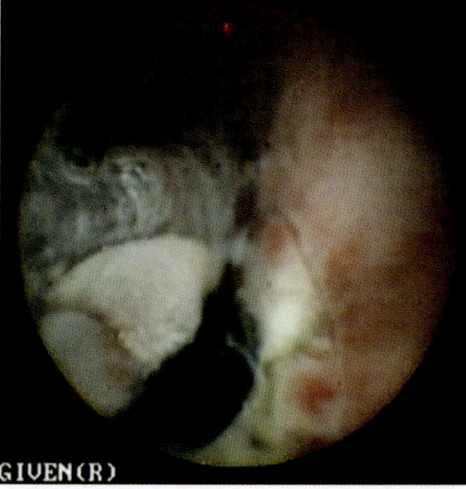

Fig. 43.23 Ligated varix with visible rubber band and ulcer

43.2.8 Tumors

Tumors of the esophagus (Fig. 43.24) are rarely seen with VCE [11].

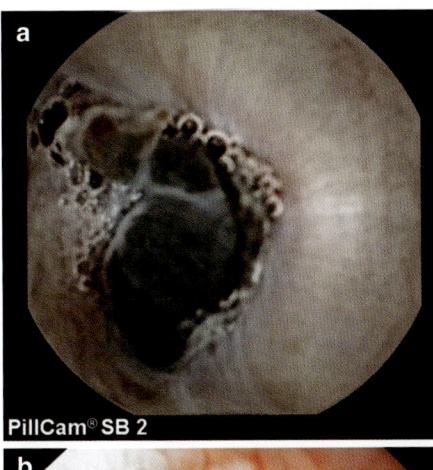

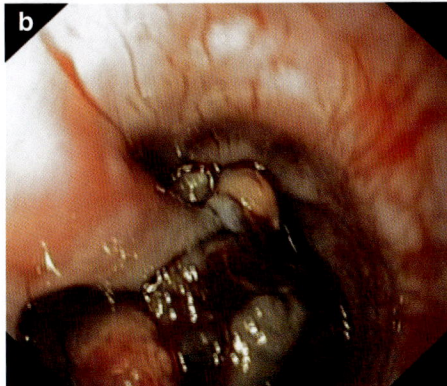

Fig. 43.24 Melanoma of the esophagus. (**a**) VCE. (**b**) Flexible esophagoscopy (Courtesy of Felix Wiedbrauck, MD)

References

1. Neu B, Wettschureck E, Rösch T. Is esophageal capsule endoscopy feasible? Results of a pilot study. Endoscopy. 2003; 35:957–61.
2. Schoofs N, Deviere J, Van Gossum A. PillCam colon capsule endoscopy compared with colonoscopy for colorectal tumor diagnosis: a prospective pilot study. Endoscopy. 2006;38:971–7.
3. Fernandez-Urien I, Borobio E, Elizalde I, et al. Z-line examination by the PillCam SB: prospective comparison of three ingestion protocols. World J Gastroenterol. 2010;16:63–8.
4. Enns R, Mergener K, Yamamoto K. Capsule endoscopy for the assessment of the gastroesophageal junction. Gastrointest Endosc. 2003;57:AB169.
5. Hong SP, Cheon JH, Kim TI, et al. Comparison of the diagnostic yield of "MiroCam" and "PillCam SB" capsule endoscopy. Hepatogastroenterology. 2012;59:778–81.
6. Simmons DT, Baron TH. Endoscopic retrieval of a capsule endoscope from a Zenker's diverticulum. Dis Esophagus. 2005;18:338–9.
7. Ferreira LE, Simmons DT, Baron TH. Zenker's diverticula: pathophysiology, clinical presentation, and flexible endoscopic management. Dis Esophagus. 2008;21:1–8.
8. Borobio E, Fernandez-Urien I, Elizalde I, Jimenez Perez FJ. Hiatal hernia and lesions of gastroesophageal reflux disease diagnosed by capsule endoscopy. Rev Esp Enferm Dig. 2009;101:355–6.
9. Ramos R, Mascarenhas J, Duarte P, et al. Capsule endoscopy "retention" permits diagnosis of eosinophilic esophagitis. Rev Esp Enferm Dig. 2009;101:228–9.
10. Van Gossum A, Hittelet A, Schmit A, et al. A prospective comparative study of push and wireless-capsule enteroscopy in patients with obscure digestive bleeding. Acta Gastroenterol Belg. 2003;66:199–205.
11. Sanchez-Yague A, Caunedo-Alvarez A, Romero-Castro R, et al. Esophageal tumor diagnosed by capsule endoscopy. Endoscopy. 2006;38:765.

Stomach and Duodenum

44

Tetsuya Nakamura, Michel Delvaux,
and Friedrich Hagenmüller

Contents

The work was first published in 2006 by Springer Medizin Verlag Heidelberg with the following title: *Atlas of Video Capsule Endoscopy*.

T. Nakamura (✉)
Department of Medical Informatics,
Dokkyo Medical University School of Medicine, Tochigi, Japan
e-mail: nakamurt@dokkyomed.ac.jp

M. Delvaux
Department of Gastroenterology and Hepatology,
Nouvel Hôpital Civil, University Hospital of Strasbourg,
Strasbourg, France
e-mail: michel.delvaux@chru-strasbourg.fr

F. Hagenmüller
1st Medical Department, Asklepios Klinik Altona,
Hamburg, Germany
e-mail: f.hagenmueller@asklepios.com

44.1   Findings in the Stomach

The distal body and antrum of the stomach are often clearly visualized by video capsule endoscopy (VCE), whereas the proximal portions are not. Changing the patient's position after capsule ingestion may increase the diagnostic yield in the stomach [1], but even so, all of the stomach cannot be reliably evaluated with VCE [2]. Nevertheless, attention should be given to any gastric pathology that may be observable at VCE, as bleeding lesions in the stomach may have been missed at prior gastroscopy [3, 4].

Normal findings are illustrated in Fig. 44.1. After the capsule has entered the stomach, it usually passes quickly to the antrum and displays the pylorus. When the camera is pointing at the pylorus, the pressure of the capsule against the pylorus can sometimes be clearly recognized (Fig. 44.2). Occasionally, the duodenal mucosa with its villi can be seen before the capsule falls back into the stomach. The time of definitive passage into the duodenum is noted for the determination of transit time.

Sometimes, the dark side of the pylorus (opposite side of the pylorus in the duodenal bulb) can be recognized (Fig. 44.3). Rarely, the dark side of the pylorus may be the bleeding spot [5].

44.1.1 Transit Abnormality in the Stomach

In patients with diabetes or strong bile reflux, the transit time of the stomach may be prolonged. Rarely, a retained capsule visualizes the process of digestion of food in the stomach (Fig. 44.4). Sometimes, bile reflux from the duodenum or operated small intestine is observed (Figs. 44.5 and 44.6).

Fig. 44.1 (**a**, **b**) Gastric body fluid-filled lumen: en face view of the gastric angle

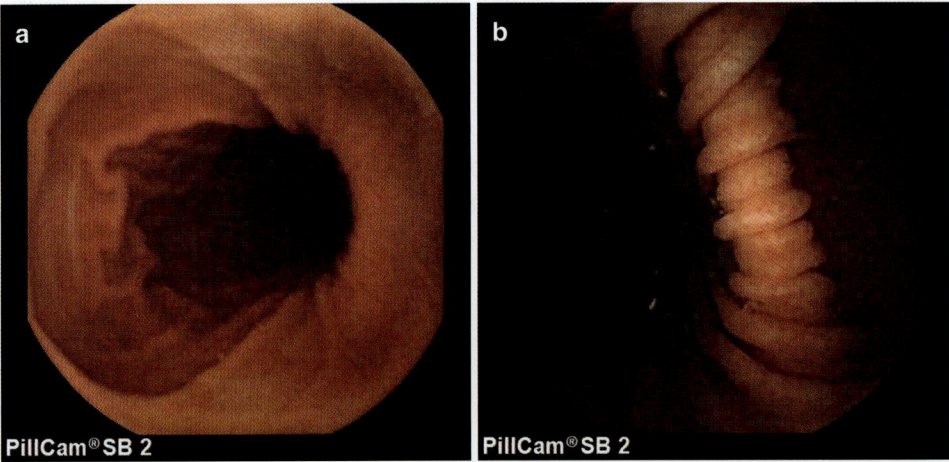

Fig. 44.2 (**a**, **b**) Pylorus compressed by the capsule

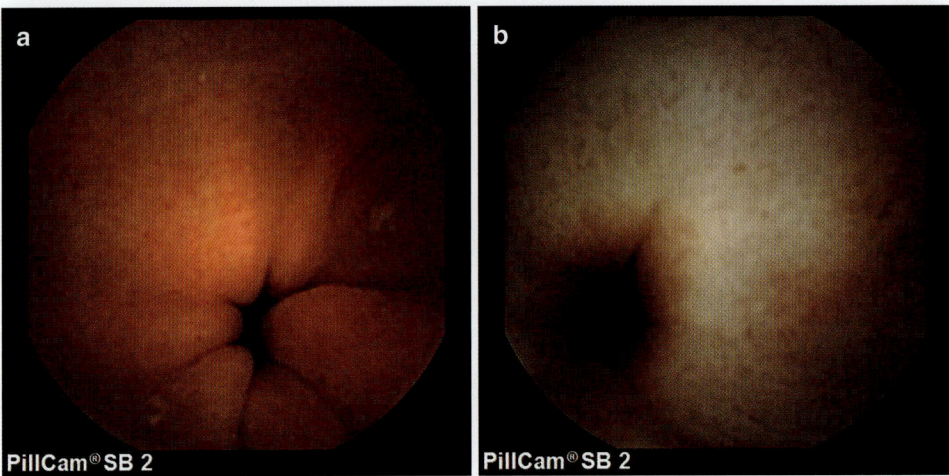

Fig. 44.3 (**a**) Dark side of the pylorus. (**b**) En face view of the pylorus in the same patient

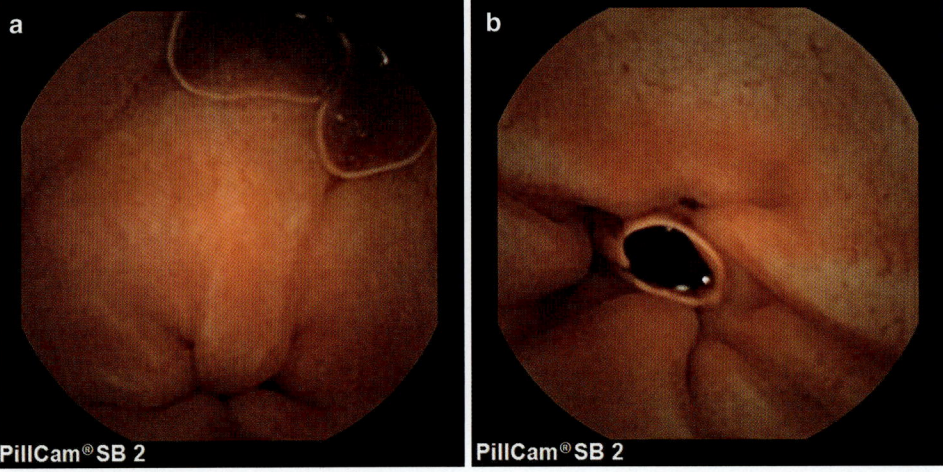

Fig. 44.4 Fried noodle in the stomach, before digestion (**a**) and after 2 h 47 min (**b**)

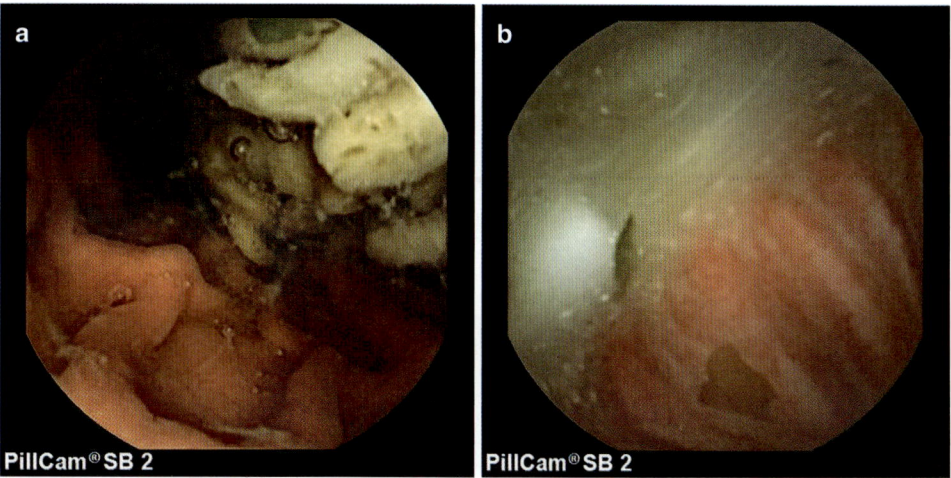

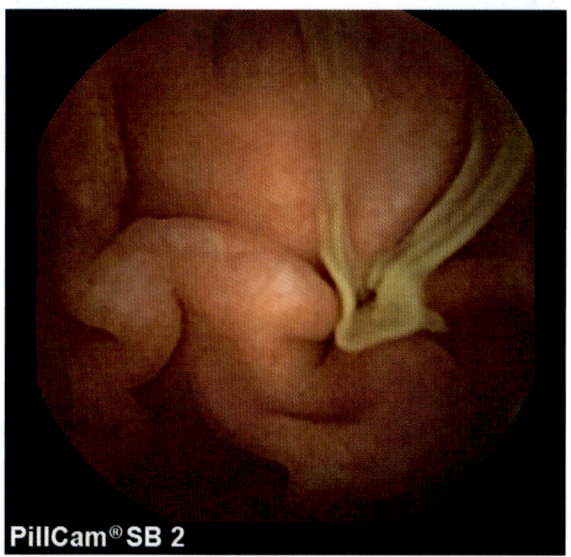

Fig. 44.5 Duodenogastric reflux (bile reflux)

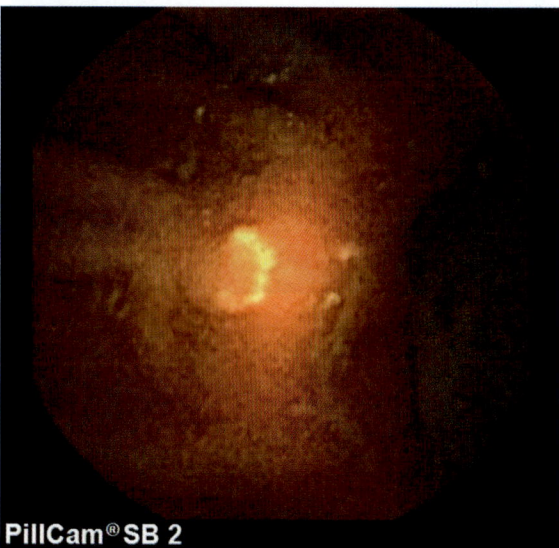

Fig. 44.6 Gastric postoperative appearance with a xanthoma

44.1.2 Gastropathy and Gastric Erosion

The absence of air insufflation and mucosal distention in VCE presents the examiner with an unaccustomed view; so, it is often difficult to interpret the images of the gastric mucosa. However, when the patient drinks some water, VCE can visualize the normal stomach and gastropathy (Figs. 44.7 and 44.8).

Gastric erosions sometimes occur in patients with *Helicobacter pylori* (*H. pylori*) infection (Fig. 44.9). However, VCE often visualizes erosions in patients without *H. pylori* infection (Figs. 44.10, 44.11, 44.12, and 44.13).

In patients with obscure gastrointestinal (GI) bleeding, VCE sometimes detects the bleeding point in the stomach (Fig. 44.14).

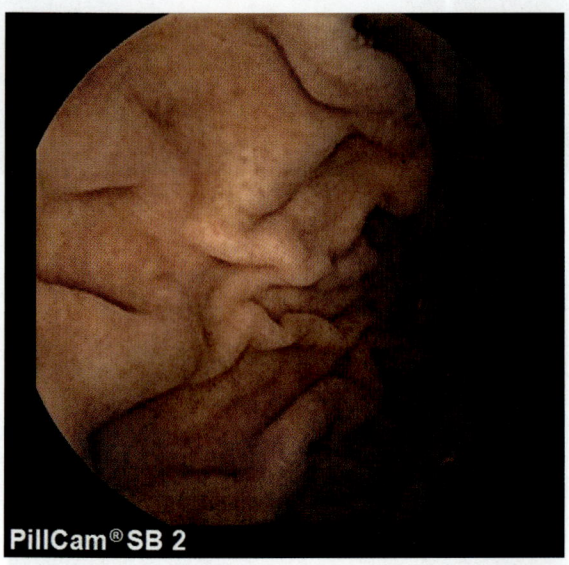

Fig. 44.7 Normal stomach (nonatrophic and negative for *Helicobacter pylori* infection)

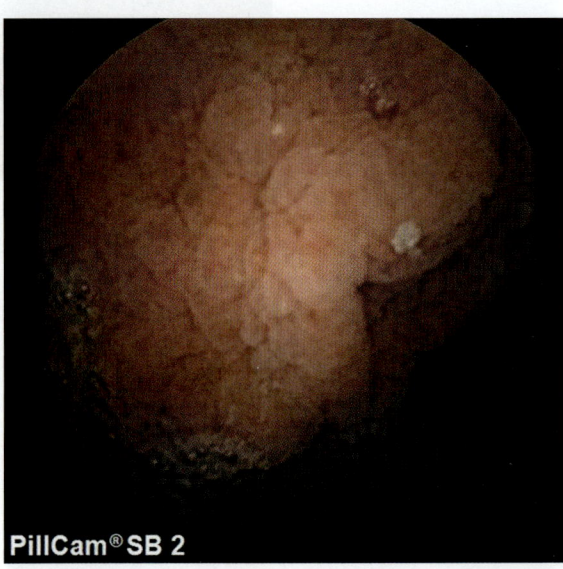

Fig. 44.8 Hypertrophic gastropathy with intestinal metaplasia (post-eradication of *H. pylori*)

Fig. 44.9 (**a**) Hemorrhagic erosive gastropathy with *H. pylori* infection, seen with VCE. (**b**) View using FICE 1 (flexible spectral imaging color enhancement setting 1)

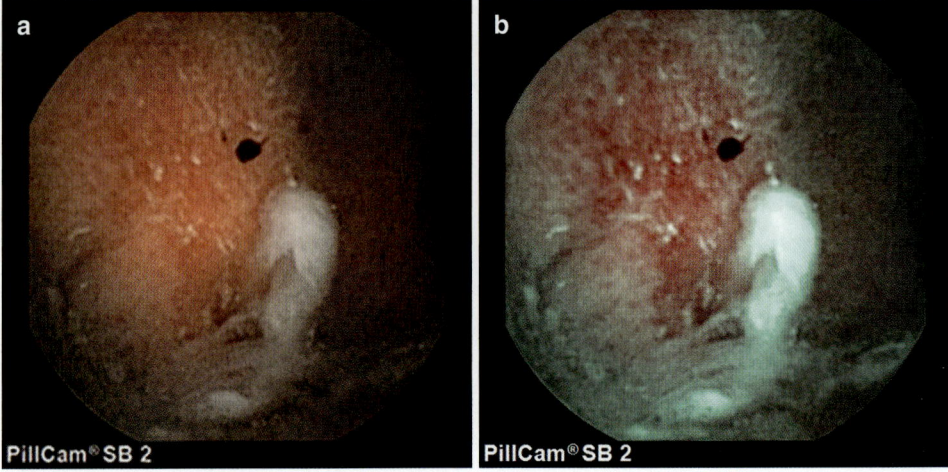

Fig. 44.10 (**a**) Hemorrhagic erosive gastropathy without *H. pylori* infection, on VCE. (**b**) View using FICE 1

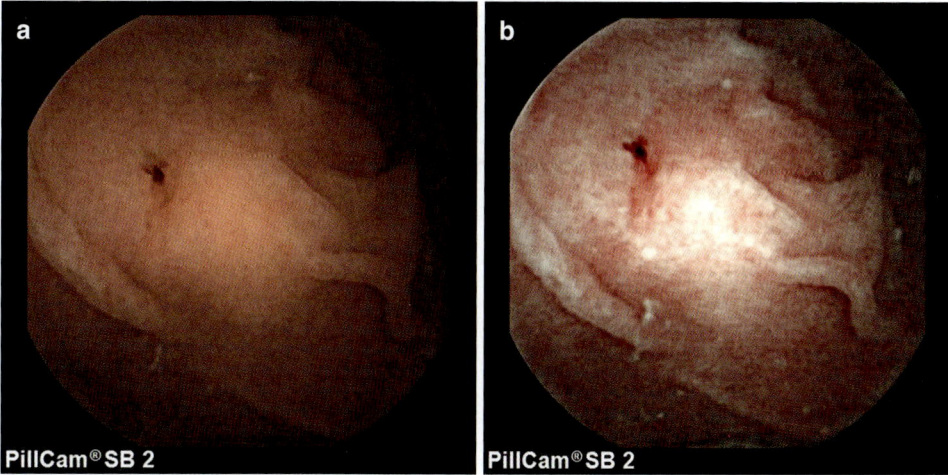

Fig. 44.11 (**a**) Erosive gastropathy (flat gastric erosions) on VCE. (**b**) View using FICE 1

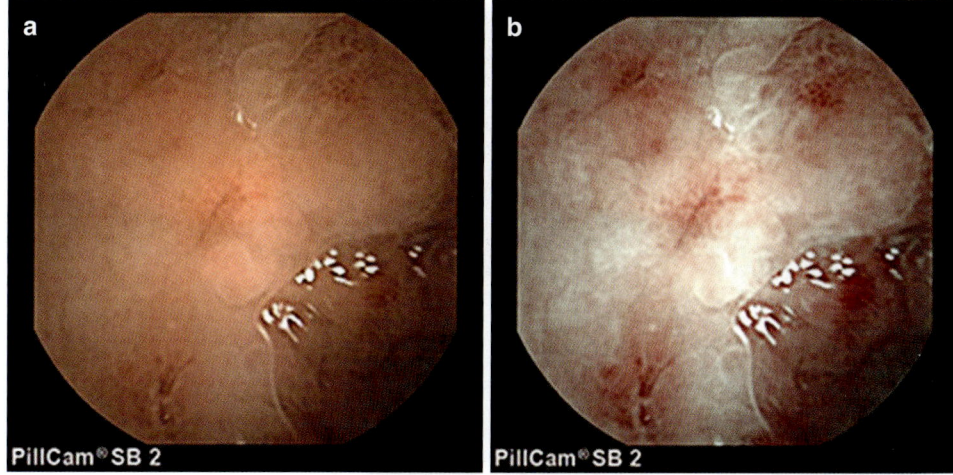

Fig. 44.12 (**a**) Erosive gastropathy (elevated erosion) on VCE. (**b**) Endoscopic image in the same patient

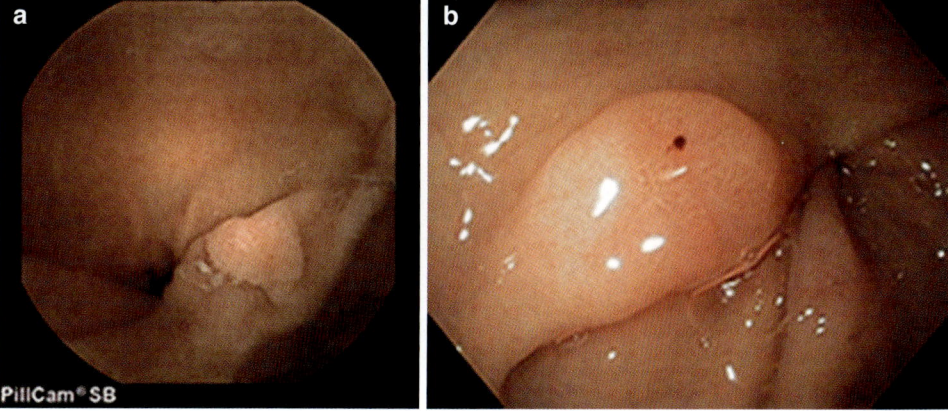

Fig. 44.13 (**a**) Erosive gastropathy (elevated erosions) on VCE. (**b**) View using FICE 1

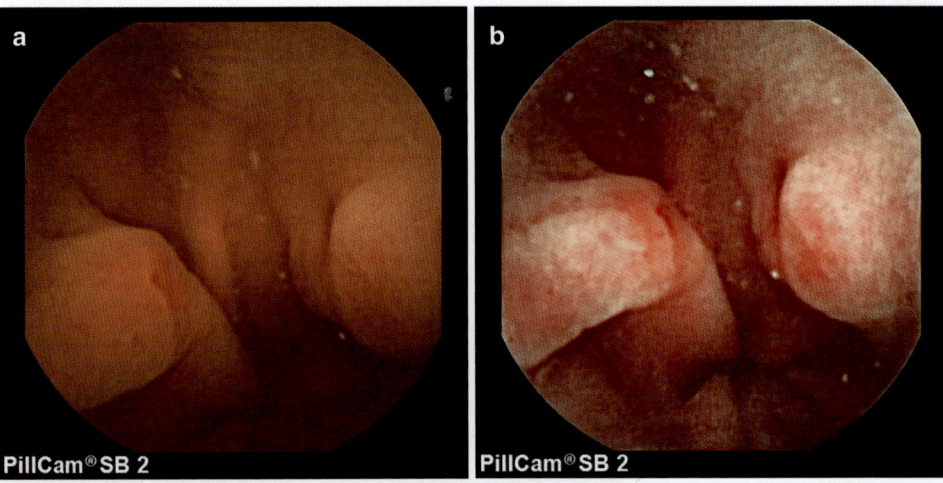

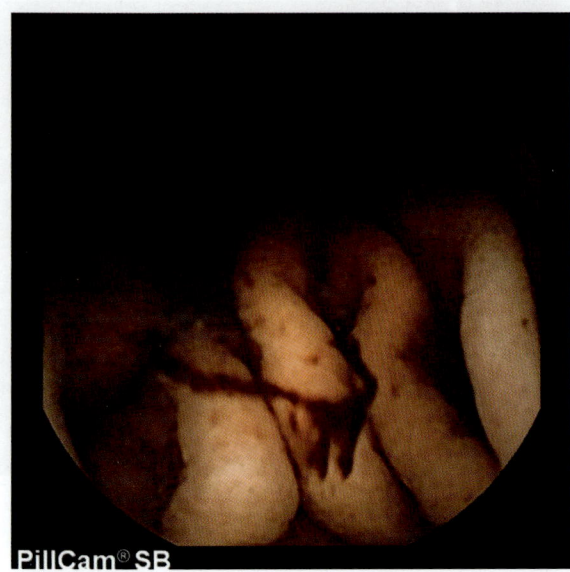

Fig. 44.14 Hemorrhagic gastropathy, seen on VCE

44.1.3 Vascular Lesions in the Stomach

Angiectasia presents as a red area in the stomach, and it is clearly visualized by FICE1 (flexible spectral imaging color enhancement setting 1; R, 595 nm; G, 540 nm; B, 535 nm; Fujifilm, Japan) (Fig. 44.15). Ordinary endoscopic and mag-

nifying endoscopic images of this lesion are shown in Fig. 44.15c, d.

Gastric antral vascular ectasia (GAVE) ("watermelon stomach") has been considered an uncommon cause of GI bleeding. GAVE is commonly missed at upper gastrointestinal (GI) endoscopy, but it is often revealed by VCE (Fig. 44.16) [6–8].

Fig. 44.15 Angiectasia of the stomach: original image from video capsule endoscopy (VCE) (**a**) and with FICE 1 (**b**); view on ordinary endoscopy (**c**) and magnifying endoscopy (**d**)

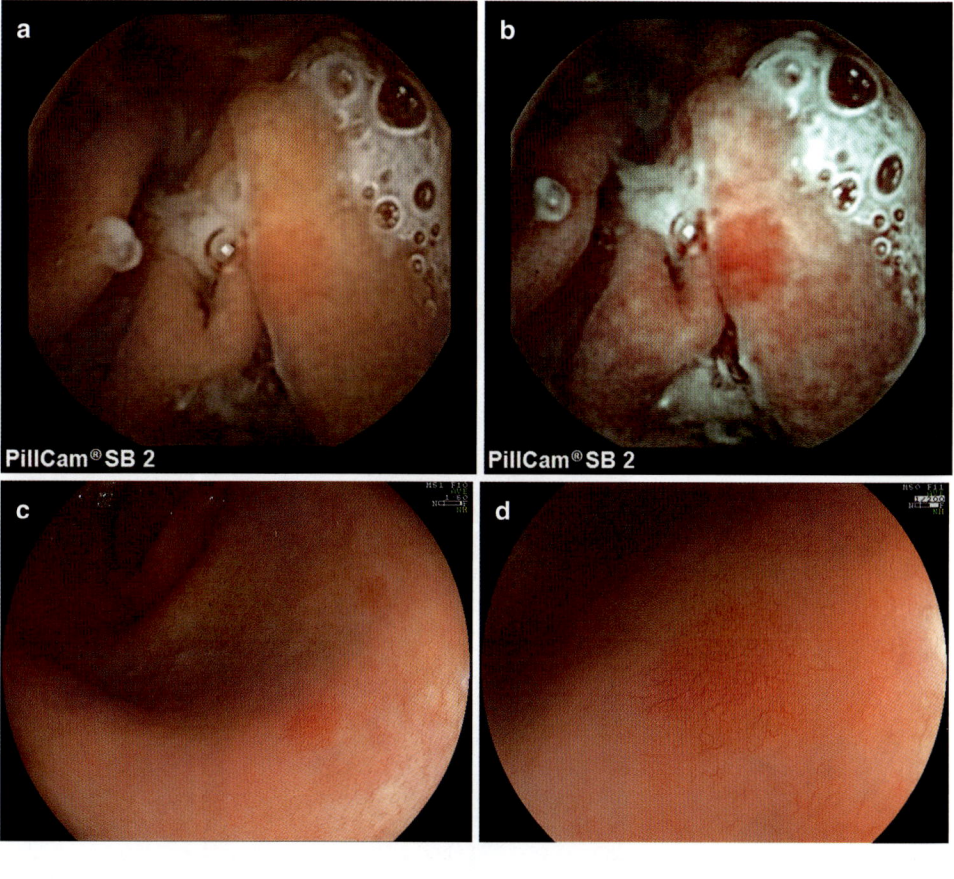

Fig. 44.16 (**a**, **b**) Gastric antral vascular ectasia (GAVE) with watermelon-like appearance in VCE

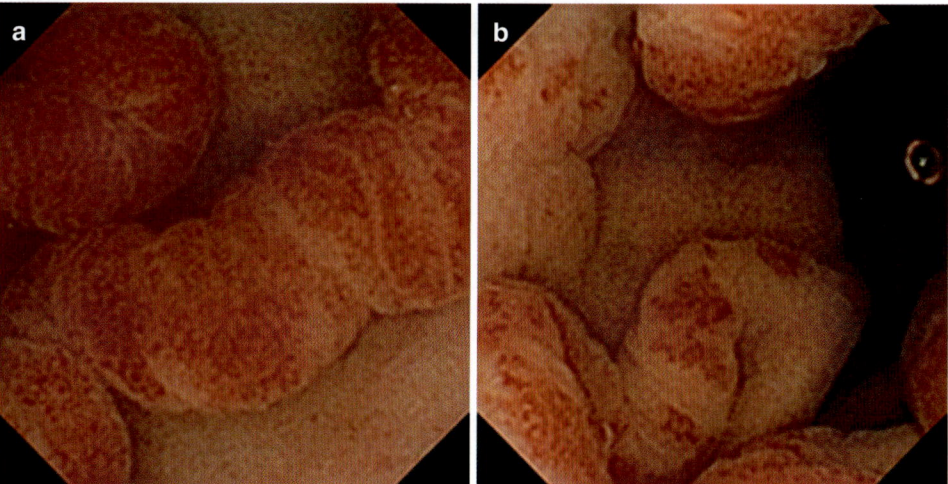

44.1.4 Gastric Tumors

Gastric tumors such as polyps, adenomas, and carcinomas occasionally may be observed at VCE. Glandular cysts can present as protruding cystic lesions with a typical thin, irregular wall. Larger size or hemorrhage is rare (Fig. 44.17). Although harmless, they may be associated with colonic adenomas. Gastric polyp is sometimes visualized by VCE, but it is defined much more reliably by conventional endoscopy (Fig. 44.18). When i-Scan (a post-processing digital filter from Pentax, Tokyo, Japan) or confocal laser microscopy is applied in the same patient, much more detailed information will be available (Fig. 44.18). VCE is less than completely reliable in detecting gastric tumors at this time. Further development of remote-controlled capsule endoscopy [9] may make early detection of gastric tumors by VCE a reality.

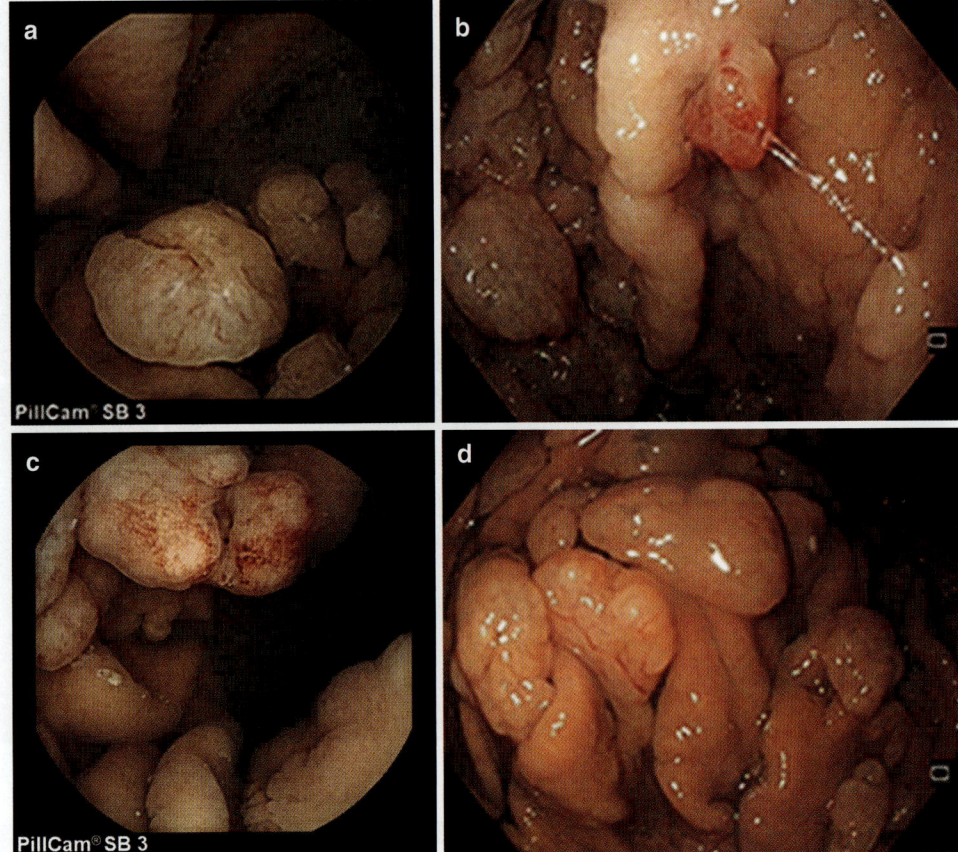

Fig. 44.17 Gastric glandular cysts, partially with intramucosal hemorrhage, viewed with VCE (**a**, **c**) and with endoscopy (**b**, **d**)

Fig. 44.18 Gastric polyp (hyperplasia of foveolar cell): (**a**) VCE original image, (**b**) endoscopic image, (**c**) image with blue mode, (**d**) i-Scan (Pentax, Tokyo, Japan), (**e**) confocal laser microscopy

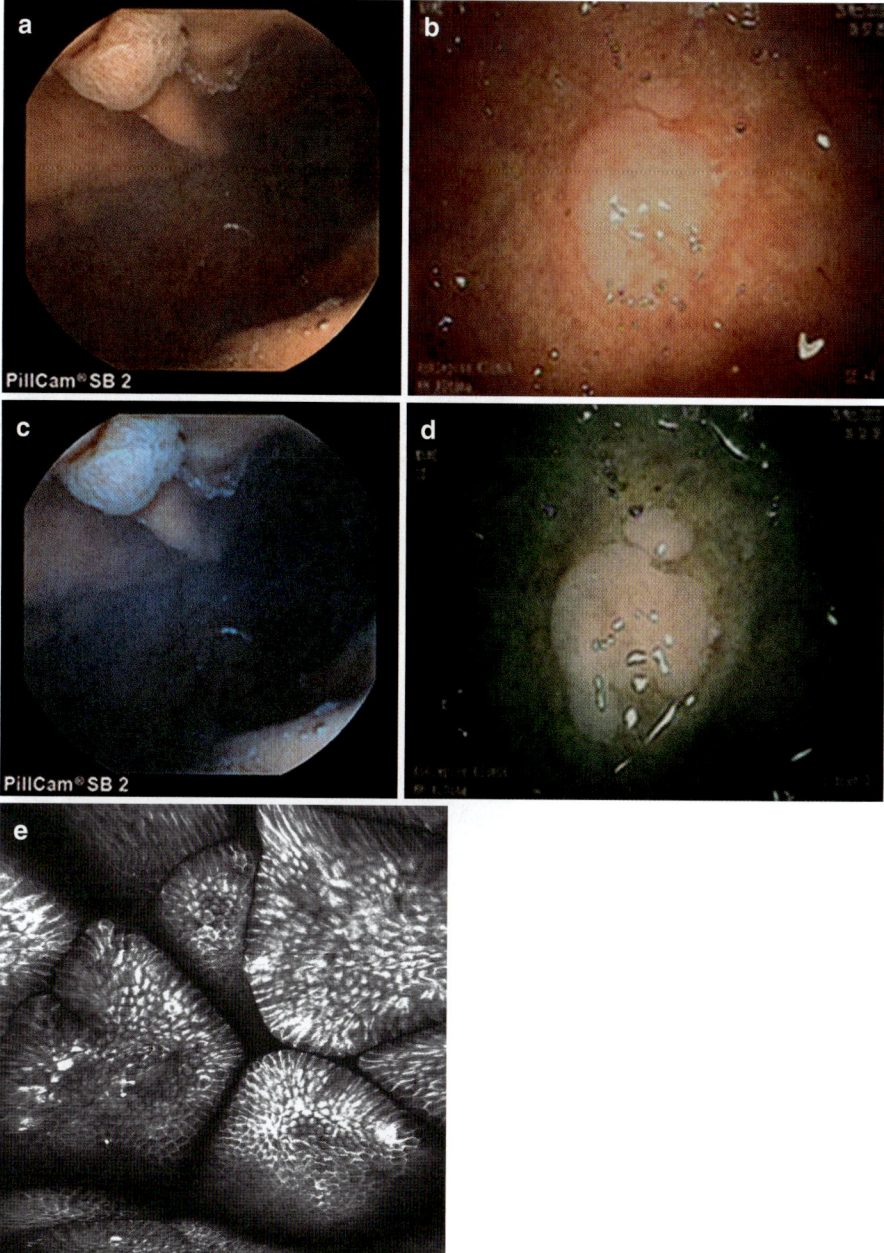

44.1.5 Rare Conditions in the Stomach

Ectopic pancreas (Fig. 44.19) and intragastric suture (Fig. 44.20) are two examples of rare conditions that may be discovered by VCE.

44.2 Findings in the Duodenum

44.2.1 Benign Lesions

Benign lesions in the duodenal bulb, such as gastric metaplasia, gastric heterotopia [10], Brunner's glands hyperplasia, and cysts, are observed at VCE. Sometimes, gastric metaplasia is suspected as benign tumor by VCE (Fig. 44.21). Occasionally, gastric heterotopia is observed by VCE (Fig. 44.22).

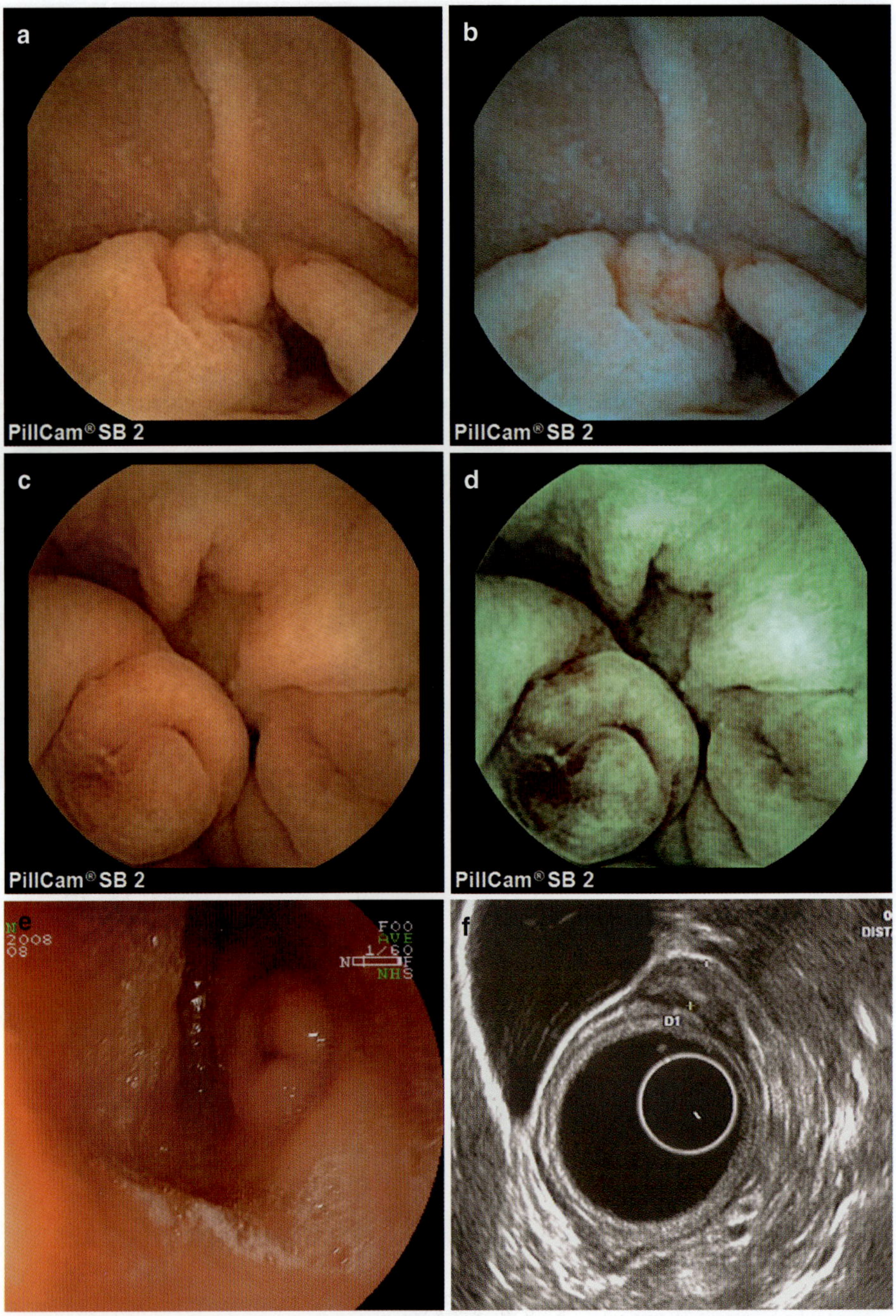

Fig. 44.19 (**a**) VCE original image, (**b**) image with blue mode, (**c**) VCE original image, (**d**) image with FICE setting 2 (R, 420 nm; G, 520 nm; B, 530 nm), (**e**) endoscopic image, (**f**) endoscopic ultrasonography

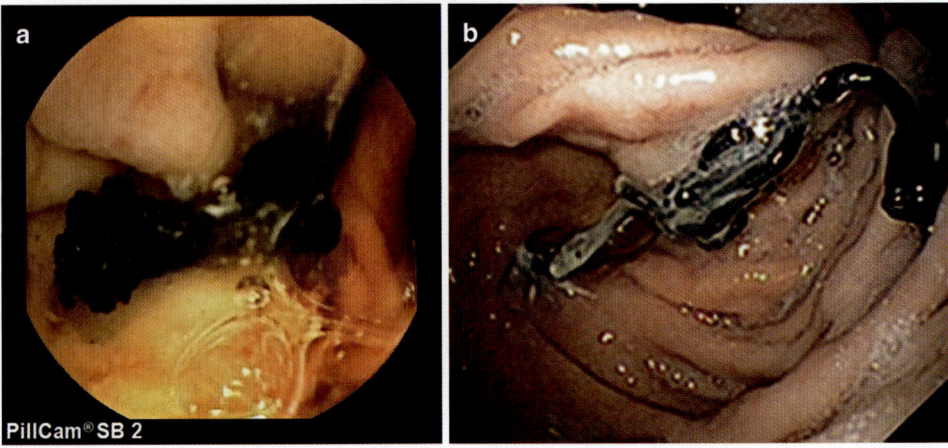

Fig. 44.20 (**a**) Intragastric suture on VCE. (**b**) Endoscopic image

Fig. 44.21 (**a**) Duodenal benign tumors (gastric metaplasias in the duodenal bulb) viewed with VCE. (**b**) Endoscopic image

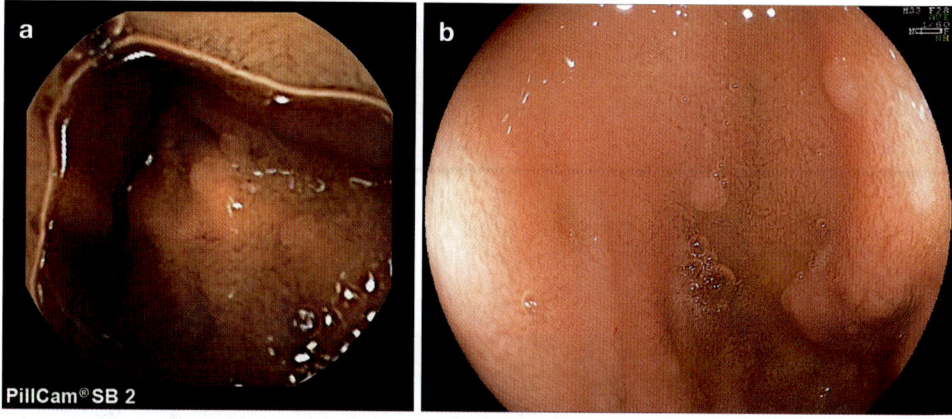

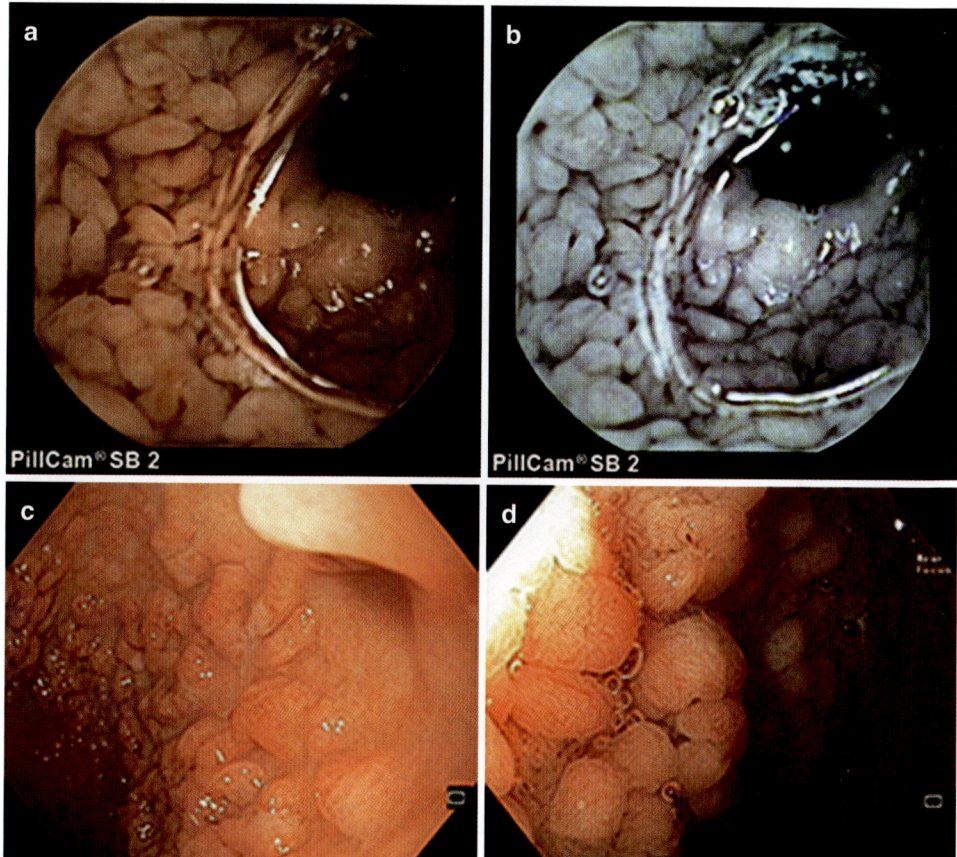

Fig. 44.22 Duodenal benign tumors (gastric heterotopia in the duodenal bulb). (**a**) VCE original image; (**b**) VCE image with *blue* mode. (**c**, **d**) Endoscopic images

44.2.2 Duodenal Ulcer

Duodenal ulcer is sometimes observed at VCE (Figs. 44.23 and 44.24). In some patients, initial upper GI endoscopy misses the lesion (Fig. 44.23).

44.2.3 Papilla of Vater and Variation of the Normal Duodenum

In most cases, the papilla of Vater is not observed at VCE, but when the camera is pointing at the oral side, the papilla can be clearly visualized (Figs. 44.25 and 44.26).

White spots of the duodenum at VCE may occur as a variation of normal duodenum (Fig. 44.27).

Fig. 44.23 (**a**) Duodenal ulcer, partially covered by inflammatory swelling of the margins viewed with VCE. (**b**) Repeat endoscopic image; the ulcer had been missed at initial upper GI endoscopy

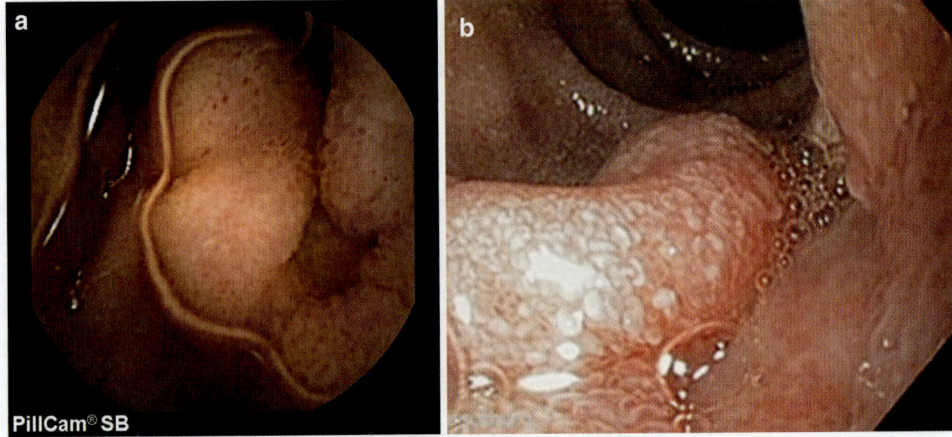

Fig. 44.24 (**a**) Duodenal ulcer (large fibrin-coated ulcer) viewed with VCE. (**b**) Endoscopic image

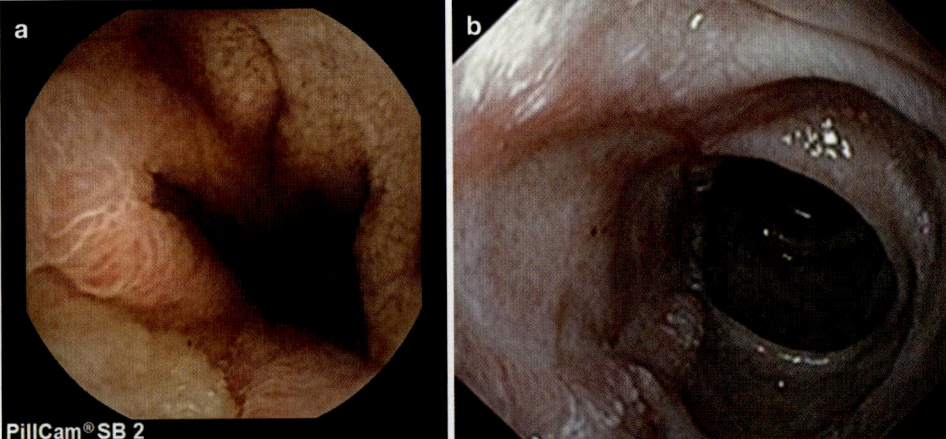

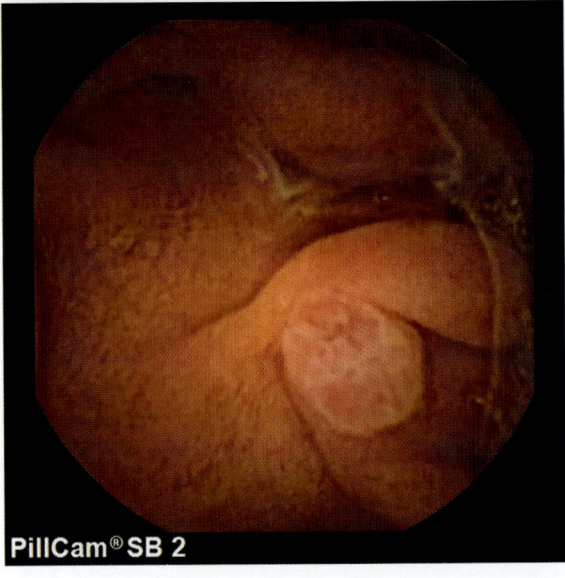

Fig. 44.25 Papilla of Vater on VCE

Fig. 44.26 Major and minor papilla of Vater seen with VCE (**a**) and side-viewing endoscopy (**b**). Detailed view of minor papilla seen with VCE (**c**) and endoscopy (**d**). Detailed view of major papilla seen with VCE (**e**) and endoscopy (**f**)

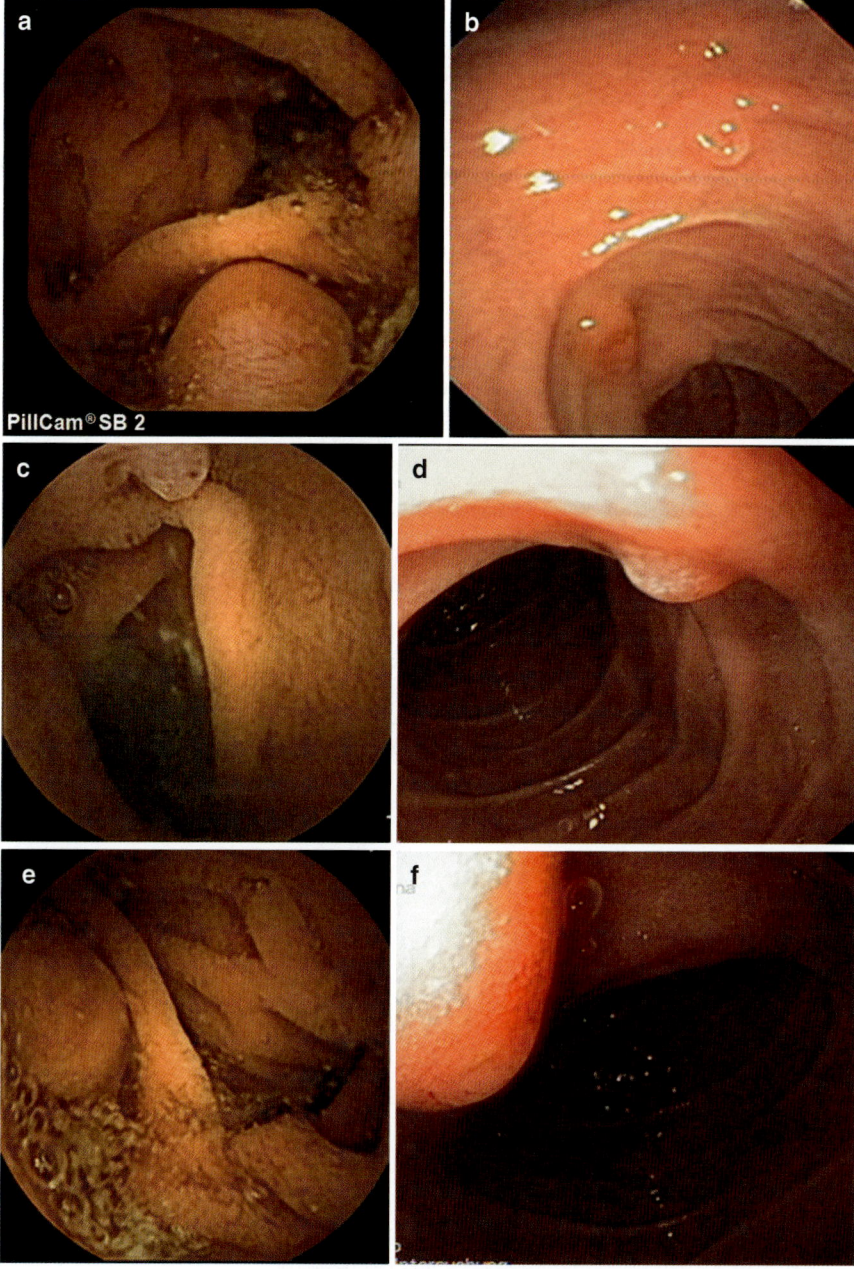

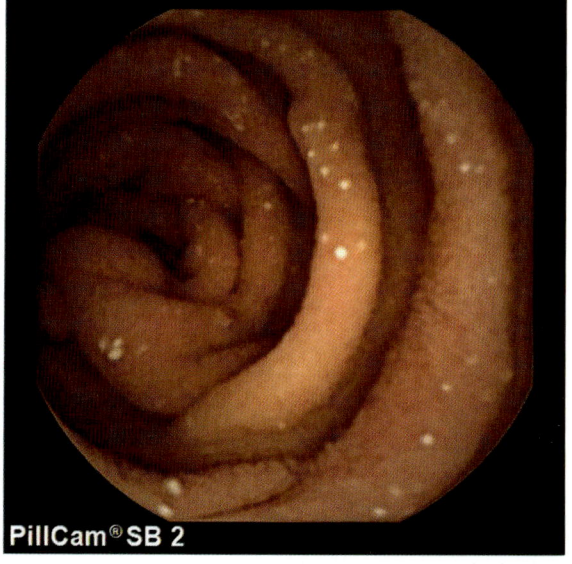

Fig. 44.27 Variation of normal duodenal image on VCE (*white spots* of the duodenum)

References

1. Adler S, Fireman T. Evaluation of the performance of the video capsule system for screening of the stomach. Gastrointest Endosc. 2003;57:AB167.
2. Kobayashi Y, Watabe H, Yamada A, et al. Diagnostic yield of capsule endoscopy for gastric diseases. Abdom Imaging. 2012;37:29–34.
3. Van Gossum A, Hittelet A, Schmit A, et al. A prospective comparative study of push and wireless-capsule enteroscopy in patients with obscure digestive bleeding. Acta Gastroenterol Belg. 2003;66:199–205.
4. Delvaux M, Fassler I, Gay G. Clinical usefulness of the endoscopic video capsule as the initial intestinal investigation in patients with obscure digestive bleeding: validation of a diagnostic strategy based on the patient outcome after 12 months. Endoscopy. 2004;36:1067–73.
5. Takahashi Y, Fujimori S, Toyoda M, et al. The blind spot of an EGD: capsule endoscopy pinpointed the source of obscure GI bleeding on the dark side of the pylorus. Gastrointest Endosc. 2011;73:607–8.
6. Kitiyakara T, Selby W. Non-small-bowel lesions detected by capsule endoscopy in patients with obscure GI bleeding. Gastrointest Endosc. 2005;62:234–8.
7. Tang SJ, Zanati S, Kandel G, et al. Gastric intestinal vascular ectasia syndrome: findings on capsule endoscopy. Endoscopy. 2005;37:1244–7.
8. Sidhu R, Sanders DS, McAlindon ME. Does capsule endoscopy recognise gastric antral vascular ectasia more frequently than conventional endoscopy? J Gastrointestin Liver Dis. 2006;15:375–7.
9. Keller J, Fibbe C, Volke F, et al. Inspection of the human stomach using remote-controlled capsule endoscopy: a feasibility study in healthy volunteers (with videos). Gastrointest Endosc. 2011;73:22–8.
10. Lessels AM, Martin DF. Heterotopic gastric mucosa in the duodenum. J Clin Pathol. 1982;35:591–5.

Colon Capsule Endoscopy: Procedure and Evaluation

45

Samuel N. Adler, Cristiano Spada, and Rami Eliakim

Contents

The work was first published in 2006 by Springer Medizin Verlag Heidelberg with the following title: *Atlas of Video Capsule Endoscopy.*

S.N. Adler (✉)
Department of Gastroenterology,
Shaare Zedek Medical Center, Jerusalem, Israel
e-mail: nasnadler@gmail.com

C. Spada
Department of Surgical Endoscopy,
Università Cattolica del Sacro Cuore, Rome, Italy
e-mail: cristianospada@gmail.com

R. Eliakim
Department of Gastroenterology, Sheba Medical Center,
Sackler School of Medicine, Tel-Aviv University,
Tel-Hashomer, Israel
e-mail: abraham.eliakim@sheba.health.gov.il

The technical aspects of performing colon capsule endoscopy may be a dry and uninspiring topic to write about, but the topic has great importance for the execution of a successful and meaningful colon capsule study. The second-generation PillCam COLON capsule (Given Imaging Ltd., Yoqneam, Israel) (Colon Capsule 2) has been equipped with a new lens that has a wider angle of view and an adjustable transmission rate of images per second to a new data recorder (DR3) (Fig. 45.1). These features have increased the sensitivity of colon capsule endoscopy by nearly 30 % in identifying patients with polyps measuring at least 6 mm [1, 2] (Figs. 45.2 and 45.3). Yet this increase is dependent on two basic premises: The bowel must be adequately cleansed and the capsule must pass through the entire colon. To achieve these two goals, it is of utmost importance to follow precise guidelines, which will guarantee adequate cleansing of the colon in 80 % of patients and a complete capsule pass rate of up to 89 % [2]. Once the study is completed, the reviewer must examine the images diligently. The best capsule technology cannot compensate for sloppy reading. Guidelines for proper reading have been formulated.

In 2011, capsule endoscopy experts met in Tarquinia, Italy, with the declared intent of defining guidelines for the performance of colon capsule endoscopy [3]. The participating physicians relied on 12 peer-reviewed, good-quality papers that covered 1,500 colon capsule studies. The level of reliability of the conclusions drawn from these studies is considered good. This chapter relates to Colon Capsule 2 procedures and omits the instructions relevant to the outdated first-generation colon capsule.

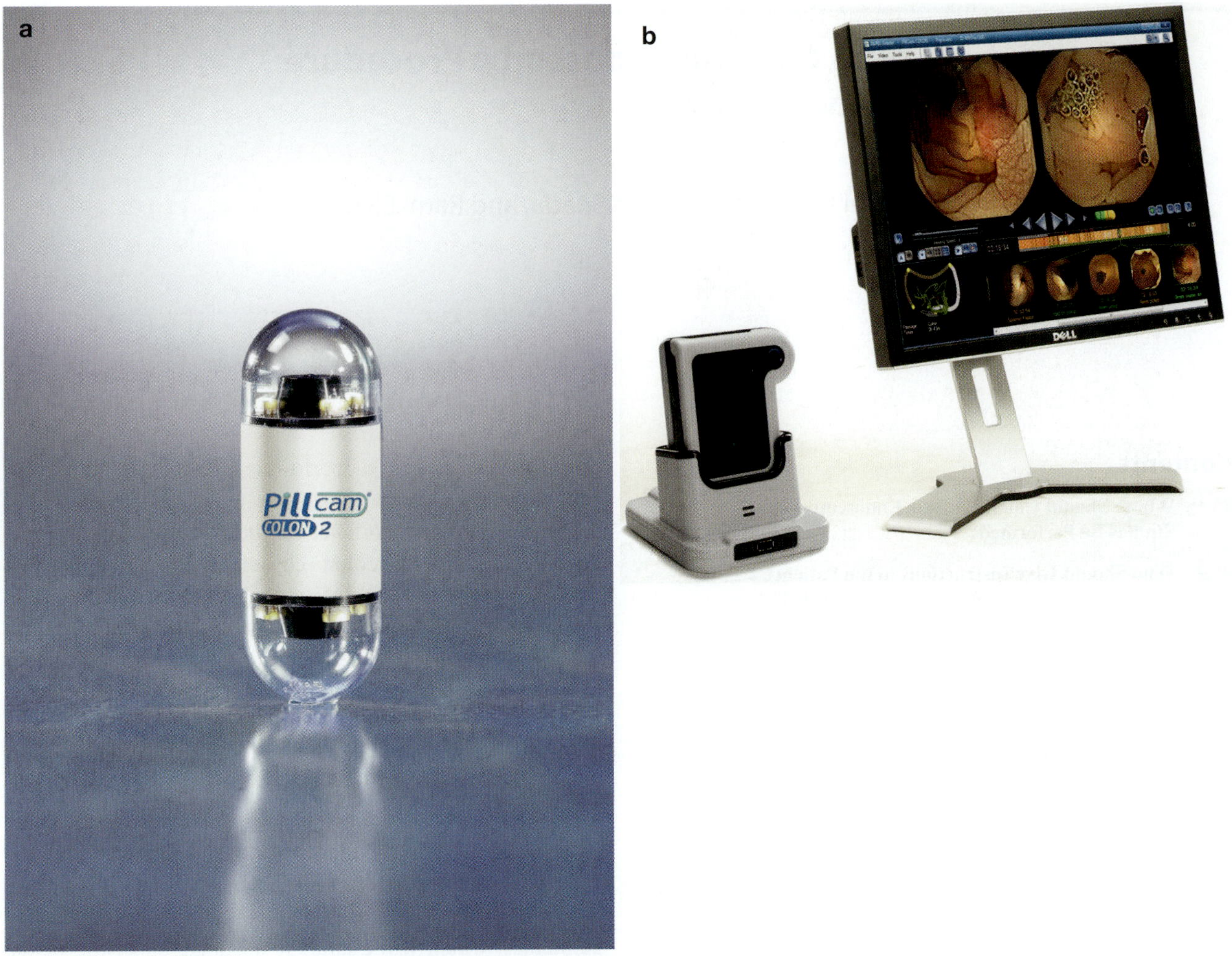

a

b

Fig. 45.1 (**a**) Second-generation PillCam COLON capsule (Given Imaging Ltd., Yoqneam, Israel). (**b**) DR3 recorder and screen

Fig. 45.2 Colonic adenoma, viewed with colon capsule endoscopy (CCE) (**a**) and conventional colonoscopy (**b**)

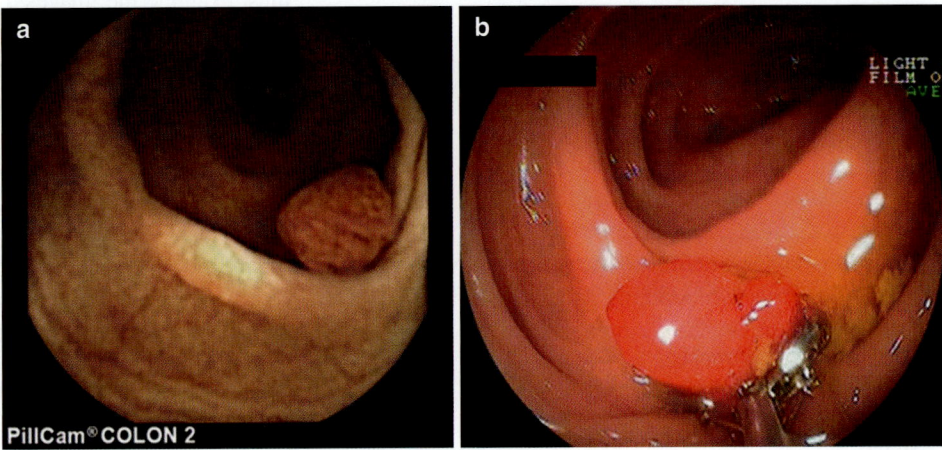

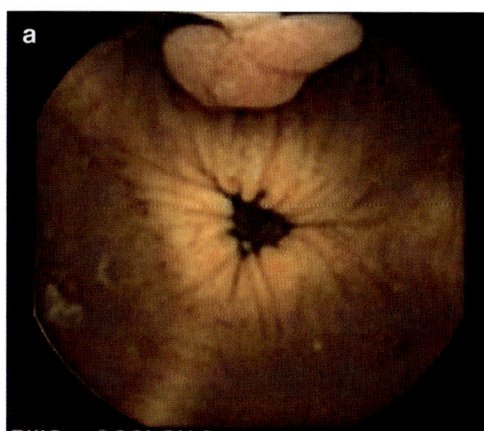

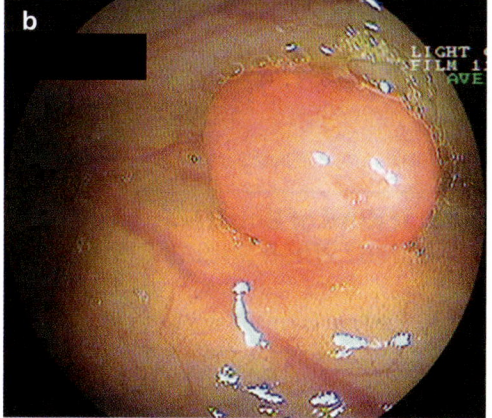

Fig. 45.3 Colonic adenoma, viewed with CCE (**a**) and conventional colonoscopy (**b**)

45.1 Where Should Colon Capsule Endoscopy Studies Be Performed?

Patients participating in a colon capsule study are required to ingest laxative boosters once the capsule has entered the small bowel. The purpose of the laxative booster is to accelerate the capsule transit through the small bowel while keeping the colon adequately clean for proper examination by the capsule. All published colon capsule studies were performed in a medically supervised outpatient setting. Therefore, this setting has been proven effective. With the advent of new technological features of the DR3, however—

specifically its autodetection mode of small bowel mucosa and the ability to inform the subject to ingest the booster laxatives—it may not be necessary to keep patients in a medically supervised outpatient setting [4]. In fact, colon capsule endoscopy has been reported to be as effective as an out-of-clinic procedure as in a medically supervised out patient setting [5]. In the future, there may be room for a home procedure, but further studies are needed.

45.2 Who Should Give Instructions to the Patient? What Kind of Bowel Preparation Is Needed?

The physician or a dedicated healthcare provider must emphasize the importance of a clean bowel for a successful study and must generate in the patient the necessary motivation and commitment to follow instructions.

All published colon capsule studies have used the bowel preparation regimen listed on Table 45.1. The day prior to the procedure, the patient must be on a clear liquid diet. The evening prior to the procedure, 2 l of polyethylene glycol (PEG) are ingested, and another 2 l are ingested on the morning of the procedure.

Although the guidelines do not recommend asking the patient whether the patient has clear bowel excretions, it may be very helpful to do so. In our experience the addition of some more laxative may be helpful if the excretions are not completely clear.

The medical personnel place the sensor array (Fig. 45.4a) or sensor belt (Fig. 45.4b) on the abdomen of the patient Fig. 45.5, who then swallows the blinking Colon Capsule 2.

Table 45.1 Bowel preparation regimen for colon capsule studies

Day prior to procedure	Clear liquid diet only
Evening prior to procedure	2 l of PEG
7 a.m. day of procedure	2 l of PEG
Ingestion of Colon Capsule 2	
Booster 1	Na phosphate or SUPREP
Booster 2 (if necessary)	Na phosphate or SUPREP
Suppository (if necessary)	Bisacodyl 10 mg

PEG polyethylene glycol

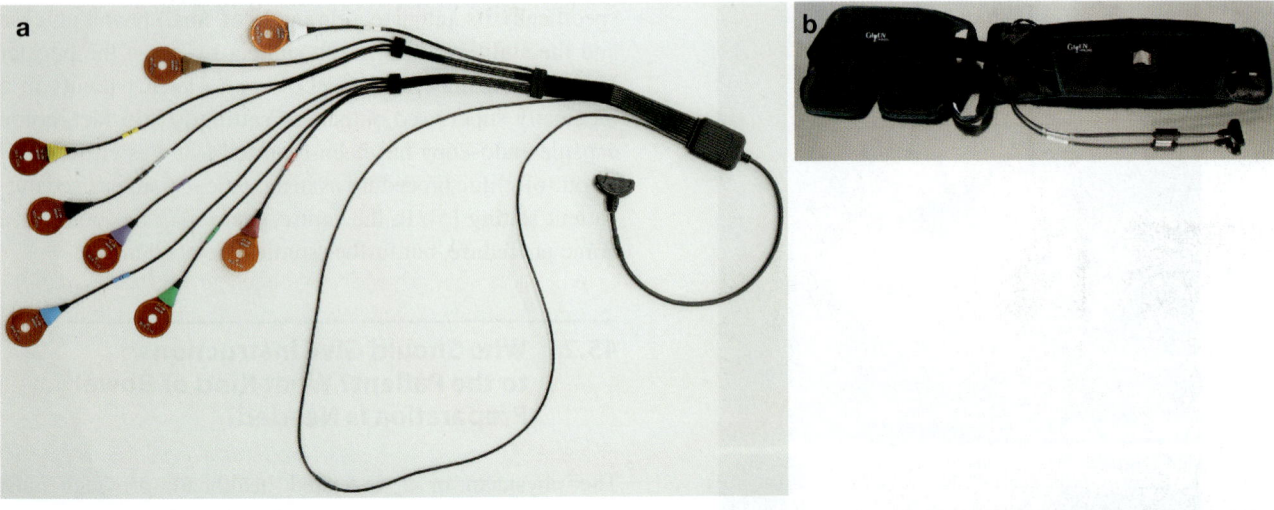

Fig. 45.4 (**a**) Sensor array. (**b**) Sensor belt

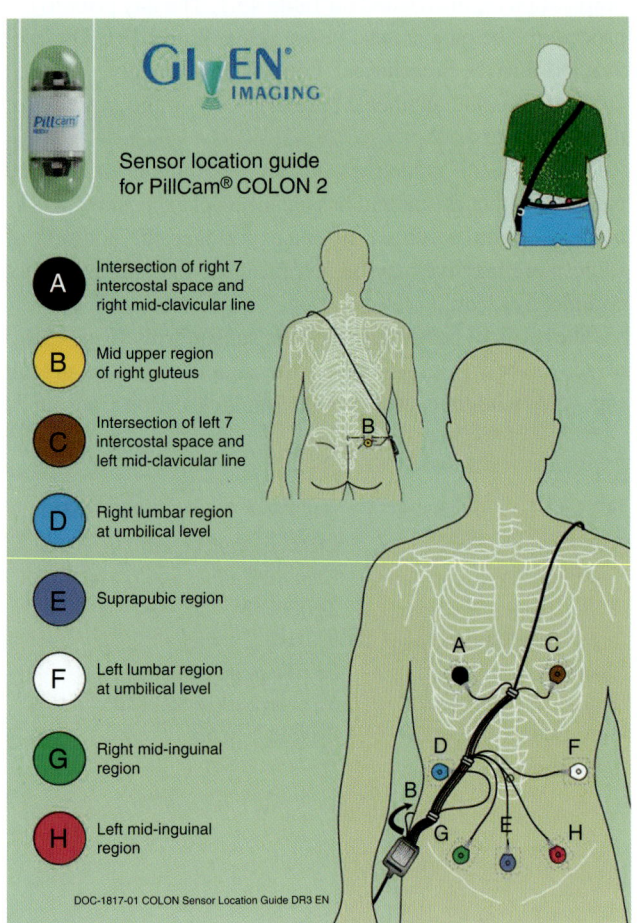

Fig. 45.5 Guide for placement of sensor arrays

45.3 What Kind of Booster Preparation Is Needed? When Should It Be Used?

If the capsule does not leave the stomach within 1 h, DR3 will sound a ringing tone, activate a vibrating device, and display on its LCD screen the digit 0 (Fig. 45.6). According to the instruction sheet (Table 45.2), the patient should then take a prokinetic agent (i.e., 10 mg metoclopramide). The intelligent features of DR3 recognize small bowel mucosa and then alert the patient to swallow the laxative booster. In the published studies, 30 mL of sodium phosphate has been used, but recently, we have successfully tried 180 mL of SUPREP (Braintree Laboratories, Braintree, MA, USA), diluted with water to 480 mL. (SUPREP is a sulfide-based laxative that has no untoward effects on renal function, according to data at the second Tarquinia meeting, 2012). If the capsule has not been passed in 3 h after ingestion of the first laxative booster alert, the patient will ingest a second laxative booster (either 15 mL of sodium phosphate or 180 mL of SUPREP, diluted with water to 480 mL). Finally, if the capsule still has not been excreted, the DR3 will display the digit 3, which indicates that the patient should insert a 10 mg bisacodyl suppository.

45.4 When Is a Study Complete?

A colon capsule study is considered complete once the blinking capsule has been excreted or the camera has transmitted images from the hemorrhoidal plexus.

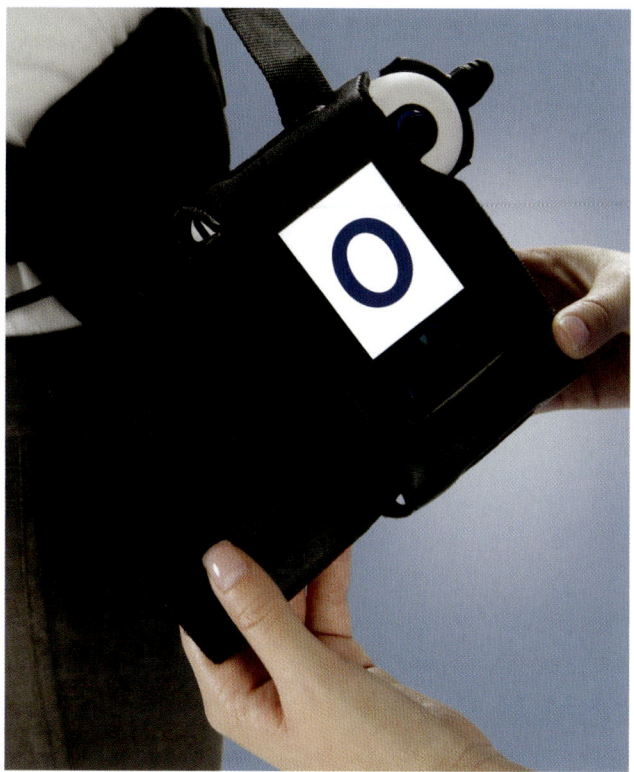

Fig. 45.6 DR3 recorder with message 0 on LCD screen (*see* Table 45.2)

Table 45.2 Instruction sheet

Alert #	Instructions
Note: Following capsule ingestion, maintain a complete fast (no drinking!) until instructed to do otherwise by the Data Recorder alerts and correlating guidelines	
0	Ingest 10 mg metoclopramide with a glass of water. Continue complete fast (no additional drinking) until next alert
1	Dilute 30 mL sodium phosphate in a glass of water and drink it. Drink at least 1 l of water over the next hour. You may resume drinking all clear liquids freely
2	Dilute 15 mL sodium phosphate in a glass of water and drink it. Drink at least 1/2 l of water over the next 30 min. You may continue drinking all clear liquids freely
3	Insert 10 mg bisacodyl suppository according to instructions in package insert
4	You may eat a meal
End of procedure. Please remove equipment from your body	

45.5 Who Should Read Colon Capsule Studies?

From small bowel capsule studies, we have learned that nurses and technical staff can identify pathology findings as well as medical doctors [6]. For this reason, there is no objection to their participation in the review process, as long as strict reading rules are followed.

All readers, including doctors, must undergo formal training and familiarize themselves with various appearances of normal and abnormal findings. The number of procedures that need to be read before proficiency can be assumed is a matter that has not been resolved. Some experts have recommended experience with 30 cases, but others have demanded higher numbers.

45.6 What Is the Proper Review Process?

First, the entire study is viewed in fast mode with the simultaneous view of both cameras. Landmarks are defined, such as first cecal image, first hepatic flexure image, last splenic flexure image, and last rectal image. Pathology findings also are recorded. Then the precise review process begins, first with one camera and then with the second camera. The frame speed should not exceed ten frames per second.

45.7 What Must the Final Report Contain?

- The indication for the procedure.
- Whether the study was complete.
- Whether the bowel was adequately cleaned in general and for each segment (cecum, ascending colon, transverse colon, and left colon).
- All findings must be mentioned, with precise description of all significant pathology (i.e., number of polyps, size of polyps, and their location).
- Diagnosis/interpretation and recommendation. (This part can only be completed by the physician in charge.)
- Adverse events (i.e., capsule retention or malfunction) and colonic transit time.

- Extracolonic findings, such as Barrett's esophagus or gastric or small bowel lesions; these findings are mentioned with a disclaimer by the reader that Colon Capsule 2 endoscopy does not provide a comprehensive review of extracolonic parts of the digestive tract.

References

1. Eliakim R, Yassin K, Niv Y, et al. Prospective multicenter performance evaluation of the second-generation colon capsule compared with colonoscopy. Endoscopy. 2009;41:1026–31.

2. Spada C, Hassan C, Munoz-Navas M, et al. Second-generation colon capsule endoscopy compared with colonoscopy. Gastrointest Endosc. 2011;74:581–9.

3. Spada C, Hassan C, Galmiche JP, et al. Colon capsule endoscopy: European Society of Gastrointestinal Endoscopy (ESGE) guideline. Endoscopy. 2012;44:527–36.

4. Adler S, Hassan C, Metzger Y, et al. Accuracy of automatic detection of small-bowel mucosa by second-generation colon capsule endoscopy. Gastrointest Endosc. 2012;76:1170–4.

5. Adler SN, Metzger YC, Sompolinsky Y, Hassan C. Capsule colonoscopy with PillCam COLON 2 is feasible as an out-of-clinic procedure. Gastroenterology. 2012;142(Suppl):s53–4.

6. Rex DK. Nurses can interpret small-bowel capsule endoscopy accurately. Dig Liver Dis. 2006;38:599–602.

Findings in the Colon

46

Mark N. Appleyard, Martin Keuchel,
and Friedrich Hagenmüller

Contents

Colonic cleansing is not routine for small bowel video capsule endoscopy (VCE), and the capsule usually is not propelled beyond the hepatic flexure, so colonic viewing is not optimal. Nevertheless, longer battery times, improved illumination, and increasing use of bowel preparation before small bowel VCE can provide relevant colonic findings. Cases with colonic findings detected during small bowel VCE but missed at preceding colonoscopy were described soon after the introduction of small bowel VCE [1]. The proportion of patients in whom colonic findings are identified during an investigation of obscure gastrointestinal bleeding ranges from 0 to 4 % [2–4]; for cohorts with all small bowel indications, the range is 0–9 % [5, 6]. Hence, it seems important to evaluate the colonic images as well.

Detection of colonic polyps is the main task of dedicated colon capsule endoscopy (CCE) (Chap. 47). The technology behind CCE studies is different from small bowel VCE (Chap. 45), but the images obtained are very similar. Thus normal colonic anatomy, variants of normal, incidental findings, and nonpolyp lesions are described together in this chapter. Different types of polyps and carcinomas are shown in Chap. 47.

In contrast to standard colonoscopy, CCE images often provide an underwater view without air distension. Though movement of the instrument can be controlled in colonoscopy, VCE has the potential advantage of a longer image acquisition time, mainly in the cecum. Occasionally better images from the proximal side of a fold are provided with the double-headed colon capsule system [7].

The work was first published in 2006 by Springer Medizin Verlag Heidelberg with the following title: *Atlas of Video Capsule Endoscopy*.

M.N. Appleyard (✉)
Department of Gastroenterology and Hepatology,
Royal Brisbane and Women's Hospital, Brisbane, QLD, Australia
e-mail: mark_appleyard@health.qld.gov.au

M. Keuchel,
Department of Internal Medicine, Bethesda Krankenhaus Bergedorf,
Hamburg, Germany
e-mail: keuchel@bkb.info

F. Hagenmüller,
1st Medical Department, Asklepios Klinik Altona,
Hamburg, Germany
e-mail: f.hagenmueller@asklepios.com

M. Keuchel et al. (eds.), *Video Capsule Endoscopy: A Reference Guide and Atlas*,
DOI 10.1007/978-3-662-44062-9_46, © Springer-Verlag Berlin Heidelberg 2014

46.1 Normal Colon

The first cecal image documents complete small bowel investigation. Images from the terminal ileum, ileocecal valve (Fig. 46.1), and appendix (Fig. 46.2) document the appropriate start of CCE in the proximal colon.

The colonic mucosa is paler than that of the ileum, has a more prominent vascular pattern, is haustrated, shows less peristalsis, and is devoid of villi (Fig. 46.3).

Sometimes the hepatic flexure can be visualized directly (Fig. 46.4a). The transverse colon presents with the typical triangular structure (Fig. 46.4b). At the flexures, the liver or spleen sometimes provides a bluish shadow visible through the colonic mucosa (Fig. 46.4c). The descending colon has a more roundish lumen (Fig. 46.4d). Because of the bends in the sigmoid colon, the capsule may be pressed against the mucosa, leading to a more pale aspect. Vessels in the rectum are often more pronounced, and the mucosa may look edematous (Fig. 46.5a). Visualization of the hemorrhoidal plexus confirms a complete colon investigation (Fig. 46.5b).

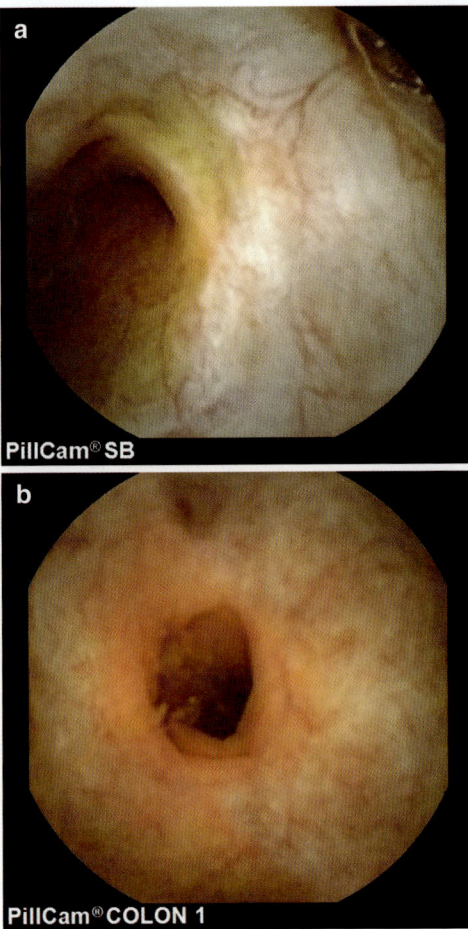

Fig. 46.2 (**a, b**) Aspects of the appendiceal orifice

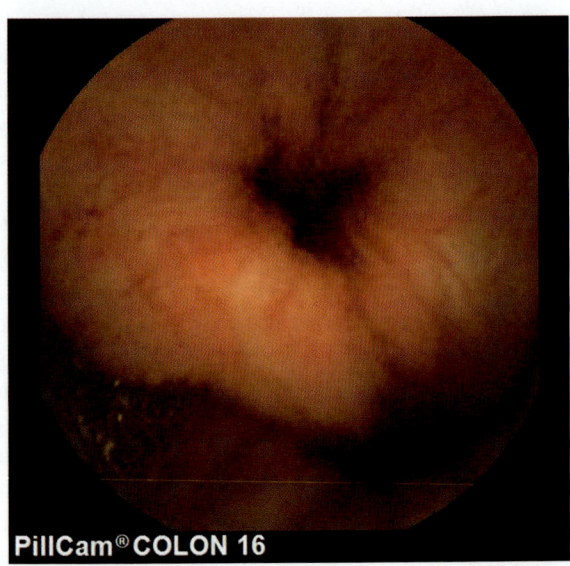

Fig. 46.1 Open lumen of the ileocecal valve seen from the cecum

Fig. 46.3 Comparison of images from the small bowel and colon as seen at video capsule endoscopy (VCE). (**a**) Small bowel mucosa is softer and folds are mobile. (**b**) Colonic haustra are more prominent, with less peristalsis, and the lumen is larger. (**c**) Small bowel mucosa is orange with less prominent vessels and with characteristic villi. (**d**) Colonic mucosa is pale with prominent vessels. (**e**) Small bowel often is filled with liquid, and air bubbles in the small bowel tend to have a more foamy appearance. (**f**) The large colonic lumen tends to be more commonly filled with air

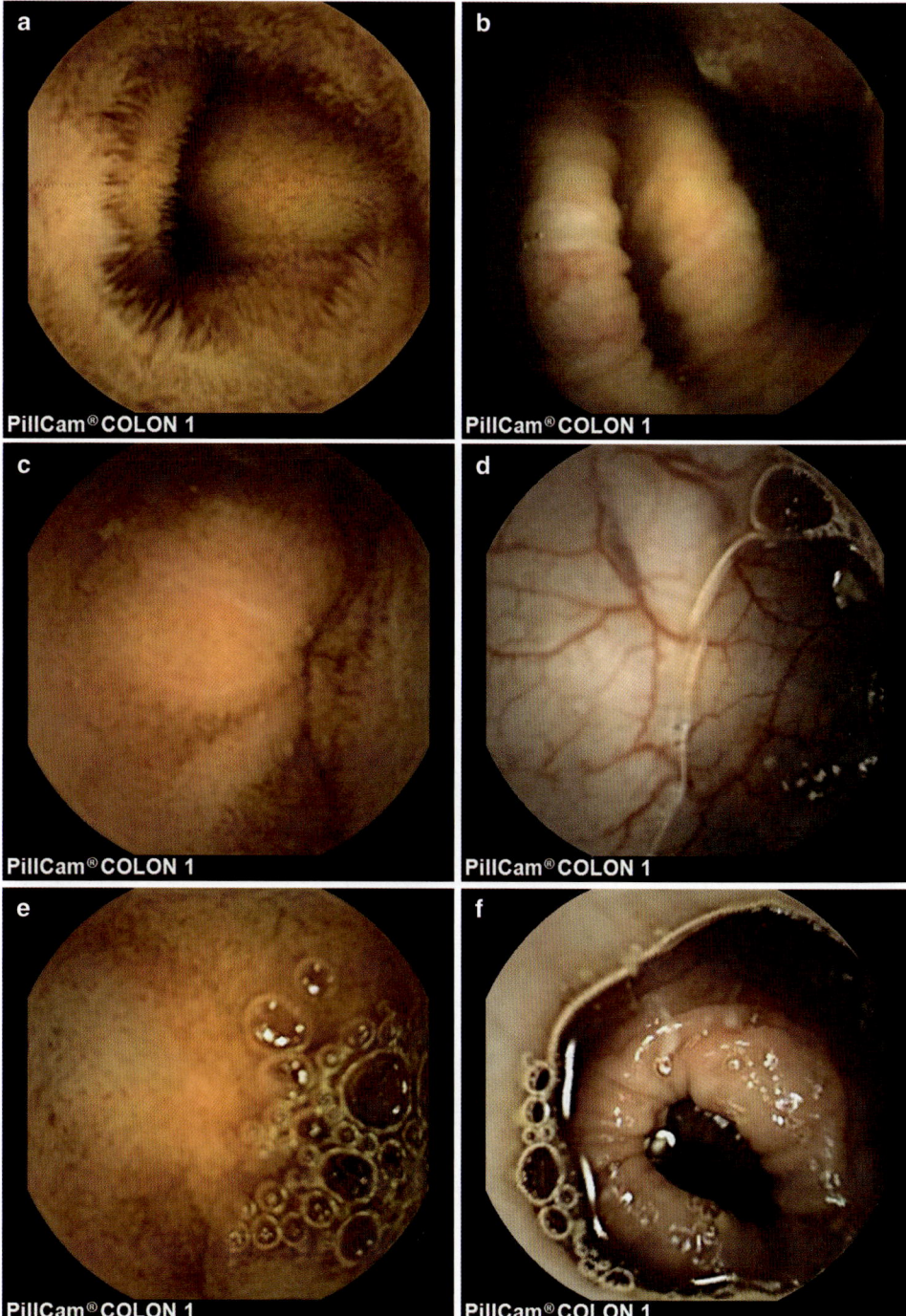

Fig. 46.4 Different areas of the normal colon seen at VCE. (**a**) Right flexure. (**b**) Transverse colon. (**c**) Spleen seen through colonic wall. (**d**) Left colon

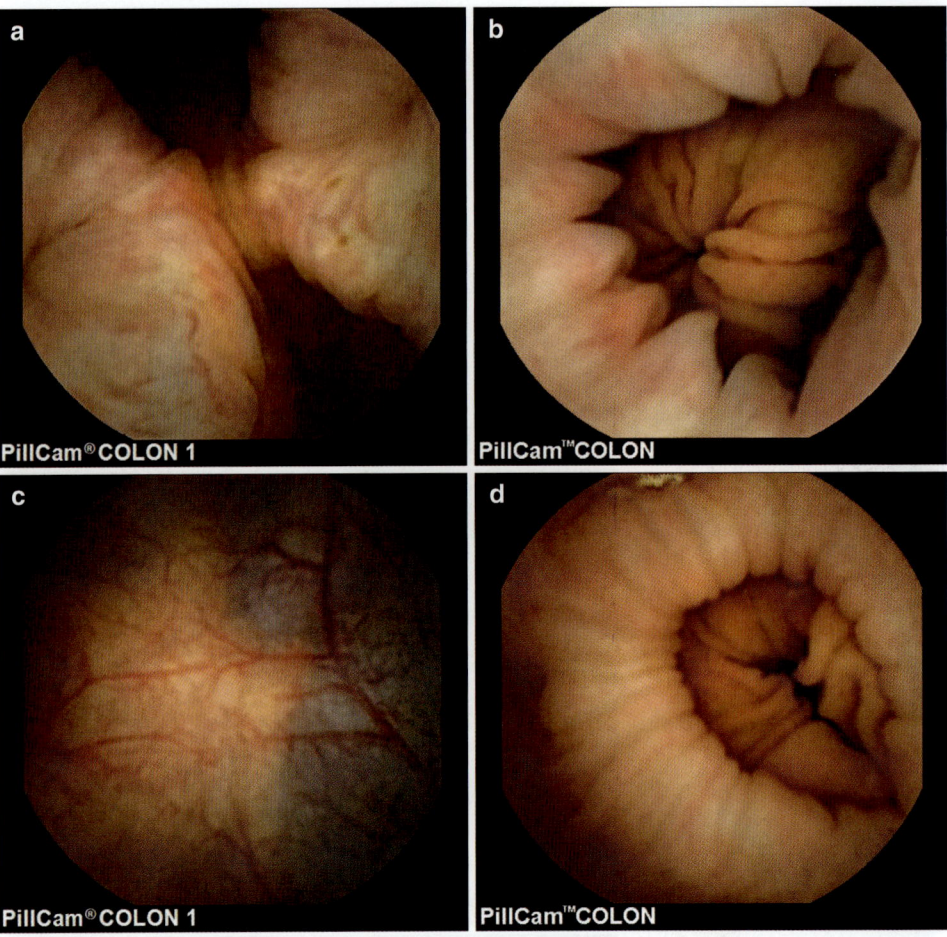

Fig. 46.5 Rectum. (**a**) Rectal mucosa with edematous aspect. (**b**) Hemorrhoidal plexus

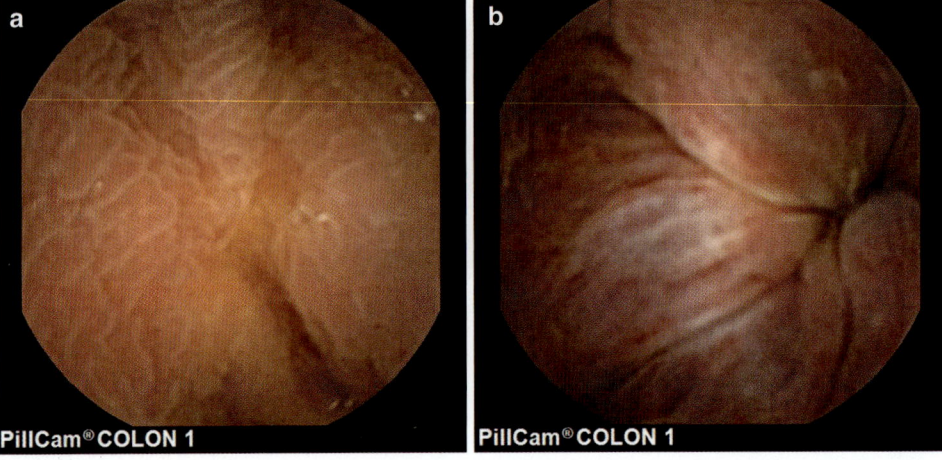

46.2 Variants of Normal

A lipomatous, thickened ileocecal valve with a yellowish, stretched mucosa should not be mistaken for a polyp (Fig. 46.6). An inverted appendiceal stump can be mistaken for a submucosal tumor (Fig. 46.7). In the sigmoid colon, diverticula are frequently seen (Fig. 46.8), especially in elderly patients. Melanosis coli with dark pigmentation of the mucosa is frequently seen in patients taking laxatives on a regular basis (Fig. 46.9). Occasionally hypertrophic anal papillae can be visualized (Fig. 46.10).

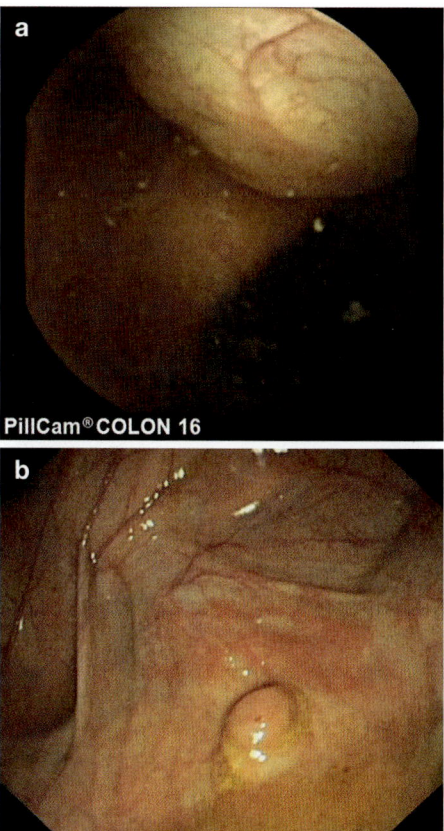

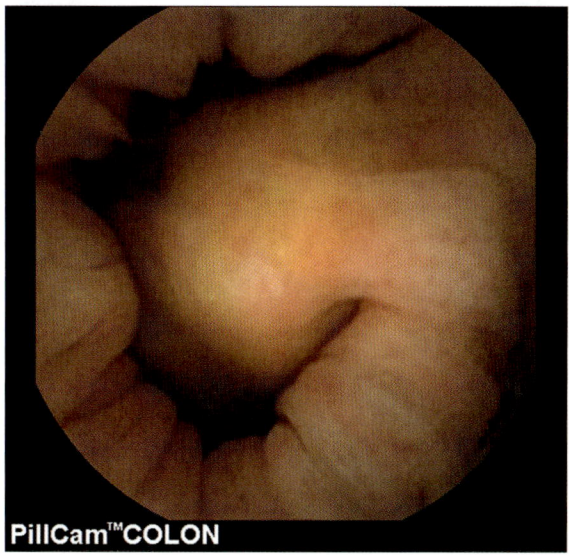

Fig. 46.6 Thickened, lipomatous ileocecal valve

Fig. 46.7 Inverted appendiceal stump, seen at VCE (**a**) and colonoscopy (**b**)

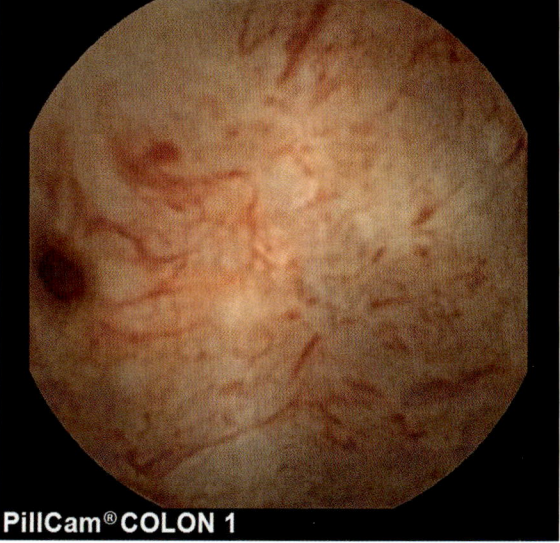

Fig. 46.8 Tiny colonic diverticulum

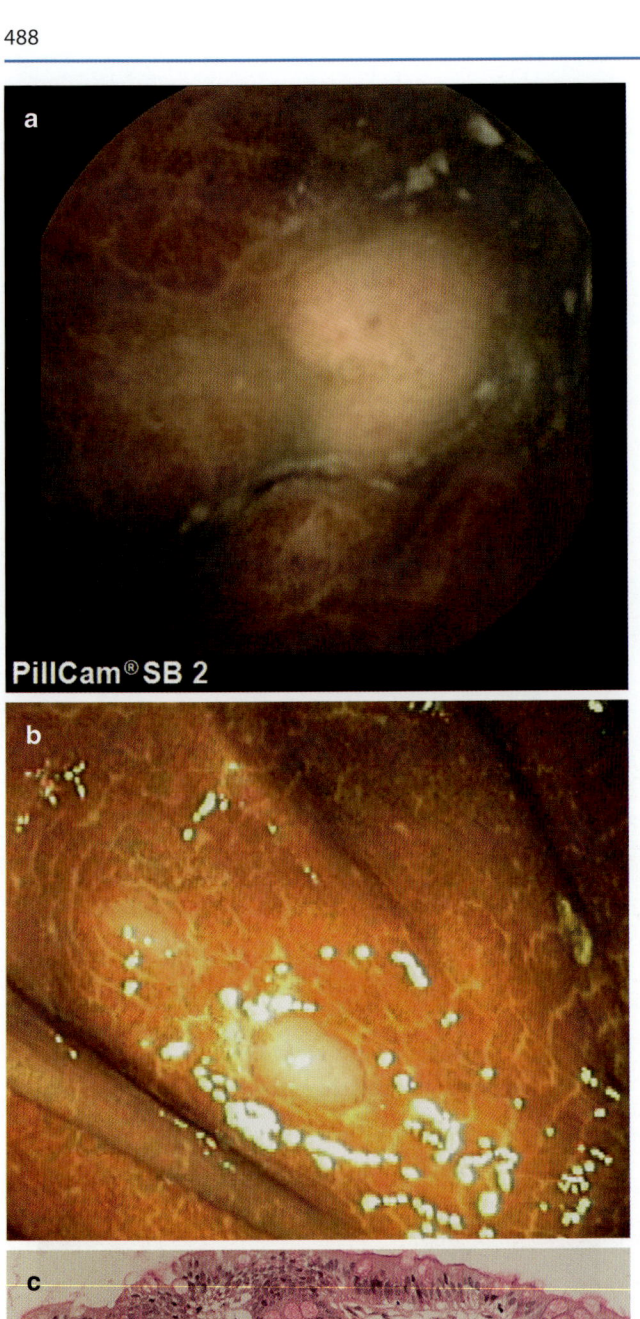

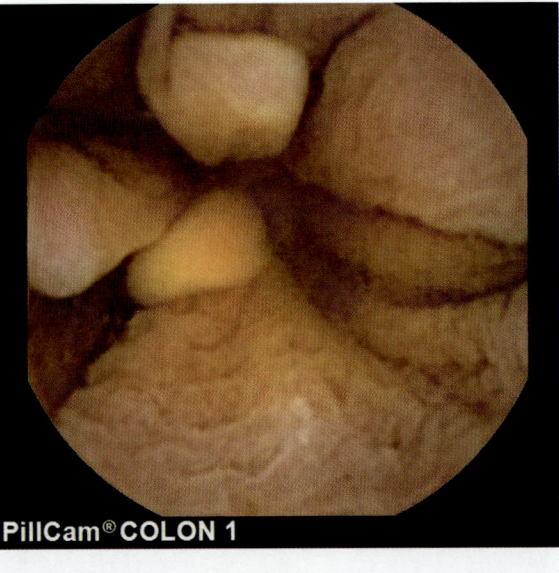

Fig. 46.10 Hypertrophic anal papillae

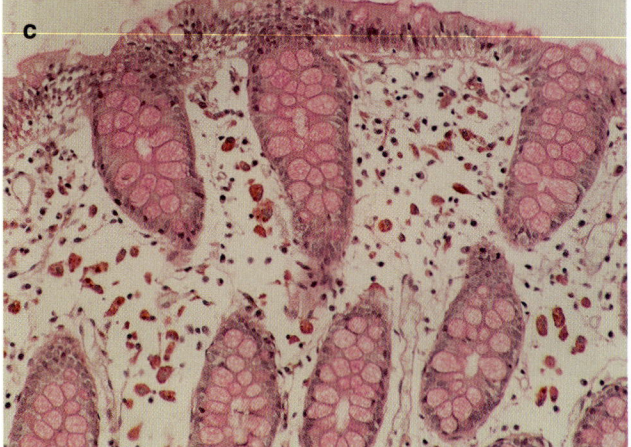

Fig. 46.9 Melanosis coli with dark pigmentation, sparing a hyperplastic polyp. (**a**) VCE. (**b**) Colonoscopy. (**c**) Histology

46.3   Pathologic Findings

Angiectasias are a common finding. Occasionally they are detected in patients after colonoscopy, especially in the cecum, where the capsule can remain for a long time and may deliver images from behind the ileocecal valve or on proximal folds that had not been obtained at standard colonoscopy (Fig. 46.11).

Diverticula of all sizes can easily be seen with capsule endoscopy, predominately in the left colon (Fig. 46.12). Erythema or edema surrounding areas with diverticula is suggestive of diverticulitis (Fig. 46.13).

Colitis can be diagnosed by VCE, although histologic confirmation is required in most cases. Patients with known colonic disease may benefit from capsule endoscopy. Capsule endoscopy in patients with problematic indeterminate colitis (Fig. 46.14a) may help differentiate a large proportion with a Crohn's disease phenotype (Fig. 46.14b) when ileoscopy and radiology have been nondiagnostic [8, 9], with obvious implications for management [10, 11]. Special issues of CCE in inflammatory bowel disorders are discussed in Chap. 48.

Polyps are a frequent finding in the colon (Fig. 46.15). This issue is addressed in detail in Chap. 47, where a wide range of different polyps are shown. Submucosal tumors may resemble polyps, but can have normal overlying mucosa (Fig. 46.16).

Even carcinomas can be missed by colonoscopy preceding small bowel VCE (Fig. 46.17). Hence, care should also be taken over colonic images obtained at small bowel VCE [2].

Pneumatosis coli is a rare disease caused by disseminated intramural air, associated with psychiatric disorders, chronic lung disease, and colitis (Fig. 46.18) [12]. Another rare finding is intraluminal colorectal endometriosis, seen as eccentric wall thickening or mucosal nodularity (Fig. 46.19) [13].

Although hemorrhoids are usually diagnosed before performing capsule endoscopy, they should be reported if detected (Fig. 46.20).

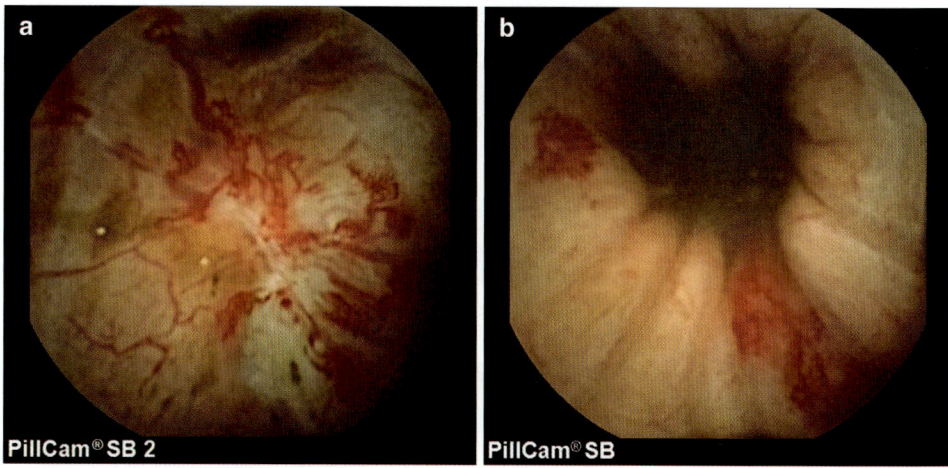

Fig. 46.11 (**a**, **b**) Angiectasias in the cecum and ascending colon detected at small bowel VCE after previously nondiagnostic colonoscopy

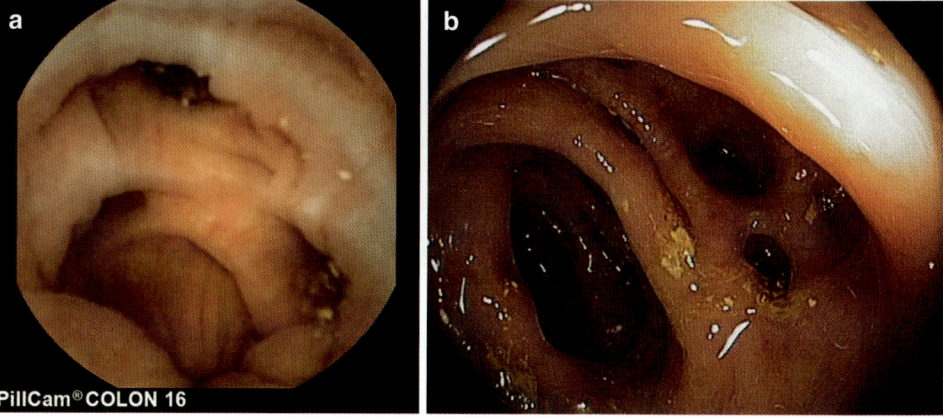

Fig. 46.12 Diverticulosis seen at VCE (**a**) and colonoscopy (**b**)

Fig. 46.13 Diverticulitis seen at VCE. (**a**) Segmental inflammation with erythema and erosions. (**b**) Red spots and stenotic lumen

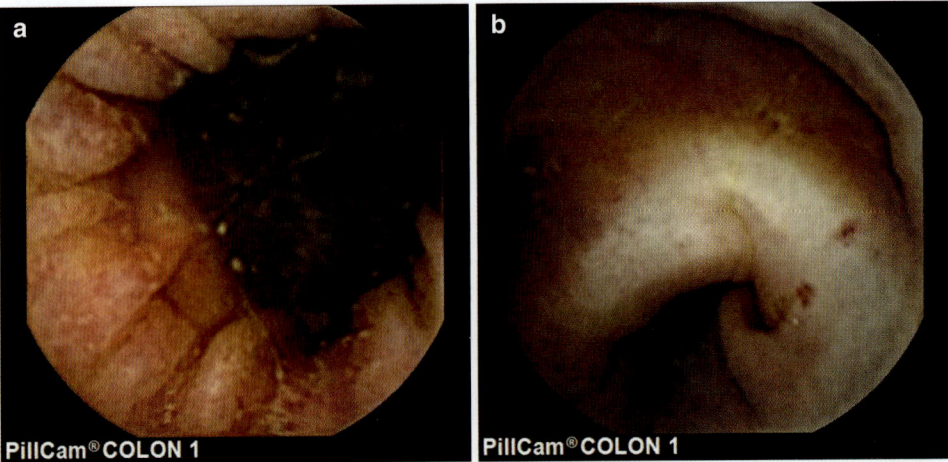

Fig. 46.14 (**a**) Cecal inflammation in a patient with indeterminate colitis. (**b**) Ulceration in the ileum consistent with Crohn's disease

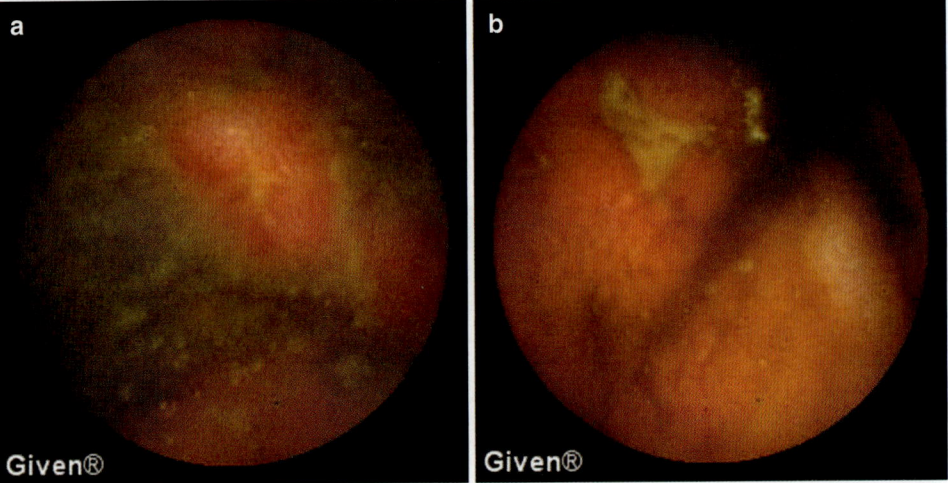

Fig. 46.15 Polyps at VCE (incidental findings at small bowel VCE). (**a**) Pedunculated polyp. (**b**) Sessile polyp

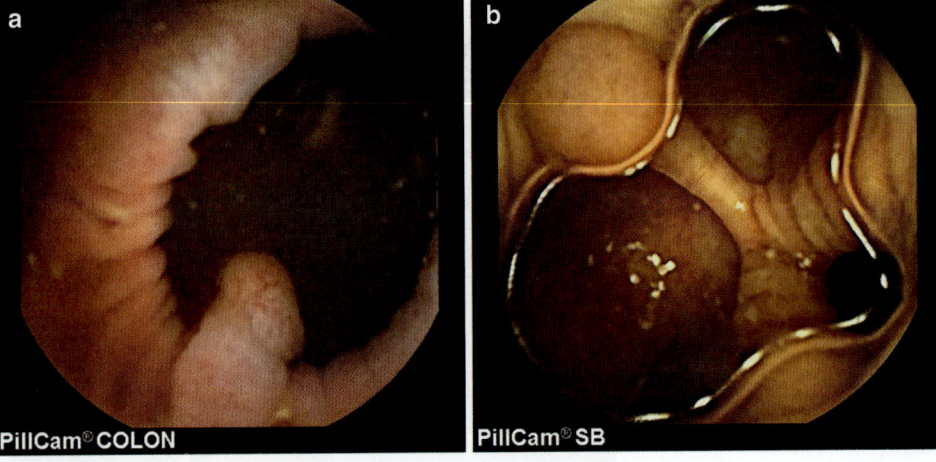

Fig. 46.16 Submucosal tumor of the colon (neurofibroma), seen at colon capsule endoscopy (CCE) (**a**) and colonoscopy (**b**)

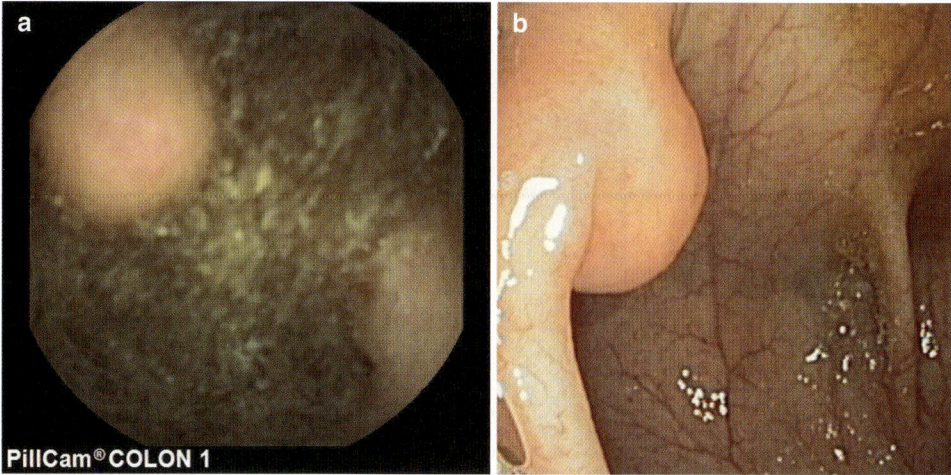

Fig. 46.17 Colon carcinoma seen at small bowel VCE. A preceding colonoscopy had been reported as normal. As anemia persisted even after hysterectomy for suspected hypermenorrhea, VCE was performed and showed normal small bowel. (**a**) A bleeding mass is seen in the colon. (**b**) The tumor is located adjacent to normal colon mucosa and to the normal ileocecal valve (ICV) with villi. (**c**) Repeated colonoscopy located the tumor to the ascending colon. (**d**) Resected specimen

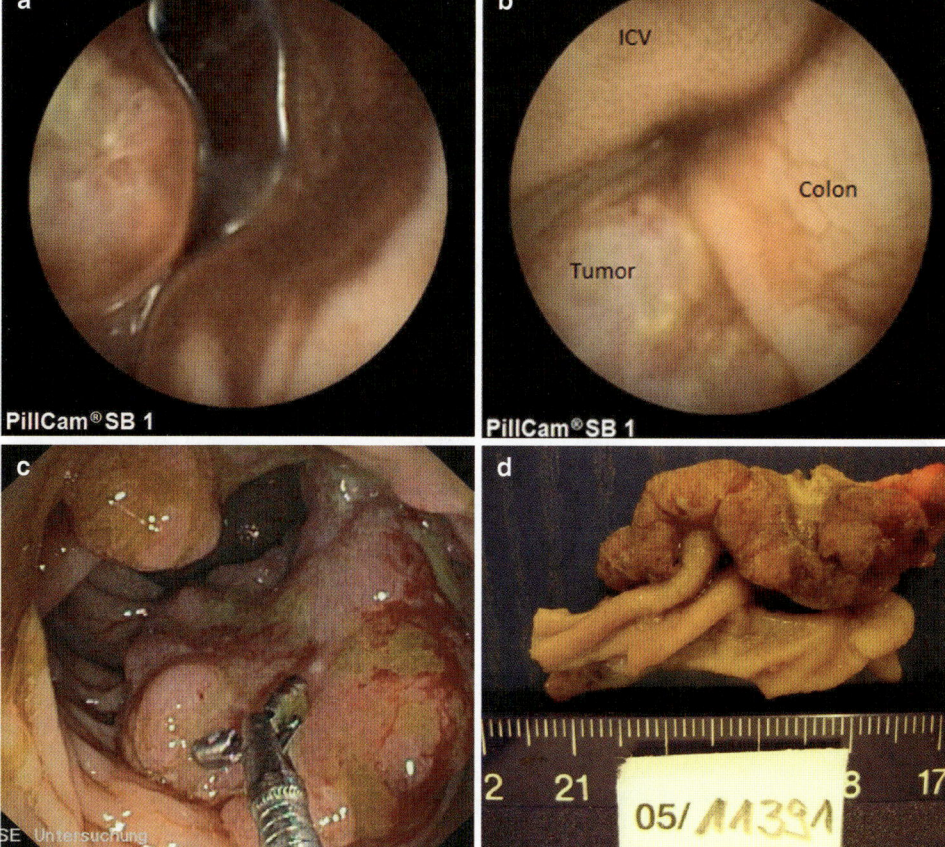

Fig. 46.18 Pneumatosis coli in a patient with previous infectious colitis. (**a**, **b**) VCE. (**c**) Colonoscopy. (**d**) After biopsy, the air-filled submucosal space is clearly visible

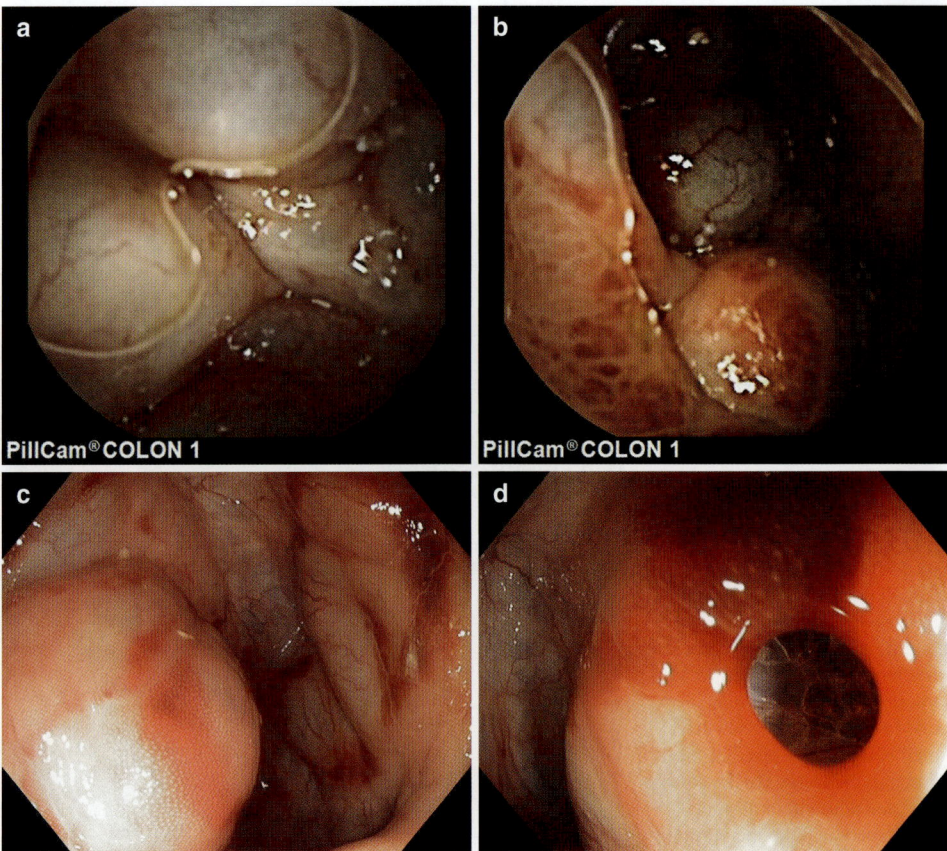

Fig. 46.19 Endometriosis of the appendix and cecum in a female patient with mild abdominal pain and anemia. Previous colonoscopy was nondiagnostic. (**a**) Small bowel VCE shows marked reddening and nodularity in the cecum. (**b**) Colonoscopy. (**c**) Chromoendoscopy. (**d**) Histology (Courtesy of Jörg Caselitz, MD)

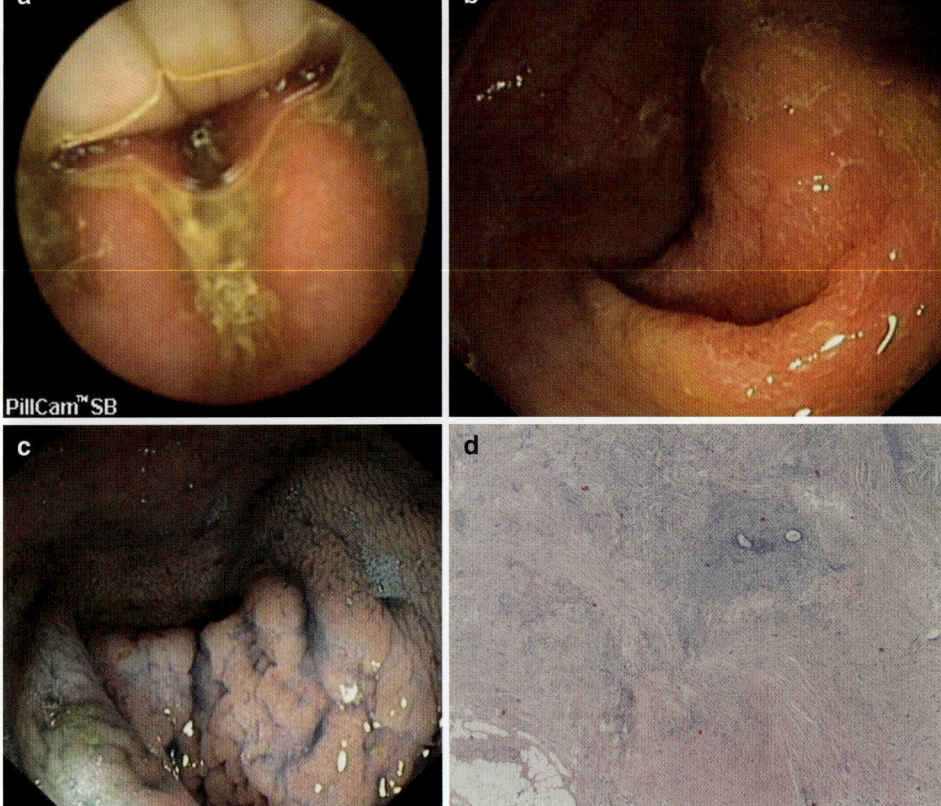

Fig. 46.20 Hemorrhoids with vasa vasorum, seen at VCE (**a**) and colonoscopy (**b**)

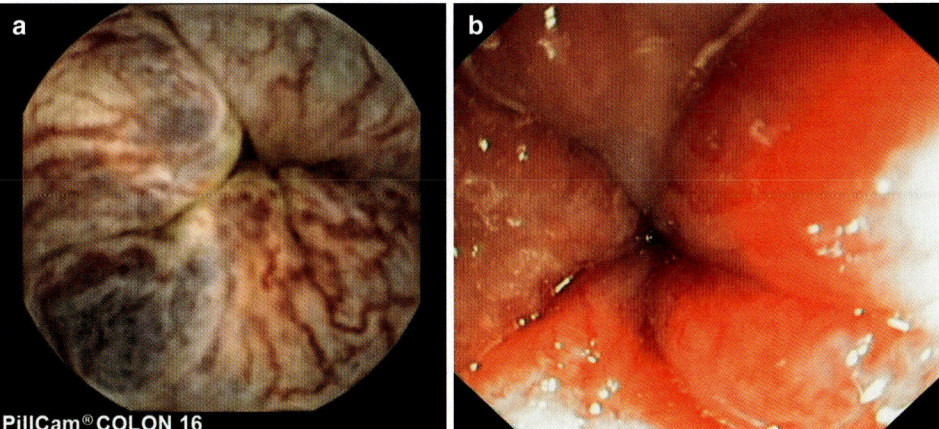

References

1. Gay G, Delvaux M, Fassler I, et al. Localization of colonic origin of obscure bleeding with the capsule endoscope: a case report. Gastrointest Endosc. 2002;56:758–62.
2. Kitiyakara T, Selby W. Non-small-bowel lesions detected by capsule endoscopy in patients with obscure GI bleeding. Gastrointest Endosc. 2005;62:234–8.
3. Pennazio M, Santucci R, Rondonotti E, et al. Outcome of patients with obscure gastrointestinal bleeding after capsule endoscopy: report of 100 consecutive cases. Gastroenterology. 2004;126:643–53.
4. van Turenhout ST, Jacobs MA, van Weyenberg SJ, et al. Diagnostic yield of capsule endoscopy in a tertiary hospital in patients with obscure gastrointestinal bleeding. J Gastrointestin Liver Dis. 2010;19:141–5.
5. Carlo JT, DeMarco D, Smith BA, et al. The utility of capsule endoscopy and its role for diagnosing pathology in the gastrointestinal tract. Am J Surg. 2005;190:886–90.
6. Rana SS, Bhasin DK, Singh K. Colonic lesions in patients undergoing small bowel capsule endoscopy. Int J Colorectal Dis. 2011;26:699–702.
7. Schoofs N, Deviere J, Van Gossum A. PillCam colon capsule endoscopy compared with colonoscopy for colorectal tumor diagnosis: a prospective pilot study. Endoscopy. 2006;38:971–7.
8. Mow WS, Lo SK, Targan SR, et al. Initial experience with wireless capsule enteroscopy in the diagnosis and management of inflammatory bowel disease. Clin Gastroenterol Hepatol. 2004;2:31–40.
9. Whitaker D, Hume G, Radford-Smith GL, Appleyard MN. Can capsule endoscopy help differentiate the aetiology of indeterminate colitis? Gastrointest Endosc. 2004;59:AB177.
10. Zhou N, Chen WX, Chen SH, et al. Inflammatory bowel disease unclassified. J Zhejiang Univ Sci B. 2011;12:280–6.
11. Gralnek IM, Cohen SA, Ephrath H, et al. Small bowel capsule endoscopy impacts diagnosis and management of pediatric inflammatory bowel disease: a prospective study. Dig Dis Sci. 2012;57:465–71.
12. Gagliardi G, Thompson IW, Hershman MJ, et al. Pneumatosis coli: a proposed pathogenesis based on study of 25 cases and review of the literature. Int J Colorectal Dis. 1996;11:111–8.
13. Kim KJ, Jung SS, Yang SK, et al. Colonoscopic findings and histologic diagnostic yield of colorectal endometriosis. J Clin Gastroenterol. 2011;45:536–41.

Colon Capsule Endoscopy in Screening and Surveillance for Polyps and Cancers

47

Hiroyuki Aihara, Hisao Tajiri, Markus Schneider,
Jean-Pierre Charton, and Horst Neuhaus

Contents

The work was first published in 2006 by Springer Medizin Verlag Heidelberg with the following title: *Atlas of Video Capsule Endoscopy.*

H. Aihara (✉)
Department of Endoscopy, Jikei University School of Medicine, Tokyo, Japan
e-mail: hiamliveinpeace@gmail.com

H. Tajiri
Division of Gastroenterology and Hepatology,
Department of Internal Medicine,
The Jikei University School of Medicine,
Tokyo, Japan
e-mail: tajiri@jikei.ac.jp

M. Schneider • J.-P. Charton • H. Neuhaus
Medical Clinic, Evangelisches Krankenhaus, Düsseldorf, Germany
e-mail: markus.schneider@evk-duesseldorf.de;
Jean-Pierre.Charton@evk-duesseldorf.de;
horst.neuhaus@evk-duesseldorf.de

Early detection and removal of precancerous neoplastic lesions are essential to reduce the risk of colorectal cancer deaths. In most cases, colorectal cancers develop from adenomas. Most early carcinomas can be curatively treated, and the 5-year survival rate is up to 90 % [1]. Therefore, early detection of adenoma and carcinoma in the context of screening programs is very important.

47.1 Screening Options and Recommendations

The current recommendation for colorectal cancer screening and surveillance is total colonoscopy [2], which seems to be the most effective modality because it allows both direct visualization and removal of colorectal neoplastic lesions [3]. The efficacy of colon capsule endoscopy (CCE) in colorectal screening was first reported in 2006 [4]. CCE is less invasive to patients than colonoscopy, which can result in abdominal pain and discomfort due to the insertion of the endoscope itself and the necessary gas insufflation. The CCE device is 31×11 mm in size, with lenses at each end for simultaneous image acquisition. A second-generation capsule (CCE-2) is now available for CCE, equipped with automatic regulation of the imaging frequency according to the capsule passage speed, a wider viewing angle (almost 360°), and a polyp size estimation (PSE) function. So far, this new capsule has been reported to have a high sensitivity for the detection of clinically relevant colorectal polypoid lesions, and it could be an adequate tool for colorectal screening. A prospective, multicenter study by Spada et al. [5] showed sensitivity as high as 84 % for polyps ≥6 mm and 88 % for polyps ≥10 mm, compared with colonoscopy.

CCE has been shown to be a safe procedure. In 1,500 procedures, no major complications were reported [6]. Moreover, CCE showed a very low rate of technical failures [6]. The excretion rate of the colon capsule is nearly 90 % [6]. CCE is still relatively invasive, in that patients should drink a lot of liquid during the examination (higher amounts than those required for colonoscopy). In addition, after ingestion of the capsule, patients take an additional dose of purgatives—a so-called booster—to facilitate passage of the capsule to the distal end of the small intestine and through the colon, so that images can be captured through the entire colon within the battery life of the device. This requirement is one of the obstacles to widespread clinical use of CCE. However, the introduction of new, lower-volume protocols for CCE preparation [7, 8] could lead to improved detection rates for colorectal cancer screening, which are currently lower than those reported in screening programs for other cancers [9].

Colonoscopy remains the standard screening procedure for colorectal carcinoma, but current studies and the guideline recently published by the European Society of Gastrointestinal Endoscopy (ESGE) show that CCE may be an alternative diagnostic option, particularly after incomplete colonoscopy or if colonoscopy is contraindicated or is refused by the patient [6, 10]. Contraindications are similar to those of small bowel capsule endoscopy: dysphagia or swallowing disorder and known or suspected bowel obstructions [6, 11]. Implanted electromedical devices (e.g., a cardiac pacemaker) are relative contraindications, as is pregnancy [6, 11]. If CCE reveals any significant finding, such as polyps or masses ≥6 mm or three or more polyps regardless of size, the patient is for colonoscopy with polypectomy [6]. If there are no significant findings, the ESGE guideline recommends control CCE or another screening test after 5 years [6].

In comparison to other noninvasive options for colorectal cancer screening, such as CT colonography and fecal occult blood testing (FOBT), the sensitivity of CCE is favorable [12, 13]. It is also important to remember that CT colonography leads to an increased risk of radiation-induced tumors [14].

47.2 Characteristic Endoscopic Appearance of Colorectal Lesions in CCE and Strategic Decision Making for the Diagnosis and Treatment

Small polyps can be identified in CCE (Figs. 47.1, 47.2, 47.3, 47.4, 47.5, 47.7, and 47.16). If one or more polyps ≥6 mm in size is detected, or three or more small polyps (<5 mm), standard colonoscopy with polypectomy is recommended. In clinical practice, this treatment strategy can be determined by using the "polyp size estimation" function.

Adenomatous polyps can be identified by a reddish mucosal surface (Figs. 47.4, 47.5, 47.6, 47.9, 47.10, 47.11, 47.12, and 47.13). However, sometimes polyps are covered by fecal residues (Figs. 47.2, 47.3, and 47.6) that hamper detailed visualization of the pit patterns at the surface of lesions. Differentiation between hyperplastic and sessile-serrated polyps by CCE is usually difficult (Figs. 47.1, 47.2, and 47.3), so serrated lesions proximal to the sigmoid colon and all serrated lesions in the rectosigmoid that are larger than 5 mm should be completely removed [15]. Complete visualization of larger neoplastic lesions is often incomplete in a single image (Figs. 47.8, 47.14, 47.15, 47.17, and 47.18). These lesions should be endoscopically evaluated, including pit pattern diagnosis and biopsy, in order to determine the feasibility of endoscopic removal.

Fig. 47.1 (**a**) CCE detected a sessile polyp in the left colon. (**b**) Colonoscopy confirmed a sessile polyp in the descending colon, 65 cm from the anal verge. The polyp was resected endoscopically. (**c**) Histologically (hematoxylin and eosin [H&E] stain), a hyperplastic polyp of the colon was diagnosed (*Courtesy of Jörg Caselitz, MD*)

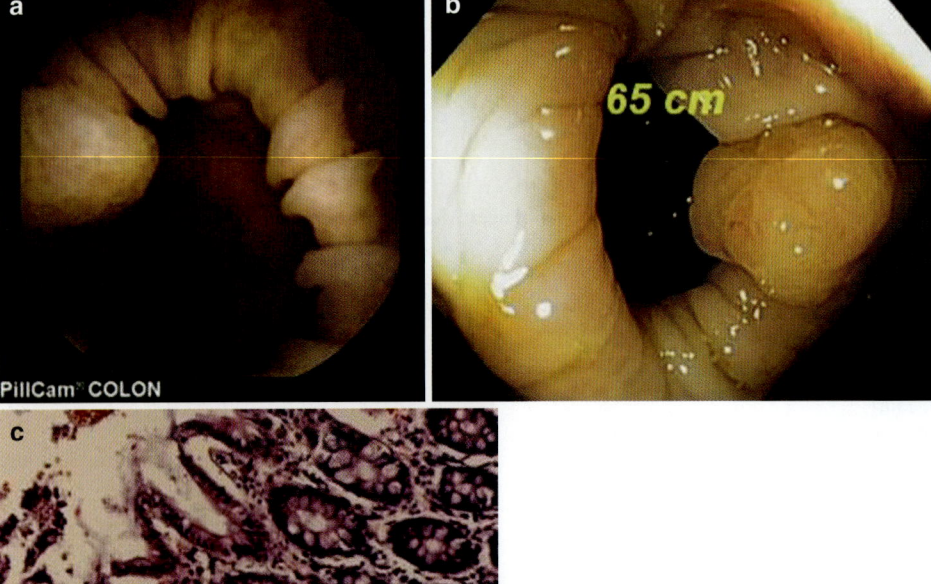

Fig. 47.2 (**a**) CCE detected an elevated lesion at the splenic flexure. (**b**) The estimated maximum diameter of this lesion was 11 mm. (**c**) The oral side of this lesion showed a finding of hyperplastic lesion (*white arrows*). (**d**) The anal side of the lesion showed an elongated and branched surface pattern. Yellowish, dirty mucus was observed attached to the surface of the lesion

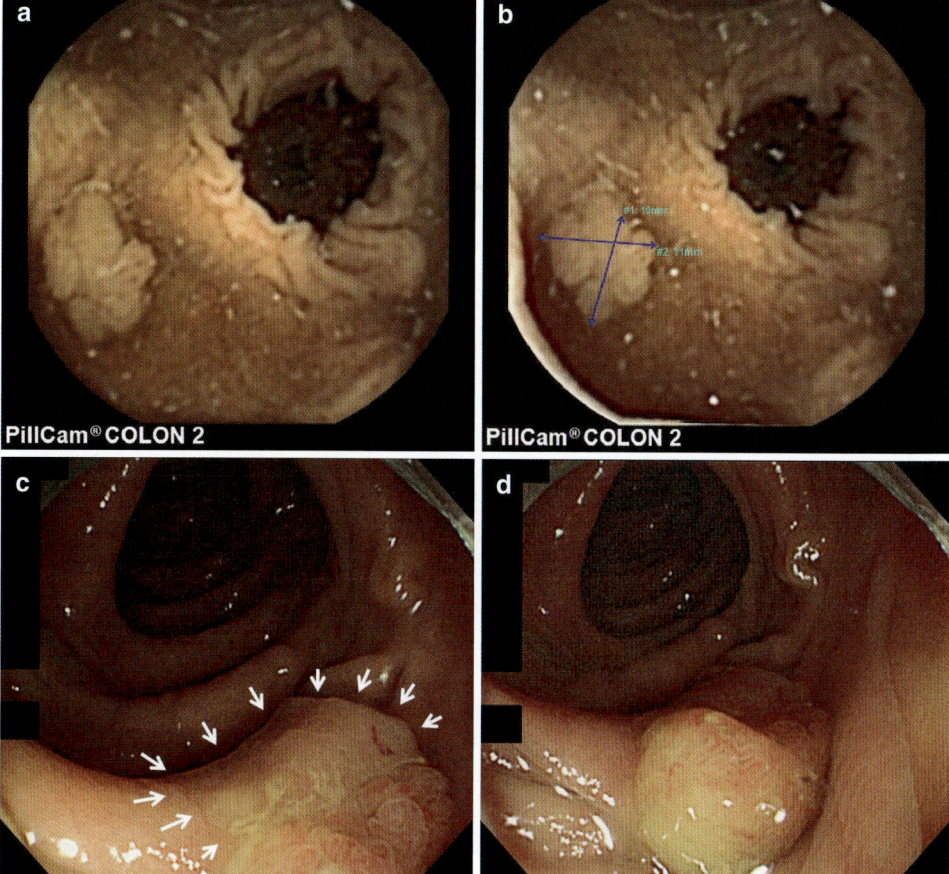

Fig. 47.3 (**a**) CCE detected a sessile pinkish lesion in the cecum. Yellowish, dirty mucus was seen adherent to the lesion. (**b**) The maximum diameter of this lesion was estimated to be 15 mm. (**c**) In WLE with indigo carmine spraying, a sessile, pinkish lesion was detected in the cecum. (**d**) Under NBI with magnification, roundly dilated crypt openings were observed. There was no surface vessel dilatation except for greenish, branched vessels running independently beneath the mucosal layer

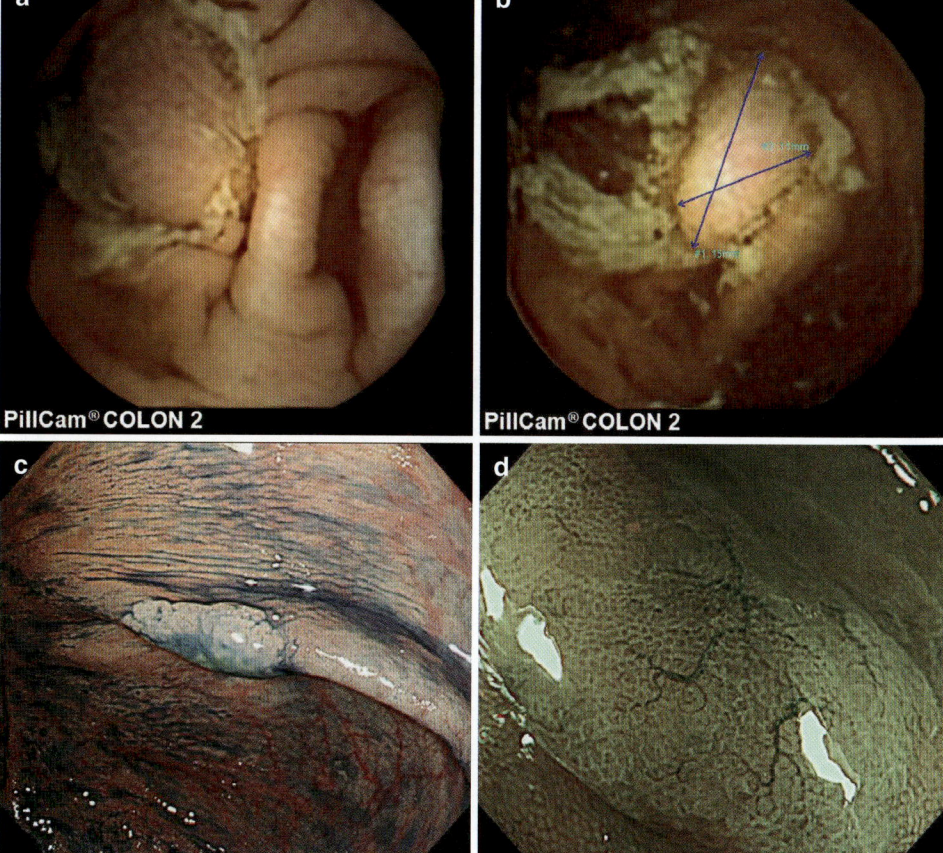

Fig. 47.4 (**a**) Colon capsule endoscopy (CCE) detected an elevated polyp in the rectum. (**b**) With the polyp size estimation (PSE) function, the maximum size of this polyp was estimated to be 7 mm. Endoscopic resection was indicated. (**c**) A small, reddish, elevated lesion was detected in the rectum with white light endoscopy (WLE). (**d**) Under low magnification with narrow band imaging (NBI), brownish dilated vessels surrounding oval crypt openings were observed

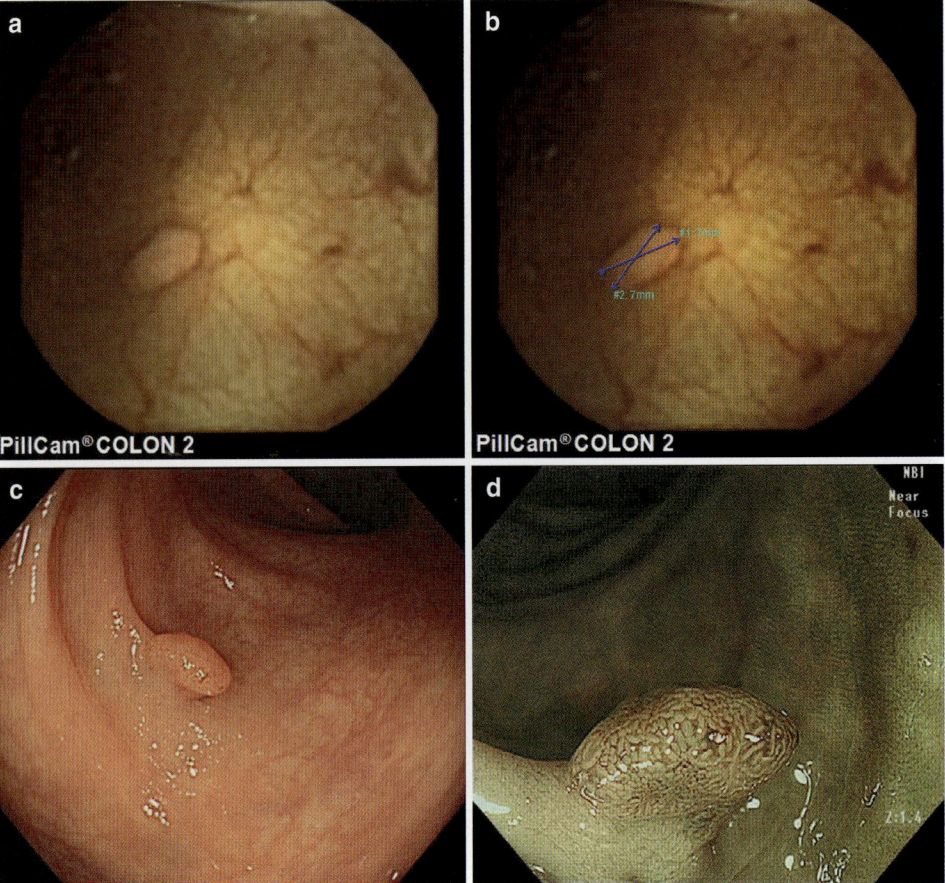

Fig. 47.5 (**a**) By CCE, a small sessile polyp was detected in the left colon (*see* also Movie 47.1). PSE estimated the size of the polyp to be 7 mm. (**b**) Colonoscopy confirmed a small sessile polyp with a diameter of approximately 6 mm in the sigmoid colon. The polyp was resected endoscopically. (**c**) The final histological diagnosis was a tubular adenoma with low-grade intraepithelial neoplasia (LGIN) (H&E) (*Courtesy of* Helmut Erich Gabbert, MD)

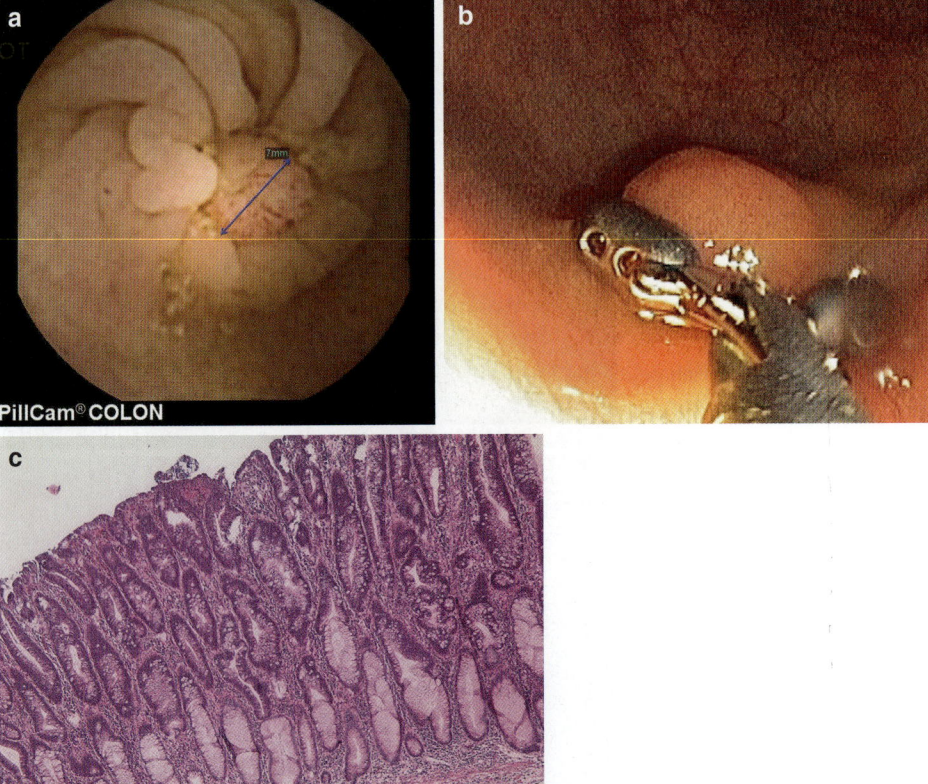

Fig. 47.6 (**a**) In CCE, a few frames showed a sessile polyp in the ascending colon. The polyp was only seen at the margin of the images, was not very well illuminated, and was covered with dirt and mucus. By PSE, its maximum diameter was estimated to be 16 mm. (**b**) Colonoscopy confirmed a sessile polyp in the first part of the ascending colon, close to the ileocecal valve. The diameter was estimated endoscopically to be approximately 15 mm. The polyp was resected endoscopically. (**c**) Histologically (H&E), a tubulovillous adenoma (LGIN) was diagnosed (*Courtesy of* Helmut Erich Gabbert, MD)

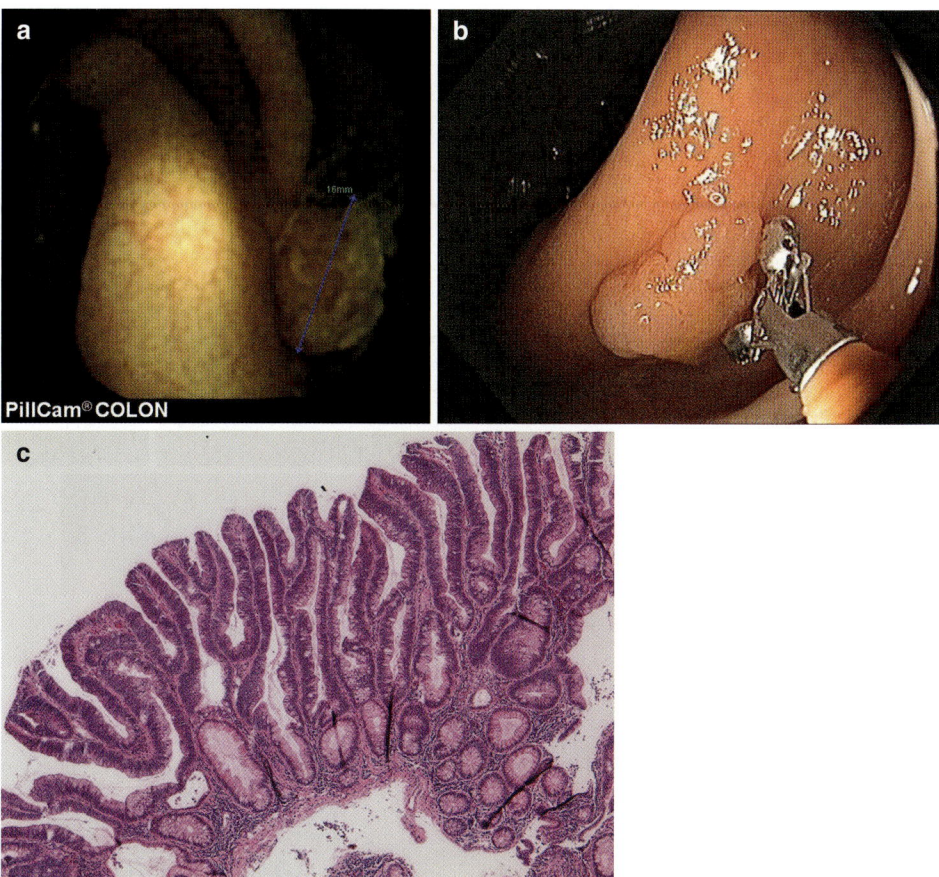

Fig. 47.7 (**a**) CCE detected a small pedunculated polyp with a maximum diameter of 7 mm (PSE) in the left colon. (**b**) Colonoscopy confirmed a small pedunculated polyp of 5 mm in the sigmoid colon. It was completely resected endoscopically. (**c**) Histology showed a tubular adenoma (LGIN) (*Courtesy of* Helmut Erich Gabbert, MD)

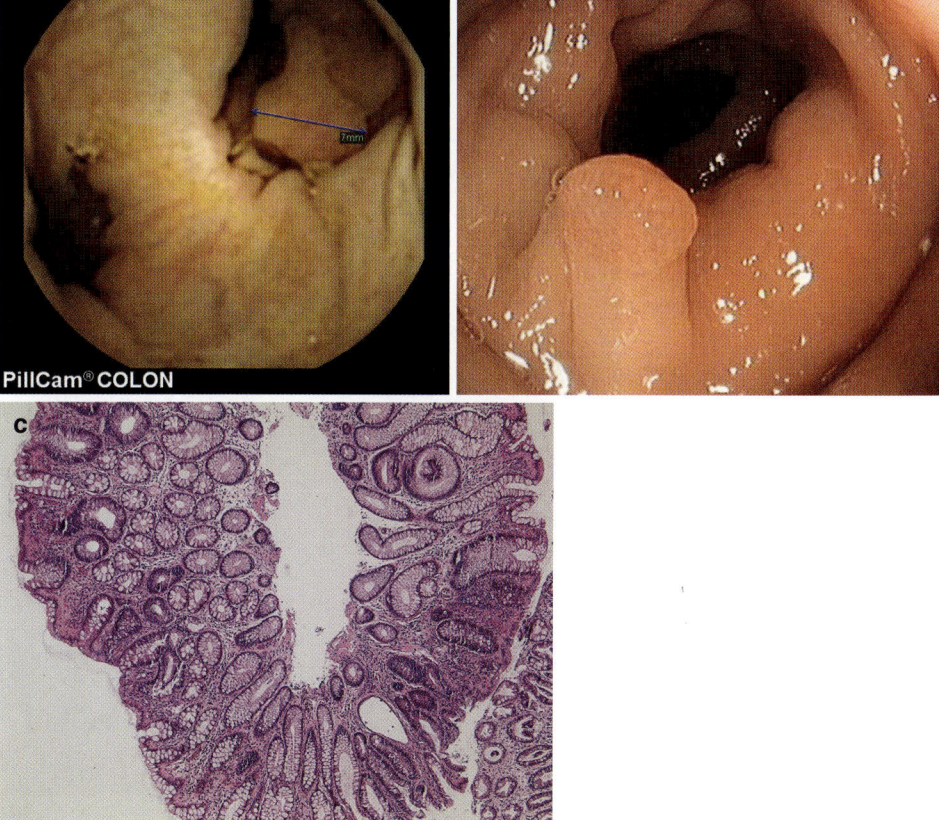

Fig. 47.8 (a) CCE detected a large, laterally spreading polyp at the ileocecal valve (*see* also Movie 47.2). The lesion is at the rim of the ileocecal valve. (b) CCE did not visualize the entire lesion, but a maximum diameter of at least 22 mm was estimated by PSE. (c) By colonoscopy, the full extension of this polyp was realized. The polyp was growing from the proximal rim of the ileocecal valve to the cecum and had a full diameter of about 30 mm. The polyp was resected endoscopically. Histologically, a tubular adenoma (LGIN) was diagnosed

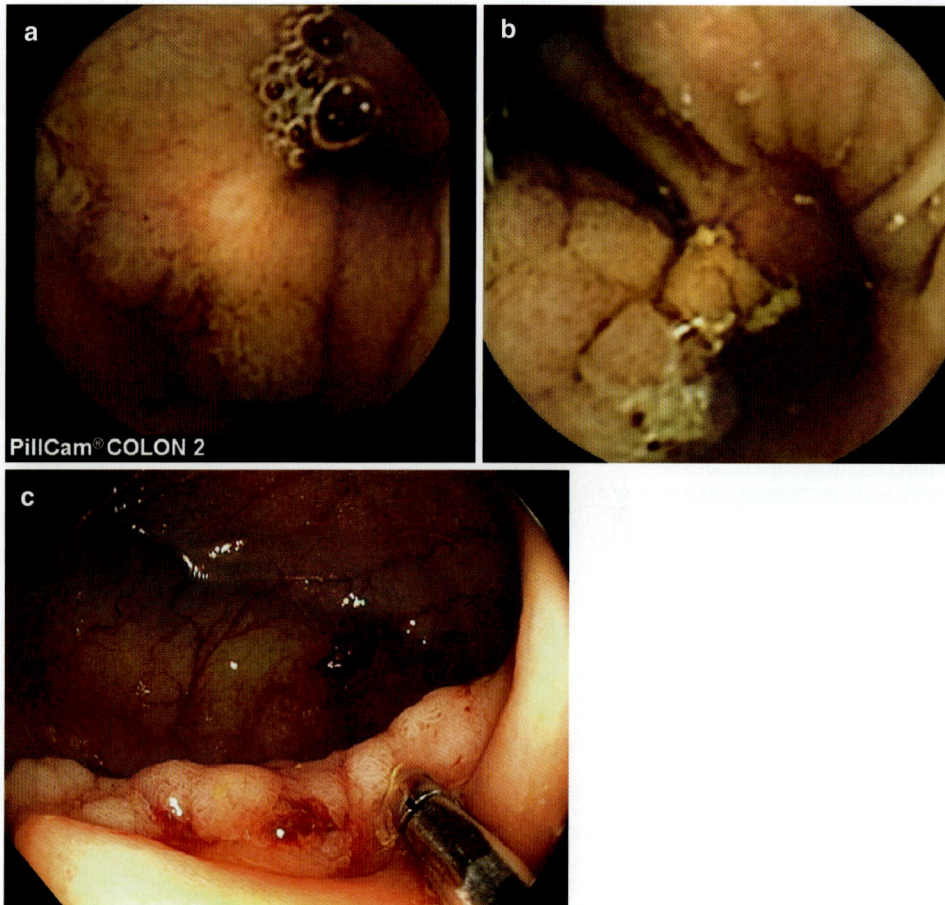

Fig. 47.9 (a) CCE detected a pedunculated polyp in the descending colon (*Courtesy of* Cristiano Spada, Rome, Italy). By PSE, the maximum size of the polyp was estimated to be 13 mm. (b) Colonoscopy confirmed the pedunculated polyp in the sigmoid colon. The polyp was completely resected endoscopically (*Courtesy of* Cristiano Spada, Rome, Italy). (c) After resection, the maximum diameter of the polyp was shown to be approximately 10 mm (*Courtesy of* Cristiano Spada, MD). (d) Histologically (H&E), a tubular adenoma (LGIN) was diagnosed (*Courtesy of* Riccardo Ricci, MD)

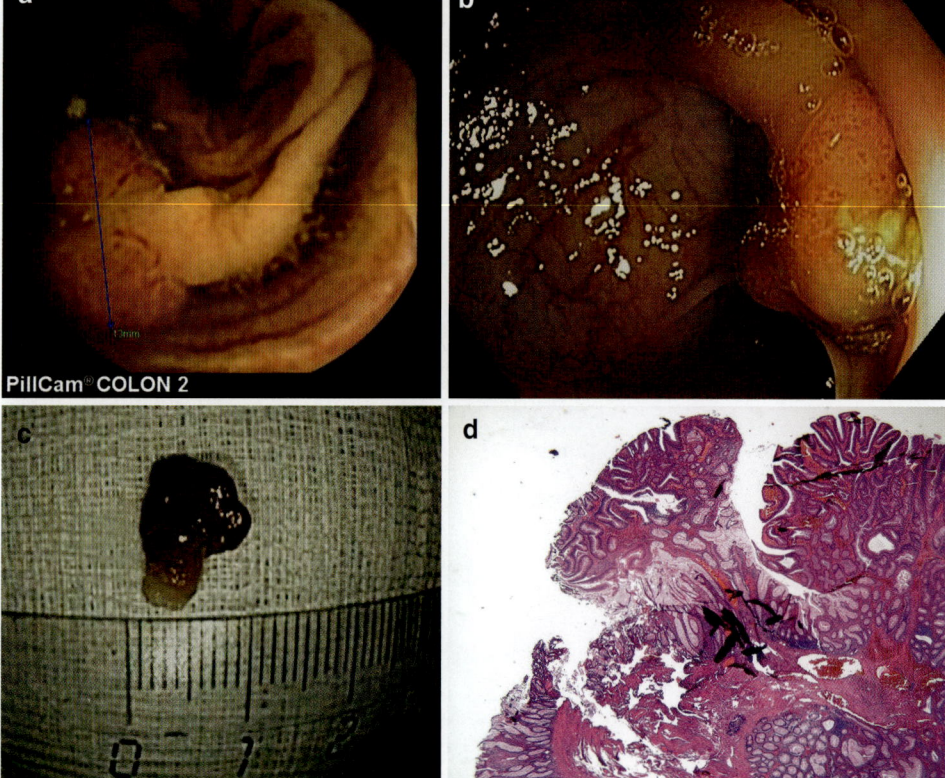

Fig. 47.10 (**a**) CCE detected a pedunculated polyp in the sigmoid colon. (**b**) The PSE function estimated the size of this lesion to be 15 mm. (**c**) A reddish, pedunculated lesion was detected under WLE. (**d**) Indigo carmine spray revealed the multilocular appearance of this lesion

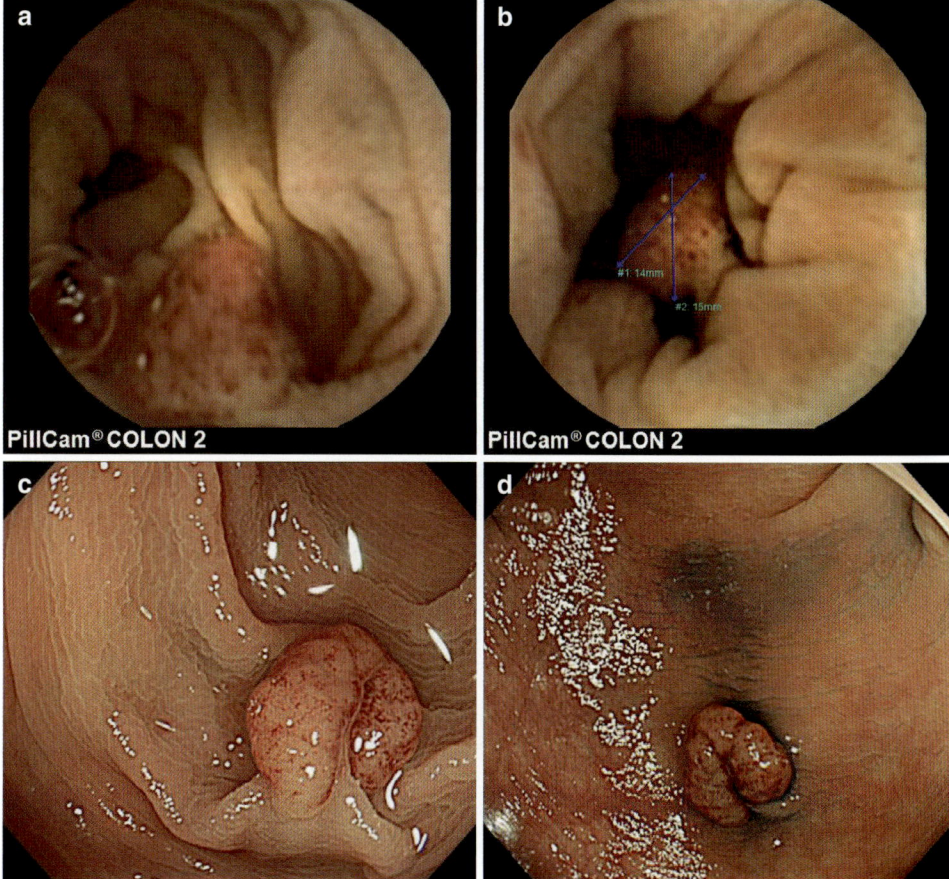

Fig. 47.11 (**a**) CCE detected a huge, pedunculated polyp in the ascending colon. (**b**) With PSE function, the maximum size of this lesion was estimated to be more than 24 mm, even though it was not visualized with entire view under CCE. (**c**) Under WLE, a huge, pedunculated lesion with a thick stalk was detected in the ascending colon. (**d**) Indigo carmine spraying and low magnifying observation revealed multilocular appearance, dilated vessels, and villous structures

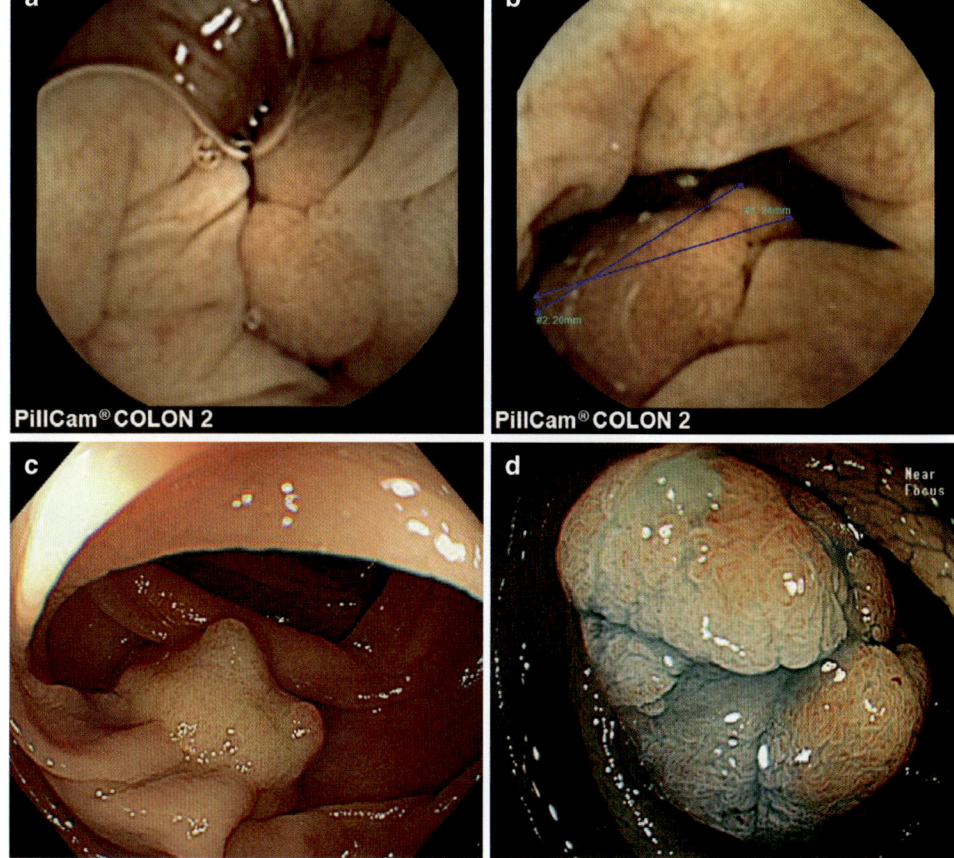

Fig. 47.12 (**a**) CCE detected a semi-pedunculated and reddish lesion in the sigmoid colon. (**b**) With PSE function, the maximum size of this lesion was estimated to be more than 15 mm, even though it was not visualized with entire view under CCE. (**c**) A dark-reddish semi-pedunculated polyp with markedly dilated vessels at the surface was detected with WLE. (**d**) Indigo carmine spraying revealed multilocular morphology and a villous surface pattern

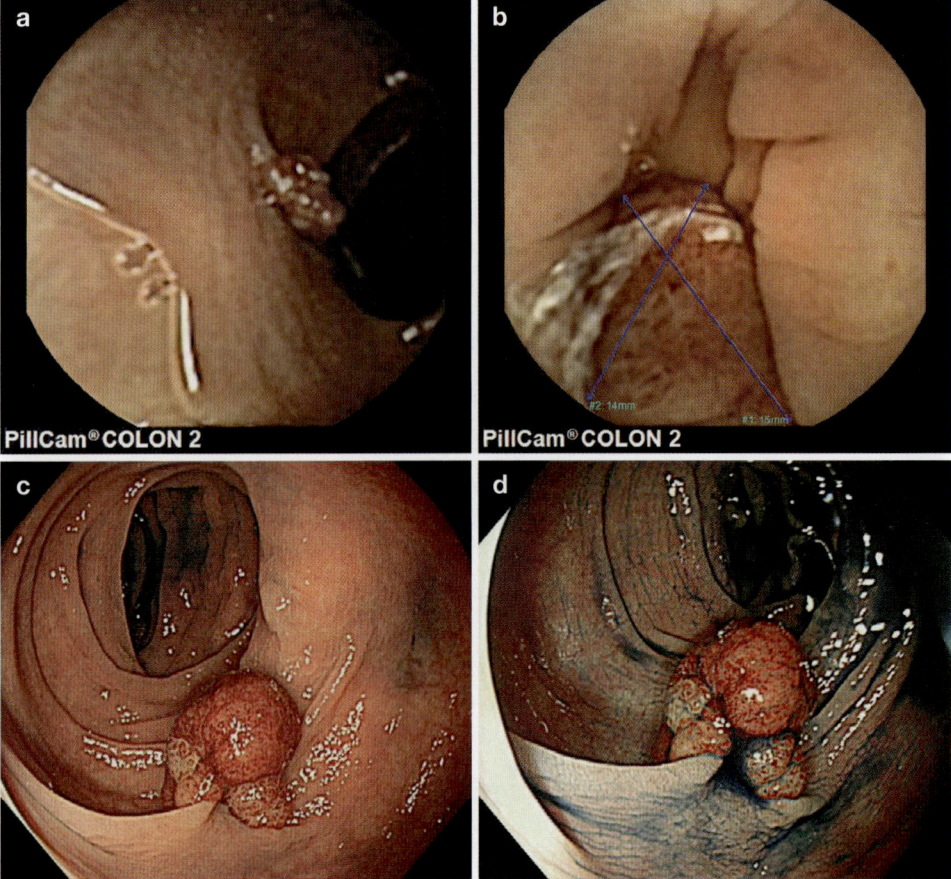

Fig. 47.13 (**a**) CCE detected a semi-pedunculated polyp in the sigmoid colon. (**b**) With PSE function, the maximum size of this lesion was estimated to be 20 mm. (**c**) A dark-reddish semi-pedunculated polyp was detected with WLE. (**d**) Indigo carmine spraying clearly revealed the villous structure of this lesion, suggesting a villous component

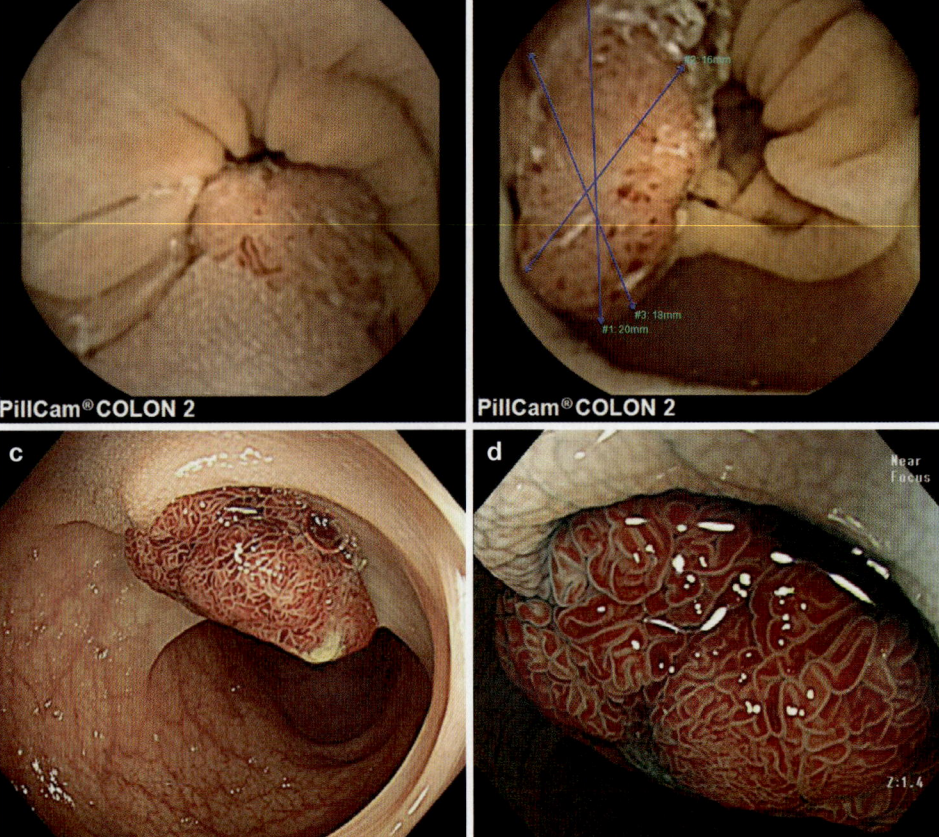

Fig. 47.14 (**a**) CCE detected a huge tumor in the rectum. (**b**) The maximum diameter of this lesion was estimated to be 25 mm. (**c**) WLE revealed a laterally spreading tumor with irregular surface. (**d**) Indigo carmine spray revealed an elongated and branched surface pattern and showed no indentation suggesting invasive cancer

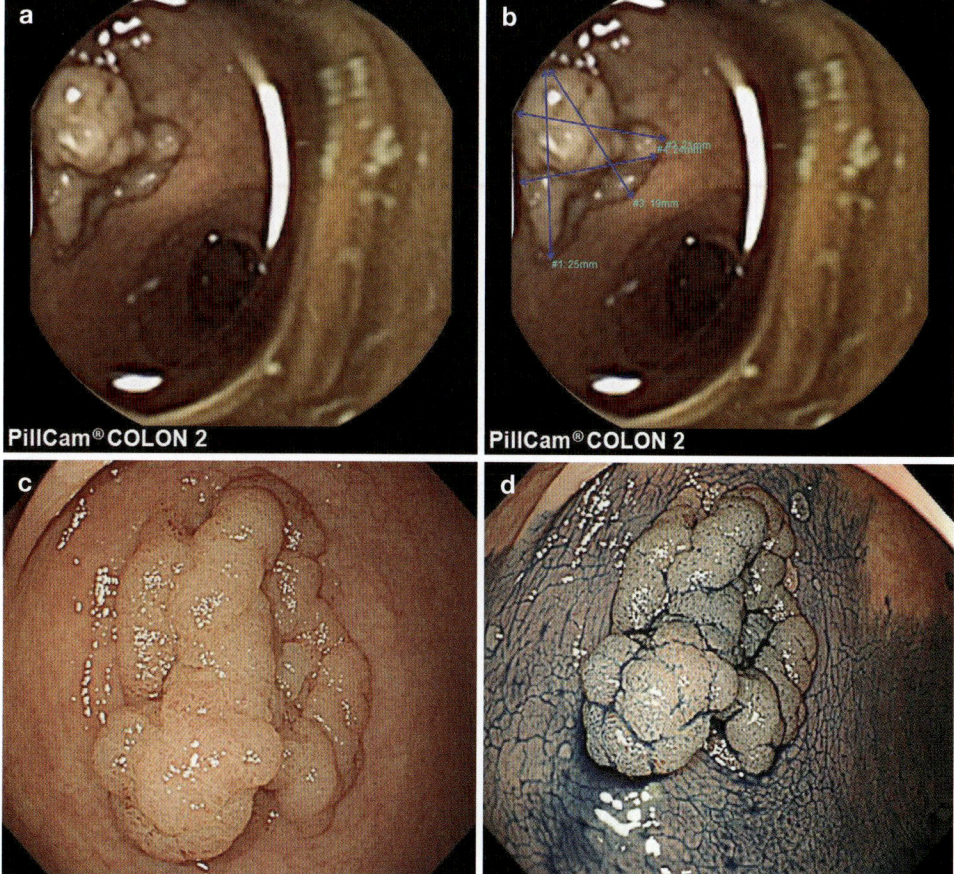

Fig. 47.15 (**a**) By CCE, a suspicious neoplastic lesion in the ascending colon was diagnosed. The mass appeared to be of almost circumferential extension. (**b**) The lesion in the ascending colon was confirmed by colonoscopy (**a**, **b**, *Courtesy of* C. Spada, Rome, Italy). Insufflation demonstrated that the real extension of the mass was only semi-circumferential. (**c**) Histologically, an adenocarcinoma was diagnosed (*Courtesy of Riccardo Ricci, MD*)

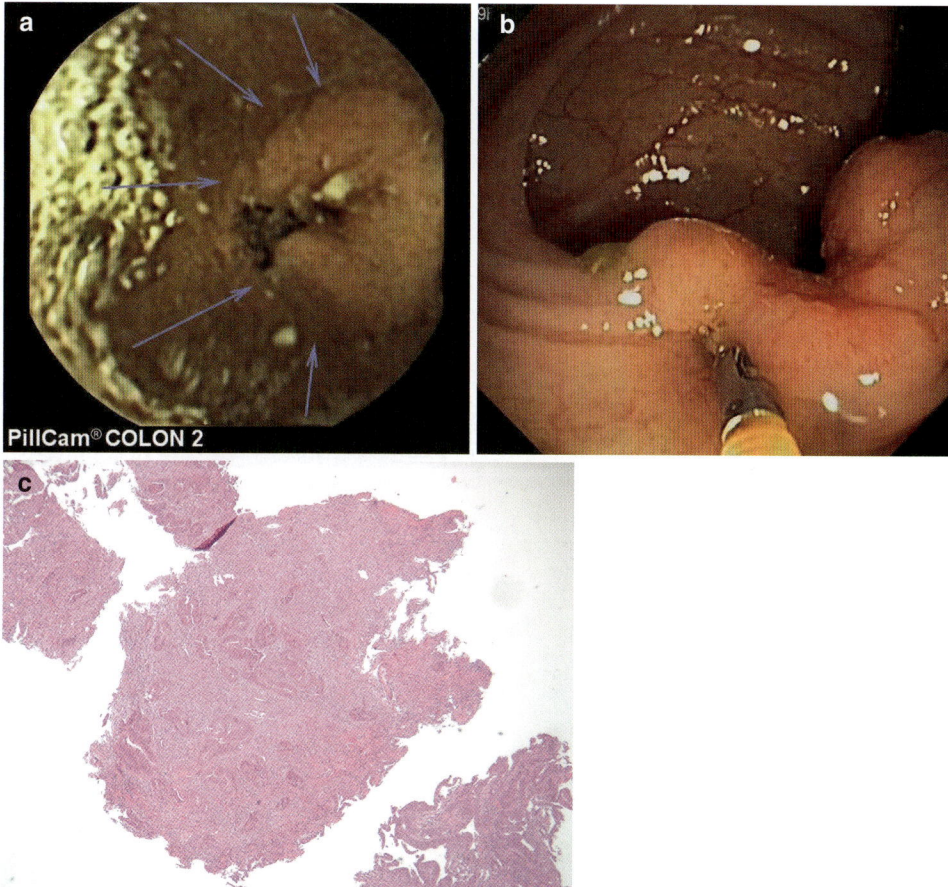

Fig. 47.16 (**a**) CCE detected a flat lesion in the descending colon. (**b**) The maximum diameter of this lesion was estimated to be 17 mm. (**c**) With WLE, a reddish and flat lesion was detected in the descending colon. (**d**) NBI with magnification revealed dilated and meshed capillaries at the surface of this lesion

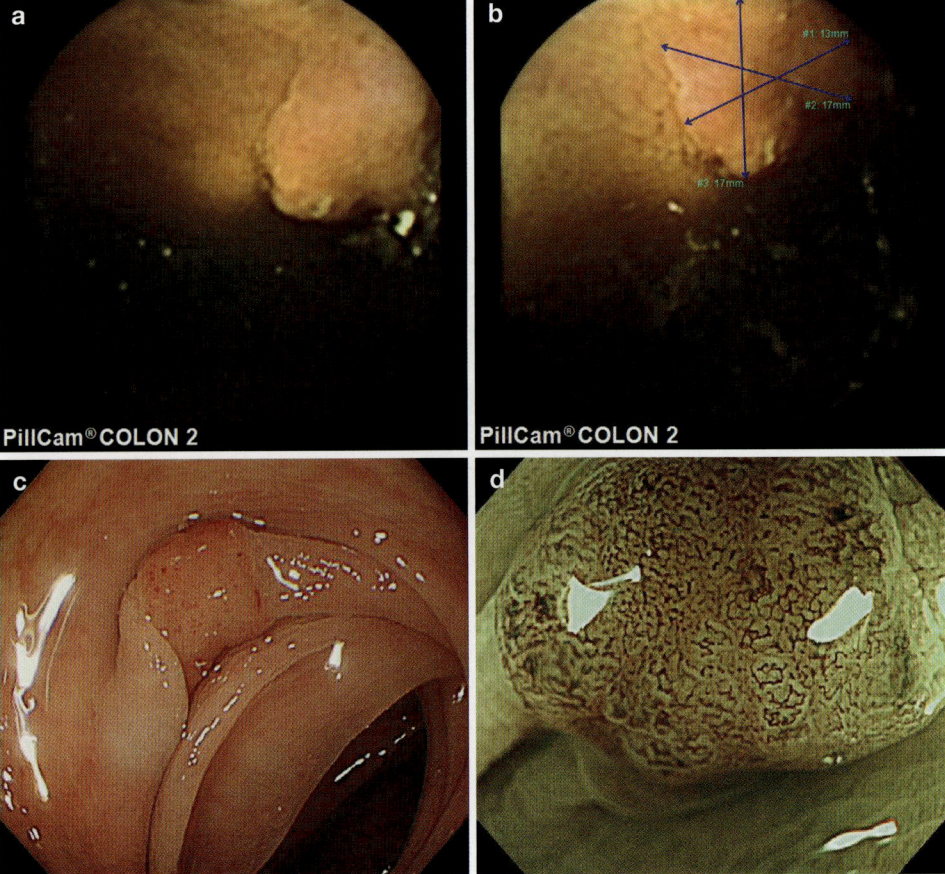

Fig. 47.17 (**a**) A partial view of a colonic lesion suggesting a huge neoplastic tumor was detected in the ascending colon by CCE. (**b**) This lesion was too large for its maximum diameter to be estimated by the PSE function. Based on the partial view, the size of this lesion was estimated to be more than 21 mm. (**c**) With WLE, a laterally spreading tumor with reddish nodules of various sizes and shapes was detected in the ascending colon. (**d**) Indigo carmine spray revealed elongated and branched surface patterns and showed no findings suggesting an invasive area

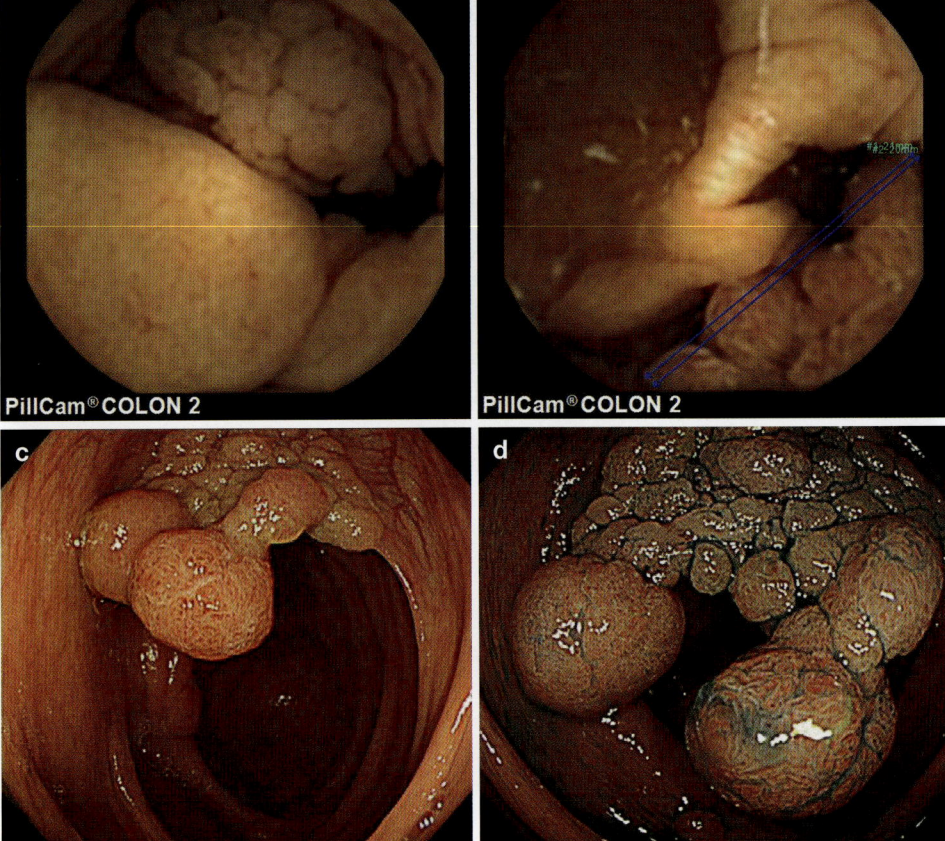

Fig. 47.18 (**a**) CCE detected a large, neoplastic colonic mass. (**b**) By colonoscopy (WLE), the tumor was confirmed; macroscopically it appeared highly suspicious for advanced malignancy (**a**, **b**, *Courtesy of* Samuel Adler, MD). (**c**) A biopsy was performed and the specimen was examined histologically. A moderately well-differentiated adenocarcinoma was diagnosed (*Courtesy of* Constantin Reinus, MD)

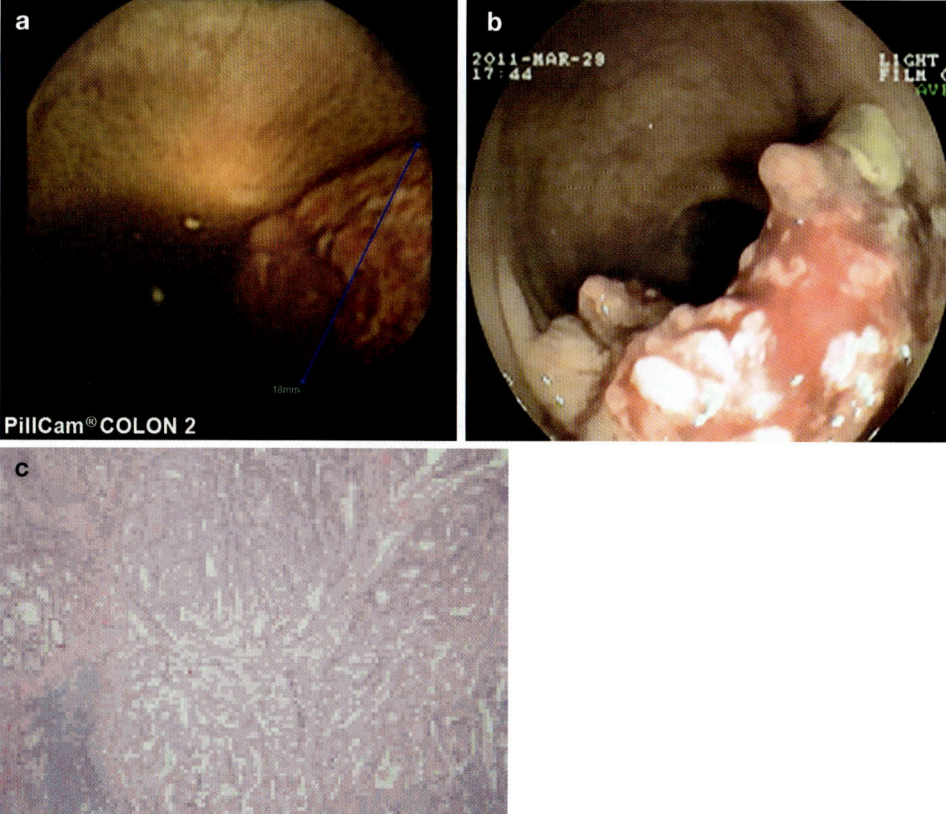

References

1. Winawer SJ, Zauber AG, Ho MN, et al. Prevention of colorectal cancer by colonoscopic polypectomy. N Engl J Med. 1993;329:1977–81.
2. Kaminska MF, Regula J, Kraszewska E, et al. Quality indicators for colonoscopy and the risk of interval cancer. N Engl J Med. 2010;362:1795–803.
3. Zauber AG, Winawer SJ, O'Brien MJ, et al. Colonoscopic polypectomy and long-term prevention of colorectal-cancer deaths. N Engl J Med. 2012;366:687–96.
4. Elliakim R, Fireman Z, Gralnek IM, et al. Evaluation of the PillCam Colon capsule in the detection of colonic pathology: results of the first multicenter, prospective, comparative study. Endoscopy. 2006;38:963–70.
5. Spada C, Hassan C, Munoz-Navas M, et al. Second generation colon capsule endoscopy compared with colonoscopy. Gastrointest Endosc. 2011;74:581–9.
6. Spada C, Hassan C, Galmiche JP, et al. Colon capsule endoscopy: European Society of Gastrointestinal Endoscopy (ESGE) guideline. Endoscopy. 2012;44:527–36.
7. Kakugawa Y, Saito Y, Saito S, et al. New reduced volume preparation regimen in colon capsule endoscopy. World J Gastroenterol. 2012;18:2092–8.
8. Hartmann D, Keuchel M, Philipper M, et al. A pilot study evaluating a new low-volume colon cleansing procedure for capsule colonoscopy. Endoscopy. 2012;44:482–6.
9. Segnan N, Senore C, Andreoni B, et al. Comparing attendance and detection rate of colonoscopy with sigmoidoscopy and FIT for colorectal cancer screening. Gastroenterology. 2007;132:2304–12.
10. Rokkas T, Papaxoinis K, Triantafyllou K, Ladas SD. A meta-analysis evaluating the accuracy of colon capsule endoscopy in detecting colon polyps. Gastrointest Endosc. 2010;71:792–8.
11. Ladas SD, Triantafyllou K, Spada C, et al. European Society of Gastrointestinal Endoscopy (ESGE): recommendations (2009) on clinical use of video capsule endoscopy to investigate small-bowel, esophageal and colonic diseases. Endoscopy. 2010;42:220–7.
12. Spada C, Hassan C, Marmo R, et al. Meta-analysis shows colon capsule endoscopy is effective in detecting colorectal polyps. Clin Gastroenterol Hepatol. 2010;8:516–22.
13. Lieberman DA. Clinical practice (screening for colorectal cancer). N Engl J Med. 2009;361:1179–87.
14. Brenner DJ, Georgsson MA. Mass screening with CT colonography: should the radiation exposure be of concern? Gastroenterology. 2005;129:328–37.
15. Rex DK, Ahnen DJ, Baron JA, et al. Serrated lesions of the colorectum: review and recommendations from an expert panel. Am J Gastroenterol. 2012;107:1315–29.

Colon Capsule Endoscopy in Inflammatory Bowel Disorders

48

Joseph J.Y. Sung and Jörg G. Albert

Contents

The work was first published in 2006 by Springer Medizin Verlag Heidelberg with the following title: *Atlas of Video Capsule Endoscopy*.

J.J.Y. Sung (✉)
The Chinese University of Hong Kong,
Hong Kong, The People's Republic of China
e-mail: joesung@cuhk.edu.hk

J.G. Albert
Medical Clinic I, University Hospital Frankfurt,
Frankfurt, Germany
e-mail: j.albert@med.uni-frankfurt.de

48.1 Indications for Colon Capsule Endoscopy

Clinical symptoms of inflammatory bowel disorders (IBDs) comprise diarrhea and abdominal pain, and inflammatory markers are often elevated in serum and stool. Ulcerative colitis (UC) and Crohn's disease (CD), the major types of chronic IBD, are characterized by episodes when symptoms flare up, followed by periods of improvement and clinical remission. The disease is lifelong and frequently manifests in the first decades of life. Detailed endoscopic visualization of the intestinal mucosa is required in these patients to diagnose or to exclude the disease. Thereby, complete investigation of the colon, the small bowel, and the upper gastrointestinal tract may be optimal to establish the exact diagnosis of IBD and to describe the distribution of the disease (Figs. 48.1 and 48.2). Colon capsule endoscopy (CCE) is convincing in combining endoscopy of the colon and of the small bowel. It could therefore become the ideal test to screen for intestinal inflammation (Figs. 48.3 and 48.4) and to monitor the effect of therapeutic measures in the small and the large bowel.

Scientific data on the use of CCE in IBD is limited, however. Capsule endoscopy with use of the small bowel capsule endoscope has been used to detect small bowel Crohn's disease [1], to define inflammatory activity in postoperative CD patients [2], to detect small bowel lesions to establish the diagnosis of CD in indeterminate findings of colitis patients [3, 4], and to predict the outcome of ileal pouch–anal anastomosis (IPAA) in UC (Figs. 48.5 and 48.6) [5].

M. Keuchel et al. (eds.), *Video Capsule Endoscopy: A Reference Guide and Atlas*,
DOI 10.1007/978-3-662-44062-9_48, © Springer-Verlag Berlin Heidelberg 2014

Fig. 48.1 Normal colonic mucosa in a Crohn's disease patient with small bowel disease. The vascular pattern is preserved in the colon, and no mucosal alterations are visible

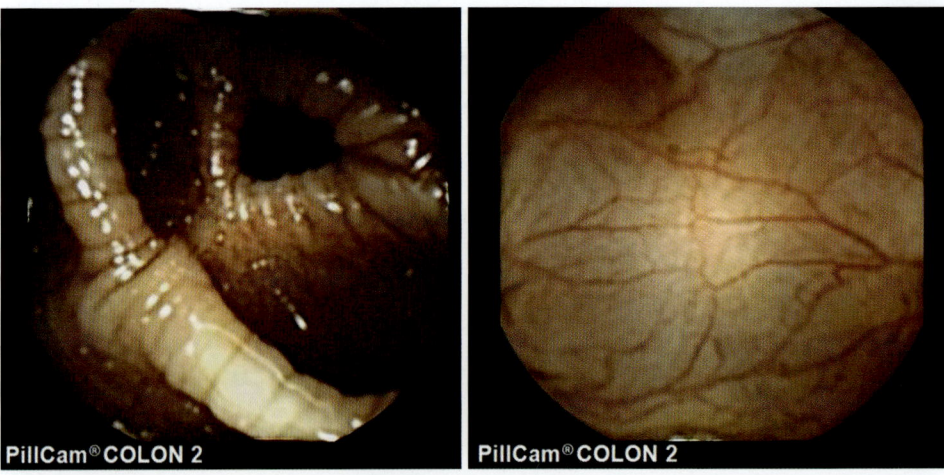

Fig. 48.2 Chronic alterations in a patient with Crohn's disease. No vascular pattern is demarcated in the colon, and some edematous swelling is suggested by the disappearance of colonic folds. No erythema or frank ulceration is detected, and the colonic findings are classified as chronic, noninflammatory alterations

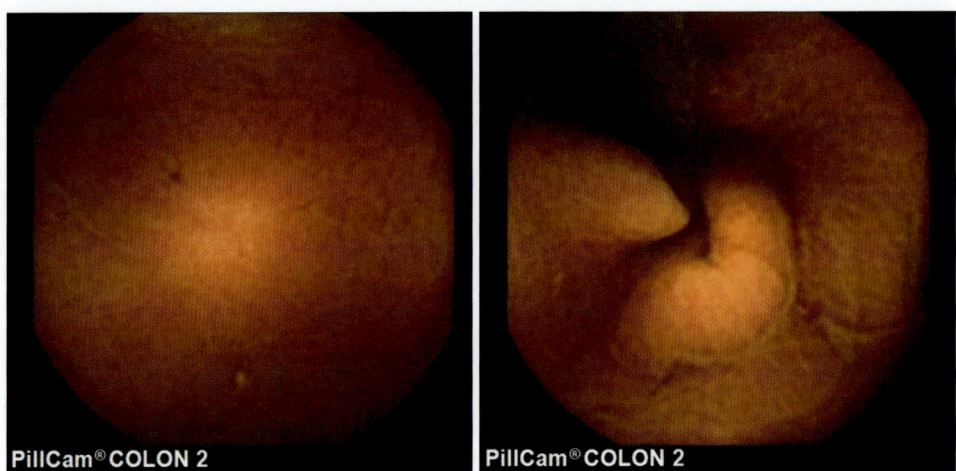

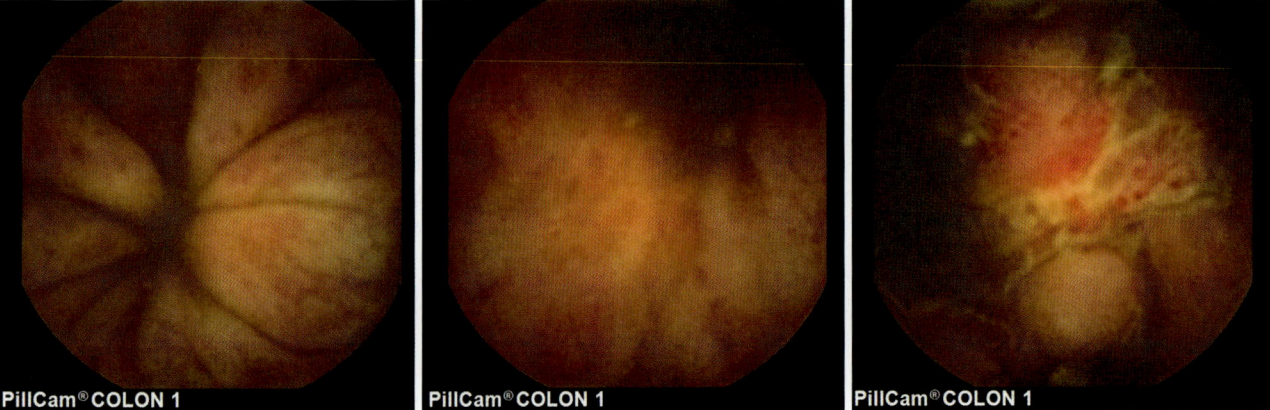

Fig. 48.3 Patchy erythema of the colonic mucosa and inflammatory pseudopolyps in Crohn's disease

Fig. 48.4 Ulcerations and stenosis from highly inflamed bowel segments in severe inflammatory Crohn's disease

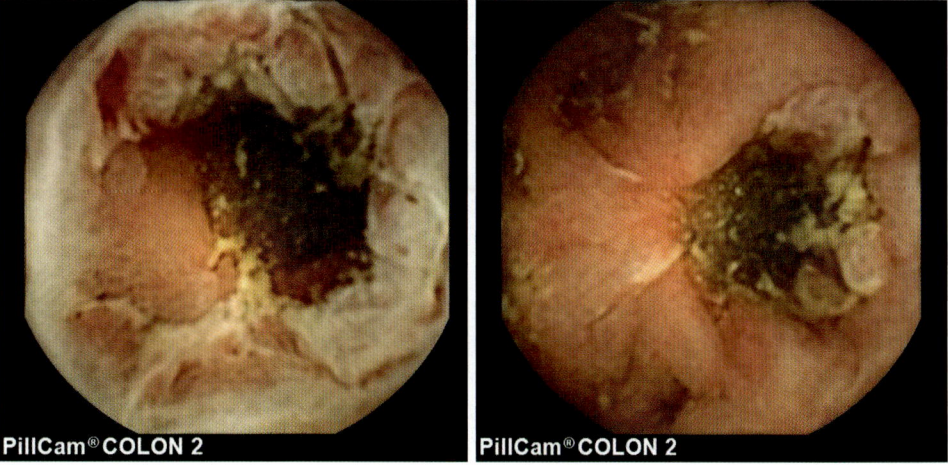

Fig. 48.5 Normal anastomotic region in ileocolonic anastomosis for stricturing Crohn's disease

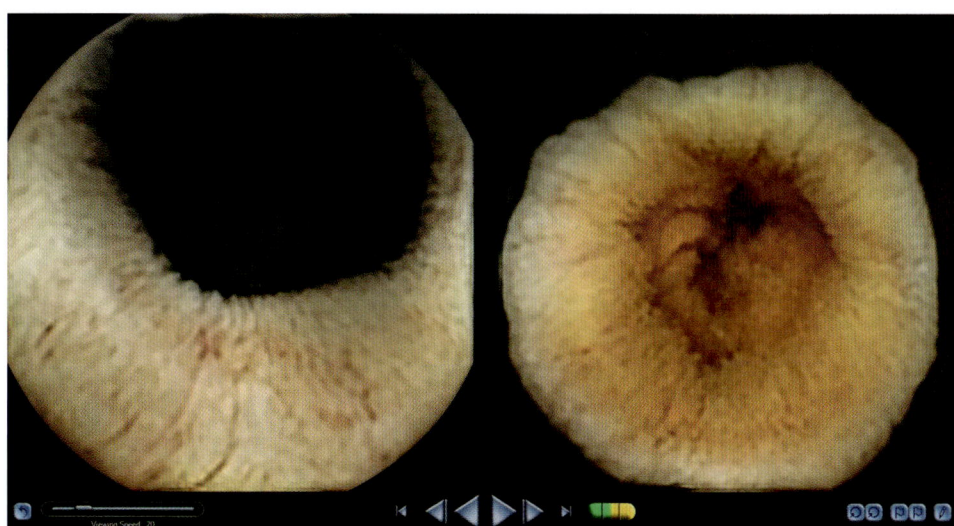

Fig. 48.6 Ileocolonic anastomosis in a patient with Crohn's disease in remission after right hemicolectomy for refractory, stricturing Crohn's disease

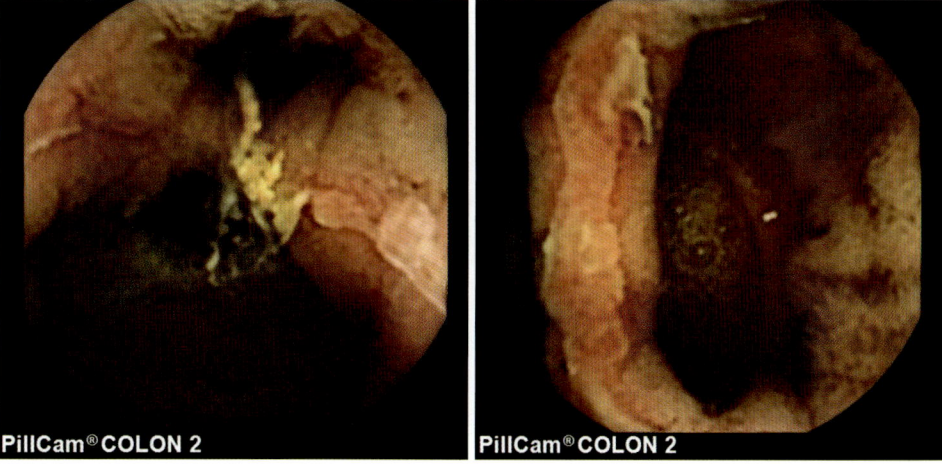

48.2 Capsule Endoscopy Compared with Other Diagnostic Techniques in IBD

In study populations, capsule endoscopy is superior to other diagnostic techniques for diagnosing nonstricturing small bowel CD. A meta-analysis found a number needed to diagnose (NND) of 3 to yield one additional diagnosis of CD compared with small bowel barium radiography and an NND of 7 compared with ileocolonoscopy [6]. Most published studies involve only about 50 patients, however, and the higher diagnostic yield of capsule endoscopy over radiologic imaging is based mostly on patients with established CD. Capsule endoscopy findings have a significant impact on the treatment of IBD patients, with a change of management in 50 % of those with established or suspected CD [7]. Capsule endoscopy is superior to radiographic and cross-sectional imaging in terms of sensitivity and negative predictive value, but there are no validated diagnostic criteria for small bowel capsule endoscopy for the diagnosis of CD [2]. Guidelines suggest performing ileocolonoscopy prior to capsule endoscopy for the diagnosis of CD [2]. As with other imaging modalities, a diagnosis of CD should not be based on the appearance at capsule endoscopy alone, but rather on a combination of clinical data, imaging, and histopathology.

Patients under surveillance after surgery for CD constitute a high-risk population prone to incur recurrence of inflammatory disease, and endoscopy is well known to reliably predict clinical recurrence [8, 9]. CCE might be helpful in detecting small bowel or colonic recurrence in these patients. Moreover, endoscopy has increasingly been used to document mucosal healing in IBD patients. Mucosal healing is recognized as important evidence for treatment efficacy and a reliable prognostic marker in patients with both CD and UC [10–12]. Today, endoscopic surveillance is used to assess disease activity, to confirm mucosal healing, and to clarify the etiology of persistent symptoms in medicated cases. Mucosal healing is now adopted as a treatment end point in clinical trials and may be used in clinical practice.

Capsule endoscopy revealed small bowel lesions suggestive of CD in 7 (28 %) of 18 patients with inflammatory bowel disease type unclassified (IBDU) or indeterminate colitis [4]. Another study group had 5 (17 %) of 30 IBDU patients reclassified as CD as a result of significant findings at capsule endoscopy [3]. There was no statistical association between preoperative capsule endoscopy findings and outcome after IPAA in patients with UC or indeterminate colitis, however, so capsule endoscopy does not appear to be necessary in the preoperative evaluation of these patients [5]. Capsule endoscopy could optimize diagnostic outcome in all patients in whom the combination of small bowel and colonic endoscopy is useful.

48.3 Use of CCE in Ulcerative Colitis and Crohn's Disease

The European Society of Gastrointestinal Endoscopy (ESGE) envisages the potential use of CCE for the diagnostic workup of patients with suspected or known IBD or in their surveillance [13]. In one study [14], the sensitivity of CCE to detect active colonic inflammation in UC patients was 89 % (95 % confidence interval [CI], 80–95 %), and the specificity was 75 % (95 % CI, 51–90 %) in comparison to colonoscopy. The positive predictive value of CCE for colonic inflammation was 93 % (95 % CI, 84–97 %), and the negative predictive value was 65 % (95 % CI, 43–83 %). No serious adverse events related to the CCE procedure or preparation were reported. The authors conclude that CCE is a safe procedure to monitor mucosal healing in UC [14]. The finding of this study was subsequently confirmed in another, smaller study showing that CCE is useful in assessing the severity and extent of UC. A significant correlation in the severity ($\kappa = 0.751, P < 0.001$) and extent ($\kappa = 0.522, P < 0.001$) of UC was found between CCE and conventional colonoscopy in another study [15], again without remarkable adverse events. Other data indicate that severity of UC may be correctly classified by CCE in optimally cleansed colon, but defining its exact extent or doing complex scoring seems more difficult for CCE (Table 48.1).

In summary, CCE can provide a significant contribution to the diagnosis and monitoring of IBD. At this stage, however, CCE cannot be recommended to replace conventional colonoscopy. More clinical data would be needed to substantiate its role in the management of IBD.

Table 48.1 Colon capsule endoscopy versus colonoscopy in detecting ulcerative colitis and defining disease extent

Study	Patients, N	Capsule	Detection	Severity	Extent
Sung et al. [14]	100	PillCam COLON[a]	Sensitivity: 89 % Specificity: 75 % PPV: 93 % NPV: 65 %	–	–
Ye et al. [15]	25	PillCam COLON[a]	–	$\kappa=0.751$ $P<0.001$	$\kappa=0.522$ $P<0.001$
Acosta et al. [16]	14	PillCam COLON 2[a]	–	$\kappa=1.0$ SE=0.0	$\kappa=0.864$ SE=0.129
Heinzow et al. [17]	13	PillCam COLON 2[a]	–	Rachmilewitz score: SC: 8.1±3.8 CCE: 5.9±3.2 $p<0.001$	–

CCE colon capsule endoscopy, *NPV* negative predictive value, *PPV* positive predictive value, *SC* standard colonoscopy
[a]Given Imaging; Yoqneam, Israel

References

1. Albert JG, Martiny F, Krummenerl A, et al. Diagnosis of small bowel Crohn's disease: a prospective comparison of capsule endoscopy with magnetic resonance imaging and fluoroscopic enteroclysis. Gut. 2005;54:1721–7.
2. Bourreille A, Ignjatovic A, Aabakken L, et al. Role of small-bowel endoscopy in the management of patients with inflammatory bowel disease: an international OMED-ECCO consensus. Endoscopy. 2009;41:618–37.
3. Maunoury V, Savoye G, Bourreille A, et al. Value of wireless capsule endoscopy in patients with indeterminate colitis (inflammatory bowel disease type unclassified). Inflamm Bowel Dis. 2007;13:152–5.
4. Lopes S, Figueiredo P, Portela F, et al. Capsule endoscopy in inflammatory bowel disease type unclassified and indeterminate colitis serologically negative. Inflamm Bowel Dis. 2010;16:1663–8.
5. Murrell Z, Vasiliauskas E, Melmed G, et al. Preoperative wireless capsule endoscopy does not predict outcome after ileal pouch-anal anastomosis. Dis Colon Rectum. 2010;53:293–300.
6. Triester SL, Leighton JA, Leontiadis GI, et al. A meta-analysis of the yield of capsule endoscopy compared to other diagnostic modalities in patients with non-stricturing small bowel Crohn's disease. Am J Gastroenterol. 2006;101:954–64.
7. van Tuyl SAC, van Noorden JT, Stolk MFJ, Kuipers EJ. Clinical consequences of videocapsule endoscopy in GI bleeding and Crohn's disease. Gastrointest Endosc. 2007;66:1164–70.
8. Rutgeerts P, Geboes K, Vantrappen G, et al. Predictability of the postoperative course of Crohn's disease. Gastroenterology. 1990;99:956–63.
9. Rutgeerts P, Van Assche G, Vermeire S, et al. Ornidazole for prophylaxis of postoperative Crohn's disease recurrence: a randomized, double-blind, placebo-controlled trial. Gastroenterology. 2005;128:856–61.
10. Regueiro M, Schraut W, Baidoo L, et al. Infliximab prevents Crohn's disease recurrence after ileal resection. Gastroenterology. 2009;136:441–50.
11. Baert F, Moortgat L, Van Assche G, et al. Mucosal healing predicts sustained clinical remission in patients with early-stage Crohn's disease. Gastroenterology. 2010;138:463–8.
12. Colombel JF, Rutgeerts P, Reinisch W, et al. Early mucosal healing with infliximab is associated with improved long-term clinical outcomes in ulcerative colitis. Gastroenterology. 2011;141:1194–201.
13. Spada C, Hassan C, Galmiche JP, et al. Colon capsule endoscopy: European Society of Gastrointestinal Endoscopy (ESGE) Guideline. Endoscopy. 2012;44:527–36.
14. Sung J, Ho KY, Chiu HM, et al. The use of Pillcam Colon in assessing mucosal inflammation in ulcerative colitis: a multicenter study. Endoscopy. 2012;44:754–8.
15. Ye CA, Gao YJ, Ge ZZ, et al. PillCam colon capsule endoscopy versus conventional colonoscopy for the detection of the severity and extent of ulcerative colitis. J Dig Dis. 2013;14:117–24.
16. Acosta MSJ, Cuesta AB, Álvarez ÁC, et al. Pillcam Colon (C2) vs colonoscopy in the assessment of colon mucosa in patients with ulcerative colitis. Endoscopy. 2012;44:A126.
17. Heinzow HS, Lügering A, Domagk D, et al. Assessing disease activity of ulcerative colitis with colon capsule endoscopy versus standard colonoscopy. Gut. 2012;61:A27.

Colon Capsule Endoscopy in Special Situations

Konstantinos Triantafyllou, Peter Baltes, and Martin Keuchel

Contents

The work was first published in 2006 by Springer Medizin Verlag Heidelberg with the following title: *Atlas of Video Capsule Endoscopy*.

K. Triantafyllou (✉)
Hepatogastroenterology Unit, Second Department of Internal Medicine and Research Institute, Attikon University General Hospital, Athens, Greece
e-mail: ktriant@med.uoa.gr

P. Baltes • M. Keuchel
Department of Internal Medicine, Bethesda Krankenhaus Bergedorf, Hamburg, Germany
e-mail: baltes@bkb.info; keuchel@bkb.info

49.1 Incomplete Colonoscopy

Traditional colonoscopy is the gold standard for evaluation of the colon for polyps, cancer, and inflammation. Applied with high expertise and a high technical standard, it is an accurate, safe diagnostic and therapeutic procedure with a high success rate, but between 4.2 and 19 % of colonoscopies are reported to be incomplete [1–3]. Considering the large number of screening colonoscopies worldwide, this percentage leads to a significant amount of incomplete procedures—such as more than 20,000 in 6 years in Ontario, Canada [4].

Women, older patients, and those with diverticulosis, prior colon resection, or long-standing colitis have a lower chance of complete colonoscopy [2]. Incomplete colonoscopies were more likely in an office setting (OR, 0.77; 95 % CI, 0.67–0.89) than in a hospital [4]. The reason for incomplete colonoscopy is often an unfavorable anatomy (Fig. 49.1); one study identified redundant colon in 46 % and diverticulosis in 40 % [5].

Exchanging the instrument for a variable stiffness, small-caliber colonoscope was successful in 15 of 16 cases of incomplete colonoscopy [1]. In 42 of 45 patients, an incomplete colonoscopy could be completed using the double-balloon technique [6]. A short double-balloon endoscope completed an incomplete colonoscopy in all of 110 patients in another report [7]; spiral-assisted colonoscopy was successful in completing the colonoscopy in 22 (92 %) of 24 patients [8], and a single-balloon endoscope was successful in 15 of 15 patients [9]. Cap-assisted colonoscopy (using a mucosectomy cap) could complete an incomplete procedure in 94 of 100 patients, but it was associated with one perforation [10].

CT colonography (virtual colonoscopy) is especially helpful in patients with colonic stenosis in order to exclude metachronous proximal lesions as well as extracolonic pathology. A recent study showed an additional diagnostic yield after incomplete colonoscopy of 11.0 % for polyps and 2.9 % for a nonsynchronous colorectal cancer [11]. Extracolonic findings with clinical consequences were detected in eight patients

Fig. 49.1 Incomplete colonoscopy due to scrotal hernia. The indication for colonoscopy was significant anemia. (**a**) Video capsule endoscopy (VCE) showing luminal narrowing. Stenosis was passed without problems. (**b**) CT scan with hernia (Courtesy of Jörg Sievers, MD)

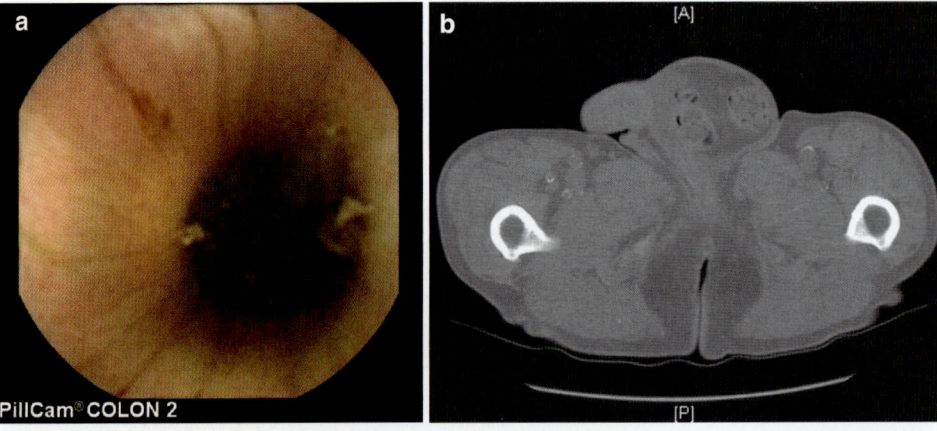

Fig. 49.2 (**a**) Visualization of a hemorrhoidal plexus proves complete colon capsule endoscopy (CCE). (**b**) Visualization of a biopsy site documents complementation of an incomplete colonoscopy

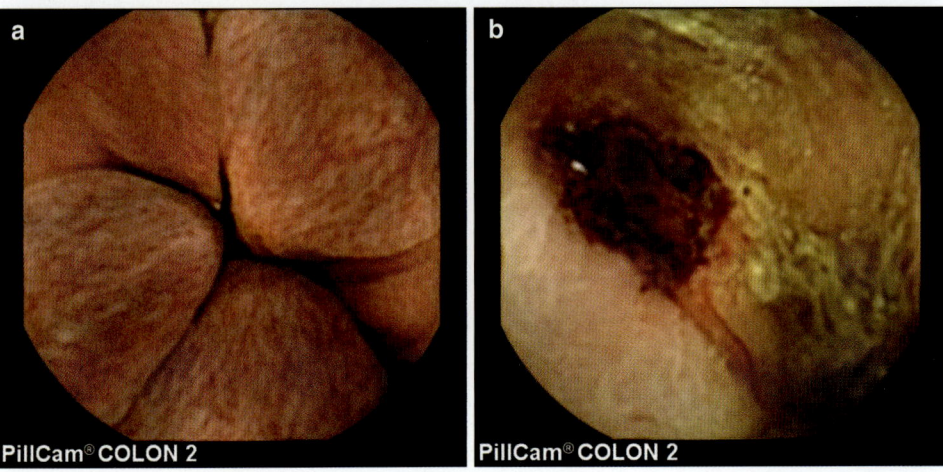

(5.9 %). MR colonography, avoiding radiation exposure, also has been shown to be feasible in complementing incomplete colonoscopy [12], but it has not entered routine clinical practice.

Astonishingly, only 29 % of patients with incomplete colonoscopy in one study had another diagnostic test within the following year [4]. In another study, only 54 % of 278 patients with incomplete colonoscopy had another test within the following 18 months. Follow-up for colorectal cancer, stenosis, anemia, inflammation, and tumor were factors positively affecting performance of a complementary method. Advanced neoplasia was missed in 4.3 % of incomplete colonoscopies [3].

49.2 CCE After Incomplete Colonoscopy

Colon capsule endoscopy (CCE) may be a feasible endoscopic tool after incomplete traditional colonoscopy in patients with adequate bowel preparation and without stenosis [13], especially in an office setting where device-assisted endoscopy is not available. CCE can be performed directly after colonoscopy or (with a new bowel preparation) after an interval. Excretion of the recording capsule or visualization of

the hemorrhoidal plexus proves complete CCE (Fig. 49.2a), whereas recognition of a landmark seen in the incomplete colonoscopy documents complementation of the procedure (Figs. 49.2b and 49.3). Detection of significant findings at CCE may lead to other procedures, including device-assisted colonoscopy or surgery (Figs. 49.4, 49.5, 49.6, and 49.7).

In a Spanish study [14] with the PillCam Colon 1 capsule (Given Imaging Ltd., Yoqneam, Israel), which enrolled 34 patients, 35 % had no relevant findings at CCE, allowing termination of diagnostics. Findings of CCE required polypectomy or surgery in seven patients (20.5 %), including one with carcinoma. One patient had initiation of therapy for Crohn's disease. However, 14 of the 34 patients had inconclusive CCE studies because of extremely fast or slow colonic transit (one patient each) or inadequate bowel cleansing (12 patients). Bowel cleanliness was good or excellent for 22 patients (64.7 %). CCE exceeded the most proximal point reached by conventional colonoscopy in 29 patients (85.3 %) (Table 49.1).

A French multicenter study [15] included 107 patients with incomplete or contraindicated colonoscopy. CCE was performed with PillCam Colon 1 after MoviPrep lavage (Salix Pharmaceuticals, Raleigh, NC, USA), either 1 day after colonoscopy or within 14 days. Bowel prep was

Fig. 49.3 Tubulovillous adenoma with high-grade intraepithelial neoplasia in the reach of an incomplete colonoscopy. (**a**) PillCam Colon 2 (image with blue mode). (**b**) Colonoscopy (the polyp was removed later)

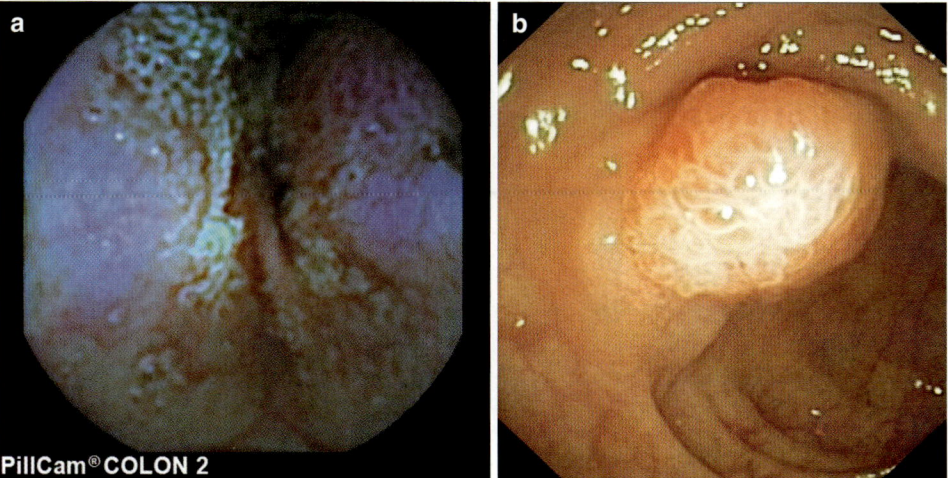

Fig. 49.4 Polyps in the right colon of a female patient with incomplete screening colonoscopy due to sigmoid adhesions. (**a**) CCE showed three small (4 mm) polyps (deemed "significant polyps" because of their number) in the right colon. (**b**) Consecutive single-balloon colonoscopy reached the cecum and confirmed three small tubular adenomas with low-grade intraepithelial neoplasia

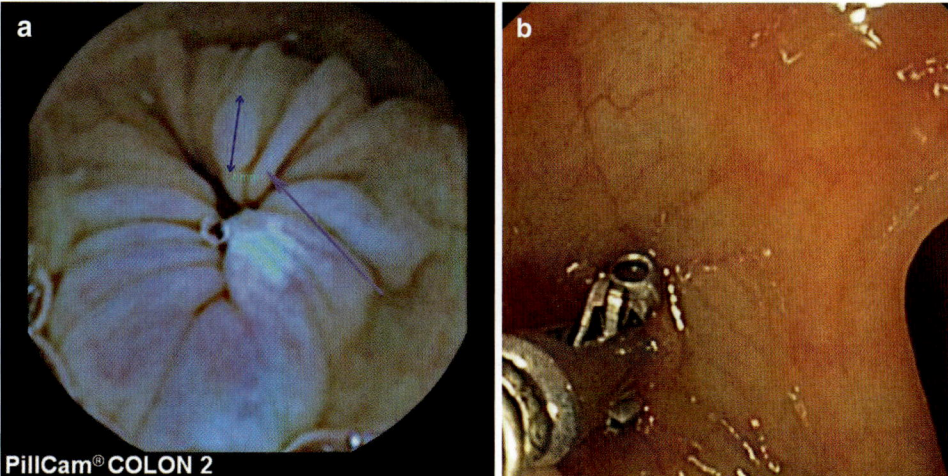

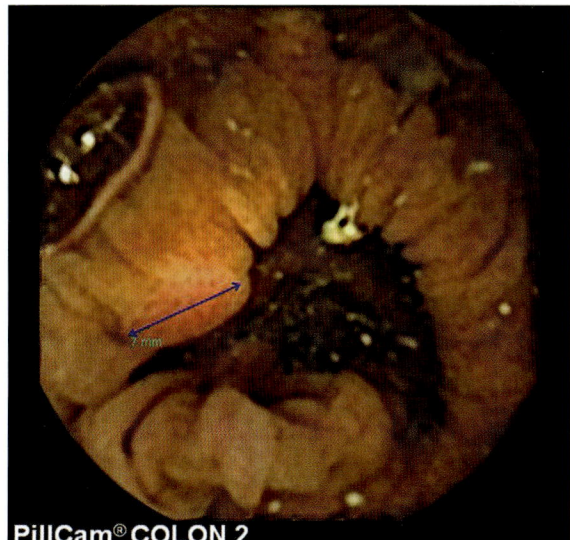

Fig. 49.5 Polyp (7 mm) in the right colon. Although significant, the polyp was not removed, as it did not explain the patient's anemia. Initial colonoscopy could not be completed because of intolerance to sedation due to severe chronic obstructive pulmonary disease

adequate (excellent or good) in 76 % of patients. The CCE procedure was not evaluable in seven patients (one recording failure; six capsules stayed in the right colon). There were no relevant complications. Additional diagnostic yield was 38.7 % in patients with symptoms and 31.6 % in the screening group. Relevant findings were polyps, one carcinoma, angiectasias, ischemia, and inflammatory bowel disorder (IBD). Of the 36 patients with additional findings, 23 subsequently underwent therapeutic intervention. Among 64 patients with negative capsule findings, nine had a complementary procedure; small adenomas were seen in only one case. No clinically evident colonic carcinoma occurred during 1-year follow-up in patients with negative CCE. The major issue with the study is that it did not report results for the incomplete colonoscopy cases ($n=75$), making comparisons with the other studies impossible.

An initial retrospective study with PillCam Colon 1 in Greece [16] included 12 patients with incomplete colonoscopy (6 stenosing left-sided tumors, 6 technical difficulties), in whom CCE was performed 4–10 days later. CCE visualized the rectum in one patient. The capsule did not reach the site where colonoscopy stopped in 6 of the 12 patients,

Fig. 49.6 Right-sided 8 mm polyp seen at CCE after incomplete colonoscopy (**a**) and confirmed at single-balloon colonoscopy. (**b**) Histology revealed hyperplastic polyp

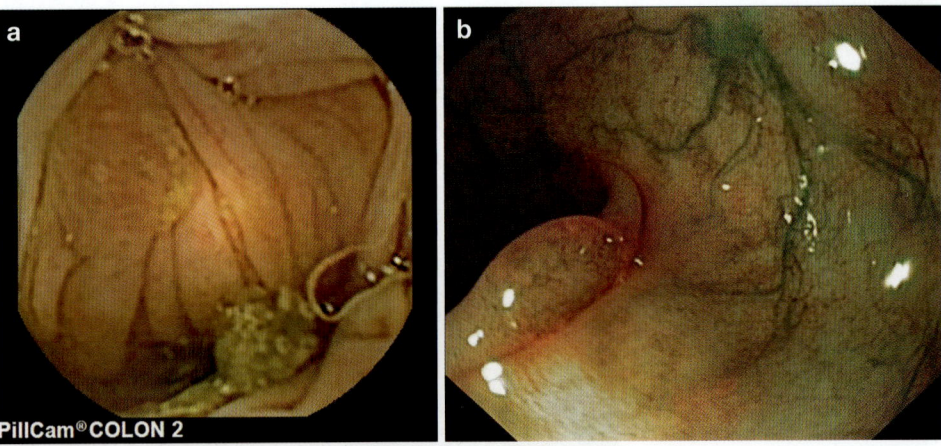

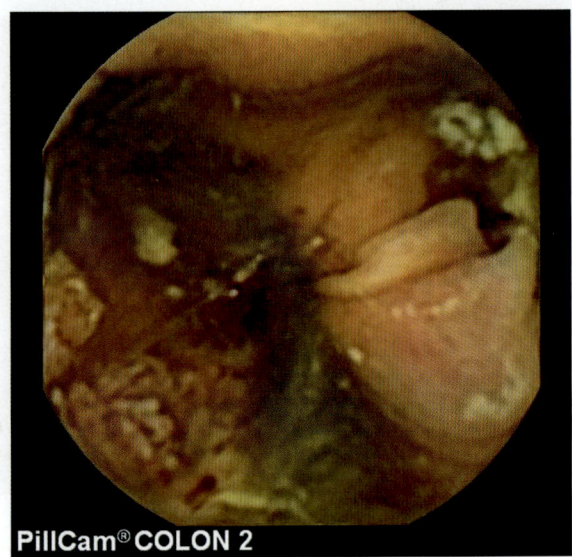

Fig. 49.7 Right-sided colon carcinoma detected by CCE after incomplete, inconclusive colonoscopy. (Courtesy of Jörg Albert, MD)

including 3 with left-sided tumors and 3 with technical difficulties. The capsule passed the site where colonoscopy stopped in three patients, but in one of these, poor bowel preparation precluded the accurate examination of the colon. Four patients underwent a third colon examination (three barium enemas and one virtual CT colonoscopy). There were no adverse events related to the CCE.

A prospective Greek trial [17] included 75 patients with colonoscopy that was incomplete because of patient intolerance (63 %), extensive looping (35 %), or stenos-

ing tumor (2 %). PillCam Colon 1 was used either directly after incomplete colonoscopy (33.3 %) or later. CCE was complete in 76 %. In 91 %, the end point of colonoscopy could be reached. Additional significant findings were obtained in 45 %, and a further workup was recommended to 23 patients (30.7 %). This study showed for the first time that CCE can be performed safely even immediately after failed colonoscopy, with high accuracy and patient acceptance, as 82 % of patients said they would be willing to undergo the same procedure again.

Data on 100 patients from an Italian multicenter comparison revealed no difference in diagnostic yield between CCE and CT colonography after incomplete colonoscopy [18]. However, there was a trend for CCE to detect more polyps than CT colonography. In almost all cases, colonoscopy could be completed by CCE.

Results of a German multicenter study [19] using PillCam Colon 2 after incomplete colonoscopy evaluated 74 patients. MoviPrep lavage produced adequate cleansing in 65 %. CCE was complete in 65 % and complemented colonoscopy in 95 %. Significant polyps were seen in 28 %, including one right-sided colon carcinoma. One capsule was retained in the small bowel, requiring surgery, and previously unknown fistulating and stenosing Crohn's disease was diagnosed as a reason for anemia (see Sect. 49.4) (Fig. 49.10).

Other causes to terminate a colonoscopy might be an increased risk of perforation in ulcerative colitis with high inflammatory activity (Fig. 49.8). Bioptic confirmation of diagnosis may be obtained from left-sided biopsy, and CCE can document the extent of disease. Systematic studies are

Table 49.1 Prospective trials on colon capsule endoscopy (CCE) after incomplete colonoscopy

Study	Patients, N	Adequate bowel cleansing (%)	Complementation of colonoscopy (%)	Complete CCE (%)	Additional findings	Remarks
Pioche et al. (2012) [15]	107	75.9	–	83.2	33.6 %	72 % incomplete colonoscopy
Alarcón-Fernández et al. (2012) [14]	34	64.7	85.3	–	23.5 %	–
Triantafyllou et al. (2014) [17]	75	60–63	91	76	45 %	–
Spada et al. (2014) [18]	50	78	98		14 % (polyps >6 mm)	Comparison to CT colonography
Baltes et al. (2014) (abstract) [19]	45	70	87	80	18	PillCam Colon2

Fig. 49.8 Severe ulcerative pancolitis. Colonoscopy was not performed beyond the sigmoid colon because of severe ulceration. (**a**) Consecutive CCE using the PillCam Colon demonstrated completely normal ileum (**b**) and diffuse inflammation of the entire colon, including the segments not visualized by conventional colonoscopy (**c**, **d**)

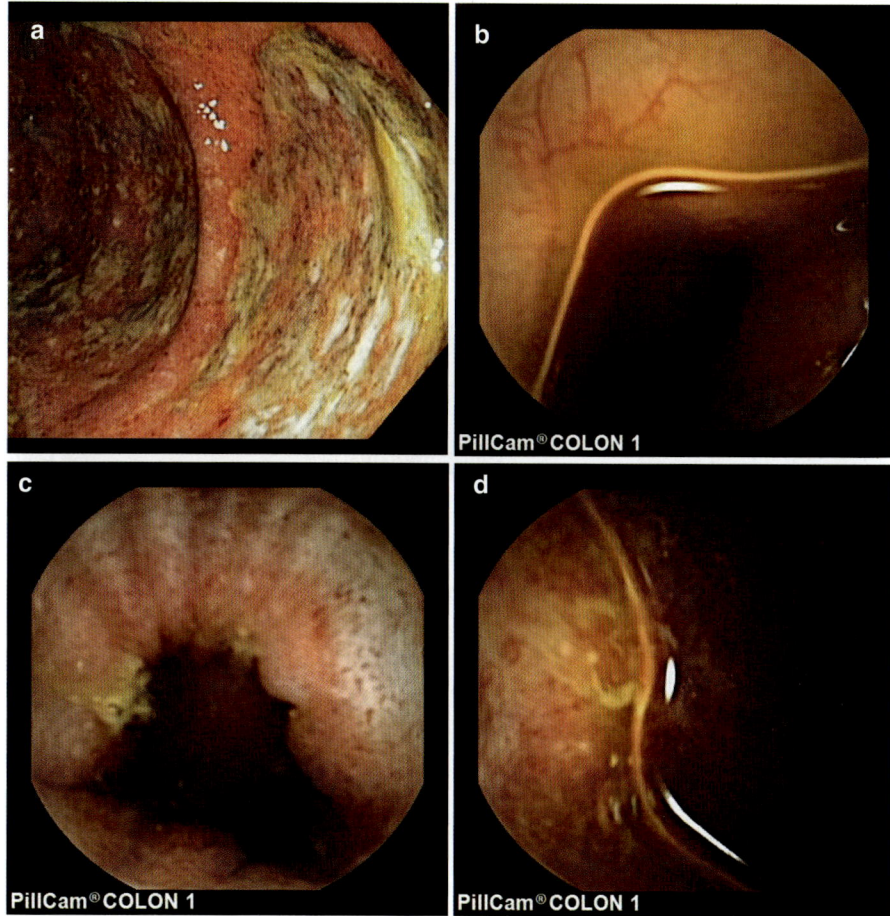

warranted. CCE also may be helpful in diverticular disease with active inflammation (Fig. 49.9), but data concerning risk of retention in this setting are missing.

Existing data suggest that the percentage of patients with inadequate cleanliness of the bowel is similar in those undergoing primary CCE and those with CCE after incomplete colonoscopy. Timing of CCE seems to be appropriate either directly after colonoscopy or following an interval, with new bowel preparation. Complementation of incomplete colonoscopy accounts for a relevant percentage of indications for CCE, with a low risk of retention and a significant additional diagnostic yield.

Fig. 49.9 CCE after incomplete colonoscopy in patients with diverticular disease. (**a**) Diverticula. (**b**) Beginning fibrosis. (**c, d**) Erythema

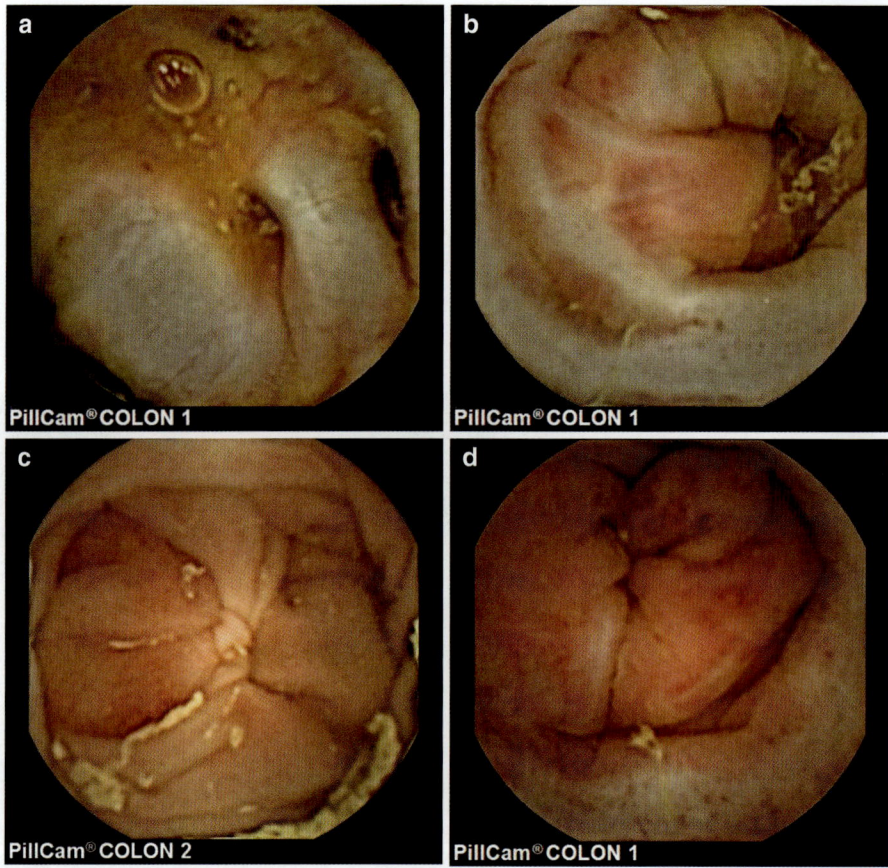

49.3 Contraindicated Colonoscopy

In a setting of clinical practice, the indication for CCE was about evenly divided between failure of colonoscopy, well-informed refusal of colonoscopy, and contraindication to colonoscopy [20].

49.3.1 Risk of Sedation

Perforation is a rare but well-known complication of traditional colonoscopy. As sedation is increasingly used, however, the complication rate of sedation is at least as high as the perforation rate, although both rates are very low. Hypotension was associated with incomplete colonoscopy [21]. In a French multicenter study [15], 26 % of included patients underwent CCE because colonoscopy with anesthesia was contraindicated because of general disease. Although

there is no need for sedation at CCE for severely ill patients, fluid challenge, including fluid boosts during CCE, is rather higher than for standard colonoscopy. This may limit the application of CCE in patients with high-grade cardiac insufficiency. Furthermore, consequences of possible CCE findings should be discussed in advance. For example, will consecutive colonoscopy or surgery be possible if significant polyps or tumors are found?

49.3.2 Impaired Coagulation

Many patients are taking thrombocyte aggregation inhibitors (TAIs). Polypectomy is considered safe with the continued use of aspirin, but it is not recommended for patients on dual platelet aggregation inhibition or those receiving oral anticoagulants [22]. An important argument in favor of traditional colonoscopy is the possibility of polypectomy in the same

Fig. 49.10 Previously undiagnosed fistulating and stenosing Crohn's disease in a 61-year-old patient with anemia. Colonoscopy reached only the left flexure because of adhesions after splenectomy 6 months previously. (**a**) Colon capsule detects stenosis, fistula, and ulcers in the terminal ileum. The capsule was retained in the small intestine (Courtesy of Michael Philipper, MD). (**b**) CT scan. (**c**) Enteroclysis. (Courtesy of Bernward Kurtz, MD)

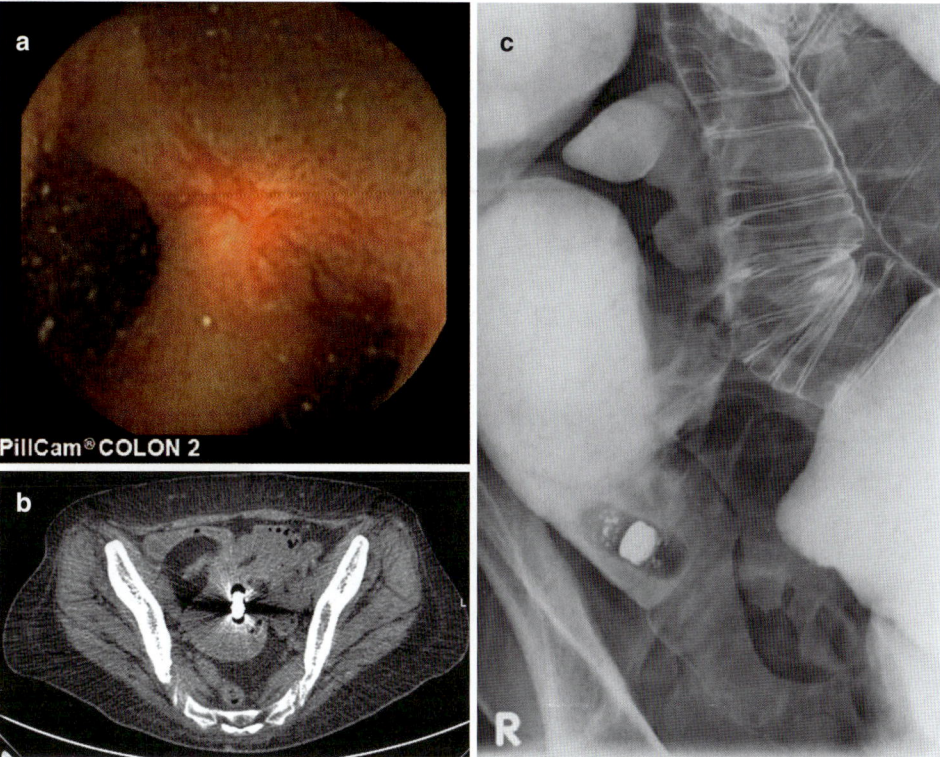

session, so the withdrawal of dual TAI and/or oral anticoagulation is often recommended before colonoscopy, but doing so can be potentially hazardous for some patients. Screening with CCE may limit the withdrawal of these medications to those patients with significant findings requiring polypectomy. This setting warrants systematic research, however.

Esophageal capsule endoscopy (ECE) has been used to screen patients receiving dual TAI therapy. Potential bleeding lesions, predominantly gastric erosions, were identified in 18 of 20 patients [23]. However, studies of CCE in patients with impaired coagulation are missing as well.

49.4 Complications of CCE

Capsule retention is not expected in healthy persons, but this rare potential complication must be considered in all clinical situations of abdominal complaints or findings such as anemia. Careful patient selection for CCE after incomplete colonoscopy should aim to exclude those with relevant stenosis. Nevertheless, capsule retention can be considered diagnostic rather than a complication in some cases of relevant new diagnosis (Fig. 49.10). Data on this issue are warranted.

The routine use of prokinetics is not recommended for the new PillCam Colon 2, as its longer battery life makes delayed gastric emptying less important. A prokinetic can be given, however, if either the software integrated in the DR3 recorder or real-time viewing recognizes that the capsule's arrival at the small bowel is delayed. Endoscopic transport with a snare holding the capsule in the middle between the two cameras (see Fig. 7.8b) is also possible, but some patients undergoing CCE may not be willing or able to undergo endoscopy. Endoscopic placement in patients with swallowing disorders is rarely appropriate; the delivery device does not accommodate the longer colon capsule securely.

49.5   Extracolonic Findings

CCE has the potential not only to complement partial colonoscopy but also to detect pathology in the proximal and mid-gastrointestinal (GI) tract. These findings may be relevant because routine esophagogastroduodenography (EGD) is not generally performed with colonoscopy. Hence, additional evaluation of the extracolonic images is advisable, although exclusion of diseases in the esophagus, stomach, or small bowel is not reliable with CCE. The colon capsule frequently visualizes the Z line because of its enhanced frame rate and the camera on both ends (Fig. 49.11). Besides suspected Barrett's esophagus or reflux esophagitis, gastritis (Fig. 49.12) and gastroduodenal ulcers should be looked for.

Small bowel lesions that may be detected during CCE include angiectasias, polyps, and tumors. In patients with suspected IBD, the potential to inspect long segments of the small bowel as well is another benefit of CCE (Chap. 48). Future technical developments may omit phases of power-saving modes associated with loss of images in the proximal GI tract, thus providing complete "one-stop-shopping" endoscopy (Fig. 49.13) from the mouth to anus ("M2A," as the first capsules were named).

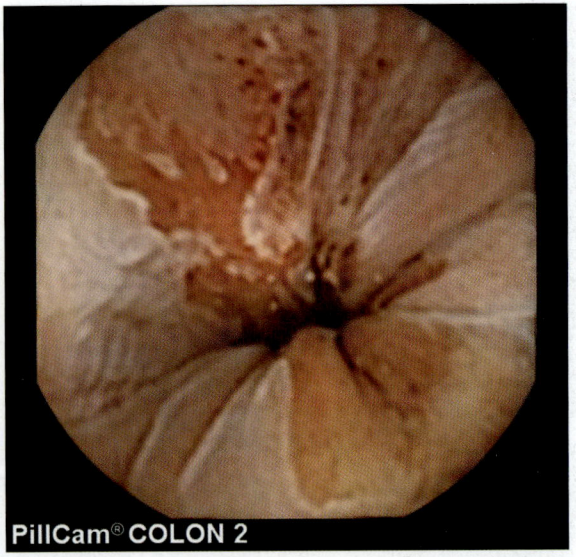

Fig. 49.11   Z line as visualized at CCE for incomplete colonoscopy

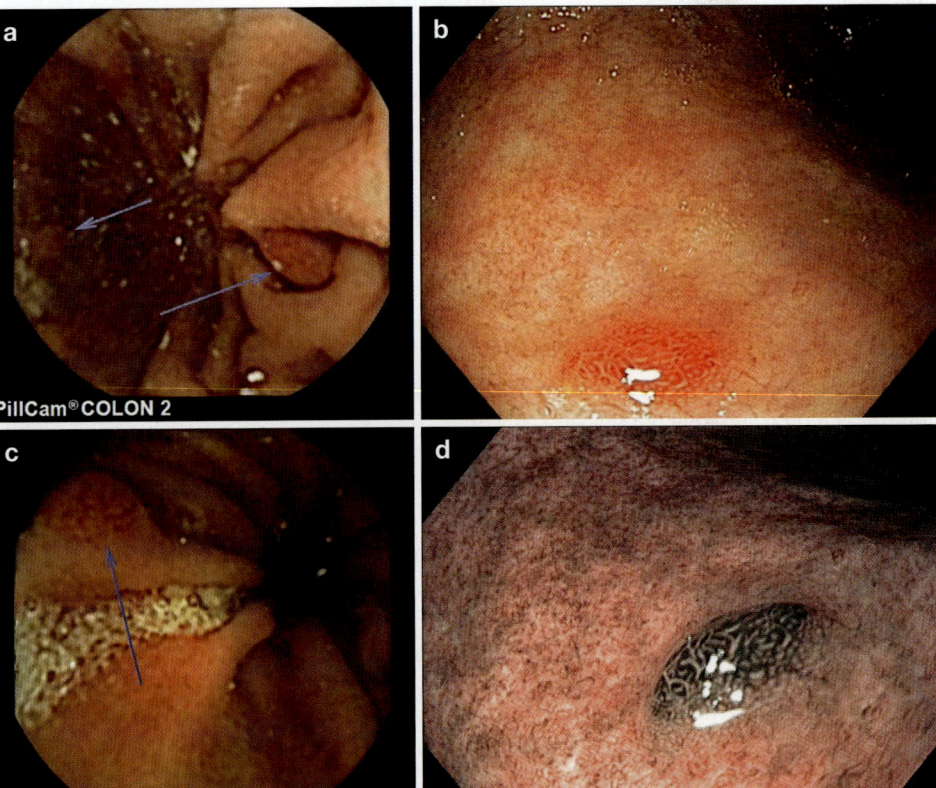

Fig. 49.12   CCE after incomplete colonoscopy in a patient without prior gastroscopy. (**a, c**) Small gastric polyps (*arrows*) seen in CCE. At consecutive gastroscopy (**b, d** [with NBI]) polyps were confirmed and resected. Histology showed pseudopyloric and intestinal metaplasia, and random gastric biopsies revealed atrophic gastritis. Subsequent laboratory tests confirmed beginning vitamin B_{12} deficiency (elevated methylmalonic acid and decreased holotranscobalamin) and positive antibodies against parietal cells. Parenteral vitamin B_{12} supplementation was initiated

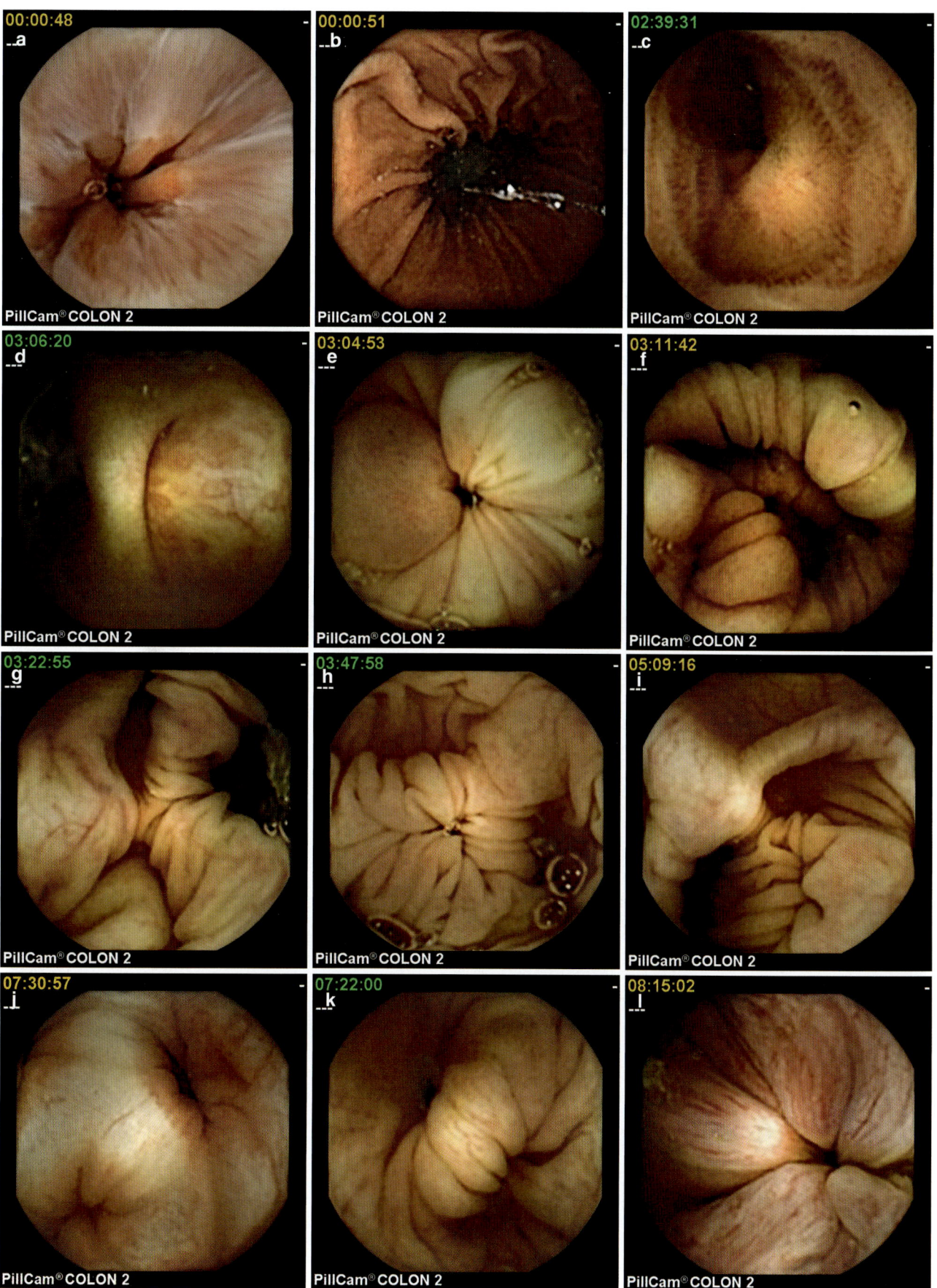

Fig. 49.13 CCE using PillCam Colon 2 after incomplete colonoscopy, showing normal passage through the gastrointestinal tract. (**a**) Z line. (**b**) Stomach. (**c**) Ileum. (**d**) Appendix. (**e**) Ileocecal valve. (**f**) Ascending colon. (**g**) Right flexure. (**h**) Transverse colon. (**i**) Left flexure. (**j**) Sigmoid. (**k**) Rectum. (**l**) Hemorrhoidal plexus

References

1. Shumaker DA, Zaman A, Katon RM. Use of a variable-stiffness colonoscope allows completion of colonoscopy after failure with the standard adult colonoscope. Endoscopy. 2002;34:711–4.

2. Dafnis G, Granath F, Pahlman L, et al. Patient factors influencing the completion rate in colonoscopy. Dig Liver Dis. 2005;37:113–8.

3. Neerincx M, Terhaar sive Droste JS, Mulder CJ, et al. Colonic work-up after incomplete colonoscopy: significant new findings during follow-up. Endoscopy. 2010;42:730–5.

4. Rizek R, Paszat LF, Stukel TA, et al. Rates of complete colonic evaluation after incomplete colonoscopy and their associated factors: a population-based study. Med Care. 2009;47:48–52.

5. Iafrate F, Hassan C, Zullo A, et al. CT colonography with reduced bowel preparation after incomplete colonoscopy in the elderly. Eur Radiol. 2008;18:1385–95.

6. Moreels TG, Macken EJ, Roth B, et al. Cecal intubation rate with the double-balloon endoscope after incomplete conventional colonoscopy: a study in 45 patients. J Gastroenterol Hepatol. 2010;25:80–3.

7. Hotta K, Katsuki S, Ohata K, et al. A multicenter, prospective trial of total colonoscopy using a short double-balloon endoscope in patients with previous incomplete colonoscopy. Gastrointest Endosc. 2012;75:813–8.

8. Schembre DB, Ross AS, Gluck MN, et al. Spiral overtube-assisted colonoscopy after incomplete colonoscopy in the redundant colon. Gastrointest Endosc. 2011;73:515–9.

9. Kobayashi K, Mukae M, Ogawa T, et al. Clinical usefulness of single-balloon endoscopy in patients with previously incomplete colonoscopy. World J Gastrointest Endosc. 2013;5:117–21.

10. Lee YT, Hui AJ, Wong VW, et al. Improved colonoscopy success rate with a distally attached mucosectomy cap. Endoscopy. 2006;38:739–42.

11. Pullens HJ, van Leeuwen MS, Laheij RJ, et al. CT-colonography after incomplete colonoscopy: what is the diagnostic yield? Dis Colon Rectum. 2013;56:593–9.

12. Hartmann D, Bassler B, Schilling D, et al. Incomplete conventional colonoscopy: magnetic resonance colonography in the evaluation of the proximal colon. Endoscopy. 2005;37:816–20.

13. Spada C, Riccioni ME, Petruzziello L, et al. The new PillCam Colon capsule: difficult colonoscopy? No longer a problem? Gastrointest Endosc. 2008;68:807–8.

14. Alarcón-Fernández O, Ramos L, Adrián-de-Ganzo Z, et al. Effects of colon capsule endoscopy on medical decision making in patients with incomplete colonoscopies. Clin Gastroenterol Hepatol. 2012;11:534–40.

15. Pioche M, de Leusse A, Filoche B, et al. Prospective multicenter evaluation of colon capsule examination indicated by colonoscopy failure or anesthesia contraindication. Endoscopy. 2012;44:911–6.

16. Triantafyllou K, Tsibouris P, Kalantzis C, et al. PillCam Colon capsule endoscopy does not always complement incomplete colonoscopy. Gastrointest Endosc. 2009;69:572–6.

17. Triantafyllou K, Viazis N, Tsibouris P, et al. Colon capsule endoscopy is feasible to perform after incomplete colonoscopy and guides further work-up in clinical practice. Gastrointest Endosc. 2014;79:307–1618.

18. Spada C, Hassan C, Barbaro B et al. Colon capsule versus CT colonography in patients with incomplete colonoscopy: a prospective, comparative trial. Gut. 2014 [Epub ahead of print].

19. Baltes P, Bota M, Albert J et al. PillCam Colon2 after incomplete colonoscopy – a multicenter study. Gastrointest Endosc 2014;79: Suppl. 5:AB477.

20. Saurin JC, Ponchon T, Gay G, et al. French multicentric experience of colon capsule endoscopy in real practice: primary results of the Colon Capsule Endoscopy Observatory "ONECC". Gastrointest Endosc. 2013;77:AB496–7.

21. Khalid-de Bakker CA, Jonkers DM, Hameeteman W, et al. Cardiopulmonary events during primary colonoscopy screening in an average risk population. Neth J Med. 2011;69:186–91.

22. Anderson MA, Ben-Menachem T, Gan SI, et al. Management of antithrombotic agents for endoscopic procedures. Gastrointest Endosc. 2009;70:1060–70.

23. Seddighzadeh A, Wolf AT, Parasuraman S, et al. Gastrointestinal complications after 3 months of dual antiplatelet therapy for drug-eluting stents as assessed by wireless capsule endoscopy. Clin Appl Thromb Hemost. 2009;15:171–6.

Practical Approach to Video Capsule Endoscopy: Frequently Asked Questions

50

Peter Baltes, Ian M. Gralnek, and Martin Keuchel

Contents

The work was first published in 2006 by Springer Medizin Verlag Heidelberg with the following title: *Atlas of Video Capsule Endoscopy*.

P. Baltes (✉) • M. Keuchel
Department of Internal Medicine,
Bethesda Krankenhaus Bergedorf, Hamburg, Germany
e-mail: baltes@bkb.info; keuchel@bkb.info

I.M. Gralnek
Department of Gastroenterology,
Rambam Health Care Campus, Haifa, Israel
e-mail: i_gralnek@rambam.health.gov.il

50.1 Technical Issues

50.1.1 What Are the Characteristics of VCE?

Video capsule endoscopy (VCE) is a "physiologic" endoscopy taking advantage of regular peristalsis without the need for air insufflation or sedation. The "underwater view" and high-resolution images allow for detailed visualization of mucosa (Fig. 50.1).

50.1.2 What Are the Components of a Video Capsule?

Within a biocompatible surface, there is an optic system with lenses and imager chip, either a transmitter or a local storage chip, batteries, and LEDs for illumination (Chap. 3).

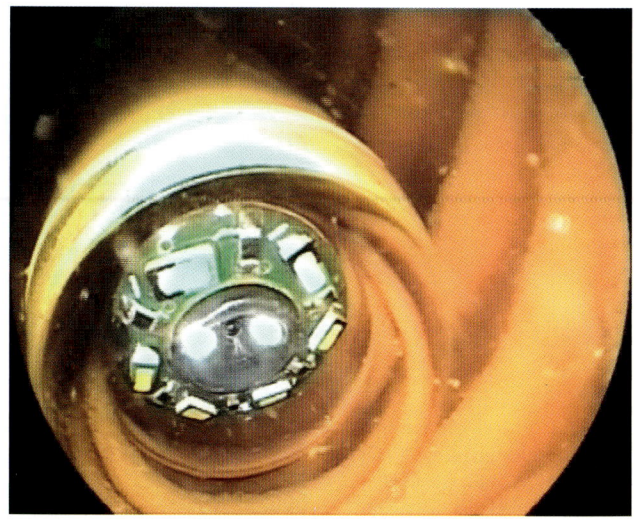

Fig. 50.1 Video capsule swimming in the liquid-filled small intestine

50.1.3 What Are the Components of a VCE System?

Besides the capsule itself, a recorder with antennas or electrodes (alternatively, an internal storage chip) is necessary to store and transfer data via a docking station to a computer workstation at the completion of the procedure. Specific software compiles data to a video for review (Chap. 3).

50.1.4 Which Capsule Endoscopes Are Commercially Available?

The first commercially available VCE system was developed and brought to market by Given Imaging (Yoqneam, Israel) in 2001. Today, Given Imaging provides an entire capsule endoscopy platform including PillCam SB2 and SB3 for the small bowel, PillCam ESO2 for the esophagus, and PillCam COLON2 for the colon. Other small bowel capsules are EndoCapsule (Olympus, Tokyo, Japan), MiroCam (IntroMedic, Seoul, Korea), OMOM (Jingshan, Chongqing, China), and CapsoCam (CapsoVision, Saratoga, CA, USA) (Chap. 3).

50.1.5 What Is the Frame Rate of Video Capsule Endoscopes?

The frame rate depends on the type and manufacturer of the video capsule. The PillCam SB2 and EndoCapsule have a single camera with a fixed rate of 2 frames per second (fps); the rate for MiroCam is 3 fps. PillCam SB3 uses an adaptive

frame rate of 2 versus 6 fps; and PillCam COLON2 uses rates of 4 versus 35 fps. The standard rate for the OMOM capsule, 2 fps, can be remotely reduced to 0.5 fps in the stomach (Chap. 3).

50.1.6 How Long Is the Operating Time of Video Capsules?

Battery life is 8–15 h, depending on the type of video capsule.

50.1.7 Do Video Capsule Endoscopes Have to Be Retrieved by the Patient?

All video capsule endoscopes are designed for single use only, are "naturally" excreted, and are not required to be collected by the patient. Patients are advised to look for the excreted capsule to confirm "natural" passage, if possible. Only capsules that store data within the capsule itself (e.g., the CapsoCam) must be retrieved to allow downloading of the endoscopy image data.

50.1.8 How Are VCE Studies Stored?

A backup copy of all capsule studies should be stored on an external hard drive, DVD, or on a safe computer network for at least 10 years or the period required by country-specific medical records regulations. If using a network storage solution, the drive should be included in the regular data backup by the IT department.

Fig. 50.2 (**a**) Bravo capsule released from introducer. (**b**) SmartPill

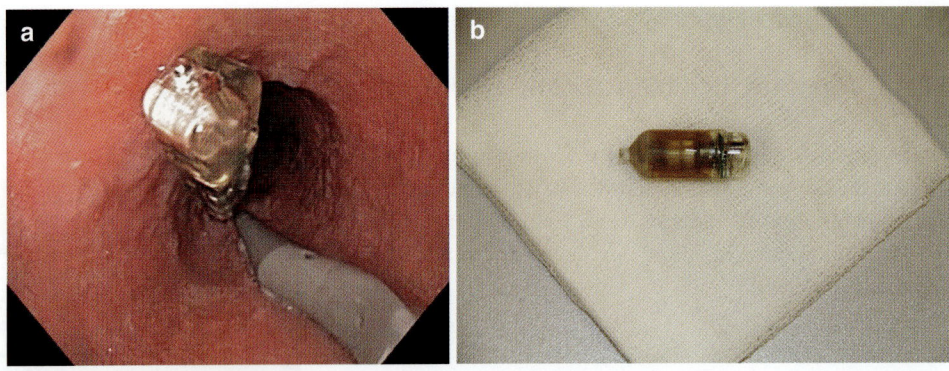

Fig. 50.3 Patient was referred for video capsule endoscopy (VCE) because of anemia. Detailed history revealed that he had no previous gastroscopy. Esophagogastroduodenoscopy (EGD) was performed instead of VCE (**a**) and detected gastric adenocarcinoma, leading to staging (**b**) and resection

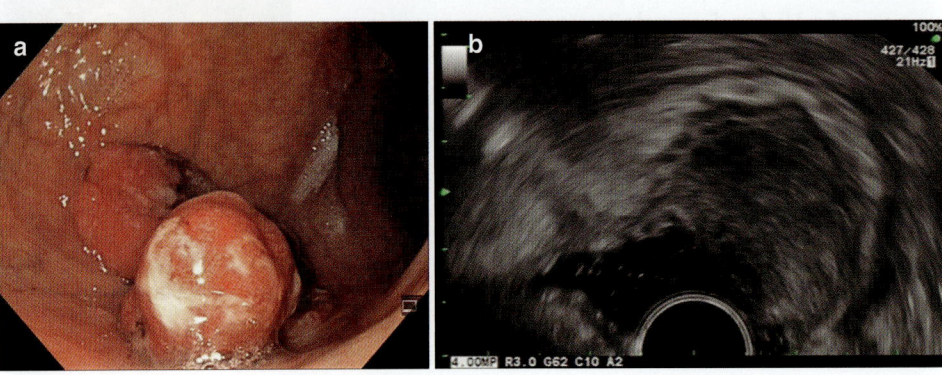

50.1.9 Are There Nonimaging Wireless Capsules?

Yes. The Bravo capsule (Given Imaging) is attached endoscopically to the distal esophagus (Fig. 50.2a) and measures pH for 48 h [1–3]. The SmartPill (Given Imaging) is naturally propelled through the entire gastrointestinal (GI) tract and measures gastric, intestinal, and colonic transit by a combination of pH, pressure, and temperature [4] (Fig. 50.2b). Data are transmitted to a recorder from both types.

50.1.10 What Future Developments in VCE Technology Are Expected?

Further enhancement of battery life, improved software with automated recognition of lesions (Chap. 52), and enhanced image quality are expected. Ongoing research is working on developments such as remote control and steering of the video capsule, tissue sampling (biopsies), and therapy such as injection, coagulation, and local drug delivery (Chap. 51).

50.1.11 Should I Start with a VCE or a "Deep" Enteroscopy System?

Sooner or later, a small bowel endoscopy service will need both methods, but it may be appropriate to start with noninvasive VCE. This first-line diagnostic tool can visualize the entire small intestinal mucosa independently from endoscopic skills and has the option to repeatedly review uncertain findings.

50.2 Procedural Issues

50.2.1 What Should I Know from the Patient's History Before VCE?

Knowledge of pregnancy, previous abdominal surgery, radiation exposure, obstructive symptoms, or swallowing difficulties is important in the search for contraindications. Antiplatelet therapy, anticoagulants, and (to a lesser extent) antidepressants are relevant in bleeding patients. The use of nonsteroidal anti-inflammatory drugs (NSAIDs) especially often goes undisclosed. Prior endoscopic therapy or biopsy may create artificial lesions, potentially confusing the interpretation of endoscopic images.

50.2.2 What Test Should Be Done Before Small Bowel Capsule Endoscopy (SBCE)?

In general, upper and lower GI endoscopy should precede SBCE (Fig. 50.3). In suspected Crohn's disease, the terminal ileum should be inspected. In obscure GI bleeding without signs of obstruction, no preceding radiographic imaging technique is required. Prior abdominal ultrasound is appropriate, however, to exclude gross pathology.

50.2.3 Should I Repeat Upper and Lower GI Endoscopy Before SBCE?

Not regularly. However, depending on the time interval and the quality of the report or investigation, upper and lower GI endoscopy may be repeated before SBCE. The diagnostic yield seems to be low if the interval is less than 6 months [5].

50.2.4 What Are the Contraindications for VCE?

Pregnancy is a contraindication due to lack of data. (Only a few cases in emergency situations have been reported [6, 7].) In intestinal stenosis, capsule endoscopy should be avoided unless surgery is scheduled. VCE is not cleared by the US Food and Drug Administration (FDA) for children less than 2 years of age. In patients with swallowing disorders, the capsule should be placed endoscopically to avoid aspiration. Implanted cardiac devices are a formal contraindication, but clinical experience does not show an increase in adverse events.

50.2.5 What Should Be Included in the Informed Consent Discussion Before SBCE?

Patients should be informed about details of the procedure, alternative methods (including deep enteroscopy or radiographic imaging techniques), and the potential risks and limitations. Risks are capsule retention (occurring in 1–16 % of patients, according to indication), which may require enteroscopy, dilation, or surgery, and aspiration, occurring in approximately 1 in 800 cases. Potential limitations are incomplete or inadequate visualization of the small intestine. During the informed consent discussion between the physician and patient, the indication and results of previous examinations should be reviewed. Information about the patient's medical history should be gathered in order to verify risk factors:

- Swallowing disorders (may need direct endoscopic capsule placement)
- Pregnancy (contraindication)
- Cardiac devices (inform patient)
- The use of NSAIDs, suspected or known Crohn's disease, prior abdominal radiation therapy, or previous small intestinal resection (increased risk of capsule retention)

50.2.6 How Should the Patient Prepare for SBCE?

The patient should stay NPO (nil per os) for at least 12 h and take a bowel preparation if recommended by his physician. Tight clothing should be avoided so that sensor arrays and wires can be placed. Body lotions may hamper attachment of sensors to the skin. MRI should not be scheduled within the next 2 weeks after VCE.

50.2.7 If an MRI Is Planned, Is VCE Contraindicated?

Patients with a scheduled MRI should not undergo VCE in the preceding 2 weeks. Once VCE has been performed, excretion of the capsule must be assured before the patient undergoes an MRI. In single cases (Fig. 50.4), patients have had an MRI with the capsule still incorporated. Artifacts jeopardized the MRI, but no clinical harm to the patient was observed [8]. However, there are no larger series, and no data are available on the influence of different MRI protocols on potential risks.

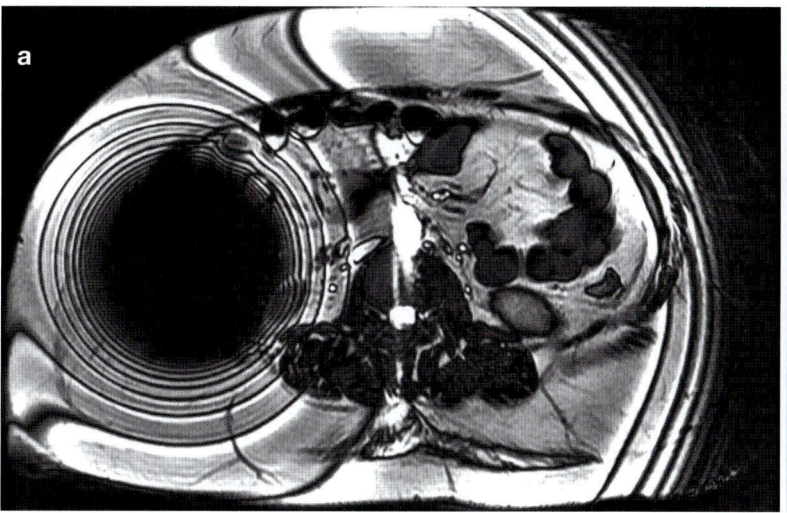
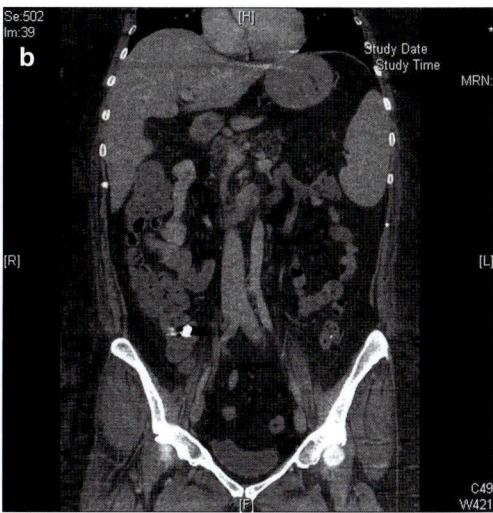

Fig. 50.4 MRI performed in a female patient. MRI shows the artifacts produced by the video capsule (**a**). A consecutive CT scan demonstrates the capsule in the cecum without any signs of injury (**b**) (Courtesy of Jörg Sievers, MD)

50.2.8 What Should I Do If GI Obstruction Is Suspected?

A qualified sonography, CT scan, or MRI can be helpful to evaluate for GI obstruction. The most effective tool to identify luminal stenosis is the patency capsule.

50.2.9 What Is a Patency Capsule?

The PillCam patency capsule (Given Imaging, Yoqneam, Israel) is designed as a "dummy" test capsule for patients with suspected small bowel stenosis. It is the same size as the SB video capsule but starts to disintegrate after about 30 h. The remaining small radiofrequency (RF) tag and external cover are designed to pass even stenotic areas. Persistence of the RF tag in the body can be identified by X-ray or an external radiofrequency scanner (Chap. 9).

50.2.10 When Should My Patient Have a Patency Capsule Test?

Patients at risk for capsule retention should be tested. Risk factors are stenosis (either suspected clinically or in an imaging test), known Crohn's disease, prior radiation, or prior resection of the small intestine.

50.2.11 How Should I Perform a Patency Capsule Test?

The test is best performed by the patient swallowing the patency capsule and retrieving the intact excreted capsule. Alternatively, a dedicated scanner can be used to prove the absence of the capsule (with its inner RF tag) before it begins to dissolve (i.e., within 30 h), though this may give false-negative results in isolated cases.

50.2.12 My Patient Has a Swallowing Disorder: Is Capsule Endoscopy Still Possible?

Prior to VCE, the patient's swallowing ability can be tested using a small piece of candy. In case of a swallowing disorder, the video capsule can be placed endoscopically directly into the duodenum using a delivery device (e.g., AdvanCE delivery device by US Endoscopy, Mentor, Ohio, USA). Capsule placement using a foreign-body retrieval net (e.g., Roth Net) may cause trauma and is not recommended (Chap. 7).

50.2.13 Is Bowel Preparation Necessary for SBCE?

SBCE is possible after the patient is NPO for 12 h, but studies have shown better visualization of the small bowel mucosa and an increased diagnostic yield when lavage is given prior to VCE. Hence, lavage is strongly recommended (Chap. 4).

50.2.14 Which Kind of Preparation Should Be Used?

The most widely used bowel prep is polyethylene glycol (PEG) or PEG with ascorbic acid. Probably a split-dose regimen (evening and early morning, at the latest 1 h before VCE) is more effective.

50.2.15 Should Simethicone Be Given Before VCE?

Yes. Studies show better visualization of small bowel mucosa when simethicone is given 15–30 min prior to VCE. Small air bubbles are thus avoided by forming large bubbles (Fig. 50.5).

50.2.16 Can I Avoid Inadequate Illumination?

Automated light control cannot be influenced. In general, it gives good results, with rare episodes of overillumination. Direct exposure to bright sunlight should be avoided [9]. Bowel preparation reduces dark images in the distal ileum. Drinking of lavage fluid after ingestion of the capsule (and passage to the small intestine) has been suggested to improve visualization.

50.2.17 What If the Patient Is Taking Oral Iron Supplementation?

Oral iron supplementation should be stopped for at least 3 days (preferably 7 days) before the capsule is ingested. The presence of ferrous oxide significantly reduces the capsule's ability to visualize the small bowel mucosa.

50.2.18 What If the Patient Is Taking Platelet Aggregation Inhibitors or Anticoagulants?

There is no need to withhold or stop platelet aggregation inhibitors or anticoagulation prior to VCE.

Fig. 50.5 (**a**) Multiple small air bubbles prohibiting adequate visualization. (**b**) Large, transparent air bubble

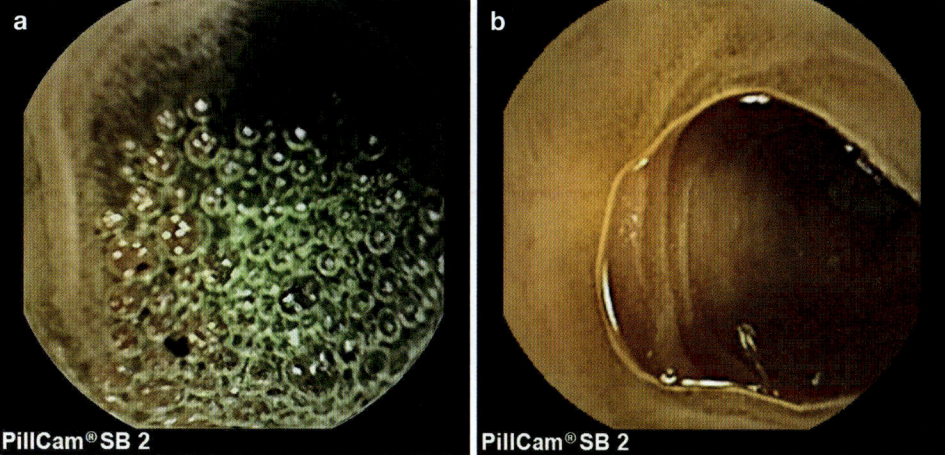

50.2.19 Is There a Need for Endocarditis Prophylaxis?

No. The smooth surface of the capsule does not cause mucosal trauma.

50.2.20 Should the Patient Take Their Oral Medications Prior to VCE?

If possible, oral medication should be withheld for about 4 h after ingestion of the capsule. Indispensable medication might be given approximately 4 h before capsule ingestion or an intravenous preparation may be used instead. Impaired mucosal visualization is most pronounced with sustained-release formulations.

50.2.21 When Should a Prokinetic Agent Be Used?

In cases of known delayed gastric emptying (gastroparesis), or when delayed gastric emptying is proven by a real-time viewer, prokinetic agents such as metoclopramide (10 mg), erythromycin (250 mg), or domperidone (20 mg) can be used. They are not recommended routinely in VCE.

50.2.22 How Should Prokinetic Agents Be Given?

Domperidone is available only for oral administration as a tablet or liquid, whereas erythromycin and metoclopramide can also be given intravenously. Oral medication may slightly reduce mucosal visualization by VCE.

50.2.23 How Long May a Capsule Stay in the Stomach?

With longer battery life, delayed gastric transit does not necessarily lead to incomplete visualization of the small intestine. Most capsules have left the stomach after 1 h; however; after 2 h, a prokinetic drug or endoscopic transport to the duodenum should be considered.

50.2.24 Which Patients Are at Risk for Prolonged Transit Times?

Potential causes of prolonged gastric transit times are diabetes mellitus, gastric emptying disorder or gastroparesis, therapy with opiates, and patient immobility. VCE directly after colonoscopy may be hampered by delayed gastric transit.

50.2.25 Does the Patient Have to Stay in the Hospital or Office During the VCE Procedure?

No. The patient may leave after swallowing the capsule. However, documentation of capsule position in the small intestine with a real-time viewer after 1 h to exclude gastric retention reduces incomplete examinations.

50.2.26 How Long Does the Patient Have to Fast After Ingestion of the Capsule?

The patient may drink clear liquids 2 h after capsule ingestion and may eat after 4 h. It may be useful to prolong these schedules in patients with known motility disorders. Once

Fig. 50.6 Chromo-capsule endoscopy in celiac disease. (**a**) Proximal small intestine with total villous atrophy. (**b**) Distal small intestine with partial atrophy

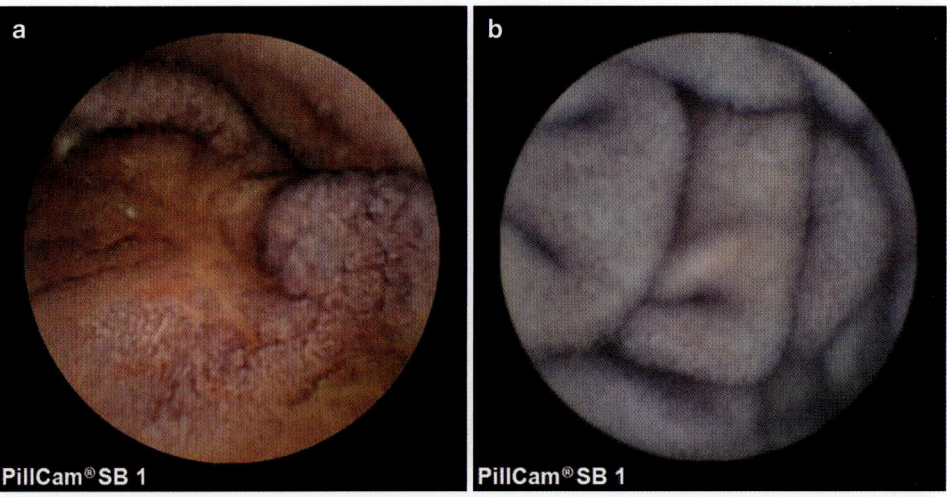

the real-time viewer verifies entry of the capsule into the small bowel, the patient may begin to drink clear liquids.

50.2.27 How Long Should the Procedure Last with Longer-Working Capsules?

Longer-lasting VCE batteries are expected to decrease the rate of incomplete small bowel examinations. This can be advantageous only if the procedure is extended to the specified working time (up to 14 h). Using a real-time viewer to document that the capsule has reached the cecum may allow the physician to terminate the procedure earlier.

50.2.28 Should the Electrodes Be Placed Differently on Obese Patients?

In obese patients, data transmission from the capsule can be impaired. It can be helpful to place the electrodes dorsally and laterally reversed. Alternatively, a capsule with local data storage, such as CapsoCam, might be considered for extremely obese patients.

50.2.29 Is Chromo-capsule Endoscopy Possible?

Yes, but it is very uncommon [10]. Chromo-capsule endoscopy of the small bowel requires prior endoscopic instillation of diluted color (e.g., 50–100 mL water with 1–2 vials of methylene blue) into the duodenum. Immediately after this instillation, the endoscope is withdrawn and reinserted again with the frontloaded capsule, which is released in the duodenum. Chromo-capsule endoscopy may enhance surface structure, such as in suspected celiac disease (Fig. 50.6), but there are

no data showing whether the diagnostic yield is improved.

50.2.30 Is Intraoperative Capsule Endoscopy Possible?

Two cases of intraoperative VCE have been described. A tube was swallowed some days before surgery, and when it was anally expelled, a capsule was tethered before pulling the tube back. Endoscopic images were displayed intraoperatively on a real-time viewer to guide surgical treatment [11].

50.3   Clinical Issues

50.3.1 What Are the Main Indications for Small Bowel Capsule Endoscopy?

VCE is helpful in diagnosing or evaluating a number of small bowel diseases. The main indication for VCE is the evaluation of obscure GI bleeding (both overt and occult) or iron deficiency anemia not otherwise explained. Moreover, VCE is also indicated in suspected or known Crohn's disease, celiac disease, polyposis syndromes, small bowel tumors, and other less common small bowel diseases.

50.3.2 What Makes a Clinical Suspicion of Crohn's Disease?

VCE has a very low diagnostic yield in patients with abdominal pain as a lone indication. The presence of additional signs and symptoms (such as fever, weight loss, diarrhea) or findings (leukocytosis, elevated C-reactive protein or erythrocyte sedimentation rate, anemia, iron deficiency, or

Fig. 50.7 (**a**) Large "sporadic" duodenal adenoma. (**b**) Small flat polyp (*arrows*) in the ileum of the same patient (flexible spectral imaging color enhancement (FICE) 3 mode)

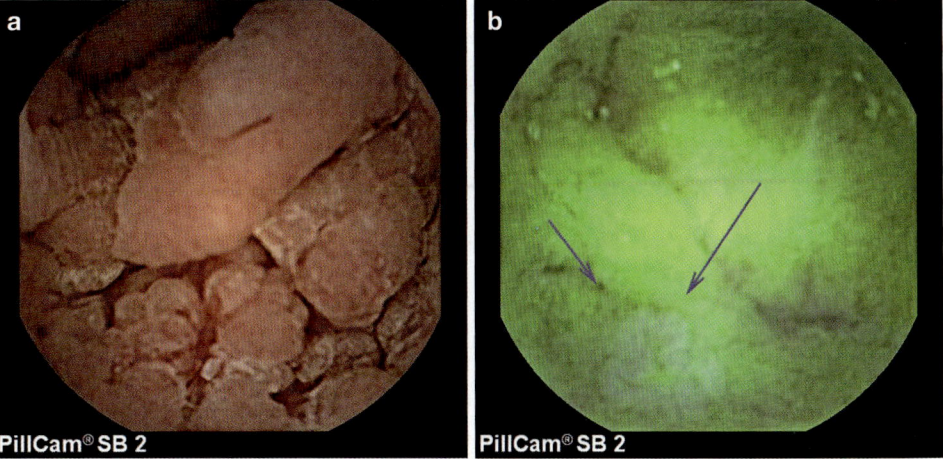

positive fecal markers such as calprotectin or lactoferrin) increases the diagnostic yield.

50.3.3 What Should I Do If VCE Is Normal in a Patient with Obscure GI Bleeding?

If VCE is normal and bleeding stops, no further tests are necessary. In ongoing or recurrent bleeding or persistent iron deficiency anemia, repeat upper and lower GI endoscopy, including ileoscopy, should be considered. CT scan may be helpful to further exclude small bowel tumor. Coagulopathy should be ruled out. The next step can be to repeat VCE or to perform device-assisted enteroscopy.

50.3.4 Is VCE Indicated in Iron Deficiency Without Anemia?

There are no data at this time for VCE in iron deficiency without anemia, so VCE is not indicated. In cases of persisting iron deficiency, celiac disease should be considered and evaluated.

50.3.5 Is VCE Indicated If a Patient Has a Positive FOBT Without Anemia?

As there are no data at this time for VCE in positive fecal occult blood test (FOBT) without anemia, VCE cannot be recommended.

50.3.6 Do the Findings on VCE Explain My Patient's Anemia?

A high bleeding potential can be assumed for angioectasias, tumors, ulcers, or large varices, whereas small erosions or singular smaller angiectasias have an uncertain bleeding potential. Venectasias or small red spots do not have a high bleeding potential, according to Saurin's classification [12].

50.3.7 Is VCE Indicated for All Patients with Familial Adenomatous Polyposis (FAP)?

No. In FAP patients without duodenal adenomas at esophagogastroduodenoscopy (EGD), including side-viewing duodenoscopy, VCE is unlikely to detect polyps in the jejunum or ileum.

50.3.8 Is VCE Indicated in Patients with "Sporadic" Duodenal Adenomas Without FAP?

VCE is not routinely recommended, although some experts do suggest it. Data are sparse; few patients may have additional polyps in the distal small intestine (Fig. 50.7).

50.3.9 Is There a Role for SBCE in the Emergency Room?

VCE has been shown to be feasible and safe in an emergency department setting for acute GI bleeding. However, the benefit of this procedure is highly dependent on the presence of trained staff and on the availability and threshold of emergency endoscopy.

50.3.10 Is There a Role for Urgent SBCE?

In patients with severe active bleeding, CT angiography is a good procedure that is easy to perform. If the actual

Fig. 50.8 During urgent VCE, this patient developed hemodynamic instability. (**a**) Red blood was seen on the real-time viewer. (**b, c**) CT angiography was performed during capsule endoscopy with only minor artifacts (*Courtesy of* Jörg Sievers, MD). (Findings are shown in Fig. 20.6)

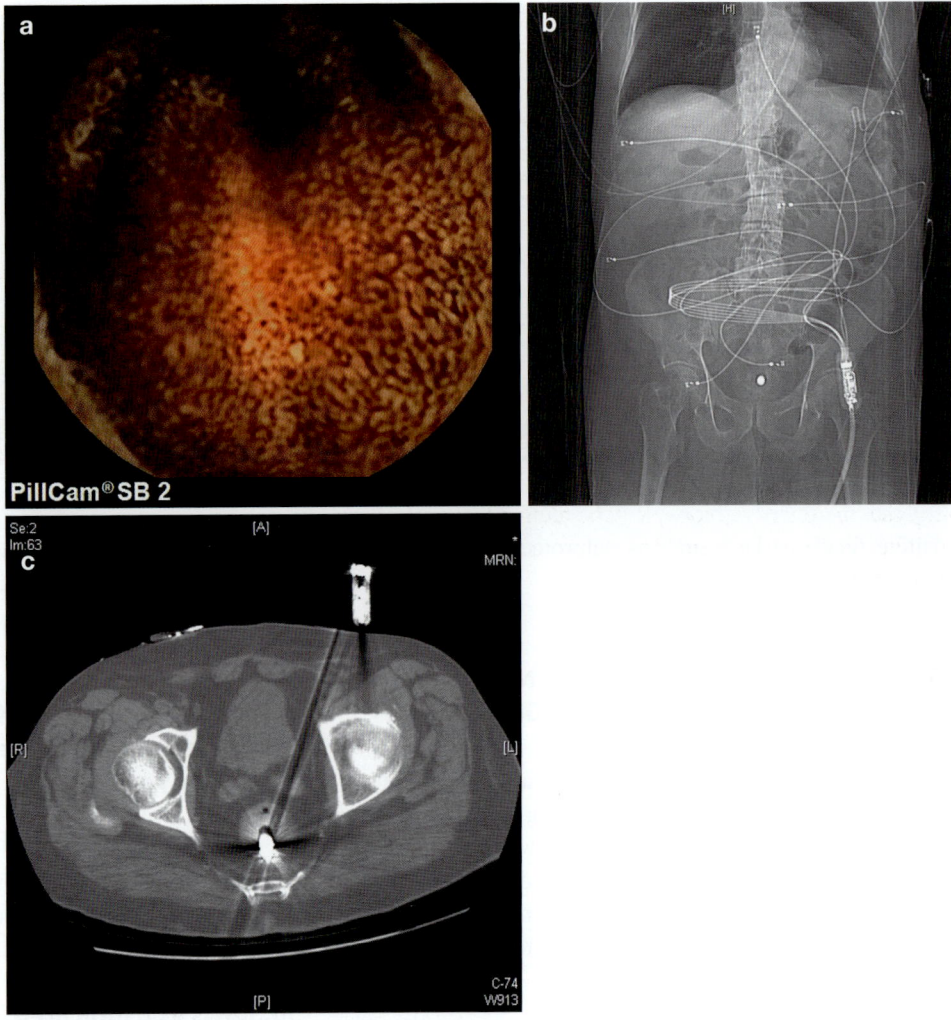

blood loss is too low for detection by CT angiography and the patient is hemodynamically stable, capsule endoscopy immediately following upper and lower GI endoscopy is often appropriate. Intermittent real-time viewing may be helpful in localizing the anatomic site of bleeding (Fig. 50.8).

50.3.11 Is VCE Justified in Patients with GI Bleeding and Only Gastric Erosions?

Not in general. Patients on NSAIDs with gastric erosions and with mild anemia will not require VCE. However, those with massive or recurrent bleeding with only small gastric erosions require further evaluation.

50.3.12 Is VCE Possible Directly After Biopsy?

Biopsies in the upper GI tract should be avoided on the day of VCE, as even small and irrelevant bleeding from biopsy sites can be very confusing. Biopsy ulcers may persist for weeks and should not be mistaken for Crohn's disease. Colon

biopsies are not problematic in SBCE as long as they are brought to the attention of the reader of the capsule study.

50.3.13 Are Imaging Studies Mandatory Before VCE for Suspected Crohn's Disease?

Imaging studies can help in identifying Crohn's disease and should be performed prior to VCE, according to a consensus statement from the World Organization of Digestive Endoscopy (OMED) and the European Crohn's and Colitis Organization (ECCO) [13].

50.3.14 Is the Patency Capsule Mandatory Prior to VCE in Patients with Known Crohn's Disease?

In known Crohn's disease, the use of the patency capsule is strongly recommended prior to standard VCE. This test is more accurate than radiographic studies in predicting intestinal patency for a video capsule.

50.3.15 Are There Contraindications to the Patency Capsule?

If a stenosis of the small intestine is long and high-grade, the use of the patency capsule (and VCE) should be avoided, as obstruction has been described with the patency capsule in selected cases. Balloon-assisted enteroscopy may then be preferred.

50.3.16 When Should Device-Assisted Deep Enteroscopy Be Used Instead of VCE?

Device-assisted deep enteroscopy is the preferred tool in patients with intestinal stenosis, or if there is a high probability that treatment or biopsy will be required. Visualization of blind loops (e.g., in Roux-en-Y anatomy) requires enteroscopy.

50.4 Diagnostic Issues

50.4.1 Who Can "Pre-read" a VCE Examination?

Capsule studies can be pre-read by nurses or endoscopy staff who are formally trained (e.g., within a curriculum of capsule endoscopy) and are assessed for competency according to national regulations.

50.4.2 Who Should Write and Sign the VCE Report?

The report should be compiled and signed by a physician with experience and competency in capsule endoscopy. Legal requirements vary from country to country.

50.4.3 Which Viewing Speed Is the Best?

The preferred viewing speed varies from clinician to clinician and also depends on the conditions of the examination. A viewing speed of 8–15 frames per second is generally recommended by VCE experts and seems appropriate. Viewing at a high speed increases the chance of missed findings.

50.4.4 How Many Images Should I Look at Simultaneously?

Most experts view one or two images simultaneously; four images are used less frequently. The number depends on personal preference. The speed should be reduced when using more images. Multiple images (mosaic, overview, map view) can provide a good orientation on the extent of lesions but are not appropriate for their detection (Chap. 5).

50.4.5 Can I Rely on Overview Modes?

The Quick View Mode (Given Imaging, Yoqneam, Israel) is a software mode designed to give an overview of the VCE examination. This mode is intended to capture the most important findings, but it does not guarantee completeness of the examination. This means that the Quick View Mode cannot and must not replace the clinician's full manual review of the VCE examination for a detailed assessment.

50.4.6 Why Is There a Color Bar?

The color bar shows the average color of all image frames, displaying the stomach as reddish, the small bowel as orange brown, and the colon as yellow green. With the color bar, the anatomic landmarks can be located more easily (Chap. 5).

50.4.7 What Is the Red Color (Blood) Detector?

Most systems come with a suspected blood detector that marks frames with red color changes. In the Rapid software (Given Imaging), this feature is automatically activated after the first duodenal image is marked. Although often helpful, this tool has only moderate accuracy (Chap. 5).

50.4.8 Is Virtual Chromo Endoscopy Helpful?

Color selection modes such as flexible spectral Imaging color enhancement (FICE) may be helpful in classifying unclear lesions that have been detected in normal viewing mode. Using these features for lesion detection may produce more false-positive findings, however (Chap. 5) (Fig. 50.9).

50.4.9 Why Should I Use Standard Terminology in My VCE Reports?

Standard terminologies such as "Minimal Standard Terminology" (actual version MST 3.0) and the specially derived "Capsule endoscopy standard terminology" (CEST) were developed to enable consistent and comparable descriptions of VCE findings. This consistency is important for study purposes and is also helpful in education and in standardizing language in VCE reports (Chap. 10).

Fig. 50.9 Subtle erosions in normal color (*left*) and with FICE 1 mode in Rapid 8 software

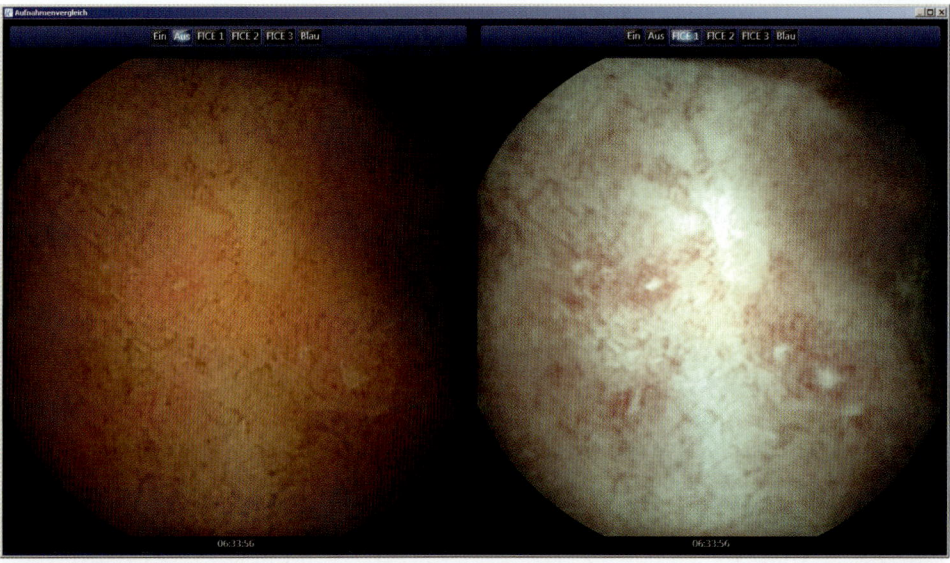

50.4.10 The Cecum Is Not Visualized on the Capsule Video: What Should I Do?

If the cecum is not visualized during VCE, the examination must be considered incomplete, and capsule retention is a possibility. Excretion of the capsule should then be verified by the patient or, if not reported after 2 weeks, by plain X-ray film.

50.4.11 Does a Normal VCE Exclude Celiac Disease?

No. Early stages of the disease without villous atrophy (Marsh stage I or II) can only be identified by histology and detection of antibodies. Furthermore, villous atrophy may be limited to the duodenum, and because the capsule often moves quickly through the duodenum, it can be missed.

50.4.12 Is It a Tumor or a Bulge?

Differentiating a tumor from a bulge on VCE can be challenging. Bulges may change their form, sometimes stretching the normal overlying mucosa. In submucosal tumors, a central umbilication, pathological vessels, ulcers, or color changes may be observed (Chap. 5).

50.4.13 What Is the Clinical Relevance of White Villi?

Single white villi do not have clinical relevance. Patchy or diffuse changes can be an epiphenomenon of

inflammatory, infectious, or malignant processes. Special attention should be paid to additional lesions. Diffuse idiopathic lymphangiectasia (Waldmann's disease) requires biopsy to rule out infection, such as Whipple's disease (Chap. 22).

50.4.14 Can I Predict Histology from a Tumor Seen at VCE?

No. Benign tumors such as lipomas, fibrolipomas, fibromas, and myomas typically present as submucosal masses, but gastrointestinal stromal tumors, neuroendocrine tumors, and even metastases (if submucosal) may look similar. An exulcerated mass is likely to be malignant (e.g., adenocarcinoma, melanoma, metastases, or lymphoma) (Chaps. 33 and 34).

50.4.15 What Is the Relevance of Invagination?

Invagination or intussusception may occur without an underlying cause (Fig. 50.10), but polyps, tumors, and celiac disease are predisposing factors that should be looked for. Device-assisted deep enteroscopy, imaging techniques, or both also can be helpful.

50.4.16 Can a Capsule Be Entrapped in a Diverticulum?

A capsule may become entrapped within a diverticulum. Permanent capsule retention in this situation is extremely rare but has been described.

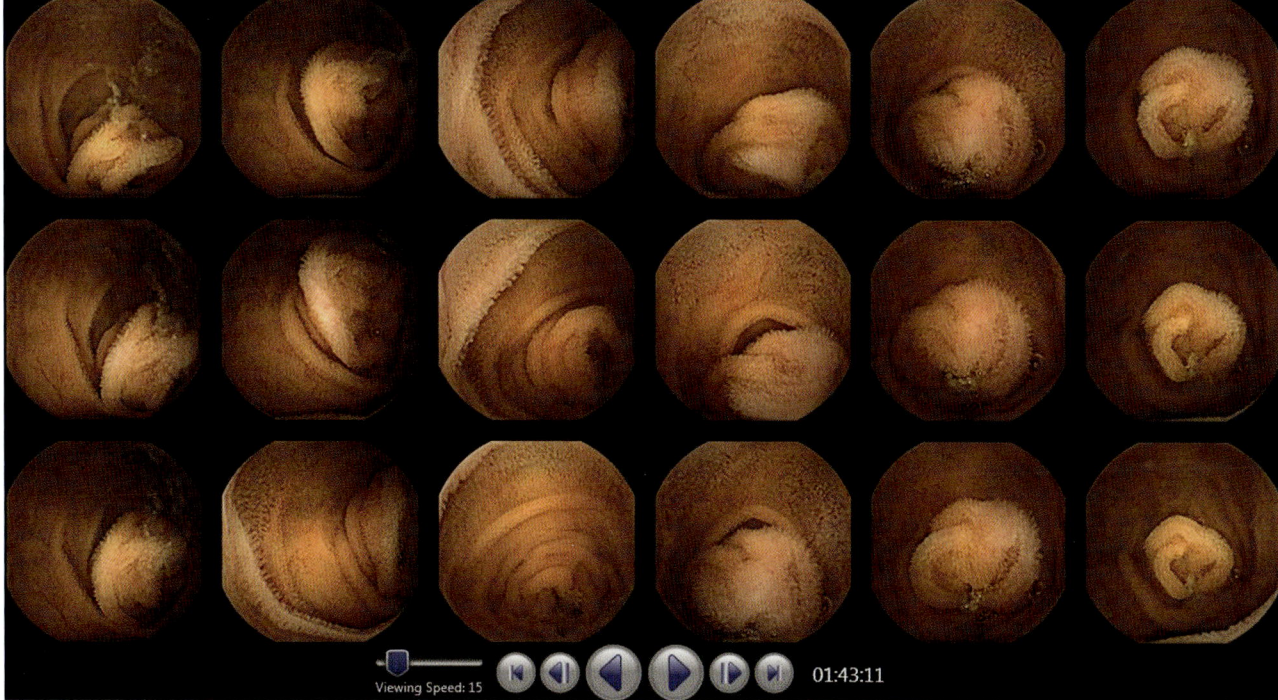

Fig. 50.10 Intussusception in mosaic view, without detectable cause

50.4.17 How Many Ulcers Equal Crohn's Disease?

There is no defined number of ulcers for the endoscopic diagnosis of Crohn's disease. Small bowel ulcerations of unknown clinical significance have also been found in "healthy" volunteers. Some studies suggest a cutoff of more than three ulcers for the definition of Crohn's disease, but these data have yet to be validated.

50.4.18 Are There VCE Findings Specific for Crohn's Disease?

Findings such as longitudinal or serpiginous aphthous ulcers are typical, but no finding is specific or pathognomonic for Crohn's disease. Differentiation from other diseases such as NSAID enteropathy is not reliable. Diagnosis should not be based solely on the VCE image (Chaps. 24 and 25).

50.4.19 How Can a Definitive Diagnosis of Diffuse Enteropathy Be Achieved?

Diffuse swelling, hemorrhage, or ulceration of small intestinal segments cannot be differentiated reliably by VCE, which may rather document the severity and longitudinal extent of the disease. Biopsies are crucial to come to a

diagnosis, together with history, microbiologic tests, serology, and extraintestinal manifestations (Fig. 50.11).

50.4.20 Is It One Lesion or Multiple Lesions?

Sometimes it can be hard to say whether a capsule passes by one lesion several times or if multiple lesions are observed. Careful observation of capsule movement as well as observation of the size and shape of the lesion(s) may be helpful in these situations.

50.4.21 How Can I Differentiate Between Iron and (Old Blood) Hematin?

Differentiating between (Old Blood) Hematin? and iron can be difficult. To avoid this problem, no oral iron supplements should be taken by the patient for at least 3 days (preferably 7 days) before capsule ingestion.

50.4.22 What Should I Do If Visualization of the Small Bowel Mucosa Is Not Optimal?

Reducing the viewing speed may decrease the probability of missed findings. The quality of the bowel cleansing should be noted in every VCE report. In cases of poor small bowel

Fig. 50.11 (**a**) Idiopathic nongranulomatous ulcerative jejunitis. (**b**) Enteritis in IgA vasculitis

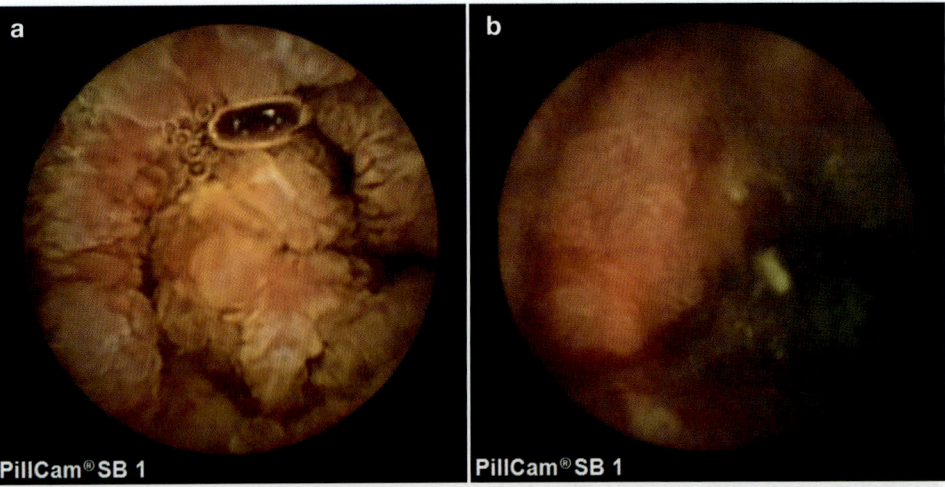

Fig. 50.12 (**a**) Small bowel carcinoma seen with colon capsule. (**b**) Cecal angiectasia detected with small bowel capsule

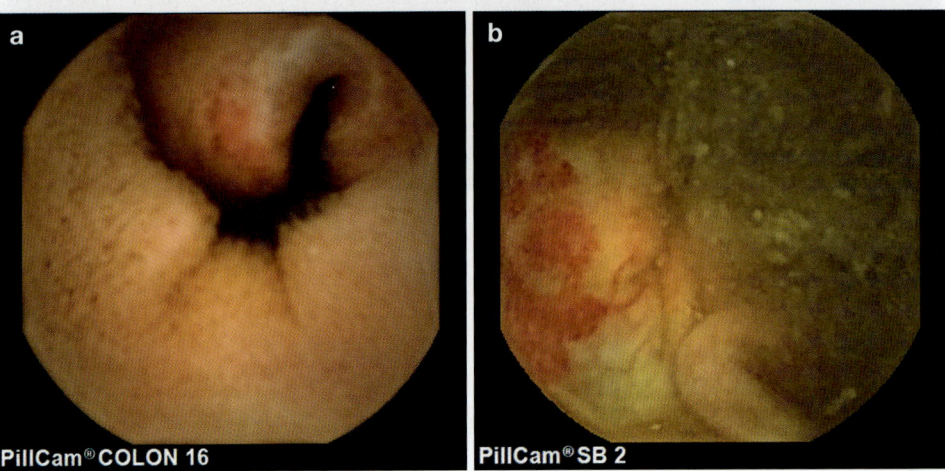

mucosal visualization, the VCE examination may need to be repeated.

50.4.23 Should I Also Look at the Upper and Lower GI Tract in SBCE?

Yes, capsule endoscopy may demonstrate findings in the upper or lower GI tract that were missed at previous inconclusive EGD or colonoscopy [14, 15] (Fig. 50.12).

50.4.24 How Is Small Bowel Transit Time Calculated If the Capsule Falls Back to the Stomach and Passes ("Ball Valves") the Pylorus Several Times?

The small bowel transit time is calculated from the time of the last passage of the capsule into the duodenum.

50.4.25 What Is a Normal Small Bowel Transit Time?

Small bowel transit times vary from patient to patient and are influenced by multiple factors, including patient age and existing medical conditions such as diabetes mellitus. VCE studies have demonstrated that previous intra-abdominal surgery also may affect the small bowel transit time. Mean small bowel transit times have been described to be approximately 235–280 min (about 4–5 h).

50.4.26 How Many VCE Studies Should I Read to Achieve Competency?

After completing a capsule endoscopy course, the first VCE examinations should be read under the supervision of a competent capsule reader. The American Society for Gastrointestinal Endoscopy (ASGE), for example,

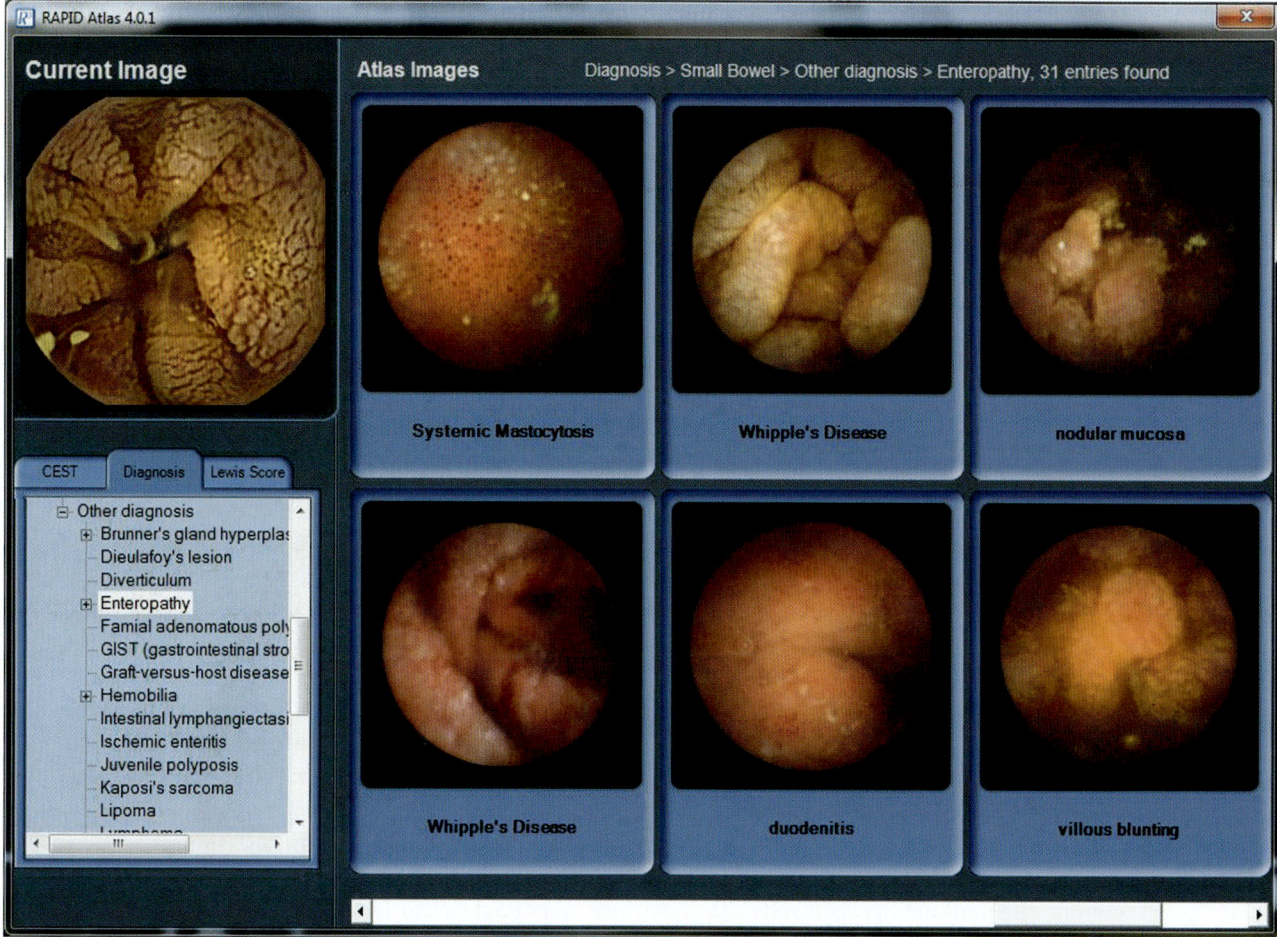

Fig. 50.13 The Rapid software atlas allows comparison of an actual image with a panel of typical and rare images (e.g., in this selection, Whipple's disease and systemic mastocytosis)

recommends 20 proctored/mentored capsule studies in order to achieve reading competency (Chap. 6).

50.4.27 How Can I Find the Next Capsule Course?

Information about capsule courses can be found on the homepage of your national or international society of gastroenterology or endoscopy. Further information can also be found on the website www.capsuleendoscopy.org.

50.4.28 Where Can I Get Help for Difficult VCE Diagnoses?

The cover pages of this book offer a direct track from description of the finding to possible diagnoses. The electronic atlas within the Rapid software allows comparison of images (Fig. 50.13). Furthermore, many capsule experts around the world will be happy to give advice, and we recommend that you reach out to them.

50.4.29 How Can I Get a Second Opinion?

Short submitted videos may provide more information than only still images and can also be sent via e-mail. In many cases, the entire capsule video on DVD will be necessary for correct evaluation. However, considering the work load, advice must be restricted to a thumbnailed part of the video.

50.5   Consequences of VCE Results and Follow-up

50.5.1 Can (Device-Assisted) Deep Enteroscopy Be Directed by Capsule Endoscopy?

Yes, capsule endoscopy can direct the type (push vs device-assisted) of enteroscopy and the approach of device-assisted deep enteroscopy. Findings on VCE localized within the first 75 % of the oral-cecal transit time or 60 % of the small bowel transit time are usually reachable by an oral approach, using device-assisted enteroscopy. Proximal small bowel findings may be reached by using "push" enteroscopy.

50.5.2 Is It Mandatory to Biopsy Small Bowel Ulcers Suggestive of Crohn's Disease?

It is advisable to obtain biopsies. If the histology is missing or inconclusive, the overall clinical, endoscopic, and serologic findings can help to make the diagnosis of Crohn's disease.

50.5.3 Is Deep Enteroscopy Mandatory Before Operating on a Tumor Found at VCE?

"Device-assisted" deep enteroscopy may provide important information (e.g., histology), but it is not mandatory in all cases. Sometimes, the findings on VCE with combined ultrasound, radiographic imaging, or both may be sufficient to initiate primary surgical treatment.

50.5.4 Should I Perform VCE Follow-up After Resection of a Small Bowel Tumor?

There are no data regarding VCE follow-up in cases of small bowel tumors. Benign tumors generally do not require VCE follow-up. For adenocarcinomas, follow-up might be scheduled according to recommendations for colon cancer.

50.5.5 When Should I Perform VCE Follow-up in Patients with Celiac Disease?

A standard VCE follow-up in patients with celiac disease is not recommended. Capsule endoscopy can be helpful if the celiac disease is refractory or the patient has new complaints in spite of adherence to a gluten-free diet (Chap. 26).

50.5.6 When Should I Perform VCE Follow-up in Patients with Small Bowel Polyposis?

Patients with Peutz-Jeghers polyposis should undergo small intestinal surveillance every second year. This can be performed by VCE or MRI or by device-assisted deep enteroscopy if there is a high probability of polyps left in the small bowel. For the other polyposis syndromes, no data are currently available on follow-up intervals (Chaps. 35, 36, and 37).

50.5.7 How Should I Care for Patients with Polyps at Colon Capsule Endoscopy?

Patients with significant polyps at colon capsule endoscopy (CCE) (one polyp of at least 6 mm or three or more polyps of any size) should undergo colonoscopy with polypectomy. A consensus statement of the European Society for Gastrointestinal Endoscopy (ESGE) recommends the next colon investigation for patients with insignificant colonic polyps (less than three and all 5 mm or less in size) should be performed after 5 years at the latest [16]. However, there are no data yet providing evidence for this extrapolation from recommendations derived from virtual colonoscopy. Hence, physicians might presently recommend colonoscopy to their patients with small polyps earlier, or even directly after CCE (Chap. 47).

50.6 Troubleshooting

50.6.1 My System or Data Recorder Crashed and I Cannot Download the Video to the Workstation: What Should I Do?

The VCE raw data are kept on the storage media in the recording device until a new patient is initialized. Therefore, it is important not to initialize the recorder again until the data are downloaded. Customer service of your VCE manufacturer can assist in downloading the data.

50.6.2 What Are the Main Adverse Events of VCE?

Capsule retention, primarily due to GI obstruction, is the main adverse event associated with VCE and occurs in approximately 1 % of patients undergoing a VCE examination. Although very rare, there are case reports about disintegrated or broken capsules and small bowel perforations with prolonged capsule retention. Aspiration is a rare (but sometimes major) adverse event, with a rate of 1 in 800 VCE examinations; therefore, swallowing disorders should be investigated prior to capsule ingestion (Chap. 40).

50.6.3 How Is Capsule Retention Defined?

Capsule retention is defined as persistence of the capsule in the GI tract for longer than 14 days with necessity of endoscopic or surgical treatment. If capsule retention leads to a new diagnosis (e.g., small bowel tumor), it is not considered a complication, but rather a diagnostic aid.

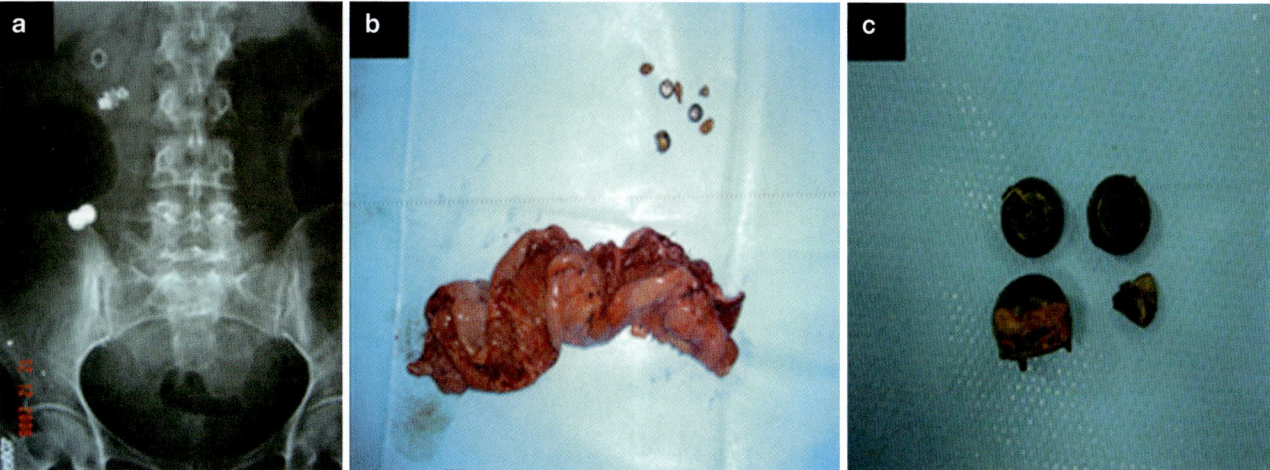

Fig. 50.14 (**a–c**) Two retained capsules, one of them fragmented. Surgery was necessary for acute abdomen (*Courtesy of* Cyrla Zaltman, MD; *Reprinted from* de Magalhaes Costa et al. [17], with permission from Elsevier)

50.6.4 How Can I Rule Out Capsule Retention If Excretion Was Not Observed?

Many patients do not see or identify the natural passage of the capsule, but if the cecum is visualized on the capsule video and prior colonoscopy was without evidence of colonic stenosis, no further diagnostic evaluations are recommended. If the patient does not observe capsule excretion within 2 weeks of ingestion and image transmission stopped before the capsule reached the cecum, retention of the video capsule can be ruled out by an abdominal X-ray (upright/supine abdominal plain film).

50.6.5 How Should Capsule Retention Be Managed?

The patient must be informed and asked about possible obstructive symptoms. MRI must be avoided. Diagnosis of the underlying disease should be attempted as far as possible by careful review of the capsule video and imaging techniques. Cases of successfully treated inflammatory stenosis with corticosteroids or biologicals and subsequent passage of the retained capsule have been reported.

50.6.6 Should a Retained Capsule Be Retrieved?

Although capsule retention in general is asymptomatic, cases of obstruction up to 6 years later [17], as well as perforation and capsule fragmentation [18] (Fig. 50.14), have been

reported. Hence, surgical or endoscopic retrieval seems appropriate even in asymptomatic patients, in order to avoid such late complications.

50.6.7 How Should a Retained Capsule Be Retrieved?

Retained capsules can be retrieved by enteroscopy. In case of bowel obstruction or when surgical treatment is indicated, the capsule can be retrieved during definitive surgery (Chap. 40) (Fig. 50.15).

50.6.8 How Can I Diagnose Video Capsule Aspiration?

Aspiration can be diagnosed clinically by coughing and dyspnea in combination with the real-time viewer showing tracheal rings and/or bronchi. If no real-time viewer is available, chest X-ray will provide the diagnosis (Chap. 40).

50.6.9 How Should I Manage Video Capsule Aspiration?

The patient may expectorate the video capsule. If the capsule is not expectorated, it must be retrieved by bronchoscopy (Fig. 50.16). Any future attempt at VCE examination in such a patient should be performed only using endoscopic capsule placement directly into the duodenum.

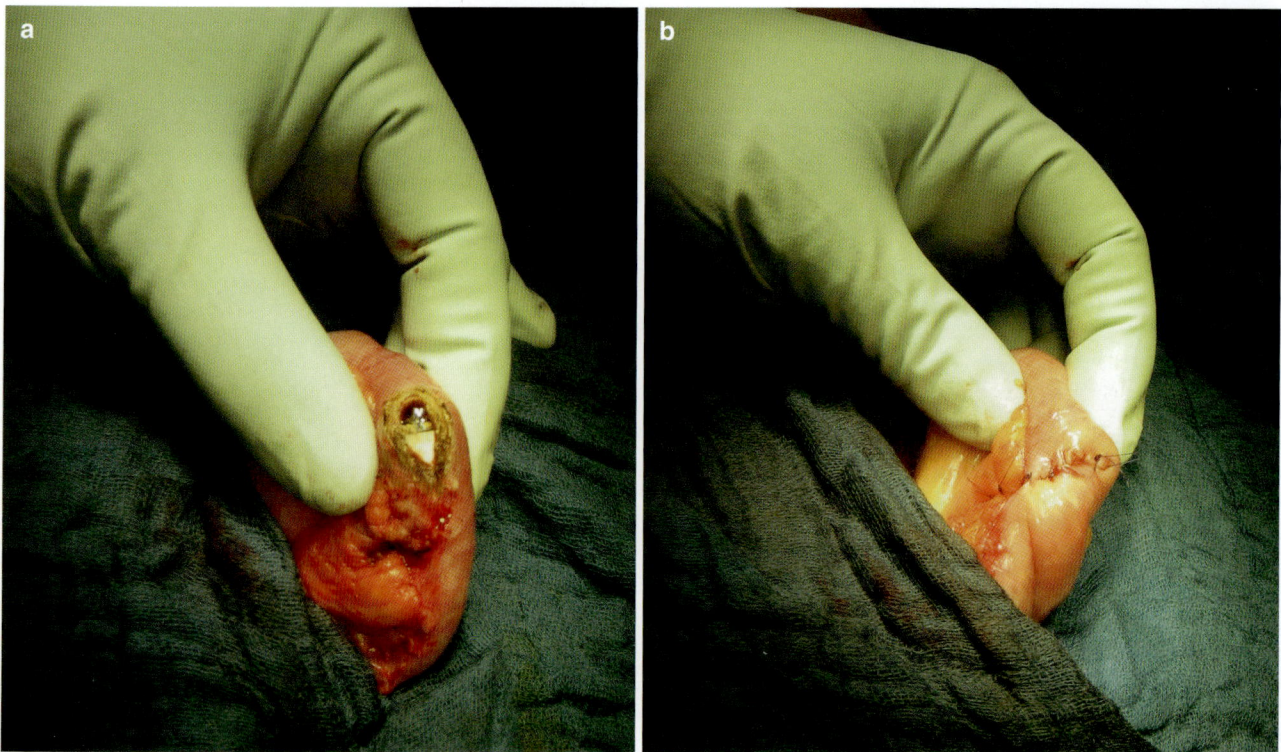

Fig. 50.15 Retained capsule in a short, fibrotic stricture in radiation enteritis. (**a**) Enterotomy and capsule retrieval using a minilaparotomy. (**b**) This procedure was combined with treatment of the stenosis by stricturoplasty (transverse suture of the longitudinal incision) (*Courtesy of* Marco Sailer, MD)

Fig. 50.16 (**a**) Aspirated capsule in the bronchial tree. (**b**) Extraction with a Roth Net during flexible bronchoscopy (*Courtesy of* Simon Panter, MD)

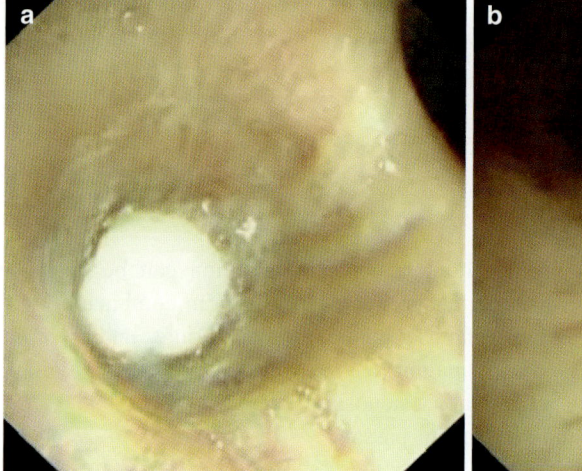
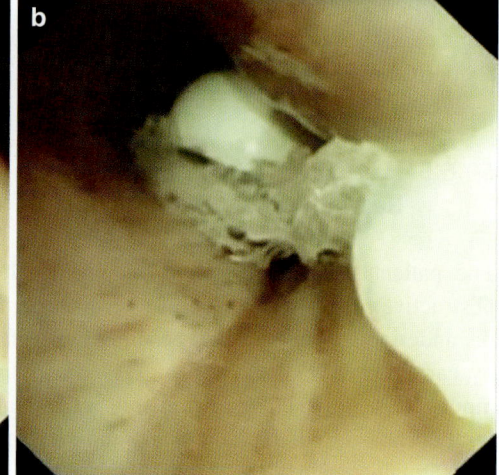

References

1. Ayazi S, Lipham JC, Portale G, et al. Bravo catheter-free pH monitoring: normal values, concordance, optimal diagnostic thresholds, and accuracy. Clin Gastroenterol Hepatol. 2009;7:60–7.
2. Ang D, Xu Y, Ang TL, et al. Wireless oesophageal pH monitoring: establishing values in a multiracial cohort of asymptomatic Asian subjects. Dig Liver Dis. 2013;45:371–6.
3. Cabrera J, Davis M, Horn D, et al. Esophageal pH monitoring with the BRAVO capsule: experience in a single tertiary medical center. J Pediatr Gastroenterol Nutr. 2011;53:404–8.
4. Tran K, Brun R, Kuo B. Evaluation of regional and whole gut motility using the wireless motility capsule: relevance in clinical practice. Ther Adv Gastroenterol. 2012;5:249–60.
5. Gilbert D, O'Malley S, Selby W. Are repeat upper gastrointestinal endoscopy and colonoscopy necessary within six months of capsule endoscopy in patients with obscure gastrointestinal bleeding? J Gastroenterol Hepatol. 2008;23:1806–9.
6. Wax JR, Pinette MG, Cartin A, et al. Cavernous transformation of the portal vein complicating pregnancy. Obstet Gynecol. 2006;108:782–4.
7. Hogan RB, Ahmad N, Hogan 3rd RB, et al. Video capsule endoscopy detection of jejunal carcinoid in life-threatening hemorrhage, first trimester pregnancy. Gastrointest Endosc. 2007;66:205–7.
8. Anderson BW, Liang JJ, Dejesus RS. Capsule endoscopy device retention and magnetic resonance imaging. Proc (Bayl Univ Med Cent). 2013;26:270–1.

9. Tang SJ, Zanati S, Dubcenco E, et al. Sunlight interference with wireless capsule endoscopy. Endoscopy. 2004;36:832.

10. Mewes PW, Foertsch S, Juloski AL, et al. Chromoendoscopy in magnetically guided capsule endoscopy. Biomed Eng Online. 2013;12:52.

11. Yamashita K, Okumura H, Oka Y, et al. Minimally invasive surgery using intraoperative real-time capsule endoscopy for small bowel lesions. Surg Endosc. 2013;27:2337–41.

12. Saurin JC, Delvaux M, Gaudin JL, et al. Diagnostic value of endoscopic capsule in patients with obscure digestive bleeding: blinded comparison with video push-enteroscopy. Endoscopy. 2003;35:576–84.

13. Bourreille A, Ignjatovic A, Aabakken L, et al. Role of small-bowel endoscopy in the management of patients with inflammatory bowel disease: an international OMED-ECCO consensus. Endoscopy. 2009;41:618–37.

14. Van Gossum A, Hittelet A, Schmit A, et al. A prospective comparative study of push and wireless-capsule enteroscopy in patients with obscure digestive bleeding. Acta Gastroenterol Belg. 2003;66:199–205.

15. Kitiyakara T, Selby W. Non-small-bowel lesions detected by capsule endoscopy in patients with obscure GI bleeding. Gastrointest Endosc. 2005;62:234–8.

16. Spada C, Hassan C, Galmiche JP, et al. Colon capsule endoscopy: European Society of Gastrointestinal Endoscopy (ESGE) guideline. Endoscopy. 2012;44:527–36.

17. Lipka S, Vacchio A, Katz S, Ginzburg L. Retained capsule extraction 6 years after wireless bowel capsule endoscopy: the importance of follow up. J Crohns Colitis. 2013;7:e271–2.

18. de Magalhaes Costa MH, da Luz MA, Zaltman C. Wireless capsule endoscopy fragmentation in a patient with Crohn's disease. Clin Gastroenterol Hepatol. 2011;9:e116–7.

Future Developments of Video Capsule Endoscopy: Hardware

51

Arianna Menciassi, Gastone Ciuti,
and Carmela Cavallotti

Contents

The work was first published in 2006 by Springer Medizin Verlag Heidelberg with the following title: *Atlas of Video Capsule Endoscopy.*

A. Menciassi (✉) • G. Ciuti • C. Cavallotti
The BioRobotics Institute, Scuola Superiore Sant'Anna,
Pontedera, Pisa, Italy
e-mail: a.menciassi@sssup.it; g.ciuti@sssup.it;
c.cavallotti@sssup.it

51.1   Introduction

Traditional endoscopic techniques (i.e. those exploiting flexible endoscopes) can be operated effectively and reliably through different districts of the gastrointestinal (GI) apparatus (the oesophagus, stomach, large bowel or colon and part of the small bowel) with diagnostic, therapeutic and surgical capabilities [1]. However, the rigidity of the instrument, due to its dimensions (diameter from 11 to 13 mm for a standard colonoscope), and the integration of actuation mechanisms running through the instrument result in limited accessibility, making endoscopic procedures significantly traumatic and poorly tolerated by patients [2]. Pain or problems with sedation make patients disinclined to undergo endoscopy, significantly limiting the pervasiveness of mass screening campaigns. A significant medical drawback of flexible endoscopy is that certain areas of the GI tract cannot be reached, such as most of the small bowel [3].

In 1981, Iddan conceived the idea of a wireless camera capsule for imaging of the entire GI tract. Limitations in available technologies prevented the development of a swallowable camera capsule, although Swain et al. performed experimental trials on a larger prototype in the mid-1990s [4]. More recently, the availability of low-power and low-cost miniaturized image sensors based on complementary metal oxide semiconductor (CMOS) technology, application-specific integrated circuits (ASIC) and miniaturized light-emitting diodes (LEDs) enabled the development of swallowable wireless camera capsules. In 2000, thanks to G. Iddan patents, the company Given Imaging Ltd. (Yoqneam, Israel) introduced "wireless capsule endoscopy" (WCE), which entails the ingestion of a miniaturized pill-sized camera that passively navigates the GI tract by means of natural peristaltic contractions and takes pictures of the surrounding wall [5]. WCE enables inspection of the digestive system without discomfort or need for sedation, avoiding the risks and poor tolerability of conventional endoscopy. In this way, WCE has the potential additional benefit of encouraging patients to undergo GI tract medical examinations, possibly increasing the success of mass screening campaigns [6].

Although WCE has entered the medical scenario as a "disruptive" technology and methodology, it still presents a number of limitations. For instance, it is not possible to actively control capsule locomotion and camera orientation, leading to low diagnostic specificity and to false-positive results (mainly in the colonic tract, owing to the collapsed anatomy). Thus, the natural evolution and future of WCE points towards integrating mechanisms for active locomotion and also providing the capsule with microsensors and microtools for advanced diagnosis and therapy [7–9]. In this regard, many research institutes and private companies are exploiting mechatronic technologies and architectures for the enhancement and improvement of WCE capabilities, ranging from simple diagnostic cameras to complete and autonomous diagnostic and therapeutic robotic platforms, thus producing innovation for the submodules of vision, telemetry, localization, power and therapeutic manipulation tools.

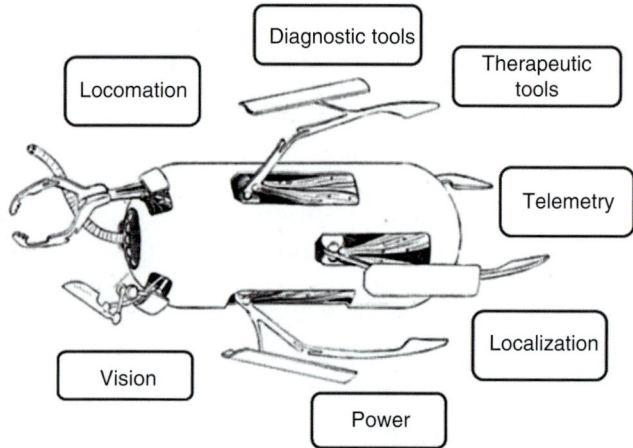

Fig. 51.1 Cartoon depicting the modules of a robotic endoscopic capsule: locomotion, vision, telemetry, localization, power and diagnostic and therapeutic manipulation tools are schematically represented (*Courtesy of* Virgilio Mattoli, PhD)

51.2 System Architecture for Endoscopic Capsules

A complete endoscopic capsule platform comprises several modules, including locomotion, vision, telemetry, localization, power and diagnostic and therapeutic manipulation tools (Fig. 51.1). Because of space constraints, however, most capsules developed to date include a subset of these modules. Each miniature module represents an engineering challenge per se, but thanks to current technological progress in microsystem development, interface and integration, devices can be designed embedding all these modules and having diagnostic and treatment functionalities. Alternatively, a possible solution may be to use several task-specific capsules that operate independently or that are self-assembled into a single, high-performance device. The following subsections of this chapter illustrate the different modules of an endoscopic capsule, with specific focus on the locomotion that is the feature distinguishing an uncontrolled probe navigating in the bowel from an innovative, teleoperated miniature robot for performing diagnostic and surgical tasks.

51.2.1 Locomotion: Active Locomotion Approaches

Locomotion represents a crucial issue for the design of a wireless endoscopic system. In this regard, WCE can be classified as passive or active capsule endoscopy, depending on whether means of controlled locomotion are present. Active locomotion is still at the research level, as passive locomotion currently dominates the WCE market. Active locomotion has the potential to enhance diagnostic and therapeutic consistency and to allow the endoscopist to manoeuvre the device for precise targeting; its main drawback is the difficulty in integrating the locomotion module into the capsule body while keeping the size small enough to swallow. There are two main strategies for providing a swallowable endoscopic capsule with active locomotion. The first involves miniaturizing locomotion systems that are integrated on board the capsule (i.e. internal locomotion); the second involves the use of an external approach where actuation, generally based on magnetic field sources, is outside the capsule (i.e. external locomotion).

51.2.1.1 Internal Locomotion

Several different internal locomotion strategies have been investigated, and the most significant solutions are discussed below, examining solutions going through the GI tract from the oesophagus to the colon.

In the oesophageal tract, active mechanisms must be developed to decelerate the rapid progression of an endoscopic capsule along the lumen. In this regard, an endoscopic robotic device with a shape memory alloy (SMA)-based anchoring mechanism has been developed; the capsule features three active, flexible legs that are provided with strain-gauge sensors for measuring the force applied onto the tissue. An on-board actuator controlled by a miniaturized, custom-made microcontroller allows the legs to be released and retracted with regard to sensor triggers (Fig. 51.2a) [10]. A mechanism that ensures the anchoring of capsules to the intestinal esophageal wall was presented by Glass et al. [11]. The mechanism consists of three actuated legs with compliant feet lined with micropillar

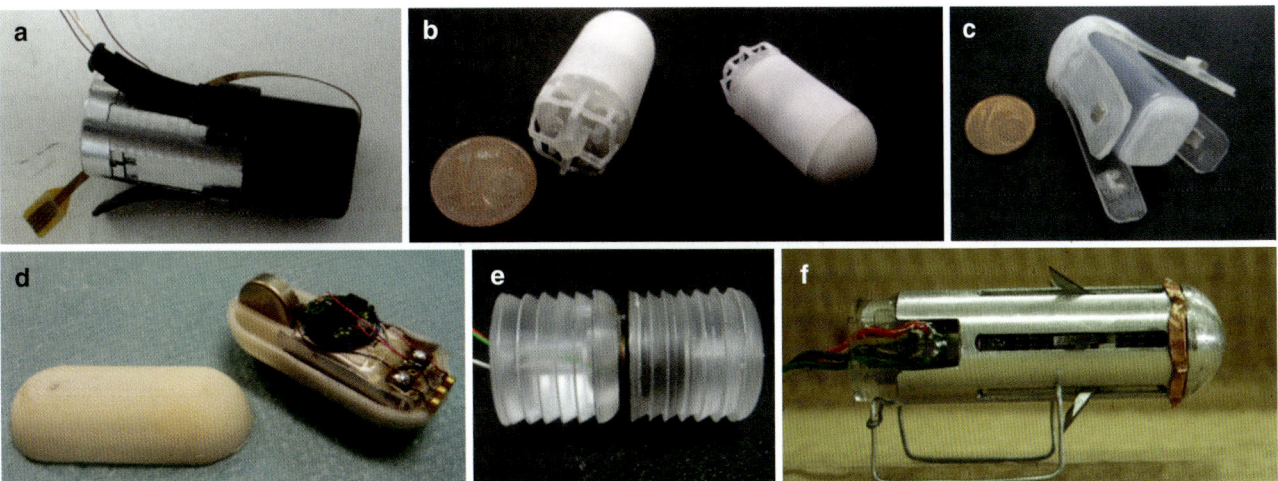

Fig. 51.2 Internal locomotion capsules: oesophagus capsules developed by Tognarelli et al. (**a**); capsules for stomach diagnosis, by Tortora et al. (**b**) and Valdastri et al. (**c**); vibrating capsule produced by Ciuti et al. (**d**); and bowel capsules developed by Kim et al. (**e**) and Park et al. (**f**) (*Courtesy of* Byungkyu Kim, PhD)

gecko-like adhesives, which are able to withstand axial peristaltic loads at a fixed location.

A promising solution for endoscopic capsule steering in a liquid-filled stomach was presented by Tortora et al. [12]. The submarine-like robotic device exploits four independent miniaturized propellers actuated by DC brushed motors that are wirelessly controlled in terms of desired three-dimensional (3D) direction and speed (Fig. 51.2b). Other possible methods of swimming in the water-filled stomach cavity include flagellar or flap-based swimming mechanisms (Fig. 51.2c) [13, 14].

A number of different internal locomotion approaches that target the entire intestine (i.e. the large and small bowel) have been developed by many research institutes, in most cases exploiting mechanisms inspired by biology. The simplest mechanism for on-board locomotion is vibratory actuation, obtained by a motor with an asymmetric mass on the rotor, which aids forward progression of the capsule along the GI tract by reducing friction (Fig. 51.2d) [15–17]. However, this approach has the disadvantages of not ensuring active orientation, change of direction and capsule fixation. Electrical stimulation of the GI muscles is a method that is able to roughly control capsule locomotion (or at least stop it) by generating a temporary restriction in the bowel [18, 19]. Other mechanisms inspired by biology have also been used, including earthworm-like, cilia-like and legged locomotion systems actuated by cyclic compression and extension of SMA spring actuators or embedded brushless motors. The mechanism proposed by Glass et al. for locomotion in the oesophagus was extended by Karagozler et al. [20], combining two of the before-mentioned anchoring modules for the development of a SMA-based six-legged endoscopic capsule that mimics a crawling motion. A bio-inspired earthworm-like intestine robot was presented by Kim et al. (Fig. 51.2e) [21, 22]; it works with cyclic compression/extension SMA spring actuators and with anchoring systems based on directional microneedles. This solution does not allow for bidirectional and oriented motion, yet the microneedles provide a passive anchoring mechanism without entailing actuators or power-demanding systems. Another bio-inspired solution exploits a locomotion system mimicking cilia extension: the capsule is composed of six SMA-actuated units (each unit with two SMA actuators to enable bidirectional motion) with two appendages for each unit [23]. A promising solution for crawling in the intestine was proposed by Park et al. [24], consisting of a paddling-based technique. The capsule is composed of multiple legs actuated by a linear actuator that travels along the entire length of the capsule. The legs are retracted at the back of the capsule, before recycling at the front, thus allowing directional propulsion (Fig. 51.2f).

Effective leg-based designs were developed by The BioRobotics Institute of the Scuola Superiore Sant'Anna (http://sssa.bioroboticsinstitute.it) over the past 10 years, demonstrating effective bidirectional control, stable anchorage and adequate visualization of the lumen without the need for insufflation. From a first solution based on SMA technology (Fig. 51.3a) [25], increasingly sophisticated legged robot prototypes, based on brushless motors, have been addressed. In particular, capsules have been developed with 4 legs [26], 8 legs [27], and 12 legs [6, 28], progressively increasing effective locomotion and complete visualization of the lumen (Fig. 51.3b). The latest design (11 mm in diameter and 25 mm in length) is able to distend tissue in a uniform manner with 6 points of contact at each end of the capsule (enhancing camera visibility and field of view); these points

Fig. 51.3 Legged capsules developed by The BioRobotics Institute of the Scuola Superiore Sant'Anna based on (**a**) SMA technology and (**b**) brushless motors. The designs based on brushless motors have been developed with 4, 8 and 12 legs

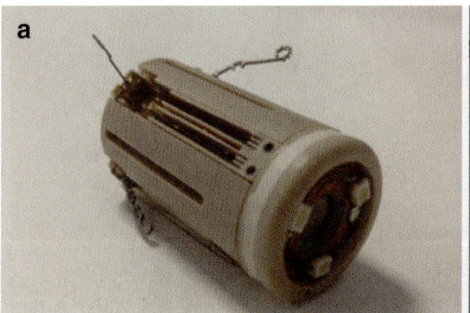
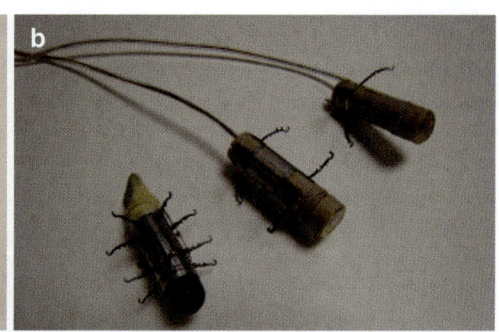

are made by 12 optimized bio-inspired legs. The capsule has the ability to travel the length of the colon at 5 cm/min, passing fully through it without insufflation in a length of time comparable with the speed of traditional colonoscopy. The total pulling force that enabled the capsule to withstand peristalsis and expand the surrounding tissue was 3.6 N.

Although internal locomotion has significant advantages, such as local distension of the tissue away from the camera and the lack of interference (e.g. from magnetic field sources), it has important drawbacks related to the presence of actuators, transmission mechanisms and high-capacity power modules that lead to excessive internal encumbrance in order to attain ingestible size (details about energy consumption for different locomotion strategies are discussed in Sect. 51.2.5.).

51.2.1.2 External Locomotion

Endoscopic capsule locomotion obtained through external propulsion has been approached by many research groups. Its path to clinical implementation appears more straightforward because it does not require the integration of dedicated miniature actuators and mechanisms. By exploiting externally generated magnetic fields, the internal available space of the capsule is increased, thus guaranteeing that most of the modules depicted in Fig. 51.1 can be included in a swallowable system. Magnetic fields that interact with internal magnetic components are normally used to provide external propulsion, imparting forces and torques to the capsule. The idea is that a large magnetic field is created near (but outside) the patient by one or more electromagnets or permanent magnets, while a much smaller magnetic source is integrated on board the capsule. The interaction between this small field and the large externally created field generates active control of the endoscopic capsule. The need for on-board actuators, mechanisms and batteries is eliminated in favour of a small on-board magnetic field generator, such as a permanent magnet. Electromagnets, as external magnetic field generators, can generate well-controlled magnetic fields, although they require bulkier equipment than external permanent magnets. Once the magnetic field allows the capsule to be reliably controlled and held in specific areas, magnetic-based solutions can be exploited for propulsion along the entire GI tract. The following description is mainly focused on the selected magnetic approach (i.e. electromagnets or permanent magnet), with some examples of capsules with external locomotion designed for specific districts. Magnetic actuation has also been exploited for other medical devices, ranging from catheters (e.g. the Niobe® Magnetic Navigation System; Stereotaxis Inc., St. Louis, MO, USA) [29] to microscale robots [30].

Among the different actuation methods, electromagnetic-based actuation has been considered by Yu et al. [31] for 3D locomotion and drilling tasks of a permanent magnet microrobot in intravascular procedures. A novel magnetic capsule endoscopy technology for gastric examination was developed cooperatively by Olympus Inc. (Olympus Medical Systems Corp., Tokyo, Japan) and Siemens Healthcare (Erlangen, Germany). The system includes an Olympus capsule endoscope (31 mm in length and 11 mm in diameter, provided with two 4 frames/s image sensors) and Siemens magnetic guidance equipment, composed of MRI and CT. The physician controls the capsule by means of two control interfaces, and the device can be moved in the stomach with five independent degrees of freedom (i.e. 3D translation, tilting and rotation) (Fig. 51.4a) [32].

Given Imaging Ltd. has investigated the use of a handheld external permanent magnet to translate and orient a capsule in the upper GI tract using a modified version of PillCam Colon, which was half filled with magnets as part of the European FP6 project called "Nanobased Capsule-Endoscopy with Molecular Imaging and Optical Biopsy" (NEMO project) [33].

A robotic magnetic navigation system (Niobe), developed for cardiovascular clinical procedures, was exploited by Carpi et al. for accurate robotic steering of a magnetically modified video capsule (PillCam, Given Imaging Ltd.). In vivo tests performed with 3D fluoroscopic localization showed an accuracy of 1° in orientation but limited translational capabilities (Fig. 51.4b) [34, 35].

Another approach to wireless capsule endoscopy has been proposed by Ciuti et al. [36, 37]. It takes advantage of active magnetic locomotion in the GI tract combined with accurate driving by an anthropomorphic robotic arm. The system combines the benefits of permanent magnets in terms of

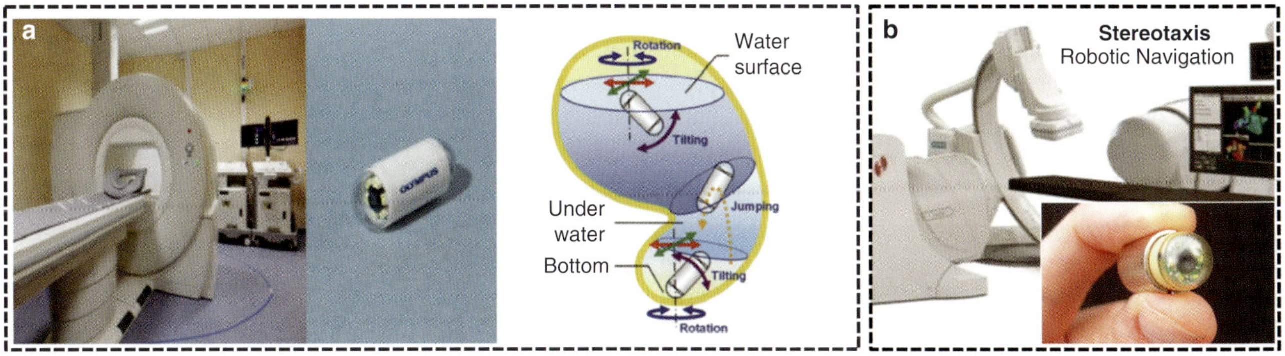

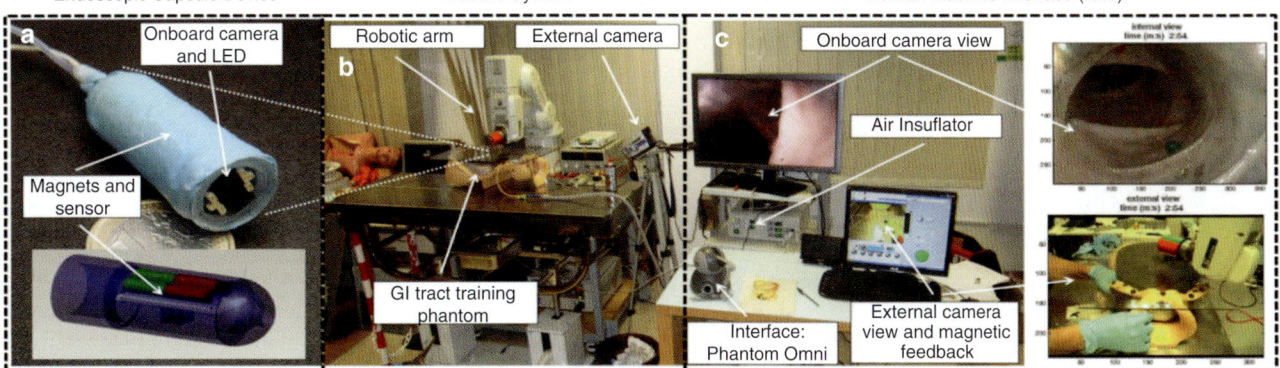

Fig. 51.4 External locomotion platforms for capsule endoscopy. (**a**) Gastric examination platform developed cooperatively by Olympus Inc. and Siemens Healthcare (*Reprinted with permission from* Siemens AG). (**b**) GI tract exploration platform developed by Carpi et al. exploiting a Stereotaxis Niobe system (*Courtesy of* Federico Carpi, PhD)

Fig. 51.5 Robotic-aided permanent magnetic platform developed by Ciuti et al., consisting of (**a**) the endoscopic device, (**b**) the robotic system and (**c**) the human-machine interface

magnetic field strength with accurate and reliable control of the magnet thanks to a robotic arm (Fig. 51.5).

A critical limitation of all these external magnetic approaches involves effective locomotion and lumen visualization of the capsule in the deflated lumen, especially in the large intestine. To overcome this problem, Simi et al. [38] developed a wireless endoscopic capsule with hybrid locomotion, as a combination between internal actuation mechanisms and external magnetic dragging. The capsule incorporates an internal actuated legged mechanism, which modifies the capsule profile, and small permanent magnets, which interact with an external magnetic field, thus imparting a magnetic dragging motion to the device. The legged mechanism is actuated whenever the capsule becomes lodged in collapsed areas of the GI tract, thus allowing modification of the capsule profile and making magnetic dragging and lumen visualization feasible and effective once again (Fig. 51.6). Another promising solution for helping tissue distension was proposed by Gorlewicz et al. [39]: a tetherless insufflation system that is based on a controlled phase transition of a small volume of fluid stored on board the capsule to a large volume of gas, emitted into the intestine.

51.2.2 Vision

An endoscopic capsule is essentially a swallowable wireless miniaturized camera for getting images from the GI tract; for this reason, image quality is a primary issue. Other considerations must be taken into account in the development of a camera system for WCE, however, such as the need for compactness (less than 2 cm³), limited power budget and data payload.

The challenge of future research and development is to overcome the current limitations by improving the image quality and the frame rate, developing a very compact, high-performance and low-powering camera module. Achieving this aim will pave the way to the on-board integration of other submodules for localization, biopsy and in situ treatments that may enhance the capsule performance.

Presently, the vision module inside a capsule comprises three distinct units with different functions: an image sensor, an LED-based illumination unit and an optical unit.

Regarding the image sensor, Given Imaging, the major worldwide industrial player in the field of capsule endoscopy, implements a CMOS imager in all its products (PillcamSB, PillcamESO, PillcamCOLON). Some competitors, such as IMC [40] and Jinshan Science & Technology Company [41], also integrate a CMOS imager, whereas the EndoCapsule developed by Olympus integrates a charge-coupled device (CCD) sensor [42]. Resolution of these systems ranges between 256×256 and 1920×1080 pixels. The frame rate (the number of frames sent wirelessly and shown in real time to the physician) ranges between 2 and 7 frames per second (fps) in continuous acquisition mode, with a peak of 35 fps for a limited time in the case of the PillcamCOLON, which integrates two cameras. All the mentioned capsules have a fixed focal length with a depth of focus in the range of 0–50 mm; they also allow a wide angle of view (over 150°).

To provide an extended depth of focus or to enable advanced vision functions such as autofocus or zoom features, the use of a deformable liquid lens was investigated by Cavallotti et al. [43] and Seo et al. [44]. Compared with other methods to change the focus of the optical system, the liquid lens solution presents some advantages; indeed, the focus is not changed mechanically but rather by applying a specific voltage, so the response is faster. Moreover, liquid lenses are low cost, low power and small (Fig. 51.7).

The illumination system of the commercial capsules comprises six or more white LEDs controlled by a pulse-width modulation (PWM) signal in order to minimize power consumption. Another innovative method to create white light is to mix monochromatic radiations from several different coloured LEDs (e.g. red, green, blue) in appropriate intensity proportions [45]. By switching on each group alternately and at high frequency, the mixed light will exhibit a spectrum that the human eye perceives as white light. This approach has been investigated in the framework of the FP6 European Project VECTOR, where a novel, low-power CMOS 320×240 active-pixel colour-RGB image sensor for capsule endoscopy was developed by Vatteroni et al. (Fig. 51.8) [46]. Electrical and optical characterizations demonstrated that targeted WCE

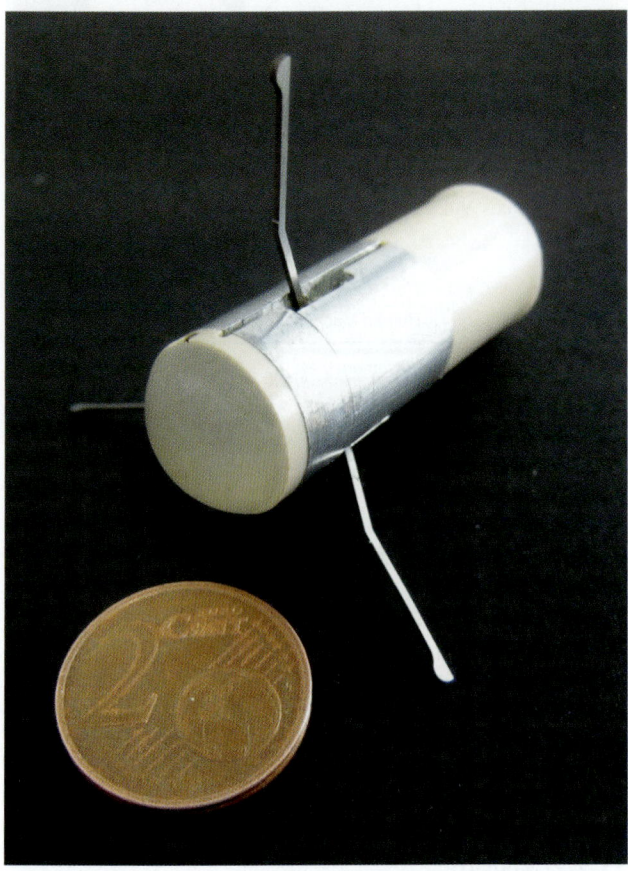

Fig. 51.6 Wireless endoscopic capsule with hybrid locomotion developed by Simi et al. (*Courtesy of* Masimiliano Simi, PhD)

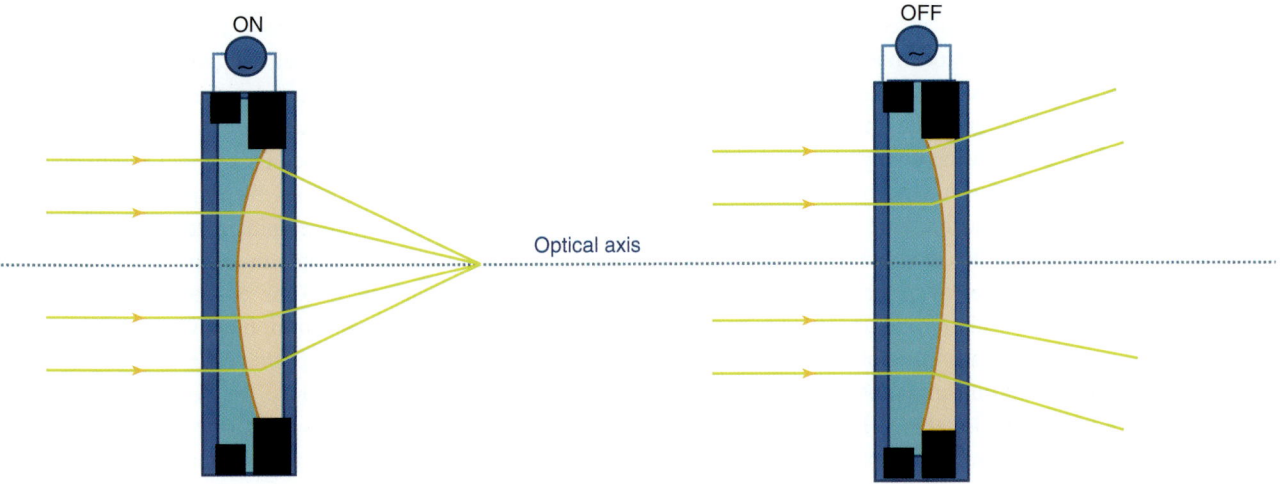

Fig. 51.7 Liquid lens working principle

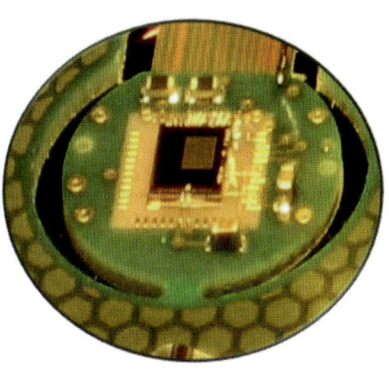 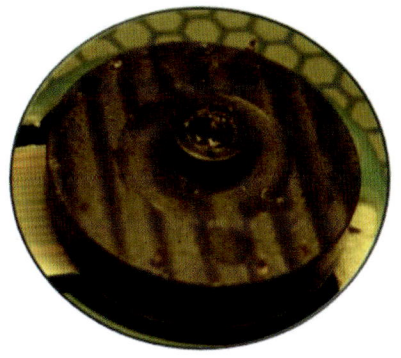 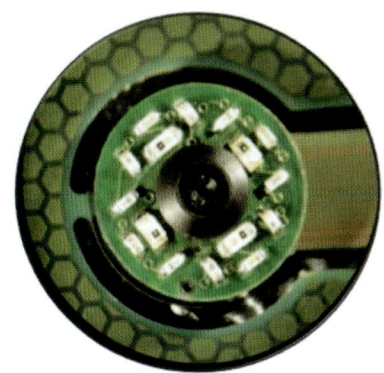

Fig. 51.8 Vision system for capsule endoscopy developed by Vatteroni et al.

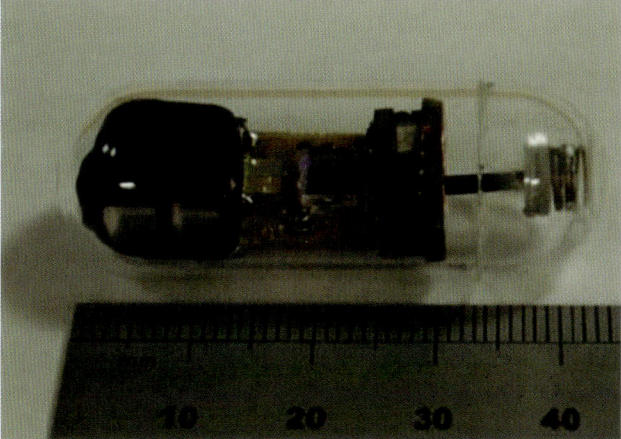 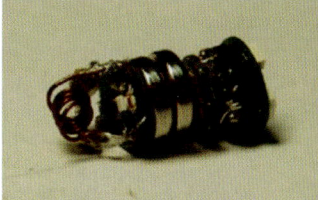 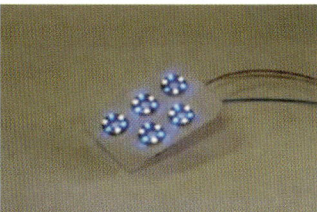 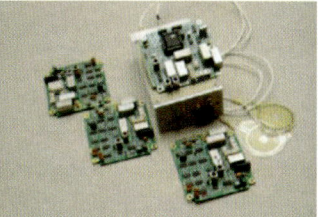 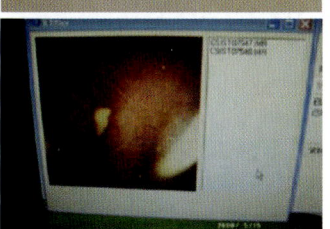

Fig. 51.9 Autofluorescence capsule (*left*) developed by Al-Rawhani et al. (*Courtesy of* David Cumming, PhD, *Reprinted with permission from* IEEE). Narrow-band imaging (NBI) capsule endoscope (*right*) developed by Dung et al. (*Reprinted with permission from* IEEE)

requirements, in terms of power consumption and high sensitivity, were met. Power consumption during normal operation was measured being less than 40 mW with a frame rate of 30 fps, which is less than half of off-the-shelf sensors, while light sensitivity was 0.32 lux at 555 nm, which makes sensor performance comparable to CCD technology for single-chip endoluminal applications. This imager was integrated in a custom vision system combined with a red/green/blue LED illumination system and a low-power field-programmable gate array (FPGA) for sensor control, image compression and interfacing with transmission. The vision system was implemented in a miniaturized electronic board able to fit into an endoscopic pill and capable of a real-time data stream up to 20 fps [47]. The novelty of this approach is that the camera setting remains fixed while the lightning control is modulated in order to set the proper amount of light for an optimum image quality in terms of chroma, light exposure and flickering effects. Moreover, the illumination is switched on only during the integration time of the optical sensor, in order to simulate a global shutter, thus minimizing image artefacts and reducing power consumption.

The combination of light with a different spectrum also enables optical-digital image-enhanced techniques, such as autofluorescence imaging (AFI) and narrow-band imaging (NBI). The AFI technique aids in the detection of smaller and earlier malignant lesions, which are not identified by white-light illumination [48, 49]. Light in the blue spectrum is used as an excitation source; when tumour tissue is irradiated with blue excitation light, the autofluorescence produced by collagen and other fluorescent substances is weaker than that produced by normal tissue. An example of a wireless capsule suitable for AFI detection was presented by Al-Rawhani et al. [50] (Fig. 51.9a). The device implements a single-photon avalanche diode, which is used for AFI detection in combination with blue LEDs. This technology seems capable of inducing and detecting autofluorescence from mammalian intestinal tissue.

With NBI, wavelengths in the visible spectrum are filtered from the illumination source, with the exception of narrow bands in the blue and green spectrum centred at 415 and 540 nm, coinciding with the peak absorption spectrum of oxyhaemoglobin; thus, blood vessels are more pronounced when viewed in NBI mode. This method is intended to emphasize the small blood vessels and minute patterns on the mucosal surface for augmented reality purposes [51]. A dedicated dual-mode CMOS sensor able to acquire one visible and one narrow-band image under inter-illumination mode at a frame rate of 2 fps was presented by Dung et al. [52] (Fig. 51.9b).

Optical-digital image-enhanced techniques, such as spectroscopy, AFI or NBI, represent potential techniques for the implementation of in situ optical biopsy on board the capsule. Such advanced diagnostic methods go beyond standard diagnostic endoscopic techniques by offering improved image resolution, contrast and tissue penetration and by providing biochemical and molecular information about mucosal disease through interactions of light and tissue.

Advanced imaging analyses also can be used during the post-processing. Several algorithms based on texture feature, local binary pattern and multilayer perceptron neural network have been implemented [53–55].

51.2.3 Data Streaming

One of the main challenges in the development of WCE system is related to the data stream versus the data payload. Indeed, data transmission bandwidth limits the performance of the whole capsule in terms of image resolution and maximum frame rate, and it is still the bottleneck for all commercial and research endoscopic capsules.

The transmission rate (TR) available at the transmitter must match the data rate (DR) from the vision module, which is calculated taking into account the resolution (number of pixels [N°Pixels]), the number of bits for each pixel (B) and the desired frame rate (FR), which should be at least 15 fps for a real-time examination. TR is expressed by Eq. 51.1:

$$TR = DR = N°Pixels \times B \times FR \qquad (51.1)$$

To minimize the DR, it is better to consider the image before demosaicing; otherwise the DR has to be multiplied by a factor 3, which takes into account the red-green-blue pixel triplet. Another possibility to reduce the DR is to consider also a compression ratio (CR), which can reduce DR by a factor of CR; however, the image quality is also decreased, and Eq. 51.1 can be expressed by Eq. 51.2:

$$TR = DR = (N°Pixels \times B \times FR)/CR \qquad (51.2)$$

51.2.3.1 Compression Algorithms

Standard state-of-the-art video compression techniques, such as JPEG, JPEG2000 or MPEG, may significantly reduce the image bit rate by their high compression ratio, but their application usually requires intensive computation and

consumes much battery power. Considering the specific application, image compression must be efficient in terms of both electrical power and time. The compression algorithms must compress images sufficiently (in the range of 5–20) for fast transmission over the wireless link, but the image quality must be preserved as much as possible for medical diagnosis. It has been reported that a minimum peak signal-to-noise ratio (PSNR) of 35 dB in the reconstructed image quality is required for accurate diagnosis [56]. The calculation of PSNR is formulated as in Eq. 51.3:

$$PSNR = 10\log\left(\frac{255^2}{MSE}\right) \qquad (51.3)$$

where MSE is the mean square error of the decompressed image.

A paper by Khan and Wahid [57] proposed a subsampling-based image compression algorithm, specially designed for wireless video capsule application. The algorithm was developed around some special features of endoscopic images, such as colour homogeneity and absence of bluish component; it consists of a differential pulse code modulation followed by Golomb-Rice coding.

Another approach was proposed by Turcza et al. [58], who developed a compressor algorithm based on integer version of discrete cosine transform (DCT). The implemented compressor sequentially performs four operations: colour transformation, image transformation, coefficients quantization and entropy coding, while the demosaicing process is performed after transmission and decompression. The achieved compression ratio is 10. An extension of the same algorithm was presented in [59]. The originality of the implementation is that image data decorrelation in the proposed algorithm is performed by an integer version of DCT.

Over the past few years, a new framework called compressed sensing (CS) has been developed for sampling and compression [60]. The CS principle is based on picking random combinations of pixels and summing their intensities; with a sufficient number of such measurements, it is possible to reproduce the original image [61]. This method has the potential to dramatically reduce sampling rates, power consumption and computational complexity. Jing and Ye [62] have proposed a CS-based video compression approach suitable for WCE, based on YUV colour space conversion, blocking, zigzag scan and CS measuring.

51.2.3.2 Transmitter

The bandwidth of the telemetry system should be wide enough to handle the transmission of image data with significant resolution and in real time. Two features should be taken into account in choosing the best telemetry system for ingested devices: (1) the power consumption should be less than 10 mW due to limited on-board energy storage and

(2) the working band should match the range of the medical band (Medical Implant Communications Service [MICS] or industrial, scientific and medical [ISM] bands [63]).

The higher the carrier frequency, the larger is the attenuation. This attenuation needs to be reasonable in WCE applications, because propagation within body thickness can reach 10–15 cm in patients who are obese.

The wireless transceiver from Microsemi (which is used inside the Given Imaging capsules), ZL70102, is MICS compatible and supports a maximum data rate of 800 kb/s [64]. A novel and simple topology for an efficient, miniaturized transmitter with low power consumption with high data rate, suitable for implanted devices, was presented by Thoné et al. [65]. The authors implemented a 2 Mbps frequency-shift-keying (FSK) transmitter, consuming 2 mW at 1.8 V and working at biocompatible frequencies. A highly efficient OOK transmitter with a high data rate also has been proposed for WCE [66]. The 440 MHz, 0dBm OOK transmitter has been fabricated using a 0.18 μm CMOS process. The OOK transmitter, consisting of the oscillator and buffer amplifier turned on/off at the same time, has been shown to achieve 40 Mb/s modulation and to operate with 860 μA current consumption from a 3 V supply.

51.2.4 Localization

The development of an efficient localization method represents an important contribution in robotic endoscopy. Knowledge of the position and orientation of the capsule allows the location of lesions and pathological areas to be determined for future follow-up treatment or more accurate diagnosis. Moreover, spatial information (e.g. absolute or relative position with regard to the GI lumen) defines the distance travelled by the capsule in the GI tract and the anatomical districts in which it is located. Finally, with a view to implement a robotic-aided platform, localization information allows for a capsule motion control loop. As a result, several research groups have approached different localization strategies with the aim of detecting the position and orientation of the capsule during its journey along the GI tract.

Magnetic sensing approaches, implemented to obtain capsule space information, represent the most reliable and effective methods for localization. The capsule, provided with on-board permanent magnets, can be detected by a three-axis magnetic sensor array (i.e. a sensorized carpet) by measuring both magnetic field strength and direction. As proposed by Hu et al. [67], the capsule can be localized with an average position error of 2 mm and an average orientation error of 1.6° when the magnet moves within the sensing area of 240×240 mm (although the overall accuracy is highly dependent on the number of external sensors used).

A promising magnetic sensor-based solution for capsule endoscopy localization was proposed by Andrä et al. [68]; here, a permanent magnet, on board the capsule, is repeatedly aligned by a vertically oriented pulsed magnetic field. Through this alignment, the position can be measured by magnetic field sensors with a position error of less than 10 mm.

None of these magnetic-based localization strategies could be used with an external magnetic locomotion approach, because the external magnetic field needed for locomotion would dramatically affect the external sensor array measurements. Kim et al. [69] implemented a position and orientation detection method for capsule endoscopes moving through the GI tract in spiral motion, with a largest position error appearing along the rotating axis of the permanent magnet of 15 mm and a maximum error of the orientation detection, appearing in the pitching direction, ranging between −4° and +15°.

A localization approach compatible with external magnetic locomotion was proposed by Salerno et al. [70]. The approach is based on a triangulation algorithm able to detect the capsule in the GI tract by recording and processing external magnetic field measurements through a custom on-board triaxial magnetic sensor. Position errors of 14 mm along the X axis, 11 mm along the Y axis and 19 mm along the Z axis were obtained (where X and Y are in the plane of the abdomen and Z is in the vertical direction as regards this plane). Salerno et al. [71] also developed an online localization method with a localization rate of 20 Hz, which combines the information of an embedded 3D Hall sensor and a 3D accelerometer with precalculated magnetic field maps describing the external-source magnetic field; the final aim is to derive online localization with 2° of freedom with a position error less than 10 mm below a distance of 120 mm between the localization module and the specific external magnet.

Alternative—but less common—approaches for localization consist of ultrasonic pulses emitted from outside the body and echoed by the internal capsule [72], or a radioactive agent placed on board the capsule and detected externally by gamma scintigraphy [73].

51.2.5 Power

The powering unit is definitely one of the main submodules inside an endoscopic capsule, as energy feeding is mandatory for all the other submodules. Commercial endoscopic capsules rely on silver-oxide coin cell batteries, which are the only batteries approved for clinical use in WCE. These batteries provide 3 V at 55 mAh for approximately 8 h, which implies an average power delivery of approximately 20 mW [74]. This amount of power is barely sufficient to transmit even low-resolution images at low data rates, and it certainly is inadequate to feed actuators for locomotion or other modules with high energy consumption. A valid alternative to batteries is inductive coupling, which significantly increases the available power by one order of magnitude, without constraints on the time of operation [75].

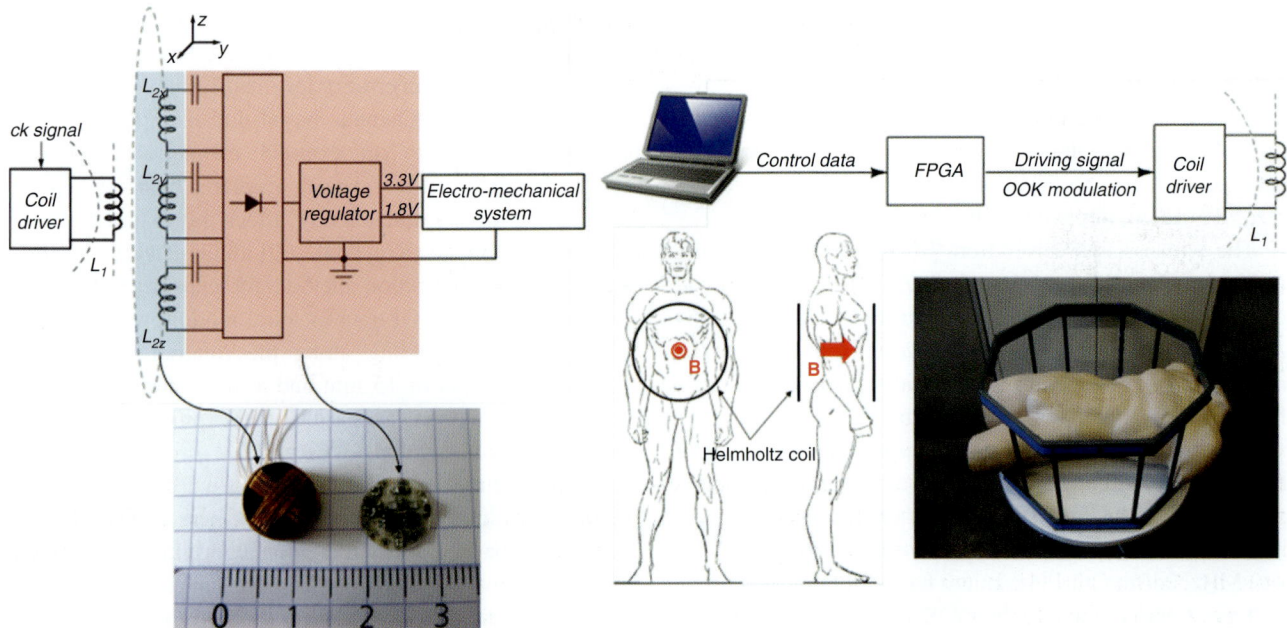

Fig. 51.10 A wireless power supply system for robotic capsule endoscopes developed by Carta et al. (*Courtesy of* Riccardo Carta, PhD)

A wireless power supply system for robotic capsule endoscopes has been presented (Fig. 51.10) [76]. An alternating magnetic field generated by an external coil around the patient's chest is partially picked up by three orthogonal coils embedded in the capsule. To maximize the received power, the three coils are tuned to resonate at the carrier frequency. Their individual contributions are added, after rectification, in order to avoid dephasing problems.

The system was integrated in a submersible capsule (the swimming capsule developed by Tortora et al. [12], described in Sect. 51.2.1.1) optimized to operate in a liquid-distended stomach. The system supplied up to 400 mW to the embedded electronics and a set of four radio-controlled motor propellers [77].

The same approach was also presented by Xin et al. [78]. The system consists of a Helmholtz primary coil outside the body and 3D multiple secondary coils inside. The Helmholtz primary coil is driven to generate a uniform alternating magnetic field covering the whole alimentary tract, and the multiple secondary coils receive energy regardless of the capsule position and orientation relative to the generated magnetic field. The safety of the electromagnetic field generated by the transmitting coil onto the human tissues was evaluated, based on a high-resolution, realistic human model [78].

51.2.6 Diagnosis and Tissue Treatment

Progress in microelectromechanical systems (MEMS) have produced endoscopic capsules with biomedical sensors (e.g. pH, pressure, blood detection and temperature), with the aim of enhancing capsule diagnostic capabilities and enabling new tasks. One of the main limitations of current capsule endoscopes is the impossibility of treating lesions during the same procedure, thus requiring a subsequent flexible endoscopic procedure. Providing clinical capsules with diagnostic, interventional and therapeutic capabilities has the potential to make capsule endoscopy a much more powerful tool. Diagnostic and tissue treatment systems can be integrated into capsules to provide accurate and reliable diagnosis and interventional capabilities, such as biopsy sampling, clip release to stop bleeding or drug delivery.

Gonzalez-Guillaumin et al. [79] developed a wireless capsule enclosing sensors for impedance and pH monitoring in the oesophageal tract for the detection and characterization of gastro-oesophageal reflux disease, using a magnetic holding solution to surgical fixation. A wireless multisensor microsystem (Lab-in-a-Pill capsule), comprising sensors for temperature, conductivity, pH and dissolved oxygen, a control chip, and a transmitter were developed by Johannessen et al. [80]. Sensors were fabricated on two separate silicon chips located at the front end of the capsule, and the system can be adapted to biomedical and industrial applications [80].

Valdastri et al. [81] developed the first therapeutic wireless endoscopic capsule able to release a clip to treat bleeding in the GI tract. The therapeutic capsule (Fig. 51.11a) is controlled by means of external magnetic-field sources and is provided with a single preloaded SMA-based clip, which can be activated and released wirelessly. Successful surgical

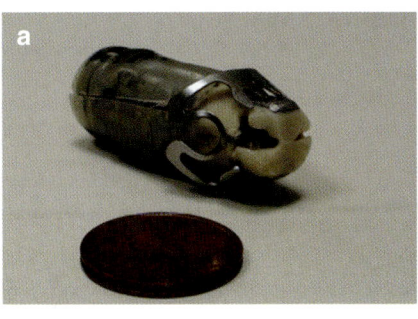 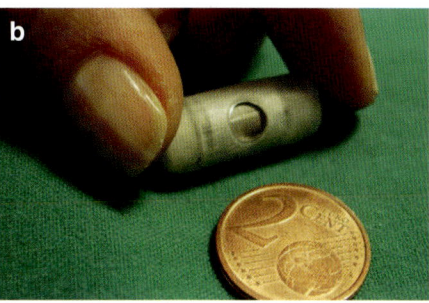 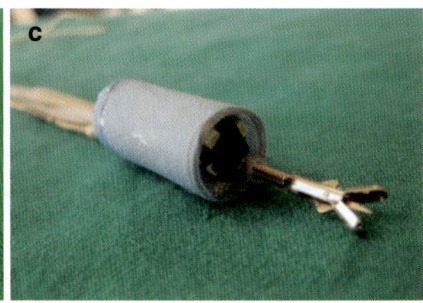

Fig. 51.11 Tissue treatment capsules. (**a**) Wireless therapeutic clipping capsule developed by Valdastri et al. [81]. (**b**) Biopsy capsule developed by Simi et al. [82]. (**c**) Soft-tethered magnetic capsule for painless colonoscopy, developed by Valdastri et al. [83].

ex vivo and in vivo experiments were performed, opening the field to a new generation of capsule devices capable of performing both diagnostic and therapeutic tasks [81].

The first example of a wireless biopsy capsule was developed by Kong et al. [84]. It consists of a rotational tissue-cutting razor fixed to a torsional spring and constrained by a paraffin block. When the paraffin block is melted by heating, the razor is released, and a tissue sample is collected. It is not yet clear, however, whether such a mechanism will be able to collect a sufficient number or volume of samples for an accurate histologic analysis, and system stabilization during sampling remains one of the main problems. A reliable and effective design, presented by Simi et al. [82], takes advantage of magnetic fields both for stabilizing the capsule during sampling and for operating the biopsy mechanism. Two couples of cylindrical, diametrically magnetized permanent magnets embedded into the capsule act as magnetic torsional springs; the external magnetic field is modulated first for stabilization and tissue penetration inside an inner chamber and then for tissue cutting. Therefore, thanks to the innovative magnetic actuation system, actuators and batteries are not required on board, allowing a more compact size of 9.5 mm in diameter and 17 mm in length (Fig. 51.11b). Because of its small dimensions, the system can be used for paediatric patients [74, 82].

To make diagnostic capsules competitive with traditional endoscopes, additional functions such as drug delivery have been considered by research groups. A device that is actuated magnetically for drug release is a soft capsule for the stomach with an axial extra degree of freedom; the capsule can perform drug injection or biopsy sampling [85]. Pi et al. [86] presented a process controlled by a microfabricated thruster able to generate a sufficient amount of gas to force medication out of the drug reservoir. Localized drug delivery was achieved by magnetic retention under biplane fluoroscopy in a study by Laulicht et al. [87], in which a drug-loaded magnetic capsule was held in a specific position in the GI tract. A future prospect for drug delivery over time is the use of drug-loaded mucoadhesives, released by a wireless capsule in specific areas of the GI tract [88].

Valdastri et al. [83] developed a novel endoscopic device consisting of a Soft-tethered magnetic capsule for painless colonoscopy under robotic magnetic steering. The capsule, provided with "front-wheel" magnetic traction, is composed of a capsule-like frontal unit and a compliant, multilumen tether allowing for gas insufflation, suction, irrigation or access for standard endoscopic tools such as biopsy forceps, polypectomy snare, retrieval basket or grasper (Fig. 51.11c). The capsule represents a trade-off between capsule and traditional colonoscopy, combining the benefits of a low-invasive actively manoeuvred capsule body with the multifunctional operating tether, which can be used for therapeutic procedures.

Conclusions

The emerging technology of WCE is producing a huge impact on the practice of endoscopy. It represents a significant advancement in medical devices enabling painless diagnosis inside the GI tract and paving the way for mass screening. As a first-generation disruptive technology, commercial WCE still has a number of limitations, namely, the inability to control locomotion, substandard image quality, no high-frame-rate real-time video capability, limited power resources, low data-rate telemetry and limited treatment capabilities. As demonstrated by recent comparative studies [89], these open issues make traditional endoscopic techniques still superior to WCE in terms of diagnostic capabilities. Several research groups worldwide are trying to overcome these drawbacks, developing new features such as active locomotion systems, which would allow the doctor to steer the capsule towards the most interesting pathological areas [37]. Examples of active locomotion in WCE range from legged to external magnetic steering [22, 25, 34]. Besides the basic functionalities and new strategies for locomotion, some advanced features have been introduced recently [5]. Because of the difficulty in miniaturizing components for integration inside the capsule, external magnetic field propulsion represents the most promising locomotion approach at medium term. [36, 37]

Despite research into the implementation of actuation, drug delivery and biopsy techniques, the imaging unit represents the core part of the system. Images obtained by the vision system are used both for diagnostic purposes and as the feedback module for autonomous steering of the capsule (e.g. facing the lumen or holding a given position against natural bowel movements). Furthermore, a real-time image stream must be processed for identification of visual clues that, together with position information, can be used as input for the locomotion controller. Autonomous active navigation, together with a real-time, high-quality vision system and treatment capabilities, would improve the state of current endoscopic platforms, producing clinical improvements and encouraging preventive mass screening.

Finally, exploitation of WCE knowledge may pave the way for the development (i.e. rescaling and redesign) of innovative probes to approach other districts and cavities of the human body, such as the vascular circuit.

References

1. Reavis KM, Melvin WS. Advanced endoscopic technologies. Surg Endosc. 2008;22:1533–46.
2. Iddan GJ, Swain CP. History and development of capsule endoscopy. Gastrointest Endosc Clin N Am. 2004;14:1–9.
3. Loeve A, Breedveld P, Dankelman J. Scopes too flexible…and too stiff. IEEE Pulse. 2010;1:26–41.
4. Swain C, Gong F, Mills T. Wireless transmission of a colour television moving image from the stomach using a miniature CCD camera, light source and microwave transmitter. Gastrointest Endosc. 1997;45:AB40.
5. Moglia A, Menciassi A, Schurr MO, Dario P. Wireless capsule endoscopy: from diagnostic devices to multipurpose robotic systems. Biomed Microdevices. 2007;9:235–43.
6. Valdastri P, Webster RJ, Quaglia C, et al. A new mechanism for mesoscale legged locomotion in compliant tubular environments. IEEE Trans Robot. 2009;25:1047–57.
7. Fireman Z, Glukhovsky A, Scapa E. Future of capsule endoscopy. Gastrointest Endosc Clin N Am. 2004;14:219–27.
8. Polla DL, Erdman AG, Robbins WP, et al. Microdevices in medicine. Annu Rev Biomed Eng. 2000;2:551–76.
9. Zahn JD, Talbot NH, Liepmann D, Pisano AP. Microfabricated polysilicon microneedles for minimally invasive biomedical devices. Biomed Microdevices. 2000;2:295–303.
10. Tognarelli S, Quaglia C, Valdastri P, et al. Innovative stopping mechanism for esophageal wireless capsular endoscopy. Procedia Chem. 2009;1:485–8.
11. Glass P, Cheung E, Sitti M. A legged anchoring mechanism for capsule endoscopes using micropatterned adhesives. IEEE Trans Biomed Eng. 2008;55:2759–67.
12. Tortora G, Valdastri P, Susilo E, et al. Propeller-based wireless device for active capsular endoscopy in the gastric district. Minim Invasive Ther Allied Technol. 2009;18:280–90.
13. Kósa G, Jakab P, Székely G, Hata N. MRI driven magnetic microswimmers. Biomed Microdevices. 2012;14:165–78.
14. Valdastri P, Sinibaldi E, Caccavaro S, et al. A novel magnetic actuation system for miniature swimming robots. IEEE Trans Robot. 2011;27:769–79.
15. Ciuti G, Pateromichelakis N, Sfakiotakis M, et al. A wireless module for vibratory motor control and inertial sensing in capsule endoscopy. Sens Actuators A Phys. 2012;186:270–6.
16. Carta R, Sfakiotakis M, Pateromichelakis N, et al. A multi-coil inductive powering system for an endoscopic capsule with vibratory actuation. Sens Actuators A Phys. 2011;172:253–8.
17. Zabulis X, Argyros AA, Tsakiris DP. Lumen detection for capsule endoscopy. IROS 2008 IEEE/RSJ International Conference; Nice, France, 2008. doi: 10.1109/IROS.2008.4650969.
18. Park HJ, Lee JH, Moon YK, et al. New method of moving control for wireless endoscopic capsule using electrical stimuli. IEICE Trans Fundam Electron Commun Comput Sci. 2005;88:1476–80.
19. Mosse CA, Mills TN, Appleyard MN, et al. Electrical stimulation for propelling endoscopes. Gastrointest Endosc. 2001;54:79–83.
20. Karagozler ME, Cheung E, Kwon J, Sitti M. Miniature endoscopic capsule robot using biomimetic micro-patterned adhesives. IEEE/RAS-EMBS International Conference on Biomedical Robotics and Biomechatronics; Pisa, Italy, 2006.
21. Kim B, Lee S, Park JH, Park J-O. Design and fabrication of a locomotive mechanism for capsule-type endoscopes using shape memory alloys (SMAs). IEEE ASME Trans Mechatron. 2005;10: 77–86.
22. Kim B, Park S, Jee CY, Yoon S-J. An earthworm-like locomotive mechanism for capsule endoscopes. IROS 2005 IEEE/RSJ International Conference; Edmonton, Alberta, Canada, 2005. doi: 10.1109/IROS.2005.1545608.
23. Li W, Guo W, Li M, Zhu Y. A novel locomotion principle for endoscopic robot. Proceedings of the 2006 IEEE International Conference on Mechatronics and Automation; Norfolk, Virginia, USA, 2006. doi: 10.1109/ICMA.2006.257445.
24. Park S, Park H, Park S, Kim B. A paddling based locomotive mechanism for capsule endoscopes. J Mech Sci Technol. 2006;20: 1012–8.
25. Gorini S, Quirini M, Menciassi A, et al. A novel SMA-based actuator for a legged endoscopic capsule. The First IEEE/RAS-EMBS International Conference on Biomedical Robotics and Biomechatronics; Pisa, Italy, 2006. doi: 10.1109/BIOROB.2006.1639128.
26. Quirini M, Menciassi A, Scapellato S, et al. Design and fabrication of a motor legged capsule for the active exploration of the gastrointestinal tract. IEEE ASME Trans Mechatron. 2008;13:169–79.
27. Quirini M, Menciassi A, Scapellato S, et al. Feasibility proof of a legged locomotion capsule for the GI tract. Gastrointest Endosc. 2008;67:1153–8.
28. Buselli E, Valdastri P, Quirini M, et al. Superelastic leg design optimization for an endoscopic capsule with active locomotion. Smart Mater Struct. 2008;18:015001.
29. Ramcharitar S, Patterson MS, van Geuns RJ, et al. Technology insight: magnetic navigation in coronary interventions. Nat Clin Pract Cardiovasc Med. 2008;5:148–56.
30. Miloro P, Llewellyn MK, Tognarelli S, et al. An innovative platform for treatment of vascular obstructions: system design and preliminary results. 4th IEEE/RAS-EMBS International Conference on Robotics and Biomechatronics; Rome, Italy, 2012. doi: 10.1109/BioRob.2012.6290758.
31. Yu C, Kim J, Choi H, Choi J, Jeong S, Cha K, et al. Novel electromagnetic actuation system for three-dimensional locomotion and drilling of intravascular microrobot. Sens Actuators A Phys. 2010; 161(1):297–304.
32. Rey JF, Ogata H, Hosoe N, et al. Blinded nonrandomized comparative study of gastric examination with a magnetically guided capsule endoscope and standard videoendoscope. Gastrointest Endosc. 2012;75:373–81.
33. Keller J, Fibbe C, Volke F, et al. Inspection of the human stomach using remote-controlled capsule endoscopy: a feasibility study in healthy volunteers (with videos). Gastrointest Endosc. 2011;73:22–8.

34. Carpi F, Kastelein N, Talcott M, Pappone C. Magnetically controllable gastrointestinal steering of video capsules. IEEE Trans Biomech Eng. 2011;58:231–4.

35. Carpi F, Pappone C. Magnetic maneuvering of endoscopic capsules by means of a robotic navigation system. IEEE Trans Biomech Eng. 2009;56:1482–90.

36. Ciuti G, Donlin R, Valdastri P, et al. Robotic versus manual control in magnetic steering of an endoscopic capsule. Endoscopy. 2010; 42:148.

37. Ciuti G, Valdastri P, Menciassi A, Dario P. Robotic magnetic steering and locomotion of capsule endoscope for diagnostic and surgical endoluminal procedures. Robotica. 2010;28:199.

38. Simi M, Valdastri P, Quaglia C, et al. Design, fabrication, and testing of a capsule with hybrid locomotion for gastrointestinal tract exploration. IEEE ASME Trans Mechatron. 2010;15:170–80.

39. Gorlewicz JL, Battaglia S, Smith BF, et al. Wireless insufflation of the gastrointestinal tract. IEEE Trans Biomed Eng. 2013;60:1225–33.

40. Bang S, Park JY, Jeong S, et al. First clinical trial of the "MiRo" capsule endoscope by using a novel transmission technology: electric-field propagation. Gastrointest Endosc. 2009;69:253–9.

41. Uehara A, Hoshina K. Capsule endoscope NORIKA system. Minim Invasive Ther Allied Technol. 2003;12:227–34.

42. Gheorghe C, Iacob R, Bancila I. Olympus capsule endoscopy for small bowel examination. J Gastrointestin Liver Dis. 2007;16:309.

43. Cavallotti C, Piccigallo M, Susilo E, et al. An integrated vision system with autofocus for wireless capsular endoscopy. Sens Actuators A Phys. 2009;156:72–8.

44. Seo SW, Han S, Seo JH, et al. Microelectromechanical-system-based variable-focus liquid lens for capsule endoscopes. Jpn J Appl Phys. 2009;48:2404.

45. Narendran N, Maliyagoda N, Deng L, Pysar RM. Characterizing LEDs for general illumination applications: mixed-color and phosphor-based white sources. Proc SPIE4445, Solid State Lighting and Displays, 137. San Diego, CA, USA, 2001. doi:10.1117/12.450037.

46. Vatteroni M, Covi D, Cavallotti C, et al. Smart optical CMOS sensor for endoluminal applications. Sens Actuators A Phys. 2010;162:297–303.

47. Vatteroni M, Cavallotti C, Valdastri P, et al. Vision system for high frame rate wireless capsule endoscope. IEEE: Sensors; 2011. doi:10.1109/ICSENS.2011.6127393.

48. Bergman J. New endoscopic imaging techniques for improved detection of early neoplasia in patients with Barrett's esophagus. Curr Gastroenterol Rep. 2004;6:343–5.

49. Matsuda T, Saito Y, Fu KI, et al. Does autofluorescence imaging videoendoscopy system improve the colonoscopic polyp detection rate? – a pilot study. Am J Gastroenterol. 2008;103:1926–32.

50. Al-Rawhani MA, Chitnis D, Beeley J, et al. Design and implementation of a wireless capsule suitable for autofluorescence intensity detection in biological tissues. IEEE Trans Biomed Eng. 2013;60:55–62.

51. Vincent BD, Fraig M, Silvestri GA. A pilot study of narrow-band imaging compared to white light bronchoscopy for evaluation of normal airways and premalignant and malignant airways disease. Chest. 2007;131:1794–9.

52. Dung LR, Wu YY. A wireless narrowband imaging chip for capsule endoscope. IEEE Trans Biomed Circuits Syst. 2010;4:462–8.

53. Li B, Meng MH. Computer-aided detection of bleeding regions for capsule endoscopy images. IEEE Trans Biomed Eng. 2009;56:1032–9.

54. Pan G, Yan G, Qiu X, Cui J. Bleeding detection in wireless capsule endoscopy based on probabilistic neural network. J Med Syst. 2011;35:1477–84.

55. Poh CK, Htwe TM, Li L, et al. Multi-level local feature classification for bleeding detection in wireless capsule endoscopy images. , 2010 IEEE Conference on Cybernetics and Intelligent Systems (CIS). Singapore, 2010. doi:10.1109/ICCIS.2010.5518576.

56. Istepanian RH, Philip N, Martini MG, et al. Subjective and objective quality assessment in wireless teleultrasonography imaging. Conf Proc IEEE Eng Med Biol Soc. 2008;2008:5346–9.

57. Khan TH, Wahid KA. Low power and low complexity compressor for video capsule endoscopy. IEEE Trans Circuits Syst Video Technol. 2011;21:1534–46.

58. Turcza P, Zielinski T, Duplaga M. Hardware implementation aspects of new low complexity image coding algorithm for wireless capsule endoscopy. Lect Notes Comput Sci. 2008;5101:476–85.

59. Turcza P, Duplaga M. Low power FPGA-based image processing core for wireless capsule endoscopy. Sens Actuators A Phys. 2011; 172:552–60.

60. Schneider D. Camera chip makes already-compressed images. IEEE Spectr. 2013;50(3):11.

61. Donoho DL. Compressed sensing. IEEE Trans Inf Theory. 2006; 52:1289–306.

62. Jing W, Ye L. Low-complexity video compression for capsule endoscope based on compressed sensing theory. EMBC 2009 Annual International Conference of the IEEE. Minneapolis, Minnesota.

63. Hanna S. Regulations and standards for wireless medical applications. Proceedings of the 3rd International Symposium on Medical Information and Communication Technology; 2009.

64. ZL70102 MICS Transceiver 2011. Available from http://www.microsemi.com.

65. Thoné J, Radiom S, Turgis D, et al. Design of a 2 Mbps FSK near-field transmitter for wireless capsule endoscopy. Sens Actuators A Phys. 2009;156:43–8.

66. Jiho R, Minchul K, Jaechun L, et al. Low power OOK transmitter for wireless capsule endoscope. Microwave Symposium, 2007 IEEE/MTT-S International. Honolulu, Hawaii

67. Hu C, Yang W, Chen D, et al. An improved magnetic localization and orientation algorithm for wireless capsule endoscope. EMBS 2008 30th Annual International Conference of the IEEE; Vancouver, British Columbia, Canada, 2008.

68. Andrä W, Danan H, Kirmsse W, et al. A novel method for real-time magnetic marker monitoring in the gastrointestinal tract. Phys Med Biol. 2000;45:3081–93.

69. Kim MG, Hong YS, Lim EJ. Position and orientation detection of capsule endoscopes in spiral motion. Int J Precis Eng Manuf. 2010;11:31–7.

70. Salerno M, Ciuti G, Lucarini G, et al. A discrete-time localization method for capsule endoscopy based on on-board magnetic sensing. Meas Sci. 2011;23:015701.

71. Salerno M, Mulana F, Rizzo R, et al. Magnetic and inertial sensor fusion for the localization of endoluminal diagnostic devices. Proc Computer Assisted Radiology and Surgery Conference, CARS, Pisa, Italy, 2012. doi: 10.1007/s11548-012-0730-5.

72. Arshak K, Adepoju F. Capsule tracking in the GI tract: a novel microcontroller based solution. Sensors Applications Symposium, Proceedings of the 2006 IEEE; Houston, Texas, USA, 2006.

73. Wilding I, Hirst P, Connor A. Development of a new engineering-based capsule for human drug absorption studies. Pharm Sci Technol Today. 2000;3:385–92.

74. Valdastri P, Simi M, Webster 3rd RJ. Advanced technologies for gastrointestinal endoscopy. Annu Rev Biomed Eng. 2012;14:397–429.

75. Lenaerts B, Puers R. An inductive power link for a wireless endoscope. Biosens Bioelectron. 2007;22:1390–5.

76. Carta R, Thoné J, Puers R. A wireless power supply system for robotic capsular endoscopes. Sens Actuators A Phys. 2010;162:177–83.

77. Carta R, Tortora G, Thoné J, et al. Wireless powering for a self-propelled and steerable endoscopic capsule for stomach inspection. Biosens Bioelectron. 2009;25:845–51.

78. Xin W, Yan G, Wang W. Study of a wireless power transmission system for an active capsule endoscope. Int J Med Robot. 2010;6: 113–22.

79. Gonzalez-Guillaumin JL, Sadowski DC, Kaler KV, Mintchev MP. Ingestible capsule for impedance and pH monitoring in the esophagus. IEEE Trans Biomed Eng. 2007;54:2231–6.

80. Johannessen EA, Wang L, Cui L, et al. Implementation of multichannel sensors for remote biomedical measurements in a microsystems format. IEEE Trans Biomed Eng. 2004;51: 525–35.

81. Valdastri P, Quaglia C, Susilo E, et al. Wireless therapeutic endoscopic capsule: in vivo experiment. Endoscopy. 2008;40:979.

82. Simi M, Gerboni G, Menciassi A, Valdastri P. Magnetic mechanism for wireless capsule biopsy. J Med Devices. 2012;6:017611.

83. Valdastri P, Ciuti G, Verbeni A, et al. Magnetic air capsule robotic system: proof of concept of a novel approach for painless colonoscopy. Surg Endosc. 2012;26:1238–46.

84. Kong KC, Cha J, Jeon D, Cho D. A rotational micro biopsy device for the capsule endoscope. IEEE/RSJ International Conference on Intelligent Robots and Systems; 2005. doi: 10.1109/IROS.2005.1545441.

85. Yim S, Sitti M. Design and rolling locomotion of a magnetically actuated soft capsule endoscope. IEEE Trans Robot. 2012;28: 183–94.

86. Pi X, Lin Y, Wei K, et al. A novel micro-fabricated thruster for drug release in remote controlled capsule. Sens Actuators A Phys. 2010;159: 227–32.

87. Laulicht B, Gidmark NJ, Tripathi A, Mathiowitz E. Localization of magnetic pills. Proc Natl Acad Sci U S A. 2011;108:2252–7.

88. Tognarelli S, Pensabene V, Condino S, et al. A pilot study on a new anchoring mechanism for surgical applications based on mucoadhesives. Minim Invasive Ther Allied Technol. 2011;20:3–13.

89. Van Gossum A, Munoz-Navas M, Fernandez-Urien I, Carretero C, Gay G, Delvaux M, et al. Capsule endoscopy versus colonoscopy for the detection of polyps and cancer. N Engl J Med. 2009; 361(3):264–70.

Future Developments of Video Capsule Endoscopy: Software

52

Pedro Narra Figueiredo

Contents

Video capsule endoscopy (VCE) is highly dependent on software. The companies that produce the capsules have upgraded their version of the reading software, but we are far from a convenient solution for some of the problems that doctors face when reporting on VCE. In fact, as a result of the type of technology used in capsule endoscopy, we expect that better software may be helpful in detecting lesions and reducing the time required to see the videos, thus reducing the cost of the procedure and making it more efficient and affordable.

Nevertheless, different problems occur when dealing with small bowel capsule endoscopy (SBCE) or colon capsule endoscopy (CCE). In SBCE, the main indication is bleeding, so the problems are how to detect the blood, how to detect the bleeding lesion (which is usually flat), and how to specify the location of the lesion. In CCE, the main indication is the detection of polyps, lesions that usually protrude in the lumen of the bowel, so the problem instead is how to detect polyps more accurately and quickly.

52.1 Detecting Blood and Bleeding Lesions

The suspected blood indicator (SBI) function (Given Imaging, Yoqneam, Israel) allows the automatic identification of red pixels. A few papers have been published [1–5], reporting that the sensitivity ranged from 20 to 56.4 % for overall lesions and from 58.3 to 93 % for actively bleeding lesions. The positive predictive value varied from 24 to 90.3 %. These results mean that the automatic detection cannot replace the doctor, who must look at the entire video, although SBI can be regarded as a useful adjunct.

Recently, some efforts to automatically inspect SBCE images were made. Coimbra and Cunha [6] measured the usefulness of a particular multimedia content descriptor for detection of a variety of events, such as bleeding, ulcers,

The work was first published in 2006 by Springer Medizin Verlag Heidelberg with the following title: *Atlas of Video Capsule Endoscopy*.

P.N. Figueiredo
Department of Gastroenterology,
University of Coimbra, Coimbra, Portugal
e-mail: pnf11@sapo.pt

Fig. 52.1 Angioectasia detected: original image (**a**); computed image (**b**)

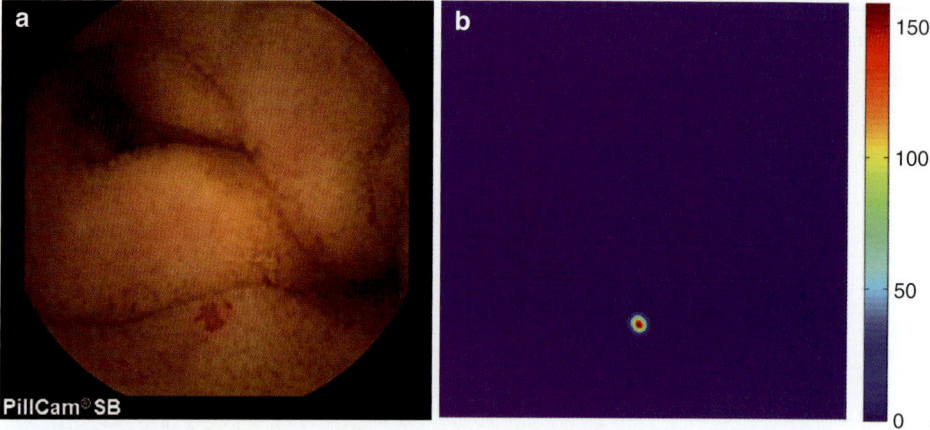

and polyps. Cui et al. [7] proposed six colour features in the hue/saturation/intensity (HSI) colour space to discriminate between normal and bleeding images. Khun et al. [8] compared the performance of colour and texture features in VCE image classification: the colour features are extracted from local colour histograms of the components of the hue/saturation/value (HSV) colour space and texture features are obtained by wavelet decomposition, on each colour component. Li and Meng [9] proposed a new idea of chrominance moment, as the colour part of the colour texture feature, which makes use of Tchebichef polynomials and illumination invariant of the hue/saturation/intensity (HSI) colour space; a combination of this moment with the uniform local binary pattern is used to discriminate between normal and bleeding regions in VCE images. Pan et al. [10] suggested a computer-aided, intelligent system based on a probabilistic neural network: colour texture features of bleeding regions, from red/green/blue (RGB) to HSI colour spaces, are extracted, and a probabilistic neural network classifier is built to recognize the bleeding [10]. In another paper, Pan et al. [11] proposed two-colour vector similarity coefficients to measure the colour similarity degree in RGB colour space; on this basis, the authors describe an algorithm for the detection of bleeding in VCE images. A method proposed by Figueiredo et al. [12] relies on enhancement techniques, for evidencing the bleeding, and segmentation, for discarding uninformative regions. This method was tested on three data sets prepared by clinicians (Fig. 52.1), and the results demonstrated that all the detectors achieved a good rate of success, evidence of promising performance for bleeding detection [12].

In an excellent review, Liedlgruber and Uhl [13] point out the limitations that exist when considering the different approaches that are published in the literature. One of these limitations is that each group uses its own databases, which makes comparisons between different methods almost impossible. Another problem is associated with the small number of images that are used in some approaches.

Interobserver discrepancies are also a difficulty when dealing with VCE, because histology is usually not available; so we must rely on visual inspection.

52.2 Locating the Lesion in the Small Bowel

Locating the lesion is an important issue in SBCE when a lesion must be treated with balloon-assisted enteroscopy or surgery. It would be very desirable to be able to measure its distance from the pylorus or the ileocaecal valve, but this problem is far from being solved [14]. A solution will probably be achieved only with the availability of a capsule that can be moved by external control [15].

52.3 Detection of Polyps in Colon Capsule Endoscopy

The main objective in CCE is to detect polyps. Computer-aided diagnosis, as in CT colonography [16], would be very helpful, as it potentially could improve diagnostic performance in the detection of polyps and masses by decreasing the variability of diagnostic accuracy among readers and probably by reducing reading time. Some efforts in this direction have already begun. An automatic image-processing algorithm to screen each image frame for potential polyps has been devised; the algorithm is based on the geometric characterization of polyps, which appear as a roundish protrusion from the surrounding mucosal surface (Fig. 52.2) [17]. The main drawback of this approach is the reliance only on the protrusion measurement of the polyp to identify the lesion. Another proposed algorithm, which labels the frame as either containing polyps or not, is based not only on geometrical analysis but also on the texture content of the frame, with good results in terms of sensitivity and specificity [18].

Fig. 52.2 Polyps detected: original image (**a**, **c**); computed image (**b**, **d**)

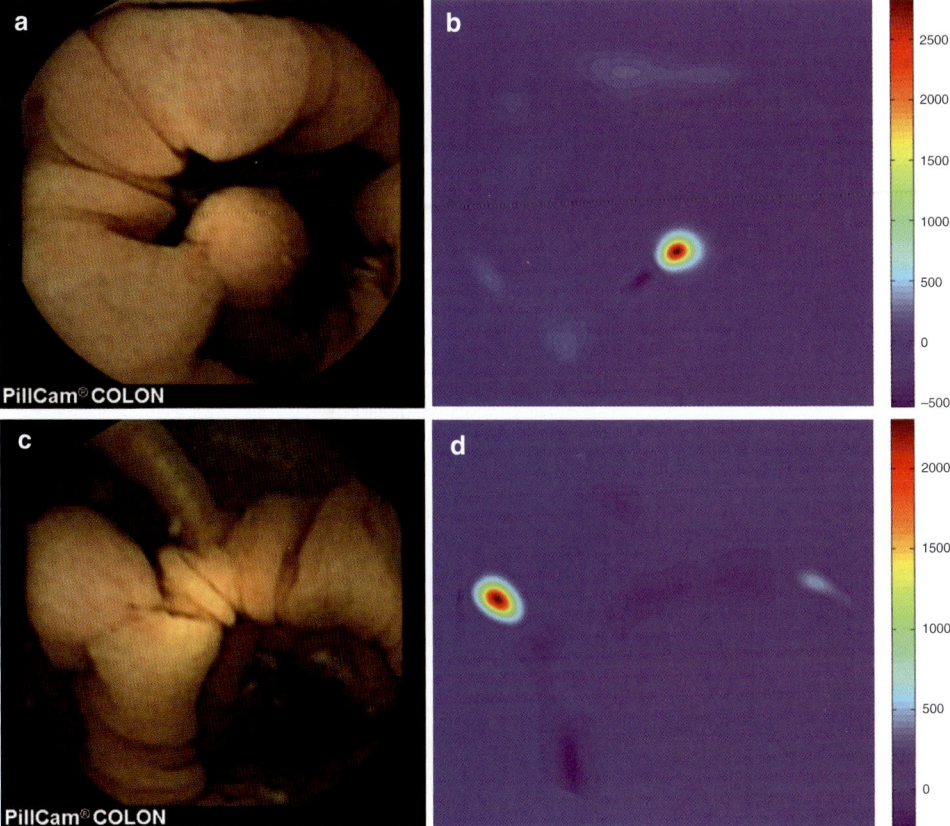

Conclusion

The software is an essential tool in VCE. The available software solutions seem to reflect the early stage of this new way of exploring the digestive tract. Nevertheless, the possibilities are huge because in VCE, unlike in flexible endoscopy, the systems are designed to process images or videos offline—that is, not in real time.

References

1. Liangpunsakul S, Mays L, Rex DK. Performance of given suspected blood indicator. Am J Gastroenterol. 2003;98:2676–8.
2. Buscaglia JM, Giday SA, Kantsevoy SV, et al. Performance characteristics of the suspected blood indicator feature in capsule endoscopy according to indication for study. Clin Gastroenterol Hepatol. 2008;6:298–301.
3. D'Halluin PN, Delvaux M, Lapalus MG, et al. Does the "suspected blood indicator" improve the detection of bleeding lesions by capsule endoscopy? Gastrointest Endosc. 2005;61:243–9.
4. Kim JY, Chun HJ, Kim CY, et al. The usefulness of a suspected blood identification system (SBIS) in capsule endoscopy according to various small bowel bleeding lesions. Korean J Gastrointest Endosc. 2008;37:253–8.
5. Signorelli C, Villa F, Rondonotti E, et al. Sensitivity and specificity of the suspected blood identification system in video capsule enteroscopy. Endoscopy. 2005;37:1170–3.
6. Coimbra MT, Cunha JP. MPEG-7 visual descriptors – contributions for automated feature extraction in capsule endoscopy. IEEE Trans Circuits Syst Video Technol. 2006;16:628–37.
7. Cui L, Hu C, Zou Y, Meng MQ. Bleeding detection in wireless capsule endoscopy images by support vector classifier. Proc IEEE Conf Inf Autom. 2010;2010:1746–51.
8. Khun PC, Zhang Z, Yang LZ, et al. Feature selection and classification for wireless capsule endoscopic frames. International Conference on Biomedical and Pharmaceutical Engineering, Singapore, Dec 2009.
9. Li B, Meng MQ. Computer-aided detection of bleeding regions for capsule endoscopy images. IEEE Trans Biomed Eng. 2009;56:1032–9.
10. Pan G, Yan G, Qiu X, Cui J. Bleeding detection in wireless capsule endoscopy based on probabilistic neural network. J Med Syst. 2011;35:1477–84.
11. Pan G, Xu F, Chen J. A novel algorithm for color similarity measurement and the application for bleeding detection in WCE. Int J Image Graph Signal Process. 2011;3(5):1–7.
12. Figueiredo IN, Kumar S, Leal C, Figueiredo PN. Computer-assisted bleeding detection in wireless capsule endoscopy images. Comput Methods Biomech Biomed Engin Imaging Vis; 2013. doi: 10.1080/21681163.2013.796164.
13. Liedlgruber M, Uhl A. Computer-aided decision support systems for endoscopy in the gastrointestinal tract: a review. IEEE Rev Biomed Eng. 2011;4:73–88.
14. Than TD, Alici G, Zhou H, Li W. A review of localization systems for robotic endoscopic capsules. IEEE Trans Biomed Eng. 2012;59:2387–99.
15. Keller J, Fibbe C, Volke F, et al. Inspection of the human stomach using remote-controlled capsule endoscopy: a feasibility

study in healthy volunteers (with videos). Gastrointest Endosc. 2011;73:22–8.

16. Bielen D, Kiss G. Computer-aided detection for CT colonography: update 2007. Abdom Imaging. 2007;32:571–81.

17. Figueiredo PN, Figueiredo IN, Prasath S, Tsai R. Automatic polyp detection in Pillcam Colon 2 capsule images and videos: preliminary feasibility report. Diagn Ther Endosc. 2011;2011:182435. doi:10.1155/2011/182435.

18. Mamonov AV, Figueiredo IN, Figueiredo PN, Tsai YR. Automated polyp detection in colon capsule endoscopy; 2013. eprint arXiv:1305.1912. Available at: http://arxiv.org/abs/1305.1912.

Index

Printing: Ten Brink, Meppel, The Netherlands
Binding: Stürtz, Würzburg, Germany